Reputation and Power

PRINCETON STUDIES IN AMERICAN POLITICS:
HISTORICAL, INTERNATIONAL, AND COMPARATIVE PERSPECTIVES

Series Editors
Ira Katznelson, Martin Shefter, Theda Skocpol

A list of titles in this series appears at the end of the book

Reputation and Power

ORGANIZATIONAL IMAGE AND PHARMACEUTICAL REGULATION AT THE FDA

DANIEL CARPENTER

PRINCETON UNIVERSITY PRESS

PRINCETON AND OXFORD

Library of Congress Cataloging-in-Publication Data

Carpenter, Daniel P., 1967–
Reputation and power : organizational image and
pharmaceutical regulation at the FDA / Daniel Carpenter.
p. cm. — (Princeton studies in American politics)
Includes bibliographical references and index.
ISBN 978-0-691-14179-4 (hardcover : alk. paper) —
ISBN 978-0-691-14180-0 (pbk. : alk. paper)
1. United States. Food and Drug Administration.
2. Pharmaceutical policy—United States.   3. Drugs—
Research—United States.   I. Title.
RA401.A3C37 2010
362.17'82—dc22
2009044230

British Library Cataloging-in-Publication Data is available

This book has been composed in Postscript Sabon

Printed on acid-free paper. ∞

press.princeton.edu

Printed in the United States of America

10 9 8 7 6 5 4 3 2 1

TO RITA

CONTENTS

ILLUSTRATIONS

TABLES

ACKNOWLEDGMENTS

MY DECADES-LONG fascination with regulation was formed from listening to two old men and a young woman. The first of the men was my grandfather, Edward R. Krumbiegel, who served as health commissioner for the city of Milwaukee, Wisconsin, from 1940 to 1973. The young woman was my mother, Kathleen (Krumbiegel) Carpenter, an accomplished and dedicated radiologist in her own right (and still young). As my grandfather reminisced about old battles won and lost, and as my mother told me stories about her father's tenure in city life, I learned that public health was an endeavor not only of science but of politics in its best and worst aspects. I learned that in his management of Milwaukee's health—in contests over fluoridation, pest control, building and residential codes and other matters—Ed Krumbiegel wore at least two faces—one benevolent, another fierce. The same generous man who could inspire his staff and the city's residents to labor with devotion for the common good could also turn his anger instantly and brashly upon city politicians and businesses who stood in the way of what he considered progress. As his grandson, I saw some of these same faces: his infectious, warm humor and his humbling dinner-table corrections.

The second man was Marver Bernstein, whom I hardly knew, but whose course in business and government I took in my final semester at Georgetown College in the spring of 1989. Bernstein was a university professor at Georgetown who had served as the first Dean of the Woodrow Wilson School at Princeton and had concluded his presidency at Brandeis six years before. A generation before I attended college, he had authored *Regulating Business by Independent Commission*, still a classic in which many precepts of what is now known as the "capture" theory of regulation first appeared. Bernstein's vigorous denial of the model of regulators as Platonic "philosopher-statesmen" in his last lecture for that course still resonates for me. Twenty years later I can still hear, even feel, his voice rising as he pounded the lectern and thundered home the point. Marver Bernstein understood, in ways that elude many scholars today, that regulators are complicated human agents embedded in organizations. They defy the portrait of neutrality and pure public-spiritedness that Bernstein had observed in the early twentieth century, and they defy as well the picture of interest-obedient and inevitably captured bureaucrats that was emerging as he wrote in the 1950s.

My initial debts in this study, then, are to the people who first inspired me to think about regulation and its politics, in ways having nothing to do with the FDA.

What follows these expressions of gratitude is not the book I set out to write. I first envisioned a rather simple story about how a plain reputation for consumer protection had shaped the regulatory behavior of a federal agency, in particular the time it took for the Administration to review new drug applications. As I waded deeper into thousands of documents from dozens of archival collections across several continents, as I interviewed and read oral histories of participants in and observers of American pharmaceutical regulation, and as I consulted a range of colleagues, I learned that "the Food and Drug Administration" meant different things to different beholders. It also became clear to me that no simple covering law ruled the political economy of U.S. pharmaceutical regulation, that many simplistic generalizations well equipped for the 1960s failed utterly in describing the 1980s or the 1940s, and vice versa. Marver Bernstein had understood this historicity in the 1950s, describing the various "life cycles" of agencies. It became my task to portray the historical complexity of an organization, its images and its governance of a vast world, while bringing some intellectual order to its reputation and its power.

Because of the complexity of the subject matter and the historicity of regulation, and because I believe that organization theory provides a crucial lens for understanding American pharmaceutical policy, what follows these measures of thanks is also an academic treatment, and unapologetically so. The research was supported in numerous ways, by archivists, collaborators, and research assistants, and perhaps most, by critics and colleagues.

For research support, I gratefully acknowledge the Center for Advanced Study in the Behavioral Sciences, an Investigator Award in Health Policy Research from the Robert Wood Johnson Foundation, the Co-Evolution of States and Markets Program of the Santa Fe Institute, the National Science Foundation (SES-0076452 and SES-0351048), and the Faculty of Arts and Sciences at Harvard University. Fellowships from the John Simon Guggenheim Memorial Foundation and the Radcliffe Institute for Advanced Study allowed me to spend a sabbatical year completing the manuscript while launching a new project on petitioning in American political development. I also benefited from support from the Deans of the Harvard Faculty of Arts and Sciences, including the late Jeremy Knowles, Mike Smith, David Cutler, and Stephen Kosslyn. My chair, Nancy Rosenblum, who understands the value of large, in-depth scholarly projects, was ever encouraging and a beacon of sanity.

For steady assistance in locating primary source materials, I thank Laura Carroll of the AMA, Marjorie Ciarlante of the National Archives in College Park, Maryland, Ken Kato and his staff at the Center for Legislative Archives at the National Archives in Washington, DC, John Swann of the FDA, Leslie Brunet at the M. D. Anderson Cancer Center, and staff members at the Mayo Foundation, the Chesney Medical Archives (Johns Hopkins), the Seeley G. Mudd Manuscript Library (Princeton), the University of Utah Archives and Special Collections, the UCSF Special Collections Library, and the Countway Medical Library of Harvard Medical School. Peter de Souza of the Indian Institute for Advanced Study facilitated access to libraries in Delhi, while Christian Bonah graciously shared some of his materials from the Archives Nationales and the Bundesarchiv Koblenz, and

Marie Villemin capably assisted in accessing materials at the World Health Organization in Geneva.

For research assistance, I thank Sarah Burg, Maureen Comfort, Anne Conlin, Abbe Finberg, Erin Fries, Alexandra Hiatt, Camilo Vidal, and Walter Wodchis. Colin Moore, Susan Moffitt, and Evan Zucker collaborated in ways both intellectual and tedious. I remain solely responsible for all omissions, errors, and characterizations.

I benefited from conversations with numerous participants in and observers of the modern pharmaceutical world. These include Matthew Herper, Donald Drakeman, Alison Lawton (Genzyme), Ed Skolnick (formerly of Merck, now of the Harvard/MIT Broad Institute), William Potter (now Merck, formerly Lilly), Steven Hyman (Harvard's Provost and former director of the National Institutes of Mental Health), Barnett Rosenberg, Lavonne Lang (then at Parke-Davis), Philip Crooker (then at AstraZeneca), Bill Smith (then at Pfizer), Frank May and B. Suresh of the Pharmacy Council of India. Current or former FDA officials Jere Goyan, David Kessler, Susan Wood, Brad Stone, William Hubbard, Fred Clounts, and Randy Levin also shared their time and insight.

FDA historians Suzanne Junod and John Swann read the entire manuscript and pressed me to think more contextually about my argument. Former FDA officials J. Richard Crout (longtime director of the Bureau of Drugs), Peter Barton Hutt (general counsel), Richard Merrill (general counsel), and Robert Temple (numerous positions and, at this writing, still at the FDA) also read essentially the entire study in draft. They saved me from hundreds of errors, all the while reflecting broadly on the contours of their agency's reputation and its power. There are still points of disagreement, on which their interpretations and explanations of American pharmaceutical regulation diverge from mine. In particular, I have strong disagreements with what I see as Hutt's narrowly legalistic approach to FDA history and behavior. Yet I am grateful to him and the others for enlightening me, and for their patience. The disagreements were as helpful as any consensus. What faults and omissions remain after these generous readings—and undoubtedly some do—are my responsibility entirely.

In the academy, my colleagues Jerry Avorn, Richard Bensel, Allan Brandt, Arthur Daemmrich, Rick Hall, Sheila Jasanoff, Arthur Kleinman, Paul Pierson, Scott Podolsky, Paul Quirk, Eric Schickler, Peter Swenson, Michael Ting, and Dominique Tobbell also read large portions or the entirety of the manuscript. I must thank two scholars in particular—Jeremy Greene and Harry Marks—for sharing their wisdom in long conversations that occurred over a several-year period on two continents. In these interactions, Jeremy and Harry provided exacting scrutiny of the broad themes and particular statements of the book. Harry in particular engaged me in numerous debates over method, argument, and footnotes; those exchanges composed an education for me.

For other helpful discussions and corrections, I thank Bruce Ackerman,

Julia Adams, Chris Ansell, Elizabeth Armstrong, David Baron, Ernst Berndt, Steven Callendar, Elizabeth Clemens, Tino Cuellar, David Cutler, Cathy De-Angelis, Christine Desan, Einer Elhauge, Arnold Epstein, W. Bruce Fye, Alan Gerber, John Gerring, Julian Go, Jacob Hacker, Chip Heath, Carol Heimer, Gregory Higby, Jennifer Hochschild, Marie Hojnacki, Scott James, Walter Johnson, Ira Katznelson, Aaron Kesselheim, Keith Krehbiel, Michael Kremer, Michelle Mello, David Moss, Mary Olson, John Padgett, Ariel Pakes, Woody Powell, Stephen Rosen, Michael Sandel, Bruce Schulman, Theda Skocpol, Stephen Skowronek, Kathleen Thelen, Richard White, and Julian Zelizer. The collegiality and endeavors of Lilia Halpern-Smith, Abby Peck, and Esther Scott render my professional life much more enjoyable.

I have been privileged to work with Chuck Myers and his capable and dedicated staff at Princeton University Press in the development and publication of this study. Leslie Grundfest simultaneously kept one eye on the clock and another on detail and quality control. Karen Verde's editing was selective, wise, and outstanding. Carol Roberts diligently indexed the book.

Many friends—John Breslin, S.J., Timothy Chafos, Kevin Esterling, Mark Gammons, Rick Hall, David Hooper, Christopher Jordan, John McCormick, David Savio, and Christopher Yannelli among them—have supported me through this last decade. Rebecca and Michael Peterson have offered the loving encouragement of a sister and brother, and my mother Kathleen Carpenter continues to sustain me with her quiet strength and wisdom. I am ever grateful for the love of my father, Jack Carpenter. Laurel Bernice and Leo Edward Carpenter came into the world as I wrote this study, and they have provided endless moments of fun. They have cathartically and cheerfully diverted the attention of their anxious dad. It is, finally, Rita Christine Butzer-Carpenter, the love of my life, a skilled scholar of agricultural economics, and the tenacious protector of a household, to whom I dedicate this study.

—Cambridge, Massachusetts, July 2009

LIST OF ABBREVIATIONS AND ACRONYMS

SUBJECT ABBREVIATIONS AND ACRONYMS

ABPI	Association of British Pharmaceutical Industries
ACOG	American College of Obstetricians and Gynecologists
ACS	American Cancer Society
ACT-UP	AIDS Coalition to Unleash Power
ADMA	American Drug Manufacturers' Association
ADR	Adverse Drug Reaction
AERS	Adverse Event Reporting System
AIDS	Acquired immune deficiency syndrome
ALL	Acute lymphoblastic leukemia
ALS	Amyotrophic lateral sclerosis
AMA	American Medical Association
AMA-COD	Council on Drugs, AMA
ANDA	Abbreviated New Drug Application (for "generic" drugs)
ASPET	American Society for Pharmacology and Experimental Therapeutics
BPPA	Bureau of Program Planning and Appraisal (FDA, 1950s)
BOM	Bureau of Medicine (FDA, 1950s and 1960s)
BRC	Bureau of Regulatory Compliance (FDA, 1960s and 1970s)
CBER	Center for Biologics Evaluation and Research, FDA
CDER	Center for Drug Evaluation and Research, FDA
CPMP	Committee on Proprietary Medicinal Products (EEC/EU)
CSTA	Committee on the Safety of Therapeutic Agents, Mayo Clinic
CTD	Common Technical Document (ICH)
EEC	European Economic Community
EMEA	European Agency for the Evaluation of Medicinal Products
EU	European Union
FDA	U.S. Food and Drug Administration
FDAMA	Food and Drug Administration Modernization Act of 1997
FSA	Federal Security Agency
GCP	Good Clinical Practice (regulations)
GLP	Good Laboratory Practice (regulations)
GMP	Good Manufacturing Practice (regulations)
HEW	U. S. Department of Health, Education and Welfare
HIV	Human immunodeficiency virus
HHS	U.S. Department of Health and Human Services
ICH	International Conference on Harmonization

IND	Investigational New Drug
MCA	Medicines Control Agency, Great Britain (1987–)
NAS/NRC	National Academy of Sciences/National Research Council
NCE	New Chemical Entity
NCI	National Cancer Institute
NDA	New Drug Application
NHL	Non-Hodgkin's lymphoma
NIH	National Institutes of Health
NLM	National Library of Medicine
NME	New Molecular Entity
NRC	National Research Council
NSAID	Non-steroidal anti-inflammatory drug
NSCLC	Non-small-cell lung cancer
NYAM	New York Academy of Medicine
ODS	Office of Drug Safety, FDA
OND	Office of New Drugs, FDA
PDUFA	Prescription Drug User Fee Act (enacted 1992)
PMA	Pharmaceutical Manufacturers Association
PhRMA	Pharmaceutical Research and Manufacturers of America
sNDA	Supplementary New Drug Application
SWOG	Southwest Oncology Group (United States)
TPA	Tissue plasminogen activator
UCSD	University of California, San Diego
UCSF	University of California, San Francisco
USP	United States Pharmacopeia, or USP Convention
WHO	World Health Organization

Source Abbreviations and Acronyms

Abbreviations are spelled out for the more commonly referenced collections and publications; for a full list of archival materials consulted, see the Primary Sources and Archival Collections.

AAMA	Archives of the American Medical Association, Chicago, Illinois
AHR	American Historical Review
AJOG	American Journal of Obstetrics and Gynecology
AmJEpid	American Journal of Epidemiology
AmJPH	American Journal of Public Health
AnnIM	Annals of Internal Medicine
ArchIM	Archives of Internal Medicine
APSR	American Political Science Review
AWHO	Archives of the World Health Organization, Geneva, Switzerland

BG	*Boston Globe*
BK	Bundesarchiv Koblenz
BullHistMed	*Bulletin of the History of Medicine*
BMJ	*British Medical Journal*
CCE	Charles C. Edwards Collection, University of California, San Diego
CFR	Code of Federal Regulations
CPRPFDA	*Consumer Protection: Regulatory Politics of the Food and Drug Administration* (Fountain Hearings, 1970)
CP&T	*Clinical Pharmacology and Therapeutics*
CR	*Congressional Record*
DIAA	*Drug Industry Antitrust Act*, Hearings before the Subcommittee on Antitrust and Monopoly of the Committee on the Judiciary, 87th Congress (Kefauver hearings, 1959 and 1960)
DRR	*Drug Research Reports* ("The Blue Sheet")
DTN	*Drug Trade News*
EKP	Estes Kefauver Papers, University of Tennessee, Knoxville, Tennessee
EMKG	Eugene Maximilian Karl Geiling Papers, Johns Hopkins University, Baltimore
FDCR	*F-D-C Reports* ("The Pink Sheet")
FDCLJ, FDCLQ, FDLJ	*Food, Drug and Cosmetic Law Journal; Food, Drug and Cosmetic Law Quarterly*, or (later) *Food and Drug Law Journal*
FOK	Frances O. Kelsey Papers, Library of Congress
FR	*Federal Register*
HWW	Harvey W. Wiley Papers, Library of Congress
ICDRR	*Interagency Coordination in Drug Regulation and Research*, Hearings before the Subcommittee on Reorganization and International Organizations of the Committee on Government Operations, 1962 and 1963
JAMA	*Journal of the American Medical Association*
JASA	*Journal of the American Statistical Association*
JCD	*Journal of Chronic Diseases*
JHE	*Journal of Health Economics*
JLG	Papers of James L. Goddard, National Library of Medicine
JHPP	Julius Hauser Professional Papers [private collection]
JRCP	J. Richard Crout Papers [private collection]
LAT	*Los Angeles Times*
LSG	Louis S. Goodman Papers, University of Utah, Salt Lake City, Utah

MAYO   Mayo Foundation and Mayo Hospital Archives, Rochester,
                Minnesota
MDAA   Archives of the M. D. Anderson Cancer Center, Houston,
                Texas
MF   Maxwell Finland Papers, Harvard Medical School
MLDT   *Medical Letter on Drugs and Therapeutics*
NA   National Archives, Washington, DC and College Park,
                Maryland
  RG   Record Group (in National Archives)
  F   Folder (in NA or other archival collection)
  B   Box
  V   Volume
NAS-DESI   Records of the Drug Efficacy Study Initiative, National
                Academy of Sciences, National Academies Archives,
                Washington, DC
NEJM   *New England Journal of Medicine*
NRDD   *Nature Reviews Drug Discovery*
NYT   *New York Times*
OP&DR   *Oil, Paint and Drug Reporter*
PBOT   *Pharmacological Basis of Therapeutics* (textbook)
RNH   Robert N. Hamburger Papers, University of California,
                San Diego
UCSF-DIDA   Drug Industry Digital Archive, University of California,
                San Francisco
UKNA   National Archives, Kew, United Kingdom
USP   Records of the U.S. Pharmacopoeial Convention,
                Wisconsin State Historical Society, Madison, Wisconsin
VTNA   Vanderbilt Television News Archives, Vanderbilt
                University, Nashville, Tennessee
WLUK   Wellcome Library, London, United Kingdom
WP   *Washington Post*
WSJ   *Wall Street Journal*

The Gatekeeper

REGULATION AND LAW currently put American citizens at second remove from therapeutic medicines. In order to use most drugs, citizens must obtain a prescription from a licensed and qualified medical authority, usually a physician. Yet before anyone can prescribe, the U.S. Food and Drug Administration must approve. No new drug can be legally marketed in the United States unless the Administration has explicitly declared it "safe and effective" for its intended uses. This authority renders the FDA the gatekeeper of the American pharmaceutical marketplace, and it sustains a battery of vast powers. Among these are the power to define medical success and shape scientific careers, the power to limit advertising and product claims, the power to govern drug manufacturing, the power to enable drug firms to generate vast riches and the power to chase those same firms from the marketplace, the power to sculpt medical and scientific concepts, and ultimately the power to influence the lives and deaths of citizens. Some of those citizens may be harmed from hazardous or ineffective therapies that the FDA has approved. Other citizens may suffer or die waiting for the agency to approve a potentially effective cure. Still others, perhaps most, may easily use a drug whose dosage, label, and chemical form have been carefully honed through the scrutiny that regulation brings. Whatever the outcome, the FDA has shaped the lives of one and all. Among the thousands of people who daily give painstaking attention to the agency's every utterance and movement, there is considerable disagreement about the Food and Drug Administration—it is venerated in one corner and bemoaned in another; it is targeted for expansion by one voice, for evisceration by a second—but there is no serious doubt about its reach or significance.

The Administration's formal powers engender a broader and more opaque set of informal forces. From one vantage, the agency's formal authority is limited to the jurisdictions and territories of the United States. It legally tends the boundaries of only one nation. From another vantage, however, the FDA rules the entire global pharmaceutical market. The United States is among the world's wealthiest nations and its pharmaceutical market is, at this time, by far the world's largest. And it has exploded in recent decades; the American market accounted for $216 billion in spending on prescription drugs in 2006, more than five times the $40.3 billion spent in 1990. At this writing, furthermore, the United States is the only major world economy without explicit pharmaceutical price controls through national health insurance. Because admission to the U.S. market is the preeminent site of profit for the world's drug companies, the FDA's veto power over entry into the American health-care system translates into global economic and scientific reach. Beyond this, the Administration carries a stature that other agencies in foreign nations consciously emulate or resist. Pharmaceutical regulators in Australia, Brazil, Egypt, France, Germany, Great Britain, India, Israel, Japan, South Korea, Switzerland, and dozens of other countries and regions model themselves upon the FDA, and in some cases contrast themselves against it.[1]

. . .

> The public has been given to believe that the Food and Drug Administration is, of its nature, a social good.
>
> —*Wall Street Journal* editorial, 1987

> Americans are justifiably proud of the regulatory system set up by the government to test new drugs.... Most consumers in this country are satisfied to rely on the FDA's time-consuming evaluations, because when that agency finally approves a drug, it is almost certainly both safe and effective.
>
> —*Washington Post* editorial, 1989

The regulatory power of the FDA became irrefutably clear in the spring and summer of 1987. Those months marked a dire, contentious moment in the industrial history of biotechnology. On the last Friday in May, an FDA advisory panel took the apparently benign step of requesting "additional data" for a drug called Activase. Activase is the trade name for a protein called tissue plasminogen activator, or TPA. At first glance, there was nothing particularly odd or daunting about the committee's request. The advisory boards counseling the FDA routinely ask for more information about the drugs they are vetting.

In the annals of American history, however, tissue plasminogen activator would qualify as something more than an ordinary drug. TPA is not a traditional "small molecule" like those that had dominated therapeutics for gen-

---

[1] As shorthand for the Food and Drug Administration I refer to "the Administration," its formal title and its referent in much correspondence over the past seven decades. In doing so, I follow U.S. statutes and legal practice. When discussing a particular presidential regime (the "Nixon administration," or the set of bureaucratic and executive appointees who served from January 1969 to August 1974), I will make the reference clear. Prescription drug spending aggregates appear in Kaiser Family Foundation, "Prescription Drug Trends" (Menlo Park, CA: Kaiser Family Foundation, September 2008).

erations. Tissue plasminogen activator is a biologically active protein found in the cells lining blood vessels; it is a "large molecule" much more complex than traditional drugs of the twentieth century. More importantly, in 1987, researchers understood that intravenous administration of TPA could dissolve clots much more quickly and with less risk of hemorrhage than previous anti-clotting drugs. Activase would thus carry the potential for treating numerous diseases in which blood clots play a role, including stroke and heart attack. With its novel mechanism of action and its potentially vast market, TPA promised "to be the first blockbuster drug in the biotechnology industry," according to the *Washington Post*. TPA was developed by the darling of the new biotech sector, Genentech, based in South San Francisco, California. A "blockbuster" is drug industry parlance for a highly lucrative drug, generally one that generates $1 billion per year or more in revenues. By reaping vast profits, a blockbuster drug like Activase can pay off hundreds of other, less fortunate wagers that a drug company has made upon promising but never-marketed therapies.[2]

In the spring of 1987, for many investors, all bets literally were off. The panel's decision on Friday, May 29, was a refusal to recommend licensing of Activase, and it presaged a more drastic event; on June 15, the Administration would reject the drug for marketing in the United States. The panel's vote on May 29 was announced after stock markets had closed. When stocks opened for trading on Monday, June 1, Genentech's share price quickly plunged by $11.50, to $36.75. In an instant, $928 million—nearly a quarter of the publicly traded value of the biotechnology industry's star company—had vanished.

American financial markets were not the only audience stunned by the FDA committee's data request and the agency's rejection of Activase. The *Wall Street Journal* editorial page—which has long positioned itself as a

[2]Examples of small molecules include penicillin, lovastatin (Mevacor, the first "statin" for high cholesterol), or even fluoxetine (Prozac, the first selective-serotonin reuptake inhibitor for depression). TPA is often expressed as tPa or tPA in the scientific literature, and is also known as alteplase. According to the *Boston Globe*, TPA would qualify as "the fledgling [biotech] industry's first major drug" ("Genentech Setback is Only Good News for Competitors," June 16, 1987). TPA also had the benefit of "fibrin specificity," in that its activity was focused on clot-bound plasminogen and it promised to lower induced bleeding in the brain that was associated with many anti-coagulant drugs. For a reasonably accessible introduction, consult Wolfram Bode and Martin Renatus, "Tissue-type plasminogen activator: variants and crystal/ solution structures demarcate structural determinants of function," *Current Opinion in Structural Biology* 7 (6) (Dec. 1997): 865–72; Richard W. Smalling, "Molecular Biology of Plasminogen Activators: What Are the Clinical Implications of Drug Design?" *American Journal of Cardiology* 78 (12A) (Dec. 19, 1996): 1–7.

On the biotechnology industry of the time, see Louis Galambos and Jeffrey Sturchio, "Pharmaceutical Firms and the Transition to Biotechnology: A Study in Strategic Innovation," *Business History Review* 72 (2) (Summer 1998): 256–60; Walter W. Powell, "The Social Construction of an Organizational Field: The Case of Biotechnology," *International Journal of Biotechnology* 1 (1) (1999): 42–67. On Genentech in particular, consult Robert Teitelman, *Gene Dreams: Wall Street, Academia, and the Rise of Biotechnology* (New York: Basic Books, 1989).

pro-business, libertarian critic of the FDA—called the advisory panel the "flat earth committee." Yet the *Journal*'s most severe criticism was reserved not for the committee but for the agency it served, "the FDA bureaucracy." In a particularly shrill essay entitled "Human Sacrifice," the *Journal*'s editorial page argued:

> Patients will die who would have lived longer. Medical research has allowed statistics to become the supreme judge of its inventions. The FDA, in particular its bureau of drugs under Robert Temple, has driven that system to its absurd extreme. The system now serves itself first and people later. Data supercede the dying....
>
> We will put it bluntly: Are American doctors going to let people die to satisfy the bureau of drugs' chi-square studies?

The *Journal*'s editorialists·were perhaps the most strident of the FDA's detractors that year, but they were not alone. The *Washington Post* ran an article entitled "TPA Foot-Dragging Costs 30 Lives a Day." Daniel Koshland, editor of the journal *Science*, wrote bluntly, "When a circus clown steps on his toes and falls on his face, it is a cause for laughter. When a regulatory agency that licenses drugs for heart attacks stumbles, it may have not only egg on its face but blood on its hands." Respected cardiologists at the National Institutes of Health, Washington University in St. Louis, Harvard Medical School, and the University of Michigan also openly disparaged the panel. Other critics pointed to France and New Zealand, among other countries, where the drug was being approved or was already launched.[3]

Like other laments about the TPA case, the *Journal* editorial targeted not a single decision but an entire regulatory structure. Why were potentially life-saving drugs being held up to the standard of narrow statistical tests and elaborately designed trials? Why was a single government agency—and not the wider and decentralized community of medical practice, or the drug marketplace—positioned as the arbiter of a drug's efficacy? To the *Journal* and many other concerned observers, modern medicine's overreliance on statistics to judge drug effectiveness was mainly the fault of the FDA. For conservative critics of American pharmaceutical regulation, quantification and bureaucracy ran together in a patient-killing, market-thwarting, unholy alliance.

---

[3] Andrew Pollack, "FDA to Get More Data on Key Genentech Drug," *NYT*, May 26, 1987. Marilyn Chase, "FDA Panel Rejection of Anti-Clot Drug Sets Genentech Back Months, Perils Stock," *WSJ*, June 1, 1987, 26. "The Flat Earth Committee," *WSJ*, July 13, 1987, 22. Marjorie Sun, "Heart Drug in Limbo: FDA Panel's Decision on TPA, an Eagerly Awaited Clot Dissolver, Stuns Doctors and Wall Street," *WP*, July 28, 1987, H7; "Human Sacrifice," *WSJ*, June 2, 1987, 30; "TPA Foot-Dragging Costs 30 Lives a Day," *WP*, Nov. 3, 1987. Daniel E. Koshland, Jr., "TPA and PDQ," *Science* 287 (July 24, 1987): 4813. For an early power-based interpretation of this controversy, see Usher Fleising, "Risk and Culture in Biotechnology," *Trends in Biotechnology* 7 (3) (March 1989): 52–7. Critics included cardiologists Eugene Braunwald (then chairman of the department of medicine at Harvard Medical School) and Eric Topol (then at the University of Michigan); two decades later, Topol would emerge as a strident drug industry critic and defender of FDA safety standards.

Matters were more complicated and uncertain than the *Journal*'s diatribe would suggest. At the core of the TPA controversy were some complex issues of causation, human pathology, and drug design. The advisory panel agreed with Genentech's claims that TPA dissolved clots, but said that there was little evidence directly tying the drug to improved survival among heart attack victims. The panel basically agreed with an FDA statistician's lament that Genentech had failed to conduct studies showing a clear and direct human benefit from the drug. The dispute over TPA's effectiveness connected to a broader debate about the value of "surrogate" markers and endpoints— variables like tumor reduction, viral load, cholesterol statistics, and clot formation that were correlated with mortality, but only partially and often misleadingly. There was also evidence—sufficiently noteworthy to cause anxiety among some financial analysts as well as FDA officials—that Genentech's proposed dose for TPA was too high, leading to bleeding in the brain. Some critics charged that the Administration had changed standards and reviewing panels midway through the approval process, a shift that was in part a reflection of TPA's odd status at the intersection of traditional drugs and biologically active proteins.[4]

So, too, did the FDA show itself to be more flexible than its detractors judged. Just five months after the panel's request for more information, TPA was licensed for marketing in the United States, based upon results from two new trials that showed a more direct link between the drug's clot-dissolving activity and improved health outcomes. At the time of product licensing, one FDA official quipped that "we are all glad that it's going to get on the market and off our backs." Just as surely as the agency's conservative and libertarian critics had piled laments upon its delay, now other critics began to wonder whether TPA had been ushered into the market too quickly and whether the drug had been overhyped. The drug's approval was seen by many critics as highly problematic, not least because TPA sold for ten times the dose price of streptokinase, the drug it aimed to replace. *Time* magazine published an article entitled "Cheaper Can Be Better" in March 1991, in which TPA's relative benefits were criticized. Sidney Wolfe, a physician with

---

[4]By contrast, the same advisory panel approved intravenous use of streptokinase for post–heart attack administration on May 29, in part because the streptokinase application was accompanied by a controlled study with over 11,000 patients that used mortality as the measured endpoint. An extensive contemporary account of these developments appears in Maggie Mahar, "The Genentech Mystique: How Much Science? How Much Hype?" *Barron's* (Jan. 11, 1988). Walter W. Powell offers an especially insightful narrative in "The Social Construction of an Organizational Field," 53–9. For other treatments, consult Baruch A. Brody, *Ethical Issues in Drug Testing, Approval and Pricing: The Clot-Dissolving Drugs* (New York: Oxford University Press, 1995); and Charles Mather, Usher Fleising, and Liam Taylor, "Translating Knowledge from Bench to Bedside: The Controversial Social Life of t-PA," *Risk Management: An International Journal* 6 (2) (2004): 49–60. Toshihiro Nishiguchi (*Managing Product Development* (New York: Oxford University Press, 1996), 240–55) and Philip Hilts (*Protecting America's Health: The FDA, Business, and One Hundred Years of Regulation* (New York: Knopf, 2003, 300–303) also offer able and engaging summaries of the scientific (and political) issues at stake.

Ralph Nader's interest group Public Citizen, argued that the flood of new and highly expensive but marginally more effective drugs was a wider problem—only 30 percent of new drugs were truly innovative, he argued—of which TPA was a poster child. TPA's success in reducing bleeding problems in the brain and other organs did not materialize. While some trials showed benefit from the drug, a series of studies published from 1989 through the early 1990s failed to find a significant aggregate difference in effectiveness and safety between TPA and streptokinase.[5]

The saga of tissue plasminogen activator is significant not merely as medical history, but as a canvas in which the politics of pharmaceutical regulation and government power are illuminated. A subtle request for information had derailed an entire industry's hopes, had erased millions of dollars in investment value, and had set in motion a wide-ranging controversy to which major national newspapers were devoting prime news and editorial pages. None of this import was lost on Genentech's executive at the time, G. Kirk Raab. Raab was hired specifically to smooth the company's journey through the regulatory process. Years later, Raab would describe regulatory approval for his products as the fundamental challenge facing his company. And he would depict the Administration in a particularly vivid metaphor.

> I've told a story hundreds of times to help people understand the FDA. When I was in Brazil I worked on the Amazon River for many months selling Terramycin for Pfizer. I hadn't seen my family for eight or nine months. They were flying in to Sao Paulo, and I was flying down from some little village on the Amazon to Manous and then to Sao Paulo. I was a young guy in his twenties. I couldn't wait to see the kids. One of them was a year-old baby, the other was three. I missed my wife.
>
> There was a quonset hut in front of just a little dirt strip with a single engine plane to fly me to Manous. I roll up and there is a Brazilian soldier standing there. The military revolution had happened literally the week before. So this soldier is standing there with this machine gun and he said to me: "You can't come in." I was speaking pretty good Portuguese by that time. I said: "My god, my plane, my family, I gotta come in!" He said again: "You can't come in." I said: "I gotta come

[5]The remark of the unidentified FDA official appears in Michael Specter, "FDA to Approve New Drug for Heart Attacks," *WP*, November 13, 1987, A16. Andrew Purvis, "Cheaper Can Be Better," *TIME*, March 18, 1991. Cardiologist Richard Smalling would summarize that "t-PA failed to lessen the risk of bleeding complications that had plagued the use of streptokinase"; Smalling, "Molecular Biology of Plasminogen Activators," 2. On the international study concluding that streptokinase had the optimal risk-benefit profile—led by Peter Sleight of Oxford and Charles H. Hennekens of Harvard Medical School—see Kathy Fackelmann, "Sizing Up the Risks of Heart-Saving Drugs," *Science News*, March 9, 1991. The International Study Group, "Mortality and clinical course of 20,891 patients with suspected acute myocardial infarction randomized between alteplase and streptokinase with or without heparin," *Lancet* 336 (1990): 71–5. Reviews of "drugs" and 'biologics" were bundled into one center—the Center for Drugs and Biologics—in 1987, but criticism from the TPA case may have led the FDA to split biologics from drug review; Marilyn Chase, "FDA Will Split Up Its New Drug Unit in an Attempt to Streamline Procedures," *WSJ*, Oct. 2, 1987, 24.

in!" And he took his machine gun, took the safety off, and pointed it at me, and said: "You can't come in." And I said: "Oh, now I got it. I can't go in there."

And that's the way I always describe the FDA. The FDA is standing there with a machine gun against the pharmaceutical industry, so you better be their friend rather than their enemy. They are the boss. If you're a pharmaceutical firm, they own you body and soul.[6]

Raab's account, taken from an oral history, waxes hyperbolic and jumbles images. The FDA is possessor ("owner body and soul") of a company, its superior ("boss"), and in the most jarring image, a gun-toting soldier. The FDA's gatekeeping power over the pharmaceutical marketplace was the reason that Raab told his allegory "hundreds of times." Like the Brazilian soldier keeping Kirk Raab from a flight to see his family, the FDA as gatekeeper separates would-be entrants from the space they wish to inhabit: the American pharmaceutical market. Even if Raab inflated the FDA's power, his exaggeration was common in industry circles at the time. Claims like Raab's, moreover, perpetuated the FDA's power in reputation by overstating it. In practice, dealing with the fact of FDA power meant a fundamental change in corporate structure and culture. At Abbott and at Genentech, Raab's most central transformation was in creating a culture of acquiescence toward a government agency. As was done at other drug companies in the late twentieth century, Raab essentially fired officials at Abbott who were insufficiently compliant with the FDA.[7]

In the context of the TPA controversy, Kirk Raab's reminiscences are telling in two other ways. First, his casual use of multiple metaphors—ownership, hierarchy, gatekeeping, gun-pointing—gestured to the many powers that he perceived in the agency's regulatory arsenal. The power of the FDA was not limited to gatekeeping alone. One of these powers, as Raab recognized, was the power to shape standards of scientific evidence and the concepts defining them. TPA received regulatory approval only after Genentech submitted trials showing a change in heart function, beyond the dissolution of blood clots. What counted as a "cure" in the treatment of heart attacks would be defined not only by a broad community of cardiologists, but also (and perhaps primarily) by an organization of government scientists and regulators.[8]

---

[6]G. Kirk Raab, "CEO at Genentech, 1990–1995," an oral history conducted in 2002 by Glenn E. Bugos, Regional Oral History Office, The Bancroft Library, University of California, Berkeley, 2003, 11–12. Genentech's market value dropped by $928 million in response to the FDA panel's decision, but a number of other biotech stocks plunged as well; "Genentech, Biotechnology Stocks Tumble After Ruling on TPA Drug for Blood Clots," *WSJ*, June 2, 1987, 3.

[7]A similar development occurred at Cetus corporation in 1990, when CEO Robert Fildes resigned under pressure from shareholders and directors after taking an antagonistic stance toward the FDA; Marilyn Chase, "Fildes Quits Top Cetus Jobs in Wake of FDA's Rebuff," *WSJ*, Aug. 17, 1990, B1. Raab remarks, "I changed the culture at Abbott to friendliness, to seeking advice, and working with the FDA"; Raab, "CEO at Genentech, 1990–1995," 12.

[8]Marilyn Chase and Joe Davidson, "FDA to Clear Genentech Drug for Blood Clots," *WSJ*, Nov. 13, 1987, 42. Of course, the FDA's definitions of curing are not independent of those in

Second, there was praise in addition to fear. In closing his discussion of the all-powerful agency, Raab extolled the very regulators who stood between his company and the marketplace. Along with its formidable status, the agency was also depicted as competent and benevolent, with a kind of compassion and service clearly impossible for the Brazilian soldier of his memory.

> I should make something very clear. There are a lot of very dedicated, capable people [who] do very important work at the FDA. Sometimes I may not agree with them or think they take too long, but I know their ultimate goal is to improve public health in the United States.[9]

This facet of the FDA's reputation clearly bothered *Wall Street Journal* editorial writers in the 1980s. Their criticism of the agency did not meet with wide agreement or public reception. The FDA was generally and broadly admired among American citizens; the deep linkage between the agency's power and its reputation was, to the *Journal* editors, a stubborn fact that needed to be challenged. "The public has been given to believe that the Food and Drug Administration is, of its nature, a social good," the editorialists observed. Two years later, in the midst of the AIDS crisis and its challenge to modern medicine and government policy, the *Washington Post*'s editorial writers noticed a similar pattern. "Americans are justifiably proud" of their system of pharmaceutical regulation, the *Post* editorial stated. Reminding readers of how, just a quarter-century before, the FDA rescued Americans from a European drug tragedy, the *Post* editorial made a bold statement about the medical and social confidence inspired by FDA regulation, as "when that agency finally approves a drug, it is almost certainly both safe and effective."[10]

. . .

The chronicle of tissue plasminogen activator leaves puzzles that beg for explanation and inquiry.[11] How is it that in the United States, long known as the land of weak regulation, smaller government, and powerful business,

---

communities of cardiology, and the advisory committee system can be seen as a set of networks that link a regulatory organization to various professional audiences for information and legitimacy; see chapters 5 and 7.

[9] Raab, "CEO at Genentech, 1990–1995," 11–12.

[10] "Drugs for the Dying," *WP*, July 11, 1989, A24. The *Journal* and other critics called for "a national debate," a re-education of the public and the national media in which the agency's image would be recast from protector to bottleneck; "TPA: Tip of the Iceberg," *WSJ*, Dec. 2, 1987, 28. It was for this reason, perhaps, that the *Journal* criticized Robert Temple, even though the agency's scientific star had not been involved in the FDA's decision on Genentech. The journal could criticize Temple, but in regulatory and scientific circles his judgment was considered rigorous and credible.

[11] What follows is a suggestive list only; I recast some of these puzzles below in the section "The Scope and Variance of Regulatory Power: Some Comparative and Historical Riddles," and in the particular analyses of the following chapters.

a regulatory agency—*any* regulatory agency—could "own you body and soul"? How could a government agency literally reshape the content and method of scientific research? How could such an agency exercise such vast sway over sectors—including financial markets and the industry of research and development—that it did not directly govern?

How in the United States—a society characterized by the distrust of government power, and at no time more starkly than in the 1980s during the presidency of Ronald Reagan—could a federal regulatory agency have an enviable public reputation that commentators on the left and right duly recognized? How could such a reputation endure through criticism by scientists, by corporations, by major newspapers? Perhaps more important, how could an agency inspire admiration from society while also being feared by some of its most powerful members?

Other puzzles are more particular to the TPA case but gesture to broader dynamics and patterns that have eluded clarity. How could a prominent drug be approved quickly in France—the exemplar of an activist regulatory state in democratic societies, and one with stringent price controls upon its drug market—but not in the United States? Why during the 1980s did the FDA clear AIDS drugs so much more quickly than it cleared TPA, which treats a disease that killed many more Americans at the time?

Finally, how did TPA's sponsor, Genentech, survive, see its child to approval and marketing, and further prosper as one of the preeminent scientific corporations of our age? How did other companies and drugs avoid TPA's fate and pass through the regulatory process smoothly? Why did thousands of other drugs (and companies sponsoring them) fail and disappear from public memory?

REPUTATION AND THE PUZZLES OF REGULATORY POWER

In a nation as purportedly anti-bureaucratic as the United States, the FDA's power in the national health system, in the scientific world and in the therapeutic marketplace is odd and telling. It is odd because the ability of an established business firm to develop and market a new product is essentially subject to veto by a federal regulatory agency. It is telling, I think, because the accretion and use of this gatekeeping power encompass a politics of reputation that suffuses numerous agencies of state—regulatory, military, security-oriented, policing, welfare—yet is rarely recognized.

The puzzle is one of economic regulation and government power. While other agencies of government have the authority to regulate a product or a firm *after* it has set foot in the marketplace—the ability to constrain a product's price, to remove large quantities from circulation by seizure, to compel factories to reduce pollution, to issue monetary fines to companies large and small—the Administration has the authority to restrict products from entering a market in the first place. Among the agencies that possess this power—

state licensors, permitting agencies—few if any have the discretion, authority, and conceptual influence of the FDA. The difference between pre-market (ex ante) and post-market (ex post) regulatory power is crucial. With fewer resources than most other government agencies, the FDA can leverage its veto authority into much greater sway over the pharmaceutical marketplace, global clinical research, multimillion-dollar advertising and sales campaigns, everyday medical practice, and other realms of the modern world.

This puzzle of power has defied the two most prominent accounts of regulation: public interest and capture theories. The rise and operation of regulatory power in American pharmaceuticals does not reflect the self-protecting initiative of drug companies in the United States. While drug companies have exercised considerable influence in the policy process and on the FDA, they have generally resisted the accrual of regulatory power to the FDA, contrary to what capture explanations suggest. When deregulatory or business-friendly measures have come to American pharmaceutical regulation, they have arrived more at the behest of scientific organizations, consumer activists, and organized patient groups than at the order of drug companies themselves. FDA regulatory decisions have not, moreover, consistently favored the largest and most powerful firms in the industry, as capture theory predicts. When patterns of industrial advantage are observed, they are generated much more by the politics of reputation than by the politics of capture.[12]

Nor does the power of American government in pharmaceutical regulation stand as a simple reflection of a democratic "popular will" or a straightforward response to a "market failure." While the FDA's power in pharmaceutical regulation has depended heavily upon broad popular support for its governing role, numerous facets of that power—authority over drug production and medical research, conceptual influence in science, and the many uses of gatekeeping—were shaped much more by regulatory officials themselves. The empowering agent for FDA behavior has been less the public or a fictional "median voter" aware of the failings of therapeutic markets than a networked congeries of audiences—pivotal professional and scientific networks, congressional committees, consumer representatives, and media organizations.

Reputation—understood as a set of symbolic beliefs about an organization, beliefs embedded in multiple audiences—comprises the central response of this study to the puzzle of American regulatory power in the global pharmaceutical world. Reputation built regulatory power in all of its facets. And power, once possessed, has been used and managed in ways that maintain reputation, and hence power itself. Power is also deployed, of course, to

---

[12]I discuss these two theoretical approaches at greater length in chapter 1. At various points in the succeeding chapters, I provide abundant evidence against modified capture accounts, such as the claim that scientific organizations and patient groups were merely doing the bidding of drug companies in the twentieth century, and thus the companies' control was all the more effective because it was indirect. Some have claimed that the past ten years provide evidence of a more captured agency, especially in pharmaceutical policy; I examine this claim in chapter 12.

advance the public health aims that animate many of the agency's members. Yet these aspirations have not arisen independently of organizational image, and the very notions of public health and public good that motivate so many federal officials have been shaped in the politics of reputation.[13]

The regulatory power of the Food and Drug Administration stems in large measure from a reputation that inspires praise and fear. Various facets of that reputation were on display in the TPA controversy—metaphors of vigilant gatekeepers, exacting FDA scientists like Robert Temple who demanded statistical rigor in new drug development, the thalidomide tragedy and the actions of Administration officials (especially medical officer Frances Kelsey) who kept it from the U.S. market, public opinion polls and journalistic writings that imparted vague but no less powerful faith to the agency and its operations. One facet of the Administration's reputation appears in its warm public image as a protector of patients and consumer safety. Another, related facet of the agency's image comes in its reputation for scientific accuracy. These positive faces of the agency's reputation have not held uniformly. As the TPA saga suggests, the FDA has been subject to withering and persistent criticism from many quarters—political, scientific, medical, and economic—over the past half-century. Indeed, the FDA's reputation for citizen protection has waned in recent years, having faded in a way that casts much of the past half-century in stark relief. Yet over the past seventy years, as the *Wall Street Journal* and *Washington Post* editorial pages both recognized in the 1980s, the FDA has generally received praise for its pharmaceutical governance from broad and often surprising quarters. Perhaps most telling, politicians, firms, doctors, and organized interests have consistently tried to use the FDA's "protector" reputation as a rhetorical tool to advance their policy objectives. In so doing, they unconsciously testify to the reputation's stability, and they reproduce its basic symbols and beliefs.[14]

If the FDA's reputation has been tarnished in recent years, this fact yields a conundrum of its own. It is puzzling politically and historically that, in the late twentieth-century United States, a federal agency could have a reputation good enough to smudge. The idea that a government organization has lost credibility presupposes, in some sense, that it possessed meaningful credibility to begin with. Except for particular periods whose exceptional nature proves the rule, national political culture in the United States has often been hostile to the idea that government agencies are to be trusted.[15]

[13]I offer a more extended definition of reputation and elaborate upon its operation in chapter 1.

[14]I discuss recent damage to the agency's reputation in chapter 12, "A Reputation in Relief." Narratives of criticisms from numerous quarters and distributed through manifold networks appear in chapters 3 through 6.

[15]For general reviews of the anti-administrative strain in American political culture, consult Richard Hofstadter, *Anti-Intellectualism in American Life* (New York: Knopf, 1963), chapters 7, 8, and 15; Stephen Skowronek, *Building a New American State: The Construction of National Administrative Capacities, 1877–1920* (New York: Cambridge University Press, 1982), chapters 1–5; Daniel Carpenter, *The Forging of Bureaucratic Autonomy: Reputations, Networks*

In its regulation of pharmaceuticals, the U.S. Food and Drug Administration marks an important exception to this pattern. In the 1970s, as public opinion on government capacity soured, the FDA and its regulatory work regularly received 70 to 80 percent or more "approval" or "confidence" from citizens surveyed; this was double or more the confidence ascribed to the federal government, to Congress and various presidents of the time in the same surveys. In the middle of the 1990s, at a time when national surveys showed that public trust of the federal government in general had fallen to about one-quarter of the American public, and that there was tepid support even for national space programs, the federal government's operations in food and drug regulation still attracted "a great deal of support" from six in ten survey respondents. In several such analyses, no other federal government agency or function scored as high as the FDA. In numerous other surveys taken over the past half-century, the FDA has consistently been named or identified as one of the most popular and well-respected agencies in government. This pattern cannot be explained by the hypothesis that Americans are ignorant of what the agency does. Aggregate survey data also suggest that Americans' familiarity with the FDA is at or near the highest among federal government agencies.[16]

Statistical data from public opinion surveys, particularly those that attempt to measure something as emotion-laden (and perhaps unconscious) as confidence in a federal agency, must be interpreted with great caution. Trust in a particular government organization can be easily conflated with norma-

---

and Policy Innovation in Executive Agencies, 1862–1928 (Princeton: Princeton University Press, 2001), introduction, chap. 2, and chap. 10.

[16]The American National Election Studies (ANES) has since 1952 asked questions about American citizens' "trust in government." The high point of the ANES index came in 1966, when 61 percent of respondents favorably answered the question: "How much of the time do you think you can trust the government in Washington to do what is right— just about always, most of the time or only some of the time?" The low point for the past half-century came in 1994, when the relevant figure had fallen to 26 percent.

In 1995 and 1997, pollsters Peter D. Hart and Robert M. Teeter and their research firms conducted two surveys for the Council for Excellence in Government, asking approximately 1,000 American adult citizens about their support for government programs. More than half of respondents expressed "strong support" for the programs identified as "Social Security" (69 percent), "The armed services" (64 percent), "Enforcing food and drug safety regulations" (60 percent), and "Enforcing environmental protection laws" (55 percent). Perhaps surprisingly, some traditionally popular functions received low marks, including "NASA and the space program" (34 percent) and "Federal law enforcement, such as the FBI," 45 percent; Council for Excellence in Government, *Attitudes Toward Government—February 1997* (Washington, DC: Council for Excellence in Government, 1997).

Another Hart-Teeter survey taken in 1999 reported that when respondents were asked to think about whether and how a particular program benefits them, 58 percent of respondents replied that "food and drug regulation" benefited them "a great deal" or "a fair amount." This aggregate outranked the statistic for "public universities" (50%) "consumer safety regulation" (56%), "medical research" (48%), "Medicare" (38%), "Environmental laws and regulations" (50%), and "Social Security" (42%). Indeed, in this survey no other federal government

tive beliefs about which policy functions of government are legitimate or desirable. Quite possibly, survey respondents will express support for the FDA because they believe that the federal government ought to be involved in protecting the nation's supply of food and drugs, even if they think that the government did a mediocre job at its task. Or perhaps survey respondents think not about the agency generally but about their own experience with product safety; if their experience has been a safe one, they might credit the agency even if the agency deserves no such tribute. Even if these limitations can be overcome, it is simply very difficult to measure the concept of trust, credibility, and legitimacy with surveys. Aggregate public opinion data are nonetheless suggestive in two senses. First, the Administration consistently ranks appreciably higher than many other agencies, including those whose policies seem to be broadly supported. Second, the data cohere with the assessments of journalists, medical journal editors, and others about the long-running public trust in the FDA.[17]

Some of the most persuasive evidence about the FDA's reputation comes from the rough and tumble of American politics, where conservatives and liberals alike heap praise upon the agency in making arguments for their favored policies. In the decades-long debate over the affordability of brand-name prescription drugs, one idea that has been consistently floated in recent years is that of "re-importing" drugs from Canada and other foreign nations where the national health system constrains drug prices. In opposing this initiative, conservative politicians and policy advocates have pointed

function performed as high; only local government functions such as "roads" (70%) and "public schools" (65%) were rated higher. *America Unplugged: Citizens and Their Government* (Washington,: Council for Excellence in Government, 1999), 14–15.

Former FDA general counsel Peter Barton Hutt cites statistics showing that FDA's "public confidence rating" was 80 percent in the 1970s, 61 percent in 2000, then declined to 36 percent in 2006; Peter Barton Hutt, "The State of Science at the FDA," *Administrative Law Review* 60 (Spring 2008), 443, citing William Hubbard and Steven Grossman, "Presentation to the FDA Alumni Association" (Apr. 11, 2007), slide 7 (in Hutt's possession). Fran Hawthorne (a senior contributing editor of the finance monthly *Institutional Investor*) remarks that "poll after poll has always shown" the FDA to be "one of the most trusted arms of the entire government"; *Inside the FDA: The Business and Politics Behind the Drugs We Take and the Food We Eat* (New York: Wiley, 2005), viii.

In 2003 and 2004, the FDA had the highest recognition among federal agencies among survey respondents who answered the following question: "I will read you a list of federal government agencies. Please say for each if you understand what it is and does, or not." 98 and 97 percent of survey respondents answered the question affirmatively for the FDA, respectively, in 2003 and 2004. "CDC, FAA, NIH, FDA, FBI and USDA Get the Highest Ratings of Thirteen Federal Government Agencies," *PRNewswire*, Feb. 6, 2007, table 1.

[17]On methodological issues affecting "trust in government" studies, consult Jack Citrin, "Comment: The Political Relevance of Trust in Government," *APSR* 68(3) (Sept. 1974): 973–88; Joseph S. Nye, Philip D. Zelikow, and David C. King, *Why People Don't Trust Government* (Cambridge: Harvard University Press, 1997), particularly essays by Derek Bok, Jane Mansbridge, David King, and the introductory essay by Nye; Steven Van de Walle and Geert Bouckaert, "Public Service Performance and Trust in Government: The Problem of Causality," *International Journal of Public Administration* 26(8, 9) (Jan. 2003): 891–913.

more to the purportedly weaker safety standards—"Canadian drugs are not FDA-approved"—than to the possible ill effects of price regulation.[18]

In a different way, liberal politicians have seized upon the agency's history of regulating drugs before their market introduction to propose a similar system for the regulation of tobacco products, especially cigarettes. Until June 2009, when President Barack Obama signed the Family Smoking Prevention and Tobacco Control Act, these efforts were unsuccessful, not least because of intransigent opposition from some tobacco companies, and in part because a March 2000 Supreme Court decision issued the unanimous opinion that Congress consciously excluded the regulation of tobacco products from the FDA's regulatory mandate. When in 1992 Commissioner of Food and Drugs David Kessler claimed authority to regulate the cigarette as a medical device, he and his allies in the effort were not so much trying to reclassify tobacco as to bring the product under broadly legitimated mechanisms of American governance and health: the FDA's gatekeeping power over new therapies. The oddity of this scheme is that there are many other agencies that could, in theory, regulate cigarettes, including the Federal Trade Commission, the Treasury Department (the Bureau of Alcohol, Tobacco and Firearms), and the U.S. Department of Agriculture. American reformers and politicians gestured to the FDA's drug approval system as a regulatory model, and in June 2009, they established that model in law.[19]

When politicians appeal to an agency's reputation, their invocation does not itself establish the organization's credibility. Yet in making arguments about how FDA pre-market judgments about drugs ought to be extended in their authority (to foreign products) or to new products (cigarettes), politicians are relying upon what they suppose that others believe. The others in question may be voters, or jurors and judges, or state and local elected officials, or physicians or pharmacists; in national politics, the important criterion is that they are numerous. Similarly, in their claim that re-importing drugs from an immediately neighboring, advanced industrial nation (one to which Americans travel by the tens of millions every year) courts health hazards, conservative politicians and other officials are relying upon public

---

[18] For a review of the claims and arguments surrounding drug safety and re-importation, see Marv Shepherd, "Drug Importation and Safety of Drugs Obtained from Canada," *Annals of Pharmacotherapy* 41 (7) (2007): 1288–91. Some of the claims made about the lower safety profile of drugs approved by the Canadian government were made by FDA leaders themselves, particularly Bush administration appointees. The aggregate effect of these claims was probably to weaken the agency's credibility; Marc Kaufman, "FDA: Canadian Drug Position Misinterpreted," *WP*, May 26, 2003, A11; Patricia Barry, "States Defy FDA on Drug Importation," *AARP Bulletin*, Oct. 2004.

[19] Kessler recounts the episode in his book, *A Question of Intent: A Great American Battle with a Deadly Industry* (New York: Public Affairs Press, 2002); Allan Brandt, *The Cigarette Century: the Rise, Fall and Deadly Persistence of the Product that Defined America* (New York: Basic Books, 2007), 391–97. Hawthorne, *Inside the FDA*, 58–60. Martha Derthick, *Up in Smoke: From Legislation to Litigation in Tobacco Politics*, 2nd ed. (Washington, DC: Congressional Quarterly Press, 2004), chapters 1, 4, and 8. The Court's decision came in *FDA v. Brown and Williamson Tobacco Corp.*, 529 U.S. 120 (2000); see chapter 12.

beliefs that the FDA is a uniquely protective institution. These appeals to the protective ability of the FDA may be insincere. Yet in the high-stakes world of pharmaceutical politics, such rhetorical appeals must be credible to be worth repeating. American politicians rarely point favorably to federal regulatory agencies other than the FDA, moreover, in their arguments for or against particular policies.[20]

The tougher surface of the FDA's protective image—the diligence of a policing regulator in constraining and at times punishing the behavior of those private entities that break basic rules of society, science, and the marketplace—is one that many citizens admire and expect. The fearsome side of the agency's reputation also appears more vividly to particular audiences in business and medicine. It emerges in the agency's capacity to dash the hopes and the expected earnings of drug sponsors, to negate tens or hundreds of millions of dollars of investment, many thousands of hours of research, and entire careers spent in the development of a new therapy. At times, the fearsome side of reputation enacts a form of power itself, as the agency relies upon different facets of its ambiguous but dreaded image to induce agreeable patterns of behavior by pharmaceutical companies, by physicians and clinical researchers, and by other regulatory agencies worldwide.

REGULATORY POWER: DIRECTIVE, GATEKEEPING, AND CONCEPTUAL

The enigma of American pharmaceutical regulation lies in the power that a national bureaucratic organization exercises over the discoverers, producers, prescribers, testers, sellers, and consumers of prescription drugs. This power is manifold; there is no one scepter that contains all of the regulatory power of the FDA. In representing regulatory power in the modern pharmaceutical world, I have chosen a threefold conception that harkens to an older tradition of inquiry in political science and sociology. The idea is that power exists not only in broad formal authority to direct the behavior of others (directive power) but also in appearances that are less obvious: the ability to define what sorts of problems, debates, and agendas structure human activity (gatekeeping power), and the ability to shape the content and structure of human cognition itself (conceptual power).[21]

[20]The methodology of inference from repeated statements that may be insincere or even false is taken from Walter Johnson's insightful study of the stock narratives repeated in lawsuits over slave sales in the antebellum slave market of New Orleans. Johnson, *Soul by Soul: Life inside the Antebellum Slave Market* (Cambridge: Harvard University Press, 1999), 12.

[21]I offer a more extended definition and discussion in the following chapter. The notion of different faces of power owes its origins to studies of Peter Bachrach, Morton Baratz, Robert Dahl, John Gaventa, and Stephen Lukes, among many others. Regulatory power is different from community power, from economic power, and from the sort of domination implied in studies of class power. My adoption of the terminology of directive, gatekeeping, and conceptual power is meant to differentiate between the kind of power that I and others see in the FDA and the kind of power that these analysts see in community elites, in organized business interests, or in the capitalist class.

All three of these faces of regulatory power appear in the Administration's regulation of therapeutic products. Directive power rests in the Administration's ability to command the various subjects of regulation—pharmaceutical and biotechnology companies; medical researchers; and pharmacies, clinics, and other stores that sell drugs. The agency is endowed by federal statute with the capacity to seize pharmaceutical products that misbranded or are otherwise deemed in violation of the law. FDA officials can order pharmaceutical makers to insert documents to their product packaging, to add or subtract language to advertisements and labels, and to alter their chemical synthesis and manufacturing processes. The Administration writes substantive regulations governing the manufacture, development, testing, submission, and marketing of pharmaceutical products, and these regulations generally carry the full force of federal law. When companies violate these regulations or the statutes on which they are based, the agency can refer cases to the U.S. Department of Justice for criminal prosecution.

The gatekeeping facet of regulatory power becomes visible only upon closer inspection of the regulatory process. It is the narrowing of decisions and deliberations to many fewer drugs (and fewer issues about drugs) than might occur if institutions were different. One reason that the drug development process does not generate more controversy in the United States is that many questionable and marginal drugs are never submitted or developed. Out of fear of rejection or stringency at the FDA, sponsors abandon hundreds if not thousands of new therapeutic ideas every year. These hard cases never appear before the Administration, and so its officials need not deal with the contentious issues they involve. The very "agenda" of drugs developed and submitted to the Administration (and numerous other drug regulatory agencies around the world) is shaped by anticipation and fear of the Administration's likely response. To be clear, this pattern is not necessarily regrettable; federal regulation prevents and deters many sub-par and unsafe therapies from entering the American health-care system.

The gatekeeping power of the Administration in the American pharmaceutical marketplace stems from its ability to veto product entry, combined with the fact that FDA approval is the only route to market for a new drug. Beyond this, the Administration's drug review decisions—to confer or not to confer rights to a sponsor to market a new drug—are, for all intents and purposes, uncontestable. Over the past half-century, if Administration officials declared a new drug "not approvable," there was little that any company or scientist could do, without great cost and low probability of success, to overturn or circumvent this decision.

From another vantage, the Administration's historical emphasis upon pre-market regulation serves to conceal many issues surrounding the safety of marketed drugs. This suppression of issues and information does not flow from a bureaucratic conspiracy of any sort, but from the way that the Administration's powers are defined and limited. So too, the definition of pharmaceutical politics in terms of "safety and "efficacy" excludes other important questions from discussion—the heterogeneity of individual responses to drug treatment, the therapeutic experience of millions of human subjects in ongoing clinical trials, the continued operation of placebo effects in markets for prescription pharmaceuticals, and the therapeutic implications of drug advertising and labeling.

A conceptual facet of regulatory power rests more quietly, but not less forcefully, in the capacity to shape patterns and terms of thought and learning. It is fair to say that the basic terms, standards, schedules, and rules of modern drug development have been fashioned by the Administration as much as by any other global entity. When scientists and physicians test a new drug in clinical studies separated by "Phase 1," "Phase 2," and "Phase 3"; when companies submit a study "protocol" to the Administration that defines hypotheses and measures before their assessment and use; when firms and physicians debate the "efficacy" and "safety" of a drug before its approval or afterward; when scientists attempt to demonstrate the "bio-availability" of a drug in a given dosage form; when legislators write laws and insurers write policies governing generic drugs that depend upon demonstrations of "bioequivalence"—in these cases and many, many others, human agents are consciously and unconsciously using terms that have been deeply and thoroughly shaped by officials of the Food and Drug Administration. In making this point, I do not claim that the Administration "invented" these terms, or that FDA officials were the only agents involved in shaping them. The narratives that follow reveal the roles of other agents in the evolution of the concepts and structures of the modern pharmaceutical world. Yet they also reveal that scientific and technical considerations have rarely if ever operated independently of national regulation in the formation of therapeutic concepts.

In the American governance of pharmaceuticals, as in other realms of political activity, organizational reputation supports regulatory power in its directive, gatekeeping, and conceptual faces. Directive power—especially legal and statutory authority—depends upon the conscious and repeated deference of legislators, judges, executive branch officials, state-level regulators, and physicians and scientists to endow the Administration with authority over the therapeutic marketplace. These decisions and nondecisions (the often unseen choices not to contest the FDA's power or its exercise) depend in large measure upon the Administration's legitimacy: its scientific esteem, its history of consumer protection, its occasionally fearsome practices of enforcement, its expressions and demonstrations of benign purpose. Gatekeeping power rests upon reputation as well. The constant monitoring of the FDA by physicians, scientists, drug companies, investors, journalists, and others testifies to the demand for information on its officials' intentions. The Administration's reputation for exacting scrutiny of new drug applications and experimental plans induces thorough documentation, caution in development, and often the wholesale discarding of new therapies. In other ways, as I hope to show, this reputation encourages a certain kind of risk-taking, leading some scientists and firms to pour much more into the experimentation and science than they otherwise would have. Regulatory power of the conceptual kind, too, is supported and shaped by reputation. The Administration is perceived as authoritative on those matters where its definitions carry sway, and in many other cases the power of the FDA has become so routine in its exercise that it is no longer meaningfully contested in law, science, or national politics.

Power does not equate to domination. Firms, professional organizations, and other actors in the modern pharmaceutical world also carry power, and they use it constantly. Moreover, the reputation-based power of any organization rests in the judgment of its audiences; those audiences have a form of power, too, as their assessments may diminish if the organization's behavior exhibits a lack of propriety, equanimity, or honesty. In the modern pharmaceutical world, medical organizations and pharmaceutical companies are both represented by vaunted and well-heeled lobbies. These lobbies have been skilled at cultivating and creating allies among large investors, organized patient advocates, universities and think tanks, and newspaper and medical journal editors. Consumer safety advocates have fewer resources and professional clout than do drug companies and organized physicians, but they enjoy widespread media access and coverage. FDA officials occasionally and properly express fear of the political clout of companies and professions—the occasional suggestion or bill or campaign to reduce the Administration's authorities or to subject the agency to greater oversight or constrain its operations. The Administration's leaders also worry about how a medical study or a new report by one of the agency's watchdogs will generate embarrassment, legislative and scientific scrutiny, emboldened challenges from the agency's subjects, and perhaps reduced authority. At some level, then, the modern pharmaceutical world involves many ongoing contests of power.

This plurality of contests does not, however, imply a pure balance of force. Over the late twentieth century, few regulatory agencies of any sort, in any nation, possessed or exercised the power held by the Food and Drug Administration. The breadth and depth of the Administration's power become clearer when its different faces are examined, and when other institutions of regulation are compared to it. The authority of the FDA to affirm and deny entry to the pharmaceutical market was innovative and, more important, globally influential in the twentieth century. Compared to other countries, particularly European regulatory regimes for drugs in the 1960s through 1990s, the United States housed much more regulatory power in its national food and drug agency. Few regulators in the United States or other countries possess such broad power to deter companies from investing in certain ideas or developing new products. Fewer still are those regulatory agencies whose concepts and structures of thought have created entire new industries and have fundamentally refashioned scientific disciplines. Even as political, economic, and scientific influence have shifted toward the organized pharmaceutical industry in recent decades, hundreds of pharmaceutical firms still take implicit and explicit orders from FDA officials on matters both minute and grand.[22]

There is nothing false or mythical about the relationship between power and reputation. To say that reputation upholds a government agency's power is not to say that power is ill-founded, unconstitutional, or illegitimate. Quite the opposite, I would argue. In a democratic republic where ultimate sovereignty rests with the people and their collective will, one might think that a government agency should have a reputation characterized by trust and expertise.

So too, to argue that the Food and Drug Administration has power is not to say that it is too powerful, or that it is necessarily more powerful than the industries and companies it regulates. I am rather interested in other questions: whether the FDA is more or less powerful over the course of time; whether the Administration bears more power vis-à-vis regulated firms, compared to other national agencies that govern the same companies. I am interested in the Administration's power compared to what it might have been, under plausibly and slightly different circumstances. The statements about power advanced in this book are historical. They are comparative across nations and organizations. They are at times counterfactual.

THE SCOPE AND VARIANCE OF REGULATORY POWER:
SOME COMPARATIVE AND HISTORICAL RIDDLES

An intensive study of one government agency may seem of limited value for understanding other organizations. Is a focused assay of American pharmaceutical regulation over seven decades a "case study" of an organization whose patterns illustrate those of other agencies, and if so, why not examine

---

[22]The contest of power is continual, so much so that the often hackneyed point about power being "essentially contested" is a truism in regulatory affairs. We see hints of such notions of "essential contest" in postmodern and conservative writings alike about the state. As Michael Oakeshott argued in his Harvard lectures, governance occurs in spheres well outside the apparatus of the state. "Governing is an activity which is apt to appear whenever men are associated together or even whenever, in the course of their activities, they habitually cross one another's paths. Families, clubs, factories, commercial enterprises, schools, universities, professional associations, committees, and robber gangs may each be the occasion of this activity. And the same is true even of gatherings of persons (such as public meetings), so long as they are not merely ephemeral or fortuitous. Indeed, it may be said that no durable association of human beings is possible in the absence of this activity"; *Morality and Politics in Modern Europe: The Harvard Lectures* (New Haven: Yale University Press, 1993), 8. Quoted in William Novak, "The American Law of Association: The Legal-Political Construction of Civil Society," *Studies in American Political Development* 15 (Fall 2001): 164, n.6. For French philosopher Michel Foucault's concept, see "Governmentality," in Graham Burchell, Colin Gordon, and Peter Miller, eds., *The Foucault Effect: Studies in Governmentality* (Chicago: University of Chicago Press, 1991), 87–104. Foucault's and Oakeshott's points (and general principles) are quite different, of course, yet they both recognize the breadth of governance outside of state realms.

these other cases as co-equal recipients of attention? Or is the FDA so unique that its analysis speaks with limited range to other settings? I think neither of these concerns has warrant. The main problem comes with the term "case study" and its all too casual use in academic work. To call something a "case study" assumes the goal of extracting universal knowledge about a population from a singular entity. A study thus amounts to a "case" only when its characteristics are representative of those shared by a larger population of research objects; a pharmaceutical regulator in the United States could, under this reasoning, represent all other pharmaceutical regulators, all other government agencies, or even all other organizations. The problems here are at least threefold. First, one might question the existence of a larger population sufficiently homogenous in so many respects that we would care to generalize about it. Is the U.S. Civil War really a "case" of a population of other "civil wars"? Many contemporary scholars assume this much in their quantitative studies of a generic phenomenon called "civil war." Yet thousands of students and scholars have examined that bloody conflict not as a "case" of a larger category, but because its occurrence more or less visibly changed so many other things in the United States and elsewhere, for decades, maybe more than a century afterward. Second, there is value in studying a singular process not because it stands in for so many others, but because it differs so radically and starkly from others, so much so that the act of comparison is itself problematic. To call a nation an "outlier" or an extreme in the path of economic development or political institutions does nothing to explain how it achieved such a distinctive place. Indeed, the assignment of "outlier" status to distinctive phenomena in the social sciences amounts to a partial or total forfeiture of the information that can be learned from these entities. A narrative may be so distinctive as to gesture to broader dynamics by casting the difference of almost all other cases in such stark relief, thereby illuminating what is normal about them.

Finally, there is value in studying a singular process not because it stands in for so many others, but because it influences so many others. The national histories of England, France, and Spain in modern global history come to mind. A narrative carries more weight when the "case" in question has become not a sample from a larger population, but indeed a model by which those other cases have evolved or have been generated. Inclusion of these phenomena in a comparative or statistical analysis—the simplistic application of John Stuart Mill's "method of comparison" to such entities—in fact commits immense errors of inference, as the independence assumptions so central to modern social science comparisons are violated when one case becomes a reputational benchmark or attractor for others.[23]

---

[23]Historian of physics Peter Galison has rendered the point with hilarity: "Imagine a book entitled *A Case Study in European History: France*. This made-up title strikes me as immensely funny, not because it purports to be a detailed study of an individual country (there are many important national histories), but because it encourages the reader to imagine a homogeneous class of European countries of which France is an instance. The absurdity rests upon the dis-

More generally, my analysis of the FDA's power and reputation is undertaken in comparison—at times explicit, at times implicit—with regulators in other settings. When these comparator institutions are viewed, it becomes clear that the U.S. Food and Drug Administration requires some historical and theoretical reckoning. On any number of dimensions, the FDA differs materially, sometimes radically, from foreign drug regulators. Perhaps the most important dimension lies in the early evolution and massive scope of FDA power. Governments worldwide now require regulatory approval of drugs before marketing, but a nationally centralized, fully administrative process of new drug review, based upon government evaluation of data from phased clinical trials, came first in the United States. The FDA has long employed more scientists and more heavily trained personnel than other agencies performing its functions, at times (in the 1970s) more so than in all the world's other drug regulators combined. Even as agencies in Europe and Asia have advanced in recent years, the United States still houses the strongest of global pharmaceutical regulators.[24]

- Why in the United States—the reputed "weak state" of the Western world, the government of what De Tocqueville, Hegel, and Marx all observed as a near "stateless" society,[25] the home of big business and small government, and the bastion of laissez-faire economic policy—has the national government displayed the world's most far-reaching and stringent regulations on medicines? Why, for most of the twentieth century, has the FDA exercised a greater degree of formal power and informal discretion over drug development and marketing than have other national regulators?

The second and more enduring puzzle comes not from difference but from similarity. Where cross-national similarities appear, they often derive from institutional mimicry. When pharmaceutical regulation in Australia, Brazil, China, Great Britain, India, Japan, New Zealand, South Korea, and Switzerland looks like pharmaceutical regulation in the United States, it is in

---

crepancy between the central and distinctive position we accord France in history and the generic position we must assume France occupies if we wish to treat it as a 'case'"; Galison, *Image and Logic: A Material Culture of Microphysics* (Chicago: University of Chicago Press, 1997), 59. For the most influential treatment of non-quantitative research in the framework of a linear regression model, see Gary King, Robert Keohane, and Sidney Verba, *Designing Social Inquiry: Scientific Inference in Qualitative Research* (Princeton: Princeton University Press, 1994). I have profitably drawn upon King, Keohane, and Verba's model in previous work, but the limits of rendering narrative research as a "qualitative regression" have become more apparent to me as I have analyzed and pondered the world of global pharmaceutical regulation. The present study stands, I hope, as an example of the value of focusing on a distinctive organization and narrative whose "independence" from other organizations cannot be maintained, even conditionally.

[24]See chapter 11 for evidence of this point.

[25]On the consensual view of the United States in the nineteenth century as a "weak state," see Skowronek, *Building a New American State*, chapters 1 and 2. For a critical review, see William Novak, "The Myth of the 'Weak' American State," *American Historical Review* 113 (2008): 752–72.

large measure because these nations have borrowed heavily from the U.S. example. The ubiquity of national pre-market review for medicines as a global phenomenon is not intrinsic to pharmaceuticals but instead postdates the FDA's powers. Among the nations regulating pharmaceutical approval, moreover, none has been more influential than the Administration in setting standards of clinical trials, drug evaluation, approval criteria, and surveillance of drugs on the market. This strong state presence in pharmaceutical regulation developed and persisted even as the United States was much less active in other realms of domestic policy: government welfare programs, the provision of social insurance and health insurance, and the regulation of occupational health and safety, agriculture, and environment. With global and national reach, the Food and Drug Administration is sometimes regarded as "the world's most powerful regulatory agency," an assessment that refers to American pharmaceutical regulation as much as any other facet of the agency.[26]

In the latter half of the twentieth century, an American model for pharmaceutical regulation has been perhaps the primary institutional export of the United States (see table I.1). It is fair to say that no other sector of global regulation—certainly not environmental or labor regulation, but also regulatory regimes in telecommunications, energy, transportation, antitrust, finance, and consumer product safety—has witnessed so great an emulation of U.S. organizational structures, procedures, and standards as has the realm of global pharmaceuticals. Nor can this pattern be chalked up to industrial dominance. American pharmaceutical companies did not dominate global drug innovation until after the period (the 1950s through the 1980s) when U.S. drug regulation became a formal and informal international standard. The regulatory dominance of the FDA in pharmaceutical regulation, in other words, is disproportionate to the scientific leadership and the economic leadership of the United States. Countries such as the United Kingdom, Germany, France, and Japan—all of them global industrial leaders in the late twentieth century, and all of them with more extensive welfare states

---

[26]Norway and Sweden preceded the United States in establishing legal pre-market regulation of drugs, and in law Sweden had an efficacy requirement for the registration of new drugs in 1935. Yet it was in the United States where a fully administrative new drug process was created (from 1938 to the 1950s), and the institutions and protocols of drug efficacy developed in the 1950s and 1960s FDA were pivotal in the subsequent development of regulatory standards throughout Europe and (through the WHO) globally. Hence, pharmaceutical regulation stands as a partial contrast to comparative portraits of the state in which the United States appears laggard, weak, or exceptional in its reliance on private mechanisms. Paul Pierson, *Dismantling the Welfare State? Reagan, Thatcher and the Politics of Retrenchment* (Cambridge: Cambridge University Press, 1994); Jacob Hacker, *The Divided Welfare State* (New York: Cambridge University Press, 2002); Monica Prasad, *The Politics of Free Markets: The Rise of Neoliberal Economic Policies in Britain, France, Germany and the United States* (Chicago: University of Chicago Press, 2006). See the judgment of Hilts, *Protecting America's Health*: "Because of its influence outside of the United States, [the FDA] has also been described as the most important regulatory agency in the world" (xiv).

TABLE I.1
Features of U.S. Pharmaceutical Regulation Adopted in Other Nations

Standardized New Drug Application (NDA) and NDA Review Process	Regulated R&D Process (Phased Studies) and Protocol Requirements	Bioequivalence and Bioavailability Regulation	Good Manufacturing Practices	Guidelines for Clinical Evaluation
Evolved 1938–1955, NDA form federally published 1955	Investigational New Drug (IND) Regulations, 1963	First regulations, 1970; final regulations, 1978	Regulations in 1956	First distributed 1971
Later adopted in: • (W.) Germany (1961) • Japan (1962) • European Economic Community (EEC) directive, 1965 • France (1967, 1978): [Demande d'Autorisation de Mise sur le Marché (AMM)] • Britain (1971) • China (1985) • Australia (1989/1990)	Later adopted worldwide, including: • Britain (1963) • European Economic Community (EEC) (1975) • Netherlands (1975) • Norway (1975) • Sweden (1975) • (W.) Germany (1978) • Australia (1989/1990) • China (1999)	Later adopted worldwide, including: • EEC and Europe (1983) • World Health Organization (WHO) directive (1975) • Australia (1990)	Later adopted worldwide, including: • Japan (1975) • European Economic Community (EEC) (1975) • Australia (1991) • WHO (1975) • Sweden (1975)	Later adopted worldwide, including: • Britain (1974, 1977) • European Economic Community (EEC) (1975) • Japan (1992) • China (1999)

Note: For sources, and other practices and standards that have diffused worldwide, including the notion of a centralized regulatory agency for foods and drugs, the concept and method of surrogate endpoints in clinical trials, and Good Laboratory Practices, see chapter 11.

than in the United States—have been laggard adopters of pharmaceutical standards when compared to the FDA.

• Why until recently has the realm of global pharmaceutical regulation been characterized by such vast emulation of the American model? Why is it that, while national regulatory policies in the realms of finance, labor safety, and environmental regulation have converged upon international governance regimes or partially voluntary standards (such as the International Standards Organization—ISO), drug regulation programs worldwide have converged upon government agencies with pre-market approval powers? Why, in other words, is there less variation across nations and regions in pharmaceutical regulation than we might expect, and why is the American model of regulation copied in the realm of pharmaceuticals when no such American model enjoys popularity or supremacy in other areas of regulation (environmental, health and safety, labor, financial, etc.)?

An additional puzzle emerges less from the comparison of the FDA to other national pharmaceutical regulators, but from comparing the Administration to other regulatory agencies within the United States.

• Why is it that, within the United States, the agency responsible for pharmaceutical regulation exercises more forceful and more discretionary powers than do national agencies regulating other sectors of the national economy?

American regulation of financial and securities markets is nearly a century old, but no national agency has meaningful discretion to review and approve each and every financial instrument or debt issue before its appearance, or to approve an industrial product before its marketing.[27] The Federal Trade Commission has governed standards of trade and the practices of advertising since 1913, but nothing in federal statute or practice permits the FTC to review and potentially veto advertisements before they appear. Since 1970, the Occupational Safety and Health Administration (OSHA) of the federal government has inspected hundreds of thousands of workplaces nationwide, while the National Highway Transportation Safety Authority (NHTSA) has responsibility for auto safety. But nothing in federal statute or regulatory practice requires businesses to receive federal approval from OSHA before starting work or production, and no federal agency is empowered to unilaterally halt the development of new automobiles before their market introduction. Like so many forms of national regulation in the United States, regulation of workplace safety and automobile safety occurs mainly after a business has already started and after a car has been produced and marketed.[28]

Even where U.S. regulatory agencies have some official veto power over

[27]Indeed, during the New Deal, the very years in which the FDA acquired its pre-market review power, the United States rejected industrial licensure. Relevant provisions of the National Industrial Recovery Act (NIRA) were voided in *A.L.A. Schechter Poultry Corp. v. United States*, 295 U.S. 495 (1935). This is not to deny the very expansive nature of the New Deal experiment; Edwin Amenta, *Bold Relief: Institutional Politics and the Origins of Modern American Social Policy* (Princeton: Princeton University Press, 1998); Jennifer Klein, *For All These Rights: Business, Labor, and the Shaping of America's Public-Private Welfare State* (Princeton: Princeton University Press, 2004). The more enduring legacy of New Deal institution-building lay in a more robust antitrust regime; Ellis Hawley, *The New Deal and the Problem of Monopoly* (Princeton: Princeton University Press, 1966).

Not coincidentally, in their analysis of regulation, economic theorists have focused almost entirely on institutions of price and quality regulation, neglecting the set of institutions that regulate R&D and/or that confer marketing rights before price and quality are shaped in a market equilibrium. See Jean-Jacques Laffont and Jean Tirole, *A Theory of Incentives in Procurement and Regulation* (Cambridge: MIT Press, 1994); this interesting book and its accompanying mathematical literature shed little if any light on institutions of pharmaceutical regulation, health and safety regulation, consumer products regulation, and occupational safety regulation.

[28]The most relevant form of federal regulation of automobiles before their market introduction comes in the Corporate Average Fuel Economy (CAFE) standards, which are loosely en-

market entry by firms—as when they must issue licenses or permits for construction, grazing, development on wetlands, or other rights to economic activity—they rarely have the power to define the parameters of product development, research, and experimentation and production. Before its demise in 1995, the Interstate Commerce Commission (ICC) regulated railroad prices for freight and passengers, railway safety, and interstate freight transport by trucks. While the ICC had licensing authority over firms, it did not directly govern the development of new transportation technologies, and it did not exercise primary force in standardization of the railroads. In the United States, federal regulation over telecommunications has been conducted by the Federal Communications Commission since 1934. While the FCC assigned and governed broadcast license rights for most of the twentieth century, its powers were circumscribed, particularly in comparison with telecommunications regulators in European countries.[29]

Another puzzle concerns federalism. Among three critical nations with domestic pharmaceutical industries and national regulatory agencies—Australia, China, and India—a more decentralized, federalist mode of regulation is observed. Such a federalist mode is also observed in the European Union, which still permits country-by-country drug approval through its "decentralized procedure." The existence of regional and subnational regulators in other countries demonstrates that there is nothing natural or inevitable about national-level pharmaceutical regulation.

- Why is pharmaceutical regulation nationalized in the United States, while other forms of regulation are not? Put equivalently, why is pharmaceutical regulation nationalized in the United States when other nations, most notably Australia and India, have had more decentralized, regional agencies that regulate medicines?

Some final puzzles concern the FDA itself.

- Why has the FDA enjoyed greater discretion, policymaking authority, and deference from other branches of government in its regulation of drugs, compared to its regulation of foods?
- What accounts for some of the intricate and counterintuitive patterns of interplay between firms, scientists, federal regulators, and social groups in the United States? And how does this most powerful agency exercise its power with such limited resources?

---

forced and which affect only the average fuel economy for a fleet. See more generally Jerry L. Mashaw and David L. Harfst, *The Struggle for Auto Safety* (Cambridge: Harvard University Press, 1990).

[29]On transportation regulation, consult Ari Hoogenboom and Olive Hoogenboom, *A History of the ICC: From Panacea to Palliative* (New York: Norton, 1976); Lawrence Rothenberg, *Regulation, Organizations and Politics: Motor Freight Policy at the Interstate Commerce Commission* (Ann Arbor: University of Michigan Press, 1994). For a clear and accessible discussion of wetland permitting, see Brandice Canes-Wrone, "The Influence of Congress and

NARRATIVE, COMPARISON, AND STATISTICS:
EMPIRICAL APPROACHES OF THIS STUDY

The world of pharmaceuticals and their regulation is a vast and complex one. I have written this book with the intent to preserve much of that complexity while giving readers a conceptual frame in which the history and some enduring patterns of political economy can be understood and rethought. My goals will have been met if the book leaves readers with an appreciation for the historical and political complications of U.S. pharmaceutical regulation as well as some general lenses through which the seemingly familiar can be viewed in a different, potentially surprising, and illuminating way.

The intensive empirical approach of this study stems not only from the complexity and ubiquity of the subject matter but from its theoretical inspiration to examine reputation. Analysis of an agency's reputation requires analysis of its audiences. Where the projections of an organization meet its audiences, where symbols engage their viewers and texts encounter their readers—this is the space inhabited by organizational image. As a reputation consists of symbolic beliefs embedded in various overlapping audiences, the study of an organizational reputation must investigate both the various symbols that represent the organization and the structure of that organization's relationships to different audiences. Both the content and the consumers of a reputation—and most vitally the nexus between them—merit systematic and enduring study.

Another reason for preserving and presenting the complexity of U.S. pharmaceutical regulation is that most attempts at simplification—and there have been many—have been misleading. There are dozens of writings on U.S. pharmaceutical regulation, and there are many, many more on prescription drugs and the American and global pharmaceutical industries. Those efforts, while collectively fascinating and occasionally enriching, often portray an all too simple landscape. In one common narrative, a government agency protects millions of citizens from unscrupulous businesses whose lust for profit vastly outweighs their concern for public health or consumer safety. In another account, much more popular in recent years, the agency has been taken over by the very companies it is supposed to govern, converted to a servant of industry. In other stories, an overzealous and illegiti-

---

the Courts over the Bureaucracy: An Analysis of Wetlands Policy," in Scott Adler and John Lapinski, eds., *The Macropolitics of Congress* (Princeton: Princeton University Press, 2006). On the American regulation of telecommunications, consult James L. Baughman, *Television's Guardians: The FCC and the Politics of Programming, 1958–1967* (Knoxville: University of Tennessee Press, 1985); Barry Cole and Mal Oettinger, *The Reluctant Regulator: The FCC and the Broadcast Audience* (Boston: Addison Wesley, 1978). Shalini Venturelli, *Liberalizing the European Media: Politics, Regulation and the Public Sphere* (Oxford: Oxford University Press, 1998).

mate government regulator, subservient either to populist, anti-technology consumer advocates or to drug companies themselves, deprives patients of medicines that would save their lives, and suffocates the innovative technology coming from one of modern capitalism's most dynamic sectors.[30]

At different moments, each of these narratives tells a partial truth. Cautious bureaucrats have bungled. Profit-thirsty firms have recklessly produced and poorly tested unsafe drugs that have killed and maimed. Pharmaceutical firms have indeed exercised more sway over regulatory affairs in recent decades. Yet in the aggregate, and over the course of decades of American and global history, these stories fundamentally mislead. More compelling and accurate truths lie not merely in between these extremes, but on other dimensions of experience. Ignoring these dimensions, these narratives divert our attention from the ongoing politics of experimentation and therapy, from the small but crucial battles over interpretation of data, over the meaning of a patient's heart attack or stroke, over the design of a medical experiment, over the image of a government agency, over the precedent and emotion induced by a particular decision. Perhaps most of all, they divert our attention from a world of immense complexity, nuance, and ambiguity.

To combine theory with narrative and other forms of empirical inquiry is to court bewilderment. Historians, journalists, and close observers of American pharmaceutical regulation may well wonder what a theory brings that they did not already know. Academics and other readers whose interest is in

---

[30]For examples of the simpler narratives, see Peter Temin, *Taking Your Medicine: Drug Regulation in the United States* (Cambridge: Harvard University Press, 1980); Marcia Angell, *The Truth About the Drug Companies: How They Deceive Us and What To Do About It* (New York: Random House, 2004); Richard Epstein, *Overdose: How Excessive Government Regulation Stifles Pharmaceutical Product Innovation* (New Haven: Yale University Press, 2007). For previous criticisms and corrections to Temin's scholarship, see Harry M. Marks, "Revisiting the Origins of Compulsory Drug Prescriptions," *American Journal of Public Health* 85 (1) (1995): 109–15; and *The Progress of Experiment* (New York: Cambridge University Press, 1997). Angell offers a revealing examination of FDA policy in recent years (see esp. 208–16), but her narrative often oversimplifies matters, particularly in discussing the FDA's drug approval standards and behavior (see pages 75–6, 93, 243 of Angell, and my notes on some of these simplifications in the chapters that follow). Minimal and misleading portraits of American pharmaceutical regulation inform some of the leading theoretical writings on regulation; Stephen Breyer, *Regulation and Its Reform* (Cambridge: Harvard University Press, 1982), 132 (characterizing FDA officials' emphasis on safety issues as induced by economic and political pressures rather than the strict and historical construction of congressional statute that many FDA officials actually followed when he wrote); in 1994, Breyer was appointed an Associate Justice of the Supreme Court. See also W. Kip Viscusi, Joseph E. Harrington, and John M. Vernon, *Economics of Regulation and Antitrust*, 4th ed. (Cambridge: MIT Press, 2005), chap. 24. Philip Hilts provides one of the more comprehensive treatments in recent years—particularly his narratives from the 1980s onward); *Protecting America's Health: The FDA, Business and One Hundred Years of Regulation* (New York: Knopf, 2003)—yet his narrative too offers a number of misleading generalizations, some of which I detail in the chapters that follow. Former FDA general counsel Richard Merrill has thoughtfully surveyed some of the criticisms and simplifications of recent decades in "The Architecture of the Government Regulation of Medical Products," *Virginia Law Review* 82 (1996): 1754–5, n.2–4.

the construction of models and simplified representations of political reality will ask why one needs detailed narratives to express what can be more simply and universally conveyed by "theory."

My hope is to explore the interface between theory and evidence in ways that are "positivist" or somewhat causally descriptive as well as interpretive. The intertwined concepts of reputation and power are intended to illuminate not only the dynamics and history of American pharmaceutical regulation, but also patterns in other forms of government regulation. In the sense of "normal science," a theoretical approach based upon organizational reputation can offer predictions and expectations that historical and empirical study can falsify or support. If this approach helps to account for the puzzles of American and global pharmaceutical regulation, then it may help in understanding other policies and their development. If it does not, then other approaches and explanations might be sought out. From this perspective, I will focus repeatedly on the sorts of expectations that emerge from a reputation-based account of pharmaceutical regulation that would not emerge readily from other perspectives.[31] The "value added" of a reputation-based account in this strict positivist sense is that it generates predictions and accounts for empirical and historical patterns that other theories cannot. It would be impossible to understand the FDA's regulatory power over the development and marketing of heart medications—and the case of tissue plasminogen activator in particular—without a narrative approach that emphasized the contingency, the ambiguity, and the unanticipated outcomes of human decision.

Yet the value of theory in studying complex phenomena is not limited to prediction and testing alone. Theory also guides interpretation. It can supply a new lens or alternative vantage point from which to re-encounter the previously familiar. It can highlight previously unexamined facets of the problem. With a theoretical lens and appropriate circumspection about what it can accomplish, an observer can make sense of otherwise puzzling patterns of behavior and action, otherwise opaque institutions and structures. Or the scholar can point to what seems sensible, expected, and tidy and suggest otherwise. Theoretical metaphors are not necessary for scholars to engage in these practices, but they can help.

Another reason for weaving back and forth between narrative and theory comes from the limitations of social science. Modern social science and statistical analysis tend to examine political and economic reality as if they were data generated in an experiment, as a sample of various cases that can be compared apple-to-apple. Like other scholars, I rely heavily upon such comparisons in this book. In some cases the comparisons are explicitly quantitative—the worlds studied are assumed to be those in which measurements are taken (a drug is approved in nine months, seven black-box warnings are added to drugs within a year, thirty votes are cast in favor of an amendment to drug legislation). In these cases, in which events and meaning

[31]These historical and empirical expectations are elaborated in the following chapter, and some of them appear more specifically in the thematic chapters (chapters 7–11).

are countable and sometimes even "commodified" such that the outcomes can be indexed by measurements (utilities, currency, other indices of value) that can be bought and sold in markets that are both implicit and explicit.[32]

The problem is that political life—and, for that matter, much of scientific life, social life and, economic life—does not often produce experimental data. And very often the assumption of countable reality does more harm than good. Quite commonly political life fashions and constrains patterns of activity and contest that cannot be understood without careful narrative and attention to contingency. The patterns of interest in pharmaceutical regulation are highly sequenced configurations of behavior in which an entire history of context and past action, combined with actors' visions, emotions, and expectations of the future, are necessary for understanding the process and the outcome. In part for this reason, close observers of (and participants in) the subject of study often see that simple scientific theories of their world do not pass what one colleague of mine calls "the dense knowledge test": Does a theoretical model generally, and an empirical account specifically, make sense to those most thoroughly and intimately aware of the action? Do quantitative analyses count up events that historians, ethnographers, and careful observers of the events would never consider comparable in the "apple-to-apple" sense? When scholars of international security claim to discover a correlation between economic growth and the incidence of "civil war," do they do so anachronistically by aggregating events (deaths, battles, patterns of ethnic strife, acts of physical, sexual, and emotional violence) that may be difficult, and perhaps impossible to compare to one another? Do these aggregations make sense of human emotions, meanings, memories, and political consequences attached to these events?

An animating principle of this study, then, is that narrative, quantitative, and comparative approaches can, indeed must, complement one another in the study of global pharmaceutical regulation and its historical development. My hope is not to attain a perfectly happy medium among the methods; indeed, the tension among the methods is itself productive. The combination is powerful when the different methods point to similar patterns, as well as when the use of one kind of method points to difficulties in what one can learn from the others.

THE SUBJECT, THE THEORY, AND THE APPROACH

Reputation and regulatory power both live at an interface—the interface of subject and audience, the interface of regulator and regulated. In studying the intertwined reputation and power of the U.S. Food and Drug Administration, I have found it necessary to examine not just statutes, rules, public

[32]The assumption of "countable additivity" to which I refer here is helpfully clarified in Patrick Billingsley, *Probability and Measure*, 3rd ed. (New York: Wiley, 1995). A more technical treatment that expands upon these notions and relates them to weak convergence concepts is Billingsley's *Convergence of Probability Measures*, 2nd ed. (New York: Wiley, 1999).

decisions, and directives, but also concepts, perceptions of action, the reception of an organization and its behavior in various audiences embedded in courts, in public opinion, in congressional committees, in journalism and its readers and viewers, in circles of professional and scientific judgment. And in the analysis of reputation and power in regulation, it is not only the regulatory official but also her audiences and subjects that merit attention (perhaps most of it).

At its core, the study concerns the administrative governance of a particular kind of commodity—the "pharmaceutical," the "ethical drug." Definitions of "drug" have changed immensely over the twentieth century, and there has always meaningful overlap between the worlds of "foods" and "drugs." An immense quantity of products officially regulated as "foods" today are profitable because they make therapeutic claims—herbal remedies, nutritional supplements (variously known as "nutri-ceuticals"), organically cultivated foods and others. The tale of how these have eluded FDA regulation is itself interesting and is taken up briefly in chapters 5 and 6. Quite differently, a range of prescription products attempts to provide nourishment—parenteral nutrition therapies form one example.

Much of the study is focused not on newer forms of medical therapies but upon a set of drugs that the FDA has called "new molecular entities." In the pharmaceutical world, two categorical distinctions are often employed to break apart the continuous and slippery space of drugs. Molecular entities are usually distinguished from "biologics." The world of biologics is often wrongly conflated with the world of "biotech," when in fact most biotechnology drugs are not vaccines or otherwise bioactive. A more pervasive difference is between "small" and "large" molecules, such that the larger molecules represent proteins and antibodies that are "biologically active," whereas the smaller molecules stand in for more traditional drugs without biological activity.[33]

Pharmaceutical regulation touches upon politics, law, medicine, science, business, and foreign affairs. In writing this book, I have incorporated methods and insights from many disciplines—history, pharmacology, political science, law, medicine, public health, mathematical finance and economics, sociology, mathematical statistics, and anthropology. To be frank, I have mastered none of these trades, and this book represents a highly imperfect combination of research methods. It is my hope that blending these different disciplines and methods—the combination of historical narrative with statistical analysis, the examination of power in agenda setting as well as in concept formation, the adoption of anthropological notions of group image

[33] "Large molecules" and "macromolecules" often refer to nucleic acids, enzyme mimetics, and monoclonal antibodies; the history of American pharmaceutical regulation with these products has not been well narrated, and the FDA's experience with such products forms a small portion of the study. Even the binary distinction of "small" versus "large" molecules misleads. The difference is often a matter of degree and of interpretation about the drug's access to target cells (a mistake I have made myself more than once). For a helpful summary review, consult Michael P. Murphy and Robin A. J. Smith, "Drug Delivery to Mitochondria: The Key to Mitochondrial Medicine," *Advanced Drug Delivery Reviews* 41 (2000): 235–50.

on the one hand, and on the other, approaches to reputations as depreciable assets in which certain forms of investment take place—will illuminate more than it obscures.

The study reported here is the result of intensive research carried out over many years in the archives of government agencies, major research and specialty hospitals, chemical and pharmaceutical corporations, the U.S. Congress and its members and committees, selected presidents of the United States and their appointees, disease and patient advocacy organizations, medical associations and scientific groups, university medical centers, and other relevant organizations and institutions. Although the subject of analysis is an organization of the U.S. government, the audiences for that organization span the globe. The study therefore relies upon primary and secondary materials from other nations and non-English languages. With a few exceptions, most of the primary sources used have never before been consulted or cited in published research. I say this primarily to convey a sense of caution. Further engagement with the materials used in this study will undoubtedly produce richer and more accurate portraits than I have elaborated here.

The world of pharmaceutical regulation is subtended by a vast number of trade reporters, newspaper reports, business and finance journals, science magazines, medical journals, and, at this writing, "web logs" available on the Internet. I have purposefully scoured a large number of these sources, in part to get a better sense of the FDA's varied images, and in part to observe the same events from different standpoints. The study often relies upon these published or written documents for narrative and statistical data. This is not the same as studying "what people say" as opposed to "what they do." For one, many of the writings and remarks are observations on others' behavior. In many other cases, the documents reveal behavior in aggregate statistics or in relatively consensual narratives of the interaction between government officers and the social and economic concerns they regulate.

I have also conducted many interviews over the past fifteen years in studying American and global pharmaceutical regulation. These have been important, though I have not taken them as the primary evidence for the study. My reliance upon documents forms a basic limitation of the book, insofar as important lessons about the FDA and other regulatory agencies have been generated from in-depth interviews conducted and interpreted by observers with long and familiar knowledge of the agency and the policies it administers.[34] A central reason for this reliance upon documents comes from what I was able to obtain from interviews and conversations. In many cases, depictions of events that I took from interviews as factual were, upon further study and reflection, simply one reading (among many) of crucial and pivotal events. As I came to do more of them, I found that interviews were important less for establishing "what actually happened" and more for getting a sense of different lenses through which the same facts, the same choices, the same rules, the same organization might be viewed. For this reason, I

---

[34]Hilts, *Protecting America's Health*; Hawthorne, *Inside the FDA*.

interviewed not only "participants" but also observers—reporters who regularly covered the FDA, physicians who testified before or who sat upon federal advisory committees, company scientists who did not deal directly with the agency but whose impressions (taken at one or more removes from those who did) were nonetheless of great value.

In the first part of the book, I offer a set of overlapping narratives in the hope of describing and explaining the evolution of the FDA's organizational reputation and its power. These powers are ever changing, but a relatively stable structure of robust directive, gatekeeping, and conceptual power had crystallized by the late 1960s. In chapters 2 through 4 I elaborate the development of reputation and power at the FDA through the thalidomide crisis of the early 1960s. These narratives embed comparisons to other realms of regulation and other nations. They show how the Administration's regulatory power developed—from legislative enactments that embodied the FDA's strong public reputation, from the acquiescence of professional and scientific bodies that ceded their powers to the FDA or allied with the Administration in their exercise, and from rulemaking and administrative behavior. In chapters 5 and 6 I discuss patterns by which the FDA's reputation in the modern pharmaceutical world were cemented and contested, not least the legitimation of broad regulatory power by American courts and the challenges to regulatory power posed by business and professional interests and by the rise of new paradigms of illness (modern cancer and AIDS and other disease-based constituencies).

The second part of the book reveals the structure of reputation and power thematically, less in the form of a progressive narrative and more in the form of a subject-based discussion of different features and realms of pharmaceutical regulation. The worlds I describe—the political economy of new drug approval (chapter 7), the regulation of clinical research and drug development (chapter 8), the advisory committee system (chapter 7), post-market surveillance (chapter 9), the dance of firms and regulators (chapter 10), and the international system of pharmaceutical regulation (chapter 11)—are not static entities. Yet in their contours, and in the way they are shaped by gatekeeping power and organizational reputation, they bear some meaningful stability. In each of these realms, moreover, a reputation-based perspective on regulatory power offers predictions and interpretations that garner the weight of evidence on numerous dimensions. I elaborate upon recent changes in chapter 12.

A more functional reading of the book is that the first part is about origins, the second about operation. The first part of the book describes how reputation and power created the modern system of pharmaceutical regulation. The second part describes the everyday operation of that system in terms of reputation and power, and it describes the mutual influence of audience and regulator in the realm of regulatory process, firms and research organizations, and the global arena.

CHAPTER ONE

Reputation and Regulatory Power

IN WAYS THAT ARE stark and in ways not easily seen, organizational reputations animate, empower, and constrain the manifold agencies of government. Reputations are composed of symbolic beliefs about an organization—its capacities, intentions, history, mission—and these images are embedded in a network of multiple audiences. From military bodies and diplomatic establishments to disaster relief outfits and regulatory commissions, government agencies are buffeted and suffused by a multidimensional politics of legitimacy. Reputations can expand or deflate the legal authority that agencies exercise by virtue of law and delegation. Reputations can intimidate or embolden the subjects of government and, in so doing, reputations can complicate an agency's tasks or render them facile. Reputations can, by assigning expertise and status to government agencies, allow them to define basic terms of debate, essential concepts of thought, learning, and activity. In its directive facets, its gatekeeping facets, and its conceptual facets, regulatory power depends profoundly upon the image of state organizations.[1]

The central concept in a reputation-based perspective on regulation is that of audience. An audience is any individual or collective that observes a regulatory organization and can judge it. Put most simply, audiences shape regulation in two ways. First, various audiences empower or weaken the regulator. Audiences such as legislatures can grant authority to the regulator. Audiences such as firms and regulated individuals can convey power by obeying the regulator's rules and suggestions, or contest power by challenging those precepts. Audiences such as scientific and professional organizations, firms, and institutions of learning can grant conceptual power to the regulator by accepting the agency's definitions of technical terms and concepts. These audiences also reproduce the regulator's definitions by using them as if they were natural or "purely" scientific, rather than as a partially regulatory creation. Second, regulatory organizations and their members adapt to their audiences. They adapt behavior and rhetoric. They adapt both consciously and unconsciously, in ways that are dynamically planned and in ways they may scarcely recognize. Patterns of anticipation and reaction to audience can in fact permit scholars to systematically interpret and explain regulatory behavior, in ways that scholars using other theories and models cannot.

---

[1] I offer a more extended definition of organizational reputation below in the section "Organizational Reputation—Performative, Moral, Technical, and Legal-Procedural Dimensions." Perhaps the classic treatment of images and state power in political science occurs in international relations; Robert Jervis, *The Logic of Images in International Relations* (New York: Columbia University Press, 1970).

Matters are of course more complicated than this simple portrait suggests. Government agencies live among numerous audiences, and these audiences overlap and blend into one another. Audiences include the political and judicial authorities who endow organizations with power; interest groups and civic associations; organizations of professional and scientific expertise; media syndicates in print and broadcast, and the mass publics who digest the information produced by these syndicates; the companies, corporations, and citizens who are governed by agencies; the clienteles who rely upon agencies for benefits and for order. In political systems like the United States—with formal separation of powers among legislative, executive, and judicial branches; with federalist structures that multiply and refract government capacity; and with pluralist political structures that often scatter the forces of business, labor, religion, race, and ethnicity—these audiences stand ever more diffuse.

Another central complication is that what one audience sees is not necessarily what another audience sees. Within and between the audiences of government there flow opaque and symbolic beliefs about the agency—its intentions, its authenticity and legality, its capacities and weaknesses, its unity or disunity, its most historic achievements and most enduring failures, its likely actions in the next day, year, or decade. In part because perception differs across audiences, so does judgment. These images and judgments shape the power of government organizations, and more broadly, the powers of the state.

The powers of government depend in enduring ways upon organizational vessels of state and their collective images. This pattern is especially relevant in government regulation of social and economic behavior. In the sort of government regulation that is practiced in democratic republics, generally small government entities undertake to shape and constrain the behavior of massive economies and institutional relationships. A regulatory agency and its diminutive staff are often charged with enforcing complex statutes over wide spaces of territory and technology; preventing and deterring consumer fraud; guarding the value, stability, and privacy of consumers and workers; compelling patterns of honesty and fair play in large, dynamic markets; establishing standards of behavior and measurement. Such an agency may facilitate its work by establishing and maintaining a name for stringency, so as to induce thoroughness and caution on the part of private actors. Such an agency may fail in its tasks if it fails to project an image of strict enforcement as a way of inducing compliance with the law and less formal policies. Such an agency may benefit from enhancing its reputation for flexibility to encourage some degree of risk-taking and, perhaps, honesty. Such an agency may preserve its political relations with representatives of producers and employers by demonstrating this flexibility. By its actions, such an agency may attract or repel members with technical skills and experience. By the oscillation of its image, it may keep or lose the persons in its employ or its circle of advice.

Because regulatory organizations include numerous individuals, offices, and activities, an organizational reputation is rarely singular. Reputations bind to the assorted capacities and actions of government agencies. A regulatory organization may be known as moderate in its enforcement behavior, stringent in its licensing, and aggressive in its development of standards. Its enforcement may be considered to be strong in administering one statute, and weak or flexible in implementing a second. An agency's governance of one marketplace or geographical region may be considered distinct from its regulation of another, perhaps so much so as to provoke questions of procedural fairness or equity. The actions of government entities, especially the more visible and controversial ones, will feed back to shape the reputations that empower and constrain them. The result of this feedback is not tautology but duality and historical reality. Expectations may be affirmed when challenges to regulatory power fail to materialize, when emotions constrain the agenda of economic and political possibility. When actions leave predictions disappointed, new images emerge and melt into the old ones, and might replace them.

REGULATION AND ITS LIMITED THEORIES

Organizational image molds government power, and perhaps nowhere more significantly than in economic regulation. Modern life is shot through with regulations and regulators, or at least it seems that way. Financial transactions and wages, radio and television broadcasts, new home construction and landscaping, the manufacturing of computers, toys, and household products, the processing and packaging of food, and the development of medicines—all of these patterns and practices of daily life, and many, many more, are shaped by government actors in the name of "regulation."[2] Not only are many things regulated, but for each entity regulated, there are often many regulators. To take one example, consider the modern automobile. The size, weight, fuel efficiency, emissions, and safety characteristics of cars—and the manner in which cars are manufactured—are all thoroughly and legally shaped by national governments, by state-level agencies and local bureaus, by courts, by industry certification programs, and by companies themselves through "self-regulation."

[2] Many forms of regulation are undertaken by nongovernmental organizations as well as by economic firms themselves, particularly as part of an alliance or cooperative effort. As an example, some of the most influential environmental regulations come in the form of standards adopted by the International Organization for Standards (ISO), which then certifies companies. See Aseem Prakash and Matthew Potoski, *The Voluntary Environmentalists: Green Clubs, ISO 14001, and Voluntary Environmental Regulations* (New York: Cambridge University Press, 2006); Cary Coglianese and Jennifer Nash, *Regulating from the Inside* (Washington, DC: Resources for the Future, 2001). See also Joseph V. Rees, *Reforming the Workplace: A Study of Self-Regulation in Occupational Safety* (Philadelphia: University of Pennsylvania Press, 1998). A reputation-based perspective may be useful for understanding these institutions, too; I discuss this possibility below.

In the United States, regulation by the national government is as old as the republic itself. Yet in nineteenth-century America regulation was more often conducted by state and local governments than by national executive agencies, and much regulation at the federal level was undertaken not through the executive branch but by the courts. As the regulatory state of the twentieth century grew—across nations and industries, and at the state, local, and national levels within the United States—academic scholars and journalists alike began to ask how regulations come about, and why the agencies that implement or enforce them behave the way they do.[3]

A century later, most of the answers to these questions seem to fall into two camps: regulations are intended to solve real problems and are implemented by neutral and public-spirited officials, or regulations are intended to redistribute (usually to the industry being regulated) and their implementing officials are kleptocrats of a sort. Regulation amounts to an endeavor toward the "public interest," or it is "captured" by the regulated industry and used as a tool to divert wealth to entrenched interests and the government itself.[4]

The Public Interest Theory as a Fictional Straw Man. At no point in the twentieth century were the various theories and narratives that we now call "public interest theory" collected into a unified, textbook account. Put differently, there is no single public interest theory. If any such theory exists, it has been synthesized much more clearly in the writings of its opponents than by any who would call themselves public interest scholars of regulation. Indeed, very few public interest accounts of regulation actually employ

---

[3]The academic literature on the evolution of regulation in the United States is large. Noteworthy treatments include Stephen Skowronek, *Building a New American State: The Expansion of National Administrative Capacities, 1877–1920* (New York: Cambridge University Press, 1982); Thomas K. McCraw, *Prophets of Regulation* (Cambridge: Harvard Belknap, 1984); Morton Keller, *Regulating a New Economy: Public Policy and Economic Change in America, 1900–1933* (Cambridge: Harvard University Press, 1990); Elizabeth Sanders, *Roots of Reform: Farmers, Workers, and the American State, 1877–1917* (Chicago: University of Chicago Press, 1999); William Novak, *The People's Welfare: Law and Regulation in Nineteenth-Century America* (Chapel Hill: University of North Carolina Press, 1999); Scott C. James, *Presidents, Parties and the State: A Party-System Perspective on Democratic Regulatory Choice, 1877–1935* (New York: Cambridge University Press, 2000).

[4]Of course many studies avoid such binary understandings, but many more do not. For a recent and influential study in economics that constrains its imagination to two possible accounts, see Simeon Djankov, Rafael La Porta, Florencio Lopes-de-Silanes, and Andrei Shleifer, "The Regulation of Entry," *Quarterly Journal of Economics* 117 (1) (Feb. 2002): 1–37. More generally, see Shleifer and Robert Vishny, *The Grabbing Hand: Government Pathologies and Their Cures* (Cambridge: Harvard University Press, 1999). A particularly strident example occurs in a 1987 article by Ann P. Bartel and Lacy Glenn Thomas, who interpret regulation as a form of predation by which larger firms destroy smaller competitors: "Predation Through Regulation: The Wage and Profit Effects of the Occupational Safety and Health Administration and the Environmental Protection Agency," *Journal of Law and Economics* 30 (1987): 239–64. Binary characterizations also dominate some major economics textbooks on regulation; W. Kip Viscusi, John M. Vernon, and Joseph E. Harrington, Jr., *Economics of Regulation and*

the term "public interest." The term is much more commonly used by capture and rent-seeking theorists.[5]

Hence, "public interest" is less a body of theory and more a descriptive
label used by critics of an earlier era's scholarship. It collects under one term
an array of views, each of which tends to render three claims about the origins and operation of regulation. These three claims combine a normative
statement of what regulation should be with a positive notion of how regulation comes about and how it operates in practice.

> First, regulation should (and generally does) serve the general interest of a society,
> in particular the welfare of consumers. Historically, consumer enrichment and
> protection are the reasons for which regulations have been created.
>
> Second (which can be read as a variant of the first), regulation serves to correct
> "market failures," such that market failures help to locate and explain the rise
> and incidence of regulation, and such that regulation in fact serves to correct or
> ameliorate these failures.
>
> Third, the administrators of a public interest regulation are, and should be,
> characterized by neutral competence in the pursuit of objectives specified in law.[6]

In the past few decades there has been little development in this literature,
at least from the standpoint of politics and political economy. The public

---

Antitrust, 3rd ed. (Cambridge: MIT Press, 2000), chap. 10, 313–33. For a classic text that
avoids many of these pitfalls, see Stephen G. Breyer, *Regulation and Its Reform* (Cambridge:
Harvard University Press, 1981). Paul Quirk, *Industry Influence in Regulatory Agencies* (Princeton: Princeton University Press, 1981), also offers a much more nuanced perspective.

[5]The straw man feature of public interest theory is in fact deeper than this. When economists
discuss the public interest theory of regulation, they usually associate it with the "externalities"
theory of A. C. Pigou (see for instance, Djankov et al., "The Regulation of Entry"). In fact, few
if any of the Progressive theorists of regulation relied upon Pigou or the theory of externalities
to make their point. It was George Stigler, animated by his fascination with the history of economic thought, who appears to have equated Pigou's writings and the public interest theory.
See Stigler, "The Economist and the State," presidential address delivered at the Seventy-
Seventh annual meeting of the American Economic Association, Chicago, December 29, 1964;
American Economic Review (March 1965); in Stigler, *The Citizen and the State: Essays on
Regulation* (Chicago: University of Chicago Press, 1975), chapters 4 and 7 (pp. 101ff.).

Public choice and capture theories of regulation also lack clarity and integrity; Michael E.
Levine, "Regulatory Capture," in the *New Palgrave Dictionary of Economics and the Law*,
vol. 3 (London: Palgrave, 1998), 267–71. Hence, my point here is one about *relative* theoretical clarity. Whatever failings the capture and interest group theories of regulation may have in
clarity and elaboration, those accounts have been far better developed over the past few decades than any variant of public interest theory. However, see Steven Croley, *Regulation and
Public Interests: The Possibility of Good Regulatory Government* (Princeton: Princeton University Press, 2008), for a compelling push in the other direction.

[6]In the field of public administration, a notion of "neutral competence" emerged that served
as something of a counterpart to public interest accounts. The essential idea was again a normative one, namely that the ideal public official—whether a regulator, a diplomat, a military
officer, a social worker, or something else—rendered decisions that were motivated not by
partisan politics or spirit, but by professional competence in pursuit of the aims of law. This
idea has its roots in the work of Max Weber and Woodrow Wilson, among others.

interest theory of regulation is mainly kept around as a punching bag for theorists of capture and rent-seeking. As critics have noticed, it is a normative portrait of what regulation ought to look like, but since it lacks an account of how regulatory politics might create regulation, it is woefully incomplete. By default, the public interest theory of regulation commits a form of theoretical naïveté.[7]

The other distinctive feature of public interest accounts is that the font of policy in these stories—the essential political decision maker or voter—is the consumer of goods and services in a modern industrial economy. Most of these studies identified consumers as the intended and actual beneficiaries of regulation. Hence the economic and political objective of regulation under the public interest view is seen to be the maximization of consumer welfare. The difficulty comes, once again, in the portrait of politics. By definition (or by the lack of it), consumers are seen to represent the mass of society, the general public. The problem with equating the public interest with the consumer interests is that consumers are often poorly organized both in the economy and in the polity, and public interest theories never specified a compelling political account of how these consumers mobilized or organized to demand regulation from their representatives.[8]

Recent Normative Accounts of Regulation: Risk and Externalities. Some recent writings might be called "public interest" views because they focus on normative justifications for regulation. The most notable of these has been the resurgence of interest in the regulation or management of risk. Analysts from law, business, and economics have identified the management of risk as the dominant form of regulatory policy, and an unappreciated form of government policy. One way of viewing government policies on environmental hazards, occupational safety, the approval of new medicines and other technologies, and other forms of regulation is that they represent public attempts to regulate risk by reallocating it across the members of society. On this view, according to some theorists, government's regulatory functions have grown because the state has a unique ability to reallocate risk in large, industrial societies.[9]

---

[7]Paul L. Joskow and Roger G. Noll, "Regulation in Theory and Practice: An Overview," in Gary Fromm, ed., *Studies in Public Regulation* (Cambridge: MIT Press, 1981).

[8]In models of pricing regulation—particularly the constraint of a firm with monopoly power—the idea is that consumer's surplus is to be enhanced (and in some cases maximized), either by reduction of the producer's surplus or by elimination of "deadweight losses"; Jean-Jacques Laffont and Jean Tirole, *A Theory of Incentives in Procurement and Regulation* (Cambridge: MIT Press, 1994).

[9]Cass R. Sunstein, *After the Rights Revolution: Reconceiving the Regulatory State* (Cambridge: Harvard University Press, 1990); Stephen G. Breyer, *Breaking the Vicious Cycle: Toward Effective Risk Regulation* (Cambridge: Harvard University Press, 1993); W. Kip Viscusi, *Fatal Tradeoffs: Public and Private Responsibilities for Risk* (New York: Oxford University Press, 1992). In a perceptive argument, David A. Moss has interpreted risk regulation as a special case of a general form of government policy called "risk management." Moss, *When All*

As with more traditional public interest accounts, however, theories of "risk regulation" falter in their portrayal of political life. Scholars can point easily to regulation of risk as a potential justification for all sorts of government policies. Yet in doing so, they leave the crucial question unanswered. What about the political system translates the existence of risk into a policy whereby government manages that risk? Why will the agents of risk regulation—what one theorist calls "risk monitors"—be expected to behave in such a way as to identify risks and manage them? If anything, the existing narratives point to a form of reputation as the decisive factor animating risk regulation: the belief that government in general, and some government bodies in particular, could smooth an unstable world. The notion that government (in general or particular) could manage risk to a degree that neither an unregulated market nor a set of social institutions could, is one shot through narratives of the origins of risk management policy in the United States, ranging from product liability to worker's insurance to environmental regulation.[10]

Today, in many analyses of regulation, and regulatory agencies, a similar sort of public interest perspective is implicitly taken, but one that is derived from microeconomic theory. The standard microeconomic analysis of regulation begins with justifications for regulation based on some notion of a market failure or externality. Conceptually speaking, an externality is a product of a transaction that affects parties who were not involved in the transaction. At least some of the externality's value is neither embedded in nor communicated by its price; hence part of the value of the product, whether negative or positive, is "external to" the price system. Modern theorists of regulation—witness any number of recent treatises or textbooks on the subject—begin with the unregulated market as a sort of "state of nature." Scholars then walk point by point through different forms of market failures and the regulations which are purported to solve them. In many cases, scholars identify nongovernmental solutions to these externalities, such as tradable permits in environmental regulations. Yet in these studies, too, the political and historical emergence of alternative forms of regulation is almost entirely neglected.[11]

Else Fails: Government as the Ultimate Risk Manager (Cambridge: Harvard University Press, 2002). The literature on risk regulation is much larger and more complex than this discussion suggests. See Moss, *When All Else Fails*, chapters 1, 2, and 10, for a clear and accessible discussion of the larger literature.

[10]The notion of insurance and risk management policy as smoothing is one taken from the realm of insurance. The limitation of political analysis in the literature on risk regulation can be seen clearly in Moss's book. As Moss admits (*When All Else Fails*, 20), his study attempts to point to risk management as a common theme of government policy; empirical or historical explanation of a particular regulation or law is beyond the point and purview of the book. In his review of justifications for different policies, however, Moss relies heavily upon the arguments of policymakers and academics, in particular legal scholars and economists. And while his evidence is only partial and necessarily suggestive, a large number of the individuals quoted express faith in the (relative) ability of government bodies to monitor and manage risks.

[11]Among the examples here, any of the published editions of Viscusi, Vernon, and Harrington,

40 CHAPTER 1

Capture and Rent-Seeking Perspectives. The producer capture argument
has become perhaps the dominant account of regulatory policy. The theory
offers both an account of formal regulation—as in laws and rules—and a
portrait of the regulatory agency that administers the formal regulation. The
legislature rewards the bribes of industry with regulatory protection because
the form of these bribes—campaign contributions or votes—assists politicians in their ultimate goal of getting re-elected. The agency cozies up to existing firms, particularly the large and stable ones, because they provide the
reason for its existence. Moreover, the agency and the industry ritually exchange personnel and thereby create an unholy "revolving door." The agency
recruits employees from the industry that it regulates. After a period of service at the relevant commission, the officials depart the agency and return to
industry for lucrative careers there. The revolving door hypothesis suggests
that industry and regulators are united not just by interests but in terms of
identity. Regulators and the regulated are one and the same people.[12]

The ultimate beneficiaries of regulation in the capture view, besides the
regulators themselves, are the incumbent firms. Because regulation is hypothesized to fatten their wallets by restricting entry of potential and actual
competitors, regulation in the producer capture view has specific implications for market structure and for the influence of regulation upon firms.
Specifically, regulation is thought to lead to greater industry concentration—
fewer firms, each with a greater market share—and a reduced rate of entry
of new products and new firms. In addition, scholars espousing the capture
view have argued that captured regulators will implicitly and explicitly favor
larger and older firms relative to smaller and newer ones in their decision
making. Licenses, grants, permits, product approvals and the like will more
likely and quickly go to established and wealthy incumbent companies.
These consequences of industrial organization and regulatory policy feed
back into regulatory politics. Whereas the public interest view suggests that
consumers should favor regulation, the producer capture view suggests that
existing and surviving firms in an industry will favor its perpetuation.[13]

Economics of Regulation and Antitrust (Cambridge: MIT Press). A classic treatment of externalities appears in William Baumol, "On Taxation and the Control of Externalities," *American
Economic Review* 62 (3) (June 1972): 307–22.

[12]As political scientist Lawrence Rothenberg writes in his exhaustive study of interstate
trucking regulation, "the view that producer dominance is the modal description of regulatory
politics remains perhaps the primary means of conceptualizing them for popular commentators
and scholars alike"; *Politics, Organization and Regulation: Interstate Trucking Regulation at
the ICC* (Ann Arbor: University of Michigan Press, 1994), 4.

On the revolving door hypothesis, see Bernstein, *Regulating Business by Independent Commission* (Princeton: Princeton University Press, 1955); Quirk, *Industry Influence in Federal
Regulatory Agencies.* For an early test of the hypothesis that sheds doubt upon its merits, see
William Gormley, Jr., "A Test of the Revolving Door Hypothesis at the FCC," *American Journal of Political Science* 23 (4) (Nov. 1979): 665–83.

[13]Viscusi's analysis of the cotton dust standards of OSHA is exemplary for its operating assumptions about the politics underlying the regulation: "The prospect for any change in the

In the past two decades, scholars have refined the capture perspective by advancing "interest-group" and "rent-seeking" theories of regulation. These views concede that producer interests are not monolithic—firm interests vary by specialization and other things—and that consumers can also organize politically. The fundamental concept in these newer theories is "rent-seeking." The pursuits of political favors, of regulatory advantage, and of market protection are lumped together under the idea. So heavily and vaguely is the term "rent-seeking" thrown around economics, political science, law, and sociology that the concept has lost much of its meaning. Properly speaking, the notion of a "rent" in economic and legal theory is that of a source of supply that only the producer owns or controls. (The vertically integrated minerals firm with its own supply of bauxite can be said to enjoy a "rent" from having this supply on hand at lower cost whereas its competitors do not.) Protection supplied by the state in the form of regulation could be conceived as a "rent," as it is an advantage that, in principle, only the incumbents in an industry can purchase through the captured political or administrative process. The difficulty here is that the ability to influence the state is, under the very notion of an implicit market for regulation, not monopolized by anyone. A vote sold to one buyer can be sold again to another, at a higher bid. Hence the equation of "rent-seeking" with lobbying misconstrues the concept of "rent" somewhat.[14]

With particular attention to organized interests under the auspices of rent-seeking models, scholars have begun to reinterpret numerous regulations as driven by interest group politics. Labor unions may favor universal occupational safety standards because they heighten compliance costs for non-unionized firms and hence reduce the relative costs of unionization in specific firms and industries. Environmental groups—who may plausibly be interpreted as a special interest because they consist of groups of voters who place higher-than-average value on clean air, clean water, and undeveloped

---

standard, however, is not great. Now that the large firms in the industry are in compliance, they no longer advocate changes in the regulation. Presumably, the reason is that the capital costs of achieving compliance represent a barrier to the entry of newcomers into the industry. This is simply one more illustration of the familiar point that surviving firms often have a strong vested interest in the continuation of a regulatory system" (*Fatal Tradeoffs*, 177). See also Stigler, "The Theory of Economic Regulation"; *The Citizen and the State*. Jordan, "Producer Protection, Prior Market Structure and the Effects of Government Regulation," *Journal of Law and Economics* 15 (1) (April 1972): 151–76.

[14] Sam Peltzman, "Toward a More General Theory of Regulation," *Journal of Law and Economics* 19 (Aug. 1976): 211–40. Gary S. Becker, "A Theory of Competition Among Pressure Groups for Political Influence," *Quarterly Journal of Economics* 98 (Aug. 1983): 371–400. Arthur Denzau and Michael Munger, "Legislators and Interest Groups: How Unorganized Interests Get Represented," *APSR* 80 (1986), 89–106. Joseph P. Kalt and Mark A. Zupan, "Capture and Ideology in the Economic Theory of Politics," *American Economic Review* 74 (June 1984): 279–300. Spiller, "Politicians, Interest Groups and Regulators: A Multiple-Principals Agency Theory of Regulation, Or, 'Let Them Be Bribed,'" *Journal of Law and Economics* 22 (April 1990): 65–101. Gene Grossman and Elhanan Helpman, *Special Interest Politics* (Cambridge: MIT Press, 2001).

land—may lobby successfully for more stringent regulation of industrial emissions. In this interpretation, environmental regulation might be seen as a form of redistribution, from industrial firms and their workers to those citizens who place greater weight upon a clean environment. Ethnic and racial minorities may favor national licensing of broadcast stations because they may receive a greater share of targeted programming than they would under an unregulated market. More liberal states may favor strong federal environmental regulations because they reduce the risk of business and capital flight to low-regulation states by mandating that these latter states beef up their environmental rules.[15]

These two accounts each have genuine contributions and limitations. The capture view recognizes that regulators—whether as individuals or as organizations—are animated by forms of self-interest. These interests often contradict legitimate public policy goals and can render ineffective an otherwise well-aimed regulatory policy. Yet capture often wrongly perceives the interests of regulators as purely material and pecuniary. While capture theory copes well with the distributive aspects of modern democratic politics—the "pluralistic" distribution of goods and services to various groups—it copes poorly with democratic and majoritarian forces, particularly the emergence of broad coalitions favoring and opposing regulation, not least the political organization and representation of consumers.[16] What the public interest view recognizes is that official regulatory missions such as environmental protection and consumer safety are hard and genuine constraints, and that those who show up for work in regulatory organizations are different and likely more dedicated to these aims. Yet the public interest view is rightly chided as naïve in that it rejects more complex and realistic human motivations, and that it wrongly identifies regulatory motivations with the public goals specified in legislation. While an organization's official mission surely

---

[15]Notice that in the example of environmental regulation as redistribution, the per se value of plants, animals, and biodiversity is ignored. This is not an issue of externality, but a matter of intrinsic valuation. Nowhere do animals and plants enter into the utility calculus other than through their effects on human welfare. For some of these examples, see Viscusi, Vernon, and Harrington, *Economics of Regulation and Antitrust*. On environmental regulation, see B. Peter Pashigian, "Environmental Regulation: Whose Self-Interests Are Being Protected?" in Stigler, ed., *Chicago Studies in Political Economy* (Chicago: University of Chicago Press, 1988), chap. 17; Pashigian, "The Effect of Environmental Regulation on Optimal Plant Size and Factor Shares," *Journal of Law and Economics* 26 (1) (1984). For other examples, see Bartel and Thomas, "Predation through Regulation"; Lacy Glenn Thomas, "Regulation and Firm Size: FDA Impacts on Innovation," *RAND Journal of Economics* 21 (4) (Winter 1990): 497–517. For a related example of environmental regulation as redistribution, see Jean-Jacques Laffont and Jean Tirole, "The Politics of Government Decision-Making: A Theory of Regulatory Capture," *Quarterly Journal of Economics* 4 (Nov. 1991): 1089–1127.

[16]This sort of inference is based on a thoroughly ahistorical and decontextualized analogy of complex regulators as another form of toll-booth collector, as if the licensing of barbers in Kansas, the management of forests in Australasia, and the approval of new medical devices in Europe were all part of the same enterprise. Shleifer and Vishny, *The Grabbing Hand*, provide the starkest example of this kind of thinking. At their simplest, these studies equate the dis-

contributes to the felt goals and perceptions of its members, official constructs and organizational missions never fully determine behavior. Just as important, particular offices and individual regulators may understand and interpret an organization's mission (or "the public interest") in different ways. Public interest accounts of regulation generally ignore these organizational complexities.[17]

Organizational Reputation and Regulation

What if the metaphor for understanding regulators is neither the automaton nor the kleptocrat? What if, instead, it is the imperfect human official motivated neither by neutral competence nor by monetary enrichment nor by raw empowerment, but by status, esteem, legitimacy, and reputation? What if we look to different exemplars—the status-conscious military officer; the error-wary intelligence analyst; the bishop or pastor who leavens his disciplinary homilies with decorum and gentility in his homilies to keep his flock attentive, respectful, and continually coming to church; the hospital administrator anxious about serving multiple constituencies (patients, community leaders, doctors and nurses, financial donors, state and federal regulators); the esteem-chasing researcher or scholar who values autonomy and professional image; or the zealous but gun-shy forester who balances love of habitat with the felt necessity for compromise with local political forces—for our regulatory analogies? Our models would then be more psychologically realistic, incorporate the complexity of politics and policymaking, attend to the historical contingencies of governance, and all the while still maintain a degree of goal pursuit and situated rationality.

The academy and the polis are in need of an alternative model for understanding regulation and regulators, one founded upon the human pursuit of esteem but one that allows for greater complexity of human motivations

---

tributive consequences of regulation with the politics of taxation, and often proceed further to equate regulation and taxation as alternative means of accomplishing the same ends; see Richard A. Posner, "Taxation by Regulation," *Bell Journal of Economics* 2 (Spring 1971) (1): 22–50. While this move has some use as a metaphor, it ignores the extensive political and economic differences between these kinds of policies—most notably the greater reliance upon bureaucratic agencies in setting and implementing regulatory policy as compared to tax policy, the more common informational designs of regulatory policy, the distinct historical origins of the two policies in many national and local settings, and the fact that the political coalitions supporting each are often quite distinct if not at odds; see R. Douglas Arnold, *Congress and the Bureaucracy: A Theory of Influence* (New Haven: Yale University Press, 1979); *The Logic of Congressional Action* (New Haven: Yale University Press, 1990).

[17]Even in cases where it would seem that public interest accounts describe the process by which individual members come to internalize the organization's values—Herbert Kaufman's *The Forest Ranger*—a closer reading gestures to the difficulties of this equilibrium. Kaufman described an agency in which far-flung personnel obeyed the aims of the central administration, but his study did not show evidence that local capture was stamped out. For a study that presents evidence of local-level political engagement by a similar agency, see Philip Selznick's classic volume, *The TVA and the Grass Roots* (Chicago: University of Chicago Press, 1947).

and understands that different political actors perceive regulation and regulators in different ways. The elaboration here is neither mathematical nor entirely formal, but conceptual. The model is not intended as a universal explanation for regulatory behavior in the sense of a covering law. It is not clear that any such explanation exists.[18]

An alternative account of regulation begins with the fact that most regulations are carried out by public organizations. Whether it is the independent commission, the parliamentary ministry, the executive department, the specialized agency, or some other bureaucratic form that is involved, many of the most important choices in regulation are undertaken by administrative officials. In fact, the dependence of regulation upon public organizations is broader than this. In numerous cases, public regulatory agencies have served as a font of regulatory legislation, have crafted the essentials of policy in interpretation and in rulemaking, and have given new meaning entirely to a regulation in their preferred patterns of enforcement.[19]

A facilitating condition for the creation of regulation in modern democratic societies is for the attentive public (and legislators in particular) to believe that whatever problems exist will be capably addressed and solved by a particular agency. In the United States and other countries, the delegation of tasks in new laws goes overwhelmingly to agencies that already exist. Regulation is no exception to this pattern; most regulations have an administrative regulator. The act of a legislature or political executive to place authority, discretion, and power in a public agency reflects, at some basic level, a belief that the agency is legitimate and effective, and that the net

---

[18]Elsewhere I have elaborated mathematically some features of this account. In doing so, I have worked with quite specific and limited applications of the theory presented here. I have doubt that a general account can be developed in the context of a single model, whether in mathematical or other form. For these more particular contributions, see "Protection without Capture: Product Approval by a Politically Responsive, Learning Regulator," *APSR* 98 (4) (Nov. 2004): 613–31; Carpenter and Ting, "Regulatory Errors with Endogenous Agendas," *American Journal of Political Science* 95 (4) (Nov. 2007): 490–505.

[19]For telling examples of partial regulatory "autonomy" in the United States, see Kelman, *Regulating America, Regulating Sweden* (Cambridge, MIT Press, 1981) (occupational safety and health); Balogh, *Chain Reaction* (New York: Cambridge University Press, 1993) (commercial nuclear power); Mashaw and Harfst, *The Struggle for Auto Safety* (Cambridge, MA: Harvard University Press, 1990) (automobile safety regulation); Carpenter, *The Forging of Bureaucratic Autonomy: Networks, Reputations and Policy Innovation in Executive Agencies, 1862–1928* (Princeton: Princeton University Press, 2001) (food and drug regulation, national forest management). Recognition of the political primacy of public agencies in economic regulation is not, however, equivalent to the conclusion that these agencies are necessarily or wholly autonomous or possess unlimited discretion. Barry R. Weingast, "The Congressional-Bureaucratic System," in *Institutions of American Democracy: The Executive Branch* (New York: Oxford University Press, 2005). Theoretical accounts of "delegation" in law and political science suggest that the degree of independent policymaking by an agency will depend on features of the agency as well as features of the political institution delegating; John D. Huber and Nolan M. McCarty, "Bureaucratic Capacity, Delegation, and Political Reform," *APSR* 98(3) (2004): 481–94. In this respect, reputation (more narrowly understood as politicians' "beliefs" about the efficacy of a particular agency) may be seen as an essential factor shaping delegation.

benefits of empowering the regulatory agency outweigh the net benefits of placing power elsewhere. In some cases, the legitimacy of the agency may make a certain regulatory policy possible, whereas with another organization it would not have been considered. Conversely, in other cases, the weakness of an agency's reputation may lead politicians to abandon regulation altogether; the presence of a weak, ineffective, or apparently corrupt energy commission may lead politicians to forgo entirely any attempt to regulate electricity networks. Even in the case of privatization, there are beliefs about the likely capacity of those private organizations that will carry out regulatory mandates, and such moves will often derive from beliefs (or doubts) about the incapacity or antagonism of the current regulator, or the weakness of current regulatory arrangements.[20]

Organizational Reputation—Performative, Moral, Technical, and Legal-Procedural Dimensions. An organizational reputation is a set of symbolic beliefs about the unique or separable capacities, roles, and obligations of an organization, where these beliefs are embedded in audience networks. The beliefs composing an organizational reputation need not be spelled out in great detail. They are usually figurative and susceptible to numerous (though limited) interpretations. The symbols that are the raw material of beliefs and reputation have inherent ambiguity, and to a degree, ambiguity coincides with robustness of the identity.[21]

Reputation forms a largely symbolic construct. A reputation is not a constitution or a statute; it is not a formalized entity. The capacity to bear reputations distinguishes organizations from rule-defined institutions, and from markets. In the main, English speakers name as "institutions" the U.S. Congress, the House of Lords, and the New York Stock Exchange only to the extent that they are organizations that can bear reputations and identities. What we call "the stock market" is less an organization than an institution; to the extent that "the stock market" has a reputation, it is probably housed in an organization such as the New York Stock Exchange or the FTSE of London. Reputations as such usually attach themselves not to rules or systems of rules, but rather to collective entities known by proper nouns. Accordingly,

---

[20]In David Epstein and Sharyn O'Halloran's study of all acts of congressional delegation to administrative agencies from 1947 to 1992, 79 percent of delegations gave laws to existing agencies, while only 21 percent of delegations were to newly created agencies (*Delegating Powers: A Transaction-Cost Approach to Policymaking under Separated Powers* (New York: Cambridge University Press, 1999), 158). On delegation "away" from an agency with a poor reputation, see the demise of administrative autonomy for the U. S. Reclamation Service; Carpenter, *The Forging of Bureaucratic Autonomy*, chap. 10.

[21]On the notion of multiple audiences see, originally, Erving Goffman, *The Presentation of the Self in Everyday Life* (New York: Doubleday, 1959). Other treatments include Goffman's *Interaction Ritual: Essays on Face-to-Face Behavior* (New York: Pantheon, 1967), and *Stigma: Notes on the Management of Spoiled Identity* (New York: Simon & Schuster, 1963). The idea receives operationalization in John F. Padgett and Christopher K. Ansell, "Robust Action and the Rise of the Medici, 1400–1434," *American Journal of Sociology* (1993): 1259–1319.

we can call the U.S. Congress and its Ways and Means Committee "institutions" largely because they are organizational; the seniority system in congressional committees is an institution in the sense of being a "rule of the game," but the seniority system as such is not an organization, and for related reasons, the seniority system lacks a reputation as commonly defined.[22]

Four dimensions of organizational image—its performative, moral, technical, and legal dimensions—comprise the structure of beliefs about an agency.

1. Organizations are often judged by their performance. Whatever the aim of the organization, its *performative reputation* expresses its audiences' varying judgments of the quality of the entity's decision making and its capacity for effectively achieving its ends and announced objectives.

A crucial feature of performative reputation lies in the organization's ability to intimidate, which depends upon the audience in question. For some audiences, such as regulated firms and industries in a political economy setting, the relevant dimension of performance may not be capacity for success, but capacity for taking drastic action that harms the interests of some of those audiences subject to the regulator's power. Some audiences may celebrate these actions even as others are horrified by them. The question concerns whether the organization can display sufficient vigor and aggressiveness in the pursuit of some of its aims so as to invite compliance, induce decisions that render the agency's work easier or less controversial, or to deter challenges to the organization's power.

2. Agencies also have *moral reputations*. Audiences may ask: does this organization have morally and ethically defensible means and ends? Does the organization protect the interests of its clients, constituencies, and members? Does the organization have a culture of ethical behavior, of transparency? Does the organization exhibit compassion for those adversely affected by its decisions or those in its environment who are less fortunate or more constrained? Is the organization flexible with respect to human needs? An organization perceived to be highly effective may nonetheless have a problematic moral reputation.

3. *Technical reputation* encompasses variables such as scientific accuracy, methodological prowess, and analytic capacity. The organization may be efficient and well-meaning, but are its representative members "expert" on the questions that confront it? In a professional or rational sense, is it "qualified" for the authority (legal and cultural) granted to it?

[22]On the distinction between organizations and markets, see Oliver Williamson, *Markets and Hierarchies* (New York: Free Press, 1983). On the notion of institutions as "rules of the game," and the resulting distinction between organizations and institutions, see Douglass North, *Institutions, Institutional Change and Economic Performance* (New York: Cambridge University Press, 1990), Introduction, and chapter 12. The symbolic character of reputation is one reason why the terms "image" and "reputation" substitute for one another in this study. Readers may fairly wonder why an institution such as the U.S. Constitution—while certainly not an organization—does not qualify for a reputation, especially since its provisions have been copied many times over worldwide. Besides the fact that a model may be copied without having a "reputation," it is fair to say that the reputation of the U.S. Constitution is in many ways the reputation of the organizations (i.e., the society, the nation, the government, the economy) that it structures.

4. An organization's *legal-procedural reputation* relates to the justness of the processes by which its behavior is generated. This is different from moral reputation because an organization may have defensible aims and ethically appropriate strategies for meeting them, but may not have followed commonly recognized norms of deliberation, procedure, or decision making. Whatever the decision, audiences (particularly courts and some scientific audiences) may ask, did the organization follow accepted procedures to come to its decision? Were its procedures thorough enough?

The different facets of organizational reputation overlap and necessarily embed some conflict. An organization can be so attentive to procedural legitimacy that it sacrifices efficiency or fails to demonstrate compassion toward those few individuals whose hopes are dashed by its decision-making process. An agency's official leaders can so zealously pursue social justice or moral rectitude that they neglect procedural concerns or betray their technical reputation. Moreover, the symbols and information that make up an organizational reputation have the property of "spillover" or transcendence. They flow across boundaries and thus impose constraints upon an agency's ability to satisfy more than one audience, to maintain an appearance of seamlessness across situations and contingencies. When this is the case, ambiguity and the possibility of multiple interpretations of symbols and actions can facilitate singularity for the organization. They can, in Goffman's words, preserve "face."

Individual Roots of Organizational Reputation: Image and Esteem. The force of reputation in organizational and public life is founded in part upon the force of image, esteem, and self-presentation in individual life. At one level, reputation is a form of identity or image. Identity in this reading has two faces: internal (the self, or "how I perceive me") and external (reputation, or how "others" perceive me). The influence of organizational identity upon individual behavior can be considered in two ways: the case where the individual is a member of the organization, and the case where the individual lies outside the organization.[23]

The idea that humans are motivated by esteem considerations—in addition to, perhaps more so than by material factors—is long held. Recent historical studies have demonstrated that human agents ranging from visual artists to monarchs took conscious and planned steps to sculpt an image for one or more audiences. Psychologists have long argued that "Individuals strive to maintain or enhance their self-esteem," and that "they strive for a positive self-concept." Yet the determinants of esteem, self-concept, and identity do not lie merely at the individual level. They also operate at the level of families, interpersonal networks, religious and geographic affiliations, organizational memberships, ethnic and racial groups to which the

---

[23]Ultimately, organizational reputation exists at the interface of the audience and the institution or structure being assessed.

individual belongs, and other shared characteristics. An important school of psychological thought, now called "social identity theory," suggests that organizational and group contexts will figure materially in the determination of individual esteem, affect, and behavior.[24]

The identity and esteem of an individual often depend upon wider social evaluations of the organization to which she belongs. A proud company employee may look to leave or shirk responsibility in response to a corporate scandal, or she may rally around her organization's identity and "stick it out." Sales representatives often acknowledge and exploit their company's brand-name identity in their pitches to potential customers. Colleges, hospitals, and military units might use their "brand name" as a sorting mechanism to attract a certain kind of member. A loyal college alumna might, upon hearing of a scandal involving a university athletic team or the college president, become disillusioned and withhold contributions or tell her daughter to attend another school. She may also neglect to tell new acquaintances about her alma mater. A grown man may carry with him the pride or shame (often both) of his family name and history.[25]

Of course, the individuals in an organization display various levels of identification with it, and different members understand the organization's identity in alternative ways. A critical variable is the individual's attachment or commitment to the organization. Psychologists have adduced considerable evidence for the hypothesis that, under conditions of a public threat to an organization's identity—a scandal or an observable episode of poor performance—less attached members may exit the organization, whereas more attached members may exhibit a combination of defensive and corrective behavior. One helpful aspect of a reputation-based perspective on regulatory organizations, then, is that it allows students to decompose these agen-

---

[24]For exemplary studies of public individuals and organizations whose consciousness of image and power governed much of their behavior, consult Jay A. Clarke, *Becoming Edvard Munch: Influence, Anxiety, and Myth* (New Haven: Yale University Press, 2009), esp. pp. 61–108; Kevin Sharpe, *Selling the Tudor Monarchy: Authority and Image in Sixteenth-Century England* (New Haven: Yale University Press, 2009). Henri Tajfel and John C. Turner, "An Integrative Theory of Intergroup Conflict," in W. G. Austin and S. Worchel, eds., *The Social Psychology of Intergroup Relations* (Monterey: Brooks-Cole, 1979); reprinted in Michael A. Hogg and Dominic Abrams, eds., *Intergroup Relations: Essential Readings* (New York: Psychology Press, 2001), 101. In social identity theory, a primary reason that individuals display preferences toward members of groups with which they identify ("in-group bias") is that group characteristics—racial identity, skin color, ethnic heritage—have positive or negative value connotations. Evaluations of one's own group are referential, that is, they rest upon an explicit or implicit comparison with another group. The idea of organizationally defined value rests upon similar foundations. For a recent synthesis of social identity theory, see Naomi Ellemers, Russell Spears, and Bertjan Doosje, "Self and Social Identity," *Annual Review of Psychology* 53 (2002): 161–86.

[25]On various responses to organizational identity threat, see Ellemers, Spears, and Doosje, "Self and Social Identity," 174–8. On identity and sorting, see Duncan Watts, "Identity and Search in Social Networks," *Science* 296 (2002): 1302–5. Also David Kreps, "Corporate Culture and Economic Theory," in James Alt and Kenneth Shepsle, eds., *Rational Perspectives on Political Science* (New York: Cambridge University Press, 1986).

cies and think about (and perhaps predict) the varying behavior of individuals within them.[26]

The commitment of an individual to an organization speaks to the attachment side of reputation. But there is another side, one that equally shapes the power and legitimacy of the organization. An ordinary citizen can hold certain beliefs, impressions, and opinions about organizations such as the U.S. Marine Corps ("the Marines"), Microsoft Corporation ("Microsoft"), the Catholic Church ("the Church"), and the U.S. Supreme Court ("the Court"). What she thinks about those organizations—literally how she conceives of them in her mind—may explain something about their political power, their social clout, and their influence over her. This is the legitimacy side of reputation. An organization or institution that is deemed legitimate, expert, or effective may enjoy deference to its decisions that is separable and independent from its more formal powers. As scholars in law and political science have long recognized, high courts in many nations depend heavily upon their perceived legitimacy for the enforcement of their decisions, as most of these judicial bodies must rely on other institutions for formal enforcement authority. In a related manner, citizens' "trust in government" is believed to shape the willingness of politicians to create, expand, or maintain government programs.[27]

An organization's reputation, then, shapes the behavior and affect of its "members," and influences the behavior of those "outsiders" who interact with it. In reality, each of these groups—members and outsiders—are manifold and complex. Within a government agency, there may be a research division, a public relations division, an enforcement division, a policy division, and so on. The same agency may face a diverse set of constituents: the business firms it regulates, the consumer groups it tries to satisfy, the legislature that funds and oversees it, the professional societies who can express faith or

[26]Naomi Ellemers and colleagues have produced a useful set of predictions by examining the intersection of (1) individual group attachment and (2) the direction or targeting of the identity threat (whether it jeopardizes individual or group image); Ellemers, Spears, and Doosje, "Self and Social Identity." J. C. Turner, M. A. Hogg, P. J. Oakes, and P. M. Smith, "Failure and Defeat as Determinants of Group Cohesiveness," *British Journal of Social Psychology* 23 (1984): 97–111.

[27]For exemplary titles in the psychology of legitimacy, see Tom R. Tyler, "Psychological Perspectives on Legitimacy and Legitimation," *Annual Review of Psychology* 57 (2006): 375–400; J. T. Jost and B. Major, *The Psychology of Legitimacy: Emerging Perspectives on Ideology, Justice and Intergroup Relations* (New York: Cambridge University Press, 2001). The literature on courts and judicial legitimacy is large. For some recent contributions, see Keith Whittington, *Political Foundations of Judicial Supremacy* (Princeton: Princeton University Press, 2007), esp. chapters 3 and 5; James L. Gibson and Gregory A. Caldeira, "Defenders of Democracy? Legitimacy, Popular Acceptance, and the South African Constitutional Court," *Journal of Politics* 65 (2003): 1–30; Gibson, Caldeira, and Virginia A. Baird, "On the Legitimacy of High Courts," *APSR* 92 (1998): 343–58. On trust in government and legitimacy, see John R. Hibbing and Elizabeth Theiss-Morse, *Stealth Democracy: Americans' Beliefs About How Government Should Work* (New York: Cambridge University Press, 2002); Joseph S. Nye, Philip D. Zelikow, and David C. King, *Why People Don't Trust Government* (Cambridge: Harvard University Press, 1998).

doubt in the technical expertise underlying its decisions, and media organizations who project an image of the agency to one or more "publics."[28]

At the core of any reputation lies a partial fiction. It is of course factually incorrect to speak of "the FDA," "Microsoft," "General Motors," "the U.S. Army," "the Marines," or "the Catholic Church" as if these were perfectly unitary things. Yet citizens do this all the time, and without giving conscious thought to it. Reputations attach themselves to entities much larger and more complex than can possibly be responsible for all of the things people attribute to them. Nonetheless, the fiction of a unitary organization gives rise to certain realities of its own. A scandal involving the abuse of military prisoners or the slaughter of innocents may have been committed by a small handful of soldiers, perhaps supported by a local culture of tolerance for such behavior. Yet even the most blameless members of the army will feel their organization's association with the scandal. A church that discovers that its priests or ministers have committed criminal acts against children will experience humiliation that will extend to its most committed members, however far removed they were from the criminal behavior. It is this very associative property of organizational and group identity that leads some individuals to exit the organization when a threat to its identity appears.[29]

Of course, symbolism, variable meaning, and embeddedness in networks can be features of any reputation, individual, aggregate, group-based, or corporate.[30] What makes a reputation "organizational"? Three things.

[28]The notion of multiple audiences owes its original formulation to Erving Goffman, "The Arts of Impression Management," in *The Presentation of Everyday Life* (London: Penguin, 1959), 208–37. Goffman's idea has been elaborated extensively in studies of organizational identity. See Jane E. Dutton and Janet M. Dukerich, "Keeping an Eye on the Mirror: Image and Identity in Organizational Adaptation," *Academy of Management Journal* 34 (1991): 517–54; Linda E. Ginzel, Roderick M. Kramer, and Robert I. Sutton, "Organizational Impression Management as a Reciprocal Influence Process: The Neglected Role of the Organizational Audience," *Research in Organizational Behavior* 15 (1993): 227–66; reprinted as chapters 10 and 11 (respectively) in Mary Jo Hatch and Majken Schultz, *Organizational Identity: A Reader* (New York: Oxford University Press, 2004). Andrew D. Brown, "A Narrative Approach to Collective Identities," *Journal of Management Studies* 43 (4) (June 2006): 731–53. For a statement of organizational identity as a "collaborative social construction" between an organization's "top management" and its audiences, see Ginzel, et al., in Hatch and Schultz, *Organizational Identity*, 242. The focus on audiences as embedded in partially orthogonal networks is from Carpenter, *The Forging of Bureaucratic Autonomy*, chap. 1.

[29]On the appearance and projection of uniformity, see Goffman's notion of consistency of self-presentation, symbolized alternatively as "maintaining "face" or "front," or "staying in character"; Goffman, "Performances," esp. 25, 32, 37–9, 45–6, 51–8, in chap. 2 of *The Presentation of Self in Everyday Life*. Stuart Albert and David A. Whetten invoked the criterion of "claimed temporal continuity" or sameness as a crucial feature of organizational image; "Organizational Identity," *Research in Organizational Behavior* 7 (1985): 263–95.

[30]It is important, in other words, to avoid "anthropomorphizing" organizations and their identity by speaking of them as if they were just larger forms of the individual human. Bryan Jones and Frank Baumgartner, *The Politics of Attention: How Government Prioritizes Problems* (Chicago: University of Chicago Press, 2005), 29.

1. Organizational reputations assign roles. They do so not just internally (that is, within the organization) but externally (that is, to audiences).

2. Organizational reputations attribute a unity ("identity") to structures, networks, and groups that may contain considerable dissimilitude, disarray, disorganization. The projection often runs ahead of the reality, but it still has causal force.

3. Organizational reputations differentiate and, by so doing, create interfaces. These symbols and functions and beliefs tell us why the FDA is different from (in some interpretations, "superior to") the American Medical Association, other agencies of government, or pharmaceutical companies. In this way, organizational identities demarcate (perhaps falsely, perhaps strategically) the boundaries of the organization.

Conceived in this way, an organizational reputation can be viewed as one facet of an organizational identity, its "external" projection. The symbols that compose this projection—a logo, a typical product, a leader, a compelling story of origins and growth, a scandal—are usually capable of multiple readings. It is for this reason that reputations, while they do not emerge exogenously, also do not admit easily of strategic design. A reputation is not something fully chosen by an organization or its leaders but is shaped as well by an organization's audiences and less authoritative members. Agency image is shaped as much by ex post responses to events as by ex ante modeling of organizational structure.[31]

Organizational Reputation and Regulatory Politics. The emergence of economic regulation follows a number of different scripts, and it is doubtful that any single theory can embed all of them. Calls for regulation may trail a corporate or industrial scandal, or organized consumers and farmers may see regulation as a tool to resist concentrated economic power. Regulation may be framed in moral and even religious terms, as a tool with which to combat the "adulteration" of products, of minds, and of society. The emergence of new technology—broadcast radio and television, or nuclear power—

[31]In this sense, my understanding of organizational reputation has deep affinities with notions of negotiated or intersubjective identity in anthropology, history, and sociology. Symbolic identity requires a degree of practical consensus on the set of symbols composing an identity, but allows for diverse interpretations of those symbols. For enduring examples of this scholarship, see Richard White's treatment of the calumet or the atonement ritual in the Great Lakes region of colonial North America; *The Middle Ground: Indians, Empires and Republics in the Great Lakes Region, 1650–1815* (New York: Cambridge University Press, 1992), Introduction, chapter 2, and chapter 7. Or consult Chrisopher Ansell's analysis of the *bourse du travail,* "Symbolic Networks: The Realignment of the French Working Class, 1887–1894," *American Journal of Sociology* 103(2) (Sept. 1997): 359–90. More generally, see James Clifford, *The Predicament of Culture: Twentieth-Century Ethnography, Literature and Art* (Cambridge: Harvard University Press, 1988), 344. This is a highly "cognitivist" notion of culture, wherein different cultures or identities consist of different "toolkits," which are variably and conflictually used; Ann Swidler, *Talk of Love: How Culture Matters* (Chicago: University of Chicago Press, 2001); Nina Eliasoph and Paul Lichterman, "Culture in Interaction," *American Journal of Sociology* 108 (4) (Jan. 2003): 735–94; Harrison White, *Identity and Control: A Structural Theory of Social Action* (Princeton: Princeton University Press, 1992).

may be met with the creation of regulatory institutions. A public tragedy such as a mass poisoning or even a terrorist attack may be followed by the creation of new institutions or the strengthening of old ones. Yet in each of these scripts, and as a more general metaphor, it is possible to conceive how organizational reputation either boosts or dampens the likelihood of government regulation.[32]

In evaluating regulation, citizens and politicians do not follow the lead of textbook economic theory by first asking whether there is a market failure and, if so, whether its solution requires government "intervention." Instead, as with other forms of policy, voters and citizens see problems that need to be addressed or solved and they perceive a set of possible solutions or policies for those problems. The set of problems arising at a given time has been the subject of extensive study by political scientists and sociologists who examine "agenda formation" or "problem definition." The determinants of policy change, in these arguments, depend in part upon politicians' preferences over given alternatives, but even more on how those alternatives are defined.[33]

Given a problem, the set of possible solutions depends heavily on existing arrangements. Here is where the reputation of a public agency figures prominently in regulatory policymaking. Existing arrangements have the advantage of familiarity and (relative) simplicity. The reputation of existing arrangements—often enough, public agencies—is therefore crucial in shaping what sort of regulatory arrangements will be entertained and created. The familiarity of existing arrangements does not mean that these arrangements will be chosen as solutions to new problems or issues. If anything, the perceived inefficacy or illegitimacy of existing arrangements may invite a search for alternatives, or may induce politicians to conclude that the problem does not admit of a governmental solution. In other circumstances, the perceived legitimacy and effectiveness of an existing public agency will lead politicians to consider favorably the organizations of the status quo in making new policies to address the problem at hand.[34]

[32]Keller, *Regulating a New Economy*; Balogh, *Chain Reaction*; Carpenter, *The Forging of Bureaucratic Autonomy*.

[33]John Kingdon, *Agendas, Alternatives and Public Policies* (Boston: Little, Brown, 1984); Frank Baumgartner and Bryan Jones, *Agendas and Instability in American Politics* (Chicago: University of Chicago Press, 1993); Jones and Baumgartner, *The Politics of Attention: How Government Prioritizes Problems*. John I. Kitsuse and Malcolm Spector, "Toward a Sociology of Social Problems: Social Conditions, Value Judgments, and Social Problems," *Social Problems* 20 (1973): 407–18; Stephen Hilgartner and Charles L. Bosk, "The Rise and Fall of Social Problems: A Public Arenas Model," *American Journal of Sociology* 94 (1988): 53–78. For an application of these ideas to regulatory politics, see Michael E. Levine and Jennifer L. Forrence, "Regulatory Capture, Public Interest, and the Public Agenda: Toward a Synthesis," *Journal of Law, Economics and Organization* 6 (Special Issue): 167–98.

[34]Some scholars have claimed that the matching of problem to solution is dependent more on the "flow" of solutions. Kingdon, *Agendas, Alternatives and Public Policies*. The familiarity of existing arrangements can create another form of state dependence, similar to the "path-dependence" described by Paul Pierson; *Politics in Time: History, Institutions and Social Analysis* (Princeton: Princeton University Press, 2004). The mechanism postulated here is funda-

Observers of the United States have historically witnessed the operation of organizational reputation most clearly in the *absence* of state legitimacy. In other nations—Western European countries form the classic examples, but Australia, Canada, Japan, and New Zealand are also notable cases—there are stronger beliefs in the efficacy and legitimacy of state, and also in specific organizational forms. In some nations, state legitimacy and bureaucratic reputations are sufficiently strong that regulation is replaced entirely by forms of public ownership. Yet within national contexts, these reputations can form the basis for new regulatory policies in which government agencies are given significant discretion over policymaking, and may be able to claim a measure of autonomy.[35]

The creation of regulatory policies depends heavily, one might say ultimately, on the actions of politicians. A large literature in political science, economics, and sociology portrays politicians in democratic systems acting in ways that are risk-averse, responding in particular to perceived threats to their interests, their ideological preferences, and their prospects for re-election. If politicians act differently under conditions of threat, then the politics of a crisis can be framed in such a way as to present an electoral threat to those who fail to act meaningfully and credibly to address the problem. It is for this reason, in part, that politicians seek to show responsiveness during times of crisis. To acknowledge this fact is not to say that politicians' responses are necessarily insincere or contrived. In fact, voters may justifiably demand near-term action on the part of politicians in times of crisis, and politicians' responses may be easily seen as an essential part of their representative function.[36]

As a general matter, then, public beliefs about the regulator will influence politicians' actions to delegate authority to regulators in making new regula-

---

mentally different, however, in that it is cognitive and cultural as opposed to institutional. I return to this important dynamic in chapter 12.

[35] Of course, public ownership as opposed to regulation can occur for reasons other than the reputation of government agencies. On reputation as the basis for policymaking and delegation to agencies, see Carpenter, *The Forging of Bureaucratic Autonomy*, and "State Building through Reputation Building: Policy Innovation and Coalitions of Esteem at the Post Office, 1883–1912," *Studies in American Political Development* 14 (2) (Fall 2000): 121–55.

[36] The role of "crisis" in regulatory politics brings into view the role of agenda-setting; Kingdon, *Agendas, Alternatives and Public Policies*; Deborah Stone, "Causal Stories and the Formation of Policy Agendas," *Political Science Quarterly* 104(2) (Summer 1989): 281–300. Risk-aversion is built into many spatial mathematical models of delegation in political science, as loss functions are quadratic (that is, they involve a squared term) and hence first-order surprises (unexpected departures from expectations) have second-order effects on the principal's utility. Keith Krehbiel, *Information and Legislative Organization* (Ann Arbor: University of Michigan Press, 1991); Kathleen Bawn, "Political Control Versus Expertise: Congressional Choices about Administrative Procedures," *APSR* 89 (1995): 62–73; David Epstein and Sharyn O'Halloran, *Delegating Powers: A Transaction-Cost Perspective on Policy Making Under Separate Powers* (New York: Cambridge University Press, 1999). But see Jonathan Bendor and Adam Meirowitz ("Spatial Models of Delegation," *APSR* 98 (2) (2004): 293–310), who show that risk-aversion is not necessary for many important results in this literature.

tory policy. As a general hypothesis, we may venture the statement than when all things are considered, the more legitimate, expert, and effective a regulator is perceived to be, the more likely politicians will be to create new regulations in policy areas that the regulator governs, and the more likely politicians will be to vest significant authority and resources in the regulator.[37]

A growing body of historical and empirical evidence points to the explanatory and interpretive value of a reputation-based account of how politicians and public agencies interact. Studies of how public agencies are created and terminated have overturned the myth that agencies live forever, and they suggest that poor reputations and evidence of bad performance are implicated when politicians take action to terminate or shrink agencies. Analyses of legislative delegation to agencies in the United States and other nations have shown that the revelation of negative evidence about an agency's performance often leads to reduced discretion and funding for the agency. Put simply, politicians do not respond to a structure fraught with three-alarm fires by supplying more fuel; they are just as likely to rid the policy of the structure altogether, or begin choosing other venues in which to vest authority and power.[38]

Externally, various audiences often attempt to evaluate or make sense of an organization by trying to define what is unique about it. Sometimes explicitly but often implicitly, audiences ask: What does this organization provide that alternatives do not? The alternatives could be a set of other agencies, or they could appear as alternative institutional arrangements. In many cases of regulation, alternative institutions may be privatization or a regulatory solution that relies upon tight statutory definition and avoids bureaucratic discretion. In matters of delegation, legislatures and their committees

---

[37]It is quite possible that, under strategic considerations, agencies will exploit this fact and use quality-based delegation as a way to shape policy in more ideological terms. For some mathematical models that explore this possibility, see Huber and McCarty, "Bureaucratic Capacity, Delegation, and Political Reform." Such a model is especially applicable to settings where the average bureaucratic agency is expected to have low capacity. Yet in most settings of industrial and post-industrial economies, this is unlikely. See also John Patty and Sean Gailmard ("Slackers and Zealots: Civil Service, Policy Discretion and Bureaucratic Expertise," *American Journal of Political Science* 51 (4) (Oct. 2007): 873–89) who discuss the incentives for an agency to signal quality and competence to legislators.

[38]David E. Lewis, "The Politics of Agency Termination: Confronting the Myth of Immortality," *Journal of Politics* 64 (1) (2002): 89–107; Carpenter and Lewis, "Political Learning from Rare Events: Poisson Inference, Fiscal Constraints, and the Lifetime of Bureaus," *Political Analysis* 12 (3) (2004): 201–32. For an account of how the U.S. Congress delegated "away" from an agency that had developed a poor reputation, consider narratives of the U.S. Reclamation Service (later the Reclamation Bureau) of the U.S. Department of Interior during the Progressive Era; Donald J. Pisani, *Water and American Government: The Reclamation Bureau, National Water Policy, and the West, 1902–1935* (Berkeley: University of California Press, 2002); Carpenter, *The Forging of Bureaucratic Autonomy*, chap. 10. For evidence on reputations and policy authority in recent years, see Jason A. MacDonald and William W. Franko, Jr., "Bureaucratic Capacity and Bureaucratic Discretion: Does Congress Tie Policy Authority to Performance?" *American Politics Research* 35 (2007): 790–807.

may seek to understand what is the "value-added" of a particular agency, particularly relative to other agencies, other possible institutional solutions to the problem, even relative to a policy of pure privatization. One implication of this politics of differentiation is that regulatory organizations will often project (intentionally or not) different identities ("faces") to different audiences. The warm glow of an agency's positive public image (broadcast to media and politicians) may differ from the harsh reception given to an organization's competitors (professions, agencies, and companies) that threaten to perform the organization's essential tasks.[39]

The effect of reputation on the creation of regulatory policy goes well beyond the mere legislative delegation of tasks and authority to a regulatory agency. Reputations can also be conceived more explicitly in terms of democratic and pluralist politics. Public agencies may have reputation-based constituencies that lobby to get them more funding and more authority, and seek to steer new policies in their direction. In some ways, this is consistent with a form of bureaucratic autonomy, as the regulatory agency becomes an active player in regulatory politics and in the creation of new statutes and formal regulatory powers. Yet this autonomy need not be equated with bureaucratic drift or legislative "abdication" of responsibilities. If the regulator is mobilizing and organizing broad social preferences that cannot be encompassed by other routes of representation—elections and legislative politics—then the regulator's political initiatives can be usefully represented as a form of republican or representative politics.[40]

Organizational Reputation and Regulatory Behavior. A reputation-based perspective can also shed useful light on the behavior of government organizations and regulatory bodies once a regulatory policy is established. Consider first the individually based motivations of government regulators. Organizations and their members in numerous walks of life aim less for profit itself, less for power itself, and more for reputation and the associated benefits that it brings: prestige, status, and authority. In many respects, as psychologists and organizational scholars have emphasized, the pursuit of these ends is not entirely conscious but instead is built into the very cognitive and emotional fabric of the organizational human. For the individual populating regulatory agencies, this logic implies that pay, budget maximization, and

[39]For pregnant examples from modern military history, see French, *Military Identities*, 334–52. For the concept of uniqueness and organizational competition in executive departments in the Progressive Era United States, see Carpenter, *The Forging of Bureaucratic Autonomy*, chapters 8 and 10. This has been observed in studies of professions as well. Professions seek to occupy a niche where their skills are uniquely held and of value. In some ways, this corresponds to the notion of rent-seeking and niche competition; Andrew Abbott, *The System of Professions* (Chicago: University of Chicago Press, 1990).

[40]For historical evidence on explicit bureaucratic incursions into legislative and partisan politics, see Balogh, *Chain Reaction*; Carpenter, The *Forging of Bureaucratic Autonomy*; J. Charles Schencking, *Making Waves: Politics, Propaganda, and the Emergence of the Imperial Japanese Navy, 1868–1922* (Stanford: Stanford University Press, 2005).

other material goods will be valued less highly than status and esteem. Hence, a reputation-based perspective directs students of regulation to look at regulators quite differently from the standard rent-seeking views of regulation. Aside from its direct value, moreover, reputation is a proximate goal that often must be achieved in order for other things to be had.[41]

Consider next the imperatives of organizational management. If an agency's reputation partially or wholly underlies its authority and power, its more authoritative and committed members may act to preserve, maintain, and enhance the reputation. This protective behavior can induce regulatory officials—particularly those more authoritative and tenured ones—to assume a more defensive posture with regard to potential or actual threats to identity. To emphasize the politics of reputation is to render regulatory agencies much more comparable (and contrast-worthy) with other organizations in modern societies: military organizations, churches and religious bodies, hospitals, law firms, intelligence agencies, scientific research units, police organizations, universities and schools, and many others. To some extent, reputational competition is brand-name competition, which shapes the fates and profits of many economic and financial entities (accounting firms, banks, rating agencies).[42]

Studies of regulatory organizations have revealed the persistence of adaptive behavior in the management of reputation. In the governance of automobile safety in the United States, the National Highway Traffic Safety Administration (NHTSA) transited from "rules to recalls." The agency began its life under 1966 legislation and relied heavily upon administrative rulemaking that governed car production. Yet largely because agency officials wanted legitimacy among their various political and legal audiences—Ralph Nader and his Public Interest Research Group, President Richard Nixon's Council on Wage and Price Stability, the U.S. Senate, and federal courts—NHTSA abandoned its rulemaking strategy in the 1970s and began to regulate by removing faulty products from the national market. This shift in regulatory strategy had the effect of moving automobile safety regulation from a "pre-market" phase (governing details of production before sale) to

[41]The classic political science argument for proximate goals taking precedence even when the ultimate goals are quite different is given in David Mayhew's analysis of the re-election incentive governing members of the U.S. Congress; Mayhew, *Congress: The Electoral Connection* (New Haven: Yale University Press, 1973). On individual-level incentives for reputation, see Murray Horn, *The Political Economy of Public Administration: Institutional Choice in the Public Sector* (New York: Cambridge University Press, 1995), 56–8.

[42]As James Q. Wilson noticed nearly two decades ago, there are numerous cases in which bureaucrats will reject more resources, in part because the resources are attached to new policies that they feel they cannot manage effectively or that depart from their basic capacities. Reputation-based concerns are thus instrumental in the frequently observed decision *not* to pursue more resources or new programs. Wilson, *Bureaucracy*. More refined statistical analyses have not found support for the budget maximization hypothesis; Daniel Carpenter, "Adaptive Signal Processing, Hierarchy and Budgetary Control in Federal Regulation," *APSR* 90 (2) (June 1996): 283–302.

a "post-market" phase (monitoring problems after sale and compelling the return or withdrawal of defective products). Similarly, in the evolution of U.S. commercial nuclear power regulation by the Atomic Energy Commission in the Cold War period, nuclear safety experts deserted the insularity of their previous administrative procedures and decision-making processes and began to "go public" by openly addressing the benefits and risks of new nuclear plants. Among broad public audiences, environmentalists, and utility and nuclear industry groups, the AEC began to invite public participation into its decisions at a much earlier stage. And in an ironic pattern of action that bows strongly to reputation-based concerns, AEC officials also consciously tried to dampen public expectations about what their agency could deliver.[43]

Organizational reputation can be differentiated from related concepts such as status and esteem in several ways. Initially, two important dimensions of a reputation are its subjectivity (a reputation almost always confers a specific trait upon an agent or organization, as in "GM has a reputation for traditionalism") and its multiplicity (an agent can have more than one reputation, as in a reputation for discipline among one's co-workers and a reputation for charity in one's residential community). Hence, at first glance, reputation lacks the one-dimensional character of status and esteem; a bureau or division or subsidiary can have "more" status or "less" esteem, but not really "more" or less reputation in the common understanding of that word. Perhaps more significant, an organizational reputation can embed individual-level status and esteem within it. Psychologists and sociologists have long recognized that group- and organization-based traits (particularly the way these traits are understood within given societies, as in a reputation) can influence individual-level identity, esteem, and mood. Just as interesting are the flows of causation that run the other way. High esteem and expectations

---

[43]The NHTSA administered the provisions of the National Traffic and Motor Vehicle Safety Act of 1966. Mashaw and Harfst, *The Struggle for Auto Safety*, chap. 9 ("Inside NHTSA"). As Mashaw and Harfst summarize, the courts in particular were an audience that legitimated one form of agency activity (recalls) while delegitimating another (rulemaking), even though the courts never forbade rulemaking: "Losses in court, stymied, embarrassed, and ultimately delegitimated the efforts of the principal proponents of aggressive rulemaking" (200). For the transformation in U.S. commercial nuclear power regulation, see Balogh, *Chain Reaction*, chap. 7 and chap. 8 See also Balogh's insightful observation on how many other professions and organizations managed reputations by diminishing expectations so as to less frequently disappoint their audiences (324–5).

There are many other examples in the United States alone. Among these are the Federal Trade Commission's efforts to restore its legal and regulatory credibility by altering its advertising enforcement decisions (Sherman, *Market Regulation*, (New York: Addison Wesley, 2007) chap. 23). Another pregnant example comes in the transformation of rulemaking for workplace safety at OSHA in the late 1970s, largely in response to federal court decisions and academic studies suggesting that its rules were somewhat ineffective by virtue of their excessive rigidity. The negative signs received by OSHA also amounted to "ridicule and derision." Sherman, *Market Regulation*, chap. 22. Gregory Huber, *Strategic Neutrality: Enforcement Behavior at OSHA* (New Haven: Yale University Press, 2007), chap.2.

among the members of the organization—what many analysts call "morale"—may be noticed by its audiences, leading these audiences to attribute a reputation for "functionality," "cohesiveness," or like traits to the entity.

In studies of regulatory agencies and other government bureaucracies there has been limited acknowledgment—and very little explicit discussion—of the politics of reputation. In quite different works, James Q. Wilson and Murray Horn both examine the importance of reputation to government organizations, seeing it as one potential motivation among many, but in neither of these works was the concept integrated into a broader theory. Economists and political scientists have written a collection of articles and papers elaborating an "external signals" account of regulation. In this approach, the regulator seeks to maximize the difference between the positive signals received from society and the negative signals received. The praiseworthy feature of these accounts derives from their recognition that external signals come into the agency, and that the agency cares about the valence of these signals. Yet in many other respects, these are dim understandings of reputation, and in no case has the theoretical discussion of the signals been accompanied by careful measurement or historical study of the signals themselves.[44]

To the extent that a reputation for protection can be thought to rise and fall, to be subject to increase and decrease, its variance and temporal structure differ from that of other indices that an agent might maximize. In some cases a reputation assumes a binary structure, as with common understandings of honesty. An organization's manager or chief executive does not gain from the impression of telling the truth "most of the time"; she is likely perceived as either "honest" or "dishonest." Other features, such as competence, ability to protect, and vigor, may admit of more fine-grained movements, in part because they embed a random component. Even the most stringent safety regulator cannot prevent all industrial accidents. Yet in general, identities are characterized by discontinuities and movements in reputation are defined by interruptions rather than flows. To the extent that organizations engage in what sociologist Erving Goffman termed "the arts of impression management," then, the calculus is entirely different from that of "profit maximization" or "rent-seeking." Organizational managers and others committed to the organization's identity may be less concerned with "maximizing" a reputation for some trait and more concerned with preventing severe damage to a reputation that already exists.

Multiple Constituencies as Multiple Overlapping Audiences: Reputation versus Pluralism. The organizations that bear reputations usually have multiple audiences. The stories of reputation to which social scientists are ac-

---

[44]Wilson, *Bureaucracy*; Horn, *The Political Economy of Public Administration*. For the classic account of an administrative agency torn among competing audiences, see Selznick, *The TVA and the Grass Roots*. For an argument in which public utility regulators demonstrated their responsiveness to different constituencies, see Paul Joskow, "Inflation and Environmental

customed often fail to appreciate this multiplicity. In economics and political science, for instance, scholars have constructed models of reputation in game theory that are premised upon the metaphor of a "chain-store" game. A chain of stores may, in a particular locality, face a threat from a competitor. In dealing with this threat, the chain store must understand that its actions in this local situation will create a reputation for its likely behavior in similar situations in the future. Other potential competitors in other localities will consider this reputation when deciding whether or not to compete in those places. Hence, an important equilibrium of these games is for the chain store to "snuff out" the first appearance of a competitor, thereby projecting a reputation for vigilance or toughness, and hence scaring off competition in other locales.[45]

Were potential entrants the only audience for the chain store, this would be a much more accurate description of reality. Yet success with one audience—inspiring fear among potential entrants—may conflict with success and legitimacy among others. A large chain store may provoke local political and economic resentment and drive customers to local stores or to another, more friendly corporate chain altogether. Or the resentment at the chain store's behavior may feed political movements for regulation of the chain.[46]

Much of the politics of reputation in modern organizations would appear to require the management of an ambiguous image among multiple audiences. This task is all the more difficult in an organizational setting, as individual agents may vary in their identification with and their devotion to the organization's reputation. Greater legitimacy among one of these audiences may imply less legitimacy among another. In many cases, the very bases of legitimacy may vary. Among the populace of a consuming public and among organizations within it, a regulator may wish to cultivate a protective reputation. Still, part of this reputation may be constructed through forcible credibility, by showing toughness even when it is not popular to do so, perhaps by negating the public's wishes at different times, or perhaps denying access to a popular material good. Among regulated entities (firms, R&D enterprises, nonprofit organizations), the agency may wish to cultivate a fearsome reputation for tough action. At the same time, the agency may also wish to preserve

---

Concern: Change in the Process of Public Utility Price Regulation," *Journal of Law and Economics* 17 (2) (Oct. 1974): 291–327.

[45]In mathematical modeling, this notion of reputation has been applied to situations of imperfect information over an organization's resolve, as in the chain-store firm or a nation-state. David M. Kreps and Robert Wilson, "Reputation and Imperfect Information," *Journal of Economic Theory* 27 (2) (Aug. 1982): 253–79. James Alt, Randall Calvert, and Brian Humes, "Reputation and Hegemonic Stability: A Game-Theoretic Analysis," *APSR* 82 (1) (1988): 445–66. These and many other mathematical models of reputation explicitly or implicitly assume a single audience and/or a single dimension of evaluation.

[46]Consider for instance the regulatory action taken against the large retailer Wal-Mart, discussed in Michael Sandel, *Democracy's Discontent: America in Search of a Public Philosophy* (Cambridge: Harvard University Press, 1996).

a reputation for fairness and flexibility. The resulting politics demands a delicate balancing of speech and action among regulatory officials.

One might wonder whether the multiplicity of audiences in the politics of reputation is just another way for diverse organized interests to make claims upon the regulator and the politicians who oversee it. What makes an audience-based account different from an account of simple distributive politics? A compelling answer must be based on the fact that in the politics of reputation, there are no contracts, and there cannot be. In contractual understandings of politics, an agency is responsive to a legislature, and perhaps a president or an interest group, because of a set of contractual relations that are either explicit (a constitution or enabling statute) or implicit (a verbal bargain or a revolving door). Yet in the politics of reputation, the relationship of a regulatory agency to professional, global, business, scientific, and public audiences cannot be so specified. For one thing, reputation—the very thing sought and fought over in the politics of reputation, the very "currency" of the realm—cannot be easily monetized and measured. For another, the very terms and turf of the politics of reputation cannot be divided and split among constituencies.[47]

Yet perhaps the most important differences emerge in what the fights are over. In the politics of reputation, groups make claims upon a regulator by threatening or enhancing an identity. If these threats are credible in the sense that the agency's reputation is both an asset to the regulator and partially malleable, the regulator will respond to these claims by adjusting her behavior after the fact or in anticipation. The asset status of reputations suggests that threats will often be more powerful than promises of enhancement. Yet whether the holder of the reputation is concerned more with "loss" or "gain," it is nonetheless possible for reputation and status to become the medium of exchanges for pluralist transactions.[48]

Once the student of regulation steps outside the politics of contracts and rent-seeking and thinks about the politics of reputation, many of the most important relationships in regulation can be reconceived. There are, for instance, at least two ways for a regulatory agency to respond to a legislature: as a contractual principal, of course, but also as an audience. Most national and territorial legislatures are not merely governing bodies. They also serve as public fora where regulators can be compelled to appear, and offer testimony under oath (perhaps with some penalty for false testimony or disclosure). Scholars of national bureaucracy in the United States have long recognized that agency personnel experience great and direct disutility from being

---

[47]Yoshiko Herrera's study of the modernization of economic statistics in Russia points to this; *Transforming Bureaucracy: Conditional Norms and the International Standardization of Statistics in Russia* (Ithaca: Cornell University Press, 2008). For an interesting and nuanced mathematical model of incontractibility in the building of government power, see Michael M. Ting, "Organizational Capacity," forthcoming, *JLEO*.

[48]I thank Paul Quirk for critical discussions on this point.

called to "the Hill" to testify, discomfort having little to do with congressional oversight or the threat of congressional action such as budget cuts after the hearing. For many agencies, a legislative setting is the forum where their decisions are most likely to be publicly revealed, discussed, and criticized, and one of the few fora in which these criticisms will be delivered face-to-face.[49]

The final and perhaps crucial difference between a politics of pluralism and a politics of reputation concerns the sort of side-payments or benefits that make pluralism work. A regulator in a pluralist world can try to appease all parties by splitting a pie of resources among them with equity or according to their power. But for a regulator in a world of reputation, the explicit assignment of benefits to some constituents may damage reputation. Scholars in the field of risk analysis and science studies have argued and demonstrated that, for instance, trust in a regulator is conditioned in part on perceptions of its relationship to the regulated industry. A regulator that gives "industry" its equilibrium share of pluralistic goods, or even a fair share, may be an agency that garners the distrust of public and legislative audiences.[50]

Faces of Regulatory Power and Their Interdependence

An understanding of reputation and its meanings among different audiences also permits new windows into regulatory power. In the United States and other countries, observers have been as likely to stress the weaknesses of regulatory agencies as they have been to emphasize the power of these organizations. In the early twenty-first century, as models of "self-regulation," standard setting, and nongovernment forms of market regulation have risen to prominence, sustained attention to the "power" of government agencies in regulating marketplaces may seem quaint or anachronistic. Yet if observers and scholars are going to perceive a fuller array of regulation's effects—whether they are induced by governments or other agents—an understanding of the facets of regulatory power is essential.[51]

[49]Christopher Foreman, *Signals from the Hill: Congressional Oversight and the Challenge of Social Regulation* (New Haven: Yale University Press, 1988); Herbert Kaufman, *The Administrative Behavior of Federal Bureau Chiefs* (Washington, DC: Brookings Institution, 1981). Audience and authority functions are of course related. Congress would not be quite the audience for agencies that it is without its status as enabler, funder, and constitutional overseer of these agencies.

[50]A. K. Weyman, N. F. Pidgeon, J. Walls, and T. Horlick-Jones, "Exploring Comparative Ratings and Constituent Facets of Public Trust in Risk Regulatory Bodies and Related Stakeholder Groups," *Journal of Risk Research* 9 (2006): 605–22; Paul Slovic, "Perceived Risk, Trust and Democracy," *Risk Analysis* 13 (1993): 675–82; M. P. White and J. R. Eiser, "Information Specificity and Hazard Risk Potential as Moderators of Trust Asymmetry," *Risk Analysis* 25 (2005): 1187–98.

[51]The tradition of power analysis to which I refer constitutes a vast literature, and grew out of analyses of poverty, class, and "community power" in studies of local politics; Robert A. Dahl,

The Distinctiveness of Regulatory Power. Much of economic regulation involves a subject acting upon an object, the governance of a "regulated entity" by the empowered "regulator." Accordingly, an agent of government
exercises regulatory power when it induces the regulated entity to behave in
a manner that it would not have behaved, absent the presence or behavior
of the regulator. Under a pattern of regulatory power, put differently, a regulated entity takes action or inaction that would not have occurred if the
regulator were not present or had behaved differently.[52]

There are many forms of power in political, economic, and social life, and
regulatory power is a limited array of these larger power dynamics. Regulatory power is much more restricted than the power that Marxist analysts
have ascribed to the "capitalist class" or the state. Regulatory power is more
akin to the "domination" that sociologist Max Weber attributes to governing entities such as states, empires, religious authorities, and political and
social leaders. When regulators and regulated firms interact, regulatory power
sometimes resembles the power that is observed among nations in world
politics.[53]

Regulatory organizations display facets of power—directive, gatekeeping,
and conceptual—that are integral to their operation and impact. These facets of regulatory power are often more forceful and more enduring in agencies of state that have the imprimatur and backing of the law and a constitu-

---

Who Governs? Democracy and Power in an American City (New Haven: Yale University
Press, 1961). For the original work on the "second face," consult Peter Bachrach and Morton
S. Baratz, "The Two Faces of Power," *APSR* 56 (1962): 941–52; and Bachrach and Baratz,
"Decisions and Nondecisions: An Analytical Framework," *APSR* 57 (1963): 641–51. The classic exposition of power's "third face" comes in Stephen Lukes, *Power: A Radical View*, 2nd ed.
(London: Palgrave, 2005; 1st ed. 1974); this second edition offers a broad overview of the literature. The decline of this tradition has occurred for many reasons, and it signifies the rise of
"rational choice" analysis in the social sciences, combined with the decline of Marxism in academic scholarship. In recent years, however, a number of important works (including several in
the rational choice and mathematical modeling traditions) have begun to turn their focus anew
to issues of power. For salient examples, see Charles Cameron, *Veto Bargaining: Presidents and
the Politics of Negative Power* (New York: Cambridge University Press, 2000); Lloyd Gruber,
Ruling the World: Power Politics and the Rise of Supranational Institutions (New York: Cambridge University Press, 2000); Terry M. Moe, "Power and Political Institutions," *Perspectives
on Politics* 3 (2) (June 2005): 215–33.

[52] The existence of regulatory power in a pattern of interaction does not imply that the regulator sees its preferred outcome realized exactly; a pattern of regulatory power can co-exist
with some degree of unintended consequences.

[53] Jack H. Nagel, *The Descriptive Analysis of Power* (New Haven: Yale University Press,
1975). The different faces of regulatory power may include the concepts of *Macht* (power) and
Herrschaft (rule) in Weber's work. On market power as a central concept in antitrust law and
economics, see Jonathan Baker and Timothy Bresnahan, "Identifying and Measuring Market
Power," *Antitrust Law Journal* 61 (1) (1992): 3–17; the idea that the FDA can set more stringent regulatory standards because it governs the largest and least price-regulated market is
consistent with a form of market power that the FDA may possess with respect to other regulators. I thank Rick Hall, Paul Pierson, Paul Quirk, and Eric Schickler for several critical discussions in which the points in this paragraph were developed and refined.

tion. Government regulators bear formal authority to confer or revoke legal rights of production, market distribution, and advertising. Government regulators can change the economic, social, scientific, and political agenda— the set of products developed, the set of issues raised in national debate, the measurements used to develop, produce, and market new products. Government regulators shape the concepts of science and economy. Whether these effects are to be praised or lamented is a topic for a separate debate. A normative discussion of whether regulatory power is insidious or desirable (or some combination of the two) should be premised upon an awareness of what powers are operating. The idea of regulatory power in its directive, gatekeeping, and conceptual facets does not enable a perfect or exhaustive listing of all relevant powers, but attention to the faces of power permits a much richer understanding of the historical force of regulation, the lives and activities affected by it, and how they are variably shaped.[54]

In its most raw form, a regulator can issue an order for a private actor to "cease and desist" from production, distribution, or marketing of a particular good. The regulator can often seize supplies of the good in question or shut down the operations of its producer or marketer. These directives have the backing of law and, while they are contestable politically and legally, they plausibly amount to power and force exercised over the subject. So too do formal decisions to confer, or take away, rights to produce and market commodities in a market. A regulator may issue a legally binding rule or edict that compels producers of a new commodity to constrain their behavior in some specific way, such as by adding pollution abatement technology to their systems of industrial exhaust. While laws and legal orders can be and are violated and ignored, it is doubtless that regulators in most societies still exercise some degree of power in their formal decisions over market entry and exit even when noncompliance occurs. These and other examples comprise directive regulatory power, a countenance based upon and expressed through formal authority.[55]

A second, gatekeeping facet of regulatory power emerges in the less visible decisions of economic producers or political combatants not to bring an idea or issue into the arena of political economy. A group of investors may decide to pull their capital from a new communications company, fearful that the firm will be too heavily regulated. Or a bank decides not to fund a new construction project out of belief that the developer's application for a new construction permit will be denied or delayed. The producer in ques-

[54]Several of these notions will be helpful to students and observers of nongovernmental regimes of regulation, not least the agenda-setting (gatekeeping) and vocabulary- and goal-shaping (conceptual) dimensions of regulatory power.

[55]Dahl's classic intuitive formulation states that "A has power over B to the extent that he can get B to do something that B would not otherwise do" ("The Concept of Power," *Behavioral Science* 2 (1957): 202–3). The concept of "getting B to do something" is crucial and has long been underspecified; at its core it involves a causal claim, but one that is very difficult to establish using standards of causal inference.

tion loses its investment and never materializes as an economic entity. The regulator in question never physically governs the firm or the builder, but the power of the regulator has been felt nonetheless. In the regulation of technological goods, such considerations can and do shape the very stock of scientific ideas and innovations which arise in academic, government, and industrial laboratories.[56]

In the political realm, regulatory organizations can be challenged in different ways, but many of these challenges never materialize out of conscious or unconscious deterrence. An opponent of the regulator who wants to weaken its powers may wish to introduce a proposal for reform. Yet the agency may have sufficient legitimacy and clout to beat back the reform proposal or even to use the proposal as an opening to expand its own powers. Alternatively, a party that is aggrieved by a regulator's decision may wish to bring suit against the agency but may fear that, in doing so, he will poison future relations with an institution whose good will he relies upon for his economic existence. This fear may be ill-founded, but in the deterrence of a political or legal challenge, the regulator has nonetheless exercised power.

A third, conceptual facet of regulatory power consists in the ability (often unconsciously exercised) of the governing organization to shape fundamental patterns of thought, communication, and learning by its formal and informal definition of concepts, vocabularies, measurements, and standards. If investment decisions are conditioned upon certain criteria (demonstrated efficacy in a Phase 2 trial, bioequivalence) that have been shaped by the regulator, then the regulator constrains the behavior of private actors even when those actors have not anticipated the regulator's behavior. If public and financial debates about a product depend heavily upon statistical measurements that the regulator has fashioned or championed (or even influenced partially), then the regulator's power is exercised and felt well outside its walls.

While the power dynamics in pharmaceutical regulation deserve some study with quantitative techniques, analysis of conceptual regulatory power requires a form of *Begriffsgeschichte*, or "concept history." If regulatory power has been exercised in the framing of scientific, medical, governmental, or social concepts, analysis of these concepts must consider the authorship of different organizations and individuals. Analysis must also consider what alternative concepts and vocabularies were possible when regulatory framing and shaping occurred, perhaps by examining criticisms of the standard model, or perhaps by considering the paths taken by other societies. At its core, the detection of conceptual power in regulation depends upon the

---

[56]I return to this theme repeatedly. For a mathematical treatment that brutally simplifies the process by which a regulatory agency's decisions feedback to influence the set of cases it considers, see Carpenter and Ting, "Regulatory Errors with Endogenous Agendas." For a mapping from veto authority to a "second face" of power, see Cameron, *Veto Bargaining*.

answer to a counterfactual query. If conceptual regulatory power has been exercised, then a regulatory authority has shaped the definition or understanding of a term or procedure such that, had the regulator not taken the shaping or framing action in question, the term or procedure would have evolved differently in substantive ways.[57]

The directive, gatekeeping, and conceptual facets of regulatory power are not distinct but depend upon one another and, in turn, upon organizational image. Formal authority buttresses the fear that constrains economic and political challenges. Fear in turn stabilizes and renders all the more natural and inevitable the agency's formal authority. A regulator's statutory capacity may allow it to mold basic terms of science and experiment. This statutory capacity may reflect widespread social and political deference to the regulator in matters where it is deemed legitimate and expert. These definitions in turn may be structured in such a way that limits the set of ideas that will be developed, thereby making difficult and contestable cases less likely to appear publicly before the regulator and its observant audiences. The absence of these challenges may serve to offer the impression that the regulatory regime works smoothly, so that its formal bases are protected from legal and political challenge.

Under a wide variety of definitions of power, a social scientist would readily detect the Food and Drug Administration's multifaceted power in the modern pharmaceutical world. When a regulator can compel a firm or university to cease activity by a simple command, directive power is exercised. When a regulator can induce a company to abandon an otherwise profitable product (or to alter the structure or content of that product significantly) without taking visible action toward that end, this is regulatory power of the gatekeeping sort. When a regulator suggests but does not dictate methods for determining the quality or safety of a product, and when firms, researchers, scientists, and other regulators follow those even when they are not required to do so, regulatory power is exercised, and it is conceptual power.

Historical and Theoretical Implications of Reputation-Based Regulation

As with other theories, reputation-based accounts of regulation offer observable implications that can be employed to assess the predictive value of the theory.

The Location of Politics. An account of regulation that features the politics of reputation will highlight certain features of regulation over others and will generate implications for behavior. Perhaps the most important of the

[57]The notion of concept history I have in mind is related to but distinct from the *Begriffsgeschichte* of Reinhard Koselleck; *Historische Semantik und Begriffsgeschichte* (Stuttgart: Klett-Cotta, 1979). The present study concentrates less upon standard intellectual history and the history of science, focusing as much upon legal and administrative texts. I am also concerned

66 CHAPTER 1

theory's lessons is its direction to look for politics in certain places. What are the fights about? What things are contested? What threats are made? What do the threats target? A theory of reputation-based regulation suggests, if nothing else, that politics will be located in struggles over identity itself. Organized interests and regulated firms will be less likely to credibly threaten an agency's budget and much more likely to render threats to its reputation and its power.

Reputation as Asset: Protection and Maintenance. Identity, and especially its reputational facet, has an asset value. Once crystallized, and once recognized, officials with authority in an organization may take measured steps to protect, maintain, and enhance it. This reputation-protection imperative has governed and animated the FDA's behavior in pharmaceutical regulation for much of the last half-century. When understood as having an "asset value," reputations may be viewed as deserving protection and maintenance. This fact changes regulatory behavior in policy realms from product review, to rulemaking, to enforcement, to patterns of reliance upon advisory committees.[58]

Even though reputations are adaptively and often strategically protected and enhanced once made, they are not instrumentally designed or chosen. Organizational reputation inevitably concerns forces that lie beyond the power of an individual to control. While managerial influence is possible, such influence is necessarily limited. There are, moreover, myriad unconscious, structural, cultural, and other forces influencing identity that lie beyond the capacities of strategic awareness or that organizational authorities are powerless to dictate. Even to the extent that organizational authorities perceive their organization to have an identity, then, and even to the extent they wish to shape or protect that identity, their attempts can at best meet with probabilistic, even ironic success.[59]

---

less with the *longue durée* of conceptual trajectories than with moments of conceptual formation and transformation in the late twentieth century. As such, I direct attention less to the formation of scientific "facts" than to methods, protocols, and bundles of concepts (e.g., bioequivalence and bioavailability) that travel together; Ludwig Fleck, *Genesis and Development of a Scientific Fact* (Chicago: University of Chicago Press, 1981 [orig. 1935]). My focus on concept formation as a power of state extends in part from the writings of James C. Scott, *Seeing Like a State: How Certain Schemes to Improve the Human Condition Have Failed* (New Haven: Yale University Press, 1998), especially Part I, "State Projects of Legibility and Simplification," 8, 11, 30-36, 80-83. The modes of conceptual power in regulation are, however, less authoritarian than the governance illuminated in Scott's studies. I thank Harry Marks for several incisive discussions of these points.

[58]Readers with a rationalist bent will more easily appreciate this portion of the argument. This is a more functional, and far from adequate, way of viewing organizational reputation. It is only one part of a larger narrative on the formation of reputation and how it shapes behavior. For more on the "asset"-like value of reputation, see Carpenter, "Protection without Capture," *APSR* (2004); "The Political Economy of FDA Drug Approval: Processing, Politics and Lessons for Policy," *Health Affairs* 23 (1) (Jan./Feb. 2004): 52–63.

[59]At least one fallacy in the design account is that, since all organizations would presumably

The study of organizational reputation in a regulatory context requires, at times, a careful differentiation among regulatory officials. A central advantage of reputation-based theory is that it allows for predictions of different behavior by different agents and different components of the regulatory agency. A corollary from the social identity theory in psychology is that protection and maintenance of the organizational reputation may be observed more commonly among higher officials within an organization, and among more attached members. Higher officials are those whose perch in the hierarchy makes attributions of organization identity more directly relevant to their status and esteem (as goes the reputation of a company, so go the status and esteem of its chief executive officer). More attached members are more likely those who have been members of the organization for a longer time, or who expect to be members for a longer time.

Risk Aversion and Irreversibility of Public Decisions. The decisions that face many regulators are decisions of timing accompanied by learning. An enforcement agency's attorneys must sift through evidence and decide whether to pursue a civil or criminal case against a private entity. An environmental agency must take a hard look at an application to build new homes in a wetlands area, a submission to re-license a new dam, or a proposal to open public lands for grazing by livestock. A pharmaceutical regulator must consider complex statistical evidence produced from various clinical studies before deciding whether to allow a product to be marketed in national commerce or to be prescribed by professionals in a national health system.

A central prediction of a reputation-based account is that, on the whole, these sorts of decisions will have an irreversibility attached to them. Once the decision is taken—once the case is litigated and a party is sued, once a wetland or a grazing permit is granted, once a product is approved for marketing—it is difficult for the regulator to go back on the decision without serious consequences for the agency's reputation. This costly reversibility has implications for how regulators will revisit their past decisions, but it also has appreciable implications for when the initial regulatory decision is made. Faced with the prospect of a regulatory decision that is irreversible for reasons of reputation, a regulator will tread even more cautiously than usual. This looks like aversion to risk, and in part it is. But it is something more. It is aversion to reputational damage. Even if the decision can be procedurally

---

want a reputation for honesty, capacity, efficiency, then if reputation were the direct and sole result of choice, all organizations would choose for themselves the best reputations, and reputations would no longer have differentiating value. From an organizational ecology standpoint, too, different organizations and individuals will compete to occupy "identity niches" (some management scholars are apt to call this "branding"); Hatch and Schultz, *Organizational Identity: A Reader* (New York: Oxford University Press, 2004). Organizations may attempt to become the "anti-Microsoft," the principal alternative to the Catholic Church, or the "front lines" military branch (consider the long-standing organizational and political conflicts between the Navy and Marines, and between the Army and Marines, in the U.S. military).

or technologically undone, the reputational damage from the appearance of an error cannot be. Indeed, the act of reversal—a product recall, the abandonment of a prosecution or litigation, the retraction of a license—will likely call the attention of different audiences to the agency's error.

This implies that familiarity and predictability are all the more important to reputation-conscious regulators. They may pursue the easy cases where guilt or liability is more facile to establish. They may grant the product applications of a trusted firm because more is known about them and the consequences of irreversibility are easier to manage.[60]

Governance through Networks. Two social facts govern the politics of organizational reputation. First, reputations are embedded in multiple audiences. Second, the bearers of reputations are complex formal organizations with somewhat flexible boundaries. In a mutual struggle for esteem, one office in the regulatory agency will relate to another office both cooperatively and competitively. Members of a firm, a professional group, a consumer lobby, and other organizations may be invited to participate in the decisions of the agency, or in councils of advice to the agency. Since many agencies in the United States and other nations rely upon advisory committees and councils, a reputation-based view of regulation offers a unique perspective on these institutions.[61]

Revisitation Constraints. The near-irreversibility of public decisions by reputation-conscious regulators has implications for their behavior after these choices are made. Once a decision has been rendered—having taken longer and having been characterized by more caution due to irreversibility concerns—the regulator will not wish to revisit it. More properly, some actors who were responsible for the decision will not wish to reopen the case. In many cases, these will be the agents who rendered the decision in the first place. In other cases, these will be actors attached to a certain vision (identity) of the organization, who may be expected to behave defensively in response to identity threats.[62]

Different Faces for Different Audiences. The politics of reputation is complicated by the fact that, much as individuals do, organizations can project a different face to different audiences. This differentiation may stem from inter-organizational competition. An organization may feel compelled to relate to its competitors by projecting fierceness; the way the FDA related to

---

[60]For a mathematical argument to this effect, see Carpenter, "Protection without Capture."

[61]In the classic account of Selznick, this governance through networks becomes a form of co-optation; *The TVA and the Grass Roots.*

[62]Ellemers, Spears, and Doosje, "Self and Social Identity." A related claim emerges from the literature on "ceremonial formalism" in organizations. As John Meyer and Brian Rowan propose in a classic article, "Institutionalized organizations seek to minimize inspection and evaluation by both internal managers and external constituents" (Proposition 6 of Meyer and Rowan, "Institutionalized Organizations: Formal Structure as Myth and Ceremony," *American Journal of Sociology* 83 (2) (1977): 340–63).

its turf competitors, such as the American Medical Association, over much of the twentieth century, provides a salient example. In other ways, differentiation of faces may reflect the functions of regulation; the warmer features of reputation occasionally must be abandoned in favor of severity. An organization's legitimacy may rest upon its "good cop" image, but the sound functioning of its policing activity may frequently require projection of a "bad cop" image to some audiences (regulated firms and industries, for example). The regulator's performative reputation of intimidation occasionally must be put to use to realize the aims of regulatory policy, to induce compliance by an otherwise unwilling firm or client.

Ambiguity. Because the very terms of organizational reputation may be vague, ambiguity attaches to the politics of reputation. Ambiguity could follow from the lack of fixity in essential terms or symbols that communicate the reputation. Or, it could follow from a sort of "mixed strategy" where the regulator behaves probabilistically in such a way as to keep firms and other audiences off balance. It is important to emphasize that ambiguity usually exists for many reasons, and that even strategic regulatory ambiguity does not imply any sort of conspiracy. It is always difficult to define an organization's identity and to pin it down.

Reputation as a Font of Regulatory Power. Another central prediction of a reputation-based perspective points to regulation's political and historical sources. The reputation of a regulator becomes a central variable in the legislative and administrative process by which new regulation gets created or older regulation gets reformed. Regulation emerges in part because organizations are seen as uniquely equipped to address a problem among one or more audiences—most concretely a national legislature, but also public, even regulated firms. This prediction differs from those of public interest accounts insofar as a clear public rationale (or externality to be solved) may exist for regulation, but a legislature may decide not to endow a regulatory organization with the authority to address the problem because the agency lacks a performative or technical reputation sufficient to warrant delegation. The prediction differs strongly from capture accounts in that regulatory power is hypothesized not to come from the regulated industry as a way of creating entry barriers. That said, a reputation-based perspective does allow for business influence, in part through the audience costs and threats that businesses and other regulatory subjects can impose upon the regulator. Even though there is not capture in many forms of regulation, business interests are not always dominated, and they often participate heavily in the making of new policy arrangements. Where broad regulatory initiatives are expected, business lobbies may fight back against these laws, and then attempt to achieve a middling result.[63]

. . .

[63]Sanders, *Roots of Reform*; for a more general notion in the context of a nuanced account,

Upon this a question arises: whether it be better to be loved than feared or feared than loved? It may be answered that one should wish to be both, but, because it is difficult to unite them in one person, it is much safer to be feared than loved, when, of the two, either must be dispensed with.... Nevertheless a prince ought to inspire fear in such a way that, if he does not win love, he avoids hatred; because he can endure very well being feared whilst he is not hated.
—Niccolò Machiavelli, *The Prince*, chapter 27

In a widely quoted section of Machiavelli's *The Prince*, modern readers have learned that it is better to be feared than to be loved. Yet even for Machiavelli, this was far too simple a conclusion. Better to have both, the political philosopher admitted. And better for the prince to restrain the image of fear so that its holder is not abhorred. Political organizations often pursue both love and fear at the same time, and the resulting tension requires a delicate pattern of equipoise.

Machiavelli's challenge to the prince came from the difficulty of uniting fear and love "in one person." Organizations may face less of this constraint, for one member can play the part of gentle cop while another plays fierce. An organization may not have to dispense with fear or love to the extent that the individual holder of a reputation does. To be sure, the flexibility of organizational behavior in the face of reputational politics is not infinite. The constraints of organizational image bind and keep many actions from consideration or execution. And these constraints have been in evidence for much of the past century of American pharmaceutical regulation.

A reputation-based account is not a panacea for all that ails the study of regulation. Reputation is not a theoretical perspective that characterizes all forms of regulation, or even all forms of regulator. Still it does govern some forms, perhaps many forms, and a complicated politics of reputation and organizational image has been a central force in the evolution of pharmaceutical regulation in the United States and other countries and continents.

An account of regulation that emphasizes reputation allows for a different portrait of politics, and a different portrait of rationality and nonrational mechanisms governing behavior by regulators and the entities they govern. A reputation-premised theory allows for strategic regulatory officials who respond to incentives of a kind. It allows for the possibility and narration of dysfunction and systematic regulatory error (including too much responsiveness to regulated industry, as well as too much cautiousness). It allows for prediction of systematic regulatory successes, including pursuit of the public interest. It can incorporate differences within a regulatory organization, and it can incorporate the multiplicity of constituencies and networks that suffuse regulatory politics. It can bring both flexibility and intellectual order to the study of regulation as it is performed by the various organizations of state.

---

see Peter Swenson, *Capitalists Against Markets: The Making of Labor Markets and Welfare States in the United States and Sweden* (New York: Oxford University Press, 2002).

PART ONE

Organizational Empowerment and Challenge

Reputation and Gatekeeping Authority: The Federal Food, Drug and Cosmetic Act of 1938 and Its Aftermath

REPUTATION AND POWER in American pharmaceutical regulation evolved jointly in an extended moment of image making and lawmaking. These crucial steps toward the interlacing of reputation and power came in the middle of the New Deal, with the Federal Food, Drug and Cosmetic Act of 1938, its subsequent enforcement by the FDA, and the Supreme Court's decision in *United States v. Dotterweich* (1943).

From the vantage of the early twenty-first century, the Act of 1938 stands as one of the most important regulatory statutes in American and perhaps global history. The Act created an original legal category—the "new drug"—and endowed the Food and Drug Administration with sole authority to reject the ex ante marketability of any new pharmaceutical product. In this statute and in crucial legal and administrative decisions that followed it, the faces of regulatory power in twentieth-century pharmaceuticals—the authoritative power to command with force, the power to veto product development and market entry, and the power to shape concepts—slowly found expression in the power of the American state.[1]

By all accounts, the Federal Food, Drug and Cosmetic Act of 1938 issued from crisis. In the midst of the New Deal and the first and second terms of President Franklin Delano Roosevelt, officials at the Agriculture Department joined with New York Senator Royal Copeland to sponsor legislation strengthening the FDA's powers to seize products and to regulate the labeling of food, drugs, and cosmetics. As their bill lay stalled in Congress in the fall of 1937, a new anti-infective drug, "Dr. Massengill's Elixir Sulfanilamide," caused 107 deaths and stoked national fears and controversy. USDA officials quickly tracked down supplies of the drug and removed it from market circulation, from pharmacy shelves, and home medicine cabinets. In the weeks following the sulfanilamide episode, Copeland and USDA officials quickly framed the events as an avoidable tragedy whose future prevention required legal change. In image and in law, the sulfanilamide tragedy of 1937

---

[1]I continually refer to the Federal Food, Drug and Cosmetic Act as "the Act of 1938" or "the 1938 Act." On the creation of novel legal concepts in the "new drug" definition, see Richard Merrill, "The Architecture of Government Regulation of Medical Products," *Virginia Law Review* 82 (1996): 1761–2. Along with the Durham-Humphrey Amendments of 1951, the 1938 Act also undergirds mandatory prescriptions for a wide category of drugs in the United States.

became an instructive moment whose essential lesson was pre-market clearance authority over new drugs.[2]

In the particular creation of modern pharmaceutical regulation, the combination of event, framing, and policy solution are well represented by the combined performative and political metaphor of a "policy tragedy." In a policy tragedy, someone has been harmed, and wrongly so. The "victim" may be individual or collective, and the latter is often represented by the former in the manner of an exemplar or "poster child." A culprit (often the system, perhaps represented by a single individual, or corporation or government actor) is responsible in a causal, nearly criminal fashion. The public (the tragedy's "chorus") points a finger at essential and observable features of the regulatory regime, the status quo, as causing or failing to prevent the harm or injustice in question. Yet in a policy tragedy, unlike the criminal or judicial realm, the culprit is less to be punished than reformed. The ultimate causal inference concerns policy, and it is drawn by the choral public and its representatives, even as it may be preceded and assisted by the lessons drawn and publicized by political elites, media organizations, and other actors. By assigning emotive weight and causal rationality to an episode—by linking the harm with a condition, and by spinning the counterfactual that the harm would not have occurred (and will not occur henceforth) with appropriate reform—the construction of policy tragedies can align problems with available solutions. Policy tragedies are historical and political products. They are complex combinations of the intended results of political framing and storytelling and the often unintended results of everyday portrayals of facts by popular media and public officials.[3]

The policy tragedy of elixir sulfanilamide established the basic lesson that undergirds gatekeeping power in American pharmaceutical policy. In the absence of a regulatory sentry at the border between drug development and

[2]Charles O. Jackson, *Food and Drug Legislation in the New Deal* (Princeton: Princeton University Press, 1970). James Harvey Young, *The Medical Messiahs: A Social History of Health Quackery in Twentieth-Century America* (Princeton: Princeton University Press, 1967). Other interpretations of the Act have been advanced, including an industry capture explanation, as scholars have argued that the rulemaking after the Act's passage largely conformed to the wishes of the organized pharmaceutical industry; Harry M. Marks, "Revisiting 'The Origins of Compulsory Drug Prescriptions,'" *American Journal of Public Health* 85 (1) (Jan. 1995): 109–15; Peter Temin, *Taking Your Medicine: Drug Regulation in the United States* (Cambridge: Harvard University Press, 1980); Paul M. Wax, "Elixirs, Diluents, and the Passage of the 1938 Federal Food, Drug and Cosmetic Act," *AnnIM* 122 (6) (March 15, 1995): 456–61.

[3]The notion of tragedy and the role of the chorus are taken from Greek literature, in particular Sophocles' *Oedipus Rex* and *Antigone*; G. M. Kirkwood, "The Dramatic Role of the Chorus in Sophocles," *Phoenix* 8 (1) (Spring 1954): 1–22. On agenda setting, consult John Kingdon, *Agendas, Alternatives and Public Policies* (Boston: Little, Brown, 1984), 94–100; Deborah Stone maintains a tighter focus on inferential patterns following the events and patterns that are interpreted, such that "causal argument is at the heart of problem definition" ("Causal Stories and the Formation of Policy Agendas," *Political Science Quarterly* 104 (2) (Summer 1989): 299). On the selective introduction or emphasis of political dimensions as akin to an act of framing, see William H. Riker, *The Art of Political Manipulation* (New Haven: Yale University Press, 1986).

market, this lesson says, people will be harmed, and massively so. In the sulfanilamide tragedy, this lesson was established vividly and commemorated in law. The first stage in the co-evolution of reputation and power came in this episode, and it underscored the dependence of regulatory power upon reputation and image. Without reputation and imagery, there was no power. Without the image of elixir sulfanilamide that an ungoverned market would kill, without the idea that an agency capable of governing that market had quickly removed the deadly elixir from American society, and without the idea that the same organization could prevent another elixir tragedy by its power to deny market entry to new drugs unless their safety had been demonstrated—without these lessons, the faces of regulatory power would not have materialized as they did.

So too, the administrative and legal aftermath of the 1938 Act established lessons that further intertwined reputation and power, less to a public and congressional audience and more to the audience of the modern business firm. Companies attempting to market new drugs soon discovered that proving safety meant proving that the therapeutic value of the drug in some sense exceeded its risks. And in the *Dotterweich* decision of 1943, drug company executives throughout the nation learned that they would be held personally and criminally responsible when their companies misbranded and adulterated medicines, even when they were not personally involved in the crime. Without the lessons established through early new drug review and fear-stoking lessons of *Dotterweich*, the Administration's power over pharmaceutical firms would have been narrower and less daunting.

Early Drug Regulation, Proprietary Medicines, and the "Right of Self-Medication"

Governments in the United States—municipal, state, and federal—have been regulating therapeutic drugs in different ways since the dawn of the republic. Yet it was not until the Biologics Act of 1902 and the Pure Food and Drugs Act of 1906 that direct and authoritative federal involvement in drug regulation was sanctioned. The first of these acts quietly established a precedent for minimal licensing power in the field of vaccines. The second established federal penalties for adulterating or misbranding medicines and strengthened a rapidly growing federal agency—the U.S. Department of Agriculture (USDA)—whose capacity for policy innovation in the Progressive Era spawned many other vital reforms. The organizational locus for early drug regulation lay in the USDA's Bureau of Chemistry, first headed by Pure Food and Drug Law founder Harvey Washington Wiley, and then from 1913 onward, by many of Wiley's appointees.[4]

The 1920s brought both renewed energy and frustration to drug regulators in the Agriculture Department. By 1927, the functions of food and drug

[4]Ramunas A. Kondratas, "Biologics Control Act of 1902," in James Harvey Young, ed., *The Early Years of Federal Food and Drug Control* (Madison, WI: American Institute for the History

regulation had become sufficiently differentiated from agricultural chemistry that regulators and regulatory chemists were moved into a separate agency called the Food, Drug and Insecticide Administration. Yet it was at this time that consciousness cemented among architects and supporters of the Pure Food and Drugs Act of 1906, who realized that their law had been an institutional success, but also something of a regulatory failure. Harvey Wiley himself worried that the law would come to nothing unless the enforcement authority and capacity of the Department of Agriculture were strengthened. In 1929, Wiley published the provocative title, *The History of a Crime Against the Food Law: The Amazing Story of the National Food and Drugs Law, Intended to Protect the Health of the People, Perverted to Protect Adulteration of Food and Drugs.* Wiley would die in 1930, but his wife Anna Kelton Wiley (who would survive him by thirty-four years), other supporters from the time, and critics of the American health economy began to press for changes to the 1906 law, including its provisions for the governance of food as well as drugs.[5]

The other agent of American drug regulation at this time was a nongovernmental actor: the Council on Pharmacy and Chemistry of the American Medical Association, established in 1905. The Council included pharmacologists, chemists, and physicians in its membership, and it published standards for drug quality. In 1930, it created a voluntary "Seal of Acceptance" program to evaluate safety and efficacy. When the Council deemed a drug unsafe, it could act to prevent the drug's advertisement in the *Journal of the American Medical Association* (JAMA). Council members also published *New and Nonofficial Remedies*, which elaborated a list of drugs whose properties attained the laboratory and clinical standards of the Council. In critical ways, FDA officials and their advisers would incorporate and build upon the Council's thinking.[6]

In the years from the Progressive Era through the New Deal, two related forces consistently opposed passage of FDA-strengthening legislation: the

of Pharmacy, 1982). The 1902 Act authorized the U.S. Hygienic Laboratory to license manufacturers, but gave limited power to the Laboratory to remove products from market, and no power to compel a series of pre-market tests. Christoph Gradmann, "Redemption, Danger and Risk: The History of Anti-Bacterial Chemotherapy and the Transformation of Tuberculin," in U. Trohler and T. Schlich, eds., *The Risks of Medical Innovation: Risk Perception and Assessment in Historical Context* (New York: Routledge, 2006), 53–70. On the 1906 Act and the USDA, see Oscar E. Anderson, Jr., *The Health of a Nation, Harvey W. Wiley and the Fight for Pure Food* (Chicago: University of Chicago Press, 1958); James Harvey Young, *Pure Food* (Princeton: Princeton University Press, 1990); Daniel Carpenter, *The Forging of Bureaucratic Autonomy: Reputations, Networks and Policy Innovation in Executive Agencies, 1862–1928,* chap. 8.

[5]Gustavus Weber, *The Food, Drug and Insecticide Administration: Its History, Activities, and Organization* (Baltimore: Johns Hopkins University Press, 1928); Marc T. Law, "How Do Regulators Regulate? Enforcement of the Pure Food and Drugs Act, 1907–1938," *Journal of Law, Economics and Organization* 22 (2) (2006): 459–89; Wiley, *History of a Crime Against the Food Law* (Washington, DC: Harvey W. Wiley, 1929). See chap. 10, "The Passing of the Bureau of Chemistry," for Wiley's critique of the 1920s enforcement regime.

[6]The Council was constituted by, relied upon, and contributed to a network of therapeutic

proprietary medicine industry, and votaries of the doctrine of "self-medication." These twin pillars of nineteenth-century health practice were mutually sustaining. The proprietary medicine industry was premised upon behavioral alternatives to professional medical practice and counsel. The
doctrine of self-medication, centuries old but waning, was viable only in the
presence of purchasable medications to which the consumer had relatively
unimpeded access.

Proprietary drugs (or "patent medicines") have long been described in
highly anachronistic terms, as "nostrums" marketed by "snake-oil peddlers,"
or as products whose manufacture and sale are equated with "quackery."
Such language might imply that the market for such medicines was a trifling
sideshow to the emergence of medically prescribed pharmaceutical products
in the economic history of the West. Nothing could be further from the truth.
The market for patent medicines in the United States grew consistently and
profitably from the colonial period through the nineteenth century and, by
the early 1900s, accounted for hundreds of millions of dollars in annual
sales. Such products accounted for millions of dollars in advertising revenue
in periodicals and medical journals nationwide, including the *Journal of the
American Medical Association*, which depended heavily upon patent medicine ads until 1905.[7]

It is difficult to demarcate patent medicines from their more legitimated
"non-patent" counterparts. "Patent medicines" were just as likely *not* to
have received a federal patent as to have one. Until the mid-twentieth century, patent medicines were commonly prescribed by fully licensed and
board-certified physicians, and they were frequently listed on official pharmacopoeia. The operative distinction became clearer in the late 1800s, when
pharmaceutical companies began restricting their advertising to doctors and
began to list the contents of their medications on the sides of the bottles.
Thus, proprietary medicines were usually distinguished by two factors: the
absence of chemical or pharmacological information on their labels, and
their heavy reliance upon direct-to-consumer advertising.[8]

Over the course of the nineteenth century, the market for proprietary
medicines—which ranged from novel concoctions to filling empty pharmaceutical containers with water or grain alcohol and reselling them—exploded in size.[9] An 1804 New York drug catalog listed some eighty or ninety
names of patent medicines, but by 1858 the number of products ranged
from 500 to 1,500, depending upon the estimate used. By 1905, *Druggist's
Circular* listed the names of over 28,000 patent medicines, and a year later

---

reformers in academic medicine and pharmacology, among other disciplines; Harry M. Marks,
The Progress of Experiment: Science and Therapeutic Reform in the United States, 1900–1990
(New York: Cambridge University Press, 1997), chapters 1 and 2.
    [7] Young, *The Toadstool Millionaires* (Princeton: Princeton University Press, 1961).
    [8] Young, *Medical Messiahs*, chap. 2.
    [9] The information in the following two pages is taken from Young, *Medical Messiahs*, chap-
ters 2 and 3, and Jackson, *Food and Drug Legislation in the New Deal*, 127–28.

congressional testimony put the estimate at 50,000. By 1859, the proprietary medicine business was valued in census figures at $3.5 million in annual revenues. By 1904, that revenue estimate reached $74.5 million, a figure which by 1912 had increased by approximately 60 percent to over $110 million. By mid-century, congressional investigators estimated annual revenues of the proprietary medicine industry at $1 billion to $2 billion.

The set of drugs marketed as patent medicines varied widely in their composition and therapeutic claims. Anti-impotence medications and sexual stimulation drugs with names such as "Persenico" and "Revivio" were very common. Within ten days of consuming "Persenico," the patient would have success "in combating neurasthenic impotence, pre-senility, low vitality and general nervous ailments, particularly . . . of sexual origin." The love-sex hormone "Revivio" offered men the chance to "improve your vigor." Those suffering from gastrointestinal constipation or "piles" could purchase, with a money-back guarantee, "Dr. Young's Rectal Dilators." The dilators purportedly used "natural methods" to strengthen rectal muscles by "imitating Nature's own process."

These medications had far more pervasive effects than might be implied by the morbid historical curiosity that they inspire today. There were at least three deleterious outcomes of the widespread marketing of these drugs. The first was equilibrium fraud. Consumers were buying products with the belief that they held curing power when in fact they usually held none or were in fact harmful to health. With the possible exception of aspirin (whose contents were usually published) and several analgesics, no widely sold patent medicine of the late nineteenth to early twentieth century was later shown to have significant clinical curative power for its consumers. Perhaps worse, many patent medicines were associated with high toxicity and other safety hazards. Most "soothing tonics" for babies and children were laced with alcohol, opium, or some combination of the two. "Gouraud's Oriental Face Cream" led to "genuine facial beauty," but government investigators later learned that it did so by imparting significant mercury to its consumers, thereby inducing skin discoloration.

The truly severe harm associated with proprietary medicines concerned not hazards in the medicines themselves but the treatment foregone by their consumption. There were at least two mechanisms that engendered such an outcome. First, knowledgeable consumers would often forgo the opportunity to consume even legitimate pharmaceutical products out of awareness of the hazards associated with fraudulent varieties. Second, and most important, for every consumer trying to reduce the risks or severity of illness by consuming a noncurative patent medicine, valuable medical treatment was forfeited. In some cases, consumers would experiment with different drug products until they found something that "worked" for them. Even in cases where they eventually happened upon a remedy with true curative value, their consumption of other patent medicines in this auto-experimental process usually implied a serious delay in effective treatment. In other cases, superstitious learning led to an even worse outcome. In cases where the consumer's ailment would have gone away on its own, the consumer often wrongly reasoned that the patent medicine had in fact cured a disease, a conclusion which induced further consumption of the drug, and then boosted consumption by others as word of the medicine's purported quality made its way through interpersonal networks.[10]

The staying power of patent medicines in the United States and other Western nations was linked to a set of beliefs about the relationship between individual agents and the curing of disease. The philosophy or ideology of "self-medication" or "auto-therapy" was centuries old and linked to organized challenges to the medical and pharmacological professions. The set of movements intertwined with these beliefs was diverse and complex, but as a general pattern, the social, economic, and political authority of organized medicine came at the expense of organized homeopathy, chiropractic practice, holistic medicine, and other movements. The emergence of a national market for proprietary drugs was in some ways akin to, in other ways vastly different from, these movements. Patent medicine makers commonly advertised their drugs as a means of avoiding the expense and personal intrusion occasioned by a visit to the doctor. This pattern helps to explain why patent medicines were popular among women living under cultural norms of Victorian domesticity, and among men seeking treatment for gonorrhea and syphilis. Yet patent medicines competed powerfully with "alternative medicine" and indeed drove out of business many nineteenth- and twentieth-century practitioners of the (non-medical) healing arts.[11]

The set of specific beliefs described by the "right of self-medication" emerged with greater cultural force during the antebellum period and continued in force through the early 1900s. At its core, claims for the primacy or privileged status of self-medication depended upon beliefs in consumer autonomy and judgment. Votaries of self-medication frequently voiced their support for stronger labeling disclosure requirements for drug manufacturers, in part out of the belief that "the intelligent layman" needed maximal information to render an informed pharmaceutical purchasing decision. Yet the supporters of auto-therapy usually disdained state and federal regulatory measures. One of the most relevant political implications of their ethic

[10] Jackson, *Food and Drug Legislation in the New Deal*, 96. For a theoretical and empirical argument that such pathological learning is common in consumer evaluations of doctor quality and pharmaceutical efficacy, see Jishnu Das, "Do Patients Learn About Doctor Quality? Theory and Evidence from India," Ph.D. diss., Department of Economics, Harvard University (2001); and Daniel Carpenter, "A Simple Theory of Placebo Learning with Self-Remitting Diseases," manuscript, Department of Government, Harvard University, 2005. R. Barker Bausell, *Snake-Oil Science: The Truth About Complementary and Alternative Medicine* (New York: Oxford University Press, 2007).

[11] Guenter B. Risse, Ronald L. Numbers, and Judith Walzer Leavitt, *Medicine without Doctors: Home Health Care in American History* (New York: Science History Publications, 1977). Alex Berman and Michael A. Flannery, *America's Botanico-Medical Movements: Vox Populi* (New York: Pharmaceutical Products Press, 2001).

was a time-honored "right of self-medication." In operation, this included the absolute liberty of the consumer or patient to purchase any and all medications for the amelioration of his or her ailments. Whatever the disease, and whatever the purported cure, the "layman" should be able to exercise his own scientific judgment in drug purchasing decisions.[12]

The proprietary medicine industry entered the twentieth century almost completely unregulated. Aside from some state-level statutes passed to regulate food in the 1880s and 1890s, no government regulation of the proprietary medicine market existed. The signal change in Progressive-Era regulation of drugs came in 1906, when Dr. Harvey Wiley of the USDA's Bureau of Chemistry successfully completed a twenty-year campaign to pass a federal food and drug regulation bill. The 1906 law gave USDA power to seize articles of manufacture deemed "fraudulent" or falsely advertised, and prodigious cooperation between Wiley and officials at the Post Office Department was successful in prosecuting hundreds of cases in the Progressive period. Yet such cases were always prosecuted after the harm had occurred, and the associated penalties were minimal. Robert Harper's marketing of "Cuforhedake Brane-Fude—a "brain food" supplement containing a dangerous combination of alcohol and acetanilid whose title subtly offered to cure headaches—eventually brought him a fine of $700. Compared with the $2 million in profits he had made on the product, it was a trifling fine.[13]

Whether due to the unevenness of state regulation or the greater staying power of self-medication ideologies in the region, Southern states provided, by the 1930s, a truly comfortable home for many firms in the proprietary medicine industry. Indeed, the proprietary medicine industry was characterized by some exclusively regional markets. Some nostrums sold in California were virtually unheard of on the East Coast, and many more drugs marketed in Southern states were generally unavailable or not widely purchased in states outside the former Confederacy.

*The Emergence of New Regulatory Alternatives: Bureaucratic
Agenda-Setting and the Power of Organized Women*

Calls for a revision of the 1906 Pure Food and Drugs Act were largely unrelated to changes in the proprietary medicine industry or to consumer tragedies of the 1920s and early 1930s. Instead, two forces—the FDA (backed by Roosevelt administration officials in the Department of Agriculture) and organized women's groups—exercised strong leverage in pressing for changes to the

---

[12] Jackson, *Food and Drug Legislation in the New Deal*, 79, 114.

[13] Anderson, *The Health of a Nation*; Young, *Pure Food*; Carpenter, *The Forging of Bureaucratic Autonomy*. Paul Quirk, "The Food and Drug Administration," in James Q. Wilson, *The Politics of Regulatory Agencies* (Washington, DC: Brookings Institution, 1980). Compounds containing acetanilid were suspected in at least 22 deaths in 1905 (Young, *Medical Messiahs*, 6). Acetanilid mimicked opiates, inducing overdoses and lending itself to addictive consumption.

1906 law. One of their principal successes was finding able legislative sponsors, principally New York Senator Royal Copeland and Tennessee Representative Virgil Chapman. From 1934 to 1937, Copeland in particular authored a succession of bills that would have substantially strengthened the FDA.

FDA officials had long been disappointed with the operation of the 1906 Act, repeatedly lamenting that manufacturers were able to exploit loopholes in the statute. Successfully prosecuted proprietary manufacturers quickly relabeled their products and entered the market again, and dangerous and worthless medications were entering commerce. Patent medicine manufacturers circumvented the labeling and fraud restrictions of the 1906 Act by veiling their therapeutic claims (hence "Cuforhedake") or by removing information from the label altogether.

The first bill addressing these problems was authored by FDA personnel, was sponsored by Copeland, and was titled "S.1944" (introduced in December 1933). Along with its successors "S.2800" and "S.5" (both introduced in 1934), Senate Bill 1944 attempted to rein in the patent medicine industry. S.1944 required disclosure of ingredients on labels, removed the 1906 Act's requirement that the FDA had to prove intent to defraud in order to seize shipments of a good, gave the FDA power to seize multiple shipments of "misbranded" goods, and rendered advertisers and manufacturers alike legally liable for fraudulent claims. The bill also gave to the FDA power over pharmaceutical advertising. S.2800 and S.5 relaxed many of these provisions, in particular by introducing judicial constraints on seizures and by relaxing the formula disclosure provisions of earlier bills. As the legislation progressed through Congress, debates over labeling, seizure, and advertising regulation would attract the greatest energy and debate.

Administrative leaders at the FDA, most notably Walter Campbell and Paul Dunbar—careerists who had trained under USDA Chief Chemist Harvey Wiley before 1910—made use of three strategies in advancing the case for strengthening the 1906 Act. First, they allied with friendly forces in the Roosevelt administration, mainly Rexford Tugwell. Tugwell was FDR's assistant secretary of agriculture and perhaps the most powerful liberal voice in the administration in the early 1930s. He desired for the pharmaceutical industry a system of industrial oversight not unlike that envisioned in the National Recovery Administration or antitrust law, where "fair and responsible competition" would be a primary policy goal. His continued support of FDA-strengthening legislation was crucial in light of a salient fact about the food and drug regulatory struggle: Roosevelt was not supportive of the FDA's or of Copeland's efforts. At a general level, the president was generally uninterested in regulatory measures and more interested in laws specifically aimed at economic recovery and national infrastructure. More specifically, Royal Copeland was a New Deal dissident, and New Dealers in Congress and the Administration resented his sponsorship of the bill.[14]

[14]Jackson, *Food and Drug Legislation in the New Deal*, 63–65, 84, 118.

The FDA's second stratagem was a skilled and indirect publicity campaign aimed at demonstrating the hazards of adulterated food and medicines to the nation's press. The FDA had been prevented from direct lobbying and publicity efforts in the Deficiency Appropriations Act of 1919, yet the FDA found creative ways to circumvent this rule, distributing pamphlets such as the one entitled *Why We Need a New Pure Food Law*, and by giving radio addresses about S.2800. FDA Information Officer Ruth Lamb successfully invited press outlets to give fresh attention to Copeland's first Senate bill (S.1944), and she used her own time and money to author a popular book on the hazards of patent medicines entitled *American Chamber of Horrors* (1936).[15]

The FDA's third strategy was one that required coordination but not persuasion. FDA officials drew upon their decades-old alliances with women's groups and organized consumer unions. Two women's groups—the General Federation of Women's Clubs (GFWC) and the Women's Christian Temperance Union (WCTU)—were instrumental in lobbying for the 1906 Act. The Federation and the Union were some of the most powerful lobbies of their time, almost single-handedly waging successful campaigns for mothers' pensions and child-labor laws. Joining the women's groups, moreover, was the increasingly assertive and powerful Consumers' Research (CR). Consumers' Research was founded in 1929 with 1,000 members and by 1933 had ballooned to 45,000 members. The organization served to coordinate sympathizers of consumer legislation in Congress and in the public at large. Rexford Tugwell found "astounding" the "receptive attitude of the general public" toward Consumers' Research.[16]

Despite the seemingly favorable circumstances—an overwhelming Democratic majority in Congress with pro-regulation impulses, a Democratic president, supportive women's groups, and a well-coordinated rhetorical campaign—several factors combined to blunt the FDA's initiative for food and drug law reform in the mid-1930s. The first was well-organized and well-represented opposition from the affected industries. As historian Charles Jackson describes the rise of opposition, "Many existing trade bodies were turned almost immediately into vehicles of resistance. Especially militant were the Proprietary Association [PA] and the United Medicine Manufacturers of America [UMMA]." The PA and UMMA sponsored protest gatherings, radio advertisements, and coordinated petition campaigns against

---

[15]See Ruth Deforest Lamb, *American Chamber of Horrors: The Truth About Food and Drugs* (New York: Farrar & Rinehart, 1935). For an informative summary of these efforts, consult Gwen Kay, "Healthy Public Relations: The FDA's 1930s Legislative Campaign," *Bulletin of the History of Medicine* 75 (2001): 446–87.

[16]The political abilities and achievements of these groups have been capably documented by Theda Skocpol and Elizabeth Clemens, among others. Skocpol, *Protecting Soldiers and Mothers* (Cambridge: Harvard University Press, 1992); Clemens, *The People's Lobby* (Chicago: University of Chicago Press, 1998); Carpenter, *The Forging of Bureaucratic Autonomy*, chap. 8. As Jackson describes the Union, "CR's influence and significance far exceeded its actual membership"; *Food and Drug Legislation in the New Deal*, 20–21.

FDA-strengthening bills. The manufacturers found able legislative defenders such as Senators Josiah Bailey of Tennessee and Arthur Vandenberg of Michigan.[17]

Two other difficulties were related less to the opponents of reform than to its supporters. Rexford Tugwell was the lightning rod of the early Roosevelt administration, was disliked by rural Democrats and conservatives, and his visible association with the Copeland bill soon become a serious liability for the FDA. Opponents of S.2800 and S.1944 sounded alarms of "Tugwellmania" and called the Copeland measure "the Tugwell bill." Yet Copeland himself was perhaps a more serious liability, at least early on. Copeland was a New Deal dissident whom Administration Democrats resented. FDR withheld endorsement for his home state's senator in the 1934 midterm elections and made no secret of the fact. Roosevelt loyalists in the Democratic Party, including Alben Barkley and other Southerners, were determined to keep Copeland an arm's length away from political or moral victories on food and drug regulation.

Opponents of reform landed an apparent deathblow in 1935, when the Senate passed Copeland's S.5, but only after attaching the infamous "Bailey Amendment" which vitiated the measure. The Bailey Amendment prohibited the FDA from regulating any aspect of pharmaceutical advertising and would give all such control to the Federal Trade Commission (FTC). From the vantage of the 1906 law, this was a step backwards for the FDA. Even under the Progressive Era statute, the FDA had at least some authority to govern fraudulent advertising and frequently assisted FTC prosecutions under the 1914 Federal Trade Commission Act. Once the Bailey Amendment was approved, S.5 passed the Senate but was doomed as a result of criticisms from the left and the right. S.5 then died in the House by an overwhelming 190–70 vote.

Roll call votes are available for three crucial votes on the Senate measure in the 74th Congress (1935–1936), and their aggregate patterns offer some insight into the political dynamics of reform before 1937. The first two votes were on procedural measures to reconsider an amendment that had been attached to S.5 during committee. Those who favored a stronger FDA wanted to revisit the committee's decisions and voted "yes" on these measures. The third vote was a vote on the Bailey amendment prohibiting the FDA from regulating pharmaceutical advertising. Proponents of reform voted "no" on this measure, while most opponents of reform voted for it.[18]

[17] Jackson, *Food and Drug Legislation in the New Deal*, 38–39.
[18] Some friends of reform who were also favorable to increased FTC jurisdiction of the economy voted for the Bailey amendment as well. The FTC had powerful friends in the House, not least among Brandeisian liberals who saw the commission as the best hope for a Progressive policy of economy-wide central management and antitrust. This was the wisdom of Bailey's measure, to have split economic liberals from the FDA by sending them headlong into an embrace with the Commission.

Statistical analysis of these Senate votes reveals some general patterns. Democrats and more liberal Senators who supported the Roosevelt administration's policies were more likely to vote in favor of these bills, just as they were likely to vote for other regulatory measures of the 1930s. Information on where UMMA firms were headquartered provides an estimate of the correlation between drug firm presence in a state and the voting record of that state's senators. Perhaps the most interesting insight from the voting patterns is that organized drug manufacturers were arrayed firmly against legislation that increased the FDA's power over pharmaceuticals. The probability of a Senator voting "yes" on the first two reconsideration measures is positively associated with the number of UMMA firms headquartered in the Senators' state (figure 2.1). For every additional UMMA firm headquartered in a Senator's state, that Senator was 10 percent less likely to vote for FDA-strengthening bills. In other words, pharmaceutical interests aligned themselves against the legislation, and their legislative representatives followed suit.[19]

The voting patterns for legislation in the 74th Congress, then, defy industry capture understandings of federal drug regulation. Indeed, a hypothesis which runs counter to the capture perspective receives strong support. Affected industries, particularly the organized pharmaceutical firms that would have benefited from removed proprietary competition, nonetheless agitated against the legislation, and their representatives were more likely to vote against FDA-strengthening measures. These measures did not contain government licensing or pre-market notification that constituted market entry restrictions, but where this possibility was raised in the 73rd and 74th Congresses, industry allies quickly scuttled the possibility.[20]

Indeed, pharmaceutical and proprietary opponents of the Copeland bill won the early battles. While the 1936 election confirmed FDR's popularity, strengthened the hand of liberals in the Democratic Party, and solidified Democratic congressional majorities, it did not generate added momentum for passage of new pharmaceutical regulation. Perhaps the most important reason was the rise of the Conservative Coalition in Congress, a cross-party alliance of Southern Democrats and Republicans that frustrated many of Roosevelt's legislative initiatives through voting and through control of the House Rules Committee. For this reason, the challenge for Copeland and FDA officials was all the greater. Some of the most steadfast opponents of

[19] Further detail on the voting regressions appears in Daniel Carpenter and Gisela Sin, "Policy Tragedy and the Emergence of Regulation: The Food, Drug and Cosmetic Act of 1938," *Studies in American Political Development* 21 (Fall 2007): 149–80. As is customary in political science analyses of these voting patterns, liberal-conservative ideology is measured by reference to the NOMINATE scores computed by Keith Poole and Howard Rosenthal; *Congress: A Political-Economic History of Roll-Call Voting* (New York: Oxford University Press, 1997). The first dimension D-NOMINATE score has a negative coefficient estimate in the first two regressions and a positive estimate in the third. Since higher scores indicate more "conservative" members, this result implies that more "liberal" senators were more likely to vote for the first two (pro-regulatory) measures and less likely to vote for the (anti-regulatory) third measure.

[20] Marks, *The Progress of Experiment*, 76.

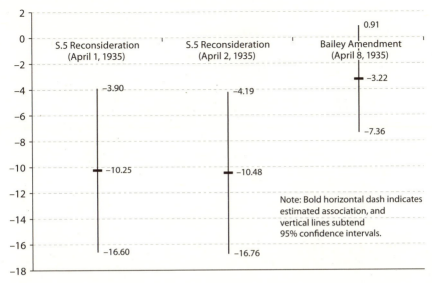

Figure 2.1. Change in Probability of Pro-Regulatory Vote for Every Additional UMMA Firm Headquartered in Senator's State

regulatory reform had just become more institutionally formidable. In the summer of 1937, Royal Copeland confided to friends and colleagues that S.5, along with other hopes for strengthening the Food and Drug Administration's power over the pharmaceutical market, was dying.[21]

The Sulfanilamide Episode of 1937

Months later, the FDA began to hear reports of several deaths in Tulsa, Oklahoma, associated with a proprietary drug called "Elixir Sulfanilamide," an anti-infective drug manufactured by the patent medicine concern Dr. Massengill, of Bristol, Tennessee. FDA officials began investigating the Tulsa deaths, but as they did so, a number of other reports of mortality and morbidity, many of them among children, were making rounds in medical and regulatory networks.

Dr. Massengill's Elixir Sulfanilamide was manufactured as part of a larger trend toward the use of sulfanilamides in the late 1930s (figure 2.2). Popular in Europe for the treatment of common colds, pneumonia, and other infections, sulfanilamide was now making its way into many medicines manufactured in the United States. FDA officials therefore suspected that the problem lay not in the sulfanilamide itself but rather in the elixir solution in which it was suspended for pharmacological delivery. Dr. Massengill's solvent, as it

[21] "Drug Law Revision Held Over Until Next Session," *OP&DR*, August 19, 1937. James T. Patterson, *Congressional Conservatism and the New Deal* (Lexington: University of Kentucky Press, 1967); Eric Schickler, *Disjointed Pluralism* (Princeton: Princeton University Press, 2001).

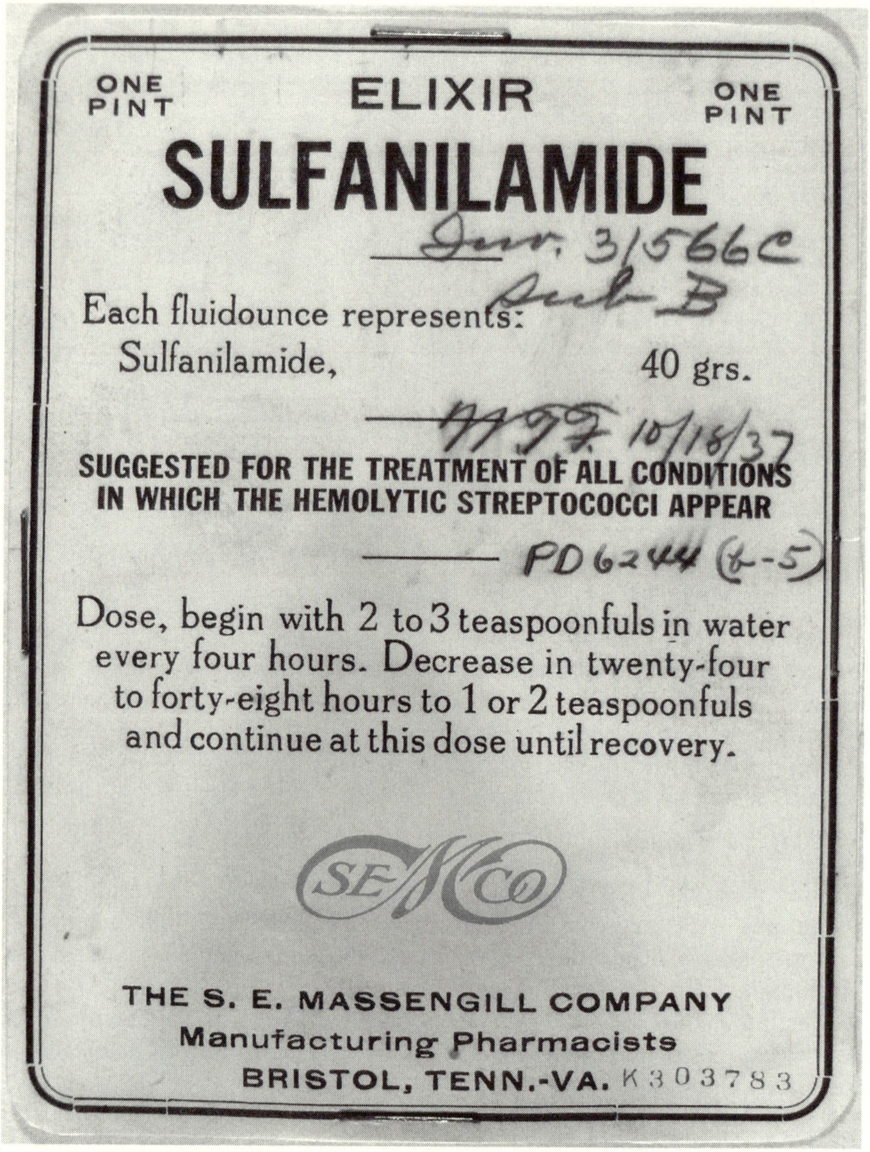

Figure 2.2. An Elixir Sulfanilamide Label, 1937

turned out, was diethylene glycol, which is similar to an essential ingredient in antifreeze and is highly toxic even in small doses.[22]

Dr. Massengill's Elixir Sulfanilamide began to ship to localities from three distribution points—New York City, Bristol, and San Francisco—in September 1937. By late October, seventy-three persons had perished in ways that doctors could directly attribute to having consumed the elixir. Another twenty deaths were suspected to be related to the drug, but the FDA and doctors lacked sufficient autopsy evidence to make a direct link in these cases. In the fall of 1937, an emergency session of the Congress called upon the Department of Agriculture to make a report regarding the deaths, and the Secretary published a highly detailed report that was cited repeatedly in the press and in congressional testimony. At the end of this document, the USDA published a map showing all of the shipment points to which the elixir had been distributed, as well as all localities in which any deaths occurred, as well as the number of deaths occurring in a locality (figure 2.3).

As it turns out, the deaths from sulfanilamide were not as widely distributed, and the public outcry was not as broad, as blunt scholarly descriptions would have us believe. Jackson reports that "Fatalities took place in fifteen states, as far east as Virginia and as far west as California."[23] Yet he fails to mention that most of the deaths occurred in Southern and "border" states, and that some states of the former Confederacy were spared relative to others. There were six deaths in East St. Louis, Illinois, and another eight in Charleston, South Carolina. Louisiana experienced no fatalities, while Oklahoma experienced eleven and Mississippi, twenty-one. Part of the problem is that the map, which is in the legislative archives of the House of Representatives, was not published with the Secretary's report. As a result, USDA officials and members of Congress saw the map, but the public probably did not. Yet the concentration of deaths (and shipments) suggests something about the mechanisms by which the drug was propagated through a large population of consumers. The prescription and consumption of elixir sulfanilamide was probably dependent upon local referral networks and the idiosyncratic practices of individual physicians.[24]

The "brute facts" of the sulfanilamide episode, then, were as follows. A product called "Elixir of Sulfanilamide-Massengill" was manufactured and distributed. Many consumed it after prescription as an anti-infective or as a

[22] Ethylene glycol was the relevant component of anti-freeze, until propylene glycol began to be substituted.

[23] Jackson, *Food and Drug Legislation in the New Deal*, 159.

[24] Aggregate statistical patterns of sulfanilamide shipments and associated deaths show that the Massengill Company was more likely to ship elixir sulfanilamide to the South, to areas where the population was less educated, and both to areas that were characterized by greater manufacturing value-added and areas with more population in rural residence. The percentage population rural variable is insignificantly related to shipments and deaths in the county-level analyses, but significantly related in the state analyses; Carpenter and Sin, "Policy Tragedy and the Emergence of Regulation," 164.

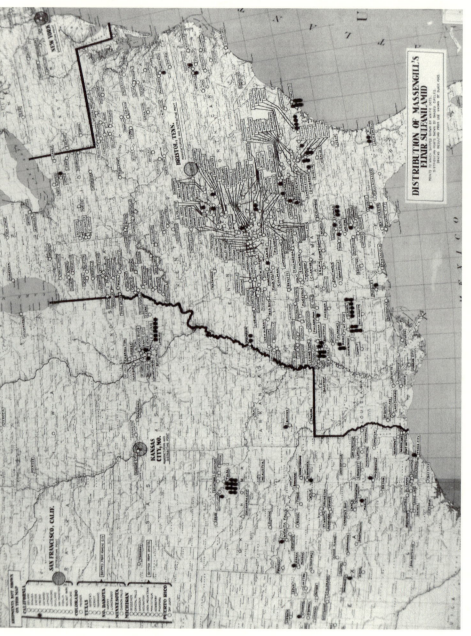

Figure 2.3. Distribution of Massengill's Elixir Sulfanilamide (USDA Report to Congress, 1937)

treatment for venereal disease. Utilization of the medicine was most common in the upper-country South (Tennessee) and in the plains Midwest (southern Illinois, Oklahoma), and appears to have been disproportionately common among African Americans. People became seriously ill from its consumption, and by late October 1937, at least seventy-three of these had died. The FDA, assisted by state and local health officials and the American Medical Association, commenced an effort to secure as much of the compound as possible before any more was consumed.

Sulfanilamide from Episode to Tragedy: The FDA and the National Media

The first reports of illness and death resulting from elixir sulfanilamide came not to the FDA but the American Medical Association. On October 11, Dr. James Stevenson, president of the Tulsa (Oklahoma) County Medical Society, sent a telegram to the AMA's Chemical Laboratory, stating that six deaths had occurred after prescription and administration of the elixir. Communications between the AMA and Tulsa area physicians continued, and the AMA Chemical Laboratory immediately requested a shipment of the Elixir, which the Massengill Company promptly sent. Upon cursory analysis and laboratory tests with experimental animals, the Chemical Laboratory concluded that diethylene glycol and not sulfanilamide was the "causative factor" in the deaths. Based upon this information, as well as new and independent reports of deaths coming from East St. Louis, Illinois, the Editor of *JAMA* issued a public warning on Saturday, October 2, then again on Monday, October 18.[25]

Three days after the initial Tulsa inquiry at the AMA, the first word of elixir sulfanilamide deaths reached the FDA on October 14, 1937. On October 16, an FDA investigator telegraphed headquarters with news that nine persons in the Tulsa area had died there from taking the elixir. From this point forward, and for about three weeks, reporting of the deaths was shared by the FDA and the American Medical Association. There was a degree of mutual dependence in this reporting. The Administration relied upon AMA reports and its own investigators; the AMA relied upon FDA reports and its own information from networks of physicians.[26]

[25] "Sulfanilamide—A Warning," *JAMA*, October 2, 1937. Paul Nicholas Leech (Director, AMA Chemical Laboratory), "Elixir of Sulfanilamide-Massengill," Special Article from the AMA Chemical Laboratory, *JAMA* 109 (19) (Nov. 6, 1937): 1531. A valuable discussion of the following narrative occurs in James Harvey Young, "Sulfanilamide and Diethylene Glycol," in John Parascandola and James C. Whorton, eds., *Chemistry and Modern Society: Essays in Honor of Aaron J. Ihde* (ACS Symposium Series 228; Washington, DC: American Chemical Society, 1983).

[26] On the AMA's dependence on the FDA, see Leech, "Elixir," *JAMA* 109 (19) (Nov. 6, 1937): 1539. On the FDA's dependence on the AMA, see *Report of the Secretary*, Sen. Doc. 124; Dunn, *Federal Food, Drug and Cosmetic Act*, 1317.

The AMA's October 18 warning was reported a day later in various newspapers, using Associated Press wire reports. The *Washington Post*'s title and subtitle were exemplary:

VENEREAL DISEASE 'CURE' KILLS 8 OF 10 PATIENTS IN OKLAHOMA

Sulfanilamide, Hailed as Remedy, Used in Fatal Preparation; Doctors Blame Other Drug; Firm Seeks to Recover 375 Cases on Market[27]

As the title of the *Post* story suggests, the very initial accounts of sulfanilamide deaths never mentioned the FDA. The American Medical Association had broken the story, and it was the manufacturer Massengill and not the FDA to which was attributed the attempt to remove Elixir Sulfanilamide from the market.

Additional insight into the deaths and their cultural reception can be gleaned from the details of these early accounts. Although the elixir had been prescribed for various conditions, early reports described it as a "Venereal Disease Cure." This was true in many cases, leading individual physicians to refuse to reveal the names of their patients to whom they had prescribed the elixir. Connected with this stigma, the early discussion of the drug and its using population also had subtle racial tones. In the initial *JAMA* report, an AMA reporting chemist noted, "In the last several days I have seen four deaths in patients using a product called "Elixir of Sulfanilamide" and sold by Massengill & Company. These patients, all Negroes, were treated by a Dr. Weathers of East St. Louis, Ill." Morris Fishbein, editor of *JAMA*, had made an implicit reference to young black males purchasing the drug as a venereal disease cure when he stated that "the association had learned of widespread purchases in one city by youths attempting to treat themselves for venereal disease."[28]

The association between black males and venereal disease was a longstanding one in white Americans' racial imagination, and the early reports of sulfanilamide mortality fed upon and strengthened that association. From death records of the victims, it would appear that a large number of the elixir sulfanilamide users (54 percent) were African Americans, but many of these were children who did not present with gonorrhea or syphilis. African Americans were also disproportionately represented among these young victims (56 percent). There was at the time no evidence that poor white males were any less likely to have contracted syphilis than poor black males. The link between Elixir Sulfanilamide, syphilis, and blackness was one established in myth, and any concentration of syphilis among black men was probably due to dislocations related to the Great War. Yet in Jim Crow

[27] *WP*, October 19, 1937, p. 3. See also "'Elixir' Fatal to 14 in West Is Seized Here," *WP*, October 20, 1937, p. 1.

[28] O. E. Hagebusch, M.D., "Necropsies of Four Patients Following Administration of Elixir of Sulfanilamide-Massengill," in "The Chemical Laboratory," *JAMA* 109 (19) (Nov. 6, 1937): 1537. Statement attributed to Fishbein in "Venereal Disease 'Cure' Kills 8 of 10 Patients in Oklahoma," *WP*, October 19, 1937, p. 3.

America, this subtle link greatly empowered the rumors and reduced the vitality and visibility of the sufferers.[29]

By the end of the week (Saturday, October 23), and certainly by the end of October 1937, the primary source of information on the sulfanilamide episode had become Campbell and the FDA. With the FDA feeding daily reports of its search and investigation activities to the Associated Press, media attention turned to the mounting death toll and whether the FDA could "round up" the medicine "in time" to save those who, with the elixir still in their medicine cabinets, were still at risk. Newspaper stories told of FDA officials working late nights and weekends to inform the public, of commandeering airplanes and academic chemists to search far and wide for remaining samples of the drug, and generally of a vast, nationwide operation centered in the FDA.

SEIZURE OF DEADLY 'ELIXIR' SAVES MARYLANDER AS U.S. HASTENS TO CHECK TOLL ALREADY AT 29

Death in Salisbury, Md., from the use of the drug "elixir of sulfanilamide" was narrowly averted yesterday while airplanes and chemists hastily drafted into service failed to save nine lives in other parts of the Nation.... From coast to coast, in large cities like New York and backwoods communities of the South, West and Midwest, field agents are desperately fighting against time to save lives of potential victims who have the elixir in their medicine cabinets.

With only four of these drug detectives available to cover Alabama, Mississippi, Louisiana and two-thirds of Texas, airplanes were chartered yesterday for the sake of speed.

"We have never had an outbreak like this," said Campbell, whose office in the south building of the Department of Agriculture is the nerve center of the life-and-death roundup. "The only thing we are concerned with is taking the compound out of circulation, removing it from wholesale houses, drug stores, homes and wherever else it may be." (*Washington Post*, October 23, 1937)

NEAR END OF CHASE FOR DEADLY ELIXIR

Government Agents Hope to Recover Today the Last of 700 Bottles.

"A nationwide race with death, seeking recovery of more than 700 bottles, mostly pints, of a new liquid medicine named elixir of sulfanilamide, which has already caused thirty-six verified deaths, was described today at the headquarters of the American Medical Association.

Every agent of the United States Food and Drug Administration is scouring the country to recover the bottles, said Dr. Morris Fishbein, spokesman of the medical association. By some time tomorrow, according to J. O. Clarke of the Food and Drug Administration, it is hoped that all the outstanding shipments will be recovered." (*New York Times*, October 25, 1937)

[29] On the racial imagining of syphilis, see Steven Epstein, *Inclusion: The Politics of Difference in Medical Research* (Chicago: University of Chicago Press, 2007), 37, and notes 26–9; Allan Brandt, "Racism and Research: The Case of the Tuskegee Syphilis Experiment," in

NURSE, HERSELF A VICTIM, SAVES SIX FROM "ELIXIR."

While 200 agents of the Federal drug office yesterday scoured the Nation for bottles of deadly sulfanilamide and diethylene "elixir" still unaccounted for, Evelyn Sharborough, a pretty 28-year old nurse in Mount Olive, Miss., was caring for six patients surviving from 13 who were treated with the mixture. . . . In Washington officials of the food and drug administration spent Sunday within reach of telephones. Dr. J. J. Durrett, chief of the drug section, said the list of verified deaths from the elixir still stood at 37. (*Washington Post*, October 25, 1937) [30]

FDA officials wasted little time in trying to frame the episode as evidence of the weakness of the 1906 laws and its patchwork of supplementary regulations. Technically nothing in the elixir sulfanilamide disaster implied that the Massengill Company had broken a single law. There was little basis in federal statute for prosecuting Bristol. The only charge against Massengill that stuck was an arcane mislabeling charge, namely that "elixir" implied alcoholic content yet "Elixir Sulfanilamide" contained no alcohol. On October 19, just the second day of media reporting on the sulfanilamide deaths, Walter Campbell noted that only a thread of the current law prohibiting misbranding allowed the Administration to round up the elixir. Campbell said that the fatalities "are new evidence of the need for tightening the Nation's food and drug laws and predicted legislation to that end will be pressed at the coming session of Congress, in spite of failure to enact loophole plugs in the last few years." [31] By the end of the week, a tidy bundle of facts and policy recommendations were consistently and almost imperceptibly bandied about news reports, including the fact that the elixir had violated federal law only by being misbranded:

Susan M. Reverby, ed., *Tuskegee's Truths: Rethinking the Tuskegee Syphilis Study* (Chapel Hill: University of North Carolina Press, 2000). The FDA did keep detailed records of the elixir sulfanilamide victims, and of the records from 72 cases that remain in FDA archives, 57 can be identified by race. Of these 57, 31 (54 percent) were identified as African Americans. Among the 23 victims aged 17 or younger whose race was recorded, 13 were identified as African American, while 10 were identified as Caucasian (10 other young victims were not identified by race). Of the 72 cases, 39 of the victims presented with gonorrhea or syphilis. Tabulation by author from Death Records of Elixir Sulfanilamide Victims, AF 1-258, v. 9, FDA Records, Rockville, MD; I thank FDA historian John Swann for his assistance with these records. See also "Elixir of Sulfanilamide-Massengill: Survey of Deaths," *JAMA* 109 (1937): 1539. On the Great War and syphilis in the 1890 to 1899 black male cohort, consult Toni P. Miles and David McBride, "World War I Origins of the Syphilis Epidemic Among 20th Century Black Americans: A Biohistorical Approach," *Social Science and Medicine* 45(1) (1997) 61-69.

[30] Gerald G. Gross, "Seizure of Deadly 'Elixir' Saves Marylander as U.S. Hastens to Check Toll Already at 29," *WP*, October 23, 1937, p. 1; "Near End of Chase for Deadly Elixir," *NYT*, October 25, 1937, p. 21; "Nurse, Herself a Victim, Saves Six from 'Elixir,'" *WP*, October 25, 1937, p. 2. A thorough review of the FDA's investigation occurs in James Harvey Young, "Sulfanilamide and Diethylene Glycol," in John Parascandola and James Whorton, eds., *Chemistry and Modern Society* (Washington, DC: American Chemical Society, 1983).

[31] Gross, "Seizure of Deadly 'Elixir' Saves Marylander," p. 1. For journalistic repetition of these arguments, almost verbatim from FDA pronouncements, see for example "Control of Drugs," *WP* [editorial], October 26, 1937. Jackson, *Food and Drug Legislation*, 156–7.

NEED FOR NEW DRUG LAWS CITED.

. . . Calling attention to the need for drastic tightening up of the Federal food and drug laws, toward which numerous bills have been introduced, but none enacted, Bureau Chief Campbell and Dr. Durrett cited the following handicaps in the present emergency:

> Intervention of the Food and Drug Administration is justified only because of the alleged misbranding, the "elixir" on the label being challenged, and not because the liquid contained poison.
>
> Even though the preparation is known to have death-dealing properties, the Federal Government cannot legally make a seizure unless it has been shipped across a state line.
>
> Confiscation of a bottle whose seal has been broken cannot be made.[32]

Along with Campbell, Durrett, and their FDA associates, there were two other voices distilling policy lessons from the sulfanilamide episode. The first was Morris Fishbein of the AMA. In the *Journal*'s editorial of October 23, he drew larger policy implications from the sulfanilamide episode: "The possibilities are unlimited because we are here concerned with a preparation not standardized by any reliable agency, semisecret in composition and apparently hastily rushed into the market to meet an overenthusiastic reception of a new remedy. This tragic experience should be a final warning to physicians relative to the prescribing and administration of this type of preparation." Despite the presence of organizational distrust between the AMA and the FDA, Fishbein himself proved to be one of the FDA's biggest supporters.[33]

A resounding political echo began to boom from the second voice, the national women's organizations who had long befriended the FDA. In a letter to her members on October 28, League of Women Voters President Marguerite M. Wells declared that the sulfanilamide events "point tragically to the need for Federal legislation ensuring a governmental check on such products before they are distributed to a helpless public." Like other women's organization officials, she blamed "special interests" for the failure of Congress to revise and strengthen the 1906 Act.[34]

One week after the first media reports of deaths, observers commonly agreed that reform was likely. Yet despite the intensive media attention to the deaths and to the FDA's hunt and chase for the elixir, nothing in the bills that had yet been floated before Congress contained a pre-market review provision of the sort to which Fishbein and Wells alluded. There was no

[32] Gross, "Seizure of Deadly 'Elixir' Saves Marylander," p. 2. James Harvey Young, "The 'Elixir Sulfanilamide' Disaster," *Emory University Quarterly* 14 (1958): 230–37.

[33] Jackson (*Food and Drug Legislation in the New Deal*, 211) describes the American Medical Association as only partially supportive of FDA-strengthening legislation throughout the 1930s. This is consistent with his account, but shows Fishbein to be an exception to the organizational pattern of the AMA.

[34] "Plea for U.S. Regulation follows 'Elixir' Deaths," *WP*, October 29, 1937, p. 9.

sustained call for a gatekeeping clause or any form of regulatory licensure. As the *Washington Post* editorial page stated the political status quo on October 26, "It seems certain that the current sulfanilamide incident will insure, at least, some improvement in food and drug regulation. The pending bill would broaden the definitions of, and put teeth into the penalties for, adulteration. It would also permit prosecution for misrepresentation, without requiring proof of fraudulent intent, as at present. It would not provide for Federal analysis and licensing of proprietary medicine as has worked so successfully in the case of vaccines. But even without this, it would be expected to prevent deaths similar to the 'elixir' tragedies."[35]

The *Post* editorial revealed how far the FDA, Congress, organized interests, and the organized public were from agreeing upon any form of gatekeeping provision. All that was certain was that "improvement" would come, but the *Post*'s best guess was that licensure of patent medicines would not be among the improvements.

Had the elixir sulfanilamide story died out in late October 1937, it is quite possible that no pre-market provision would have accrued to the FDA in the 1930s. Yet the sulfanilamide story endured, for several reasons. First, the deaths had occurred while Congress was out of session, and when the second session of the 75th Congress resumed in November 1937, FDA officials and Royal Copeland seized an opportunity to place the episode and its tragic meaning at the center of the legislative agenda. Second, the reports of deaths were still trickling in, creating something of a news cycle and fastening reporters to FDA officials week after week.

Ironically, the first synthesized "report" on the elixir sulfanilamide deaths was issued not by the FDA but in the *Journal of the American Medical Association* on November 6, 1937. The AMA's Chemical Laboratory, under the direction of Paul Nicholas Leech, commissioned a team of investigators from the University of Chicago and Johns Hopkins and assessed the physiological effects of administration of three treatments: (1) diethylene glycol alone, (2) sulfanilamide alone (not suspending in diethylene glycol), and (3) repeated dosages of Elixir Sulfanilamide-Massengill. The results were unequivocal; diethylene glycol and not sulfanilamide was to blame for the deaths and illnesses.[36] Yet Leech (and probably Morris Fishbein) added language extolling the FDA's effort in securing unconsumed shipments of the elixir

> Deaths and clues of deaths were reported to the American Medical Association headquarters by various press services, by information received from physicians, and chiefly clues from the Food and Drug Administration. The latter organization placed a tremendous force of inspectors in the field. It obtained a list of approximately 700 shipments from the manufacturer. The inspectors then traced every shipment to its final destination. If the bottle had been opened, they inquired to

[35] "Control of Drugs," *WP* [editorial], October 26, 1937.
[36] Leech, "Elixir," *JAMA* 109 (19) (Nov. 6, 1937): 1531–39.

whom it had been dispensed. It was in this manner that most of the deaths were traced after the original reports from Tulsa and East St. Louis.[37]

Leech and Fishbein's acknowledgment was more than symbolic, for it pointed to a wider transformation in public responsibility for information provision in the wake of the elixir deaths. By the second week of November, when the Senate had reconvened and had asked (in Senate Resolution 194) the Secretary of Agriculture to issue a report on the deaths resulting from use of the elixir, the FDA's role in information provision about the episode had eclipsed that of the AMA. News reports of the elixir episode now mentioned the FDA almost exclusively, the AMA hardly at all. And the AMA, too (as Leech's editorial thanks to the Administration suggests) also relied heavily upon the FDA's reporting for its analysis. By November 1937, the agency had secured a near monopoly on information about the deaths and the elixir.

Walter Campbell and the Wallace Report. From the very earliest stages of the sulfanilamide episode, Walter Campbell and his FDA associates saw an opportunity to add a pre-market licensing provision to the nation's food and drug statute. On October 19, Campbell issued a press release advocating for a "Governmental licensing system." The release was largely ignored at the time, but Campbell kept up his campaign more quietly. In correspondence with Clark Gavin, managing editor of *National Consumer News*, Campbell confided on October 28:

> In my opinion, full and complete public protection can be guaranteed against the preparation and sale of harmful medicines only by the adoption of proper preventative measures. Such products, in my judgment, should be marketed under Governmental supervision. This would require legislation authorizing control by the issuance of licenses.... a Governmental licensing system, at least for new and potent medicines, probably will be required if the tragic experiences growing out of the ale and use of this poisonous elixir of sulfanilamid are not to be repeated.[38]

To underscore the point that support and publicity from mouthpieces such as Gavin's magazine and other consumerist outlets would be necessary for passage of FDA-strengthening legislation, Campbell added a sober prognosis of the prospects for near-term reform. Citing "powerful opposition to the enactment of a food and drug bill," he argued that "The promptness with which legislative action may be contemplated, and the adequacy of the law passed, will depend in large measure, if not entirely, upon the extent and the aggressiveness of consumer interests displayed."[39]

[37]Ibid., 1539.

[38]Campbell to Clark Gavin, Managing Editor, *National Consumer News* (New York), October 28, 1937; USDA-FDA Press Release, "Death-Dealing Drug," October 19, 1937; enclosure in Campbell to Gavin letter. National Archives I, RG 46, HR75A.

[39]Campbell to Clark Gavin, Managing Editor, *National Consumer News*, October 28, 1937; RG 46, HR75A, NA.

Campbell's next stratagem was to turn to Royal Copeland and the U.S. Senate. On October 26, Copeland wrote Campbell and asked whether S.5 as currently written would have prevented the elixir sulfanilamide episode. On October 29, Campbell replied with a vivid and reasoned negative.

To seize these hastily concocted and untried preparations after discovery of their lethal effect, or to prosecute the manufacturer criminally, is not enough. It is our view that the bill [S.5] should be amended to require a license from the Government preliminary to the distribution of all drugs containing any potent ingredient or combination of ingredients, the use of which has not become well established in medical practice.

In the interest of safety, society has required that physicians be licensed to practice the healing art. Pharmacists are licensed to compound drugs. Even steam-fitters, electricians and plumbers are required to have licenses. Certainly a requirement that potent proprietary medicines be manufactured under license can be justified on the ground of public safety.[40]

Campbell then closed the letter with a promise of full cooperation in drafting appropriate legislation.

I recognize the extreme difficulty that there may be in drafting suitable language for the amendment I am recommending. We shall be glad to make ourselves available for any help we can be of to you, to the Legislative Counsel, or to others whom you may ask to work on the problem.[41]

The next event, perhaps the crucial step as far as Congress and much of the reading public was concerned, was the release of Secretary of Agriculture Henry A. Wallace's report on the deaths. From the very first page of the report, Wallace and his FDA colleagues distilled one overwhelming lesson from the tragedy: the absolute necessity of pre-market review of drugs to assess their safety profile:

Before the "elixir" was put on the market, it was tested by the firm for flavor but not for its effect on human life. The existing Food and Drugs Act does not require that new drugs be tested before they are placed on sale.

...Since the Federal Food and Drugs Act contains no provision against dangerous drugs, seizures had to be based on a charge that the word elixir implies an alcoholic solution, whereas this product was a diethylene glycol solution. Had the product been called a solution, rather than an elixir, no charge of violating the law could have been brought.

...The fatal "elixir" was rushed onto the market without adequate test to determine whether or not diethylene glycol may be safely used as a solvent for sulfanilamide, despite previously published reports in scientific literature showing that diethylene glycol might be dangerous when taken internally. A few simple

[40]Campbell to Copeland, October 29, 1937; NA, RG 46, HR75A. Underlining in original.
[41]Ibid.

and inexpensive tests on experimental animals would have quickly demonstrated the toxic properties of both diethylene glycol and the "elixir."[42]

Wallace's report began with this "executive summary" of the sulfanilamide story. The implied causal inference was clear. Not only did elixir sulfanilamide cause at least seventy-three deaths, but deficiencies in the process by which the drug was brought to market, which were equivalent to deficiencies in the 1906 law, also caused those deaths. Just as clear as the implied causal story was the counterfactual: "A few simple and inexpensive tests," the sort that would be performed by the company before marketing and analyzed in a pre-market review process by the FDA, would quickly have evinced the elixir's "toxic properties." Translation: with a pre-market review process, none of this would have happened.

The structure of the Campbell-Wallace report also laid bare the nature of the tragedy and the FDA's intended policy solutions (see table 2.1). It proceeded, not unlike a court brief, from facts to conclusions in a near deductive manner. The USDA report started on its strongest footing, dealing first with those facts of a scientific character, then the facts of historical and legal ones. It then proceeded methodically to limitations of the 1906 statute and suggestions for reform. It was also succinct, at twenty-three pages of double-spaced courier type.

For several reasons, the Campbell-Wallace report rendered the sulfanilamide tragedy even more evocative and memorable than it had been. First, USDA officials and news reports connected the deaths together in a way that wove the entire affair into a single narrative, making it ready for consumption by news-hungry reporters and editors. Some portions of the narrative were particularly vivid, even visually so. Only a few deaths were among young children who had taken the drug to combat an infection. Yet one of these was the single most publicized death, both in congressional debates, in USDA reports, and in newspaper coverage of the sulfanilamide episode. The most widely known story was prompted by a letter from Mrs. Maise Nidiffer of Tulsa—whose six-year-old daughter Joan died from taking the drug—to President Roosevelt. Nidiffer wrote of her daughter's harrowing death, "her little body tossing to & fro... & that little voice screaming with pain and it seems as tho it drive me insane [sic]." She pleaded with the president to "take steps to prevent such sales of drugs that will take little lives & leave such suffering behind and such a bleak outlook on the future as I have tonight." Along with the letter, she enclosed a photograph of her smiling but now deceased child, a print that made its way into several newspaper reports and into the USDA report on the tragedy (figure 2.4). In the entire

[42]U.S. Department of Agriculture, *Report of the Secretary of Agriculture on Deaths Due to Elixir Sulfanilamide-Massengill, Submitted in Response to Senate Resolution 194 of November 16, 1937*, Senate Document No. 124, 75th Congress, Second Session (Washington, DC: GPO). Original typescript in NA, RG 46, SEN75A-F674; parts reprinted in Dunn, *Federal Food, Drug and Cosmetic Act*, 1317, 1319. The paragraphs above (except for the last) appear on the first page of the original typescript.

TABLE 2.1
Subject Headings in the USDA's Report on Elixir Sulfanilamide (November 1937)*

HOW THE "ELIXIR" WAS PRODUCED

THE FOOD AND DRUG ADMINISTRATION STEPS IN

THE PROBLEM BEFORE PHYSICIANS AND PHARMACISTS

EFFECTS OF THE DRUG

ACTION UNDER THE LAW

LIMITATIONS OF THE LAW

RECOMMENDATIONS FOR LEGISLATION

*These headings are reported as they appear in the typescript version sent to Congress, which appears in the Senate Committee files, typescript *Report to the Secretary of Agriculture on Deaths due to Elixir Sulfanilamide-Massengill*, NA, RG 46, SEN75A-F674. All words were in capitals and all titles were center-justified as they appear here.

reporting on the deaths due to elixir sulfanilamide, the Joan Nidiffer story did not surface until the Wallace report.[43]

Maise Nidiffer's letter and the photograph of her daughter impelled and expressed the conversion of episode to tragedy. Together, text and image took what had been a series of scattered deaths among "patients"—faceless subjects who in the American racial imagination were syphilitic black men—and purged it of blackness, of sexual maturity, and of social isolation. The victim of American policy failure was now a daughter connected to a mother and a loving family, a smiling white child who could not be said to have courted the agony that sulfanilamide wreaked upon her body.

In the pages immediately following the Nidiffer letter and the photo of the elixir's adorable young victim, the FDA turned immediately to the decisive action it took under the current law and the existing limitations of that law. Then, bringing the report to its culmination, Wallace issued four policy recommendations.[44] The Department first offered an explicit argument for licensure, not of firms, but of products. And the Wallace report reflected the carefully chosen words of Walter Campbell in his letter to Copeland of a month earlier.

[43] Maise Nidiffer to President Roosevelt, November 8, 1937; copy in typescript *Report of the Secretary of Agriculture on Deaths due to Elixir Sulfanilamide-Massengill*, NA, RG 46, SEN75A-F674. Jackson (*Food and Drug Legislation in the New Deal*, 163) reports that the Nidiffer story was "widely distributed," and that by the spring of 1938 it "had even become part of the [Agriculture] Secretary's report to Congress on the drug disaster" (184). In fact, the USDA's inclusion of the photo seems to have preceded popular media coverage of the girl's death; see Jackson's discussion of the May 1938 issue of *Survey Graphic*, which reprinted the letter (184).

[44] These appear on pages 21–24 of the typescript in the Archives. Reprinted in Dunn, *Federal Food, Drug and Cosmetic Act*, 1326–7.

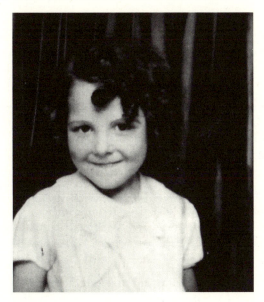

Figure 2.4. The Joan Nidiffer Photo, in *Report of the Secretary of Agriculture*, 1937

1. License control of new drugs to insure that they will not be generally distributed until experimental and clinical tests have shown them to be safe for use.

...It is the Department's view that no other form of control will effectively safeguard the public from the dangers of premature distribution of new drugs. To increase the penalties for violations and to require label disclosure of ingredients would be helpful, but by no means fully adequate.

In the interest of safety society has required that physicians be licensed to practice the healing art. Pharmacists are licensed to compound and dispense drugs. Electricians, plumbers and steam engineers pursue their respective trades under license. But there is no such control to prevent incompetent drug manufacturers from marketing any kind of lethal potion.

The first USDA suggestion seemed innocent enough, but it stood as the most far-reaching licensure provision to be enacted for any agency during the New Deal. The bills leading to the National Industrial Recovery Act of 1933 had proposed licensure of firms prior to market entry, but this idea was scrapped long before the bills came to a vote. Beyond this, the pre-market review provision that Wallace was calling for would give Congress (and ultimately the FDA) power to define what a new drug is.

However broad the power to define new drugs would be, there was a problem with relying on pre-market review alone. Drugs already on the market were not coverable under a licensure statute. So Wallace asked for FDA authority to prohibit these outright.

2. Prohibition of drugs which are dangerous to health when administered in accordance with the manufacturer's directions for use. This would provide a more appropriate basis of action than that on which proceedings were instituted against the "elixir." A number of dangerous drugs are not on the market against which not even a trivial charge of violation can be made.

When passed, this provision and the pre-market review procedure would foretell the deathblow of the patent medicine industry in the United States. Not long in following were stringent labeling requirements, such that every adverse effect of which the manufacturer had prior evidence must be stated on the label.

3. Requirement that drug labels bear appropriate directions for use and warnings against probable misuse. Much injury results from insufficient directions and from lack of warning against overdosage, or administration to children, or use in disease conditions where the drug is dangerous, or the possibility of drug addiction.

Finally, FDA officials received their long-sought wish of a compulsory disclosure requirement for all ingredients (inactive as well as active) on the label of the drug. Diethylene glycol, after all, had not been the active ingredient in "Elixir Sulfanilamide-Massengill," just a solvent. And as the report stated, this provision was intended to serve as much as a control on foreign firms as on domestic patent medicine manufacturers.

4. Prohibition of secret remedies by requiring that labels disclose fully the composition of the drug. Many foreign countries now impose this requirement. Many drugs manufactured in the United States are exported to such countries under labels bearing such disclosure. The same drugs are sold to our citizens under labels that give no hint of their composition.

The Campbell-Wallace report has long since disappeared from public memory, relegated to congressional and USDA archives and the appendices of aging legal histories of the 1938 legislation. Yet it is no understatement to say that Campbell and Wallace's document forms the originary basis of modern pharmaceutical regulation in the United States and much of the industrialized world.[45] The four enumerated powers—(1) pre-market review and notification, (2) prohibition (or withdrawal authority), (3) labeling reg-

[45] See chapters 3 and 11 for a discussion of the regimes of efficacy regulation in Scandinavian countries, particularly Sweden, Denmark and Norway. By 1940, these countries had something of an "efficacy requirement" for drug listing on national pharmacopoeia, but not a developed pre-market review process as the United States possessed from 1938 onward. In crucial respects, what the Wallace report offered was a set of policy prescriptions that a number of groups, muckrakers, Harvey Wiley and his allies and other FDA personnel had been advocating for years. Wallace's report, understood properly in context, brought these various concerns and ideas together in a central act of agenda-framing and stunningly effective rhetoric. See Kay, "Healthy Public Relations: The FDA's 1930s Legislative Campaign," and Lamb, *American Chamber of Horrors.*

ulation, and (4) compulsory disclosure of all drug contents (active and inactive)—have become assumed and core legal features of pharmaceutical markets ranging from European national economies and the European Union to Japan, India, Australia, Canada, and South Africa. While crucial provisions and procedures have been added to these powers, the origins of government gatekeeping authority over the pharmaceutical marketplace can, in many respects, be traced to this document.

More immediately, Wallace's report occasioned the biggest single flood of news reporting since the original deaths were reported. Headlines from New York and Washington area papers were noteworthy in their attribution of a "drive" or "demand" for new legislation that the Wallace report, the elixir deaths, and the FDA's successful "roundup" of the drug had now created.

COPELAND ASKS CURB ON ELIXIR. Joins Wallace in Move for Tighter Law. AIMS TO PROTECT PUBLIC. Secretary of Agriculture has 4-Point Program to Guard Lives.

FEDERAL ROUNDUP OF ELIXIR REVIVES DRUG BILL DRIVE. Copeland Backs Wallace Rules as Secretary Tells How Deaths Were Stopped.

Elixir Deaths Result in Demand for Law.[46]

On the House floor, Republican Edward Herbert Rees of Kansas complained that "newspapers and periodicals are crowded with information and of incidents where individuals and companies have taken advantage of people by the hundreds and the thousands, by falsification of advertising and adulteration as well as misbranding of foods and medicines."[47]

In this respect, the reaction to the disaster was not simply confined to the actual deaths but also to fear of numerous medications marketed under the title of "Elixir," as well as fear of other sulfanilamide drugs that were not suspended in a diethylene glycol solution. Worried consumers flooded FDA investigators and county and state medication societies with questions about whether they had taken a deadly medication, or whether anything in their medicine cabinet was safe. For this reason, the pattern of *shipments* of Elixir Sulfanilamide-Massengill was just as important politically as the pattern of deaths it caused. Virtually every town that received at least one shipment of the Elixir later hosted several or more FDA investigators, state food and drug regulators, members of state and local presses, and visitors from local and state medical societies.[48]

The success of the FDA in quickly ridding the country of the elixir shipments was celebrated and widely noted. By December 1937, FDA officials

[46]Story headings taken, respectively, from *New York Sun*, November 26, 1937; *New York Post*, November 26, 1937; *Washington Daily News*, November 26, 1937, p. 28. Copies of all three stories are available from clipping in Copeland Papers, Bentley Historical Library, University of Michigan, Ann Arbor.

[47]CR 83 (Nov, 24, 1937): 549–50; reprinted in Dunn, *Federal Food, Drug and Cosmetic Act*, 771–2.

[48]Jackson, *Food and Drug Legislation in the New Deal*, 159–60.

had removed 99.2 percent of the 240 gallons of the elixir that were originally sent out in September. Fred B. Linton published a pamphlet entitled
*Federal Food and Drug Laws—Leaders Who Achieved their Enactment and
Enforcement*.[49] Linton's pamphlet offered a horrifying counterfactual: had
the entire shipment of Dr. Massengill's Elixir Sulfanilamide been consumed,
and had deaths occurred in the same proportion as they had to earlier levels
of consumption, over 4,500 persons would have died from the elixir.

The Sulfanilamide Tragedy and the Passage of the Food, Drug and Cosmetic Act of 1938

The media reporting in the wake of the Wallace report bespoke a much
deeper transformation. In late October 1937, even with the national news
craze over the mounting death toll and the FDA's pursuit of the remaining
elixir bottles, no discussion of a gatekeeping provision had occurred. Yet
USDA officials, in concert with newspaper editorial boards and women's
groups, pointed to the pre-market clearance of vaccines under the Biologics
Act of 1902 as a successful policy that needed emulation in the world of
pharmaceuticals.[50]

The Wallace report did not introduce the possibility of a pre-marketing
regulatory check on drugs; its main effect was to establish the idea as the
dominant alternative to the status quo. The USDA report tied the threads
from news coverage, private experience (Joan Nidiffer), medical investigation, regulatory detail, and other features together into a story that made
sense, a story in which the moral of policy reform followed narratively from
the apparently brute facts. Media coverage of the momentum for new legislation now attributed the "demand" and "drive" for a new law to the elixir
deaths, the Wallace report, and the quickness with which federal agents had
tracked down the sulfanilamide supply and had removed it from the marketplace.[51]

In this light, Royal Copeland's introduction of a pre-market review provision was a reaction to the USDA's proposals, not a forerunner. Wallace's
report was the first official proposal for gatekeeping authority. None of
Copeland's bills before the report contained a pre-market review provision,
and Copeland's first bill after the report, wrote the USDA's recommendations in to a proposed law.

[49] Ibid.

[50] *League of Women Voters Newsletter* 3 (19), October 28, 1937; Accession No. 52A-86
(Records of the Office of Committee on Legislation, 1927 *Federal Food, Drug and Cosmetic
Act*, 1940), B5, RG 88, NA.

[51] "'Elixir' Deaths Result in Demand for Law," *Washington Daily News*, November 26,
1937, p. 8; "Federal Roundup of Elixir Revives Drug Bill Drive," *New York Post*, November
26, 1937; "Copeland Asks Curb on Elixir," *New York Sun*, November 26, 1937. All in scrapbooks, Royal Copeland Papers, Bentley Historical Library, University of Michigan. To be clear,
some licensing proposals had been floated in the 73rd and 74th Congresses, only to be shot
down in committee; Marks, *Progress of Experiment*, 75.

On December 1, 1937, Copeland introduced a new measure to replace S.5. Copeland's S.3073 had many of the provisions of S.5, but added the pre-market review provision in a new "Section 505," which remains today the basis for FDA review of new drugs. The bill required manufacturers to supply the USDA with records of their clinical and nonclinical experiments, a list of the drug's ingredients, a plan for manufacturing practices, and examples of labels. The Secretary of Agriculture would then certify the drug for sale or give a reason why the drug was refused marketability. A proprietary trade journal warned that under S.3073, "the Food and Drug Administration would become absolute dictator, the overlord of the drug industry." The *Drug Trade News*, at the time one of the two dominant trade journals covering the pharmaceutical trade, broadcast a more dire warning in capitals on its front page, a "drastic control of drug firms," including the specter of "licensing" and a "guarantee of safety" before marketing.[52]

In February 1938, Copeland's S.3073 was again considered in the Senate. Women's groups and public health leagues now lobbied intensively for its passage, and their rhetoric made clear the centrality of the Wallace report in the new deliberations. The Public Health Federation recorded itself as "heartily in favor of the recommendations of the Secretary of Agriculture, to protect the public against drugs like elixir of sulphanilamide."[53] It passed the Senate again, and again unanimously, and was combined with S.5 into a new S.5, and went to the House, where the Commerce Committee, chaired by California Democrat Clarence Lea, again stalled the bill. The Lea Committee reported the House's version of the bill in April 1938, but with at least two significant differences from the Senate version. First, the Senate version provided explicitly for the regulation of combination drugs—bundles of drugs which were individually already on the market, but which were possibly new as a combination—whereas the House did not provide for regulation of these products. Patent medicine interests could exploit this loophole, it was feared, by selling combination products which, by virtue of their components' previous marketing, would bypass the FDA review process.

The second amendment to emerge from the Lea Committee was something of a poison pill, and it threatened the entire measure. Lea's committee attached a provision requiring the Secretary of Agriculture to respond to any suit against any regulation by withholding the entire enforcement of the regulation until court review, and conduct public hearings in response to any suit brought by a private party. The ostensible source of this amendment was the apple-growing interests of Washington State, who had been burned by tightened restrictions on lead arsenic in their pesticide sprays. It was later claimed by the *St. Louis Post Dispatch* that patent medicine makers

[52] "67 Deaths Kindle Campaigns for Drastic Control of Drug Firms," *DTN* 12 (23), November 8, 1937.

[53] Bleecker Marquette (Executive Secretary, Public Health Federation, Cincinnati, Ohio) to Chairman, Committee on Commerce, U.S. Senate, February 21, 1938; NA, RG 46, SEN 75A-E1, "Papers relating to specific bills," "with respect to S. 3073."

and Washington farmers had secretly agreed to the court review provision as a means of killing the entire Copeland legislation. The minority of the House committee, led by Tennesee Democrat Virgil Chapman, expressed its fear that "the bill, if enacted with this [court] review provision," would fail to offer "any substantial improvement over the terms of the present law." An *Emporia Gazette* editorialist lamented that "it is a pity the good things in the bill have no chance of being put into operation." Women's groups again wrote Congress and produced pamphlets indicating their displeasure with the bills before the House, and they outlined alternative measures with gatekeeping provisions. Reform supporters now seemed convinced that the court review provision had vitiated entirely the gatekeeping procedures of the bill. As a coalition of fourteen women's groups put it, "We are convinced that this proposal for judicial review of regulations more than offsets the improvements over the present law contained in this bill." Concluded Washington Rep. John Coffee: "If the right to sell poison unbranded is a vested right—since when?"[54]

In the House debate in April and June 1938, the elixir tragedy loomed large. Coffee of Washington invoked the "excellent recommendations" of the Wallace report of the previous November and lamented that the bill reported by the Lea Committee had followed Wallace's suggestions "but in part." He gestured poignantly to "such utterly needless and inexcusable tragedies" as the elixir disaster: "Shall we have to wait for another hundred deaths before we get proper preventative measures?" Montana Democrat Jerry Joseph O'Connell, with echoes of Maise Nidiffer's letter, shifted the focus from apple-grower interests to the elixir victims.

> This [court review] section, as written, is decidedly for the benefit of the producer and not for the consumer.
>
> It has been stated that the issue here is whether you are going to wipe out the investment of these poor apple growers, but I contend that the issue in this court review section and the issue in this bill is whether you are going to permit these young children and men and women to be killed by spurious patent medicines and by all the fake drugs and cures that are flooding the market today, which are far more involved in this bill than the question of the production of apples.
>
> The question further is whether little children are going to die in vain and whether all this agitation over such poisonous deaths is to be in vain. The question

---

[54] *Minority Views to Accompany S.5.*, April 21, 1938; House of Representatives, 75th Congress, Third Session, Report 2139, Part 2; reprinted in Dunn, 834. William Allen White, "The Drug Pirates," *Emporia Gazette*, April 21, 1938; in Extension of Remarks by John H. Coffee, CR 83 (May 20, 1938), appendix, p. 9515; reprinted in Dunn, *Federal Food, Drug and Cosmetic Act*, 839. On the continued attention of women's groups to the progress of the bill, see Mrs. William Dick Sporborg, "Organized Women Keep Close Watch on Food-Drug Act," *New York Tribune*, April 10, 1938. National Federation of Independent Business and Women's Professional Clubs, *The Food and Drug Act: Its Status, Arguments For and Against, and Alternative Measures* (New York, 1938); Accession No. 52A-86 (Records of the Office of Committee on Legislation, 1927–1940), B5, RG 88, NA. "Food and Drug Laws to be Discussed by Women Voters," *New York Herald-Tribune*, March 20, 1938.

is whether we are going to wipe all that out now in order to help a few apple grow-
ers in this country. I maintain that human life is far more important than profits.

Are we going to legislate for the great benefit of the American people and for the
consumers of the United States or are we going to legislate for this little group?[55]

S.5 passed the House with the court review provision intact. The end result
of the provision, had it passed both chambers, would have been a wholesale
shakeup in U.S. administrative law. No longer would courts be limited to reviewing administrative rules ex post; instead, rules would have to survive court
review before they could ever take hold. USDA officials rightly foresaw that
the court review provision was an invitation to endless delay of effective regulation by interminable lawsuits and complaints. In a composite letter of April
22, 1938, and sent to the House, representatives of fourteen women's groups
threatened to lobby President Roosevelt to veto the measure entirely.[56]

The FDA, Wallace, and Copeland saw their final triumph in the House-
Senate conference committee that reported a consensual version of the bill
on June 11, 1938. The court review provision was dropped, and the confer-
ees made it clear that the Secretary of Agriculture could promulgate regulations to define combination drugs as new drugs. After unanimous passage in
both chambers, Roosevelt signed the bill into law on June 25, 1938.

For purposes of legislative history, the essential puzzle is this: Why did
Congress move from unanimous Senate support of a weaker bill in the first
session of the 75th Congress (May to August 1937) to a generally unanimous approval of a stronger bill in the second session of the 75th Congress
(April and June 1938)? There are several possible explanations other than
the sulfanilamide tragedy, not least a host of possible narratives connected
to the 1936 general election and perhaps the impending 1938 midterms. It
is clear that the 75th Senate passed a weaker version of regulation in its first
session (1937), and a stronger version of regulation with gatekeeping authority for the FDA in its second session (1938). In both cases the House
served to defeat or delay passage of the Senate legislation. What changed
was not voting patterns but the *content* of the proposed legislation. What is
needed to explain the 1938 legislation and its difference from 1937 bills,
then, is not voting analysis but narrative.[57]

[55]Coffee, in Dunn, *Federal Food, Drug and Cosmetic Act*, 873. O'Connell, in Dunn, *Federal Food, Drug and Cosmetic Act*, 946–7.

[56]Wallace: "It is the Department's considered judgment that it would be better to continue the old law in effect than to enact S.5 with this provision." Women's groups: "Unless this sec-tion providing for judicial review is struck out, the undersigned organizations must oppose the enactment of the measure." (Letter reprinted in House debate; Dunn, *Federal Food, Drug and Cosmetic Act*, 845). On the veto threat, see remarks of John Coffee in the *Congressional Rec-ord*, reprinted in Dunn, ibid., 876; also Richard L. Stokes, "Dispute Over Alleged Joker in Drug Act in Conference May Cause Measure to Fail," *St. Louis Post-Dispatch*, June 8, 1938; reprinted in Dunn, ibid., 1012.

[57]And because the 1938 bill became *more* legally stringent than the 1937 bills, median voter dynamics (a softening of the legislation from the first to the second session of the 75th Con-gress) cannot explain the transformation.

TABLE 2.2
Comparison of S.5 before and after Tragedy and Wallace Proposal

Bill	S.5 (1937)	Campbell-Wallace Proposal	S.5 (1938)
Congress	75th	75th	75th
Session of Congress	First	Btw 1st and 2nd	Third
Final passage in Senate	Unanimous	NA	Unanimous
Provision for Cosmetics Regulation	Yes	Kept	Yes
Advertising Regulation	Yes	Kept	Yes
Primary Advertising Regulation with FTC	Yes	Kept	Yes
Multiple Seizure Authority (all commodities)	Yes	Kept	Yes
Pre-market Review Provision [Section 505 (a)–(c)]	No	Proposed	Yes

Perhaps the starkest comparison can be conducted between the 1937 version of S.5 and the 1938 version of S.5. This is something of a test of the effects of sulfanilamide—and in particular the Administration's framing of the episode—upon the legislation of the 75th Congress.

As the comparison in table 2.2 suggests, virtually nothing else changed in the legislation from the S.5 passed in 1937 to the final 1938 Act. The electoral composition of the legislature was identical, the leadership of Congress and that of the relevant committees were identical, the votes were identical, and all of the other provisions affecting food, cosmetics, inspection, and seizure authority remained the same.

The tabular analysis, then, allows us to answer the counterfactual evidence posed earlier. In the absence of the sulfanilamide tragedy—the episode framed by the FDA and converted into a tragedy with specific political lessons—the 1938 Food, Drug and Cosmetic Act would not have contained a pre-market review provision.

What of the 75th Congress? Several possibilities related to the 1936 election are evident as partial explanations for the 1938 legislation, in the sense that the composition of the 75th Congress may have been a necessary condition for the 1938 Act's passage. It is noteworthy that the 75th Congress was famous not for its liberalism but for its conservatism, namely the institutional emergence of the Conservative Coalition and its hostile takeover of the House Rules Committee. This coalition effectively frustrated many of

Roosevelt's New Deal initiatives. Yet analysis of measures of congressional ideology that are directly comparable over time suggests that the Senate became only marginally more liberal in its voting propensity from the 74th Congress to the 75th Congress. This difference, moreover, is not statistically significant.[58]

Of course, these ideological shifts can only provide context. The 75th Congress, after all, passed a weakened reform initiative in 1937, before the sulfanilamide tragedy. So, too, Roosevelt had lashed out at the Copeland measure in a press conference on February 23. The Commerce Committee had dramatically weakened S.5 and, while it then passed the Senate, it did so over the objections of Copeland, the FDA, and consumers' and women's groups. To make matters worse, the Senate in March 1937 passed the Wheeler-Lea Act, giving control over all advertising regulation to the Federal Trade Commission. In the House, meanwhile, Copeland's much-weakened Senate measure was pigeonholed in the Commerce Committee there. The upshot of these developments is that the 75th Congress was, until the sulfanilamide tragedy, acting more conservatively on matters related to pharmaceuticals than was the 74th.

FDR's broadsides against the Copeland measure in February 1937—Copeland was among the most outspoken Senate opponents of the President's court-packing plan—suggest one other thing. The shift in legislative fortunes for FDA-strengthening legislation was not one induced by FDR's warming to the Copeland bill. If FDR did warm to stronger FDA regulation of patent medicines and pharmaceuticals, this was a shift directly related to the fall 1937 tragedy.

Bailey's Deathblow: The Geographic Burden of Elixir Sulfanilamide. While it appears that the sulfanilamide episode registered on a nationwide consciousness and agenda, it is also true that the sulfanilamide deaths were somewhat geographically concentrated. In a way that seems symbolic now but was evident to few at the time, the pattern of elixir shipments, deaths, and subsequent FDA visits struck in the very region that housed the most vocal defenders of the right of self-medication, and of the patent medicine industry. *Newsweek* reported that FDA officials were morbidly "jubilant" over the fact that the elixir was produced in the district of Tennessee Republican Carroll Reece, a consistent and vocal opponent of FDA-strengthening legislation. The concentration of sulfanilamide deaths in Tennessee was also noted by Senator Josiah Bailey, a Senate foe of Copeland's measure who received mail asking him to change his stance on regulation "so to make impossible a repetition of the recent Sulfanilamide tragedy."[59]

[58]The congressional ideology measures are chamber medians from the DW-NOMINATE score. Indeed, the Democrats of the 75th Congress were, by the DW-NOMINATE measure, less liberal in their voting behavior in the 75th Congress than in the 73rd (and the 72nd), during which Copeland's bill was under consideration. Nor is there appreciable change in the Republican median.

[59]*Newsweek*, November 22, 1937; FDA Scrapbooks, vol. 17. Cited in Jackson, *Food and*

There is some narrative evidence to support a more specific hypothesis, namely that the sulfanilamide deaths may have peeled more liberal members of the anti-regulatory coalition from its ranks and sent them into an embrace of FDA control. In the last, very brief Senate debate on S.3073 in May 1938, Arthur Vandenburg still expressed his reservations about the measure, but Josiah Bailey, who was the most vociferous and public opponent of earlier reform bills, did not (even though he was apparently on the floor). Bailey's home state of Tennessee suffered an above-average share of sulfanilamide deaths and, it is worth pointing out, was the point of manufacture and principal point of shipment of the deadly product. Bailey was, moreover, hardly the conservative ideologue that Vandenburg was.

An explanation centered upon the framing of sulfanilamide plausibly accounts for the shift in votes from a divisive battle over a weak bill to stronger support for a vigorous law. It does, moreover, perform better than the available alternatives, which are irreconcilable with the anti-regulatory posture struck by the early 75th Congress. It is possible that the tragedy convinced a broad swath of the public—whether their constituency was affected or not—that additional regulation was needed. The symbolic character of the tragedy made a gate-keeping provision more palatable to all those who had previously opposed strengthening the FDA, in part because neither Copeland nor Tugwell nor anyone else had written such a provision into any seriously considered bill. Yet this symbolic character of the tragedy was not exogenous to regulatory politics but incipient to it. At least in part, the tragedy had been intentionally framed, emphasized, and presented to the organized public and Congress by Agriculture Department officials.

Hard-core opponents of FDA authority continued to speak out against the Copeland legislation, implying that the unanimity observed in the vote was not indicative of a full embrace of the 1938 Act by all those who voted for it. Although the final House margin of passage was "overwhelming" (but also unreported), FDA opponents there continued a vigorous defense of the right of self-medication and loudly voiced their worries about the continued accretion of bureaucratic power to federal agencies.

Lessons of the Policy Tragedy of Elixir Sulfanilamide

New regulations often follow tragedies, but not reflexively so. The reason that scholars and pundits call some adverse events "tragedies" and that others fail to enter the annals of popular and recorded history is that active political agents seek to frame and reinterpret episodes into tragedies. Of course, this process is loaded with unintended consequences and is rarely one in which any single agent takes full control. But because the Administration possessed a near monopoly on information relating to sulfanilamide and the

Drug Legislation in the New Deal, 165. Letter to Bailey: Mecklenburg [TN] Medical Association to Bailey, March 20, 1938; Bailey Papers. Cited in Jackson, ibid.,163.

deaths resulting from it, the conversion of sulfanilamide from episode to tragedy was in large measure the effective work of a single organization.

Perhaps the strongest conclusion that emerges from close analysis of the 1938 law is a negative one. Rent-seeking and industry capture explanations of the 1938 Food, Drug and Cosmetic Act fare poorly in explaining either the process of agenda-setting or the votes on regulatory legislation. Indeed, it is not merely that affected industries were uninvolved in buying protection from the legislative process, but that affected industries, including and especially those who stood to profit from entry barriers that would be created in the 1938 Act, were opposed to new regulation.

This is not to deny the importance of the organized pharmaceutical industry and patent medicine associations in shaping the legislation and (perhaps) its administrative implementation. The emergence of American pharmaceutical regulation did witness business influence, particularly in successful attempts by industry allies before the fall of 1937, to weaken, sidetrack, or altogether gut the USDA's legislative proposals. Yet if business influence is observed, industry capture—the rigging of regulation by economic "incumbents" in order to restrict competition and create a marketplace with rents—is not.[60]

A second lesson comes in the timing of the sulfanilamide tragedy, which allows its historical observers to gain some perspective on its precise contribution to the new regulation. The sulfanilamide deaths occurred *after* FDA leaders had, through steady and entrepreneurial political action, established an FDA-strengthening measure as the dominant alternative to the status quo. By the autumn of 1937, there was already a relatively structured debate between those who favored the existing body of law accumulated from the 1906 Pure Food and Drugs Act (or a slightly modified version thereof that would have given the Federal Trade Commission more power), and those who favored a bill that would have given the FDA broader regulatory authority over cosmetic and pharmaceutical products. Many features of the regulation had been proposed and refined before the deaths occurred. It was because of this context, not in spite of it, that the 1938 law passed.[61]

With attention to the timing of the reform, the substantive political move that centers the narrative of American pharmaceutical regulation can also be understood. The most significant feature of the 1938 Act was its inclusion of a gatekeeping provision—allowing the FDA to reject the introduction of any drug intended for introduction into interstate commerce. Comparing

[60]David Vogel, *Fluctuating Fortunes: The Political Power of Business in America* (New York: Basic Books, 1989); Daniel Carpenter, "Protection without Capture: Product Approval by a Politically Responsive, Learning Regulator," *APSR* 98 (4) (Nov. 2004): 613–31.

[61]In other words, the sulfanilamide tragedy did not "spur elected officials to promulgate governmental regulation," as Lawrence Rothenberg has characterized many such episodes; *Politics, Organizations and Regulation: Interstate Trucking Regulation at the ICC* (Ann Arbor: University of Michigan Press, 1994), 40. The regulation and the plans were largely already present; the crisis served to grease its passage through the chokehold of American institutional politics.

legislation passed by one house of Congress, and before the tragedy, to legislation passed after the tragedy, reveals a crucial difference in the appearance, for the first time, of a provision for pre-market review of pharmaceuticals. Underlying voting patterns did not shift appreciably. It is the content of the bill that changed.

Because the FDA was successfully able to frame the sulfanilamide episode as exemplary of the defects of existing law, and as an instance in which the agency acted quickly and forcefully within its limited capacities, the sulfanilamide tragedy induced a change in the policy agenda. The form of regulatory legislation considered by Congress changed unalterably, as House and Senate leaders, at the prompting of FDA officials, attached a gatekeeping provision (Section 505(a)-(c)) to the food and drug bill. The tragedy also shifted preferences among previously reluctant Southern Democrats and conservative Republicans, leading them to abandon the rhetoric of self-medication, to drop their resistance to FDA-strengthening legislation, and to take up and pass the core legislation comprising the 1938 Act. Since 1937–38 coincides with the emergence of a "conservative coalition" of Southern Democrats and Republicans in Congress, the timing of the tragedy was particularly powerful.

Yet it is also worth reflecting on the historical context. The sulfanilamide tragedy occurred when the Senate and House were already well informed about alternative regulatory measures facing them. In both chambers of Congress, the FDA had found able and energetic sponsors for drug reform (Copeland and Tennessee Rep. Virgil Chapman). Much of the costly work of building coalitions behind legislation had already been accomplished. Had the sulfanilamide tragedy occurred at another time, when FDA regulation as the dominant alternative to the status quo was not advanced by bureaucratic leaders, the Act either would not have passed or would have taken a much different form. In this respect, it is possible to confidently reject the counterfactual that, had the sulfanilamide tragedy not occurred, regulatory reform in food and drugs would not have been on the agenda in the 75th Congress. Such reform was indeed on the agenda of the 75th Congress in the spring of 1937, even though that legislature did not warmly embrace pharmaceutical regulation. What the sulfanilamide tragedy did, once distilled by USDA-FDA rhetoric, was to change the specific legislative agenda from regulation without licensure to regulation with licensure.

Framing: The Inversion of Victimhood, the Admixture of Race and Innocence. The third conditional feature of the tragedy concerns not its timing but its framing. In part due to the thorough and relentless efforts of FDA officials to turn and frame the sulfanilamide episode to the agency's advantage, in part due to media coverage (which relied heavily upon the FDA's information), two social facts became attached to the sulfanilamide episode. These facts and the episode created a unique match between an evocative event and its political framing, a match that propelled a more muscular version of FDA-strengthening legislation through the 75th Congress. First, the tragedy was seen as a nationwide disaster affecting primarily white victims, especially children. In fact, most of the sulfanilamide deaths occurred in the upper-country South and lower Midwest, and in the early public imagination of the tragedy it was African Americans who were disproportionately affected by consumption of the elixir.[62] Second, the FDA acted quickly to remove the entire product supply from the market, and its trumpeting and careful presentation of this action both vaulted its reputation and left politicians and consumer advocates decrying weaknesses in the earlier (1906) law. These were not fully consistent tenets, and the ultimate success of the FDA's activity was to bundle them into a logical, sense-making whole.

Perhaps the most striking reframing of the episode came in the way that first the USDA, then the 75th Congress and the American media, inverted the status of chemical victimhood and reframed the "target population" of pharmaceutical regulation. Whereas the early medical reports described a drug popular among mature men, many of them black, many of whom were seeking a quick and private treatment for syphilis, the Administration had, by the late autumn of 1937, morphed the exemplar of a sulfanilamide victim, and the visible casualty of policy failure, into the darling face of Joan Nidiffer. The victimhood of American policy failure had been inverted, from black, male, and possibly sexually licentious, to white, virginal, and deserving. The contribution of the Nidiffer story to the Act's passage is impossible to know with causal precision, but it merits reflection that in the debates before Congress in 1937 and 1938, not one of the black male, rural male, or syphilis patient consumers of sulfanilamide was mentioned as a tragedy.

It is important, then, to consider how other advocates interpreted the sulfanilamide tragedy and how they read its lessons into rather different policy implications and statutory proposals. One of them was embedded in Charles Wesley Dunn's proposal to add another misbranding charge to any medicine that had not, before its market entry, proved its therapeutic claims. This would have changed the FDA's authority and the basis of a "misbranding" charge, but federal regulation of medicines would still have been regulation ex post approval, as it was from 1906 to 1938. Dunn's alternative proposal would have recognized the severity of the sulfanilamide episode but would not have gleaned from the tragedy the necessity of explicitly preventative measures.

Another set of alternative framings—admittedly less concrete and quite manifold—were all the other versions of the Copeland bill that had received serious consideration before October 1937. When the *Washington Post* and other news outlets waxed prophetic on the likelihood of new legislation, their editors had in mind the S.5 that had passed the Senate in the first session

[62] Again, the precise extent of Elixir Sulfanilamide use by African Americans is unknown. The key to this narrative is not that African Americans were in fact disproportionate users of Elixir Sulfanilamide, but that in early newspaper accounts of the tragedy, reporters and physicians mentioned their African American patients more than white patients.

of the 75th Congress, but which had stalled in the House. That bill, too, lacked a gatekeeping provision.

There is nothing in the primary evidence suggesting that anyone in the Agriculture Department or the FDA deliberately or consciously misrepresented any feature of the sulfanilamide episode. Some features of the sulfanilamide affair were in fact tailor-made for re-interpretation. Some facts and sequences lend themselves to the production of lessons more than others do. Throughout, the FDA was constrained by some "factual" features of the sulfanilamide episode. What its officials did—quite skillfully, it now appears—is to emphasize some features of the episode more than others.

As with other forms of reputation, however, the power observed in the sulfanilamide episode rested not merely with the narrator. The tragic framing of the episode was, throughout, dependent upon audiences in medical journals, in national and regional newspapers, and, most important, in Congress. Like the choruses of Sophocles and Euripides, these were not passive audiences. Morris Fishbein and Royal Copeland actively inserted their judgment and energy into the struggle over food and drug law reform. Yet the fundamental reshaping of the narrative of elixir sulfanilamide was accomplished by federal officials in the U.S. Department of Agriculture. The crucial features of the USDA's framing were three: its exposure of apparent weaknesses in existing law; its conversion of pharmaceutical victimhood from black to white, from maturity to childhood; and its equation of such undeserved sulfanilamide deaths with tragedies that could and must be explicitly prevented through licensure.

The endeavors of Walter Campbell, Royal Copeland, and Henry Wallace are forgotten now. Yet they shaped the American and global history of medicine and pharmaceutical development for decades in ways that have yet to be appreciated, and perhaps never will. Their actions amount to a form of political innovation, a feat shared in this case between a career bureaucrat (Campbell), an administrator emerging as a national politician (Wallace), and a career legislator (Copeland).[63] The saga of American pharmaceutical regulation and its origins demonstrates that political innovation and entrepreneurship, in its most powerful and enduring moment, consists in symbolic politics—in the interpretation, framing, and public distillation of observable history.

The Construction of Processes and Standards

The 1938 statute compelled FDA administrators and scientists to construct from scratch an entirely new system of processing and evaluation. An applied chemistry bureau now had to solve a problem that was jointly regulatory and administrative—the review of hundreds of requests to market a

[63]Sheingate, "Political Entrepreneurship, Institutional Change, and American Political Development"; Stephen Skowronek and Matt Glassman, *Formative Acts: American Politics in the Making* (Philadelphia: University of Pennsylvania Press, 2007).

novel legal and commercial entity known as a "new drug." Two medical officers—Theodore Klumpp and J. J. Durrett—inaugurated new drug review at the Administration, and their experience with the first novel therapeutic compound submitted under the law—sulfapyridine—expressed important patterns of evaluation that would be applied to later drugs.

Merck's sulfapyridine—submitted to the FDA in October 1938—was the latest in the celebrated class of sulfa drugs that had revolutionized anti-infective therapy in the 1930s. Merck submitted the drug as a treatment for pneumonia, in part because the severity of the disease and the inefficacy of existing anti-pneumonia serums meant that the benefit-to-risk profile of the drug would be higher than if it were submitted for another indication. Like other sulfa drugs, sulfapyridine was highly toxic to the liver and to red blood cells, and this fact was evident from the animal studies submitted with the application. The question that Klumpp and Durrett explicitly considered was whether the therapeutic effects of the drug made the drug's "margin of safety" sufficiently tolerable for approval. From the very first moments of sulfapyridine's review, and hence from the very first moments of the 1938 Act's application, medical officers considered questions of "therapeutic value" in new drug review.[64]

In their assessment of sulfapyridine and other drugs, FDA medical officers borrowed heavily from existing practices of pharmacological evaluation, particularly toxicity studies in animals of multiple species. Yet thorough protocols for extensive animal studies and for clinical studies in human subjects were not established. In their experiment with new drug review, Klumpp and Durrett thus rendered as systematic as possible a procedure that fundamentally lacked consistent and predictable structure. In the absence of clinical trial information, they examined nearly 2,000 cases in which patients were treated with the drug, and they consulted an informal network of researchers who had worked with the compound and interviewed these men at length. By February 1939, when they concluded that their existing data were insufficient for a decision, they interviewed another forty-five clinicians about the drug. Pressures for sulfapyridine's release began to grow, and on February 23, 1939, Theodore Klumpp issued a letter indicating the agency would not withhold the drug's approval.[65]

[64] John E. Lesch, *The First Miracle Drugs: How the Sulfa Drugs Transformed Medicine* (New York: Oxford University Press, 2007). Writers as early as the 1940s were celebrating the class; see Iago Galdston, *Behind the Sulfa Drugs: A Short History of Chemotherapy* (New York: D. Appleton-Century, 1943). This discussion of the sulfapyridine review relies almost entirely on Harry Marks' excellent analysis in *Progress of Experiment*, 83–97, and an earlier version of this chapter, "Playing It Safe: Federal Drug Regulation After 1938," presented at the Session on Scientific Languages and Political Cultures, Organization of American Historians annual meeting, April 1994.

[65] For a glimpse into the standard pharmacological practices used by academically trained physicians of the time, consult Louis Goodman and Alfred Gilman, *The Pharmaceutical Basis of Therapeutics: A Textbook of Pharmacology, Toxicology and Therapeutics for Medical Students*, 1st ed. (New York: Macmillan, 1941); also John Parascandola, *The Development of*

Klumpp and Durrett actually knew early on in the sulfapyridine review that the drug would eventually be approved; the question was not whether to approve, but when, and under what conditions as expressed in the drug's labeling. Much of the early practice of drug review became an exercise in regulating the label. The Administration was less likely to reject new drug applications themselves than to disallow labeling claims and to delay the clearance of the drug until labeling claims could be settled.[66]

Pharmaceutical and chemical firms reacted to the new law and to the patterns of administration by adapting their research and development strategies. Many firms had trained pharmacologists and clinical investigators on their staffs or in consultation. Merck, like many other firms of the period, consulted extensively with academic pharmacologists and clinicians at university medical schools and research hospitals. What changed for firms like Merck was less the fact of pharmacology than its intensity; the rigor and thoroughness of the work expected had increased so much as to upset established patterns of laboratory work and division of scientific labor. Hans Molitor, head of the Merck Institute, reported that as a result of regulatory expectations—enforced by the Administration's inspectors—he was compelled to keep a wider variety of test animals (including goats, sheep, and pigs in addition to rats and dogs) at his laboratories as compared to previous years. Noting an "unforeseen increase of work" in the early spring of 1939—from 1938 to 1939 alone, Merck's experimental work increased 62 percent—Molitor then described how the fear of regulatory derailment had led him to heighten the quantity and quality of his supervision of the Merck Institute's pharmacology and toxicology work.

> [Our] work includes not only regular pharmacologic bioassays, but also ... investigations into the variation in toxicity of certain standard material, and such apparently uninteresting and "routine" experiments, as determination of acute and chronic toxicity; irritating properties; hypnotic, analgesic, local anesthetic effects; etc. The latter type of work, often (but without justification) regarded as a "necessary evil," is undoubtedly one of the most important responsibilities of our laboratory and requires painstaking execution and closest supervision, since an error or oversight is liable to cause the discarding of a possibly valuable compound or the continuation of work which should have been abandoned after the first few trials. For these reasons I am anxious to control these investigations personally

---

American Pharmacology: John Jacob Abel and the Making of a Discipline (Baltimore: Johns Hopkins University Press, 1992). On the 2,000-case analysis and the survey of clinical investigators, see Marks, *Progress of Experiment*, 86–9. See also Marks' conclusion that "the medical-scientific community ... originated the principles under which the FDA operated" (93); as I suggest in the following two chapters, FDA officials played a co-equal role in procedural and methodological innovation in new drug evaluation from the late 1940s through the 1960s.

[66] Marks, "Playing It Safe," n.41. Examples of drugs whose labeling claims were rejected and substantially altered include sulfathiazole, and sulfadiazine, and the companies in play included some of the central players, including Lederle Laboratories, Parke Davis, Winthrop, Sharp & Dohme, and Merck; Marks, "Playing It Safe," n.39.

and to entrust their execution to workers whom I have trained myself and of whose absolute dependability I am certain.[67]

For every firm like Merck whose transition to the new regime was "anxious" but relatively smooth, dozens of other companies large and small found the new terrain of American pharmaceutical development profoundly uncertain and frustrating.

From Therapeutic Value to Efficacy. FDA officials had supported the regulation of a drug's curative powers since before the 1938 Act. In the battle over the 1938 legislation, pharmaceutical industry representatives, particularly proprietary manufacturers, were able to successfully beat back an efficacy provision in the statute. Yet it was a matter of months after the Act went into law that FDA officials were openly discussing the matter of efficacy in their review of new drug applications. These unalloyed practices of evaluation became increasingly systematized, in part by the annealing of experience, and in part by patterns of cooperation between FDA medical officers and the American Medical Association's Council on Pharmacy and Chemistry. In the mid-1940s, in the rhetoric of Walton van Winkle, a more programmatic idea of efficacy regulation began to take shape. In a report prepared by van Winkle and his colleagues Robert Herwick and Herbert Calvery—and conspicuously co-authored with Austin Smith, then Secretary of the Council on Pharmacy and Chemistry—FDA officials drove an important public wedge between the concepts of "toxicity" and "safety." The Van Winkle report was subsequently published in the *Journal of the American Medical Association* on December 9, 1944. It was presented gently to *JAMA* readers as a sort of guidance document, "a pattern and not a regulation," but it sent a clear message to practicing physicians and drug makers that FDA physicians did not intend to confine their pre-market review of drugs to toxicity issues alone.

> Two factors enter into the decision with regard to the merits of the drug: (1) Is it efficacious? (2) Is it dangerous? Neither of these factors can be separated from one another and considered alone. That has been emphasized by van Winkle in discussing the evaluation of new drug applications submitted under the new drug provisions of the Federal Food, Drug and Cosmetic Act. It has been emphasized that there is no arbitrary standard of safety; it is a relative matter in which the

[67]John Swann, *Academic Scientists and the Pharmaceutical Industry: Cooperative Research in Twentieth-Century America* (Baltimore: Johns Hopkins University Press, 1988). *Merck Institute Seventh Annual Report* (1939), January 22, 1940, prepared by Hans Molitor (quote from pp. 3–4); FF 41, B 16, Alfred Newton Richards Papers, University of Pennsylvania. Among the growing research inquiries were investigations of sulfapyridine; Molitor and Robinson, "Toxic Manifestations after Oral Administration of Sodium Sulfapyridine," *Proceedings of the Society for Experimental Biology and Medicine* 41 (June 1939). On academic-industrial cooperation in the 1940s and 1950s, see Dominique Tobbell, "Pharmaceutical Networks: the Political Economy of Drug Development in the United States, 1945–1980," Ph.D. diss., University of Pennsylvania, 2008.

toxicity of the drug must be weighed against the therapeutic benefits which its use will bring about.

The van Winkle article of December 1944 briefly discussed expectations for chronic toxicity studies and mentioned the possibility that the different investigations into a drug's safety and efficacy could be systematically phased. The co-authorship of the article was significant for its symbolism—readers of the *Journal of the American Medical Association* understood that the central concepts had developed at the intersection of the AMA's Council and the Administration, and that the precepts of the article had the official blessing of both organizations. The cooperation between the two organizations that was evinced in the sulfanilamide episode was not evident in the production of method.

Judicial Legitimation of Industry Fear: The Dotterweich Decision of 1943

If there was a weak or improbable link in the regulation-building measures of 1938, it lay in the U.S. Supreme Court's uncertain reaction to the new law. The federal judiciary had not greeted the Pure Food and Drugs Act of 1906 with much favor—the Supreme Court invalidated crucial provisions in *United States v. Johnson* (1911)—and many of Roosevelt's state-building initiatives in the early 1930s also went down to defeat in judicial challenges. The mid-century legal challenge to American pharmaceutical regulation came when FDA investigators charged the chief executive of the Buffalo Pharmacal Company with violation of the 1938 Act's Section 301(a), which prohibits the "introduction or delivery for introduction into interstate commerce of any drug that is adulterated or misbranded." Buffalo Pharmacal's president was charged with a federal misdemeanor. The federal circuit court reviewing the case argued that the individual penalized was at sufficient remove from the "crime" to invalidate his conviction. But in a five-to-four decision whose consequences would reverberate through corporate boardrooms for decades afterward, the Supreme Court sided with the Administration, and offered a stunningly broad interpretation of the scope of the 1938 law.

> The Food and Drugs Act of 1906 was an exertion by Congress of its power to keep impure and adulterated food and drugs out of the channels of commerce. By the Act of 1938, Congress extended the range of its control over illicit and noxious articles and stiffened the penalties for disobedience. The purposes of this legislation thus touch phases of the lives and health of people which, in the circumstances of modern industrialism, are largely beyond self-protection. Regard for these purposes should infuse construction of the legislation if it is to be treated as a working instrument of government, and not merely as a collection of English words.... The prosecution to which Dotterweich was subjected is based on a now familiar type of legislation whereby penalties serve as effective means of regulation. Such legislation dispenses with the conventional requirement for criminal conduct—awareness of some wrongdoing. In the interest of the larger good, it

puts the burden of acting at hazard upon a person otherwise innocent but standing in responsible relation to a public danger.[68]

The Dotterweich decision applied to a small, undistinguished outfit that had sold a modernized patent medicine, yet its potential reach extended to the largest, most distinguished and professional of research-based corporations then in existence. With the *Dotterweich* decision, pharmaceutical and chemical executives could now be called to account for introducing a misbranded drug into interstate commerce. Criminal responsibility for regulatory violations was placed upon those individuals with the greatest degree of authoritative power in the modern corporation. The Administration now had legal authority to place responsibility for regulatory violations at the highest level of the firm.[69]

. . .

Unlike the sulfanilamide episode, the *Dotterweich* decision was scarcely visible to the American mass public, having been drowned out by news of European war and by other court decisions. Yet for a particular set of audiences—the industries and companies regulated by the FDA's pharmaceutical specialists—the power of the Administration grew significantly even as the specter of its forcible action became more fearful. Reputation and power in the sulfanilamide episode were general and public. In the sulfapyridine review and later moments of administrative practice, and in the *Dotterweich* decision, the audiences, the reputation, and the regulatory force of the Administration were particular and targeted, but no less vast.

[68] *United States v Dotterweich*, 320 U.S. 277 (1943); quoted section appears at 320 U.S. 281.

[69] Daniel F. O'Keefe, Jr., and Marc H. Shapiro, "Personal Criminal Liability under the Federal Food, Drug and Cosmetic Act: The Dotterweich Doctrine," *FDCLJ* 30 (1) (January 1975): 5–80.

The Ambiguous Emergence of American Pharmaceutical Regulation, 1944–1961

> It has been my experience in the past that when such differences arose between ourselves and the New Drug Division, we were told to go get the needed data— and did, because we knew that if we didn't we damn well wouldn't get our NDA approved. I don't see how you can get more power than that, and it's being used now—and boy, are they asking for minutiae!
>
> —Searle medical director I. C. Winter, December 1960

THE BUREAUCRATIC regulation of pharmaceuticals arrived not starkly in new laws, nor in scientific and medical upheavals, but continuously, haltingly, and ambiguously in regulatory practice. It came in administrative conflict and the symbolic lessons that citizens, journalists, scientists, company officials, and federal policymakers drew from those struggles. In tilts between competing visions of scientific experiment, between alternative views of the relationship between medicine and business, between brash pharmaceutical firms and newly cautious medical reviewers—in these battles the regulatory system of the past half-century was created. There was no designer, no founding moment. Instead, a slow, publicly imperceptible clash of administrative practices, scientific debates, business strategies, and individual agendas issued in a set of alternative understandings of regulation, industry, and science. These understandings were increasingly codified on paper, reflecting a broader impulse toward protocol.

In these post-War developments was established the interlacing of reputation and regulatory power in American pharmaceuticals. The Administration's identity was partially recast—less and less as a market cop or field enforcer, more and more as a health protection agency whose fundamental capacity lay in the governance of new drugs. The first face of regulatory power was sculpted in the 1938 Federal Food, Drug and Cosmetic Act, and it began to crystallize in federal rules and guidelines issued in the 1950s. Yet the intertwining of reputation and power came most forcefully in the second and third faces of regulatory power—the ability to set research and develop-ment agendas and induce obedience through reputation, and the ability to shape the vocabularies of the modern pharmaceutical regime, its commer-cial, scientific, professional, and political debates.

Beginning in 1957, the confluence of several events—Senator Estes Ke-fauver's hearings on the pharmaceutical industry, the tragedy of the sedative thalidomide, and an internal FDA push for regulation of efficacy and clini-cal development—transformed U.S. pharmaceutical policy and thrust a new facet of the FDA into the public spotlight. Doctor Frances Oldham Kelsey arrived to the FDA and began processing Richardson-Merrell's new drug application for Kevadon (thalidomide), a sedative already widely used in Europe. Kelsey found flaws in the application and delayed Kevadon's intro-duction into the United States. Only two years later would the wisdom of her judgment be so horrifically confirmed, as thousands of infants were born limbless, earless, and dead in Europe and Australia from complications re-sulting from thalidomide use. Thalidomide was pulled from the worldwide market, and Kelsey was soon celebrated as a national heroine in the United States. Estes Kefauver and President John F. Kennedy, in different ways, drew upon the thalidomide story to create lasting statutory change. The 1962 Kefauver-Harris Amendments replaced an earlier requirement for pre-market notification of new drug introductions to a dispositive mandate for pre-market FDA approval, and the amendments added an "effectiveness" requirement to the Act of 1938. In theory and at law, drugs now had to prove curative power as well as safety before entering the U.S. prescription market.[1]

In the public chronicles that are still with us, Frances Kelsey's triumph and Estes Kefauver's lawmaking are depicted as liberation from a dark de-cade, an abrupt departure from a "disastrous era" of "non-regulation of prescription drugs." The 1950s Commissioner of the FDA, George Larrick, is portrayed alternatively as a bumble or an industry sop. Images abound of drug company officials walking unimpeded through the agency's corridors, setting up informal residence and hounding medical reviewers. Medical re-viewers like Barbara Moulton complained that their cautionary stances to-ward new drugs were being overruled by their industry-humbled superiors, and prominent medical academics like Cornell's Walter Modell lampooned the FDA's decisions. Famed journalists like Morton Mintz saw (and de-picted) the agency in utter disarray. Rendered this way, the standard history of the FDA is not unlike the Christian history of the world, neatly spliced into epochs of "Before Thalidomide" and "After Kelsey." Consider Philip Hilts' telling:

[1] A crucial context for these developments—especially changes to the FDA's public reputa-tion—lay in the consumption-based society of the mid-twentieth century United States. See Lizabeth Cohen, *A Consumers' Republic: The Politics of Mass Consumption in Postwar Amer-ica* (New York: Basic Books, 2003); Meg Jacobs, *Pocketbook Politics: Economic Citizenship in Twentieth-Century America* (Princeton: Princeton University Press, 2004).

In sum, during the 1950s and early 1960s the drug companies were occasionally policing themselves in the new pharmaceutical market, while the FDA was struggling to catch up. After the Kefauver hearings, thalidomide and the new law, the FDA was now seen as a potential serious force, one that could protect the public in an emergency.[2]

As with many "before and after" histories, these binary narratives mislead. Their focus on individual events and personalities, while necessary, obscures a set of pivotal and organizationally embedded developments that together made the modern regime of pharmaceutical regulation. A more informative and accurate understanding of the origins of modern pharmaceutical regulation—one that peers behind the limelight and grandstanding of congressional testimony and newscasts, one that focuses not only upon the legislative process but also upon regulation as it is made in political struggles between regulators, companies, scientists, politicians, and consumer advocates—starts not with Kefauver, Kelsey, and thalidomide but much earlier. It centers upon a slowly changing organization, the FDA's Bureau of Medicine, which in the late 1940s and early 1950s began to greet new drugs with more conscious and more procedurally *orchestrated* scrutiny than ever before. The arrival of procedural drug regulation happened not merely in science, not merely in business, and not merely within the confines of an agency. It happened at the interstices of state, medicine, and market. In a set of far-reaching procedural and behavioral changes surrounding federal drug evaluation, these three realms overlapped and hosted a subtle but vast and durable shift in American pharmaceutical policy.

Our existing chronicles also miss a set of at least three more continuous and emergent changes in U.S. pharmaceutical regulation. First, FDA officials developed a set of uncoordinated practices and rationales for efficacy regulation and pharmacological evaluation in the late 1940s and early 1950s, at least eight years before Frances Kelsey arrived to the agency. Indeed, Kelsey's very matriculation to the FDA was an historical product of a preexisting agency ideology, one thoroughly expressed in hiring practices and networks. The ideology included not only regulation of "therapeutic value" for drugs submitted to the FDA, but also a focus on long-term safety and the regulation of drugs in their clinical trial phase. In this respect, Kelsey's skepticism for thalidomide was a legacy of broader, older patterns in the organization she inhabited. So too, the problems surfacing at the FDA—Barbara Moulton being overruled, industry friendliness, Walter Modell's complaints—were as much a product of the new regulatory outlook

[2]Hilts, *Protecting America's Health: The FDA, Business and One Hundred Years of Regulation* (New York: Knopf, 2003), 163. Morton Mintz, *By Prescription Only* [originally published as *The Therapeutic Nightmare*] (Boston: Houghton Mifflin, 1967), Preface ("disastrous era" of "non-regulation") and passim. For other accounts see Richard Harris, *The Real Voice* (New York: Macmillan, 1964). Temin, *Taking Your Medicine*, chapters 4 and 5, ignores the 1950s developments entirely; for a cogent critique of some of these omissions, see Marks, "Revisiting 'The Origins of Compulsory Prescriptions.'"

and the way that it challenged older patterns of business-government relations as they were a signal of an underlying, static reality.[3]

Second, the fundamental change was not statutory revision, but a joint shift in perception and in practice. One set of changes saw the congealing of beliefs among professions and disciplines, U.S. and European companies, politicians and a media-saturated public. Among these diverse audiences, new views formed about government capacity, specifically, the ability and role of the FDA in governing thousands of new drugs. Combined with these shifts in perception—in some ways fueling them, in other ways reflecting them—were changes in regulatory behavior. Federal officials, company scientists, and clinical investigators at hospitals and universities began to apply novel standards of assessment to all new drugs: protocols for a sequence of experiments, more exacting and lengthy toxicology studies, multiple species in animal trials, randomization of human subjects, placebo arms, exact testing for dose-response relationships, stability and physiological availability of the drug in the bloodstream, and more. FDA officials began to shape almost every facet of the ethical drug industry and much of medicine—clinical experimentation, manufacturing, labeling, promotion, and prescribing behavior—through the new drug approval process. Clinical researchers and FDA officials together imposed stringent new standards—from the rapidly changing disciplines of toxicology, "pharmacodynamics," and "clinical pharmacology"—to drugs and the firms that produced them. Even as they sired new compounds by the hundreds, drug companies, domestic and foreign, raced to keep up with the new standards and the FDA's implementation of them. Firms varied appreciably in the speed and skill with which they adapted. Some withered, others prospered, and some converted their skill in navigating the regulatory maze into the primary basis of their corporate value.

The multiplicity and ambiguity of these perceptions and practices should not be understated. There were variable readings of the FDA in different quarters of American industrial society, images of the regulator that ranged from cooperative enforcer to vigilant purity cop to industry bully to vanguard assessor to bought-off corporate servant. Yet a common element in most of these perceptions was a growing belief in the capacity of the Administration—the potential and fundamental benevolence of the agency, its need for greater funding and authority, the general promise of the direction in which it was moving. In many respects, these different understandings of the

[3] One element of this argument has been entertained before by scholars—Harry Marks and John Swann most notable among them—who have noticed that efficacy considerations were entering into FDA drug regulation before 1960. Swann, "Sure Cure: Public Policy on Drug Efficacy before 1962," in Gregory J. Higby and Elaine C. Stroud, eds., *The Inside Story of Medicines: A Symposium* (Madison, WI: American Institute for the History of Pharmacy, 1997), 223–62; Marks, *The Progress of Experiment* (New York: Cambridge University Press, 1996), 78–97. Perhaps the first legal scholar writing after 1962 to have noticed that efficacy regulation predated the 1962 Act was Vincent Kleinfeld, in "Commentary," in John B. Blake, ed., *Safeguarding the Public: Historical Aspects of Medicinal Drug Control* (Baltimore: Johns Hopkins University Press, 1970), 182.

FDA corresponded to different audiences of early Cold War American society. For many elite physicians and pharmacologists, great possibilities resided in the agency, along with trusted colleagues there. For many of these same voices, FDA regulation was an experience in frustration and lack of predictability. For consumer advocacy groups, the American regulatory system was described as too weak, but even among these voices the FDA became the only agent truly capable of protecting American consumers, and the only genuine quality control process in the public health system. In the consumer public and the media, images abounded of the FDA as less a pharmacological assessor and more of a cop. The diversity of these understandings among different audiences was not ephemeral but relatively stable, and the very ambiguity that characterized the FDA's reputation served to make the agency's esteem ever more robust. The FDA's identity was hard to pin down. Yet the agency exuded a warm public glow, a disciplinary stance toward firms and clinical researchers, and a cool diffidence to the American Medical Association even as it embraced smaller, newer, and more specialized medical and scientific societies.

Third, the symbolic and practical emergence of the modern FDA was equivalent, in large part, to the departure of other organizations from important policy niches in early Cold War U.S. politics. Among these, chief was the waning of the American Medical Association and its role in evaluating drugs. As the political and scientific niche of "drug evaluation" evolved, the FDA's Bureau of Medicine came to possess a procedural monopoly on the activity. So too, the federal regulation of labeling, promotion, dispensing, and prescription patterns and distribution networks incurred deeply into the turf of organized pharmacists, particularly the American Pharmaceutical Association. In addition, the warm glow associated with the Administration contrasted with the harsh public light being shed upon two behemoths that were seen as increasingly intertwined: the AMA and the American pharmaceutical industry, particularly its political spokesman, the American Pharmaceutical Manufacturers' Association.[4] Just as the FDA was coming to be viewed as the generally benevolent but congressionally ill-equipped guarantor of public safety, the AMA was being hit for its weakened neutrality and its continuing status as a "doctor's trust," and the pharmaceutical industry was being targeted for its contribution to national inflation.[5]

The context of early Cold War America provided not just multiple audi-

---

[4]The Pharmaceutical Manufacturers' Association has its own history during this very period, having been produced by a merger of the American Drug Manufacturers Association (ADMA) and the American Pharmaceutical Manufacturers' Association (APMA). "Pharmacy Law Interest, Participation Urged at Rutgers," *OP&DR*, May 20, 1957, 7. "PMA Officially in Existence; Papers on File in Delaware," *OP&DR*, April 7, 1958, 7; also *OP&DR*, April 21, 1958, 5.

[5]On the role of professions in this sort of niche competition, see Andrew Abbott, *The System of Professions* (Chicago: University of Chicago Press, 1992). Harrison White, *Chains of Opportunity* (Cambridge: Harvard University Press, 1970).

ences and shifting professional fates, but an environment in which government claims to scientific authority and capacity could meet with public belief. The atomic age was under way, in policy and in myth. The contributions of physical and biological science to American economy, culture, and society were tangible and real. With the Hill-Burton Act of 1946, the federal government became active in the construction and design of hospitals and their research facilities. The National Science Foundation launched in 1950, and throughout the 1940s and 1950s, the National Institutes of Health was launching new centers and programs for heart disease, arthritis, and neurological diseases, mental health, and cancer chemotherapy. These federal programs forever altered the relationship between government and academy, and they greatly expanded the breadth and capacity of America's research universities. Perhaps most important, the federal government's far-reaching involvement with science—ranging from the Manhattan Project to fledgling commercial nuclear power programs, from the National Cancer Institute to the Mercury and Apollo programs and other responses to the Russian government's Sputnik launch of 1957—had attracted public attention and enthusiasm. The increasing professional and scientific legitimacy of the FDA drew energy from these broader trends.[6]

Frances Kelsey's triumph, then, was neither an exogenous historical pivot nor the inevitable outcome of the clash between business and the state. Her prescience formed a powerful symbol for those in American society who favored a more systematic and rigorous approach to drug development and regulation, and those outside of the agency who saw its regulatory functions as essential protections for a consumer-based society. It solidified an emergent set of scientific, professional, and public judgments that were made of a government agency, and it helped to cement a strong set of organizational identifications within the FDA's ranks. Yet what appears as culmination was not. A set of competing beliefs about regulation, the FDA, medicine, and business—beliefs that suffused the politics of U.S. pharmaceutical regulation in the 1950s—was narrowed well before Kelsey took her post in September 1960.

[6]Brian Balogh, *Chain Reaction: Expert Debate and Public Participation in American Commercial Nuclear Power, 1945–1975* (New York: Cambridge University Press, 1993). See in particular Vannevar Bush's pathbreaking report, *Science: The Endless Frontier* (1945); and David M. Hart's argument that Bush's influence, while genuine, has been overestimated. Hart locates crucial shifts in national science policy in the 1920s through the 1940s; *Forged Consensus: Science, Technology, and Economic Policy in the United States, 1921–1953* (Princeton: Princeton University Press, 1998). Jessica Wang, *American Science in an Age of Anxiety: Scientists, Anticommunism, and the Cold War* (Chapel Hill: University of North Carolina Press, 1999); Don K. Price, *Government and Science: Their Dynamic Relation in American Democracy* (New York: NYU Press, 1954); Bruce L. R. Smith, *U. S. Science Policy Since World War II* (Washington, DC: Brookings Institution, 1990); Daniel J. Kevles, "The National Science Foundation and the Debate over Postwar Research Policy, 1942–1955," *Isis* 68 (241) (1977): 4–26; David Guston and Kenneth Keniston, eds., *The Fragile Contract: University Science and the Federal Government* (Cambridge: MIT Press, 1994).

*The Severity of Procedural Scrutiny: Organizational Change
and Bureaucratic Learning*

In the wake of the 1938 Food, Drug and Cosmetic Act, a collision of forces brought pharmaceutical companies, academic researchers, and regulators into a new world. A new generation of chemical therapeutics was changing the practice of medicine, the conduct of public health, and the nature of pharmaceutical development and production. At the same time, academic medicine was being influenced by the development of rational therapeutics and clinical pharmacology, both emphasizing the prospective, statistical, and experimental evaluation and utilization of medicines and alternative treatments. Rising public and professional awareness of chronic illnesses and the possibilities for treating these maladies—including cancers, arthritis, diabetes, mood disorders and mental illnesses, and bacterial infections targeted by broad-spectrum and fixed-combination antibiotics—supported a broad interest in drugs for long-term stockpiling and use. And not least, the 1938 Act, the evolution of medical and chemical science at the FDA, and the responsibilities of the Administration during the World War had created organizational capacities that lay yearning for new policy applications. Within the FDA and the emergent scientific networks of clinical pharmacology, government and academic scientists perceived serious inadequacies in new drugs coming to market and in the processes used to develop, test, and manufacture them.[7]

The vibrancy of regulatory politics during the 1950s belies the "dark decade" image that Philip Hilts, Morton Mintz, and others have given to the time. Some of the most familiar players in that drama, most notably FDA Commissioner George Larrick, occupied a set of much more complicated positions and carried and vocalized a more diverse range of views than the recent chroniclers have described. In the writings of Hilts and Mintz, Larrick and the 1950s FDA are seen as tied too closely to industry, resistant to change, and all but incapable of responding to the complex new world of rational pharmaceuticals. While there is some truth to these portrayals, the reality is much more complicated. FDA officers acutely perceived the new world of therapeutics, and indeed some of them assisted in its creation. In diverse ways, these federal officials adapted an outmoded regulatory apparatus to meet the dilemmas contained in that world. In this way, some of the very "triumphs" and hardest-wired "lessons" of the early 1960s—the perils of investigational drugs, the public health problems posed by inefficacious medicines, the teratogenic potential of drugs for chronic conditions, the lack

[7]For useful summaries, see Thomas Maeder, *Adverse Reactions*, chap. 2; John Swann, *Academic Scientists and the American Pharmaceutical Industry*; Dowling, *Medicines for Man*. Marks, *The Progress of Experiment*. John Parascandola, *The Development of American Pharmacology: John Jacob Abel and the Shaping of a Discipline* (Baltimore: Johns Hopkins University Press, 1992), has a very useful epilogue (146–52) outlining the development of "classical" versus "clinical" pharmacology in the late twentieth century.

of rigor and completeness in studies conducted by pharmaceutical companies—were premised upon behaviors that emerged and were legitimized in the 1940s and 1950s. George Larrick was an organization man caught between these two worlds. The older world of regulation by inspection and enforcement—in which Larrick had been trained, and in which the public enemies of note were the "cancer quack" and the drug adulterer—was giving way to a new reality of molecular pharmaceutical development, an art that even the wealthiest and most equipped of companies could not master.[8]

FDA Recruitment and the Regime of Pharmacology. The post-War vision of drug regulation emerged from a congeries of factors, not least administrative experience, the chemotherapeutic revolution in pharmaceuticals and the rise of molecular drugs for chronic conditions, and the increasing prominence of toxicology and clinical pharmacology at university medical faculties and in the FDA itself. It stemmed from the advocacy of a coterie of new physician-bureaucrats, including Ralph G. Smith, Ralph Weilerstein, Albert "Jerry" Holland, Barbara Moulton, Irvin Kerlan, Gordon Granger, and others. Smith was head of the New Drug Branch and responsible for policy development; he was the agency's pioneer in articulating and orchestrating the use of efficacy considerations into new drug review. Smith rendered explicit and conscious less formal patterns of efficacy evaluation that prevailed from 1938 through the 1940s. Weilerstein was a San Francisco-based inspector who spoke with ever greater force during the 1950s and eventually became Associate Medical Director (in 1957) and then Medical Director of the FDA (in 1961) before returning to the West Coast. Holland was FDA Medical Director in the mid-1950s, the agency's most talented spokesman, and with Ralph Smith, a major force in recruiting pharmacological and medical talent to the agency. Moulton was among the most radical of the new medical officers in Washington, and responsible for the agency's aggressive posture in critical new drug applications such as Altafur. Kerlan headed the BOM's Research and Reference Branch and is perhaps the individual most responsible for the FDA's contemporary adverse events reporting system.[9]

[8] On the "molecular revolution," see L. Kay, "Life as Technology: Representing, Intervening and Molecularizing," *Rivista di Storia della Scienza*, series II, 1 (1993): 85–103. For a useful collection of essays, see Soraya de Chadarevian and Harmke Kamminga, *Molecularizing Biology and Medicine: New Practices and Alliances, 1910s–1970s* (Amsterdam: Harwood Academic Publishers, 1998). John P. Swann, *Academic Scientists and the U.S. Pharmaceutical Industry: Cooperative Research in Twentieth-Century America* (Baltimore: Johns Hopkins University Press, 1988). Jonathan Liebenau, *Medical Science and Medical Industry: The Formation of the American Pharmaceutical Industry* (London: Macmillan, 1987). Temin, *Taking Your Medicine*, chap. 4; Alfred Chandler, *Shaping the Industrial Century: The Remarkable Story of the Evolution of the Modern Chemical and Pharmaceutical Industries* (Cambridge: Harvard University Press, 2005).

[9] For a list of BOM personnel and their associated positions, see *Department of Health, Education and Welfare Telephone Directory* (Washington, General Services Administration, January 1958); DF 306.3, RG 88, NA. Holland became Medical Director in April 1954 (*FDCR* 16 (43) (Dec. 4, 1954): 10–11) and resigned in December 1958 (*FDCR* 20 (50) (Dec. 15, 1958): 3–5).

The other voice of the procedural regime in the 1950s FDA was Albert "Jerry" Holland, Jr., formerly of the New York University College of Medicine and Armour Laboratories, where he had been medical director. Holland had also spent pivotal years at the Atomic Energy Commission, where he had forged ties with Allan Gregg. Following Erwin Nelson's tenure as medical director of the FDA, Holland was appointed to the post in March 1954.[10]

The cohort of significance at the FDA was not restricted to the Bureau of Medicine but also populated other offices (table 3.1). Perhaps the most consequential developments occurred in the Division of Pharmacology, which in 1949 began publishing landmark treatises on methods for the evaluation of safety in chemicals found in foods, drugs, and cosmetics. At the head of these efforts was Arnold J. Lehman, M.D., director of the Division from 1946 on. Upon his appointment Lehman reorganized the division, and he conducted a further reorganization of the Division in 1952. Along with O. Garth Fitzhugh (the agency's chief toxicologist), Lehman constructed an "experimental program" for safety appraisals that applied simultaneously to drugs and to food additives. Then in 1955 and 1958, the Pharmacology Division issued a new manual—*Appraisal of Safety of Chemicals in Foods, Drugs and Cosmetics*—that combined and standardized methods for the different targets of regulation under the 1938 Act.[11]

At the intersection of drug regulation and food additive regulation, Lehman's group reshaped the concept of "chronic toxicity" and authored the notion of planned sequences of experiments that could assess it. From these studies, the Division of Pharmacology began looking into food additives and inactive ingredients in drugs and cosmetics, particularly coal-tar dye colors. Yet Lehman and his colleagues also focused new and more systematic attention on the active ingredients of drugs. In a review of his Division's work in 1953, Lehman stated that he was particularly interested in reactions of drugs with enzymes, and more generally in "improved methods and criteria for evaluation of safety of drugs," including both the "therapeutic and toxic consequences" of medicines. He also believed that the agency's pharmacology division had broken immense new ground since 1938. The work

[10]Holland to Lloyd C. Miller (Director of Revision, USP), February 26, 1954; B179, F6, USP. From 1946 to 1950, Holland served as director of the Office of Research and Medicine for the AEC's Oak Ridge, Tennessee operations, and was tied to the Rockefeller Foundation and Alan Gregg. *FDCR* 20 (50) (Dec. 15, 1958): 3–5; "Albert Holland Jr., 69, F.D.A. Medical Chief," *NYT*, June 12, 1988.

[11]Lehman was appointed to fill the vacancy left by the sudden death of Herbert O. Calvery in September 1945; *FDCLQ* 1 (1946): 278. Lehman et al., "Procedures for the appraisal of the toxicity of chemicals in foods," *FDCLQ* 4 (1949): 4121–34, 1949. See also Lehman, "Proof of Safety: Some Interpretations," *Journal of the American Pharmacological Association* (Scient. Ed.) 40 (1951): 305–8. The main investigator of chronic toxicity was Fitzhugh; among many other publications, see Fitzhugh, Arthur A. Nelson, and C. I. Bliss, "Chronic Oral Toxicity of Selenium," *Journal of Pharmacology and Experimental Therapeutics* 80 (1944): 289–99. FDA Division of Pharmacology, "Appraisal of Safety of Chemicals in Foods, Drugs, and Cosmetics," *FDCLJ* 10 (1955): 679; *Appraisal of Safety of Chemicals in Foods, Drugs, and Cosmetics* (Washington, DC: FDA, 1958).

TABLE 3.1
Selected Members of the Post-War Cohort at the U.S. Food and Drug
Administration, 1947–1963

Division/Bureau of Medicine

Ralph G. Smith, M.D. (started 1950; Director)

Albert "Jerry" Holland, M.D. (Medical Director 1954–1959)

Ernest Q. King, M.D. (Medical Director before Holland)

William Kessenich, M.D. (started 1955; Medical Director after Holland)

Irvin Kerlan, M.D. (medical officer, and head of Drug Reference Branch)

Julius Hauser (started 1930s, became Assistant to Director)

Earl L. Meyers, Ph.D. (pharmacologist)

Claudia S. Prickett, Ph.D. (pharmacologist)

Eugene R. (Dick) Jolly, M.D., D. Pharm., Ph.D. (started 1957; eventually asst chief
of New Drug Branch)

Eugene M. K. Geiling, M.D., Ph.D. (consultant, medical officer, 1959–1963)

Barbara Moulton, M.D. (medical officer)

Bert Vos, M.D., Ph.D. (medical officer, 1957– ; student of Geiling)

Frances Oldham Kelsey, M.D., Ph.D. (medical officer, 1960– ; Geiling student)

Bureau of Field Administration

Kenneth Milstead (Chief, BFA)

George T. Daughters (Chief, Chicago District)

E.C. Boudreaux (Chief, New Orleans District)

Ralph Weilerstein, M.D. (San Francisco District)

Division/Bureau of Pharmacology

Arnold J. Lehman, Ph.D. (Director, Division of Pharmacology)

Bert J. Vos, Ph.D. (Assistant Director, Division of Pharmacology)

O. Garth Fitzhugh, Ph.D. (Chief, Toxicology Branch)

Edwin I. Goldenthal, Ph.D. (Chief, Pharmacodynamics Branch)

Robert S. Rose, Ph.D. (Director, Bureau of Pharmacology [after Lehman])

Geoffrey Woodard, Ph.D. (pharmacologist)

M. R. Woodard, Ph.D. (pharmacologist)

F. Ellis Kelsey, M.D., Ph.D. (pharmacologist, 1960–)

TABLE 3.1
cont.

Commissioner's Office, and General Counsel's Office

John L. Harvey (Associate Commissioner)

William Goodrich (General Counsel)

Kenneth Kirk (Associate Commissioner for Compliance)

Malcolm Stephens

Sam Fine

Bureau of Biological and Physical Sciences

Robert S. Roe, Ph.D. (Director)

Division of Antibiotics

Henry Welch, M.D. (Director)

Except where noted, all of these individuals arrived to the agency before Estes Kefauver launched his investigation of the drug industry in 1959 and before the submission of thalidomide in 1960. Some of them arrived well before 1947; see chapter 2.

of the Division under the early years of the 1938 Act had been uncoordinated and underequipped, and it lacked the hallmark of modern scientific organization—a division of administrative and intellectual labor. "Although the various projects of acute, chronic and skin toxicity, biochemical, pharmacodynamic and bioassay studies were separate entities," Lehman acknowledged, "the personnel of the [Pharmacology] Division had not yet reached this stage of specialization and were assigned to the various projects and shifted when necessary to those problems where the pressure was greatest at the time." Moreover, Lehman regarded the standards of chronic toxicity testing after the 1938 Act as insufficient. Among the many products that escaped rigorous attention were the coal-tar colors, whose widening use demanded "a re-evaluation of [their] innocuousness... and must be established on a more critical basis than occurred 15 years ago."[12]

---

[12]Lehman, "Some Functions of the Division of Pharmacology of the Food and Drug Administration," typescript dated May 13, 1953, pp. 7, 9; Accession 58-A277, B16, F 11, RG 88, NA. Lehman also stated that in the 1930s, the division was not doing "scientific investigations" or developing new standards but instead the work "was almost entirely of a regulatory nature."

As much as he systematized and advanced his Division, Lehman also exploited methodological advances that were occurring in the five years before his arrival. In a pivotal 1942 study, Fitzhugh and co-authors showed that feeding of ergot induced rat tumors only after a year or more of exposure; Arthur A. Nelson, Fitzhugh, and H. J. Morris, "Neurofibromatous Tumors of the Ears of Rats Produced by Prolonged Feeding of Crude Ergot," *Cancer Research*

Just as the Pharmacology Division was re-examining coal-tar colors, it began revisiting drugs approved in the late 1930s and early 1940s. Part of the reason was that Lehman's division was better staffed; in 1953, FDA Pharmacology had fifty-eight full-time members, including twenty-six with professional degrees. In other respects, however, Lehman and his colleagues became aware that the sort of strict toxicity tests that shed valuable light on common remedies and compounds—two-year toxicity studies, using multiple species, and extensive pathology examinations of animal subjects—needed application to new drugs. FDA pharmacologists studied anti-malaria drugs, both those widely used in the war and those under development. They re-examined digitoxins, sunscreen and suntanning creams, muscle relaxants and topical anesthetics, antiseptic mouthwashes, and abortifacients. In doing so, they created, borrowed, implemented, and advanced a set of tools that had not been available to the medical officers examining drugs in 1938 and 1939.[13]

The regulatory logic behind chronic toxicity tests was manifold. At its core, it signaled a broad departure from the anti-infective model of drug evaluation. Studies of chronic toxicity increasingly pointed to an important but little recognized connection between food additives and drugs. The

---

2 (1) (1942). For a general review of methods used in the early 1940s, which the authors admittedly saw as "incomplete," see Woodard and Calvery, "Acute and Chronic Toxicity—Public Health Aspects," *Industrial Medicine* (Jan.1943).

For a summary of the state of knowledge on chronic toxicity in the mid-1950s, see J. M. Barnes and F. A. Denz, "Experimental Methods Used in Determining Chronic Toxicity: A Critical Review," *Pharmacological Reviews* 6 (1954): 191–242. Barnes and Denz locate the earliest wave of new methodological studies in the mid-1930s, and their review cites dozen of studies published by FDA authors (C. I. Bliss, Calvery, Draize, Fitzhugh, Lila Knudsen, Lehman, and Woodard). The earliest pharmacology paper cited by Barnes and Denz is also FDA-authored: C. O. Johns, A. J., Finks, A. J. and Carl L. Alsberg, "Chronic Intoxication by Small Quantities of Cadmium Chloride in the Diet," *Journal of Pharmacology and Experimental Therapeutics* 21 (1923): 59–64.

[13]One strong impetus for the turn to renewed investigations of drugs was the Second World War, during which time FDA pharmacologists began examining the chronic toxicity of anti-malarial remedies, especially quinidine (atabrine) and chloroquine. Fitzhugh, "The Chronic Toxicity of Atabrine," paper presented at the District of Columbia Section of the Society for Experimental Biology and Medicine, December 7, 1944; Accession 54-A477, B4, F6, RG 88, NA. Fitzhugh, Nelson, and Holland, "The Chronic Oral Toxicity of Chloroquine," *Journal of Pharmacology and Experimental Therapeutics* 88 (2) (June 1948): 147–52. On surface-active agents, including quaternary ammonium salts used in muscle relaxants and anesthetics, consult the following: Woodard and Calvery, "Toxicological Properties of Surface-Active Agents," *Proceedings of the Scientific Section of the Toilet Goods Association* 3 (June 1945) (the maximum length of exposure in the Woodard-Calvery study was 180 days (cf. table 2)); Fitzhugh and Nelson, "Chronic Oral Toxicities of Surface-Active Agents," *Journal of the American Pharmaceutical Association* 37 (1) (Jan. 1948): 29–32; J. H. Draize, "Appraisal of the Toxicity of Suncreen Preparations," *AMA Archives of Dermatology and Syphilology* 64 (Nov. 1951): 585–7; Lehman, "Subacute and Chronic Toxicity of Quaternary Ammonium Surfactants," *Quarterly Bulletin of the Association of Food and Drug Officials of the United States* 18 (2) (April 1954): 18. Related to surface-active agents, FDA physicians such as Ralph W. Weilerstein of the San Francisco District were concerned over abortifacient pastes imported from Europe; Weilerstein, "Intra-Uterine Pastes," *JAMA* 125 (May 20, 1944): 205–7.

drugs for chronic conditions being developed in the 1950s would, like synthetic food additives, expose humans to potentially toxic substances over many years through weekly or daily consumption. Hence, regulatory questions of "safety" shifted from short-term to long-term use. Yet another central driver was that chronic toxicity studies always created possibilities for examining "therapeutic effectiveness" or even "therapeutic efficiency," which invited comparisons across drugs. FDA pharmacologists had routinely joined the examination of therapeutic effect to chronic toxicity since the mid-1940s. In a January 1950 speech to the Commercial Chemical Development Association in Chicago, FDA Medical Director Erwin Nelson argued that "each [new drug] application should carry a sound pharmacological and toxicological study." Numerous questions could be addressed by such studies, not least the relationship between the "toxic dose" and the "effective" dose. Nelson termed this the "margin of safety," while other pharmacologists called it the "therapeutic index."

> Is it effective in reasonable amounts? What is the margin of safety, or relationship between effective dose and toxic dose? How does this ratio compare with other substances of similar therapeutic action? If the substance is to be given at frequent intervals, what is its toxicity when so given? Chronic toxicity determinations, so called, are particularly important when the drug may be given for long periods of time. How is the drug test absorbed? How is it excreted? Does it possess local irritating properties? Is it sensitizing? What effects follow overdosage? How may these be treated? These illustrate but do not delimit the information required from the laboratory, from work on laboratory animals.[14]

By the late 1950s, industry trade reporters described the Division of Pharmacology as the center of regulatory innovation at the agency. "While Lehman and his Pharmacology Div. do not establish FDA regulatory policy," wrote one reporter, "they have rapidly become the single most powerful factors in determining the direction of govt. food, drug and cosmetic controls." Lehman had begun making announcements and writing regula-

[14]The linkage of efficacy questions to the anti-infective model was explicit in earlier FDA writings; see van Winkle, Herwick, Calvery, and Smith, "Laboratory and Clinical Appraisal of New Drugs," *JAMA* 126 (15) (Dec. 9, 1944): 958 ("In dealing with chemotherapeutic agents, these preliminary observations consist usually of tests of the efficacy of the agent in combating or preventing some experimental infections"). On the link between chronic toxicity and efficacy studies, consult Fitzhugh et al., "The Toxicities of Compounds Related to 2,3-Dimercaptopropanol (BAR) with a Note on Their Relative Therapeutic Efficiency," *Journal of Pharmacology and Experimental Therapeutics* 87 (4) (Aug. 1945): 23–7. Nelson, "Development of New Drugs," *FDCLJ* 5 (1950): 247. Some of Nelson's concepts appear in earlier writings, not least Van Winkle et al., "Laboratory and Clinical Appraisal of New Drugs," 959–60 (see chapter 2 for a discussion of this piece). Yet Nelson tied these methods to FDA requirements in a way that van Winkle, Herwick, and Calvery had not. Lehman and his co-authors, moreover, put forth much more detailed methods for appraisal of safety, and much more than earlier FDA writers, his group focused upon chronic toxicity tests as the central criterion of new drug evaluation. Compare the brief discussions of chronic toxicity in van Winkle et al. (p. 958) to the safety monographs of Lehman and colleagues in 1949, 1955, and 1958.

tions that required particular kinds of chronic toxicity studies, and industry audiences saw bold new departures. In the fall of 1960, Administration officials announced a Lehman-inspired policy that by January 1963, all submissions for new color additives to lipstick would need to be accompanied by two-year toxicity tests. The Pharmacology Division added new testing facilities for examination of coal-tar dyes, and began targeting products at the borderlands between foods, cosmetics, and drugs. Lehman stoked front-page coverage in trade reports when he drew concrete and public links between cosmetics and food colors and drugs. In a series of remarks to reporters and industry audiences, he contended that some colors and cosmetics (including hormone creams and ointments) could be regulated as pharmaceutical agents. He expressed his doubts about the effectiveness of vitamin A and D drugs, due to skin absorption. And he tied chronic toxicity studies to efficacy concerns when he argued that over-the-counter drugs should have a dosage-toxicity ratio (the ratio of toxic dose to therapeutic dose) of twenty-to-one, as opposed to the minimum four-to-one ratio usually required for prescription drugs.[15]

In implementing much of Lehman's program, agency medical officials began to tie chronic toxicity tests to emerging practices of testing for absorptions and "physiological availability." Medical officers demanded data on drug metabolism, especially for drugs with sustained-release and delayed-release dosage forms. And new chemical assays were required, including data on the stability of new drugs when stored on pharmacy or consumer shelves for months or years at a time. Each of these new questions gestured to the porous conceptual boundaries between chronic effects, chronic toxicity, and therapeutic efficacy. Even as they announced specific requirements and expectations, Administration medical officers refused to commit ahead of time to a particular protocol. Instead, medical officers would reserve the right to delay and refusal of a new drug application during formal review. As Nelson argued, the agency "has expressed its general views with respect to what is covered by a thorough study, but does not ordinarily like to comment on a specific program in advance for the reason that it thereby would be committed to approval of the program as completed."[16]

In other areas of the agency, new outlooks were also emerging. F. H. Wiley headed the Division of Pharmaceutical Chemistry and also took an

[15]FDCR, February 9, 1959, 4. Lehman, "Some Functions of the Division of Pharmacology of the Food and Drug Administration," manuscript of May 13, 1953; Accession 58-A277, B16, F 11, RG 88, NA. On the two-year toxicity tests for new colors, see FDCR, November 21, 1960, 9; these tests were estimated to cost $20,000 to $200,000 per color. Link between drugs and cosmetics; FDCR, February 9, 1959, pp. 1–2, 4, 6. In response to Lehman's fusillade, the cosmetic industry perceived that its regulatory fate would follow that of drug regulation in imposition of new FDA controls. Consequently, industry observers noticed an attempt by cosmetics companies to reinvent their common public identity as a "research-based" enterprise; FDCR, February 16, 1959, 10. On OTC preparations and their dosage-toxicity ratios, see FDCR, May 18, 1959, 23.

[16]Referring to Lehman's 1949 paper, Barnes and Denz would write that "The standard pub-

increasingly active consultant-like role in new drug approval. In the enforcement bureaus, J. Kenneth Kirk headed the Boston District and joined an activist force of inspectors who launched upon an "anti-quackery" initiative. Lila Knudson became one of the most notable women's voices in the practice of government statistics.

This emergence of what might today be called a procedural reform cohort at the 1950s FDA was not anticipated or induced by changes in Congress, the White House, or other FDA clientele. The Citizens' Advisory Committee, for instance, was concerned mainly about aggregate staffing levels, not about what professional sorts of staff ought to be hired.[17] And Lehman, Smith, Kerlan, Holland, Nelson, Weilerstein and other protagonists in the pharmacological regime came to the agency years before the Advisory Committee was created. The Eisenhower administration, for its part, paid little attention to the FDA, and only later in the decade (after the cohort had arrived, crystallized, and cemented itself) did Senator Estes Kefauver of Tennessee play a significant oversight role in pharmaceutical regulation. While national politics did play a crucial role in the display of the FDA's organizational identity, it did not materially affect hiring except through aggregate resource shifts. Indeed, the early tenor of the Eisenhower administration and the Congresses of the 1950s was one of punitive and shrift treatment for the FDA, as FDA staffing dropped by 155 positions (13 percent) from 1950 to 1954. It was not until Oveta Culp Hobby's 1955 creation of a Citizens'

lication on the toxicity test is that of Lehman and his colleagues"; "Experimental Methods Used in Determining Chronic Toxicity," *Pharmacological Review* 6 (1954): 191–242. The four-stage sequence of toxicity studies developed by Lehman and Fitzhugh started with examination of the drug's chemical and physical characteristics, and then proceeded to acute toxicity studies (where for instance LD 50 levels were determined), to sub-acute toxicity studies, then finally to chronic toxicity studies. Lehman's notion of sequential experimentation would also become encoded in the vision and preferences of the Bureaus of Pharmacology and Medicine, and would contribute pivotally to the notion of three-phased experiment concretized in federal regulations in 1963. See chapter 4.

For legislative attention to food additives, see *Federal Food, Drug and Cosmetic Act (Chemical Additives in Food): Hearings before a Subcommittee on Interstate and Foreign Commerce*, 84th Congress (Washington, DC: GPO, 1956). These hearings and other initiatives resulted in new legislation and regulations governing food additives, in particular the Food Additives Amendment of 1958 (Public Law 85-929); Lars Noah and Richard A. Merrill, "Starting from Scratch? Reinventing the Food Additive Approval Process," *Boston University Law Review* 78 (2) (April 1998): 329–443. On the demand for data on metabolic rate of drugs in NDA review, see *FDCR*, March 6, 1961, 25. The "Pink Sheet" surveyed many of these new announcements and developments in the spring of 1959; *FDCR*, March 9, 1959, 21 (on delayed-dosage tests, which agency officials declared a valuable addition to their regulatory toolkit); *FDCR*, April 13, 1959, 28; *FDCR* May 4, 1959, 23, and *FDCR*, May 12, 1959, 24 (demand disintegration data in vivo, and in artificial intestinal and gastric juices); *FDCR*, June 8, 1959, 7–9 (demands increased stability data in new drug clearances); Nelson, "New Drug Development," *FDCLJ* 1950, 247.

[17] *Report of the Citizens' Advisory Committee on the U.S. Food and Drug Administration*, (Washington, DC: Department of Health, Education and Welfare, 1955); typescript copy, Folder "Special Data, 1955," 0272-08, Bureau of Investigation Files, AAMA. See also assorted

Advisory Committee on the Food and Drug Administration that the FDA's staffing budget began to increase appreciably.[18]

Pharmacology was not unknown to FDA drug regulation before the 1950s, yet its involvement in the 1930s and 1940s was one of official distance. A Division of Pharmacology previously separated all "pharmacologists" from "doctors" in the Division of Medicine (later Bureau of Medicine). What changed was the merger of a set of new pharmacological practices into what was previously known as "medical evaluation" of drugs. This merger transformed both the status of the FDA "medical officer" and the meaning of applied pharmacology itself. It also reflected ongoing changes in pharmacology at the university level, mainly the emergence of clinical pharmacology (the uneasy merger of experimental therapeutics and the rise of a new science of drug evaluation) and claims from prominent university pharmacologists that the new pharmacology could serve as a "basis" for rational therapeutics.

The late 1940s and 1950s witnessed the slow, piecemeal, and only half-intentional establishment of networks of information exchange, referral, and consultation among FDA officials and pharmacology faculties at university medical centers. The central figures included University of Chicago's Eugene M. K. Geiling, Harvard's Maxwell Finland, University of Utah's Louis Goodman, Louis Lasagna at Johns Hopkins and Rochester, and Walter Modell at Cornell. It appears that Geiling had the most pronounced effect upon hiring at the FDA. Geiling was arguably the most prominent student of John Jacob Abel, and was a leader in pharmacology and toxicology. With Abel he had pioneered methods in the crystallization of insulin. When Abel died in 1938, it was Geiling who wrote his obituary for *Scientific Monthly*. Yet Geiling was better known to the general medical profession as the principal university scientist consulting for the FDA and the AMA in the sulfanilamide affair. For this reason, he was familiar to FDA officials in the Commissioners' Office, familiar to Morris Fishbein and the AMA, and celebrated among applied pharmacologists and toxicologists. And not unlike Abel, whose penchant for training students he took note of, Geiling was a

---

documents from the Citizens' Advisory Committee Files and Other Records, 1950–1969; FRC Boxes 1-6, RG 88, NA.

[18]*Report of the Citizens' Advisory Committee*, typescript copy; F "Special Data, 1955," 0272-08, AAMA. Staffing data from FDA Project data archive, Department of Government, Harvard University; and Peter Barton Hutt and Suzanne White, "A Statistical History of the U.S. Food and Drug Administration, FY1938-FY1990," unpublished manuscript (1992), FDA History Office, Bethesda, Maryland. Charles Goodman, a psychology professor at American University in Washington, DC, also noted that the growth of personnel from 1956 to 1959 created personnel issues at the agency; Goodman, "A Survey of Employee Attitudes Toward their Employment with the U.S. Food and Drug Administration," 1960, in *ICDRR*, 340. By 1962, Commissioner George Larrick would acknowledge that two-thirds of his agency's staff "has been acquired within the last one-eighth of its history"; Larrick to Secretary of HEW, "Annual FDA Management Improvement Report—Fiscal Year 1962," August 30, 1962; *ICDRR*, 398.

skilled mentor whose manner and style were infectious and inspired a quiet devotion from his younger colleagues. His skill and demeanor had placed him at the center of worldwide networks in clinical pharmacology and toxicology. As the director of military radiation laboratory remarked in the early 1960s, there were "no important committees or movements in toxicology" that lacked one of Geiling's "people" on it.[19]

So fluid was the recruitment conduit between Geiling's pharmacology center at Chicago and the FDA that Geiling began to worry that the federal agency would siphon away the quantity and quality of his talent. As early as 1939, Geiling complained to University of Chicago officials that "Only last summer the Food and Drug Administration offered posts to four of our men." In September of that year, the Administration lured away Chicago pharmacology instructor Bert Vos, Geiling's most promising junior colleague and an active participant in Geiling's ongoing research on endocrine systems in whales. What Geiling, his students, and his colleagues offered was a combination of basic medicine, up-to-date pharmacological training, specialty knowledge in toxicology, and professional esteem.[20] And like many pharmacologists of their day, Geiling, Finland, Modell, and Lasagna consulted with the FDA and in some cases often worked directly for the agency. Geiling continued a pattern of "consultancy" with the Administration on matters of toxicology and pharmacology, a relationship that culminated in 1959 with a four-year full-time appointment at the FDA. Geiling's move from Chicago to the FDA in 1959—he took over as head of the new Pharmacodynamics Branch of the Division of Pharmacology—was greeted with HEW press releases, university news attention, and scientific fanfare.[21]

Because Arnold Lehman, Ralph Smith, and Albert Holland were doing the hiring, and because Geiling was an important conduit and reference (and, near the end of the decade, an FDA employee himself), recruitment to

---

[19] John Parascandola, the principal biographer and historian of Abel's influence on American medicine, refers to Geiling as Abel's "protégé" who "worked regularly" with his mentor in the 1920s; *Development of American Pharmacology* 157, n.1, 56, respectively. On Abel and Geiling's research in the 1920s (including that on insulin crystallization), see ibid., 56–61; also B. Holmstedt and G. Liljestrand, *Readings in Pharmacology* (New York: Macmillan, 1963), 333. The central article is J. J. Abel, "Crystalline Insulin," *PNAS* (Washington) 12: 76–80. Geiling's obituary: "Professor John J. Abel: President of the American Association for the Advancement of Science," *Scientific Monthly* 34 (Feb. 1932): 182–86. Kenneth P. DuBois (Director, USAF Radiation Laboratory, Chicago, Illinois) to Geiling, February 26, 1964; B 503518, F "Univ of Chicago," EMKG, Johns Hopkins University.

[20] It was not just the FDA that had Geiling worried. "The passage of the new Food, Drug and Cosmetic Bill, and also the European situation," he wrote, "has caused a considerable increase in the demand for trained pharmacologists, and of course the recent death of both Dr. Plant and Dr. Dawson will leave two professional vacancies." Geiling memorandum to Alan G. Gregg (Rockefeller Foundation), October 24, 1939; Box 33, Folder 12, "Presidents' Papers, 1940–1946," University of Chicago Special Collections. The whale endocrinology research was funded by the Rockefeller Foundation; Geiling to Miss M. L. David, Comptroller's Office, May 6, 1937. Box 106, Folder 13, "Presidents' Papers, 1940–1946," University of Chicago Special Collections.

[21] Geiling's full-time appointment appears to have been arranged by A. J. Lehman and by

the Bureau of Medicine and the Division of Pharmacology reflected the growing field of "clinical" pharmacology as opposed to its "classical" past, which focused heavily upon animal experimentation and applied molecular chemistry. The newer members of the FDA medical cohort held not just medical degrees, but also doctorates in pharmacology or extensive postgraduate training in clinical pharmacology. Geiling's former Chicago colleague Bert Vos was now Assistant Director of the Bureau of Pharmacology. Among the pharmacologically trained arrivals in the late 1950s were John Archer, John Palmer, and Geiling himself. In 1960 and 1961, specialists Christian Wingaard, David Davis, and Arthur Ruskin joined the Bureau of Medicine, and Geiling's students Frances Oldham Kelsey and F. Ellis Kelsey joined the Bureau of Medicine and the Bureau of Pharmacology, respectively.[22]

The shift in FDA recruitment was accompanied by a transformation in the form and practice of pharmacology at numerous university medical schools. One of the cleanest markers for this transformation was the 1955 publication of Louis Goodman and Alfred Gilman's *The Pharmacological Basis of Therapeutics; A Textbook of Pharmacology, Toxicology, and Therapeutics for Physicians and Medical Students*. Goodman and Gilman were enormously influential, not merely through their textbook but also through their prominent research. Gilman was later awarded the Nobel Prize in Medicine (in 1994), and Goodman is today recognized as a pioneer in the chemotherapeutic treatment of cancer. It is fair to say that Goodman and Gilman's *Pharmacological Basis of Therapeutics* was the most widely used and assigned book on pharmacology in the twentieth century. Goodman and Gilman had published the first edition of their textbook in 1941, but the second edition added almost 450 pages of new material, which reflect a stunning transformation of knowledge in the ensuing fourteen years.[23]

PHARMACOLOGY AND THE IMPULSE TO PROTOCOL

Along with a focus on new types of drugs, clinical pharmacology brought to its classical forebear an emphasis on prospective study designs, a study protocol, and centralized administration of experimental assignment. In

Robert Roe (Director, Bureau of Biological and Physical Sciences). Lehman to Geiling; August 28, 1959; EMKG. Roe to Geiling, May 21, 1959; Box 503520, Folder "Personal Correspondence—R," EMKG. On Geiling's appointment, see Folder "Personal Material I"; HEW Press Release, and *JAMA* (10/17/1939), EMKG.

[22]"Summaries of Professional Background of Members of the Staff of the New Drug Division, Food and Drug Administration," in *ICDRR*, Exhibit 32, 193–4.

[23]On the differentiation in the 1950s between "classical" and "clinical" pharmacology, see the perceptive essay that concludes John Parascandola's *The Development of American Pharmacology*, 147–52. Louis Goodman and Alfred Gilman, *The Pharmacological Basis of Therapeutics; A Textbook of Pharmacology, Toxicology, and Therapeutics for Physicians and Medical Students* (New York: Macmillan, 1955); hereafter *PBOT* in footnotes. The Goodman and Gilman volume is still in use in medical schools today. From 1941 to 1955, the size of

addition to these hallmarks of rationalist therapeutics, cutting-edge clinical pharmacology in the 1950s—led by the "Cornell school" of New York's Walter Modell—brought several new emphases and concepts. Where earlier pharmacology studies had examined outcomes using radiology-based measures, clinical pharmacologists now wished to supplement these measures with full "case reports" summarizing numerous measures that were or were not the object of study. Where earlier a centralized assignment mechanism was deemed necessary to eliminate bias from clinical studies, clinical pharmacologists and other "reformers" now focused upon randomized assignment as the cure for bias. And, piqued by the writings of Henry K. Beecher, chief of anesthesiology at Massachusetts General Hospital, academicians and general practitioners alike began to worry about the contaminating influence of placebo effects in human clinical experiments, and how to account for them in medical research.[24]

Like much of the new pharmaceutical world, clinical pharmacology was a set of people and practices that lay at the intersection of the market, state, and science. The emergence of randomized controlled trials as a science began in England, with the trial of streptomycin by the United Kingdom's Medical Research Council as a standard-setting reference point. In the United States, where the term "clinical pharmacology" was first used, much of the early funding for clinical pharmacology units at medical schools came from grants from the National Institutes of Health, and much additional funding came from the pharmaceutical industry itself. The American Society for Pharmacology and Experimental Therapeutics (ASPET) spanned the formally economic, medical, scientific, and regulatory realms. At the same time that Ralph Smith became the face of the American state in clinical pharmacology, Walter Modell, Eugene Geiling, and Louis Goodman (among others)

PBOT went from 1,387 pages to 1,831 pages. From that point forward the pace of expansion was much slower; by the 1990s, the Goodman-Gilman book had been taken over by Gilman's son, Alfred Goodman Gilman, and it numbered just over 2,000 pages. Goodman's exhaustive notes for revision for later editions of *PBOT* are housed in Boxes 11, 20–49, LSG. On concern for case reports and randomization, see Marks, *The Progress of Experiment*, 124, 132.

[24]On the ideas of "rationalist therapeutics," see Marks, *Progress of Experiment*, 124 (on case reports and multiple observable outcomes), 127–32 (on randomization) and chap. 5, passim (on statistics in medicine). Randomization in experimentation possesses its own history and owes much to R. A. Fisher's influence in statistics and his early studies in agronomy. On the evolution of placebo research, consult Anne Harrington's perceptive opening essay of her edited volume, *The Placebo Effect: An Interdisciplinary Exploration* (Cambridge: Harvard University Press, 1997). Among the early articles, see Stewart Wolf, "Effects of Suggestion and Conditioning on the Action of Chemical Agents in Human Subjects—The Pharmacology of Placebos," *Journal of Clinical Investigation* 29 (1950): 100–109; L. Lasagna, F. Mosteller, J. M. von Felsinger, and H. K. Beecher, "A Study of the Placebo Response," *American Journal of Medicine* 16 (1954): 770–9. The most influential publication appears to be Henry K. Beecher, "The Powerful Placebo," *JAMA* 159 (1956): 1602–6. None of the three concepts—case reports, randomization, or placebo accounting—receive mention in the 1941 *PBOT* or the 1947 Oldham, Geiling, and Kelsey volume, *Fundamentals of Pharmacology*. From the period 1955 to 1960, all three concepts enter into the mainstream of the academic literature in clinical pharmacology.

began to represent the discipline. Pharmaceutical companies were adding clinical pharmacologists to their staffs by the dozens. Few if any could match Eli Lilly's expertise. Lilly's pharmacology unit was led by K. K. Chen, an Abel student and former ASPET president whom Goodman saw as "the true elder statesman" of the American Society and who had decades-long relations with university and government scientists. Clinical pharmacology's rise to dominance at the FDA coincided, then, with the development of pharmacology faculties at American and British university medical centers and American, British, and German pharmaceutical companies.[25]

In addition, American regulatory officials kept their eye on legal precedents for the regulation of drug "efficacy" in Sweden and, to a lesser extent, Norway. In these nations, drugs could not be administered without the approval of local boards of health and national ministries of public health. Norway had been governed by national drug legislation since 1928, Sweden since 1934. The Swedish law created a royal Board of Pharmaceutical Specialties. This Board advised the national state and established an official list of "registered" drugs permitted to be marketed. When a manufacturer wanted to introduce new drugs, a manufacturer representative would notify the royal Board, would send a sample of the drug along with details on its composition, accompanied by relevant chemical, clinical, and biological information. The Board's evaluations were based upon efficacy, safety, accuracy of promotion, and limits upon pricing. It was partially with an eye to the Swedish standards that Walter Campbell and Henry Wallace tried to add efficacy requirements to the pre-market review authority of the Administration in 1937 and 1938. The other central precedent lay in the American government's regime for licensing of biologics and vaccines, founded in the Biologics Act of 1902. Campbell and Wallace failed in 1938, but the Administration's hunger for efficacy regulation did not wane. Administration officials continued to study Swedish law, to invite Swedish regulators to the United States, and to lecture audiences on the virtues of Sweden's system.[26]

[25]Thomas C. Chalmers, "Medical Intelligence: Clinical Pharmacology as an Academic Discipline," *NEJM* 270 (3) (Jan. 16, 1964): 140–41. A. Bradford Hill, "The Clinical Trial," *British Medical Bulletin* 7 (1951): 278–82; Hill, "The Clinical Trial," *NEJM* 247 (July 24, 1952): 113–19; Hill, *Controlled Clinical Trials*, Conference of Council for International Organizations of Medical Sciences (Oxford: Blackwell Scientific Publications, 1960). H. Gold, "The Proper Study of Mankind is Man," *American Journal of Medicine* 12 (1952): 619–20. Kenneth L. Melmon and Howard F. Morelli, *Clinical Pharmacology: Basic Principles in Therapeutics*, 2nd ed. (New York: Macmillan, 1978), 7–17. On ASPET, see Louis Goodman to Dr. and Mrs. K. K. Chen, July 27, 1971; Goodman to Chen, January 15, 1963; Folder 19, LSG. K. K. Chen, *The American Society for Pharmacology and Experimental Therapeutics—The First Sixty Years, 1908–1969* (New York: ASPET, 1969). On Chen's career at Lilly, see *The Lilly News*, February 16, 1963. On pharmaceutical company support for clinical pharmacology centers, see Dominique Tobbell, "Pharmaceutical Networks: The Political Economy of Drug Development in the United States, 1945–1980," Ph.D. diss., University of Pennsylvania, 2008.

[26]Philip R. Lee and Jessica Herzstein, "International Drug Regulation," *Annual Review of Public Health* 7 (1986): 218–19. For legal addresses given in Sweden, Denmark, West Germany, and Great Britain, see Charles Wesley Dunn, *The Food and Drug Law in the United States*

There were two crucial differences between American efforts and Swedish efforts. First, the Swedish system relied not upon administrative discretion but upon professional counsel to the crown. The Board of Pharmaceutical Specialties did not continually regulate drugs but instead established an official approved list, or pharmacopoeia. After drugs were registered, they were marketed in accordance with the regulations; at this point, most regulatory authority and activity shifted to local health boards. In addition, the state pharmaceutical laboratory was separated from the Board, whereas investigative and evaluative functions were fused in the United States. The second and pivotal difference came in the centrality of pharmacology in the United States and its relative absence in Sweden. Swedish officials relied extensively upon the pharmacopoeia of other nations, as well as the work of the Nordic Pharmacopoeia Commission established in 1948. The royal Board of Pharmaceutical Specialties did not establish or promulgate standards of drug evaluation and did not demand pharmacological investigations, while the American regulatory system relied heavily upon pharmacology and toxicity. The standards of testing and evaluation in the United States generated real and durable contrasts in regulatory outcomes, contrasts that were visible in food regulation. The FDA required the certification of many more food additives than did Sweden, Germany, and other European countries, and the agency was far more aggressive in excluding commonly sold food additives from its domestic market. Swedish regulatory specialist Ernst Abramson noted in 1954 that the United States was the most restrictive Western country in its regulation of synthetic food coloring, particularly food dyes extracted from coal tar (table 3.2), licensing only nineteen color additives in comparison with the twenty-six authorized by his home country. Months after Abramson spoke, the FDA de-listed several more colors. By 1959, food, drug, and industry watchers lamented that the number of coal-tar-based colors allowed by the agency had fallen to thirteen, with another about to be withdrawn.[27]

(Chicago: Commerce Clearing House, 1955). Another important network of cross-national standard setting came in a pharmaceutical "study group" sponsored by the WHO in 1956; Bernard L. Oser, "The Scientists' Forum," *FDCLJ* 13 (1958): 192–205.

[27] On Swedish reliance upon pharmacopoeia, see Daniel Banes, "International Drug Pharmacopoeia," *FDCLJ* 23 (June 1968): 322–8, esp. 324. The U.S. Pharmacopeia was established in 1906 but from the late 1920s on, FDA officials often regulated drugs independently of it. The coal-tar colors FD&C Orange No. 1, FD&C Orange No. 2, and FD&C Red No. 32 were withdrawn from certification; *Food, Drug Cosmetic Law Reports* 152 (Jan. 11, 1955). The United States was the only country among the four listed in table 3.2 without a certified coal-tar dye for black food coloring. Fritz Eichholtz, "The Chemical Preservation of Foods and Its Importance for Human Health: Pharmacological Comments," *FDCLJ* 10 (April 1955): 206–14; Eichholtz notes the particularly "progressive," possibly "paternal" character of American food regulation, in contrast with that of Europe. See, more generally, Walter Waitz, *Lebensmittelrechtliche Regelungen von Zusatzstoffen in 18 europäischen Staaten* (Wiesban and Berlin: B. Behr's Verlag, 1957). On reductions in the late 1950s, see *FDCR*, November 14, 1960, 8–9.

TABLE 3.2
Variants of Coal-Tar Dyes Permitted in Marketing, by Country, 1954

United States	West Germany	Sweden	Switzerland
19 (13 by 1960)	22	26	28

Sources: Ernst Abramson, "Food Legislation in Sweden," address to the Food Law Institute, 1954; reprinted in *FDCLJ* 10 (1) (Jan. 1955): 18–19. *FDCR*, November 14, 1960, 8–9.

These changes in science and standards cannot be seen as antecedent to changes in drug regulation. Indeed, one of the principal causes of change in academic and research pharmacology was the growing demand for pharmaceutical evaluation, occasioned more than anything else by the gatekeeping provisions of the 1938 Federal Food, Drug and Cosmetic Act and their aggressive interpretation in the 1950s. As the Food and Drug Administration came to evaluate more and more medicines, more and more university scientists and clinicians were pulled into its regulatory orbit. This was not inevitable, but the explicit result of choices made by FDA officials Walton van Winkle, Erwin Nelson, Ralph Smith, and Jerry Holland. Debates about drug evaluation were central to federal regulation as they were central to academic medicine.[28]

The pharmaceutical world of the 1950s United States, then, was one where diversely organized drug firms were producing thousands of new products for "conditions" which were just coming into existence; where clinical pharmacology was splitting more rapidly from its classical heritage; where medicine was becoming more specialized and more dependent upon prescription drugs; and where proving "therapeutic value" for new treatments was essential, but where nobody could agree on one method for doing so.[29]

Administrative practice increasingly reflected the steady dominance of pharmacological principles in the new drug review process. This worked in two ways, one intra-organizational and one inter-organizational. With the Bureau of Medicine, medical officers were increasingly trained in pharmacology and routinely examined reports from the medical and pharmacological literature in their reviews, particularly from the foreign literature.[30]

[28]See for instance the pivotal publication of clinical pharmacologist Walter Modell in 1958, "Factors Influencing Clinical Evaluation of Drugs with Special Reference to the Double-Blind Technique," *JAMA* 167 (Aug. 30, 1958). As I demonstrate here, FDA officials were mandating these features in clinical studies well before Modell's article and other pivotal publications. For an early example of FDA officials consulting academic clinicians and pharmacologists in the review of sulfapyridine, see Marks, *Progress of Experiment*, 83–9.

[29]On the definition of disease as a process contingent upon new drug marketing, see Jeremy A. Greene, "Releasing the Flood Waters: Diuril and the Reshaping of Hypertension," *Bulletin of the History of Medicine* 79 (4) (2005): 749–97.

[30]FDA Division of Pharmacology, "Appraisal of the Safety of Chemicals in Foods, Drugs and Cosmetics," *FDCLJ* 10 (Oct. 1955): 679; Smith, "Food and Drug Administration Requirements for the Introduction of New Drugs," presented at the Symposium on Clinical Evaluation

Second, informal but regular patterns of consultation arose between the Division of Medicine and the Division of Pharmacology and the Bureau of Pharmaceutical Sciences (BPS). So transformative were the relations between pharmacology, pharmaceutical chemistry, and drug review that BPS Director Robert Roe felt compelled to prepare a long memorandum on the subject in October 1958, explaining the new state of affairs. In the BPS, Roe worried, NDA review had been consuming an ever greater fraction of pharmacologists' energy: "the work load in reviewing NDAs has been increasing appreciably both in volume and complexity, particularly in the Division of Pharmacology."[31]

In the 1940s, pharmacology chief Lehman recalled, "new-drug applications were made effective without requiring animal work and no regular review of applications was made by the Division of Pharmacology." With the arrival of Ralph Smith and Ernest Q. King to the Bureau of Medicine, this changed irreversibly. King began to scrutinize animal studies as early as 1954, and to refer new drug applications to the Division of Pharmacology. Pharmacology personnel asked for larger sample sizes in animal tests and for longer periods of administration for evidence of toxicity. An informal pattern of consultation developed, which steadily evolved into a standardized practice.

> Dr. Vos believed that NDA's were first sent to the Division by Dr. Ernest King, and originally this was done primarily to provide the Division with information as to the new drugs that were being produced. In sending the NDA's over Dr. King invited comments. From time to time members of the Division did review and comment on the applications and gradually this developed into a regular routine. Often comments were handled by telephone in a rather informal manner.[32]

By the late 1950s, Bureau of Medicine officials were clear that this pattern of consultation with pharmacologists was an unprecedented state of affairs, but one that was thoroughly entrenched in regulatory practice. One driving force behind consultation was the increasing long-term use of medicines for chronic conditions such as high blood pressure.

> [I]n recent years there have been developed high blood pressure drugs, anticonvulsant drugs, arthritis preparations, and other drugs that are in the category of "maintenance" drugs, to be used over long periods of time—perhaps for a lifetime. These recently developed drugs are obviously in a different category than

of New Drugs, Albert Einstein Medical Center, Philadelphia, PA, April 8, 1959; typescript of address, p. 6; DF 505.5, RG 88, NA.

[31]Robert S. Roe, Memorandum of Conference, Subject "Review of New-Drug Applications by Division of Pharmacology," October 22, 1958; Roe, Memorandum of Conference, Subject "Review of New-Drug Applications by the Division of Pharmaceutical Chemistry," October 23, 1958; DF 505, RG 88, NA.

[32]Ernest Q. King, Acting Medical Director, to Raymond J. Braun, Specific Pharmaceuticals, Inc., February 12, 1954; Roe, Memorandum of Conference, Subject "Review of New-Drug Applications by Division of Pharmacology," October 22, 1958; DF 505, RG 88, NA.

the usual drugs of 15–20 years ago, which were expected to be used perhaps only once or twice in the treatment of a particular illness. The need for information on toxicity and the likelihood of chronic toxicity effects obviously become important in the case of drugs that are to be employed continuously or over long periods. Hence the development of requirements for residue data and more animal experimentation in pharmacology.[33]

It was not simply the pattern of consultation that had changed, but the capacities, methods, and protocols of the FDA Division of Pharmacology. The earlier generation of agency pharmacologists—Herbert Calvery, Geoffrey Woodard, Garth Fitzhugh, and others—were doing quite different studies and were not consulting on new drugs. Hence, the methodological and procedural tools for chronic toxicity and "safety in use" questions being used in the 1950s were unavailable (either conceptually or administratively, usually both) to the FDA Division of Medicine in 1938 and the years immediately following the law. As a result, FDA pharmacologists began revisiting drugs that were already widely sold or that the agency had long ago approved, such as lithium or syrup of ipecac. Lithium chloride was being tried for psychosis in the late 1940s, but was also manufactured as a commercial salt substitute. On the basis of extensive tests for chronic toxicity, physiological distribution, excretion, and other properties of lithium chloride, the agency banned the substance in 1949.[34]

So too, when the Division of Medicine began examining new anti-infective drugs such as those of the chloroquine series in the late 1940s and 1950s, it was often the case that agency pharmacologists had already tilled some of the toughest ground. By the time the new drug application for chloroquine (Aralen) was submitted to the New Drug Division in 1949, FDA pharmacologists had already completed two-year chronic toxicity tests on the compound a year earlier. By contrast, when FDA medical officers examined

[33] Smith, "New Drug Applications, General Principles and Details," December 12, 1952; King to Braun, February 12, 1954; Roe, Memorandum of Conference, October 22, 1958; DF 505, RG 88, NA. Greene, "Releasing the Flood Waters: Diuril and the Reshaping of Hypertension," 778–84.

[34] Jack L. Radomski, E. C. Hagan, Henry N. Fuyat, and Arthur A. Nelson, "The Pharmacology of Ipecac," *Journal of Pharmacology and Experimental Therapeutics* 104 (4) (April 1952): 421–6; Radomski, Fuyat, Nelson, and Paul K. Smith, "The Toxic Effects, Excretion and Distribution of Lithium Chloride," *Journal of Pharmacology and Experimental Therapeutics* 100 (4) (Dec. 1950): 429–44; Radomski's lithium studies entailed much greater reliance on blood analysis and electrocardiography than had previous research in pharmacology. On the basis of Radomski's experiments, the FDA had banned lithium chloride products from the market in February 1949; "The Case of the Substitute Salt," *TIME*, February 28, 1949. In a clear criticism of some tracks in the new clinical pharmacology, Radomski and his colleagues wrote in 1950 that "the history of lithium chloride as a salt substitute is an excellent example of the danger involved in releasing a substance for use on the basis of clinical trials alone without a thorough understanding of its toxicology and pharmacology" (443). At some level, Radomski's research involved the reassertion of classical pharmacology, but in other ways it marked the changing standards of evaluation, particularly for long-term toxicity studies and for blood, absorption, and distribution analyses.

Merck's sulfapyridine in the fall 1938, they were compelled to survey academic and clinical researchers for information about its safety and efficacy. Chloroquine's advance study was uncommon for most drugs at the time—and such in-house scrutiny certainly was not required of NDAs—but it gestured powerfully to the future. With chloroquine as with many other new drugs of the 1940s and 1950s, the FDA's laboratories had carried out more thorough toxicology tests on the compound than had the drug's sponsors.[35]

If FDA officers could write lucidly about the reality of the new pharmacology, they were less clear about its implications. Neither a change in statute nor a change in political direction, but the evolving practice of pharmaceutical evaluation now demanded that new drug applications pass a higher hurdle before market entry. "The requirements for acceptance of NDA's have increased," Robert Roe wrote in 1958. "This change has to some extent been subtle and has occurred gradually as with experience it has been found desirable to ask for more information and additional tests." The typical review "might consume many days of literature research and review by pharmacologists, microbiologists, nutritionists, and chemists, as well as other members of the technical staff." Administrative protocols developed by the Division of New Drugs now specified a new division of labor in new drug review. Not merely a medical officer but also a chemist reviewed the entire new drug application, and active consultation with Divisions of Pharmacology and Microbiology were officially encouraged.[36]

Roe concluded that increased laboratory work was a necessary element of any new drug review. "We are not now doing laboratory work in connection

[35]The two chloroquine molecules cleared by the Division of Medicine in the postwar period were chloroquine phosphate (NDA 6-002, Aralen) which was approved October 31, 1949; and hydroxychloroquine sulfate (NDA 9-768, Plaquenil), approved April 18, 1955. Three years before the Aralen NDA was cleared, FDA pharmacologists had commenced long-term toxicity studies on the drug, albeit in a single species only. Nelson and Fitzhugh, "Chloroquine [SN-7618]: Pathologic Changes in Rats Which for Two Years Had Been Fed in Various Proportions," *Archives of Pathology* 45 (April 1948): 454–62. For the sulfapyridine comparison, see Marks, *Progress of Experiment*, 86–7. Erwin E. Nelson remarked in 1948 that the inclusion of long-term chronic toxicity studies in new drug applications was occasional but rare; "The Federal Food, Drug and Cosmetic Act and New Analgesic Drugs," *Annals of the New York Academy of Sciences* 51 (1) (Nov. 1, 1948): 131.

[36]FDA officials advertised this pattern of consultation between medical officers and pharmacologists to several audiences, including firms, members of Congress, and the Commissioner himself. See Holland's letter to Minnesota Rep. John Blatnik, Chair of the Subcommittee on Legal and Monetary Affairs of the Committee on Government Operations, March 5, 1958; DF 505, RG 88, NA. Roe, Memorandum of Conference, October 22, 1958; Holland to Hart E. Van Riper, Medical Director, Geigy Pharmaceuticals (Yonkers, New York), September 26, 1957; DF 505, RG 88, NA. As Roe saw matters, the new state of affairs was a necessary but painful drain upon the Bureau's resources: "The increased demands and the increased requirements and complexities result in more and longer conferences with drug company representatives and technical advisers, not only after submission of NDA's but even before submission, also. Such conferences have added appreciably to the workload of NDA reviewers." Memorandum from John D. Archer, M.D. (Division of New Drugs) to Larrick, Subject "Review of New Drug Applications," March 20, 1962; DF 505.5, RG 88, NA.

with the NDA reviews to test out or check methods of analysis, etc. We think that this would be advisable and that we should make provision for it in our expanding program." Most of the NDAs routed to Pharmacology were sent to Eugene Geiling's former Chicago colleague, Bert Vos, who coordinated the Division's reviews and checked them for uniformity of governing criteria. Vos' job was subsequently given to Edwin Goldenthal, who was prized for his "ability to make sound appraisal of NDA's and pesticide petitions and successfully deal with industry representatives." Goldenthal's stringency in demanding and examining chronic toxicity tests contributed materially to the perceived NDA slowdown of the late 1950s. A number of new drug applications began taking longer than six months for clearance because of Goldenthal's insistence on longer trials in both animal and human subjects, with monthly examinations of blood and urine and extensive pathology studies upon sacrifice of the subjects. Among these was the anti-anxiety medication chlormezanone (Trancopal) (figure 3.1), submitted for approval by Winthrop Laboratories on April 1, 1958. After Goldenthal expressed his concern about the brevity and weakness of Winthrop's toxicity studies for the Trancopal application—his reasoning was that Trancopal's indications required "long-term therapy"—the company was compelled to conduct new and tightly controlled toxicity studies of a year's duration. Trancopal was not cleared until May 20, 1960, an administrative review that consumed over two years, or four times longer than the statutory limit for pre-market review of new drugs.[37]

As of 1958, the FDA's Division of Pharmacology was consulting on more than 200 original new-drug applications per year. Often the consultations were on the most novel and least studied of molecules. The pattern of internal referencing also extended to the Division of Pharmaceutical Chemistry, headed by Dr. F. H. Wiley, which reviewed about 150 per year. These networks of consultation were administratively indigenous. The new cooperation had never been ordained in statute, in regulation, or in official medical practice. In part for this reason, FDA physicians and others who lacked a doctorate in pharmacology began to resent the dominance of pharmacologists in FDA decision making. John Nestor, elaborating his laments with new drug approval before the Humphrey Senate hearings in 1963, gestured to the dominance of his agency's pharmacologists and lamented that "men trained in other scientific disciplines are not qualified to make final medical decisions." One month later, Robert P. Fischelis, former Secretary of the

[37]Roe, Memorandum, "Review of New-Drug Applications by Division of Pharmaceutical Chemistry," October 23, 1958; RG 88, NA. E. I. Goldenthal to Sandmeyer, April 28, 1958; Sandmeyer handwritten notes, October 2, 1958; NDA 11-467 (Chlormezanone [Trancopal]), FDA. The application was rendered "conditionally effective" but for final labeling and test reports in October 1959. Scientists at Merck also noted the lengthening of required toxicity tests; see "Scientific Operations Committee Meeting Minutes," January 6, 1960 (for sustained-release penicillin); "Minutes," 2/17/1960 (diallylhextrol); Minutes, April 27, 1960, p. 2 (Amprol); FF31, A. N. Richards Papers, University of Pennsylvania.

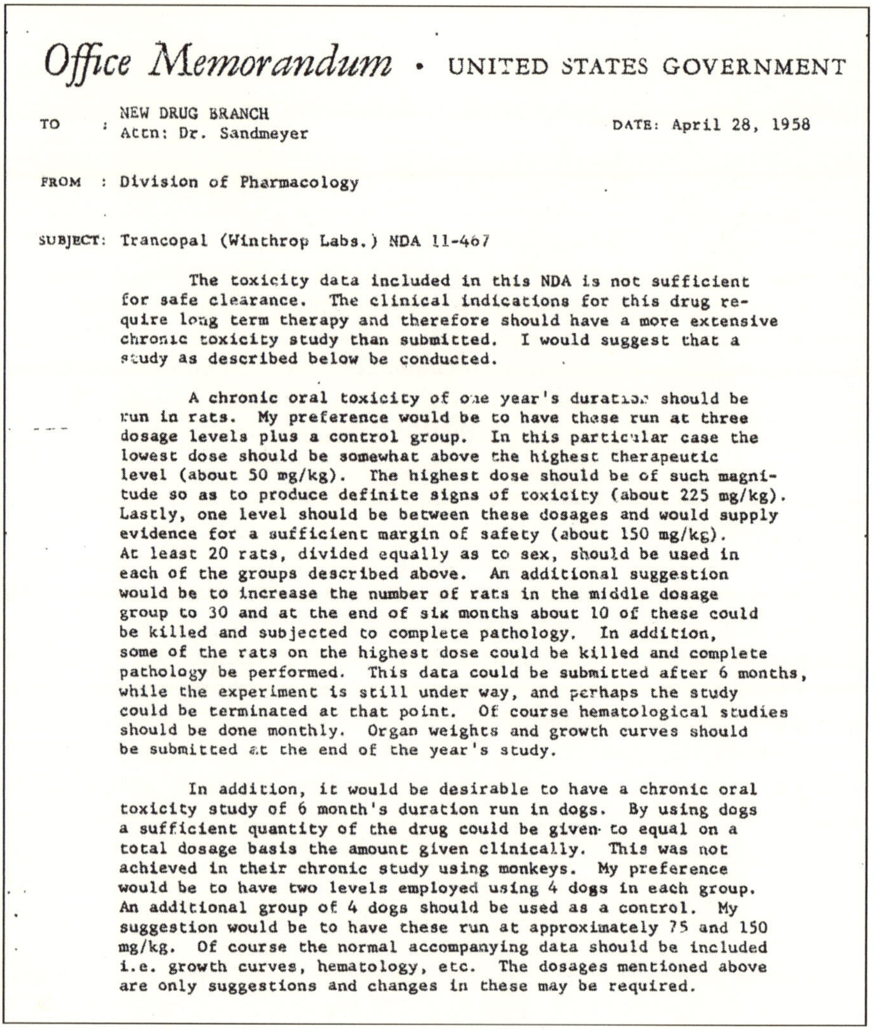

Office Memorandum • UNITED STATES GOVERNMENT

TO   : NEW DRUG BRANCH
          Attn: Dr. Sandmeyer   DATE: April 28, 1958

FROM   : Division of Pharmacology

SUBJECT: Trancopal (Winthrop Labs.) NDA 11-467

       The toxicity data included in this NDA is not sufficient for safe clearance. The clinical indications for this drug require long term therapy and therefore should have a more extensive chronic toxicity study than submitted. I would suggest that a study as described below be conducted.

       A chronic oral toxicity of one year's duration should be run in rats. My preference would be to have these run at three dosage levels plus a control group. In this particular case the lowest dose should be somewhat above the highest therapeutic level (about 50 mg/kg). The highest dose should be of such magnitude so as to produce definite signs of toxicity (about 225 mg/kg). Lastly, one level should be between these dosages and would supply evidence for a sufficient margin of safety (about 150 mg/kg). At least 20 rats, divided equally as to sex, should be used in each of the groups described above. An additional suggestion would be to increase the number of rats in the middle dosage group to 30 and at the end of six months about 10 of these could be killed and subjected to complete pathology. In addition, some of the rats on the highest dose could be killed and complete pathology be performed. This data could be submitted after 6 months, while the experiment is still under way, and perhaps the study could be terminated at that point. Of course hematological studies should be done monthly. Organ weights and growth curves should be submitted at the end of the year's study.

       In addition, it would be desirable to have a chronic oral toxicity study of 6 month's duration run in dogs. By using dogs a sufficient quantity of the drug could be given to equal on a total dosage basis the amount given clinically. This was not achieved in their chronic study using monkeys. My preference would be to have two levels employed using 4 dogs in each group. An additional group of 4 dogs should be used as a control. My suggestion would be to use these run at approximately 75 and 150 mg/kg. Of course the normal accompanying data should be included i.e. growth curves, hematology, etc. The dosages mentioned above are only suggestions and changes in these may be required.

Figure 3.1. Edwin Goldenthal's Halting of the NDA for Trancopal, April 1958

American Pharmaceutical Association, penned an essay with the title "Who Should Decide to Release a Drug?" for the *American Druggist*. Fischelis concluded that "when new drug regulatory control in FDA is finally placed in the hands of the medical profession, the medical staffs of drug manufacturers will also come into their own, because it will be necessary for industry to match medical control with equally competent medical service."[38]

[38] "Sixty to 70 percent of the NDA's received in Pharmacology are referred by Dr. Vos to various members of the Division for study and preparation of comment and conclusions. These are then reviewed by Dr. Vos to see that reasonably uniform and equitable requirements are being proposed by the various Division reviewers." Roe, Memorandum of Conference, October

PHARMACEUTICAL REGULATION, 1944-1961   145

Fischelis and Nestor's rendering of drug approval as a "medical decision" was a re-assertion of professional boundaries, but in 1963 they were too weak and too late to invert a hierarchy that had been fixed. By the late 1950s, it was assumed among leading drug firms and elite medical professionals that drug testing would involve not just any physician, not just any scientist, but a pharmacologist. Leading drug firms such as Lilly, Merck, Sharp & Dohme, Schering, and Hoffmann-La Roche were actively employing pharmacologists in the research and development divisions and aggressively expanding their chemical and pharmacological laboratories. In amplified announcements, companies began promoting pharmacologists and toxicologists to top positions. These firm expansions were not mere exogenous shifts in "research and development," but were in many cases anticipating the changed regulatory and technical requirements for new drug development.[39]

Pharmacology's advance posed challenges and opportunities not just to drug manufacturers but also to American medicine. At the root of both classical and clinical pharmacology there lay a pervasive institutional distrust of the capacities of the mid-century American physician, who was perceived (sometimes correctly, sometimes not) as a general practitioner without any training in statistics, pharmacology, or toxicology. Combined with the chemotherapeutic revolution, the average physicians' incapacity to assess the quality and hazards of drug treatments meant that thousands of new molecular treatments were cascading upon a population of undertrained professionals who did not know how to use and prescribe them. This lack of trust in physician capacity engendered another set of doubts about "the medical marketplace." With their eye on placebo effects, the "dynamic nature" of the "disease state," and the psychological "biases" of the doctor-patient relationship, clinical pharmacologists felt that only long-term animal

---

22, 1958; RG 88, NA. Nestor remarks in *ICDRR*, 781. Senator Hubert Humphrey repeated this concern, ibid., 803. Fischelis, "Who Should Decide to Release a Drug?" *American Druggist*, April 1, 1963; *ICDRR*, 813.

[39] When asked by Colorado Senator John Albert Carroll (at the first Kefauver hearings) what sort of person would perform the testing on a new drug, AMA President Hugh Hussey replied that it "could be done by a pharmacologist working in a university. It could be done by a pharmacologist in a drug manufacturing establishment" (*DIAA*, I, 56). See also Chen, *The American Society for Pharmacology and Experimental Therapeutics*. Among the many pharmacologists and toxicologists rising through firm hierarchies was Dr. Robert C. Anderson, head of toxicology for Eli Lilly. In 1957 Anderson was elected vice president of the AAAS and chairman of its pharmaceutical sciences section; *OP&DR*, February 25, 1957, p. 7. Vannevar Bush advised Merck from the early 1950s onward, and ascended to a leadership position at Merck in 1957; *OP&DR*, December 23, 1957, p. 3. Alfred Newton Richards had advised Merck since 1940. Other moves at Merck were less publicized but just as important; "Merck Elects 4 Scientists to High Administrative Posts," *OP&DR*, May 5, 1958, p. 7.

On plant expansions in the 1950s, mainly for construction of new labs for individual company scientists, see the series of stories in *OP&DR* in the late 1950s: April 8, 1957, p. 7 (Warner-Chilcott); November 4, 1957, p. 5 (Ciba); November 25, 1957, p. 5 (Pfizer); February 24, 1958, p. 5 (Geigy); June 16, 1958, p. 3 (Schering); September 15, 1958, p. 3 (Squibb); October 5, 1959, p. 7 (Norwich); April 25, 1960, p. 7 (Parke-Davis).

studies and controlled clinical trials could permit an accurate assessment of the efficacy and safety of drugs new and old. Hence, their larger point about methodology was strengthened by the chemotherapeutic revolution but was somewhat independent of it. Clinical pharmacology's insistence upon clinical trials and "rational therapeutics" would have applied to any market, no matter how small the trickle of new therapies arriving.[40]

These problems were not ethereal and academic but real and tangible in the FDA's confrontation with a slew of new and largely untested products. As slippery a concept as "efficacy" was, it became all the more indefinable for some of the new products that combined molecules in fixed or variable propositions, such as combination antibiotics. Henry Welch's Division of Antibiotics had been certifying batches of antibiotics since its work with penicillin in 1949 as part of the War effort. As of 1957, there were a dozen antibiotics in regular clinical use, including penicillin, bacitracin, chloramphenicol, erythromycin, neomycin, carbomycin, polymyxin, tetracycline, chlortetracycline, oxytetracycline, and streptomycin. Welch's Division and antibiotics researchers had developed methods for testing the potency of antibiotics in laboratory samples. Yet the emergence of combination products in which erythromycin was mixed with penicillin posed unique problems. How could the FDA determine even the microbial action of one antibiotic if another was simultaneously operative and perhaps conflicting with it? More to the point, how could it be concluded that the combination worked "better"—had more "activity" or more "therapeutic action"—than either of the two drugs alone? Did these products have the jeopardy, as Harvard's Maxwell Finland had suggested in the 1950s, that resistant bacteria were developing more quickly than before because pathogens were exposed to two or more molecules at once? Combination antibiotics served as a metaphor of sorts for relative value comparisons. They led the FDA much more directly and openly into issues of relative safety, relative efficacy, and comparative value.[41]

Organizational Learning through Adversity. The emerging regime of procedural pharmacology in regulation was accompanied by some difficult lessons from the late 1940s and early 1950s. The process of organizational learning that occurred from the late 1940s through the 1950s was in many

[40]Goodman, *DIAA*, I, 243: "That is why experts talk in detail about controlled clinical experiments; that is why the individual practicing doctor cannot be the judge." On placebos: "I could make a fortune and support our entire medical center if I could market placebos, and that is why we have controlled studies" (241). Kefauver echoed the concern that doctors "can't keep up" with the medical literature on new drugs (9). Administration personnel carried this skepticism of general practitioners and preferred that studies in support of a new drug application include specialists; NYAM, Public Health Committee, "The Importance of Clinical Testing in Determining the Efficacy and Safety of New Drugs," *Bulletin of the New York Academy of Medicine* 38 (June 1962): 415; *ICDRR*, 536.

[41]B. Arret, M. R. Woodard, D. M. Wintermere, and A. Kirshbaum, "Antibiotic Interference Thresholds of Microbial Arrays," *Antibiotics and Chemotherapy* 12 (10) (Oct. 1957): 545–8.

ways inseparable from the process by which the Administration's identity was transformed. Along with the arrival to power of a new cohort of regulators, a series of memorable, sometimes jarring interactions between the FDA and drug companies occurred. These episodes upset older categories and shook loose a set of cozy assumptions and relationships. At the core of these interactions were important political, economic, and social lessons about the new world of pharmaceuticals. Established and reasonably trusted firms presented just as much a problem as did fly-by-night operations. NDAs were being abused and the investigational phase of drug development was being commercially hijacked. Drugs were being sold without effective NDAs or in a structure materially different from their approved form. And as FDA officials perceived it, companies large and small were less than forthcoming about the risks of their products and the ways in which they were tested and manufactured.

The FDA had issued six total market recalls in the late spring of 1948, leading one trade journal to report that "Leaders of the Drug Industry have reason to feel disturbed over the flurry of activity being directed against some of its products by the [FDA]. Something seems to have gone haywire in the industry." What made the safety problems of the late 1940s and early 1950s different and troubling is that they were characterized less by the mistakes of smaller drug companies and more and more often by the slips of established and respected pharmaceutical laboratories. A glucose and saline mixture manufactured by Cutter Labs of Berkeley had killed several patients and injured dozens more in four southern states. Abbott Laboratories' "Nembutal" suppositories, used as a sedative for small children, had induced days of sleep by pediatric patients. Abbott had collected data on the adverse events but had not informed the FDA about the problem. For industry observers, the magic purveyed by manufacturers had quickly outpaced the ability of drug firms to deal with its risks, and the FDA was sending a message. "It is apparent," as the *Oil, Paint and Drug Reporter* reported in 1948, "that something has gone wrong and that the Food and Drug Administration expects the industry to take proper notice of it."[42]

D. C. Grove and W. A. Randall, *Assay Methods of Antibiotics: A Laboratory Manual* (New York: Medical Encyclopedia, 1955). For a review of some of the known uses of the various antibiotics available as of 1950, see Henry Welch, Charles N. Lewis, and Chester S. Keefer, *Antibiotic Therapy* (Washington, DC: Arundel Press, 1951). On Finland's cautionary statements regarding antibiotic therapy, see James Whorten, "Antibiotic Abandon: The Resurgence of Therapeutic Rationalism," in John Parascandola, ed., *The History of Antibiotics: A Symposium* (Madison, WI: American Institute of the History of Pharmacy, 1980), 129–130; also Finland, "Clinical Uses of the Presently Available Antibiotics," *Antibiotics Annual* (1953–1954): 10–26; Hobart A. Reimann, "The Misuse of Antimicrobics," *Medical Clinics of North America* 45 (1961): 849–56. For a useful essay that sets antibiotic resistance into a larger public health and medical context and discusses Finland's role in some of these controversies, see Scott H. Podolsky, "The Changing Fate of Pneumonia as a Public Health Concern in 20th-Century America and Beyond," *American Journal of Public Health* 95 (2005): 2144–54.

[42] *OP&DR*, August 9, 1948; RWW, "Drugs Are Not Always What They Seem," NA, RG 88, Accession 54A-477, B11, F7.

Another feature of the emerging regulatory agenda was the twice transformed nature of quackery. Quackery began to explicitly and publicly target much more severe diseases such as cancer for which partially effective treatments had been developed. Whereas prior to 1950, therapeutically useless products were associated primarily with pain medication or mental disease, a number of quack medications in the 1940s and 1950s began to explicitly target tumors, not as part of a catch-all list of indications, but specifically. These included Illinois physician Andrew Ivy's Krebiozen and Hoxsey's Cancer Cure. In the main, these FDA efforts involved the old-line capacities of enforcement and protestation. Yet cancer changed the meaning and stakes of quackery. Regulatory combat with Hoxsey and Krebiozen led FDA officials such as Shelbey Grey, Ralph Weilerstein, Gordon Granger, E. C. Boudreaux, and Jerry Holland to formulate a set of cohesive and structured rationales for why "more products" in the drug sphere did not necessarily translate into greater value or health for the "American consumer" or the "patient."[43]

Perhaps the most startling information came from the Administration's dealings with an established pharmaceutical firm—Parke-Davis and Company—over its antibiotic Chloromycetin. Chloromycetin was approved by the Administration in January 1949 and was one of the broad-spectrum antibiotics revolutionizing infectious disease medicine at the time. Yet Chloromycetin (chloramphenicol) had a little noticed but pervasive and deadly side effect. It induced blood dyscrasia—a "turning of blood into water" that depleted red and white blood cells in many who took it. Affected patients were denied cellular nutrition and could not fight off the simplest and otherwise most benign of infections.[44]

Along with Eli Lilly of Indianapolis, Detroit's Parke-Davis was one of the most trusted names in American pharmaceuticals. The FDA at first reacted

---

[43]For changes in regulatory posture, see Shelbey T. Gray (Director, Division of Program Planning, FDA), "Economic Adulteration and Misbranding: Why the Food and Drug Administration's Regulatory Programs are Restricted," delivered at the 39th annual meeting of the Central Atlantic States Association of Food and Drug Officials, June 2, 1955; Grey to Margarethe Oakley (Bureau of Laboratories, State Department of Health, Maryland), undated; DF 505, RG 88, NA. Gordon A. Granger, M.D., "Unorthodox Cancer Remedies," *Medical Annals of the District of Columbia* 24 (2) (Feb. 1955): 73–80; presented in absentia at the Medical Society of the District of Columbia, October 13, 1954. On the agency's campaign against the Hoxsey Cancer Cure, see William W. Goodrich (Assistant General Counsel for Foods and Drugs, HEW), "Judicial Progress in 1957," presented before the 13th annual meeting of the Section on Food, Drug and Cosmetic Law, New York Bar Association, January 29, 1958; DF 505, RG 88, NA.

Harry Hoxsey, *You Don't Have to Die* (New York: Milestone Books), 1956. James Harvey Young, "The Persistence of Medical Quackery in America," *American Scientist* 60 (3) (May–June 1972): 318–26. Young, *The Medical Messiahs: A Social History of Health Quackery in Twentieth-Century America* (Princeton: Princeton University Press, 1967), particularly chap. 17, "The Most Heartless."

[44]Thomas Maeder, *Adverse Reactions* (New York: William Morrow, 1994); see the chapter "Turning Blood into Water."

cautiously and deferentially to reports of dyscrasias, alerting P-D executives. Yet investigations by FDA pharmacologists, including a separate bioassay and animal experiment conducted by Jack Radomski and presented at a Chicago medical conference, suggested that the problems with chloramphenicol and dyscrasias were much deeper. Larrick joined forces with his pharmacologists and demanded a relabeling of the product, complete with a visceral warning attached to every package. As Thomas Maeder aptly summarizes the "lesson," it was one learned not merely by the Administration but also by its audiences.

> A faint shudder passed through the pharmaceutical industry. As *F-D-C Reports*, the food, drug and cosmetic industry newsletter, also known as the *Pink Sheet* because of the color of its paper, remarked, the FDA announcement implied important developments for all manufacturers. Observers deduced that FDA planned to refine and expand its nationwide hospital survey technique for use whenever reports of serious reactions came in, that the FDA would keep a closer watch for reactions to new drugs, that National Research Council expert committees would play a greater role in the future, and, perhaps most critically, that the FDA would more closely scrutinize New Drug Applications, having realized that drug dangers do not always surface until after the drugs are in wide distribution.[45]

For the FDA's post-War generation, the troubling lessons of chloramphenicol did not stop there. Radomski's work was attacked by Parke-Davis officials and others in Chicago, and P-D executives personally complained to Larrick. Henry Welch—whose judgment was increasingly compromised by his ownership of the journals for which he served as editor—published Radomski's work only after a lengthy delay; he allowed Parke-Davis men a 33-page rebuttal that took just two months to process. In San Francisco, Weilerstein was visited by detail men from Parke-Davis and, in what he described as a "questionable detailing call," was told of "negligible" blood problems and side effects results from chloramphenicol use. The Chloromycetin episode was one of several jarring episodes in the 1950s where Administration officials lost trust in representatives of one of the nation's most esteemed pharmaceutical companies.[46]

The Procedural Recasting of Pharmaceutical "Efficacy"

As the pharmacological regime began to populate and govern FDA drug regulation, its officers transformed the standards by which new drugs were reviewed. The most visible and durable of these shifts was the stable emergence of an efficacy standard in new drug review years before Congress explicitly authorized FDA rulings on pharmaceutical "effectiveness" in the Kefauver-Harris Amendments of 1962. Considerations of efficacy and therapeutic value had been in play since the first drug reviews following the

[45]Ibid., n.41.
[46]Ibid., 215–16.

1938 Act. What changed was the emergence of protocol – a systematic, planned, and sequentially ordered assay of efficacy issues in drug development and new drug review.

Having unmoored "safety" from acute toxicity and "potentiality for harm" in the late 1930s and early 1940s, FDA officials slowly and ambiguously nudged the concept toward the inclusion of "therapeutic effect" issues. This happened in public speech, in administrative practice, and in rulemaking. In 1948, the Administration issued rules claiming that no degree of restrictive labeling was sufficient to qualify inert glandular substances under the 1938 statute. The reason, FDA officials wrote, is that it was "obviously" impossible to write good directions for "safe use" of an ineffectual drug. Combined with new standards issued in 1949 for "proof of safety" by Lehman's Division of Pharmacology, the agency began to develop a procedural basis for the joint examination of safety and efficacy, particularly for drugs used in long-term therapy.[47]

Astride these developments internal to the FDA, the agency received a powerful vote of confidence from the federal judiciary in 1948. In seizing the arthritis remedy Nue-Ovo as adulterated and misbranded, FDA had premised its action upon the company's efficacy claim. Statements made for Nue-Ovo were "false and misleading in this, that such statements represent and suggest and create in the mind of the reader thereof the impression that the article of drug, Nue-Ovo, is effective in the treatment of arthritis, rheumatism, neuritis, sciatica, and lumbago, whereas, the article is not effective in the treatment of such conditions." The defendant drew upon the 1902 McAnnulty Supreme Court decision, in which the Court invalidated the Post Office Department's fraud claim against a magnetic healing company. Justice Rufus Wheeler Peckham wrote for the McAnnulty majority that "As the effectiveness of almost any particular method of treatment of disease is, to a more or less extent, a fruitful source of difference of opinion, even though the great majority may be of one way of thinking, the efficacy of any special method is certainly not a matter for the decision of the Postmaster General.... Unless the question may be reduced to one of fact, as distinguished from mere opinion, we think these statutes cannot be invoked for the purpose of stopping the delivery of mail matter." The McAnnulty decision was applied to drug misbranding in another pivotal Supreme Court case, *United States v. Johnson* (1912). But in 1948, the Ninth Circuit Court of Appeals refused to apply the McAnnulty logic to the FDA. The crucial difference was

[47]On the battle over efficacy in the 1930s, see "Drug Law Tightening Seems Sure to be an Echo of Kefauver Hearings," *OP&DR*, June 13, 1960, p. 3. Van Winkle statement in *JAMA*, December 9, 1944; *DIAA*, I, 76. On the glandular substances rule, see *FR* 13 (March 18, 1948): 1406. See also Charles Wesley Dunn and Vincent Kleinfeld, *Federal Food, Drug and Cosmetic Act* (n. 36), 756–7; cited in Marks, *The Progress of Experiment*, 96. The joint AMA-FDA statement of 1944 reveals one other fact that waned in the ensuing fifteen years—the open cooperation of the AMA with FDA officials in advancing regulation of therapeutic value.

one of the professional and scientific capacity of the regulating agency. Writing for the Circuit, Judge Francis Arthur Garrecht held that "In contrast to the meager technical facilities for the determination of medical questions possessed by the Postmaster General—at least at the time the McAnnulty case was decided—we find that the Federal Security Agency has at its disposal almost unlimited professional resources with which to carry out its investigations in the enforcement of the Federal Food, Drug and Cosmetic Act." In the Administration, Congress had established "a well-equipped Federal agency capable of arriving at a professional conclusion as to the adulteration or misbranding of drugs 'when introduced into or while in interstate commerce.'" The *Research Laboratories* decision of 1948 related not to new drug review, but to FDA enforcement of drugs deemed misbranded and distributed in interstate commerce. Yet in its praise of the agency's capacity and in its direct attack on the question of efficacy, the federal courts had now affirmed the Administration's legitimacy in pharmaceutical matters.[48]

Then, in a February 1949 speech to the American Pharmaceutical Manufacturers' Association, Erwin E. Nelson, Chief of the FDA's New Drug Section, explicitly and publicly deduced that "safety in use" required an evaluation of efficacy. So intimate was the connection between safety and efficacy that, as a matter of good pharmacology, medical investigators and ethical drug manufacturers were now *expected* to assess "efficacy" in their new drug applications and to focus on the procedures by which efficacy could be assessed.

> We believe that an application should contain a sound pharmacological study.... Besides observations in these early studies on efficacy and toxicity, the clinical trials must at an early stage define the procedures to be employed in more extensive studies by those who are chiefly interested in therapeutic efficacy. . . While the fundamental concern of the new drug application is with the evidence for safety, the law also has a requirement to the effect that direction for use must be supplied. And these will have to do with both the safest and the most efficacious way of using the drug. In other words, the reports of the clinical trials will properly include not only observations on freedom from untoward reactions, but also evaluations of efficacy. As a matter of fact few investigators are willing to make studies of safety alone. *Safety without efficacy is of little significance.*[49]

To be sure, FDA officials were often reluctant to speak openly and aggressively about a formal efficacy calculus in drug review. When Winton VanWinkle's successor Robert Stormont addressed the American Drug

---

[48]The Administration's original claim against Nue-Ovo related to its advertisements and the appearance of a claim for effectiveness. *Research Laboratories, Inc., v. United States* 167 F.2d 410 (1948), Ninth Circuit Court of Appeals; *United States v. Johnson* 221 U.S. 488 (1911); *American School of Magnetic Healing v. McAnnulty* 187 U.S. 94 (1902).

[49]Nelson, typescript of February 1949 speech to the American Pharmaceutical Manufacturers' Association; DF 505.1, RG 88, NA. Emphasis in original.

Manufacturers' Association in 1950, he felt that his agency could no longer include explicit efficacy considerations in new drug review. By at least one account, Stormont's capitulation marked the end of the FDA's fusillade for efficacy standards, leaving the battle to other reformers housed primarily within academic networks. Yet from Nelson's February 1949 speech onward, the public wedding of efficacy to safety was maintained even as explicit discussion of separate efficacy standards fell silent. In the procedural regulation of "long-term therapy," chronic toxicity, and "safety-in-use," FDA officials were undermining Stormont's statement in practice even as it met the ears of his audience in 1950.[50]

The Administration's power—and the reach of its Bureau of Medicine and Pharmacology—were also indirectly strengthened by the passage of the Durham-Humphrey Amendments in 1951. The Durham-Humphrey law cemented the distinction between prescription drugs and over-the-counter drugs and gave the FDA the power of "administrative listing" for which drugs were available to the consumer by prescription only. The Act was a defeat for the American Pharmaceutical Association, the dominant trade organization of American pharmacists, and for the pharmacy profession generally.[51]

In the decade following Erwin Nelson's address and Robert Stormont's expression of reluctance, FDA officials in the Bureau of Medicine regulated efficacy through several related tactics. First, they sought to change regulations, and they actively modified the meaning of "safety." These two strategies were necessarily intertwined since rulemaking changes were often founded upon the precedent of administrative practice. Writing to Weilerstein, Erwin Nelson, no longer in charge of the New Drug Branch but still toiling in the Division of Medicine, expressed his intentions to change regulations as early as 1951.[52]

---

[50]Stormont, "Our Mutual Responsibilities in the Regulatory Control of Drugs," *American Drug Manufacturers' Association, Proceedings of the 38th Annual Meeting* (1950), 139–44; quoted in Marks, *The Progress of Experiment*, 97 (n.114). In the postwar period, Marks writes, the Administration's "circumspection" left "reformers" with no other choice but to "turn once again to the profession's scientific elite to take the lead in reforming therapeutic practice"; *Progress of Experiment*, 97. Marks' otherwise fine and detailed research is constrained by two factors. First, he devotes a large amount of analysis to labeling regulations and the prescription status of drugs, generally sidestepping lower-level administrative practice. Second, his narrative seems to peter out after 1950, which is precisely the point at which Ralph Smith and colleagues launch anew their efficacy regulation initiative.

[51]The Amendments appear at 65 Stat. 648, and altered Section 503(b)(1) of the FFDCA. David F. Cavers, "The Evolution of the Contemporary System of Drug Regulation under the 1938 Act," in John B. Blake, ed., *Safeguarding the Public: Historical Aspects of Medicinal Drug Control* (Baltimore: Johns Hopkins University Press, 1970), 160–63. John P. Swann, "The FDA and the Practice of Pharmacy: Prescription Drug Regulation before 1968," *Pharmacy in History* 36 (1994): 55–70. Karin Shieh, "Prescriptive Boundaries: Pharmacy's Battle for Social Control and Professional Authority, 1940–1955," Harvard College Senior Thesis, 2005.

[52]Nelson to Weilerstein (San Francisco District), October 22, 1951; DF 505.5, RG 88, NA. I have not been able to locate the original memo from Weilerstein. Underlining in original.

I want to assure you that the need for certain modifications in the 505(i) regulations has been very much on our minds. Members of the New Drug Section have actually discussed certain proposals with Regulatory Management and with General Counsel....

I cannot go along with the position that it would be desirable to limit investigations to safety alone. In the first place what must be established is not safety in any absolute sense, but *safety for use when used as directed*. In the second place no investigator, or at least very few, is going to use his time and facilities for an investigation solely of safety. Why should he, assuming that he could? The good investigators, on whose reports most new drug applications are based, base their interest in the drugs in the hope or expectation that they will serve a useful purpose, have therapeutic value.

Nelson and other FDA officials intended to communicate expectations to clinical investigators about the need to examine efficacy in their new drug applications. These expectations could be communicated as matters of professional standards and norms of experiment, and outside of the constraints of the law. Yet norms were not the only conduit for efficacy policy. The agency's rulemaking, too, began to suggest a tie-in between safety and efficacy as early as February 1952, when proposed regulations required a complete and documented specification of seven different properties of the therapy and the properties of its "use":

(1) Statements of all conditions, purposes, or uses for which such drug or device is intended by its manufacturer, packer, distributor, or seller, including conditions, purposes, or uses for which it is prescribed, recommended, or suggested in its oral, written, printed, or graphic advertising, and conditions, purposes, or uses for which the drug or device is commonly used....

(2) Quantity of dose (including quantities for each of the uses for which it is intended and quantities for persons of different ages and different physical conditions).

(3) Frequency of administration or application.

(4) Duration of administration or application.

(5) Time of administration...

(6) Route or method of administration or application.

(7) Preparation for use.[53]

As a matter of labeling, drug firms now had to make explicit and documented claims about which conditions would be treated by their products. To this the Administration added an important caveat. "Such statements" as were made on the label, the FDA held, "shall not refer to conditions, uses or purposes in which the drug or device is unsafe for use except under the supervision of a practitioner licensed by law to administer it or direct its use for which it is advertised solely to such practitioner." In other words, some uses of a drug could be safe, and other uses could be dangerous. The relative

[53]*FR* 17 (Feb. 5, 1952): 1130.

character of safety had transited from a concept to a set of procedural recognitions, increasingly enshrined in the *Federal Register*. In the regime of protocol, drug safety depended upon "use," hence upon dosage, prescribing patterns, labeling, and whatever other human elements might mediate between the manufacture of a drug and its use in treatment.[54]

Perhaps no administrative officer in the Bureau of Medicine offered a better public articulation of the safety-efficacy nexus than Ralph G. Smith. In his 1952 address to the American Proprietary Association, Smith offered one of the first and most durable rationales for bundling efficacy to safety considerations: safety could only be considered in the context of dosage. The plant-based "galenical" products of the early twentieth century were characterized by "doubtful efficacy" because they were highly diluted. The medical profession and clinical investigators in particular had since become "more demanding in their requirements for clearly defined efficacious action." For this, "Dosages which produce definite physiologic changes are required and it must be established that these dosages have adequate safety margin with respect to side effects and toxicity." Attention to efficacy was equivalent, in Smith's view, to a detailed analysis of the pharmacological action of the drug, including its composition, its metabolism, its "target" ("the tissues on which the drug has its primary action"), and toxicity. A new drug application would now need to spell out a theoretical mechanism of action, not only chemical but also physiological. This specificity in new drug application requirements—all of it specified through administrative practice later codified in rulemaking—amounted to yet another (indirect) mechanism for regulating therapeutic value.[55]

If anything, Smith felt, the "pure" and "potent synthetic" compounds that had arrived with the chemotherapeutic revolution necessitated even more "thorough investigation" than the generation of therapies that had come before it. In a statement about the centrality of protocol, Smith reasoned that "the process of the new-drug application is an assurance that this is conducted." So emerged a vision of regulation in which the central act, the central document, and the central instrument of force in drug regulation was one of administrative procedure: the new drug application.

Smith would echo these themes with ever greater clarity as his tenure progressed. Three years later, speaking to the Association of Food and Drug Officials at their Atlantic City meeting, Smith argued that safety and efficacy were inseparable in pharmaceutical evaluation. Because "Safety is a relative term," drug evaluators were inevitably drawn into a risk-benefit analysis. "The efficacy or value of a drug is drawn into the general picture of safety.

[54]Ibid.

[55]Smith, "New Drug Applications: General Principles and Details," delivered to American Proprietary Association, December 12, 1952; DF 505, RG 88, NA. Smith, "Food and Drug Administration Requirements for the Introduction of New Drugs," presented at the Symposium on Clinical Evaluation of New Drugs, Albert Einstein Medical Center, Philadelphia, PA, April 8, 1959; typescript of address, pp. 3–4; DF 505.5, RG 88, NA.

The degree of safety must be viewed in light of the value of therapy." This procedural approach to regulation was called for not merely by the progress of medical science, but also by the uncertainty attached to the new generation of molecular therapies produced in the past several decades. "The organic chemist is presenting to the pharmacologist, the manufacturer and ultimately to the physician ever increasing numbers of compounds with widely varying structures and of unknown and unpredictable toxicities." The uncertainty bedeviling pharmacologists and manufacturers was a bare fraction of the uncertainty experienced by physicians, two generations of whom were bereft of pharmacological understanding and lacked training in clinical therapeutics.[56]

The procedural inseparability of safety and efficacy—an inseparability expressed in the requirements and format of the new drug application—persisted for the remainder of the decade. Ralph Smith earnestly repeated the logic in addresses to professional audiences, in correspondence with firms, and in lunchtime conversations with New Drug Branch physicians and reviewers. As Smith admonished his audience at the Albert Einstein Medical Center in April 1959, the known standards of safety and efficacy carried obligations for clinical research in new drug applications, obligations that were not being met by researchers. "Clinical studies with controls are received all too infrequently," which was worrisome because such controls would allow for "evaluation not only of efficacy but of safety and side effects." Smith revealed that his Division officers engaged quite explicitly in the practice of weighing trade-offs between safety and the concepts of "necessity" or "therapeutic value."

> We must decide whether the drug is safe if it is used as directed and provided that the physician has all the information furnished in the labeling. A decision must be made with the recognition that safety is relative. No drug is entirely safe. There are a number of drugs on the market which involves [sic] a definite hazard in their use. In this connection consideration is given to the value of a drug as a therapeutic agent. If it is an agent which is life-saving or if it is palliative in a serious condition for which there is no effective remedy, some degree of hazard can be tolerated, certainly to an extent which would not be acceptable for a drug useful in controlling simple headache or for a cathartic. Between these situations there is a broad field with gradations of necessity and safety.[57]

Smith's language eventually diffused upward, to the Commissioner's Office and the directorate of the Bureau of Medicine. George Larrick, a man

[56]Smith, "Problems Raised by New Drugs," presented at the Annual Meeting of the Central States Association of Food and Drug Officials, Atlantic City, NJ; in *Association of Food & Drug Officials of the United States*, 19 (4) (Oct. 1955): 148.

[57]Smith, "Food and Drug Administration Requirements for the Introduction of New Drugs," presented at the Symposium on Clinical Evaluation of New Drugs, Albert Einstein Medical Center, Philadelphia, PA, April 8, 1959; typescript of address, p. 6; DF 505.5, RG 88, NA. It is apparent from later reporting that by the late 1950s, Smith was one of the most

thought by many contemporaries and more than a few FDA historians to have been intimidated by the pharmaceutical industry, declared, in a 1957 address to the Annual Meeting of the APMA, "Since safety and efficacy are so intimately related, it follows that if the evidence for a new use justifies a major promotional effort, it should also be sufficient for a supplemental application." As with the 1952 rules, then, Larrick wanted firms to provide evidence and documentation for new uses for their drugs, not voluntarily, but as part of the new drug application process. William Kessenich, who took over as Medical Director of the Bureau of Medicine in 1959, amplified Ralph Smith's rhetoric with new aggressiveness. Kessenich admonished industry officials for their "worthless" clinical reports, and called upon firms and doctors alike to adopt a "proper perspective" in promotion and marketing, one tailored not to "the common lure of the market place—financial gain" but to "the welfare and benefit of society."[58]

The notion of "efficacy" and the means for regulating that entity were robustly ambiguous. The battery of terms floating through pharmaceutical regulation—"safety in use," "effectiveness," therapeutic value," "necessity"—were at times equated with the evolving concept of efficacy, but not necessarily so or in a monotone fashion. The trade-off between "value" and "safety" was conscious, but something less than explicit and formalized. The new regulatory posture envisioned a world in which the FDA would regulate not just the market entry of drugs, not just the marketing itself, but the development of therapies in their "investigational phase." And implicit in this posture was the necessity for federal regulators to make judgments about pharmaceutical firms. In one respect, this meant differentiating good from bad new drug applications, and differentiating trustworthy from untrustworthy companies, even though there were no statutory provisions or legal basis for doing so. In another respect, it meant prodding a transformation among U.S., European, and Japanese pharmaceutical companies. In this transformation, the sort of regulatory scrutiny that emergently characterized the Bureau of Medicine would be built in-house within pharmacology, clinical development, and regulatory affairs units placed prominently within corporate structures.[59]

---

powerful individuals in the Administration, in part because Commissioner George Larrick had openly and confidently delegated broad authority to Smith in matters medical and scientific; Nate Haseltine and Morton Mintz, "Safety of Birth Control Pill Questioned: FDA May Ask Study by Outside Experts," *WP*, December 23, 1962, A1.

[58] George Larrick at the Annual Meeting of the American Pharmaceutical Manufacturers Association, May 29, 1957; DF 505.1, RG 88, NA. Kessenich, "The Challenge of New Drugs to the Food and Drug Administration," presented to the Antibiotic Symposium, Washington, DC, November 4, 1959, p. 6; DF 505, RG 88, NA. On Larrick's purported intimidation by the pharmaceutical industry, see Hilts, *Protecting America's Health*, 119–20.

[59] RGS, "New Drug Applications, General Principles and Details," December 12, 1952, p. 8; DF 505, RG 88, NA. FDA officials outside of the Bureau of Medicine noticed that "masses" of efficacy data were accompanying NDA submissions. William Weiss, "Long-Range Planning in the Scientific Areas," attachment to memorandum from BPPA chief Shelbey Grey to "Directors

THE PROCEDURAL UNITY OF PHARMACOLOGY-BASED REGULATION: NDA AT CENTER

Federal officials exercised increasing procedural power over the new pharmaceutical world largely with an administrative instrument: the New Drug Application (NDA) form. Smith, Weilerstein, Holland, Lehman, and Irvin Kerlan saw not a clash between an old regime of inspection and a new regime of pharmacological science, but for the need to fuse the two. The emergent vision of regulation saw the NDA form as the central document of federal control over the development, manufacturing, and distribution of prescription drugs. As it grew in size and importance, the NDA form contained many requirements that the statutes did not, and Bureau of Medicine officials were as quick to include an NDA form in correspondence as they were to insert copies of the 1938 Act and regulations.[60]

In September 1955, the blank schematic for filling out a new drug application—Form FD 356—was published in proposed rulemaking in *Federal Register*. The form had been distributed before, but never so publicly standardized. The form was later revised before becoming finalized in 1956 (see figure 3.2).

In their essence, the regulations of 1955 and 1956 rewrote fundamental portions of U.S. pharmaceutical regulation. Whereas the new drug section of the 1938 Act—section 505(b)—had required a demonstration that drugs would be "safe for use," FDA rules now provided for summary rejection as "incomplete" any new drug application that did not contain detailed, individualized data and a report on "therapeutic results observed."

> An application may be incomplete or may be refused unless it includes full reports of adequate tests by all methods reasonably applicable to show whether or not the drug is safe for use as suggested in the proposed labeling. The reports ordinarily should include detailed data derived from appropriate animal or other biological experiments in which the methods used and the results obtained are clearly set forth. Reports of all clinical tests by experts, qualified by scientific training and experience to evaluate the safety of drugs, should be attached and ordinarily should include detailed information pertaining to each individual treated, including age, sex, conditions treated, dosage, frequency of administration, duration of administration of the drug, results of clinical and laboratory examinations made, and a full statement of any adverse effects and therapeutic results observed.[61]

---

of Bureaus, Divisions and Districts," subject "PPA Presentation at 1961 Bureau, Division and District Directors' Conference," October 16, 1961. "That the drug companies tacitly agree that FDA is concerned with the measurement of efficacy is evidenced by the masses of data they submit to demonstrate efficacy"; *ICDRR*, 374.

[60]Ralph G. Smith to Ivan Merrick (Horrigan, Merrick, Peterson, and Merrick; Pasco, Washington), May 26, 1954; DF 505.1, RG 88, NA. See also the schematic for review procedures sketched in John D. Archer, M.D. (Division of New Drugs) to Larrick, "Review of New Drug Applications," March 20, 1962; DF 505.5, RG 88, NA.

[61]*FR* 20 (175) (Sept. 8, 1955): 6586; *FR* 21 (143) (July 25, 1956): 5578. Paragraph (1)(a) of

3692

Form FD-356—Rev. 1956

Department of Health, Education, and Welfare, Food and Drug Administration.

ORIGINAL ☐ OR SUPPLEMENTAL ☐ APPLICATION

Name of applicant _____
Address _____
Date _____
Name of new drug _____
(If this is a supplemental application see Item (8))

To the Secretary of Health, Education, and Welfare,
For the Commissioner of Food and Drugs,
Washington 25, D. C.
Dear Sir:

The undersigned, _____ submits this application with respect to a new drug pursuant to section 505 (b) of the Federal Food, Drug, and Cosmetic Act. Attached hereto, in duplicate, and constituting a part of this application are the following:

(1) Full reports of all investigations that have been made to show whether or not the drug is safe for use.

(a) An application may be incomplete or may be refused unless it includes full reports of adequate tests by all methods reasonably applicable to show whether or not the drug is safe for use as suggested in the proposed labeling. The reports ordinarily should include detailed data derived from appropriate animal or other biological experiments in which the methods used and the results obtained are clearly set forth. Reports of all clinical tests by experts, qualified by scientific training and experience to evaluate the safety of drugs, should be attached and ordinarily should include detailed information pertaining to each individual treated, including age, sex, conditions treated, dosage, frequency of administration, duration of administration of the drug, results of clinical and laboratory examinations made, and a full statement of any adverse effects and therapeutic results observed.

(b) The complete composition and/or method of manufacture of the new drug used in each submitted report of investigation should be shown to the extent necessary to establish its identity, strength, quality, and purity if it differs from the description in parts (2), (3), or (4) of the application in any way that would bias an evaluation of the report.

(c) The unexplained omission of any reports of investigations made with the drug by the applicant or submitted to him by an investigator he supplied with the drug that would bias an evaluation of the safety of the drug constitutes grounds for the refusal or suspension of an application.

(2) A full list of the articles used as components of the drug. (This list should include all substances used in the synthesis, extraction, or other method of preparation of any new-drug substance, regardless of whether they undergo chemical change in the process. Each substance should be identified by its common English name or complete chemical name, using structural formulas when necessary for specific identification. If any proprietary preparation is used as a component, the proprietary name should be followed by a complete quantitative statement of composition. Reasonable alternatives for any listed substance may be specified.)

(3) A full statement of the composition of the drug. (This statement should set forth the name and amount of each ingredient, whether active or not, contained in a stated quantity of the drug in the form in which it is to be distributed; as, for example, amount per tablet or per milliliter, in addition to a representative batch formula. Any calculated excess of an ingredient over the label declaration should be designated as such and percent excess shown. Reasonable variations may be specified.)

(4) (a) A full description of the methods used in the manufacture, processing, and packing of the drug. (Included in this description should be full information on the following, in sufficient detail to permit evaluation of the adequacy of the manufacturing, processing, and packing methods to determine the identity, strength, quality, and purity of the drug:

(i) The methods used in the synthesis, extraction, isolation, or purification of any new-drug susbtance. When the specifications and controls applied to such substance (described in part (4) (b) of this form) are inadequate in themselves to determine its identity, strength, quality, and purity, the methods should be described in sufficient detail, including quantities used, times, temperature, pH, solvents, etc., to determine these characteristics. Alternative methods or variations in methods within reasonable limits that do not affect such characteristics of the substance may be specified.

(ii) The methods used in processing and packing each proposed dosage form of the new drug, including a description of the container or other packaging material.

(iii) If the applicant does not himself perform all the manufacturing, processing, and packing operations for any new drug substance or the new drug, his statement identifying each person who will perform a part of such operations and designating the part and a signed statement from each such person, fully describing the methods he uses directly or by reference.

(b) A full description of the facilities and controls used for the manufacture, processing, and packing of the drug.

(Included in this description should be full information on the following in sufficient detail to permit evaluation of the adequacy of the described methods, facilities, and controls to preserve the identity, strength, quality, and purity of the drug.)

(i) A description of the physical facilities including plant and equipment used in manufacturing, processing, packing, and control operations on the new drug.

(ii) If the applicant does not himself perform all the manufacturing, processing, packing, and control operations, his statement identifying each person who will perform a part of such operations and designating the part; and a signed statement from each such person, fully describing the facilities and controls he uses in his part of the operations directly or by reference.

(iii) Precautions to insure proper identity, strength, quality, and purity of the raw materials, whether active or not, including the specifications for acceptance of each lot of raw material.

(iv) Whether or not each lot of raw materials is given a serial number to identify it, and the use made of such numbers in subsequent plant operations.

(v) Method of preparation of formula card, and manner in which it is used.

(vi) Number of individuals checking weight or volume of each individual ingredient entering into each batch of the drug.

(vii) Whether or not the total weight or volume of each batch is determined at any stage of the manufacturing process subsequent to making up a batch according to the formula card and at what stage and by whom it is done.

(viii) Precautions to check the actual packaged yield produced from a batch of the drug with the theoretical yield.

(ix) Precautions to insure that the proper labels are placed on the drug for a particular lot, including provisions for label storage and inventory control.

(x) The analytical controls used during the various stages of the manufacturing, processing, and packing of the drug, including a detailed description of the collection of samples and the analytical procedures to which they are subjected. If the article is one which is represented to be sterile, the same information should be given for sterility controls. Include the standards required for acceptance of each lot of the finished drug.

(xi) An explanation of the exact significance of any batch control numbers used in the manufacturing, processing, and packing of the drug, including any such control numbers that may appear on the label of the finished article. State whether or not any of the numbers appear on invoices and describe any other methods used to permit determination of the distribution of any batch if its recall is required.

(xii) A complete description of and the data derived from studies of the stability of the drug. If the data indicate that an expiration date is needed to preserve the identity, strength, quality, and purity of the drug until it is used, a statement of an expiration date.

(xiii) Additional procedures employed which are designed to prevent contamination and otherwise insure proper control of the product.

(5) Three finished market packages of the drug, and other samples of the drug or its components on request.

(When finished market packages of the drug are not available to submit with the application, state that finished market packages conforming to the description under part (4) (a) (ii) and labeled as provided in part (6) of the application will be submitted as soon as available and prior to the marketing of the drug. In case the drug is available only in limited quantity, state the extent to which samples of the drug and its components will be available on request.)

(6) Five copies of each label and other labeling to be used for the drug.

(a) Each label, or other labeling, should be clearly identified to show its position on, or the manner in which it accompanies, the market package.

(b) The labeling on or within the retail package should include adequate directions for use by the layman under all the conditions for which the drug is intended for lay use, or is to be prescribed, recommended, or suggested in any labeling or advertising sponsored by or on behalf of the applicant and directed to laymen.

(c) The labeling on or within the retail package, or a brochure or other printed matter specifically identified on such label or labeling and made available to practitioners, should contain adequate information for use of the drug by such practitioners under all the conditions for which the drug is intended or is to be prescribed, recommended, or suggested in any labeling or advertising sponsored by or on behalf of the applicant.

(d) Labeling bearing adequate information for use of the drug by practitioners should be a part of the retail package of injections and any other drug that may be unsafe for the intended use unless such information is immediately available to the practitioner.

(e) Typewritten or other draft labeling copy may be accepted for conditional consideration of an application, provided, a statement is made that final printed labeling identical in content to the draft copy provided for in the application will be submitted as soon as available and prior to the marketing of the drug.

(7) State whether the drug is (or is not) limited in its labeling and by this application to use under the professional supervision of a practitioner licensed by law to administer it.

(8) If this is a supplemental application, full information on each proposed change concerning any statement made in the effective application.

(After an application is effective, a supplemental application may propose changes. The supplemental application may omit statements made in the effective

Figure 3.2. The Published New Drug Application Form of 1956

The September 1955 new drug rules are generally forgotten now, super-seded as they were by the 1962 Kefauver-Harris Amendments and 1963 Investigational New Drug Regulations. Yet much of what would happen in 1962, 1963, and afterward—the procedural overhaul of American drug de-velopment, the cleaving of research into distinct phases, the necessity of producing data not only in statistical summaries but also in replicable form—was an appreciable echo of the Administration's 1955 rules. Through the new drug application, Smith and his New Drug Branch could now gov-ern clinical experimentation and its reporting, scrutinize the training and fitness of scientific investigators (for both animal and human tests), require that drug companies essentially hand over their data in individual form (so that it could be re-analyzed), require analysis of dose-response functions and blood distribution of the drug, and compel a reporting of "therapeutic results," or, in other words, "efficacy" considerations.[62]

The core differences between the procedural regime of the 1950s and the regulatory activities of the early 1940s emerge most starkly in the contrast of two documents. Before 1955, the most notable attempt to elaborate a vision of regulation and development came when Walton van Winkle, Her-bert Calvery, and Austin Smith published their article on drug evaluation in the *Journal of the American Medical Association*. In December 1944, the rules of the modern pharmaceutical world were issued jointly by medical lead-ers and regulatory officials, and they were published as suggestions in the flagship journal of the world's largest physicians' association. By contrast, the rules of 1955 were published without the official co-authorship of the AMA (indeed, without the official imprimatur of any other professional associa-tion). They were published in the *Federal Register*, the American state's organ of regulatory governance from the late New Deal onward. They were pub-lished in the form of an administrative document, a procedural submission

---

Form FD-356 marks the first time in the twenty-year history of the *Federal Register* that any of the phrases "full reports of adequate tests," "by all methods reasonably applicable," and "ther-apeutic results observed" had ever appeared. FDA officials had used the "incomplete designa-tion" since 1938, but the 1955 rules greatly expanded the set of criteria on which FDA medical officers could refuse to consider an NDA. Of the 13,623 NDAs received by the Administration from 1938 to fiscal year 1962, 2,379 (or 17.5 percent) were declared incomplete; John L. Har-vey (Deputy Commission of Food and Drugs) to Sen. Hubert Humphrey, November 14, 1962; *ICDRR*, 461. The Bureau of Medicine would draw upon the "full statement of adverse effects and therapeutic results" clause as a primary regulatory strategy used to refuse marketing to drugs about which medical officers had skepticism, including Wallace & Tiernan's Dornwal and Merrell's Kevadon (thalidomide); *ICDRR*, 522, 526–7. I thank Peter Barton Hutt for valu-able perspective in developing this point.

[62]It is worth noting, in this light, that the 1955 rules were drafted and the Administration's philosophy was elaborated several years before some of the most influential publications ap-peared calling for double-blinded and controlled clinical trials with a placebo arm as the basis of drug evaluation. Walter Modell and R. W. Houde, "Factors Influencing Clinical Evaluation of Drugs with Special Reference to the Double-Blind Technique," *JAMA* 167 (18) (Aug. 30, 1958): 2190–9.

form whose completion was required for the marketing of a new pharmaceutical commodity. From a medical journal article in 1944 to a proposed rule in 1955, the procedural regime of American drug regulation had passed from rhetorical to the tangible, from the hortatory to the compulsory.

The 1956 rules occasioned much commentary from industry quarters and from the trade press, yet what observers noted chiefly about the new rules were not their statements, but their silences. The ambiguity of the rules became evident on two issues: the lapsing of new drug status and changes to a drug's brochure. On the first, the "Pink Sheet" noticed that the "FDA ducked the question of 'When is a new drug no longer new' in the regs, partly because important segments of the industry opposed spelling out when a 'new drug' is no longer in NDA status." On another issue, however, the agency had sounded a warning to industry. Any change in a drug's brochure that departed from the approved brochure (the one submitted with the original new drug application) could bring a suspension of the drug's NDA.[63]

Regulatory Inspection in the Awkward Service of the NDA. Perhaps the most surprising effect of this new regime was its reassignment of organizational roles. The Administration's field operations staff now oriented their work increasingly to the needs of the Bureau of Medicine, to the lacunae left by staffing holes there, and to the sanctity of the NDA itself. FDA Division officers were increasingly charged with regulating a drug in its investigational phases, to check on the accuracy of information presented in new drug applications, indeed to go beyond the NDA itself. As the FDA's official regulatory program put it, "Since the New Drug Section of the Act places a heavy responsibility on the FDA in evaluating the safety of new drugs, it is essential that investigations be made in the field to insure that the new drug applications (NDA's) are factual, [and] that information pertinent to evaluation of safety has not been withheld." Indeed, because the Bureau of Medicine was "not yet adequately staffed to initiate all investigations desirable at this stage," the agency's regulatory program counseled that "Inspections should not be limited to those requested by the Administration." The field officers were given wide latitude to prioritize their inspections, allocating time and attention to the newest drugs in a firm's pipeline and giving "prime importance" to the composition of the drug and, not least, "its labeling (including advertising)." All of the questions asked of these facets of the drug were premised upon the NDA. Because the revised regulations now required firms to supply "Full reports of all investigations that have been made to show whether or not the drug is safe for use," field officers were now expected to examine all "investigational facilities" and required to "list any experts who are not M.D.'s." In effect, the Bureau of Medicine was employ-

[63] *FDCR* 18 (25) (July 30, 1956): 11. The agency avoided spelling out a formal procedure for the end of an NDA, creating the uncertain state that "there is no way for a manufacturer to know whether a drug is still on NDA status unless he specifically asks FDA"; *FDCR* 19 (38) (Sept. 23, 1957): 13–14. *ICDRR*, 989–91.

ing field officials to regulate investigational drug research as well as advertising. Field officers began to consult with firms on how to complete a new drug application.[64]

The process by which FDA field operations were subsumed within the regime of regulation-by-new-drug-application was not always a smooth one. In March 1954, FDA inspectors descended on the Cincinnati, Ohio operations of William S. Merrell & Co., in an effort to assess quality control. Merrell was, in the early 1950s, one of the more trusted and familiar of firms that the FDA dealt with, both at the field level and in the Bureau of Medicine. Far from being a new or fly-by-night operation, Merrell was closely connected to one of America's oldest and most established chemical companies (Dow Chemical), and included a full array of medical officers and pharmacologists who had regularly appeared before the FDA. In March 1954, however, Merrell officials resisted the FDA inspectors at every turn, blocking access to portions of the plant, refusing to turn over documents on production and quality control, and abjectly declining to give information on the scientific qualifications of Merrell employees. When the inspector insisted that an employee transferring potent drugs from one part of the laboratory plant to another "should be a trained pharmacist," Merrell officials balked at such a brash assertion of regulatory authority over a company's hiring decisions and staffing patterns.[65]

[64]FDA Bureau of Program Planning and Appraisal, *New Drugs, Human Use* (Regulatory Program, Commodity Code 47), pp. 6, 11; March 1, 1957; DF 505, RG 88, NA. The FDA's Division of Field Operations had created a career ladder for chemists replete with a "probationary year," a "broadening period," a "personal development stage," and only then a transition to managerial activity or "advanced investigational activity." Frank A. Vorhes, Jr., "Training of Chemists," prepared for delivery before sectional meeting of the Association of Food and Drug Officials, Philadelphia, May 5, 1949; DF 505, RG 88, NA. For an application of these principles to one firm, see Thomas H. Riggs, "Memorandum of Conference, Subject Glutavene and Glutavene K (NDA 11-616, 11-650, 12-036, 12-037, Inj. 362)" with representatives of Crookes-Barne Laboratories, Wayne, NJ, July 2 and 14, 1959; DF 505.3, RG 88, NA. On field officers consulting activity, see Francis J. Fiskett, "Memorandum of Interview" with Bernard Kirshbaum, M.D., and Joseph DiPietro, Ph.D., Philadelphia, PA, May 23, 1961; DF 505.5, RG 88, NA. These activities partially belie Morton Mintz's claim that "For twenty-four years [after the 1938 Act] FDA failed to decide what an 'expert' is, its principal justification being a reluctance to interfere in the practice of medicine" (*By Prescription Only*, 148).

[65]"I recalled to Dr. Kreider the inspection of the Merrell establishment undertaken by Inspector Charles A. Armstrong on March 17 and 18, 1954, and told him that I had some concern about it. I wished to learn, if possible, whether the manifestations of company policy with respect to withholding certain information were a considered position or whether they might represent decisions of the moment." John L. Harvey, "Memorandum of Interview (Dr. Henry R. Kreider, Associate Director of Scientific Laboratories, The William S. Merrell Co. Research Labs, Cincinnati, Ohio)" (1954); DF 505.5, RG 88, NA. The Merrell inspection was part of a growing pattern of FDA field forces investigating "field issues" with new drug application, including whether pharmacy chains were selling drugs without approved NDAs. See Harvey, Memorandum to "Chiefs of Districts" from "Administration," January 6, 1954, subject "Improper Sale of Prescription Legend Drugs under 503(b)(1)(c)"; DF 505 (also 500.67), RG 88, NA.

The March affair in Cincinnati was an embarrassment to both the FDA and Merrell. It prompted a visit from Merrell's scientific director, Henry Kreider, to FDA headquarters, including a meeting with Deputy Commissioner John Harvey, who had asked to see him. In Harvey's view, Merrell's resistance to the March inspection was upsetting not merely because it interfered with the regular activities of field officers, but primarily because it hindered cooperation between the field divisions and the New Drug Branch in Washington. A significant portion of the inspectors' work was being done in service of the New Drug Branch, gaining information relevant to the review of Merrell's NDAs and determining whether "the obligations assumed under a new drug application [were] being met." In Harvey's view, Merrell had shown disrespect and rudeness not merely to the Cincinnati District inspectors, but to the entire organized program of drug regulation. Fieldwork and new drug review were inseparable, both centered upon the new drug application.

> I told him that I was particularly concerned that inspectors have a full opportunity to see and study the papers and records maintained incident to manufacture of drugs and new drugs, and, in the case of the latter, that they have all opportunity necessary to be fully satisfied either that the terms and conditions of the new drug application were being followed in actual practice or that they be able to ascertain precisely any variations that are being practiced.

A related point of controversy was whether inspectors could see complaints and records of adverse events and complaints from pre-market testing. The FDA had no clear rights to these documents in the 1950s, and Merrell was willing to allow FDA inspectors to see everything in their possession *but* these "complaint files." Kreider's explanation for this discrepancy focused not upon a direct rationale for the proprietary restrictions on complaint files but on a bold interpretation of what the FDA really wanted. Kreider "said that he rather understood from people in the New Drug Branch that we [the FDA] were not really concerned with seeing the actual complaints that were received about a product but more nearly concerned with what the company does about the complaints that they received."[66]

Harvey was rendered speechless by this remark. Kreider's implied claim—that a Merrell official knew the FDA's interests better than the agency's own deputy commissioner did—was a source of genuine "puzzlement" to Harvey, but he was powerless to combat the assertion. He "was not prepared to agree or disagree," and could only promise to contact Bureau of Medicine officials and find out "what our New Drug people had in mind." The awkward exchange showed that, while Harvey and other FDA officials viewed inspection work as a projection of the image and practices of the Bureau of Medicine, some firms were rejecting this equation.[67]

[66] John L. Harvey, Memorandum of Interview with Kreider June 2, 1954, p. 2; DF 505.5, RG 88, NA.
[67] Ibid.

Kreider and Harvey departed from their meeting with "mutual assurances of good will," but the next interaction between officials of FDA and Merrell was not so pleasant. When the Cincinnati District decided to make another inspection at Merrell, they first sent the District's chief, Chester T. Hubble, for a meeting with Merrell officials in August 1954. The discussion quickly turned to the events of the preceding March. Merrell openly defended its decision not to provide "full and complete information," arguing that since its products were in regulatory compliance, FDA inspectors neither needed nor were entitled to more information. When Hubble asked them about the qualifications and training of an employee transferring materials from one part of the plant to another, the men engaged in a "lengthy and heated discussion" over what qualifications Merrell employees were to have, and what say FDA was to have in such a matter.[68]

Perhaps Merrell officials' bluntness was a form of "home style"; the meetings with inspectors took place in Cincinnati on Merrell property. Yet the series of 1954 interactions showed that while Merrell officials were inclined to show considerable respect to top FDA officials and the New Drug Branch, they would display confrontation to field officers. In behaving this way, Merrell and other company officials were differentiating between two organizations (Field Administration and Medicine) and two functions (inspection and new drug review) that FDA officials had procedurally and metaphorically fused.[69]

As Merrell and other companies soon learned, the functionaries of FDA field operations division operated with a new charge. They were not the "rat-turd counters" of lore but medical officers, chemists, and "reviewing officers" as well as standard inspectors. Everything from semi-annual visits to manufacturing control was subsumed into a vision of regulation that was, for middle-level officials such as Smith, symbolically and procedurally unified. After a seminal conference between the Division of New Drugs and the Bureau of Field Administration in May 1961, chemists at various FDA districts were actively employed in replicating and assessing the analytical methods that firms used in their new drug applications. To some degree, the 1961 conference legitimized patterns of consultation that had occurred before, but now field officers and Bureau of Medicine officials (and not least, drug company officials themselves) were consciously aware that the hundreds of regulatory employees outside of the New Drug Branch and the

[68]Chester T. Hubble, Memorandum of Meeting with Merrell Officials, August 6, 1954 (duplicate in Washington office files); DF 505.5, RG 88, NA.

[69]Hubble asked Merrell officials "what was their basis for not desiring to furnish full and complete information, inasmuch as we have examined scores of their products and apparently are finding all of them to be in compliance with the requirements of the act." Hubble, Memorandum, August 6, 1954. Kessenich expressed the same puzzlement when Merrell officials complained of slow treatment for their thalidomide application in May 1961; "Memorandum of Interview" between "F. Jos. Murray, M.D., Robert H. Woodward, and William Kessenich, M.D.Medical Director [FDA]", May 10, 1961; *ICDRR*, 94.

Division of Medicine, and hundreds of miles from Washington, would be involved in the scrutiny of new drug review.[70]

The public face of the agency's legal battles in the 1950s lay in other cases. The endless Hoxsey Cancer cure prosecution and the Tri-Wonda case consumed national press headlines. The tumor therapy of Harry Hoxsey was the preeminent quack treatment of the decade, while the Tri-Wonda case involved a three-drug combination arthritis therapy that had been around since the 1920s. In these cases and others, however, FDA investigators focused on either the lack of a new drug application, the deficiency of the application, or material that was not strictly labeling but which accompanied it. Industry personalities—not just those in the proprietary medicine industry, but those working for large manufacturers—took fearful and sometimes angry notice. When FDA inspectors in 1960 seized vitamin supplements on the basis that material used in sales training qualified as "accompanying labeling," Squibb general manager J. J. Toohy decried the action. Noting that the seizure was based not on identified deficiencies but upon marketing claims, Toohy claimed it was the first such enforcement against sales training material in the FDA's "100-year history."[71]

Behind the limelight of the Tri-Wonda and Hoxsey cases, the Administration was more active in seizing products that were being marketed without a new drug application, destroying the product lines, shutting down the labs and factories used to make them, and (especially late in the decade) pressing criminal charges against the manufacturer. Drug recalls observed a steady pace of about thirty per year, but starting in 1954 they, too, were increasingly concentrated upon products that lacked a new drug application. From 1950 to 1953, one drug—E. S. Miller's "Hormestrin-T"—was recalled from the American market for lacking an effective NDA. In 1954, three drugs were withdrawn for lacking a new drug application, and Lederle Laboratories' "Triethylene Melamine" was withdrawn because Lederle had changed the formula slightly but had not amended its NDA. Then in 1959, the agency took the rare step of requesting an involuntary recall from Upjohn—one of the nation's most prestigious and oldest firms—because its "Kaopectate with Neomycin" product had an over-the-counter label but Upjohn had not

[70]*New Drugs, Human Use*, p. 8; March 1, 1957; DF 505, RG 88, NA. Memorandum of Conference between Division of New Drugs and Bureau of Field Administration; Memorandum from BFA to Directors of Districts, Subject "District Testing of NDA Analytical Methods," June 8, 1961; DF 505.5 (500.31) (651.7), RG 88, NA. On Smith's vision for the incorporation of manufacturing control regulation under a regime of pharmacological guidance, see RGS, "New Drug Applications, General Principles and Details," December 12, 1952; p. 8; DF 505, RG 88, NA.

[71]Ronald W. Lamont-Havers, "Arthritis Quackery," *American Journal of Nursing* 63 (3) (March 1963): 94. The central argument in the Tri-Wonda case entailed the Administration's attempt to limit the makers' claims, especially regarding the efficacy of the three-drug combination in ameliorating arthritis. Industry observers saw the FDA's enforcement initiative against advertising as a novel development; *FDCR*, August 22, 1960, 15. Relatedly, there were increasing seizures of vitamin manufacturers (*FDCR*, Oct. 18, 1960, 25) including Squibb (*FDCR*, Dec. 5, 1960).

yet secured nonprescription status for Kaopectate through the new drug application process.[72]

Regulating Labels and Promotion through NDA Control. FDA medical officials shrewdly perceived another tactic for regulating therapeutic value: control over labeling. Drawing from the older adulteration theory of regulation, a product was held to be in violation of the law if it was misbranded. The connection of misbranding and false labeling with the moral concept of "adulteration" continued through the New Deal and was centrally expressed in the 1938 legislation. What changed was the procedural link between labeling regulation and the new drug application. While they slowly discarded the Progressive talk of adulteration, FDA officials of the 1950s spoke of "truthful labeling" as labeling consistent with the original new drug application. Such labeling was a matter of "responsibility" and "honesty." Backing up this rhetoric, the regulation of labeling (and the consistency of the label and other promotion with the new drug application) quickly assumed primary importance in post-approval activity. Quite "apart from the consideration of inherent safety of the drug," Jerry Holland told a House subcommittee in 1958, "the labeling assumes primary importance to the physician and to his patient." Product labeling was "inseparably linked to safety for it is only through truthful informative labeling that the physician becomes aware of the usefulness, the limitations, and the potential side effects and contraindications to its use." The procedural regulation of the label allowed for the safety-based regulation of therapeutic value.[73]

The expanse and jeopardy of Holland's vision became apparent when he elaborated the totality of information that would fall under the designation "label." Labeling had been defined in the 1938 legislation as "any printed, written or graphic material which accompanies the product." This included the labeling on the retail package and the official brochure, which were "subject to detailed review, sentence by sentence and even word by word, by our New Drug Branch." Yet in Holland's reading, labeling also included "any promotional literature which reaches the physician or consumer in possession of the drug." This included "promotional and educational literature to physicians" as well as "so-called direct mail" to consumers. Even as Holland admitted that his Bureau possessed neither the literal authority nor

[72]Prosecution and other enforcement data from Larrick statement to Kefauver Committee, 1960, Appendix, table 1, "Regulatory Record Since January 1, 1950 on 32 Firms Appearing in the Record of Hearings by Subcommittee on Antitrust and Monopoly," and Table 3, "Record of Legal Actions Involving Composition of Drugs (Control) since January 1, 1950." Recall data from Larrick statement, Appendix, Tables 8–17, "Drug Recalls." Copy of Larrick address and unpublished appendices in Historical Health Fraud and Alternative Medicine Collection, Folder 0273-01, AAMA.

[73]Statement of Holland "Before the House Subcommittee on Legal and Monetary Affairs of the House Committee on Government Operations," February 18, 1958; DF 505, RG 88, NA. Holland's successor William Kessenich cleaved to the same theory of labeling regulation; "The Challenge of New Drugs to the Food and Drug Administration," presented to the Antibiotic Symposium, Washington, DC, November 4, 1959; DF 505, RG 88, NA.

the resources to attempt it, he reminded his listeners of the possibility that all literature sent to physicians was potentially reviewable by regulatory authorities *prior* to its distribution. Gatekeeping authority over drugs might, he intimated, translate into gatekeeping authority over advertising and other forms of firm communication.[74]

Holland's rhetoric soon emerged as a procedural reality. The Administration began modifying requirements for new drug applications, mandating that all NDAs include a finished sample of the drug product along with any brochure. While the Bureau of Medicine could not survey advertising and promotion in far-flung markets, the field enforcement divisions could. With this appreciation of the possibility for field divisions to serve the aims of medical officials, FDA leaders floated new promotion regulations in 1959 and 1960. Whereas the previous requirement for brochures in new drug application was informal, Medical Bureau leaders now supported a brochure requirement in the *Federal Register*, while staff members in the General Counsel and Commissioner's Office were more reluctant. Proposed regulations were published in July 1960, and they met with immediate and detailed complaints. In October 1960, the AMA began asking for a delay in the promotion regulations, and the Pharmaceutical Manufacturers' Association began complaining about the regulations and asked agency staff for modifications. The FDA-PMA talks quickly broke down, however, amid what an industry trade reporter called an "atmosphere of suspicion." Despite repeated AMA calls for further delay in the promotion control rules, the Administration published final regulations in December 1960—the election of John F. Kennedy as president the previous month had eliminated much uncertainty about whether political authorities would support the regulations—and told industry trade reporters of their desire to "make an example" of the first companies that were found in violation. More publicly, new FDA Medical Director William Kessenich expressed a strong view of the regulations and their enforcement. Shortly before Kennedy took office in January 1961, Kessenich reorganized the Medical Bureau into three sections, separating those agents who cooperated with postal enforcement from drug and device personnel. The upshot of the reorganization, as industry observers detected it, was to shift resources and emphasis to the regulation of promotion. The Administration had greatly extended its control over drug promotion, not directly but indirectly, by repartitioning the Medical Bureau and modifying the NDA form.[75]

[74]Statement of Holland, February 18, 1958; DF 505, RG 88, NA; *FDCR*, February 16, 1959, 3.
[75]On the promotion control regulations, see *FDCR*, March 9, 1959, 20. In a speech to the New York Pharmaceutical Advertising Club, Hoffmann-La Roche general counsel Raymond McMurray argued that drug advertising and promotion pieces could now be brought under FDA control; *FDCR*, November 30, 1959, 7. The proposed "promotion control" regulations were published in *FR* 25 (142) (July 22, 1960): 6985–7; the revised rules appear at *FR* 25 (239) (Dec. 9, 1960): 12592–95. Industry concerns about the regulatory initiative were expressed in

It is perhaps tempting to see the FDA's new vigor with drug regulation as a result of the 1955 study of the Citizens' Advisory Committee on the Food and Drug Administration. In March 1954, after several years of budget cuts at the hands of the House Appropriations Committee and New York representative Charles Taber, Eisenhower administration officials lobbied the Committee to have FDA activities reviewed by "a representative citizens' advisory group." Congress provided funding for the Committee in July 1954. HEW Secretary Oveta Culp Hobby appointed the fourteen-member board in the fall, and the committee held its first meeting the following February, issuing its report in June 1955. Well before its report was published and presented to Hobby, industry trade reporters noted that the Committee's basic purpose was less to investigate the agency and more to "provide support for a drive to raise FDA's budget."[76]

The composition of the Citizens' Advisory Committee reflected an exercise in corporatism. The body had representatives from the "fields" of law, courts, medicine, and science, from labor, from "consumers and consumers groups," and from regulated industries. A substantial fraction (six of fourteen) of the Committee's "citizens" were in fact executives from regulated companies—including General Mills, Hoffmann-La Roche, Heinz, American Home Products, and Chanel. The "consumer" voices on the panel could as easily have been labeled women's group representatives: Grace Nichols of the General Federation of Women's Clubs and Catherine Dennis of the American Home Economics Association. The medical and scientific representatives were highlighted by Harry Dowling, a University of Illinois physician with standing at the AMA's Council on Drugs.[77]

The Citizens' Committee did not make headline news, but its report was widely read on Capitol Hill, in the pharmaceutical trade, and in Washington

---

a series of Pink Sheet stories in the fall of 1960; *FDCR*, December 14, 1959, 25; August 22, 1960, 18; August 29, 1960, 11; September 19, 1960, 25ff.; September 26, 1960, 12; October 3, 1960, 7. On the AMA's response and call for delay, see *FDCR*, October 24, 1960, 15–17. See also *FDCR*, October 24, 1960, 18–19 (Smith, Kline & French comments about regulation of efficacy claims for specific diseases); October 31, 1960, 14 ("collapse" of FDA-PMA talks, due to "atmosphere of suspicion"); December 12, 1960, 19, 23 ("making an example," Kessenich's strong view); December 19, 1960, 24 (possibility of indirect control over advertising in medical journals); January 2, 1961, 31 (reorganization). Kessenich appointed Howard I. Weinstein, a thirteen-year career employee, to head the Drug and Device Branch; Denis McGrath served as head of the Branch's Drug Section.

[76] *Report of the Citizens' Advisory Committee on the U.S. Food and Drug Administration to the Secretary of Health, Education and Welfare* (Washington, DC, HEW; June 1955), pp. 3–4; typescript copy in "Special Data, 1955," Folder 0272-08, AAMA. Citizens' Advisory Committee Files and Other Records, 1950–1969; Records Series A-1, E-16, FRC Boxes 1-6, RG 88, NA.

[77] *Report of the Citizens' Advisory Committee on the U.S. Food and Drug Administration*, (n.p., Washington, DC, June 1955). G. Cullen Thomas (Vice President of General Mills) was the Committee's chairman. The Committee also included Frank W. Abrams, retired Chairman of the Board for Standard Oil, and Charles Wesley Dunn of the Food Law Institute, arguably the most distinguished and influential of food and drug lawyers in the nation at that time.

policy circles. Appointed by Hobby and serving the Eisenhower administration, the Committee was seen as relatively nonpartisan though somewhat favorable to the pharmaceutical industry. The principal aims of the report were to describe the agency's meager resources, explain its reduced regulatory activity, and make the case for a bold increase in funding. So threadbare were essential resources, the Committee claimed, that "inadequacy of funds was the underlying cause of almost all other shortcomings." The committee focused most of its energy upon the problem of inadequate resources, and it called for a potential fourfold increase in the agency's budget and legal staff in order to "provide adequate protection for the American consumer." In a statement that was eagerly rehearsed to congressional appropriations committees by Albert Holland, the Committee concluded that "The stature, prestige and salaries of the professional personnel who must bear the burden of passing on new drugs should be increased." The Committee's report noted the weak status of research operations and applied science at the Administration.[78]

The Report's legacy was manifold and paradoxical. Industry observers had noted the Committee's implicit purpose of raising the FDA's budget, and whether the Committee was cause or symptom of the FDA's funding initiative, the agency's total budget multiplied several times over the years following the committee's report. Here the paradox was that many of the new positions accruing to the FDA in the late 1950s were used to strengthen agency muscles that the Citizens' Committee had ignored. Ralph Smith and Albert Holland were using the funds to hire not just medical doctors, but scientists with training in pharmacology and toxicology, and giving them laboratory resources as well.[79]

In reality, the shift toward more exacting and systematic pharmaceutical regulation had begun in the decade before the Citizens' Committee report.

[78] *Report of the Citizens' Advisory Committee on the U.S. Food and Drug Administration* (n.p., Washington, DC, June 1955), 15, 76. Criticism of the 1955 advisory committee was modest in comparison to that directed at the Second Citizens' Advisory Committee, which issued its report in 1962 and was overshadowed by the thalidomide affair, the Kefauver hearings, and the new law. See "Drug Safety," *Consumer Reports*, March 1963, 134–7.

[79] *Report of the Citizens' Advisory Committee on the U.S. Food and Drug Administration*, June 1955, pp. 42, 59. Bureau of Medicine officials eagerly recited the Committee's recommendations regarding "stature, prestige and salaries" in communication with Congress. Albert Holland, Jr., to Minnesota Rep. John Blatnik, Chair of the Subcommittee on Legal and Monetary Affairs of the Committee on Government Operations, March 5, 1958; DF 505, RG 88, NA. "FDA Citizens Cmte.," *FDCR*, July 4, 1955. The boosts in FDA funding in the late 1950s were noticeable, all the more so because Eisenhower's "economy program" meant cuts for many other government agencies. "President Asks More Funds for FDA Enforcement, Control of Pollution, Medical Study," *OP&DR*, January 21, 1957, 3. "FDA's Big Build-Up Program May Be Chopped Down as Ax Swings from Budget Bureau," *OP&DR*, September 16, 1957, 3. "FDA Wins Battle of Budget, Gets Back All of Its Money," *OP&DR*, September 30, 1957, 3; *OP&DR*, January 5, 1959, 3. "FDA to Get $2.8 Million More Next Year," *OP&DR*, August 24, 1959, 5. "FDA in Line for Whopping 16.7 Percent Fund Boost," *OP&DR*, January 25, 1960, 5.

And, ironically enough, the Committee's report provides some of the best documentation of this shift, though the Committee seems to have ignored most of its own data. From 1947 to 1954, the FDA had suffered several unexpected budget hits, not least the chill on agency appropriations placed by Charles Taber in 1952. Yet as the FDA's staffing resources continued their chaotic slide, the agency's legal actions shifted decisively away from food regulation and toward pharmaceuticals (figure 3.3). From 1949 to 1954, the number of prosecutions in drug regulation had almost doubled, from 80 to 152, and the number of injunctions had more than tripled from four to fourteen. At the same time, similar activities in food regulation had been scaled back, prosecutions falling from 256 to 108 and injunctions falling from thirteen to two over the same period. The new vigor in drug policing was all the more noteworthy because the complement of attorneys general had been halved over the same five years. The data on criminal injunctions tell the story most starkly, with the ratio of drug-related to food-related injunctions having been essentially reversed in just seven years.[80]

As the Administration's enforcement arms began to center their activities upon the new drug application, the NDA form itself was strengthened. In new regulations and practices that were announced in the summer and fall of 1960, NDAs were required to include a version of the product (a "new drug sample") at the beginning stage of the application. Abbott Laboratories declared in a filing with the agency that the "NDA sample" regulation departed from the agency's historical policy of "restraint and discretion" in requesting samples from manufacturers at the time of new drug review. The sampling regulation, Abbott felt, also transgressed "beyond the territory contemplated by Congress when it enacted the drug law." The brochure and sample requirements for new NDAs were enforced by the second face of regulatory power; the Medical Bureau simply threatened to withhold approval or delay approval of an NDA to induce compliance. Industry observers noted that most companies were sprinting to ensure that their promotional strategies complied with regulations that had not yet been finalized. Administration officials used the threat of an "incomplete" filing for NDA application to survey promotional material ahead of marketing, to scrutinize product samples, and to compel investigators to disclose "unfavorable" reports from clinical trials and toxicity studies as well as the central data being put forth for approval. And in December 1960, agency official Julius Hauser argued that "good evidence" of efficacy was needed in "virtually

[80]Citizens' Advisory Committee Files and Other Records, 1950–1969; Record Series A-1, E-16, FRC Boxes 1–6, RG 88, NA. The number of attorneys general serving the agency rose from 17 in 1947 to 21 in 1950, then plummeted to 12 in 1954. As enforcement aggregates depended upon both field enforcement activity and legal action undertaken by executive branch attorneys, it is difficult to tie these trends simply or causally to shifts in resource allocation, especially with data so sparse and aggregate. So too, many of the attorneys general serving FDA were housed in the Department of Health, Education and Welfare. Source: Appendix P-1, *Report of the Citizens' Advisory Committee on the Food and Drug Administration*, June 1955.

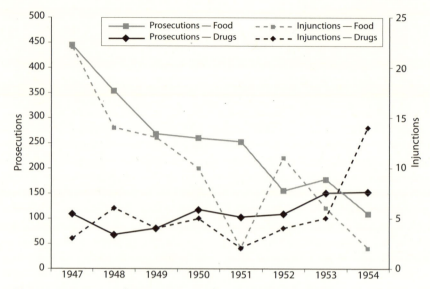

Figure 3.3. FDA Food versus Drug Enforcement, 1947–1954

all" new drug submissions. Claiming his agency's "right to inquire into the efficacy of a new drug," Hauser again wielded the rhetorical threat of an incomplete designation where such "good evidence" was lacking.[81]

The regulatory obsession with new drug applications—their thoroughness, their instrumentality in governing the entire realm of pharmaceuticals—soon made its way to promotion. By no later than 1957, Ralph Smith's Bureau was requiring that *any form* of information produced by the firm about the drug must be consistent with the approved new drug application and the studies supporting it. In the new administrative apparatus, then, the agency's field operations units served as a functional and symbolic appendage to the Bureau of Medicine, scrutinizing labels and advertisements for consistency with the new drug application. Regulatory practice all but required inspection of manufacturing facilities before the clearance of an NDA. And in December 1960, FDA officials quietly let it become known that, absent the explicit written promise that a company would not go beyond the labeling in the original NDA, the Bureau of Medicine would regard an application as "incomplete." As with drugs lacking effective NDAs, labeling issues began to consume a greater and greater proportion of market

[81] On the new NDA form requirements and trade reporters' nervous reaction to them, see *FDCR*, September 26, 1960, 18; October 3, 1960, 8, 23; October 24, 1960, 25; October 31, 1960, 29. Extensive meetings were held between the AMA and the FDA over the brochure regulation, and USP officials offered their services for brochure evaluation; *FDCR*, December 5, 1960, 14. The regulations were delayed, but trade reporters noticed that their principles were nonetheless enforced; *FDCR*, October 10, 1960, 28. On strong firm compliance before regulations were finalized, see *FDCR*, February 13, 1961, 22. Industry officials saw the NDA revisions as connected to the Holland-Smith efficacy initiative; *FDCR*, March 6, 1961, 19; March 27, 1961, 18. For Hauser's statement, see *FDCR*, May 9, 1960, 16.

recalls. Only once before 1950 had labeling-related recalls exceeded 15 percent of the total amount, as low-potency and sterility issues dominated. As the regulatory initiative progressed, the volume of labeling-related recalls doubled from two per year in the 1950–55 period (7 percent of all recalls) to over four annually from 1956 to 1960 (16 percent of all drug recalls). Finally, control over the NDA and control over labeling through the NDA soon brought issues regarding the specificity of clinical tests. By 1961, A. J. Lehman of the Pharmacology Division and John O. Nestor of the Bureau of Medicine had proposed new rules to require "not for pediatric use" labels upon all drugs where the clinical tests did not explicitly examine and support the safety of pediatric dosages.[82]

The realignment of organizational roles even repositioned the "mother discipline" of pharmacology itself. FDA pharmacologists oriented their laboratory efforts toward NDA review. Perhaps concerned that field personnel were conducting work of which his staff was capable, Bureau of Biological and Physical Sciences chief Robert Roe wanted his scientists to replicate and check methods of analysis in NDAs: "We are not now doing laboratory work in connection with the NDA reviews to test out or check methods of analysis, etc. We think that this would be advisable and that we should make provision for it in our expanding program." Roe's proposal—which would amount to an incursion on the turf of the U.S. Pharmacopeia and the AOAC—would become part of the Kefauver Committee's agenda in 1959 and 1960.[83]

. . .

By expanding the uses and reach of the New Drug Application, FDA officials were ensuring that the entire pipeline of drug development was coming under the active and official watch of the Administration. Ralph Weilerstein's vision of the new drug application as a document integrating the entire apparatus of pharmaceutical regulation was beginning to take shape, though not in ways that he had intended or planned. This regulatory outlook allowed FDA officials to engage in regulatory practices that were not statutorily authorized until the Kefauver-Harris Amendments of 1962 and subsequent regulations.[84] The explicit regulation of "investigational new drugs"

[82]Recall data from Larrick statement, Appendix, tables 8–17, "Drug Recalls." Copy of Larrick address and unpublished appendices in Historical Health Fraud and Alternative Medicine Collection, Folder 0273-01, AAMA. "FDA's New Pediatric Look at Drug Uses and Doses May Result in "Not for Pediatric Use' Labeling in Absence of Specific Work," FDCR, September 25, 1961; ICDRR, 973–4. On inspection requirements for NDAs and required promises, see FDCR, December 12, 1960, 25.

[83]Robert S. Roe, "Memorandum of Conference: Review of New-Drug Applications by the Division of Pharmaceutical Chemistry," October 23, 1958; DF 505 (001.2), RG 88, NA.

[84]This is not, of course, to say that the FDA's actions were beyond the bounds of the law. The ability of regulation to incorporate considerations not explicitly discussed in authorizing statutes could have rested within the agency's administrative discretion as intended by Congress. Alternatively, as an executive branch agency, FDA could have engaged in its own construction

and separate phases of clinical studies would come in federal rules published in 1963. Yet it is evident from correspondence and administrative memoranda that Bureau of Medicine officials were consciously using NDA review to regulate drugs in their investigational phase several years before. When confronted in May 1961 with the complaint of a prominent young pharmacologist at Johns Hopkins that the investigational phase of drug development was being "widely abused," Medical Director William Kessenich replied that while the agency had no direct authority to regulate investigational drugs, new drug review did allow FDA reviewers to consider "all the factors which go to make up the value of a study." These included "the design and accomplishment of the protocol," the "thoroughness" and "completeness" of the study, and the "training and stature of the investigator," including the quality of the facilities available. In August 1961, Bureau of Medicine pediatrician John Nestor formally asked Kessenich to change FDA regulations to require inclusion in the New Drug Application of a brief biography or curriculum vitae of each clinical investigator, so that "we can form some idea of the value of his contribution in establishing the safety and efficacy of the drug." Later that year, Deputy Commissioner John Harvey made public the equation that clinical investigators had already feared: regulation of safety and efficacy *implied* the regulation of investigators and their reports. "In evaluating reports of safety and efficacy," Harvey wrote to a Mississippi psychiatrist, "the physicians and pharmacologists of [the] Administration evaluate the qualifications of the investigator as well as the credit and weight to be given to the report." Beyond this, Harvey and his colleagues refused to spell out standards or minimal requirements. In ambiguous response after response, FDA officials cited the impossibility of a "completely precise determination" of what a qualified and competent investigator was. Decisions that disqualified investigators or their reports would continue to flow from the agency, but on a case-by-case basis, and without commitment to formal criteria.[85]

The simultaneous ambiguity and fear-provoking stance of investigational regulation was, in part, FDA officials' manner of expressing and maintaining the agency's gatekeeping role, even as they did not fully comprehend it. The New Drug Application became a symbol of unified regulation, a building block of a new organizational image. The FDA's identity as "protector" (of the public, of consumer welfare, of patient safety) was well and ambiguously established in public and professional audiences. Yet increasingly, the early Cold War generation of FDA officials and national politicians saw the protectorate and gatekeeper identities as one. Consumer protection would

---

of the statute and its powers for enforcing it; Keith Whittington, *Constitutional Construction* (Cambridge: Harvard University Press, 1999).

[85]Kessenich to Fredrick Wolff (Assistant Professor of Medicine, Division of Clinical Pharmacology, Johns Hopkins Hospital), June 23, 1961; DF 505.5, RG 88, NA. Nestor memo to Kessenich, "Change in Regulations to Require Inclusion of Essential Biographical Data of Medical Investigators in Each New Drug Application," August 30, 1961; *ICDRR*, 815. Harvey to A. T. Butterworth (Psychiatrist-in-Chief, The Earl Johnson Sanatorium, Meridian, Mississippi), November 7, 1961; DF 505.1, RG 88, NA.

follow only partially from vigilance and efforts against adulteration. Protection of the consumer, the citizen, and the patient would occur *through* pharmaceutical gatekeeping. As Kefauver casually elaborated the vision in 1961:

> [W]e are confronted with a situation where nobody wants an entirely useless drug on the market that may be actually harmful.... There is a period of testing or experimentation which is authorized, and, after that is over, then comes the test whether a drug is worth anything at all or not, and somebody has to pass on it, or ought to pass on it, for the protection of the public. We set up the Food and Drug Administration to be the public protector. So they pass on it.[86]

Regulation of Clinical Development through NDA Control. The Eisenhower era transformation at the Food and Drug Administration, then, witnessed a fusion of the "gatekeeper" and "protector" roles that had come to the agency from the New Deal and Progressive eras, respectively. The New Drug Application published in 1956 projected this symbolic fusion, as did the emerging population of documents that regulated the investigational phase and established "phases" of clinical development. Back in the 1950s, before the creation of forms for Investigational New Drugs (later called "IND forms"), federal officials were compelled to use the NDA as a blunt instrument for regulating clinical development. Investigators were sufficiently aware of the agency's new posture that they openly expressed their worries that their clinical reports would not be accepted if they did not abide by the letter of the "guidelines" that the agency had elaborated. The gatekeeping role over medical and investigational practice was now legally implicit but politically conscious. The FDA enforcement bureau eagerly and explicitly made examples of firms that distributed drugs without an effective NDA or that commercialized the investigational phase.[87]

Acting Medical Director Irvin Kerlan saw the principle more clearly as his tenure progressed. In 1954, he openly advocated a change in federal rules, one that would allow direct FDA regulation of investigational drugs and that would encourage if not completely require the independent scientific publication of clinical data used for NDAs. But he acknowledged that no such authority was forthcoming soon.

> An additional requirement imposed on the manufacturer is that he submit to the Food and Drug Administration complete reports of all clinical and experimental investigations undertaken with a drug, in establishing its safety, before it is introduced into interstate commerce.

[86]Kefauver in *DIAA* I, 88.

[87]Thomas H. Riggs, "Memorandum of Conference, Subject Glutavene and Glutavene K (NDA 11-616, 11-650, 12-036, 12-037, Inj. 362)" with representatives of Crookes-Barne Laboratories, Wayne, NJ, July 2 and 14, 1959; DF 505.3, RG 88, NA. "The result of these two interviews was to make it clear to the firm that effective new drug applications must be obtained before the drugs manufactured and labeled as proposed can be legally distributed." M. L. Yakowitz, leader in the development of new enforcement strategies at the Bureau of Enforcement, was also present at these meetings.

This Administration cannot require that the reports submitted to us in fulfill-
ment of the requirements of the new drug section of the law be made available in
scientific publications. We would certainly endorse such practices, but this is again
a determination which can only be made by the supplier of the drug.[88]

Administration officials were keenly aware of the vacuum in federal regulations on regulatory method. This was a constraint, but also an advantage.
On one hand, officials could not ask willy-nilly for any test and state unequivocal authority to do so. On the other hand, the lack of regulations meant
that Administration officials were free to develop drug-specific standards for
evaluation of tests. As pharmacologist J. H. Draize wrote in April 1954,
"there are no government regulations, per se, on methods to appraise safety
of individual products. Each new drug application is judged on the nature and
type of data submitted to establish safety for use."[89] The ad hoc nature of
regulatory development imparted discretion and ambiguity to FDA medical
officials. Yet it also left drug research phases (and hence some of the FDA's
.power) vulnerable to those firms bent on hijacking research as a form of
physician advertisement. Albert Holland openly targeted the Code of Federal Regulations for revision.

> Until this Section [130.3 of the new drug regulations] is substantially revised, the
> Food and Drug Administration will not be in a position to effectively regulate
> those firms that commercially exploit their products in the investigational stage,
> with apparent literal compliance with the conditions for exemptions."[90]

The move toward broader regulation of clinical development was spurred
by concerns about exploitation of the investigational stage of drug research.
Bureau of Medicine staff were convinced that firms were commercializing
the clinical testing process, equating investigation with detailing, and distributing their products well beyond legitimate clinical investigators. To many
FDA officials, these patterns exposed a wider problem: the agency's regulatory vision and its gatekeeping power simply did not extend to drugs as they
existed *before* the submission of a New Drug Application. Some of these
concerns were amplified from within; William Kessenich lamented in one
memorandum that his agency lacked "any regulatory program in the field of

[88]Irvin Kerlan, Acting Medical Director, to Austin H. Kutscher, D.D.S., Columbia University, April 23, 1954; DF 505.5 (023), RG 88, NA. Albert H. Holland, Jr., M.D., Medical Director, Bureau of Medicine, testimony "Before the House Subcommittee on Legal and Monetary
Affairs of the House Committee on Government Operations," February 18, 1958; DF 505, RG
88, NA.

[89]Draize to Dr. Albert M. Kligman (Department of Dermatology and Syphiology, University
of Pennsylvania Hospital), April 19, 1954; DF 505.5, RG 88, NA.

[90]"Inspector's Manual 47.0-1, Regulatory Program, New Drugs, Human Use," March 1,
1957, p. 1; RG 88, NA. Albert Holland, "Current Drug Problems under the Federal Food,
Drug and Cosmetic Act," paper presented at the Annual Meeting of the Division of Food, Drug
and Cosmetic Law of the American Bar Association, August 28, 1956, Dallas, TX; Earl L.
Meyers, Raw Material Control in New Drug Applications," paper presented at the Parenteral
Drug Association, New York City, January 27, 1956.

investigative drugs." Yet other worries came from established university medical centers with distinguished pharmacology faculty. In May 1961, Frederick Wolff, Assistant Professor in the Division of Clinical Pharmacology at Johns Hopkins, expressed his worries to Kessenich. At the moment, Wolff thought, the use of these drugs "appear to require nothing but the signature on the investigator's form," leaving experimental drugs vulnerable to "commercial exploitation." Doubts were settling in about both legally qualified physicians and established drug firms.

> In my view, and in that of my colleagues, there is considerable abuse in this field partly due to insufficient information having been obtained by drug houses prior to early clinical trials, or, on the other hand, by physicians not requesting such additional information as should be obligatory prior to giving drugs to man.[91]

Wolff called for Kessenich and the FDA to address this problem via rule-making. Kessenich responded that many would question the legitimacy of the "Federal Government" regulating "who may and who may not receive a drug for investigation." He argued that general rules regulating investigational work would be very difficult to draw up, even more difficult to enforce. But he did offer his judgment that new drug application review would allow for his staff to claim a partial check on investigational work.[92]

Rigor versus Testimony. The sort of evidence that the New Drug Application called for was not entirely clear. As of 1956, nothing in the established regulations for a new drug application required a randomized, placebo-controlled, multi-center clinical trial. As a result, FDA officials found themselves reading documents that bridged (often dishonestly, other times inadvertently) the older patent-medicine world of promotional advertising and the newer realm of sponsored, controlled clinical research. Drug companies sent "investigational" samples of their product to practicing physicians and asked for "reports" of its safety and effectiveness. Among the most common forms of "data" submitted for regulatory approval were the casually summarized notes of physicians that the product "worked wonders" in their patients. The notion of research as "testimonial" came in for frequent and increasingly bitter complaint at the FDA. In regulatory talk a "testimonial" could mean several things, from advertisements to poorly summarized and executed research. What is clear is that FDA staff in the emerging regime of protocol increasingly equated the two. As Smith had remarked to drug firms in 1952, "a great difference exists between detailed reports and a short letter in which the investigator states in effect that the drug has been used successfully with no toxic effects, and that he thinks it should be marketed. The latter is merely a testimonial." Smith's language was repeated incessantly in public and professional fora by his colleagues and superiors, as well as his peers in

[91] Frederick Wolff, M.D. (Assistant Professor of Medicine, Division of Clinical Pharmacology), Johns Hopkins Hospital, to Kessenich, May 22, 1961; Kessenich to Wolff, June 23, 1961; DF 505, RG 88, NA.

[92] Kessenich to Wolff, June 23, 1961; DF 505, RG 88, NA.

university settings. FDA medical officers and university pharmacologists alike increasingly lamented the predominance of "pervasive anecdotes" and "worthless testimonials" in all sorts of firm activities, including supposedly scientific communications with physicians.[93]

The assessment of drug efficacy meant that FDA officials were slowly projecting their own vision of clinical study design onto the development and research plans of drug companies and university academics. FDA medical reviewers in 1960 criticized a company's study of its anti-cholesterol drug for failing to include a "no treatment" arm—the cholesterol might have fallen naturally by virtue of a "regression to the mean," they reasoned, for those with the highest serum levels at the beginning of the trial—and for failing to acknowledge the possibility of placebo effects. This internally conscious drive for protocol was a central concern of officials in the agency's Bureau of Program Planning and Appraisal (PPA), which was the central storehouse of the FDA's statistical talent. In January 1961, PPA chief Shelbey Grey outlined his vision that companies' clinical trial protocols should be vetted and even partially planned by agency medical officers. "The FDA is confronted with the problem of evaluating the efficacy of many new drugs. This can be done only by the conduct of strictly disciplined investigations which have to be initiated and supervised by FDA physicians." Grey worried that many companies' studies were so poorly designed that agency medical officers were "forced to gamble" in their evaluation of "mass data."

Shelbey Grey spoke of an emerging pattern of consultation and facilitation that was already well under way. When the PPA Bureau's William Weiss reflected on the capacities of the agency's drug review division in 1961, he noted that FDA medical reviewers and statisticians had already been assisting companies in the design and execution of double-blinded, randomized controlled trials with a placebo arm. For the handful of cases in which new drug applications were premised upon a blinded and randomized trial, the Division of New Drugs was in the habit of keeping the "code" that dictated assignment of patients to the treatment or control arms of the study.

> The "double-blind" control experiment is a research design that is presently the standard evaluative technique for drug effect testing. For example, in research currently being conducted for FDA, a clinician has received many numbered bottles

[93]RGS, "New Drug Applications, General Principles and Details," December 12, 1952, p. 7. Smith, "Food and Drug Administration Requirements for the Introduction of New Drugs," presented at the Symposium on Clinical Evaluation of New Drugs, Albert Einstein Medical Center, Philadelphia, PA, April 8, 1959; typescript of address, p. 6; DF 505.5, RG 88, NA. Winton B. Rankin, Memorandum of Conference, NDA 12-343 (Parstelin), Officials of FDA and Smith, Kline and French, March 23, 1962, p. 5; DF 505.5, RG 88, NA. Kessenich, "The Challenge of New Drugs to the Food and Drug Administration," presented to the Antibiotic Symposium, Washington, DC, November 4, 1959; DF 505, RG 88, NA. Kessenich's 1959 speech appears to lift a number of phrases and terms from Smith's earlier texts. Louis Goodman would express the same concern about the prevalence of "anecdotal" material in new drug applications to the Kefauver Committee in 1959; *DIAA*, I, 213.

of pills, with the bottles to be distributed to patients selected for a study of claimed appetite depressant. Half of the bottles contain placebos—similar in appearance and taste to the pills containing the test drug. The clinician has no way of knowing whether a particular patient is receiving an inert compound or the drug under test, since FDA holds the key to the code. At the conclusion of the experiment, when the code is broken, the comparison of results for the placebo group and those on the test compound will provide an unbiased measure of the effect of the drug. This research technique is well known and accepted; yet it rarely appears in the studies submitted in support of New Drug Applications.[94]

Reputation and Irreversibility: The Public and Administrative Meanings of Approval. Even as the Cold War regulatory regime codified practice and advanced protocol, it continued to display opacity in decision making on new drug applications. Because FDA decisions to render a new drug application effective had been used for decades by pharmaceutical firms who sought to brandish FDA "approval" as a seal of legitimation for their new product, the agency began to publicly back away from assigning any meaning to its new drug reviews. In correspondence, Smith questioned the ability of his agency to approve new drugs, saying only that distribution in interstate commerce was illegal unless and until an application became "effective" for the product. Hence as Smith saw it, the FDA allowed products on the market but never "approved" the products or the claims made for them.[95]

Perhaps the most salient feature of the new drug review process was the avowed "conservatism" that it embedded. As Smith explained his Division's approach to the American Proprietary Association in 1952:

> [W]here real differences of opinion arise it must be remembered that in allowing a new-drug application to become effective, we also are assuming a responsibility for the safety of the drug. We feel that this responsibility cannot be taken lightly.

[94] U.S. Department of HEW—FDA (Shelbey Grey, author), "10-Year Objectives in Food, Drug, Cosmetic, and Therapeutic Device Protection—January 1961"; reprinted in *ICDRR*, 362. Weiss, "Long-Range Planning in the Scientific Areas," attachment to memorandum from Grey to "Directors of Bureaus, Divisions and Districts," subject "PPA Presentation at 1961 Bureau, Division and District Directors' Conference," October 16, 1961; *ICDRR*, 374. This extensive pattern of assistance was made possible in part by the expansion of scientific personnel at the agency; according to Grey's report, the FDA's research budget grew from $1.051M to $2.962M from 1957 to 1961, and the number of research positions grew from 155 to 331; *ICDRR*, 361. On a related expansion of pharmacology lab facilities, which FDA officials undertook with the express purpose of revisiting and possibly revoking the approval of previously approved drugs, see *FDCR*, August 16, 1960, 21.

[95] A series of administrative decisions in 1954 by Ralph Smith, then the Acting Medical Director of the Bureau, had reshaped the NDA form. The Division's NDA form required "data derived from studies of the stability of the drug" and a proposed expiration date. Smith to Ivan Merrick (Horrigan, Merrick, Peterson & Merrick), Pasco, Washington; May 26, 1954; Smith to J. Berk (Bryant Pharmaceutical Corp.), New York; June 24, 1954; DF 505.1, RG 88, NA. Smith, "Food and Drug Administration Requirements for the Introduction of New Drugs," presented at the Symposium on Clinical Evaluation of New Drugs, Albert Einstein Medical Center, Philadelphia, PA, April 8, 1959; typescript of address, p. 6; DF 505.5, RG 88, NA.

Naturally this results in a conservative attitude which at times the applicant may consider unwarranted. However, the mistakes which we make on the side of liberality and the criticism to which we are consequently subjected does not tend to make us less exacting.[96]

In the New Drug Branch as Ralph Smith perceived it, medical reviewers and regulators lay claim to a sense of ownership over an approved drug. Drug approval was, in Smith's vision, an irreversible decision in two dimensions. One of these dimensions was ethical; the FDA assumed responsibility for the safety of a drug once it was approved. A second was related but more explicitly political. Even in 1952, Smith hinted, his office could face criticism for approving a drug later shown to be unsafe. That the New Drug Branch's response to such criticism was to err more on the side of procedural conservatism was a practice that Smith openly acknowledged and defended. "In the conduct of investigations to determine the relative safety of a drug coincident with the preparation of a new-drug application," he noted, "many applicants with a background of experience may be, on the whole, just as demanding as the Administration. In other instances, however, applications on first submission are found to be incomplete or inadequate. The possibility of certain hazards may not be realized by the applicant, or he may feel justified in making certain assumptions which we are unwilling to make."[97]

Ralph Smith's rhetoric revealed a much deeper and ongoing pattern of deliberation with new drug applications. At about the same time as Smith and his colleagues released the new drug regulations and their embedded NDA form in 1955, the distribution of approval times began to look quite different from the steady and predictable world that characterized the agency work from 1939 to the early 1950s. The slow (and at its time, nearly imperceptible) shift can be seen retrospectively in figure 3.4. For each year from 1950 to 1964, figure 3.4 displays different "quantiles" of the approval time distribution for new molecular entities—novel molecules never before seen in drugs marketed in the United States, either alone or in combination—submitted to the FDA in that year. The first quartile represents the time (in months) at which 25 percent of the drugs submitted in that year are approved, the median the time at which half of the drugs are approved.

[96]RGS, "New Drug Applications: General Principles and Details" (p. 4) delivered to American Proprietary Association, December 12, 1952; DF 505, RG 88, NA.

[97]Smith, address to the American Proprietary Association, 1952, p. 4. Smith, "Food and Drug Administration Requirements for the Introduction of New Drugs," presented at the Symposium on Clinical Evaluation of New Drugs, Albert Einstein Medical Center, Philadelphia, PA, April 8, 1959; typescript of address, pp. 4–5; DF 505.5, RG 88, NA. A New York Academy of Medicine report would also underscore the frequency with which NDAs were incomplete; NYAM, Public Health Committee, "The Importance of Clinical Testing in Determining the Efficacy and Safety of New Drugs," *Bulletin of the New York Academy of Medicine* 38 (June 1962): 415. Relatedly, industry observers noted that by 1961, in a development they saw as novel, two FDA medical reviewers were regularly checking every NDA review, reviewing not only the drug application but also each other's work; *FDCR*, February 20, 1961, 23.

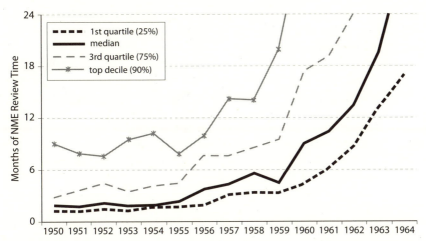

Figure 3.4. Quantiles of the Approval Time Distribution for New Molecular Entities, 1950–1964 (by year of submission)

Until 1954, the first quartile had never exceeded two months, but from 1955 to 1960 (all years before the thalidomide episode) it rose steadily to over four months. Put differently, as of 1960, fully three-quarters of all drugs could be expected to last more than four months in the FDA's new drug review process.

The trends in median and upper quantiles suggest that, with selected therapies, FDA officials were taking the discretion to give much more detailed and elaborate scrutiny to some new drugs. From 1950 through 1954, the median review time was two months or less, and the third quartile (the time at which 75 percent of drugs submitted were approved) was four months or less. From 1955 to 1959—years in which the FDA's staff was growing rapidly—both of these quantiles doubled, the median rising to four and one-half months, the third quartile to over nine months. And the outer tail of the review time distribution was exploding, from an average of eight months in the 1950–54 period to a year and a half or more by 1959. During this entire stretch of time the statutory deadline for new drug review—beyond which point the agency was supposed to request an extension—remained at six months.

Which drugs were receiving more elaborate scrutiny? Examining the twenty-two molecules submitted in 1957 and 1958 that took a year or more to approve reveals some surprising patterns. For one, prominent and larger firms were well-represented in this sample, including Pfizer, whose Visine solution took over thirteen months to approve, and Smith, Kline & French (whose allergic rhinitis remedy Temaril took twenty-two months to approve). Even trusted industry regulars such as Eli Lilly (Brevital Sodium; 24.6 months) and Parke-Davis (Petritrate SA; 28 months) could not escape a delay of greater than two years in the NDA process for their submitted products. Year-long delays for arrhythmia medicine—Abbott's Endrate (edentate sodium) and Purdue Frederick's Cardiquin (quinidine polygalac-turonate)—were quite common.[98]

As the distribution of new drug review changed, so did its behavioral structure. The review process quietly incorporated a time of reading and reflection during the first few months of a drug's submission, during which medical officers would consult the medical and pharmacological literatures widely (usually in many languages). If the drug was approved overseas, they would assess medical reports of any hazards associated with its use. As a result, the cycle of approval resembled less a process of rubber stamping and more and more a process of learning where the Bureau of Medicine's "ownership" of a new drug and irreversibility of its approval decisions were clear.

The change in the structure of FDA review behavior can be represented statistically and graphically using an intuitive statistical technique that com-pares the structure of the review cycle for different "periods" or "regimes." Figure 3.5 displays approval hazard ratios retrieved from a flexible statisti-cal model of drug approval times. In each month of the review cycle, the hazard rate is the conditional probability of approval in that month, given no approval to date. The approval hazard ratio is then the ratio of hazard in the selected month of review, divided by the average hazard for all drugs in all months, where the "average hazard" is determined by the full comple-ment of variables in the model. In figure 3.5, the approval hazard is listed (in solid lines) for the period 1950–55, the period 1956–61 (before the Kefau-ver amendments and the thalidomide episode), and the period 1962–68. Confidence intervals are represented by "minus signs" for lower intervals and "plus" signs for upper. The approval hazard ratio can be interpreted as a multiplier, or a number by which the general rate of approval is multiplied during the month of the review cycle in question.[99]

Beginning in 1955 and 1956, the chances of extremely quick review (an approval in the first several months of the review cycle) plummeted. From approval hazard ratios of 10.6, 7.0, 4.0, 4.4, and 6.0 in the first five months

[98]At Merck's Scientific Operations Committee, advisers noticed that Canada had become quicker in new drug clearance than the FDA. See the discussion of Amprol in "Scientific Op-erations Committee Meeting Minutes," May 18, 1960, p. 2: FF31, Alfred Newton Richards Papers (UPT50/R514), University of Pennsylvania.

[99]Specifically, the model whose estimates are reported in figure 3.5) is a Cox proportional hazards regression of the new molecular entity approval time (in months) upon the aggregate staff of the Division/Bureau of Medicine in the year in which the drug was submitted, a battery of review-month-specific indicator variables, and a "frailty" (or "random effect") term that specifies a different distribution for each group of drugs that target a different disease (techni-cally, a different primary indication). The frailty distribution is assumed to be a gamma distri-bution with mean one, hence it enters the model multiplicatively. The basic structure of the estimator is reported in Terry M. Therneau and Patricia M. Gramsch, *Analysis of Survival Data: Extending the Cox Model* (New York: Wiley, 2002). I estimated all Cox models in S-Plus version 6.2.

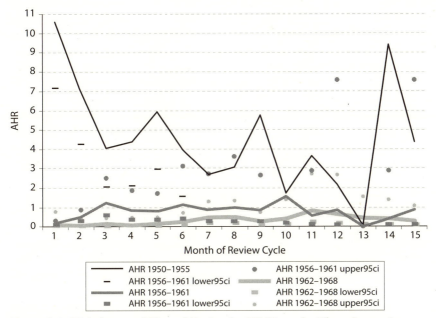

Figure 3.5. FDA Approval Hazard Ratios for NMEs under Three Successive Regimes, 1950–1968

of the review cycle for the 1950–55 period, the ratios for the same five months of the review cycle in the 1956–61 period fell to 0.2, 0.5, 1.2, 0.8, and 0.8, respectively. In other words, whereas approvals were more likely in the earliest months of the review cycle in the 1950–55 period, they were specifically less likely during the same months of the review cycle from 1956 to 1961. Quick reviews became scarce, and new drug approval was increasingly characterized by a "waiting period" in the first moments of the process.[100]

The estimates also show that a further deceleration of review occurred from 1962 onward, a slowing impelled by the thalidomide example, by changes at the FDA, and by statutory reforms. Yet when the approval hazard ratios for the first two months of the review cycle are compared for the 1956–61 and 1962–68 period, there is no statistically detectable difference. In other words, there is no statistical evidence that the approval rate in the

[100] A crucial feature of the statistical technique employed is that the month-specific approval hazards of the different regimes (1950–55, 1956–61, and 1962–68) are estimated jointly. Hence, the approval hazards for different months can be compared within regimes and, more importantly, across them, using a chi-squared statistic. Comparing the AHR for the first month of the cycle for the 1950–55 period and the AHR for the first month of the review cycle for the 1956–61 period yields a chi-squared value of 102.3 ($p < 0.0001$). The AHR for the second cycle month for the 1950–55 period and the AHR for the second cycle month of the 1956–61 period $\chi^2 = 30.9$; $p < 0.0001$), and similar differences hold for the third $\chi^2 = 4.26$; $p = 0.0391$), fourth $\chi^2 = 6.65$; $p = 0.0099$), and fifth $\chi^2 = 9.62$; $p = 0.0019$).

first few months of the review cycle slowed after 1961, relative to the previous six years. What this means is that the FDA's behavioral shift toward the scarcity of quick review occurred not with thalidomide, but in fact five years before thalidomide was even submitted.[101]

These patterns were not lost on industry observers, but they were variably interpreted. Tracker Paul DeHaen told an October 1960 meeting of the Parenteral Drug Association that the agency's "NDA slowdown" was a "principal factor" in the reduction of single chemical entities reaching the market in 1959 and 1960. Pointing as much to pharmacology chief Arnold Lehman as to the Division of Medicine, DeHaen in particular argued that the FDA had "stiffened its requirements for data on toxicity studies." Other industry voices saw not Lehman and pharmacological standards behind the slowdown, but Kefauver and the pressure of public opinion. Still others saw not so much long-term developments at the FDA, but the replacement of Jerry Holland with thirty-four-year-old William Kessenich, who had far fewer contacts among industry officials. Indeed, industry observers increasingly expressed fears of a social "vacuum" at the FDA in the late 1950s, worrying about their lack of familiarity with the new cohort of pharmacologists and physicians hired. In a December 1960 meeting between industry men and Kessenich—at which the FDA Medical Director sat curiously distant from the others in the room, not unlike a "leper," as he later confessed to a trade reporter—Searle medical director I. C. ("Icy") Winter expressed his vision of the specter of regulatory power.

> It has been my experience in the past that when such difference arose between ourselves and the New Drug Division, we were told to go get the needed data— and did, because we knew that if we didn't we damn well wouldn't get our NDA approved. I don't see how you can get more power than that, and it's being used now—and boy, are they asking for minutiae!"

Meanwhile, William Kessenich said that there was no conscious slowdown. Instead, Kessenich made the odd argument that the abundant new staff in the Division of Medicine actually permitted greater scrutiny; "we have been giving NDAs a review in depth that perhaps was not available when we had fewer people."[102]

[101] Comparing the AHR for the first review cycle month in the 1956–61 period to that for the 1962–68 yields a χ^2 statistic of 0.20 ($p = 0.6580$). The statistic for the second month is 3.72 ($p = 0.0537$). Only for the third $\chi^2 = 8.10$; $p = 0.0044$), fourth $\chi^2 = 4.29$; $p = 0.0383$), and fifth months $\chi^2 = 4.34$; $p = 0.0373$) is the difference between the two regimes statistically significant.

[102] FDCR, October 31, 1960, 29. DeHaen also said that a more important reason for the NCE slowdown was the "temporary halt" that seems to have been taken in pharmaceutical research for "reflection and for the development of really new ideas." Kessenich's explanation and Winter's complaint appear in FDCR, December 19, 1960, 18; see also FDCR, February 27, 1961, 27. On industry worries of a social vacuum, in which Kessenich's lack of familiarity with industry interacted with congressional concerns about drug company pressure on medical reviewers, consult FDCR January 2, 1961, 10–13.

"In Use" and Efficacy in New Drug Review:
Hepasyn, Altafur, and the Pill

In many respects, Ralph Smith's vision of efficacy regulation was more clearly articulated in theory than in the practice of new drug evaluation by his subordinate medical officers. FDA medical officers usually refrained from direct appeals to "efficacy" alone in their reviews and in their correspondence. Still, the resurgence of "therapeutic value" judgments from the 1940s, and the dominance of pharmacology's protocol-driven vision, were unmistakable in 1950s new drug review.

The procedural regulation of efficacy came to the fore in the Bureau of Medicine's 1955 review of Hepasyn (arginase), essentially the liver enzyme that helps to hydrolyze the amino acid arginine. Hepasyn was touted as a cancer cure by its sponsor Wesley Irons, a departed academic dentist who developed and distributed the drug from the San Francisco College of Mortuary Science. Geoffrey Woodard, the reviewing pharmacologist who had been an integral collaborator in the FDA's pharmacological network, worried about the effective sample size of the studies supporting Hepasyn and expressed the characteristic worry about the "testimonial" quality of new drug application data. Having turned to issues of pharmaceutical potency in his recent research, he also worried about the lack of an identifiable or measurable mechanism behind Hepasyn: "It seems to me that without some measure of the activity of the product, it is impossible to establish an effective dose and therefore impossible to establish a safe dose." FDA reviewers found the application technically "incomplete," even though there was substantial agreement that the compound was "non-toxic." After repeated delays in FDA decision making, Iron's secretary complained that "too much stress" was being laid "upon efficacy when it is safety that is involved under the New Drug section of the law." A wide range of individuals based both in Washington and the field—Barbara Moulton and Ralph Weilerstein—contributed their doubts to the case. The Hepasyn NDA was deemed not approvable in the spring of 1957 and was never resubmitted. Because the Bureau had repeatedly delayed an essentially "safe" medicine for reasons of an incomplete NDA and efficacy concerns, Albert Holland recognized Hepasyn as a "precedent-setting case."[103]

[103]John Swann, "Sure Cure: Public Policy on Drug Efficacy before 1962," in Gregory J. Higby and Elaine C. Stroud, eds., *The Inside Story of Medicines: A Symposium* (Madison, WI: American Institute for the History of Pharmacy, 1997). Woodard had been an active participant in the FDA's internal pharmacological network, authorizing studies with other researchers from the cohort of 1938–39. For his engagement in the Division of Pharmacology's research community, see the collection of his papers in the publication file for "Geoffrey Woodard, Division of Pharmacology," Accession Number 54-A477, B 12, F 10; and earlier files from Accession Number 58-A277, B 19, F 11; RG 88, NA. For Woodard's comment on "effective dose," see Woodard, "For Comment," 18 January 1954, NDA 9214, Misc File IV; cited in Swann, "Sure Cure," n.112. Woodard also communicated with Barbara Moulton regarding the Hepasyn

The agency's ability to employ efficacy criteria received some support in the wake of its December 1960 suspension of Eaton Laboratories' Altafur Tablets, an antibiotic purported to be effective against "serious and life-threatening infections." Suspension of a new drug application was equivalent to market withdrawal, and the notice of suspension explicitly stated lack of evidence for efficacy as the basis of the finding that the drug was "unsafe for use under the conditions of use upon the basis of which the application became effective." In particular, the FDA found that "the drug is of little or no value in the treatment of serious and life-threatening infections," that "Altafur is not sufficiently efficacious in the treatment of infections" to justify its risks, and that the evidence in a supplemental new drug application failed to demonstrate safety because they had failed to demonstrate efficacy. Beyond this, the agency was backdating its evidence base—reasoning that "methods not deemed reasonably applicable" when furaltadone was cleared had since demonstrated its lack of therapeutic value. For companies and regulatory conservatives, this move set a disturbing precedent: the specter that drugs previously approved by the agency could be removed from the market because later and more advanced tests demonstrated insufficient efficacy.[104]

At the administrative hearing on Altafur, the Administration lined up an impressive series of specialists, headlined by Maxwell Finland, to make their case to HEW Examiner Edward B. Terkel. In October 1961, Terkel not only affirmed the FDA's ruling in all particulars, he also stated that relative and "comparative efficacy" were proper and fully legitimate dimensions of judgment, and he appeared to castigate the FDA for allowing the Altafur NDA to become effective in the first place. As the trade press reported it, Terkel's decision "embraced" the concept of comparative efficacy, "a nasty phrase in American Medical Association and pharmaceutical industry quarters." So worried were Eaton and its allies about this outcome that, for the first time in recorded administrative history, a firm appealed the suspension of its NDA. The issue went to Deputy FDA Commissioner John Harvey, who sided with the agency.[105]

The Altafur suspension reverberated vividly and strategically in industry

review (Woodard to Moulton, 5 May 1955, NDA 9214, Misc File IV; Swann, n.112). On Moulton and Holland's thoughts and concerns, see notes 121 and 122, Swann, "Sure Cure."

[104] Altafur's NDA suspension was first proposed in a notice of hearing issued December 27, 1960; *FDCR*, January 2, 1961, 25.

[105] Deputy Commissioner of Foods and Drugs (John L. Harvey), Notice of Hearing, FDC-D-62, suspending NDA No. 11-965; Department of HEW, *In the Matter of "Altafur Tablets," Eaton Laboratories, Division of Norwich Pharmacal Co., Norwich, N.Y.,* October 25, 1961. "Altafur NDA Ordered Suspended by HEW Examiner Who Finds FDA Can Consider Comparative Efficacy; He Criticizes FDA and Eaton," *FDCR*, November 6, 1961; "FDA Orders Suspension of Eaton Laboratories' New Drug Application Covering Altafur Tablets," *DTN*, September 3, 1962; *ICDRR*, 504–8, 945–55. Eaton Laboratories argued in its appeal that "Therapeutic efficacy should not have been a consideration in determining the safety of Altafur tablets"; *DRR* 4 (24) (Dec. 27, 1961): 15–6.

circles. The second face of regulatory power showed as companies began to enter talks with the FDA over the possible withdrawal of older treatments based entirely on their lack of evidence for efficacy. In January 1961, Roche voluntarily withdrew its antidepressant Marsilid (iproniazid) after discussions with the Bureau of Medicine. Trade reporters who narrated the Marsilid withdrawal for their data-hungry readers interpreted Roche's move as new evidence for the aggressiveness of the FDA's efficacy initiative. The Marsilid suspension "confirms [the] view that FDA is conscious of benefits-to-risks ratios of older drugs" when new alternatives become available, a "Pink Sheet" reporter wrote. "FDA-ers deny this is a consideration when passing on new NDAs," but "Marsilid, Chloromycetin and Altafur make it difficult for FDA-ers to deny, convincingly, that they have something like this in mind when looking over the really potent drugs already on the market."[106]

"In use" considerations also arose when G. D. Searle and Company submitted its application for norethynordrel/mestranol (trade name Enovid). Later to become the first oral contraceptive marketed in the United States and throughout the world, Enovid was submitted first not for fertility but for irregular menstruation (amenorrhea, dysmenorrhea, menorrhagia, and endometriosis). Searle hoped to gain a relatively quick and noncontroversial approval for a narrow indication and then file a "supplemental" application for more lucrative markets. When in 1959 Searle told the FDA that it intended to file a supplemental NDA for Enovid as an anti-fertility drug, Administration officials recognized the moral and political issues at stake and acknowledged publicly that "our consideration has to be confined to safety for intended use." Among the many ironies of this pronouncement is that Searle's investigational data—from 1,500 women in Puerto Rico—were prospectively and overwhelmingly designed to address efficacy questions. Safety issues were a tangential feature of the research design. The new drug application was assigned to Jose DeFelice, a newly minted doctor who was still in residency in obstetrics and gynecology. Over the next several years, in his review and in his correspondence with Searle, DeFelice repeatedly concerned himself with the eventual utilization patterns of Enovid, even though the review was pronounced to be an examination of safety alone.[107]

[106]*FDCR*, January 30, 1961, 22. Medical officers also targeted procaine injections, acknowledging a clear demonstration of safety but maintaining that the product's "rejuvenation claim" was unsupported; *FDCR*, August 29, 1960, 14.

[107]Each 10-mg tablet of Enovid contained 9.85 mg of norethynodrel and 0.15 mg of mestranol. These compounds were synthetic forms of estrogen and progesterone (progestin/progestogen), two hormones critical in ovulation and the menstrual cycle. The claimed advantage of a synthetic estrogen-progestin combination for endometriosis was that the drug simulated pregnancy by creating a larger predecidua in the stromal lining of the endometrium. The subsequent menstrual flow would be stronger, and this "more satisfactory shedding of the endometrium" would induce "a more normal uterine lining during the next cycle." R. W. Kistner, "The Use of Newer Progestines in the Treatment of Endometriosis," *AJOG* 75 (Feb. 1958): 264–78; M. C. Andrews, W. C. Andrews, and A. F. Strauss, "Effects of Progestin-Induced Pseudopregnancy on Endometriosis: Clinical and Microscopic Studies," *AJOG* 78 (Oct. 1959): 776–85. See proposed labeling for Enovid

Despite the abnormality of its politics, Enovid was reviewed in ways that expressed a changing regulatory order at the FDA. First, the review was long. In a manner that was surprising and annoying to Searle and political sponsors of "the pill," DeFelice and his colleagues at the Bureau of Medicine took ten months to review Enovid-10 (the 10-milligram dose), and two years for the 5-milligram dose, Enovid-5. By comparison, the agency took only sixty days to approve the original Enovid application for menstrual irregularities. Second, the Enovid application brought a wide range of Administration officials into the review orbit, including William Kessenich (then the FDA's Deputy Medical Director), Gordon Granger (head of the Drugs and Devices Division), Ralph Weilerstein and Morris Yakowitz from field operations, Deputy Commissioner John Harvey, and Commissioner George Larrick himself. Third, the practice of informal consultation within medical specialties was extended in the act of sending a questionnaire on Enovid to seventy-five obstetrician-gynecologists throughout the United States, including Planned Parenthood Clinic chief Dr. Edward Tyler. FDA officials and field officers sought out Tyler's advice on the drug, personally interviewed him about his use of Enovid in his practice, and sought and used records from his practice in reviewing the Enovid application.[108]

The consultation standards, the time consumed, and the regulatory orbit were part of a larger review process in which standards, methods, language, and assumptions had changed. DeFelice drew upon "in use" considerations when he required Searle to submit a separate supplemental NDA for Enovid's lower dose. Searle officials protested that the Bureau of Medicine had already found Enovid-10 safe, hence the lower dosage form of Enovid-5 should be assumed safe, since a lower dose must be safer than a higher dose. DeFelice and Deputy Medical Director William Kessenich replied that prescription and utilization patterns might differ across the doses in a way that would render Searle's monotone logic invalid. Although Enovid-5 was eventually approved, it took fully two years for Searle's cheaper yet equally ef-

---

in NDA 10976, V 124; RG 88, NA. Sharon Snyder, "The Pill: 30 Years of Safety Concerns," *FDA Consumer* 24 (4) (Dec. 1990); Suzanne White Junod, "The Pill at 40," *FDA Consumer* 34 (4) (2000): 36; Junod and Lara Marks, "Women's Trials: The Approval of the First Oral Contraceptive Pill in the United States and Great Britain," *Journal of the History of Medicine and Allied Sciences* 57 (April 2002): 117–60. For announcement on the principles governing the review, see Deputy Commissioner John L. Harvey's letter to Senator Leonora K. Sullivan, NDA 10976, V 21, FDA Records; cited in Junod and Marks, "Women's Trials," 130, n.33.

[108] See "Exhibit 35: Food and Drug Administration Chronological Summary and Memoranda on the New Drug Application for Enovid," in *ICDRR*, Part 2, 233ff. See the correspondence for the Enovid new drug application, NDA 10976, V 14 and 15, RG 88, NA; see also the notes in Junod and Marks, "Women's Trials," passim. On the questionnaire, see Junod and Marks, p. 131; NDA 10976, RG 88, NA. Junod and Marks argue that the FDA's consultation with medical professionals and academic scientists on the Enovid application was a "result" of DeFelice's residential status and the Bureau of Medicine's resource constraints ("Women's Trials," p. 130). In fact, the pattern of liaison and informal consultation was common throughout this period, certainly not isolated to the Enovid review.

fective dosage form to reach the American market. The "in use" logic was rehearsed by Kessenich and the Bureau of Medicine in justifying Enovid's approval to Commissioner George Larrick. "Altogether in the series of clinical cases," Kessenich wrote, "897 women representing 801.6 women-years and 10,427 cycles have been studied." Sociologist Nelly Oudshoorn has deftly recognized that this rhetoric mapped female subjects onto a women-time axis, thus understating individual experiences and overstating statistical power. Yet the representation of patients in terms of patient-years was a common practice in the pharmacological study of drugs for chronic illnesses. Wittingly or not, Larrick, Kessenich, and Bureau of Medicine officials were borrowing from the "life-table" methodology that was increasingly used in the FDA to analyze time-to-event and survival data. That methodology, and the "woman-years" concepts that it implied, were a statistical bow to the concern that standard conceptions of clinical samples—an "N" of "300 subjects"—were flawed in the evaluation of drugs that, intentionally or not, would be used continually for chronic conditions. Throughout the review, whether it was DeFelice or Kessenich talking, or Weilerstein and Granger questioning established obstetricians, or top officials rehearsing the rationale for Enovid's approval, the notion of value "in use" was consistently (through variably) invoked. The concern for utilization patterns also led agency officials to regulate the prescription interval for oral contraceptives; Enovid was the first drug approved with an enforced time limit upon its prescription.[109]

When it came time to announce approval of Enovid as an oral contraceptive, Administration officials hedged their rhetoric and described the approval in the narrowest of procedural and legal terms. The pill had already created new social and political divides, and FDA representatives wanted to avoid even the appearance of having visited these dimensions of the drug. Perhaps appropriately, the first announcement of Enovid's approval as an oral contraceptive was made not by Larrick, but by Associate Commissioner John L. Harvey, who announced that "our own ideas of morality had nothing to do with the case." And, despite the administrative reality of the

[109] J. Crosson (Searle) to William Kessenich, November 11, 1961, V 16, NDA 10976, RG 88, NA; DeFelice to Kessenich, February 15, 1961, V21, NDA 10976, RG 88, NA. Cited in Junod and Marks, "Women's Trials," p. 144 (n.82), p. 145 (n.85). Memorandum from Bureau of Medicine to Larrick, May 11, 1960, *ICDRR*, 234. Nelly Oudshoorn, *Beyond the Natural Body: An Archaeology of Sex Hormones* (London, 1994). Oudshoorn (ibid., 132) and Junod and Marks ("Women's Trials," 139) wrongly attribute this statement to Larrick, though perhaps Larrick might have rehearsed the statement in another context. For an example of life-table methodology being used in an office close to the Office of the Commissioner, see Rose Sachs, FDA Bureau of Program Planning and Appraisal, "Life Table Techniques in the Analysis of Response Time Data from Laboratory Experiments on Animals" (1958); B 24, F 42, Accession 62A-379, RG 88, NA. On the enforced time limit for Enovid prescriptions, see "Searle's 'Enovid' Okayed for Contraceptive Use," *OP&DR*, May 16, 1960, 3. FDA historian Suzanne White Junod is the first to have noticed this precedent; Junod, "The Pill at 40," *FDA Consumer* 34 (4) (2000): 36.

Enovid review, despite the preponderance of Searle's data for Enovid which spoke to questions of efficacy and not to safety, and despite the public fora in which FDA regulation of efficacy was being openly discussed and admitted, Harvey avoided any mention of therapeutic value criteria: "Approval was based on the question of safety."[110]

The Administration's clearance of Enovid for contraceptive use was quickly noted and exploited in oral and written arguments to the Supreme Court for the landmark case of *Griswold v. Connecticut*. Planned Parenthood counsel Harriet Pilpel wrote in an amicus brief that the Administration's clearance of the supplemental NDA "only last month" stood as evidence of "a consensus of medical opinion" supporting the use of contraceptives to protect women's and infants' health. In their reference to the FDA's decision, Pilpel and other contraception advocates were relying not upon a safety calculus but upon the agency's efficacy judgments on Enovid.[111]

An Ambiguous Statement of Fact: Efficacy Politics
at the First Kefauver Hearings

In December 1959, Tennessee Senator Estes Kefauver commenced hearings on issues of drug pricing and monopoly profits before his Subcommittee on Antitrust and Monopoly. By the time they concluded in 1962, Kefauver's hearings had issued in landmark revisions to the 1938 Act, and Kefauver's attention to pharmaceutical issues is credited with making possible fundamental and lasting change in pharmaceutical development and regulation in the United States. Still, in the summer of 1961, when Frances Kelsey was still holding up the Kevadon application, and months before German and Australian investigators began to tie the torrent of global birth defects to thalidomide use, Estes Kefauver was little interested in drug safety. His was an antitrust committee, and with national inflation dominating the politics of the 1950s and early 1960s, Kefauver's principal target was drug pricing and marketing. Pricing issues, too, were what most stirred the anxieties of pharmaceutical companies, who had been nervously watching Kefauver for signs that he might turn his attention from steel and automobiles to pharmaceuticals.

In the aftermath of the 1960 elections, the specter of new government regulation only swelled further. If the anxious buzz from trade reporters of the 1950s is any guide, though, industry fears were stoked not by the Food and Drug Administration but by Kefauver and the legislation he was brewing in the Senate. Among American corporations, moreover, Kefauver was

---

[110]"FDA Approves Pill for Use in Birth Control," *Chicago Tribune*, May 10, 1960, A11; *FDCR*, February 20, 1961, 23, 28.

[111]On the citation of Enovid's approval in *Griswold* argumentation, see *FDCR*, March 6, 1961, 15. *Griswold v. Connecticut*, 381 U.S. 479. Briefs of *amici curiae*, urging reversal of the Connecticut Supreme Court's decision, were filed by Pilpel, Morris L. Ernst, and Nancy F. Wechsler for Planned Parenthood.

perhaps the most despised and feared politician of the Cold War era. American pharmaceutical executives approached the 1959–60 Kefauver hearings with dread. In addition to the negative publicity entailed in the hearings, Kefauver had surpassed his earlier efficacy proposals and had recommended two new aggressive planks that would regulate drug advertising by the Federal Trade Commission (FTC) and would limit patent life. The first of these prospects so frightened the Pharmaceutical Manufacturers' Association that its officials had spoken out in favor of FDA control over drug advertising, so as to keep such authority out of the hands of the Commission. The drug industry, the PMA's Austin Smith declared in December 1960, was suffering from acute "Kefauverrhea."[112]

Yet the clearest lesson from Kefauver's first antitrust hearings had nothing to do with industry concentration or pricing. The hearings revealed that U.S. drug approval had been irrevocably changed, not by Kefauver, but by the Administration. Kefauver's hearings only gradually alighted on the issues facing new drug review at the FDA, but when they did, they revealed a fact to which everyone seemed to have accustomed themselves but which had never been discussed in a public forum. The standards of drug review had changed, and they had changed through regulatory practice. No longer did anyone in Washington, in the pharmaceutical industry, in organized medicine, or in academic pharmacology doubt that organizational practice at the FDA had stepped well beyond the narrow statutory concept of "safety." The occasion for the hearings was Kefauver's introduction of S.1552 into the Senate chamber. S.1552 was a radical measure that would have required FDA officials to make a determination of efficacy in new drug applications. The witnesses at Kefauver's first hearings that year—Physicians' Council President Julius Richmond, Cornell's Walter Modell, *Pediatrics* editor Charles May, Rochester's Louis Lasagna, the AMA's Hugh Hussey, University of Illinois' Harry Dowling, University of Utah's Louis Goodman, Massachusetts General Hospital's Allan Butler, Harvard's Maxwell Finland, and George Larrick himself—were manifold and diverse. Yet to a tee, every one of these individuals acknowledged that Bureau of Medicine decisions were actively and necessarily incorporating "efficacy" considerations already, and that pharmaceutical companies had already adapted their research and development to this fact. And despite heated dissent from Senators Everett Dirksen and John Hruska on Kefauver's proposal to authorize efficacy reviews *in statute*, not one of Kefauver's witnesses denied either that efficacy regulation was in practice *or* that it was legitimate and legally permissible. "It is," as Utah's Louis Goodman put it, "no wonder to me that the FDA has found it necessary, over the years, to expand its program so that it does, in fact, examine conditions of recommended use and

---

[112]The Kefauver hearings of 1959–61 and the legislative content of reform bills are discussed at greater length and depth in chapter 4. Many in Congress took credit for the new policies that had actually commenced in regulatory practice (Humphrey, "I believe I played somewhat of a role in accomplishing that objective," *ICDRR*, 776). *FDCR*, December 16, 1960, 14.

claims for therapeutic efficacy in making decisions concerning the safety of a drug product."[113]

The wide agreement on the FDA's existing pattern of efficacy regulation was all the more notable because the parties contending over Kefauver's bill sought to exploit the fact to their advantage. Kefauver himself claimed that since the FDA was already regulating efficacy "through the back door," his bill was simply a formal encoding of established and legitimated practice. Opponents such as AMA President Hussey pointed to the same fact as a reason that obviated the need for any new legislation.

> SENATOR KEFAUVER: If you want a drug to be efficacious before it is placed on the market, why not make that a condition as to placing it on the market? I do not understand.
>
> DR. HUSSEY: It seems to me it is a condition under existing practice before it is placed on the market.
>
> SENATOR KEFAUVER: But if that is what the law means now, then why do you object?

A later exchange with John Hopkins pharmacologist Louis Lasagna revealed the reputational basis of efficacy regulation. Not only was the FDA already governing efficacy, it was doing so in a way that elite academic pharmacologists found admirable and feasible. Goodman perceived that the medical profession was confident that drugs had been "appropriately scrutinized" by federal regulators. Charles May found no reason to have his "confidence shaken" in the FDA and their performance of "whatever duties they may have," and Lasagna thought that current efficacy regulation was marked by "efficiency." All the more reason, Kefauver pointed out, to entrust the FDA with formal authority for efficacy regulation. Yet Republican counterparts to Kefauver highlighted the same set of facts and wondered again why S.1552 was needed.

> SENATOR KEFAUVER: It has been our understanding that the Food and Drug Administration has had very satisfactory experience in evaluating the efficacy as well as the safety of antibiotics and diabetic drugs, is that so?
>
> DR. LASAGNA: Yes, sir.
>
> SENATOR HRUSKA: If that is true, why do we need another law?[114]

---

[113]U.S. Senate, *Drug Industry Antitrust Act*, Hearings before the Subcommittee on Antitrust and Monopoly of the Committee on the Judiciary, 87th Congress, First Session (Washington, GPO, 1961), passim. See the remarks of Hussey (p. 54), Howard (75), Goodman (213), Lasagna (283, 288), Butler (351–2), Richmond (373), Finland (436), Larrick (78, 80–81, 86), and Kefauver himself (82, 88, 421).

[114]U.S. Senate, *DIAA*, 77 (Kefauver-Hussey exchange), 79 ("back-door method"), 205 (May on "confidence"), 217 (Goodman on "appropriately scrutinized" drug), 288 (Kefauver-Lasagna-Hruska exchange, and Lasagna "efficiency" statement). Lasagna vouched for a new efficacy requirement outside of the hearings as well; *FDCR*, April 13, 1959, 27. In response to pointed questioning from Hruska, Goodman offered a vigorous defense of the efficacy-safety bundle. "And you say, 'Let the Food and Drug Administration operate as it does; don't freeze it into law;

The concerns of FDA opponents were genuine and subtle. The stated objection of industry and AMA officials was that, with a statutory imprimatur, the FDA would step well beyond and assess the relative efficacy of new drugs: How well did the compound under examination compare to those therapies already marketed for the condition? Industry officials and pharmacologists knew that Ralph Smith's bureau was asking this question already, but they wanted to avoid legitimating such practices.

The other concern was that of turf. It was clear to the American Medical Association's Hussey and its Council of Delegates, who expressed vocal opposition to the effectiveness provisions of Kefauver's 1960 bill, that further FDA regulation of effectiveness would put the AMA's drug evaluation business "out of it." This did not bother Kefauver, who characterized the AMA's previous attempts to examine efficacy as a "hit-or-miss operation," and worried that even if the Association found a drug to be without therapeutic effect, no penalty could be leveled because "All you are is an advisory group." Partly in response to the Kefauver proposal and partly to wrest back some symbolic turf from the FDA, the AMA trustees had authorized and advertised a "drug information program," to be run in cooperation with the Pharmaceutical Manufacturers' Association. Yet even as enthusiastic an AMA spokesman as Hussey was compelled to acknowledge that his organization had essentially bowed out of competition with the Administration.[115]

By 1960, it was clear to every interested observer in Washington that "the Administration's regulations [had] gone far beyond the exact words of the 1938 Act." As if to echo the Kefauver hearings, Julius Hauser (now assistant to the Medical Director) stated in a May 1960 speech at St. John's College of Pharmacy that "virtually all new drugs" required substantial evidence of efficacy. Efficacy regulation, to which most pharmaceutical companies had already adapted, had arrived through a vague combination of "administrative directive" and FDA "practice." It came as little surprise to industry and FDA observers in the spring of 1960, then, when Kefauver began drawing up his first efficacy regulation bill, with considerable help from the Administration. As the *Oil, Paint and Drug Reporter*, breaking news of the Kefauver draft, put it, "Persons in the drug industry who have spent the last twenty-five years keeping in touch with the FDA's activities will be quick to

---

talk only about safety.' And I claim, sir, that you cannot make any valid statement, any meaningful statement, about safety without taking recommended use, conditions of use, into consideration—and this immediately gets you into the area of therapeutic claims" (*DIAA*, 239).

[115]U.S. Senate, *DIAA*, Hussey (54, on relative efficacy worries), (65, "out of it" statement); Kefauver insult to AMA at 63. On the AMA's program, which was slow to get off the ground, see Don R. Swanson, "Draft Report of the Subcommittee on Data Collection, Evaluation and Retrieval," and Don R. Swanson memo to L. T. Coggeshall (Chairman, Commission on Drug Safety), "Subject: Communication of Drug Information," May 14, 1963; Archives of the AMA-COD, F 3909; AAMA. The details were also discussed at joint meetings of the AMA and FDA leadership. See "Agenda, FDA-AMA Meeting," and "FDA-AMA Meeting" (minutes), August 7, 1963, AMA Headquarters, Chicago; Archives of the AMA-COD, F 3909; AAMA.

recognize these proposals as recommendations which have long been favored by FDA."[116]

Does the rise of efficacy regulation then speak to issues of bureaucratic autonomy? It is possible that a more politically germane bureaucratic autonomy founded in political and social networks was operating, though the relevant networks for the mid-century FDA were not as manifold as they were for Harvey Wiley a half-century earlier.[117] More important and more informative than questions of bureaucratic autonomy are questions about the mechanisms of regulatory change. For FDA officials and their audiences in medicine, public health, and pharmacology, efficacy regulation was not an aim unto itself, but part of a broader transformation of regulation in which the agency's self-understanding as "protector" merged with its role as "gatekeeper." Efficacy regulation was not a mere epiphenomenon of "science" or "clinical pharmacology"; it was an organizational achievement, one positioned at the interstices of market, state, and science. Those interstices were, moreover, located in the new drug review process. The transformation of efficacy regulation demonstrates a growing pattern of the post–New Deal American state: federal rulemaking and statutes frequently encode administrative practices that were established years before.[118]

The other notable pattern about the rise of efficacy regulation was the ambiguity attached to the term and related concepts. In some respects the ambiguity was a result of FDA operating procedure and a cultivated strategy. As easily as they admitted at the Kefauver hearings that an efficacy standard was implicitly governing new drugs, Administration officials explicitly rejected that any particular drug had been denied on the basis of efficacy considerations. When Bureau of Medicine officials approved Richardson Merrell's drug MER/29—a drug later removed from the market—the approval letter to Merrell stated that no review of the drug's efficacy had been undertaken. Two years after witnesses at the Kefauver hearings testified that efficacy regulation was established as regulatory custom, prominent voices such as a New York Academy of Medicine review panel would concur that efficacy regulation was *not* a practice of the FDA. Trade jour-

---

[116] "FDA Does Require Evidence of Efficacy to Clear New Drugs: Speech by FDAer Replies to MD Critics at Kefauver Hearings," *FDCR* 22 (19) (May 9, 1960): 16–17. "Drug Law Tightening Seems Sure to be an Echo of Kefauver Hearings," *OP&DR*, June 13, 1960, p. 3.

[117] A large literature in political science attempts to tie the concept of autonomy to delegation. In previous scholarship, I have argued that the terms "discretion" and "autonomy" are conceptually separable and should be kept distinct. Carpenter, *The Forging of Bureaucratic Autonomy: Reputations, Networks and Policy Innovation in Executive Agencies, 1862–1928* (Princeton: Princeton University Press, 2001), chap. 1.

[118] Swann concludes that "By the time Senator Kefauver began the hearings that ultimately ended with a new drug law that embraced efficacy, the latter was already an established component of public health in America" ("Sure Cure," 250). My principal concern with Swann's interpretation is that it downplays the robust ambiguity of efficacy regulation. Ambiguity governed new drug review precisely because it was *not* "established," at least not established clearly and officially in public discourse.

nals had noticed that Administration officials had become fond of making policy not through formal rulemaking, and not through lawmaking proposals to Estes Kefauver or other legislators, but through public addresses and "informal" policy statements in the *Federal Register*.[119]

Yet in other ways, the very word "efficacy" defied precise or formulaic meaning at the time. Witnesses at the first Kefauver hearings—whether they supported or opposed a pre-market efficacy requirement, as the FDA and Kefauver had proposed—confessed their ignorance of how to define the term. Was "efficacious" the same as "useful," "curative," "valuable"? Did efficacy mean the same thing when comparing drug treatments as when comparing drug treatments to surgical interventions? If regulation of efficacy was the goal, how should it be achieved? By labeling restrictions? By regulation of advertising and medical promotion? By raising the bar for drug approval in the first place? Or by some combination of these strategies?[120]

In practice and in rulemaking, the Bureau of Medicine was calling for "pharmacological studies" planned and conducted by "qualified investigators," presumably a trained pharmacologist. Yet nowhere—not in government, not in industry, and certainly not in academic medicine—was there general agreement on the meaning of these terms. The very by-laws of the American Society for Pharmacology and Experimental Therapeutics (ASPET) underscored the difficult in defining "pharmacology":

> This is the most difficult [term] to define and is the area in which greatest difference of opinion has existed. Most Committee members have firm subjective ideas as to what constitutes classical pharmacology, but these ideas break down rapidly in borderline cases. In recent years we have seen a greatly increased interest in biochemistry, toxicology, endocrinology, anesthesiology, and clinical applications. There has been a definite effort on the part of recent Councils to enlarge and broaden the Society. Hence, pharmacology in a classical sense (whatever the individual's idea as to what that is) is no longer a rigidly applied criterion.[121]

Exactly what role ambiguity played in the emergence of the FDA's new reputation, and in the arrival of efficacy regulation, is not clear. It is facile to imagine that very elaborate standards of review, spelled out in the *Federal Register* or in proposals for statutory revision, would have met with concerted

[119]See John Nestor's complaint about the inconsistency in this FDA statement at *ICDRR*, 786; NYAM, Committee on Public Health, "The Importance of Clinical Testing in Determining the Efficacy and Safety of Drugs," *Bulletin of the New York Academy of Medicine* 38 (June 1962): 415. "FDA Gives Clue to Thinking Via Informal Policy Statements," *OP&DR*, December 9, 1957, p. 4. See also the report on the FDA's new advisory service for food and drug law; *OP&DR*, December 2, 1957.

[120]For deliberation and confusion on the meaning of "efficacy" and "efficacious," see the remarks of the following at the first Kefauver hearings: Hussey (45, 51), Kefauver (63), Majority counsel Chumbris (72), Louis Goodman (220), Wallace (278), Lasagna (281), Hruska (287); *DIAA*, I.

[121]ASPET, "Notes on the Procedures of the Membership Committee," [1960]; Folder "Pharmacol. Soc.," LSG.

resistance. The terms of FDA efficacy regulation had a different sort of legitimacy. By the late 1950s, "efficacy," "safe for use," "pharmacology," "qualified investigator" and other terms had the imprimatur not of law, but of familiarity in use.[122]

The other feature of policymaking by ambiguity was a consistent and repeated denial of jurisdiction—or the wish for it—over more controversial dimensions of health and medical policy. This came in Albert Holland's 1957 insistence that the FDA was "not anxious to get into the field of actively policing promotional literature between manufacturers and the doctors," or in George Larrick's reminder to the Kefauver Committee in 1961 that the "the Food, Drug and Cosmetic Act does not deal with the economics involved in drug development and merchandising," and hence that "we disclaim any expertise in these areas. Neither are we a price-fixing agency." Larrick's distancing of the Administration from issues of drug pricing was a common agency strategy throughout the period, and a shrewd one. General inflation—particularly in prescription drug prices—was among the most pressing issues in American electoral and congressional politics in the 1950s. Several years before he set his sights on the pharmaceutical industry, Kefauver had held Senate hearings on price-fixing in the auto and steel industries. By stepping astride the drug prices debate, the Administration kept to its more secure policy turf and avoided cries of medical socialism that advanced as European countries began to regulate drug prices. Yet the agency's plea of incapacity in the face of rising drug prices also kept it from guilt by association over spiraling medical inflation. As drug prices and hospital costs skyrocketed in the 1950s, two symbolic entities—the pharmaceutical industry, publicly despised for its high profit margins, and the AMA, known widely as "the doctor's trust" since the antitrust battles of the 1940s—came in for most of the public criticism. Neither the Administration nor its drug regulations was ever tied to the problem.[123]

[122]For a theoretical approach to how the familiarity of rehearsed government language and symbolism can induce a form of steady, predictable obedience, see Lisa Wedeen, "Killing Politics: Official Rhetoric and Permissible Speech," chap. 2 in *Ambiguities of Domination: Politics, Rhetoric and Symbols in Contemporary Syria* (Chicago: University of Chicago Press, 1999), 33–66. The primary difference here, of course, is that while Administration officials were the primary voices repeatedly speaking these concepts (without defining them), the FDA did not possess a legal monopoly on discussions on pharmacology or drug evaluation during this period. Hence the process by which repetition, recirculation, and rehearsal make otherwise radical concepts familiar is not one that the state could "control," though it was certainly a process in which the state participated.

[123]"Tranquilizer Ads Don't Hurt Doctors Too Much; Government Can't Hear Them Cry 'Ouch'," *OP&DR*, March 3, 1958, 5. Text of Larrick statement before Senate Committee on Antitrust and Monopoly of the Senate Committee on the Judiciary, pp. 2–3; copy enclosed with letter of Kenneth L. Milstead to Oliver Field, June 7, 1960; AMA Historical Health Fraud and Alternative Medicine Collection, Box 273-01, AAMA. On inflation politics at mid-century, see Meg Jacobs, "Pocketbook Politics in an Age of Inflation, 1946–1960," chap. 6 of *Pocketbook Politics*, esp. 246–61. Estes Kefauver, *In a Few Hands: Monopoly Power in America* (New York: Pantheon, 1957). Lizabeth Cohen, "Reconversion: The Emergence of the Consumers' Republic," chap. 3 in *A Consumers' Republic*.

The Kefauver hearings also exposed a broad and generally warm nexus of associations between the networks of academic pharmacology and the FDA. Some of the most highly respected pharmacologists of the period—Charles May, Louis Goodman, Louis Lasagna, Walter Modell—spoke highly of the agency and its scientific staff. In other cases, officials' rhetoric belied an affiliation with FDA officials that Kefauver himself and the pharmaceutical industry could barely fathom. In commenting on Kefauver's proposal to strengthen antibiotics certification, Lasagna deftly noted that, in talking to colleagues in the Administration, there was simply no need for such a provision, and that administrative and regulatory resources were better directed elsewhere. "Some friends in the FDA informed me that there are other drugs which are much more likely to provide problems in regard to quality control. The examples I have been given are the reserpine family and ACTH."[124]

An Emergent Reputation, Multiply Refracted

The Administration's emerging identity was neither simple nor seamless. While pharmaceutical firms, state and federal inspectors, specialty medical professionals, and academic researchers were beginning to rationalize, legitimate, and otherwise come to terms with a new regime of pharmaceutical regulation, public audiences and industry observers continued to see—and FDA officials continued to project to them—an older image of pharmaceutical policy as inspection, enforcement, and a "hot war against medical quacks." George Larrick distinguished between his agency's "old business" and its "new business," but the enforcement of laws against quackery still took center stage in press releases, industry trade reports, and popular publications.[125]

The Citizens' Advisory Committee report was also significant in organizational image building, especially for the image of pharmaceutical regulation it projected to Congress and to media organizations. Here the Committee was influential even where, frequently enough, it misled. The Committee's defense of its recommendation to bolster the FDA's scientific capacity invoked a deferential separation of science from regulation. "Although the FDA is primarily a regulatory agency," the Committee conceded, science was still important for determining methods of assessing safety. In its view,

---

[124]Lasagna statement at *DIAA*, I, 293.

[125]"What Constitutes Interstate Commerce?" *FDCR*, May 17, 1952; "Delivery for Interstate Sale," *FDCR*, September 20, 1952; "Drugs Sold in Interstate Commerce," *FDCR*, October 18, 1952. FSA-FDA Press Releases, "For P.M. Papers" and "For Release to Medical Journals," February 20, 1953; Folder 0272-07, "Special Data, 1953–1954," AAMA. "Restitution Issue," *FDCR*, November 20, 1954; Larrick, "Our Unfinished Business," address to Eastern Section of the American Pharmaceutical Manufacturers' Association, Waldorf-Astoria Hotel, New York, December 8, 1954; Folder 0272-07, "Special Data, 1953–1954," AAMA. Roger Greene, "Just How Good Are the 'Revolutionary' Remedies?" *Louisville (Ky) Courier-Journal*, January 19, 1958; the Greene article, copied in the AAMA, appears to have been syndicated through the Associated Press.

science would serve the interest of consumer protection. Yet the report missed the changing reality of regulation, ignoring entirely the agency's developed capacities in drug evaluation and pharmacology. The report also bypassed the behavioral shift in FDA enforcement activities that had concentrated more fire upon drugs and less upon food (figure 3.3).[126]

The other legacy of the Committee report was the echo it provided about the underlying strength and benevolence of the Administration. Whatever problems existed with U.S. pharmaceutical regulation were weaknesses in the law, not weaknesses in the "public protector" charged with enforcing it. Put differently, the fault of weak food and drug regulation lay with Congress, not with the FDA. When Patricia Williams, a Vermont high school senior, wrote to the AMA Bureau of information in 1958, she succinctly described the purpose of her fall term paper. "I am trying to show how the Pure Food and Drug Law is weak," she wrote, and asked for any information that the AMA could provide to that end. AMA Information Director Oliver Field replied, "while the law is not overburdened with weaknesses," its "most glaring weakness" lay in "the fact that the Food and Drug Administration does not have jurisdiction over advertising." General newspapers and industry trade reporters repeated the judgment on a near-weekly basis; the problems with the FDA were problems of institutional neglect: too little nurturing from its caretakers in Congress.[127]

The agency's public reputation for pharmaceutical protection also received a boost from scientific review committees—particularly a NAS/NRC committee that reviewed the FDA's drug regulation, one chaired by University of Chicago's Philip C. Miller, hence known as "the Miller Committee." The essence of the Miller Committee's report was that the agency possessed high organizational and analytic capacity, but that "certain weaknesses inherent in the existing law and current staffing and budgetary support hamper the FDA in its task of protecting the public health." Perhaps most notably, the Miller Committee report stated openly that "The FDA should be given statutory authority to require proof of efficacy, as well as the safety, of all new drugs." HEW Secretary Arthur Flemming concurred in this recommendation, and industry trade reporters highlighted the efficacy proposal to their concerned readers. *Saturday Review* editor Jonathan Lear printed the full text of the Miller Committee report in his magazine, and the report quickly diffused through intellectual, political, medical, and scientific networks. Phar-

---

[126] *Report of the Citizens' Advisory Committee on the U.S. Food and Drug Administration* (n.p., Washington, DC, June 1955) p. 15, Appendix P-I.

[127] Patricia Williams (Jacksonville, VT) to Oliver Field (Director, Bureau of Information), AMA, September 23, 1958; Field to Williams, October 27, 1958; Historical Health Fraud and Alternative Medicine Collection, Folder 11, "Food and Drug Administration, U.S., Federal Security Agency, Correspondence 1940–1959," Box 272; AAMA. "There is little, if any, reason to believe that the Food &Drug Administration has not been doing all that it possibly can effectively do to administer the patchwork of statutes with which it is entrusted. There is some reason to believe that it does not have the power or the personnel to do a completely satisfactory job." "For Better Drugs," *OP&DR*, June 13, 1960, p. 9.

macologist Chauncey Leake wrote to Miller that his committee's report would
well serve "the first-class agency of the Food and Drug Administration,"
and he celebrated the *Saturday Review*'s printing, which would ensure "its
wide appreciation by intelligent people all over the country, and may result
in real backing and support for the best kind of effort on the part of the
Food and Drug Administration for the protection of our people's health."
In the months following the Miller Committee report, representatives of four
women's and consumers' groups—the National Council of Jewish Women,
the American Home Economics Association, the American Association of
University Women, and the Consumers' Union—visited FDA headquarters
and endorsed the committee's proposals and Secretary Flemming's recommendations.[128]

THE PUBLIC FACET OF REPUTATION: PROTECTION THROUGH POLICING

Steady public criticism of pharmaceutical regulation was part and parcel of
the FDA's emerging reputation, but most of this lament had a built-in ex-
cuse for the agency. The unspoken assumption that ran through so much
criticism of the agency was that of basic and abiding trust in the capacity
of the career organization. The agency's problems were tied to poor resources, "inadequate" laws, and in some cases poor appointed leadership.
"Despite legislative advances," Dr. Bruce Andreas wrote to *Blue Cross Digest* readers, "the fraudulent and misleading promotion of drugs and cosmetics is on the increase, for the FDA is still hampered by lack of funds,
equipment, and personnel, as well as by the inadequacy of many prevailing
laws." The doctor's inference was a common one in press coverage of the
late 1950s. Whatever failures the FDA was experiencing were failures of
Congress, failure of national politicians to adequately equip, with "manpower" or with "legislation," the scientist-regulators at the Administration. The counterfactual was clear: Left to their own devices, and given

[128]The full title of the Miller Committee report is *Report of September 27, 1960, by a Special Advisory Committee of the National Academy of Sciences-National Research Council to the Secretary of Health, Education and Welfare on the Division of Antibiotics and the New Drug Branch of the Food and Drug Administration together with Subsequent Comments by Secretary Flemming*; reprinted in *ICDRR*, 341. On industry concern over the report's efficacy rec-ommendation, see *FDCR*, November 21, 1960, 14. Leake (Professor of Pharmacology, and President, American Association for the Advancement of Science), to Miller, November 1, 1960; F24, B2, MF. The Miller Committee report also endorsed the agency's promotion control and disclosure regulations of July 22, 1960. The Committee included Maxwell Finland; John H. Diegle (preventive medicine, Western Reserve University); Colin M. MacLeod, (medicine, New York University); Karl F. Mayer (director emeritus, George Williams Hooper Foundation, UCSF); John B. Paul (preventive medicine, Yale); Carl F. Schmidt, (pharmacology, University of Pennsylvania); and Wesley W. Spink (University of Minnesota). On the December 1960 con-sumer groups' visit, see Paul L. Day, Ph.D., "Long-Range Program for the Food and Drug Administration," address before the Animal Nutrition Research Council, October 12, 1960; *ICDRR*, 356.

proper resources and discretion to perform their work, FDA medical officers and pharmacologists would get it right.[129]

General practitioners in the medical profession saw a similar image, one
that worried some as the American Medical Association seemed to disappear from regulatory prominence. As the Hoxsey case drew slowly to a conclusion in 1957, and as the agency successfully concluded its market removal of the quack arthritis remedy Tri-Wonda, most medical professionals
still associated FDA activities with drug policing and anti-quackery initiatives. Combined with controversial decisions on cranberry marketing and
food additives, the Hoxsey and Tri-Wonda cases occasioned a surge of popular media coverage of the FDA during the late Eisenhower administration
and early Kennedy administration. Yet in this new wave of media coverage,
only certain facets of the FDA's operations were presented. Drug "regulation" was witnessed, but not new drug review. Policing and enforcement
functions were emphasized in news to general practitioners and "public"
media of the medical profession, but new drug evaluation and the gatekeeper function were virtually hidden from view.[130]

U.S. FOOD-DRUG AGENCY HAS BROAD POWERS

[*New York Times*, November 15, 1959]

TOUGH FDA PROMISES TO GET TOUGHER IN FUTURE

The Food and Drug Administration flexed its muscles this year, and promises to
get downright tough in the future. The secret behind this increasing power is public support. The American people seem to be getting angry over deceptive trade
practices, attractive but unfilled packaging, counterfeit drugs, watered orange
juice, nutritional quackery, synthetic Swiss cheese and unlabeled poisons. [*Washington Post*, December 25, 1961]

As the *Times* projected the FDA's image with industry, "there is rather
healthy respect for the agency among the industry groups subject to its supervision." "While the F.D.A. is able to police only a tiny fraction of its
beat... its vigilance and integrity have earned it the respect of industry and
a quiet sort of fame within the Government." Like other narratives in the
popular media, the *Times* emphasized a positive, "integrity"-based image
for the FDA, but it was still the image of a cop: "the great bulk of its work

---

[129]Bruce F. Andreas, M.D., "On the Alert," Blue Print for Health Series, *Blue Cross Digest*
(Summer 1958), 10–13. "Food and Drug Administration," *Atlantic City* (NJ) *Press*, June 4,
1955; T. R. vanDellen, M.D., "How to Keep Well," *Chicago Tribune*, June 17, 1958 and September 2, 1959; "The FDA: Guardian of the Nation's Health," *Today's Health* (June 1959),
36–43.

[130]"Drug and Device Seizures," *JAMA* 172 (18) (April 30, 1960): 167/2097; "Quack Devices
Seized By Food, Drug Agents," *AMA News*, June 13, 1960; "FDA Wins Long Battles; Hoxsey,
Tri-Wonda Hit," *AMA News*, October 3, 1960; "Sales Stopped by Seizure," *JAMA* 174 (2)
(Sept. 10, 1960): 186; "Government Wins Battle Against Arthritis Remedy," *JAMA* 174 (12)
(Nov. 19, 1960): 1642; "Larrick Outlines FDA Activities," *JAMA* 176 (8) (May 27, 1961): 17.
Annabel Hecht, "Hocus-Pocus as Applied to Arthritis," *FDA Consumer* (Sept. 1980).

is in ferreting out contaminated or adulterated food and drug products." A similar characterization governed the *Washington Post*'s discussion. Although a waxing of "public support" for the agency was evident, this seems to have been an appreciation for the agency's police functions, aimed at counterfeiting, adulteration, nutritional, and medicinal "quackery." The *Washington Star* described the FDA as Larrick's "policing agency." And the July 9, 1956 issue of *Time* magazine reported that "A policeman is rarely popular, but reputable makers and marketers of foods and drugs are deeply grateful to FDA for bringing peace and order to a once chaotic business." In story after story of this type, drug review and regulation of research was mentioned only in passing, and the agency's pharmacology capacities not at all.[131]

Yet if general public and media outlets were rehearsing the older language of policing and adulteration, trade journal and nested observers in the chemical and pharmaceutical industries saw something subtly different: a protocol-stacked regulatory offensive aimed at new drugs. The *Oil, Paint and Drug Reporter* of November 30, 1959, noted the anti-quackery initiative, too, but it broadcast a different image of the Administration, one that readers of the national news were not seeing.

FDA DECLARES OPEN WARFARE ON MEDICAL QUACKS AND FRAUDS; NEW DRUGS ARE FIRST TARGET

Food & Drug Administration has declared war on medical quackery and frauds. The opening gun is a tightening of its enforcement program on the marketing of new drugs. The objective is to give closer supervision to claims of the therapeutic values of new products and the promotional efforts of manufacturers and distributors. The stepped-up efforts are part of an overall program that is currently being worked up by the government to improve the lot of the older-age population.

Another part of FDA's program will be the introduction of legislation probably during the next session of congress, that will apply the principle of pre-testing for safety the new drug and therapeutic devices that have been coming onto the market.

The *Oil, Paint and Drug Reporter*'s story revealed several facets of the Administration's behavior and identity that were hidden from view in urban press and general physicians journals' depictions of the agency. First, it discussed a legislative initiative designed to regulate clinical development of drugs and devices directly in addition to powers exercised through new drug approval. Second, the article acknowledged that federal regulators were intent upon regulating claims of "therapeutic value." Few if any such allusions appear in popular press accounts of the period. Finally, the article discussed the support of the Federal Council on Aging for the FDA's new programs. The Federal Council's assertions were more than Ralph Smith

---

[131]Cabell Phillips, "U.S. Food-Drug Agency Has Broad Powers," *NYT*, November 15, 1959. Nate Haseltine, "Tough FDA to Get Tougher in Future," *WP*, December 26, 1961. "There Ought to Be a Law," *Time* (July 9, 1956), 60.

could have wished for. Noting that drug therapies were increasingly target-ing "diseases of older persons" and "degenerative processes," the Council urged a form of efficacy regulation: "This agency must take steps to assure that such drugs are pure and potent; that they are properly labeled with adequate directions for use and, where appropriate, with warnings against misuse."[132]

Reputation to Industry: Paternalism, Doubt, Vigor

As Frances Kelsey situated herself within her new bureau, established phar-maceutical firms also noticed an unpleasant change of affairs. In a series of phone calls and letters from 1959 to 1961, officials from Smith, Kline and French asked FDA leadership why their new drug applications were being rejected, and why they were taking longer to review. While an evolving set of concepts and symbols and standards had emerged within the Bureau of Medicine, there was much less clarity outside of the FDA. Presidents and vice presidents of major manufacturers asked for personal conferences with Larrick and his subordinates, asking why their NDAs were getting rejected at twice or three times the rate they had experienced in the 1950s, and asking why the approval time for applications had more than doubled, with many NDAs languishing a year or more without decision.[133]

Officials from numerous companies—Smith, Kline and French, Mead Johnson, Ives-Cameron, Merrell, and many others—were puzzled. Why, they asked, would applications get rejected as "inadequate" or "incomplete" be-cause some of the cases are reported in a sketchy manner? How could the sponsoring firms possibly be held responsible for this failure, when it was a clinical investigator who had failed to perform thorough duty? Ralph Smith's response to Smith, Kline and French (SKF) officials was simply to represent the regulatory vigor as part of established and standardized practice. "Our Medical Officers indicated that this is exactly the way we operate." SKF's executive Francis Boyer wanted full and open discussions between company scientists and FDA medical officers. Smith took this into consideration sepa-rately from Larrick and considered this but, writing to Larrick a month be-fore the Kefauver hearings and the Mintz story, forbade such meetings until the review was completed. Smith's policy fell far short of what company of-ficials wanted, as it did not address the problem of delay in NDA review.[134]

---

[132]"FDA Declares Open Warfare on Medical Quacks and Frauds; New Drugs Are First Target," *OP&DR*, November 30, 1959. For other reports noting the shift in pharmaceutical policy, see *FDCR*, November 20, 1954, 18; "FDA's D-H Enforcement Actvity," *FDCR*, Decem-ber 24, 1956, 11.

[133]Winton B. Rankin, Memorandum of Conference, NDA 12-343 (Parstelin), Officials of FDA and Smith, Kline and French, March 23, 1962; DF 505.5, RG 88, NA. Francis Boyer, Chairman of SKF's Board, and J. Kapp Clark, SKF Vice President for Research and Develop-ment, were both in attendance at this conference. FDA attendees included Larrick, William Kessenich, and Deputy Commissioner Winton B. Rankin.

[134]Kessenich, Memorandum of Conference with E. R. Jolly, representing Ives-Cameron, Sep-

Worse yet, company officials detected a troubling scent of regulatory paternalism in the FDA's new posture. "SKF thinks that there is a growing tendency by the FDA to decide the kind of medical practice to be followed in the United States even to the point of using the price of a drug as a basis for evaluating it. The firm thinks that this is not right. The firm thinks that when we find a drug to be safe and see that the doctor gets full information this is as far as the Government should go." FDA officials replied that since numerous alternative treatments were available in the pharmaceutical world, they were in no way intervening in medical decision making.[135]

Pharmaceutical companies detected these changes slowly and with considerable uncertainty and anxiety. One set of changes occurred in their research and development programs, while another was observed in their political dialogue. In their internal correspondence and communications with clinical researchers, pharmaceutical firms showed increasing apprehension about demonstrating "usefulness," "value," and "efficacy" to the FDA, even for minor applications such as dosage form changes. In February 1957, Abbott Laboratories approached Otto Guttentag, the University of California homeopathic doctor who had become something of an authority on obesity and its treatment. Abbott had already developed Desoxyn (methamphetamine hydrochloride) for obesity treatment, and had received its first approval for the drug in December 1943. Taking Desoxyn required that patients ingest three tablets per day at different times. Abbott now wished to test a "long-acting" preparation of its popular drug, and amid growing reports of the FDA's increasing scrutiny to sustained-release, delayed-release, and long-acting dosage forms in the late 1950s, company officials lined up the best researchers possible, asking Guttentag to examine its "usefulness." When Guttentag agreed to test the Desoxyn formulation, Abbott's clinical investigation chief George Berryman sent him 500 tablets of the drug. Berryman repeatedly reminded Guttentag that Abbott was about to submit an amended NDA, and he primed Guttentag to report favorable evidence on the long-acting version. "If therefore, you will be in a position to send a report on six or more patients indicating that a single dose of the long-acting form is equivalent to two doses of the conventional form, this will be very helpful for that purpose."[136]

tember 21, 1961, Subject "NDA 13-026 (Trecator); DF 505.5, RG 88, NA. Smith, "Memorandum of Interview" with Mead Johnson Officials, October 10, 1961; Winton B. Rankin, Memorandum of Conference, NDA 12-343 (Parstelin), Officials of FDA and Smith, Kline and French, p. 3; March 23, 1962; DF 505.5, RG 88, NA. Smith memorandum to Larrick, "Discussion of NDAs with applicants re letter of April 27, 1962, to Mr. Francis Boyer, SKF, from Mr. Larrick," July 25, 1962; DF 505, RG 88, NA.

[135] Winton B. Rankin, Memorandum of Conference, NDA 12-343 (Parstelin), Officials of FDA and Smith, Kline and French, March 23, 1962; DF 505.5, RG 88, NA.

[136] George H. Berryman, M.D. (Head of Clinical Investigation, Abbott Laboratories) to Guttentag, February 20, 1957; Berryman to Guttentag, March 13, 1957, enclosing Abbott Laboratories Shipping Memorandum 74063; Guttentag to Berryman, April 5, 1957; Berryman to Guttentag, August 7, 1957; Guttentag Papers, MSS 90-35, C 17, F "A"; UCSF Archives. Desoxyn was NDA 5378, approved December 31, 1943.

Guttentag's study was a casual one, without controls, but he launched it quickly, giving the new tablets to three patients in his private practice. Even before he began observing his patients, however, he expressed doubt about the logic behind Abbott's new formulation: "it seems to me that taking a drug orally three times a day instead of once is rarely more than a negligible inconvenience." Indeed, Guttentag found the existing regimen of Desoxyn "therapeutically preferable" to the new, longer-acting version because the thrice-daily regimen was a memory aid. To change existing practice, further-more, required a valid study, and Guttentag feared that "with the tremen-dous influence of psychological factors, a reliable answer to the problem can only be given on a very large statistical basis."[137]

Abbott officials persisted. They wanted a form of testimony from a well-known obesity researcher, and they wanted it for FDA approval on the basis of efficacy. Guttentag went to work prescribing his new Desoxyn tablets, but when he wrote back to Berryman he did not report the positive results that Abbott desired. Of the five patients (of eight original) who reported back to him, two preferred the original formulation, two saw no difference and "had no preference," and one preferred the long-acting formulation. Guttentag concluded with a note of apology: "I am sorry that I cannot provide you with a more favorable report." Despite Guttentag's reservations, Berryman spun the doctor's results positively. "Despite your feeling that these data are not as favorable as we should both like," he wrote Guttentag,

> I consider that the information will be helpful anyway. It seems to me that the two patients who preferred the two tablet arrangement may have found the "string around the finger" aspects desirable for appetite reducing purposes, as we have discussed. If so, their preference for the two tablets does not necessarily reflect the ability of the long-acting form to release the drug slowly. The remaining three, it seems to me, can be considered to have found the one tablet regime satisfactory.[138]

Under Berryman's criteria of interpretation, *any* data would have been favorable to a showing of efficacy for Desoxyn. The fact that Berryman rep-resented Abbott Laboratories, which was among the most established re-search enterprises in the global pharmaceutical industry of the time, and whose officers were mild supporters of strengthened testing requirements for drug firms, highlights the premium that companies placed upon testi-mony from credible researchers. Yet Abbott's development of single-dose Dexosyn also highlights the ambiguity attached to the concept of efficacy, and how little developed the methods for demonstrating efficacy were.

[137]Guttentag to Berryman, June 19, 1957; Guttentag Papers, UCSF.

[138]Guttentag to Berryman, August 28, 1957; Berryman to Guttentag, September 9, 1957; Guttentag Papers, UCSF. For the view of other Abbott officials on drug development, see the remarks of Dr. Edward J. Matson, director of scientific relations for Abbott, expressed at the annual meetings of the Association of Food and Drug Officials of the United States in Louis-ville, KY, in 1957. "Drug Laws Seen as Big Need," *OP&DR* May 13, 1957, 4.

More broadly, the political and organizational spokesmen for the industry were expressing their concern about the near future. With their eye on Estes Kefauver and his antitrust energies and observing the new caution at the FDA, they consistently pleaded for more organizational unity, both among companies themselves and between companies and organized health professionals such as doctors and pharmacists. The worries about a new regulatory posture were voiced as early as 1957, two years before the Kefauver hearings started. "The pharmaceutical economy must resist any piecemeal impairment of its institutional integrity," inveighed Frank T. Dierson, associate counsel of American Pharmaceutical Manufacturers' Association. Robert B. Fiske, vice president in charge of public relations for American Cyanamid Company, New York spoke ominously of the impending "dangers to pharmacy." Fiske warned organized pharmacists to be watchful of those who, "cynical of the justifiable profit motive which provides the means to fuel the system," are "prepared by demagoguery and innuendo to slow—if not to stop—the momentum which is even now attacking the great unsolved areas of human mystery."[139]

Complicating matters for drug companies was the Janus-faced character of the Administration's image. The gentler, more discriminating façade of the FDA's public identity—suppression of quacks, consumer protection, sifting good from bad drugs—differed from the façade exposed to industry. When the Citizens' Advisory Committee convened again in 1962, it expressed its "particular concern with the current status of FDA-industry relationships." Those relationships, the Committee worried, were founded not upon "common understanding, trust and respect," but upon "fear, questioning of basic motives, and lack of opportunity for discussion before drastic action is taken on violations, many of them minor and not related to health hazards."[140]

The persistent irony in the Administration's emergent image had traditional policing functions of food and drug regulation receiving the attention of the popular press and general medical practitioners, while less familiar pre-market regulation and evaluation functions were occupying the attention of the pharmaceutical industry, the academic pharmacology, and clinical research network. In both of these frames the FDA was portrayed as a potential guardian or protector of sorts, but an increasingly disciplinary face was apparent to many in industry and clinical research. In the general public image, protection came through policing; in the agency's internal

[139] Among the many occasions in the mid- to late-1950s where such cautionary remarks were made were the Sixth Annual Rutgers Pharmaceutical Conference at the New Jersey State University in New Brunswick. "Pharmacy Law Interest, Participation Urged at Rutgers," *OP&DR*, May 20, 1957, p. 7.

[140] Citizens' Advisory Committee, *Report to the Secretary of Health, Education and Welfare on the U.S. Food and Drug Administration* (October 1962), p. II-7; in White House Subject Files, Papers of President John F. Kennedy, John F. Kennedy Memorial Library, Boston, MA.

understanding and in the fears of pharmaceutical companies and medical researchers, protection came through gatekeeping and all that this power implied.[141]

George Larrick stood astride these developments, neither leading them nor passionately resisting them. Throughout the 1950s, he spoke of the needs and successes of his "policing agency" and regularly trumpeted the work and triumphs of his inspectors and legal team. Yet he also acknowledged that "subpotent drugs" were a major policy issue, thereby offering implicit support for regulation of therapeutic value and efficacy.[142]

DIFFERENTIATION: THE AMA, PHARMACISTS, AND THE ETHICAL DRUG INDUSTRY

The empowerment of the Administration in drug regulation came at the partial expense of the American Medical Association's turf and authority. The AMA had long been at the center of organized medical efforts to aggregate and pass along information about new drugs to physicians. AMA headquarters had used numerous publications for this purpose, not least its *Journal of the American Medical Association*, a simplified annual entitled *New and Nonofficial Drugs*, and the Association's drug evaluation reports. In the early 1940s, state regulators as well as FDA officials relied continually and thoroughly upon these AMA outlets for information about drug risks, just as the FDA had relied upon AMA reporting in the early stages of the sulfanilamide episode in 1937. Yet by the 1950s, medical opinion leaders, therapeutic reformers, and Administration officials had come to harbor severe doubts about the traditional channels of information flow. Labeling itself came under suspicion, as did the ability of a decentralized, physician-based system of AMA reporting to detect drug risks.[143]

[141] "What Constitutes Interstate Commerce?" *FDCR*, May 17, 1952; "Delivery for Interstate Sale," *FDCR*, September 20, 1952; "Drugs Sold in Interstate Commerce," *FDCR*, October 18, 1952; Bruce F. Andreas, M.D., "On the Alert," Blue Print for Health Series, *Blue Cross Digest* (Summer 1958); 10–13. New drug review is far down the list of powers that Andreas enumerates in his essay.

[142] On Larrick and the reception of his rhetoric in news accounts, see "Quackery and Fake Cures Rising in U.S., Official Warns," (Washington) *Evening Star*, March 17, 1955, p. A-26.

[143] For the AMA's role in the sulfanilamide episode, see the previous chapter. See the FDA's drug alert of May 6, 1948 for "Code CM8164 of 5% Glucose in Normal Saline." Weilerstein reports that the initial reports for the Cutter Laboratories product came from the AMA's Chicago headquarters; RWW, "Drugs Are Not Always What They Seem" (1948), NA, RG 88, Accession 54A-477, B 11, F 7 (DF 505). For the insertion of labeling scrutiny into the new drug application review procedure, see Memorandum (author, William H. Kessenich, M.D., Medical Director, Bureau of Medicine) from Bureau of Medicine to Commissioner, November 28, 1960, Subject "Revised New Drug Procedure." Administrative and enforcement experience had reinforced this conclusion. Memorandum of Conference between Walter Hoskins, Vice President, Crookes-Barnes Laboratories, Inc., Wayne, NJ, and M. L. Yakowitz, B. E. [Bureau of Enforcement] and Thomas H. Riggs, B. M., New Drug Branch, July 2 and July 14, 1959;

The Administration's programmatic response to these concerns was to develop, in social concert with professional organizations, a new agenda for post-market circulation of safety information. Once again identity was negotiated through networks even as it created them. Irvin Kerlan was then serving as head of the drug reference and research branch of the Bureau of Medicine, a position that brought him into liaison with Helen McGuire of the American Association of Medical Record Librarians and George Archambault of the American Society of Hospital Pharmacists. In 1954 and 1955, Kerlan, Archambault, and several of McGuire's staff met in Washington and began to sketch out plans for a central national repository of data on adverse drug reactions. The program would utilize not the AMA but instead a complex of U.S. hospitals, a network emboldened and expanded by recent federal legislation, most notably the Hill-Burton Act. Kerlan invited hospital officials into his program even as he assured them that the Administration had no jurisdiction over them. A pilot program, launched in 1956, involved five hospitals. By 1960, Kerlan had become the agency's Associate Commissioner and the "FDA Drug Adverse Reaction Reporting Program" had been established in the Bureau of Medicine. A year later, the Administration's efforts to rationalize data aggregation and analysis found homes in a new "Statistical Analysis Program." Separately, the Divisions of Pharmacology and Pharmaceutical Chemistry launched individually honed statistical programs and data indexation. When the FDA examined its information aggregation and retrieval systems in 1962, after the thalidomide episode, it found that numerous reforms were already under way in the Bureau of Medicine, but beneath the Bureau's leadership and at a very decentralized level.[144]

The relationship was one of distance on some issues and cooperation on

Subject "Glutavene and Glutavene K (NDA 11-616, 11-650, 2-036, 12-037, Inj. 362)" DF 505.3, RG 88, NA.

[144]McGuire and Archambault served as president of their respective organizations in the 1950s. McGuire, "Medical Records in Therapeutics," *The Prescriber* 2 (January 1955): 4–6. Holland, "Drugs, Records, and You," *Journal of the American Association of Medical Record Librarians* 26 (April 1955), 109–14. Kerlan was head of the Bureau of Medicine's Research and Reference Branch from 1954 to 1958; Kerlan, "Reporting Adverse Reactions to Drugs," *Bulletin of the American Society of Hospital Pharmacists* 13 (July–August 1956): 311–14. As Kerlan and Holland began planning for a new FDA system, Harry Alexander and Chauncey D. Leake added public calls for a national initiative for reporting drug experiences; Leake, "Drug Allergies," *Postgraduate Medicine* 17 (February 1955): 132–9; Alexander, *Reactions with Drug Therapy* (Philadelphia: Saunders, 1955). See chapter 9 for further discussion of the historical evolution of the Adverse Event Reporting System. DRAFT Portion of Report of FDA Committee on Scientific Information, November 29, 1962, p. 8; FOK, B11, F13. John Archer would note the organizational improvements, but would call attention to their scattered nature: "The present procedure for updating and modernizing information handling systems depends upon the initiative and ingenuity of the individual organizational unit to identify its own needs and suggest its own improvements. Up to this time, most efforts to improve have been centered at the Division or Branch level." Memorandum from John D. Archer, M.D. (Division of New Drugs) to Larrick, Subject "Review of New Drug Applications," March 20, 1962; DF 505.5, RG 88, NA.

others. When it came to quackery, there was the appearance of an ongoing and friendly relationship of cooperation between the Association and the Administration. The two organizations held a mutual Congress on Quackery in October 1961, and they continued to press for public recognition of the links between nutritional and medicinal quackery. Both forms of quackery targeted the "consumer," creating a much larger problem of "public health." So too, in matters of "over-the-counter conversions"—where drugs were made available without requiring a physician's prescription—Albert Holland consulted regularly with AMA officials Robert Stormont (formerly of the FDA) and Norman deNosaquo.[145]

As the procedural regime of regulation developed, the FDA and AMA silently crossed swords over new drug evaluation. All the while the Administration was developing novel principles of drug evaluation and rolling out new tools to monitor drugs after NDA approval, the AMA was at once publicly asserting itself in the drug review field and, operationally, ramping down its drug evaluation operations. This duality of messages led to metaphorical confusion. In some respects, the Administration and the Association were considered united, but FDA officials in the Bureau of Medicine maintained an arm's-length relationship, and rarely discussed their cooperation with officials from the Association's Chicago headquarters. AMA official Oliver Field privately complained that while the Association carried on a "close liaison with the federal agency" at the level of operations, and cooperated with FDA officials on matters requiring federal investigation, "it is true that these matters do not get publicity, nor are we portrayed by the federal agency as an organization that has been of help to it in its program." Indeed, AMA officials felt that they had the worst of both worlds: distance from the FDA in the latter's more glorious activities, and accusations that the Association was conspiratorially involved in the agency's more aggressive and unpopular actions. "Our quacks uniformly blame the American Medical Association when the federal agency proceeds against them or their products," wrote Field in 1959. When it took unpopular stands, the FDA's problems mapped onto the "medical trust." In this respect, the agency benefited from the widespread distrust toward the Association in the 1950s and 1960s.[146]

[145]K. L. Milstead, "The Food and Drug Administration's Program Against Quackery," delivered to the Yonkers Academy of Medicine, May 16, 1962; "Federal Food and Drug Administration," Historical Health Fraud Collection, FDA Special Data 1959–1969, Folder 0273-02, AAMA. Holland to Stormont (regarding lotions containing hydrocortisone and hydrocortisone acetate), January 19, 1957; Irvin Kerlan to deNosaquo (regarding tripelennamine hydrochloride), October 16, 1957; H. D. Kautz, M.D. (Secretary, AMA Committee on Research) to Kerlan, November 22, 1957; AMA-COD, Correspondence 1957, Binder T-Z, AAMA.

[146]Dwight Murray, M.D. (President, AMA), "The AMA and FDA: A Story of Cooperation," delivered before the 50th anniversary program of the Pure Food and Drug Act, Washington, DC, June 27, 1956; copy of typescript in AAMA. Starr, *Social Transformation of American Medicine*. Oliver Field (Director, Bureau of Information, AMA) to Dr. M. Howard Rapp (Auburn, NY), November 30, 1959; "FDA Correspondence 1959–1972," Folder 0273-04, AAMA.

General practitioners and specialist physicians alike who were allied with the American Medical Association read these articles with interest, and also some alarm. The spate of new articles never mentioned the AMA in their discussions of drug safety regulation.[147]

On matters of drug evaluation, however, the FDA and the AMA increasingly diverged. The AMA's Council on Drugs (previously the Council on Pharmacy and Chemistry) had long provided public and professional judgments about the efficacy and safety of new drugs coming to market. The Association's publication, *New and Nonofficial Drugs*, had functioned for decades as a guide to new medications for the tens of thousands of American physicians who lacked training or any sort of familiarity in pharmacology. And for much of the twentieth century, when the AMA's Council on Drugs was under the leadership of Torrald Sollman, and the *Journal* was under the direction of Morris Fishbein (1922–1949) or Austin Smith (1949–1959), FDA officials carried on rather warm relations with the Association. Yet even in the mid-1950s, the Association had begun a slow departure from the activity of dispassionate, institutionalized pharmaceutical evaluation, one noticed in the United States and even overseas by German observers of American health policy. In 1952, the Council on Drugs had abandoned *Useful Drugs*, and later that year the AMA stopped distributing *New and Nonofficial Drugs* at no cost to all physicians. In 1954 and 1955, in successive administrative moves dictated from AMA's Chicago headquarters, the Council on Drugs lost authority over advertising in the *Journal of the American Medical Association*. This authority was placed in a new "advertising evaluation department." The Council on Drugs then terminated its "seal of acceptance" procedure for new drugs on February 15, 1955. Prominent physicians and university researchers decried the move.[148]

[147]M. Howard Rapp, M.D. (Auburn, NY), to "Dept. of Queries and Answers," AMA, November 16, 1959; Folder 0273-04, "FDA Correspondence 1959–1972," AAMA. On the important role of specialist physicians in the AMA at mid-century, see Elton Rayack, *Professional Power and American Medicine: The Economics of the AMA* (Cleveland: World Publishing, 1967). My analysis of FDA-AMA relations was greatly assisted by the reading and criticism of Peter Swenson.

[148]On termination of seal of acceptance, see *JAMA* 157 (Feb. 15, 1955): 664–5. For contemporary German perceptions on the AMA and drugs, including a comparison to the FDA, see Gerhard Kärber, "Grundsätze des Council on Pharmacy and Chemistry der American Medical Association für die Anerkennung von Arzneimitteln," *Pharmazeutische Zeitung—Nachrichten*, 17 (1952): 423–7. Walter Modell criticized the drug Tenuate and *JAMA*'s acceptance of Tenuate advertising (*DIAA*, I, 160–61). For other criticism of the termination of the seal of acceptance program, see remarks of Louis Goodman in *DIAA*, I, 241–2: "I think the seal program under the AMA was one of the finest things they ever did, and I regret that it was dropped." The Council on Drugs continued a pattern of informal drug evaluation, on a case-by-case basis as letters arrived. See J. H. Barnebee, M.D. (Corsicana, TX) to "Department of Pharmacy and Chemistry," AMA, April 13, 1957; Robert T. Stormont (Director, Division of Therapy and Research, AMA) to Walter G. Benjamin, M.D. (Pipestone, MN), May 13, 1957; AMA Council on Drugs, Correspondence, 1957, Binder A-C, AAMA.

Then, in 1959, Georgetown University Medical School Dean Hugh Hussey became AMA President and began openly embracing drug advertising in the *Journal*, defending the practice before Congress. In a move whose symbolic importance the Association seriously underestimated, the AMA demoted its Council on Drugs and booted several prominent pharmacologists, including Torrald Sollman, from its membership. Leaders in the clinical pharmacology community, including E.M.K. Geiling, were incensed. As Geiling wrote to Sollman, "We still feel a little hurt at the way the A.M.A. treated you after so many years of outstanding service, and you may be sure that all of us will remember your kindness and patience and noble way in which you accepted this insult." Geiling went on to trash Hussey as a "first class 'bull in the China shop'" who quickly "rushes into print without having the facts or having the wrong information." Editors at other medical journals, including the *New England Journal of Medicine*, shared this uncharitable view of Hussey. Sollman took the dismissal nobly at the personal level but expressed his deep concern for the direction of AMA drug evaluation.

> Like yourself, I view the changes in the Council, office personnel, executive and facilities, with doubt and apprehension. I do not know what is behind the scenes, but it seems to me a striving for the "new outlook," taken over from "big business"; a shift from the old emphasis on good tradition and personality, and special knowledge and qualifications in a given field, to an "integrated" pyramid of supposed executive efficiency, without special experience in the particular field. This may give quick results in business, but it does not seem to me to make for genuine advance, not for devoted loyalty. I regret very much the changes in the personnel of the Council. Those who were dropped all contributed something special, personal, which it will be difficult to replace & which will be sorely missed. Of the new members I know only Haag and [Harry] Dowling, who will make good additions.[149]

Sollmann's dismissal in 1959 coincided with another rough patch for the AMA's reputation and relations with the Administration. By the time Estes Kefauver launched hearings into antitrust issues in the drug industry, and introduced a bill, the AMA's leadership was openly and publicly opposed to the statements and stances of its own Council on Drugs. AMA President Hugh Hussey strongly voiced his concern that, "Although physicians do not want useless drugs cluttering up the practice of medicine and although it is difficult for physicians to become familiar with all of the drugs which have become available during the past two or three decades, we are convinced that the Food and Drug Administration cannot solve these problems for us." In May 1961, the AMA's House of Delegates voted unanimously to pass a resolution expressing opposition to any FDA efficacy requirement, and in May 1961 the Association's Board of Trustees, fearful of being

---

[149] Geiling to Torrald Sollman, January 20, 1960; Sollman to Geiling, January 26, 1960; Box 503521, Folder "Correspondence S," EMKG.

eclipsed by the Administration, proposed a new "AMA Drug Information Program."[150]

To two quite different audiences—academic pharmacologists and Kefauver himself—the AMA's opposition was unpersuasive. No less an authority than Louis Goodman—president of the American Society for Pharmacology and Experimental Therapeutics (ASPET), at that time the world's largest scientific society for pharmacology, and co-author of the most widely used pharmacology textbook on the planet—publicly urged the AMA to abandon its stance and wondered aloud to the Kefauver Committee why he and other members of the AMA's own Council on Drugs were not consulted before the Association announced its position on the efficacy provisions of the Kefauver bill.[151]

The FDA's political diffidence with the AMA was not extended to most specialty medical societies, however. Bureau of Medicine officials actively and publicly sought alliances and consultation with what they termed "the leading medical specialties." From 1951 onward, these included a set of committees co-appointed with the American Academy of Allergy, the American Academy of Pediatrics, the American Congress of Physical Medicine, the American Diabetes Association, and the American Rheumatism Association. All the while Administration leaders actively publicized these overtures.[152]

The other arm's length relationship that the Administration maintained in the 1950s was with the American Pharmacists' Association and, relatedly, the U.S. Pharmacopeia. Among the litany of complaints reaching American physicians, drug companies, and federal officials in the 1950s was the bewildering complexity of trade names for new drugs. Cornell pharmacologist Walter Modell publicly lampooned the "detergent-like names" that companies were bestowing on their drugs. State medical societies, the American College of Apothecaries, and pharmacists' associations had all expressed their frustration with the multiplication of proprietary names that were difficult to remember and as uninformative as they were catchy. The USP and the AMA had long sought to standardize a set of nonproprietary "generic" names for drugs, but both organizations relied upon "wholly voluntary" arrangements for securing these names. When the AMA terminated its seal of acceptance program, furthermore, it lost a bargaining chip in its negotiations with companies. As one AMA official admitted in a letter to Robert P. Fischelis, Secretary of the American Pharmaceutical Association and the most recognized leader among organized pharmacists, "I can say without

---

[150]Hussey remark at *DIAA*, I, 44. "Proposed AMA Drug Information Program," Exhibit A, *DIAA*, I, 47.

[151]Goodman remarks in *DIAA*, I, 212 (ASPET), 215 (opposition to AMA stance), 234 (wonders why AMA did not consult him).

[152]FSA-FDA, "Allergy Group Named to Consult with Food and Drug Administration," June 14, 1951; Folder 0272-06, "FDA, U.S. Federal Security Agency, Special Data, 1941–1952," AAMA.

reservation that nomenclature is the greatest single source of specific complaint that we hear from both pharmacists and physicians."[153]

In the spring of 1957, the FDA began to enter the fray. It did so innocently enough, with Albert Holland proposing merely that the Administration host a conference on the standardization of nonproprietary generic names. Why, trade reporters asked, would the FDA's Division of Medicine be interested in this subject? Because review of new drug applications was becoming confused and delayed by multiple submissions of drugs with identical or near-identical proprietary names. Hence the centrality of the new drug application became, for Holland and Smith, a reason for the agency to step into drug nomenclature as well. AMA, APA, and U.S.P. officials were willing to cooperate with the World Health Organization, with the American College of Apothecaries, and with other interests, but hearing news of FDA "interest" in nomenclature from the trade presses greatly concerned AMA and U.S.P. officials. As Lloyd Miller, Director of Revision for the U.S. Pharmacopeia, complained to Fischelis:

> It seems to me that there is in existence sufficient machinery for selecting suitable non-proprietary names for drugs that it should be unnecessary for the Food and Drug Administration to take a part. The fact that the Administration is expressing a lively interest in this subject simply means that some of us are not doing all we should to work out the problems before us. Some aspects of these problems are intimately tied up with our highly cherished system of free enterprise and I am sure that we would all want to make certain that we agree on our objectives and on the areas where a compromise would be fruitful.[154]

Organized pharmacists, general practitioners, and industry voices were receptive to Miller's worries. Under Fischelis's leadership, the American Pharmaceutical Association had already acted by passing a resolution which recommended that "the selection of nonproprietary names of new drug products be made a matter of cooperation between the American Medical Association, the U.S. Pharmacopeia, the National Formulary, and the International Pharmacopoeia." The absence of the FDA from this resolution was

---

[153]Lloyd C. Miller (Director of Revision, USP) to Robert P. Fischelis, July 25, 1957, p. 4; AMA-COD, Correspondence (1957), Binder T-Z, AAMA. Modell remark at *DIAA*, I, 323.

[154]"FDA Plans to Pin Down Habit-Forming Drug Names," *OP&DR*, August 26, 1957, 3. Lloyd C. Miller (Director of Revision, USP) to Robert P. Fischelis, July 25, 1957, p. 4; AMA-COD, Correspondence (1957), Binder T-Z, AAMA. With respect to the conference, Miller noted, "we have had no recent word, although there has been an item or two in the pharmaceutical press on the F.D.A. plans which indicate a considerably broader scope than was first announced"; Miller to Harold D. Kautz (Secretary, AMA), August 8, 1957; AMA-COD, Correspondence (1957), Binder T-Z, AAMA. Miller had other basis for concern; the FDA's Frank Wiley, head of the Bureau of Pharmaceutical Chemistry, had begun questioning the rigor of USP assays for a wide range of new medicines, placing Miller and his organization on the defensive. See Wiley to Miller, June 19, 1953; A. G. Murray to Miller, September 8, 1953; Miller to Larrick, July 23, 1957; Wiley to Miller, December 17, 1959; B179, F 6, USP.

intentional and noticeable, and Fischelis urged the Pharmacopoeia and the American Medical Association to act quickly upon the resolution. When Estes Kefauver included an FDA nomenclature provision in one of his early reform bills, the AMA weighed in with public opposition. Some industry voices—Theodore Klumpp of Winthrop Laboratories—went still further and defended the idea of "distinctive trade names" as uniquely capable of permitting consumer differentiation of drugs.[155]

By November 1960, as the nation's attention was focused on the presidential election, and as Kelsey was settling in to her new position and was just starting her review of the Kevadon application, and the broadcast horrors of thalidomide babies lay a year or more in the future, the Bureau of Medicine announced new procedures for new drug application review. The reasoning in part concerned public attitudes and the possibility of a bad approval, one with irreversible damage to the Administration's image. "One of the obvious steps to reassure against any such possibility is a procedure that would require checking at a supervisory level of conclusions reached by the individual medical officers responsible for the action taken on applications. It is obvious that in the past we were too understaffed to contemplate any such check operations. . . . We now recognize that present staffing permits and public attitudes require check procedures that may reduce the basis for false alarms about the adequacy of our new drug review." Procedures for duplication of review by chemists as well as medical officers, each writing up separate reports, and patterns of supervision of medical officers by Division and Bureau directors, the latter functioning as an additional check and veto upon the approval decisions of the former, now became codified in administrative practice.[156]

Inspectors, confessed their stark confusion about whether the policy of regulating efficacy had become official, and just how broadly it was applied. Field officers openly wrote Ralph Smith, stating that they "would like to know if the New Drug Branch has now established a firm policy of requiring proof of efficacy before making effective any new drug application." Even though the FDA's field divisions were largely on the same page as that of the New Drug Branch, misunderstanding persisted, in part because the New

[155]Resolution of the House of Delegates of the American Pharmaceutical Association, April 28, 1957; reported in Robert P. Fischelis to George F. Lull, M.D. (Secretary, AMA), July 10, 1957; H. D. Kautz (Secretary to Lull) to Fischelis, July 18, 1957; AMA-COD, Correspondence (1957), Binder D-I, AAMA. As Hugh Hussey told the first Kefauver hearings, "we believe that the problems which remain in the field of drug nomenclature can and should be solved by the profession itself" (*DIAA*, I, 43). "Medicinals Under Brand Names? That's The Only Way, Says Klumpp," *OP&DR*, April 20, 1959, 7. Klumpp was one of the first drug reviewers to work on new drug applications in the days after the 1938 Act passed; by this time, he was president of Winthrop Laboratories and spoke in an address to the College of Pharmacy at St. John's University, Brooklyn.

[156]Memorandum from John D. Archer (Division of New Drugs) to Larrick, Subject "Review of New Drug Applications," March 20, 1962; DF 505.5, RG 88, NA.

Drug Branch's attempts at efficacy regulation in the late 1950s were so bold and continual.[157]

In early 1962, the procedural regime of regulation would stir up anger and confusion in one Stuart Symington, Democratic Senator from Missouri, who placed a call to Ralph Smith on January 3. He drew Smith's attention to the following day's conference between Symington and representatives from Philips Roxane, Inc., based in Symington's home state.

> The Senator inquired why, in handling this application, we had restricted the indications to three conditions rather than nine. I explained that it was on the basis of the lack of investigative reports adequate to show the safety of the drug in certain of these conditions. The Senator inquired whether it was not just a lack of evidence of efficacy since he knew that Secretary Ribicoff had testified that we did not have authority to withhold a drug from the market on the basis of lack of efficacy. I tried to explain that these two factors, safety and efficacy, could not be clearly separated. . . .
>
> The Senator questioned the propriety of one man, Dr. DeFelice, being given authority to make a final and arbitrary decision in connection with the introduction of a new drug. I explained that his decision was not final and that the letter from Dr. DeFelice was considered as a letter from the Food and Drug Administration. Senator Symington inquired who was in control in the Food and Drug Administration and I told him that the Commissioner was Mr. Larrick. The Senator requested that in any case we give his constituent every consideration. I assured him that we would do so but stated that we had no basis for doing anything at the present time unless they submitted more material for our consideration.[158]

This, then, was the state of affairs in American pharmaceutical regulation in January 1962, when efficacy regulation lay dormant in the Senate, fully six months before Morton Mintz wrote his history-altering front-page story, and nine months before the enactment of the Kefauver-Harris Amendments. FDA reviewers and pharmacologists were adding six months to two years to the development time of new drugs by asking for stiffer chronic toxicity tests (explicitly designed to answer safety and efficacy questions as bundled concepts). Efficacy had moved from a concomitant requirement of "proof of safety" to a publicly announced and expected feature of new drug applications. Medical officers were standing up to U.S. Senators. A single medical officer was becoming a veto player in the complex game of drug develop-

[157]Harold F. O'Keefe (Division of Case Control), Memorandum to Bureau of Medicine, "Attention: Ralph Smith & Others," June 29, 1961; DF 505.1, RG 88, NA.

[158]Ralph G. Smith, "Memorandum of Telephone Conversation," between RGS and Senator Stuart Symington, January 3, 1962; DF 505.5; RG 88, NA. Symington's intervention was not an isolated occurrence. Four months after Symington's tirade, Florida Senator George Smathers intervened to allow Nathaniel Klien of Miami-based Key Pharmaceuticals a discussion with Larrick. Larrick, "Memorandum of Interview" with Nathaniel Klien, Key Pharmaceuticals, Miami; NDA 12-368 (Proternol), May 10, 1962; DF 505.5; RG 88, NA.

ment, so much so that interested outsiders wondered who was actually in control of the agency.

Kelsey and Thalidomide in Context

We come, finally, to thalidomide. The story of thalidomide has many times been chronicled, and its outlines are well known if not established as a sort of public myth. In September 1960, the William S. Merrell Company of Cincinnati, Ohio, submitted a new drug application for thalidomide (trade name Kevadon), a sedative that would substitute for the barbiturate-based sleep medications then in use. Available in West Germany without a prescription as Contergan, it was taken by 3 million people nightly within the first year of its introduction there. The Kevadon application was assigned to Frances Kelsey, and it was her first new drug application as an FDA medical officer. Kelsey recognized serious problems in the application and refused to approve Kevadon despite repeated visits and pressure from Merrell officials. By November 1961, Contergan had been tied to an epidemic of birth defects in Europe and Australia, and it was withdrawn from the European market. The U.S. public remained unaware of Kelsey's refusal to approve thalidomide until a quiet Sunday morning in July 1962, when Morton Mintz penned the story of the "heroine of the FDA" in a front-page article in the *Washington Post*. President John F. Kennedy gave her a Distinguished Medal for Civilian Service and asked homemakers everywhere to clean out their medicine cabinets. Hubert Humphrey and Estes Kefauver invited her testimony before Congress and celebrated her example. Frances Kelsey became, literally, a household name. In a much more horrific way, so did thalidomide. Robust new regulations—a statute establishing an "efficacy" standard for FDA drug review in 1962, and new rules regulating clinical trials in 1963— quickly followed.[159]

So oft-rehearsed is Kelsey's triumph in the annals of journalism and popular history that its historical and organizational context has been largely forgotten. No account of the making of modern U.S. pharmaceutical regulation can dispense with this event. Yet instead of narrating the history of pharmaceutical regulation using thalidomide as a breaking point, it is worth starting the thalidomide narrative much earlier and stopping it at the point where public fears about the drug exploded and before Kelsey's decision was publicized and she was elevated to the status of American heroine. In other words, it is worth considering just how much Kelsey's matriculation to the FDA and her behavior at the agency bespoke an already emerging administrative reality.

Frances Kelsey arrived not randomly to the FDA but through the auspices (and at the behest) of one of America's most distinguished pharmacologists:

---

[159]The thalidomide tragedy and the 1962 Kefauver-Harris Drug Amendments are the subject of chapters 4 and 5.

Eugene Maximilian Karl Geiling. Geiling had studied under John Jacob Abel, now viewed as the "Father of American Pharmacology," and had studiously followed Abel's career and his example. After launching his clinical and research career at Johns Hopkins, Geiling left in 1935 to head up a new pharmacology faculty at the University of Chicago medical center. Under Geiling's mentorship, Frances Oldham had conducted research on drug evaluation in the 1940s at the University of Chicago. Specifically, she had investigated the teratogenic effects of drugs on animal newborns and fetuses. She had taught as professor of pharmacology at South Dakota State University from 1948 to 1960. And with her husband F. Ellis Kelsey and Geiling, she had published *Essentials of Pharmacology*, a widely used introductory textbook that went through multiple printings in the 1940s. Kelsey was not, then, an unknown medical reviewer but something of a young known entity when she arrived to the Administration.[160]

Yet the Kelseys were somewhat disenchanted with their experience in South Dakota, and Frances made a habit of sending long, confessional handwritten letters to Geiling. Geiling responded with sympathy, and actively encouraged his colleagues in pharmacology and regulatory work to hire his "brilliant" young student who could "write so well." It is historically significant, then, that Geiling himself preceded Kelsey by several years in arriving to the FDA, first as consultant in 1957 then as full-time head of the new Pharmacodynamics Branch in 1959. For FDA officials who had long known Geiling and yearned to recruit him to Washington, appointing the University of Chicago star was not a new departure but confirmed an earlier pattern of "consultantship."[161]

Although direct evidence is scarce, it is almost certain that Ralph Smith and Albert Holland consulted with Geiling in their decision to interview and recruit the South Dakota professor. Smith himself had consulted Geiling on recruitment matters since at least 1957, and the two men had met at professional conferences to discuss Geiling's recommendations for FDA hiring. Geiling was, moreover, actively promoting his young colleague Frances Oldham Kelsey in the networks he knew, including those in Washington. In fact, food and drug regulation was not the only possibility for Frances Oldham Kelsey in Washington in 1960; Geiling had suggested several others. Along with her

[160]For Geiling's assorted notes and writings on Abel's career, see Folder "Welch Papers, Biography. Abel, Dr. John Jacob, 1857–1938" EMKG. "Dr. E.M.K. Geiling to Leave Hopkins," *Baltimore Sun*, December 21, 1935. On Abel, see John Parascandola, *The Development of American Pharmacology: John J. Abel and the Shaping of a Discipline* (Baltimore: Johns Hopkins University Press, 1992). See the announcement in *JAMA* (Oct. 17, 1939); "Safety and Skepticism: Thalidomide," *Modern Medicine*, October 15, 1962, p. 36.

[161]See the four- to six-page single-spaced handwritten letters in Box 503520, Folder "Correspondence K II," EMKG; e.g., FOK to Geiling, October 2, 1956. No such elaborate letters issued from Kelsey's husband F. Ellis Kelsey. On FDA officials' understanding of the Geiling appointment, see Robert S. Roe (Director, Bureau of Biological and Physical Sciences) to Geiling, May 21, 1959; Box 503520, Folder "Personal Correspondence—R," EMKG.

husband, Kelsey also considered the National Institutes of Health and its Research Grant Division. Once the Kelseys decided to move to Washington, they enlisted Geiling as a reference for their children's private school.[162]

Kelsey was one of several new arrivals to the Bureau of Medicine, and perhaps the most prominent feature of the new arrivals was formalized, procedural scrutiny in new drug review. Frances Kelsey spoke often of the value of "scrutiny" and told a reporter early in her career that "My job is to pick these new-drug applications to pieces." A *Modern Medicine* reporter characterized the data priorities of the FDA reviewers in portraying a scheme of evaluation that had been solidifying for more than a decade: "Generally, the quality rather than the size of clinical trials is more significant to the medical officer. Testimonials that provide no data are considered useless, and fragmentary or partially detailed reports may be cause for finding an application incomplete."[163] As her colleagues had learned in the years before her arrival, Kelsey also shrewdly detected shoddy applications and openly worried about the incentives of doctors testing new drugs. The late 1950s and early 1960s also witnessed publicity about fraud in privately conducted clinical research, including the highly publicized conviction in 1960 of a Philadelphia testing company (Wyanel Laboratories) for falsifying safety and potency tests to small manufacturers. Kelsey's procedural approach to the clinical and animals studies submitted in NDAs put her at odds with older members of her organization.[164]

Beyond this, Kelsey expressed a characteristic distrust of self-medication, especially for sedatives, hypnotics, antihistamines, and other drugs commonly taken in oral form, and over the counter. As she wrote in a May 1961 review of a new antihistamine drug, "I do not feel that an antihistamine of the ethanolamine class could be safely labeled for O.T.C. use because of the sedating properties." Later, reviewing new data for the same application, she worried that "patients are prone to disregard directions and [equate] the drug with aspirin." Kelsey drew upon recent writings in pharmacology journals that cautioned physicians about the sedating properties of some antihistamines and warned that patients would be insufficiently informed to judge their own degree of likely sedation. This was part of a larger concern voiced

[162]Smith to Geiling, January 4, 1957 and January 18, 1957; Box 503521, Folder "Correspondence S," EMKG. FOK to Geiling, February 24, 1960; "I too had the feeling that F & D offered more of a challenge. However, I should have an opportunity to explore the Research Grants Division as I am flying East on March 8th & will spend the 9th & probably part of the 10th at Bethesda. Our friend Harry Clausen is arranging it so that on the 9th I will be able to sit in on several board meetings & see just what they do do." Box 503520, Folder "Correspondence K II," EMKG.

[163]"Safety and Skepticism: Thalidomide," *Modern Medicine*, October 15, 1962, p. 28.

[164]On Wyanel laboratories, *FDCR*, January 11, 1960, p. 28; "On clinical trials, an FDA official recently expressed great concern about doctors who receive a fee to perform a test but either do not test or rig the test to fit a predetermined result" ("Safety and Skepticism: Thalidomide," *Modern Medicine*, October 15, 1962, p. 32).

about the ability of patients to self-medicate with the increasingly complex compounds being released on the market. The FDA's new generation had major concerns about this. It was a common concern in pharmacological circles but not in circles of family practice.[165]

And, characteristic of those in her generation, Kelsey subjected every claim possible, even the most minute and innocuous, to test by means of literature review. Such consultation with the existing medical and pharmacological literature had occurred in the 1940s, of course, but the *degree* of consultation with the clinical research literature, in particular the pharmacology literature, was unprecedented. Kelsey even subjected claims about aspirin and caffeine to literature reviews. She worried that "the tremendous influxes of new drugs and developments following World War II" had necessitated a much "better and faster exchange of scientific information." Her faith in pharmacological medicine and rational therapeutics bespoke a social distrust of the analytic capacities of American physicians in general practice.[166]

Like other medical reviewers, Kelsey was concerned about the quality of clinical investigations, frequently distrusting small-time research operations and foreign studies. As she bluntly put it in an October 1961 review of an antihistamine, "The german work cannot be considered as we do not know the investigator." In other reviews, she expressed bald skepticism about the statistical claims of company new drug applications.[167]

In the language of a later account, these disagreements amounted to a "civil war" within the Bureau, one in which Kelsey had taken sides. Kelsey, wrote *New York Post* writer Barbara Yuncker, "is a partisan in a small civil war inside the Bureau of Medicine between the 'old turks,' who are comfortable with and respectful of drug tycoons, and a few 'young turks,' who administer the law with zeal"; Yuncker, "Pills and You—Is the Kefauver Bill Enough?" *New York Post*, September 16, 1962. Corroborating portraits appear in Stephens Rippey, "FDA's Leadership is Having Trouble," *Drug Trade News*, September 17, 1962, p. 2; *ICDRR*, 625–6.

[165] "Summary" of Review of NDA 12-831, Ambodryl Hydrochloride Compound (CI-477), May 12, 1961; FOK, B11, F9. Dale G. Friend, "Current Drug Therapy," *Clinical Pharmacology and Therapeutics* 3 (Sept.–Oct. 1960): 557–60: Antihistamines "frequently cause sedation which in certain patients, is of sufficient severity to present a hazard to those in positions or activities requiring alertness or close attention. Since the degree of sedation varies with the individual, it is absolutely essential that the physician carefully instruct and see that each patient understands this and ascertains his reactions to the drug before placing himself in situations where serious harm to himself or others might occur." Based upon Kelsey's review, FDA did not allow over-the-counter sales of Ambodryl at the time. Summary of NDA 12-831, Bodryl Compressed Tablets—Ambodryl hydrochloride, October 24, 1961; FOK, B11, F9.

[166] "Summary" of Review of NDA 12-831, Ambodryl Hydrochloride Compound (CI-477), May 12, 1961; FOK, B11, F9. "In respect to the claims about the value of caffeine, it is difficult to see how a dose of 15 mg could exert any effect on an average adult. Further as the *Medical Letter* March 17, 1961, points out, there have been no controlled studies to show that the aspirin, phenacetin and caffeine combination has any greater analgesic effect than aspirin alone." FOK to FDA Historian John Swann, October 12, 1995; FOK, B11, F13. On foreign medical literature, see "FDA Letter to Humphrey Subcommittee on International Drug Data," *DRR*, November 28, 1962.

[167] "Summary of NDA 12-831, Bodryl Compressed Tablets—Ambodryl hydrochloride," October 24, 1961; FOK, B11, F9.

I hardly believe the observed drowsiness was a placebo effect since it increased greatly eg 4% in patients taking one q.i.d. x 2 and 21% in those taking one q.i.d. x 3. If extended studies did prove it to be a placebo effect then I would question whether the drug had any antihistamine effect at the dosage level used since it is chemically related to benadryl and therefore, highly likely to have side effects.[168]

ADMINISTRATIVE CONTINUITY IN KELSEY'S REVIEW OF THALIDOMIDE

Frances Kelsey's approach to thalidomide expressed and continued broader patterns of regulatory practice. In at least three ways, her behavior was characteristic of that of other medical officers in her cohort. First, Kelsey gave express and detailed scrutiny to the research design and the statistics of the safety studies submitted by the Merrell company. Second, she consulted both published literature and the unpublished judgments of peers in government and pharmacology networks. Kelsey examined dozens of medical journal articles on the drug and similar compounds, giving some weight to studies of its chemical composition and stability, but even more to medical reports and clinical experience. And she was assisted throughout her review by a chemist and two pharmacologists. Third, she kept a watchful eye upon the claims made by the company, continuing a sort of social examination of Merrell and its credibility. In this respect, Kelsey was continually assessing not only the drug, but also the competence and moral status of company executives, scientists, and physicians.

Kelsey began her review by subjecting the Kevadon NDA to a searching examination, particularly with regard to the statistical quality of the data presented. Here she found some initial reason for hesitancy. As Kelsey later confided to a Spanish researcher, "the basic experimental work was inadequate. There were, for example, very little data regarding the absorption, distribution, metabolism, and excretion of the drug." In her first letter to Merrell officials in November 1960, Kelsey judged the application "incomplete." She elaborated a host of problems with the application, ranging from statistical power to chemical precision to foreign-language translation.

> It fails to report the animal studies in full detail. . . .
> It fails to report the clinical studies in full detail. . . .
> Many of the cases reported in the application are in summary form without the necessary details included. In addition . . . insufficient cases have been studied. Many of the 3,156 cited cases are in foreign literature reports and in many instances the reports do not represent detailed studies to determine the safety of the drug. The reports should contain more cases in which detailed studies have been done. . . .

---

[168]Ibid.

218

CHAPTER 3

The chronic toxicity data are incomplete and therefore, no evaluation can be made of the safety of the drug when used for a prolonged period of time. . . .

The first paragraph on page 463 titled "Production Method" is rather confusing, and not an accurate translation of the original German. . . .

The application contains rather limited stability data. . . .

The brochure fails to bring out the chemical and pharmacological relationship between Kevadon and glutethimide. . . .

We feel that the side effects are passed over too lightly in the brochure.[169]

All the while scrutinizing every sentence of the application, Kelsey also consulted a wide medical literature and a network of specialists in central nervous system drugs. Her review of the literature was in ways routine, but no less pivotal for the fact. There had been renewed attention to issues of teratogenicity—the tendency for drugs to harm the developing fetuses of expectant mothers—in pharmacology and obstetrics and gynecology circles in the 1940s and 1950s, and Kelsey was well aware of this literature. In her purview she included studies of "therapeutic abortions" induced by drugs, and the "masculinization" of female infants after their mothers had taken oral progestins. "When the thalidomide application was understudy," she later remarked,[170]

> there was developing an increasing interest in the effects of the drugs and other environmental hazards on the human fetus and newborn all of which contributed to our caution in evaluating the application. This subject had previously been somewhat neglected despite the rather extensive animal studies undertaken in this field by such investigators as Werkany, Ingalls, and Fraser. However, in 1940, Gregg recognized the adverse effect of the virus of German measles on the human fetus and the teratogenic effect of aminopterin was described by Thiersch in 1952, while in 1958 Wilkins described the occurrence of non-adrenal pseudohermaphroditism in female infants born of mothers who received synthetic progestine during gestation.[171]

Evidence from administrative records and her contemporaries suggests that Kelsey's memory of the review was not that of an optimistic reminiscence. Kelsey knew well of the Gregg and Thiersch and Wilkins studies and had

---

[169]FOK to E. Iwarchiaha [Barcelona-12, Espana], October 15, 1962; FOK. FOK to Wm. S. Merrell Company ("Attention of Dr. F. Jos. Murray"), November 10, 1960; in *ICDRR*, 81. Something of an administrative and legal chronology appears in *ICDRR*, 75–81.

[170]M. M. Grumbach, J. R. Ducharme, and R. Moloslok, "On the Fetal Masculinisation Action of Certain Oral Progestins," *Journal of Clinical Endocrinology* 19 (Nov. 1959): 1369–80. J. B. Thiersch, "Therapeutic Abortions with Folic Acid Antagonist, 4-aminopteroyl-glutamic Acid (4-amino PGA) Administered by Oral Route," *American Journal of Obstetrics and Gynecology* 63 (1952): 1298–1304. R. Courrier and A. Jost, "Intersexualite foetale provoquee par la Pregneninilone au cours de la grossess," *Compt Rend Soc de Biol.* 136 (June 13, 1942): 395–6.

[171]FOK, "Problems Raised for the FDA by the Occurrence of Thalidomide Embryopathy in Germany, 1960–1961." Presented at the 91st Annual Meeting of the American Public Health Association, Kansas City, MO, November 14, 1963; FOK.

read them carefully. She had noted the drug's adverse effect upon spermato-genesis in males. She targeted her reading to studies of the effect of thalido-mide and like compounds on the central nervous system of animals and humans. She noted in a 1960 study that thalidomide "does antagonize the effects of well-known central stimulants on spontaneous activity of rodents in a 'jingle cage,'" and she circled and noted two animal studies on the cen-tral nervous system effects of thalidomide and on the absorption of thalido-mide in the rat. She took particular note of a physician's letter to the *British Medical Journal* in 1959 describing the "disorientation" experienced after his patient took thalidomide. She scrutinized carefully any study touted by Merrell officials, criticizing one of their central articles for lacking a placebo control. And characteristic of her rigor in evaluating statistical research, she circled a study submitted by one Doctor Ray Nulsen of Cincinnati (who provided what Richardson-Merrell officials saw as some of their best "clinical evidence" for thalidomide) and noted her concern that Nulsen's safety esti-mate was based not on controlled trials but merely on "avail. Reports."[172]

Kelsey's perusal of current literature eventually brought her to a Decem-ber 1960 letter in the *British Medical Journal* from British physician A. Les-lie Florence, entitled "Is Thalidomide to Blame?" Florence noted the appear-ance of "marked paraesthesia," "pallor," "coldness," and "numbness" in the feet and hands of four of his patients who were taking thalidomide. The med-ical term for this bundle of conditions was peripheral neuropathy (or pe-ripheral neuritis), a loss of sensation in the limb extremities. Florence noted cautiously that "Thalidomide is generally regarded as being free of toxic ef-fects, but in this instance the drug was stopped." The report piqued Kelsey's curiosity and concern, for she knew that the "general regard" for thalido-mide's lack of toxicity was not premised upon studies in the vein of clinical pharmacology.[173]

Kelsey consulted not merely a web of literature but also a network of col-

---

[172]Johns Hopkins University pediatrician Helen Taussig wrote several articles in 1962, and she intimated that Kelsey had developed concerns about the possible teratogenicity of thalido-mide early on, based upon her knowledge about teratogenicity from animal studies from her work with Geiling at the University of Chicago; Taussig, "The Thalidomide Syndrome," *Scien-tific American* 207 (2): 29–35. On the disoriented patient, see *BMJ* 2 (Oct. 3, 1959): 635. Among other studies from which Kelsey had taken notes in 1960 and 1961 were F. Coulston, A. L. Beyler, and H. P. Drobeck, "The Biological Actions of a New Series of bis(dichloroacetyl) diamines," *Toxicology and Applied Pharmacology* 2 (1960): 715–31; Louis Lasagna, "Tha-lidomide—A New Nonbarbiturate Sleep-Inducing Drug," *Journal of Chronic Diseases* 11 (6) (1960): 627–31; C. G. Heath, D. J. Moore, and C. A. Paulsen, "Suppression of Spermatogen-esis and Chronic Toxicity in Men by a new Series of bis(dichloroacetyl)diamines," *Toxicology and Applied Pharmacology* 3 (1961): 1–11. From the Heath, et al., article, Kelsey noted: "Sup-presses sperm output & motility & alters sperm morphology. Depression of spermatogenesis." B1, F2, FOK. Her concerns about the Nulsen's studies were first expressed in November 1960; Kelsey to Wm. S. Merrell Company, November 10, 1960; *Interagency Coordination*, 82.

[173]*BMJ* 2 (Dec. 31, 1960): 1954. Denis Burley of the Distiller Company (the British firm marketing thalidomide as Distaval in the UK) acknowledged Florence's report and urged mon-itoring of patients taking it for longer than six months; *BMJ* 3 (Jan. 14, 1961): 130.

leagues in government and academic institutions. Throughout her review of thalidomide, even after it was clear that the drug would not enter the "U.S. market, Kelsey maintained contact with a diverse group of scientists and clinicians who were conducting animal research into thalidomide or had specialties in teratogenic side effects of drugs. These included John Nestor, who had joined the Bureau when Kelsey did, and who later introduced her to Helen Taussig of Johns Hopkins and who arranged for meetings between FDA and NIH scientists in 1961 on another Merrell drug, MER/29. Kelsey asked frankly for judgments not merely of Kevadon's potential safety profile, but also for its therapeutic value. On both dimensions, she received blunt and largely negative assessments. Donald Tower of the federal Institute for Neurological Diseases and Blindness confided to Kelsey that "He knew of no similar toxicity for other drugs, and had not heard of this drug but did not feel it offered much." Moreover, "in view of the chronic use this drug was advocated for, the toxicity was important and could well be underestimated." Kelsey's husband F. Ellis Kelsey, then working in the FDA Pharmacology division, had even harsher things to say. The section of the NDA comparing thalidomide to a similar drug (glutethimide), he wrote, "is an interesting collection of meaningless, pseudoscientific jargon, apparently intended to impress chemically unsophisticated readers." A proposed comparison of the two drugs was "absurd," and a study of thalidomide's absorption was so heavily weakened by an "either undescribed or inadequate" experimental procedure as to render the data "completely meaningless as presented." Richardson-Merrell's statement that thalidomide exhibited no LD50—no lethal dose—induced a mocking F. Ellis Kelsey to write: "No other substance can make *that* claim!" So too, when comparing glutethimide and thalidomide, Richardson-Merrell's application used a dosage for thalidomide that matched a common dosage form for glutethimide. This F. Ellis Kelsey found "absurd" and infuriating.

> The last sentence in this section is an almost classic example of the widely used irrelevancy of size-of-dose comparisons between drugs. Weight is never a determinant of activity or toxicity; this is a property of each drug. For example one gram of a great many drugs is very much less toxic (or effective) than one-hundredth of a gram of a large number of other drugs. Since this is an elementary concept of pharmacology I cannot believe this to be honest incompetence.

The discussions between Kelsey and her consults in 1960 and 1961 reflected two dimensions of judgment that lay outside the official purview of the law. The first dimension was efficacy. Tower's doubts about the drug were not just safety-based, but were expressed in relation to the drug's apparently poor profile of therapeutic benefit. Kelsey herself may have echoed this theme when she allegedly expressed doubt to Murray about the need for "a new hypnotic."[174]

[174]Kelsey, "Summary of Substance of Contact" with Dr. Donald B. Tower—Chief of Clinical

At its core, though, Kelsey's thalidomide review was essentially and self-consciously a moral appraisal of Merrell. Thus a second dimension of judgment entailed a mix of the competency of the investigation and the honesty of Kevadon's presentation. Kelsey's doubts were piqued early on by the vagueness of the application and the grandiosity of its claims. The claims were just too glowing—"too good to be true," and the clinical reports in the NDA were "really more testimonials than scientific studies." These initial judgments were echoed by her husband, who openly called into question the honesty of Merrell officials after reading their application. What cemented these doubts in Kelsey's mind was the company's failure to notify her of the peripheral neuritis reports coming from Britain. Merrell officials could not honestly plead ignorance of these, for officials from Distillers (the British marketer of thalidomide) had written the *BMJ* in January 1961 to address A. Leslie Florence's report and, in so doing, acknowledged other reports of peripheral neuropathy they had received "early in 1960." Even so, when speaking by phone in February 1961, Merrell's F. Joseph Murray did not acknowledge the peripheral neuropathy reports until Kelsey confronted him with the Florence letter. Kelsey was dismayed by the omission and her distrust deepened. Her memoranda and writings on the Kevadon application were shot through with frank appraisals of whether company officials were behaving in ways that were "honest," "frank," "trustworthy," or "competent." Most telling are her troubled but routine write-ups of meetings with Richardson-Merrell officials, for instance that in March 1961.

> Mr. Jones and Murray came in to discuss the Kevadon application in view of their recent visit to England and Germany. They maintained the toxicity incidence was low and rapidly reversible. Brief perusal of a report by Cohen in California indicated this was not always the case. They displayed British and German labeling that drew attention to the toxicity. They kept urging me to say we would pass the drug with similar cautions. I pointed out we would have to study the submitted material in detail before reaching any conclusions as we felt that the field of usefulness of the drug was such that untoward reactions would be highly inexcusable. *I had the feeling throughout the day that they were at no time being wholly frank with me and that this attitude has obtained in all our conferences etc. regarding this drug.* I may have been partly prejudiced by their advanced publicity (*Medical Sciences* March 52, 1961 [sic]) in which they featured work by Lester which we indicated was inadequate and in which they compare Doriden [glutethimide] and Kevadon chemically after they had previously mentioned they

Neurochemistry Laboratory, Institute of Neurological Diseases and Blindness; June 28, 1961; FOK. Oscar E. Schotté, Professor of Biology, Amherst College, to FOK, September 5, 1962; FOK, B1, F2. For F. Ellis Kelsey's memoranda, see Memorandum from F. E. Kelsey to F. O. Kelsey, December 23, 1960, Subject "Comment on information concerning Kevadon submitted by W. S. Merrell Co., December 9, 1960," in *ICDRR*, 85. See also Insight Team of the Sunday Times of London, *Suffer the Children*, 75. Ralph G. Smith, Handwritten "Memo of Telephone Interview," NDA 12-611 (Kevadon), April 13, 1961: "Dr. Murray stated that in a previous

were entirely different drugs, and by their failure to notify us of the British reports of toxicity.[175]

What Kelsey's notes reveal in brutal honesty is that, for much of 1960 and 1961, she doubted thalidomide because she doubted its sponsor. While Kelsey's famed "stubbornness" appears well evinced in these notes, so does her substantial discomfort in her meetings with Merrell. Repeatedly she talked with other government officials, other university clinicians and researchers, even her husband, to check her gut instincts that she was being misled.

Kelsey's ethical doubts about Merrell officials were representative of other concerns that had spread through her organization since the Cincinnati imbroglio of 1954. When the company submitted an NDA for its cholesterol inhibitor MER/29 on July 21, 1959, it expected a quick and positive review. Merrell's new drug had generated considerable excitement in academic medical and cardiology networks. Yet less than two months after Merrell submitted MER/29, the application was deemed incomplete "since the data submitted shows a low margin of safety for a drug which would receive chronic use." The agency requested additional studies of the drug's toxicity in animals. When those tests came back, Edwin Goldenthal reviewed them and found them satisfactory for questions about toxicity over a several-month period but nonetheless recommended against approval. Echoing the global and long-term view of the FDA's pharmacological regime, Goldenthal urged that "Before we release this drug for general distribution... the company should submit results of well controlled extensive clinical studies in which the individuals have received the drug for periods of years." Yet the level of trust in Merrell's products was higher in the Bureau of Medicine than in the Division of Pharmacology, and MER/29 was made conditionally effective on April 19, 1960.[176]

The Bureau of Medicine's judgment on MER/29 in April 1960 would soon be revisited and doubted by external audiences. The year-old *Medical*

---

interview with Dr. Kelsey, she had doubted the need for a new hypnotic"; FOK; see also *ICDRR*, 91. On Nestor's introduction of Kelsey and Taussig, see Jonathan Will, "The Feminine Conscience of FDA—Dr. Frances Oldham Kelsey," *Saturday Review*, September 1, 1962, 41–3; *ICDRR*, 779. "Memorandum from Senator Hubert H. Humphrey on Background to Exhibits on MER/29," ibid., 820.

[175] Kelsey oral history (Rockville, MD), May 30, 1974, NLM; cited in Richard McFadyen, "Thalidomide in America," *Clio Medica* 11 (2) (July 1976): 80. Kelsey, Handwritten memorandum in thalidomide file, February 23, 1961; *ICDRR*, 87. Kelsey, "Summary of Substance of Contact" and "Memo of Interview," March 30, 1961; FOK, B1. In narrating the Kelsey review, journalists from the *Sunday Times of London* have claimed that the crucial phone conversation of February 23, 1961, "can be seen to mark the end of Richardson-Merrell's chances of ever marketing thalidomide in the United States" (*Suffer the Children*, 76). There is little evidence to suggest that this phone call represented a form of turning point. If anything, rather substantial doubts appear to have settled in Kelsey's mind much earlier.

[176] "Proceedings of the Princeton, New Jersey, Conference on MER/29," December 16–17,

Letter on Drugs and Therapeutics, founded in 1959 by Arthur Kallet of Consumers' Research fame, expressed open doubts about the drug's efficacy, suggesting that "the drug should still be reserved for experimental trial." Reports of diabetic complications in MER/29 patients, including a high rate of cataract formation, began to flow into the agency from numerous sources, most prominent among them the Mayo Clinic. These concerns were then echoed by the American Medical Association's Council on Drugs, which published a November 1961 editorial in *JAMA* that stopped short of calling for market withdrawal but concluded that MER/29 be limited to severe cases of atherosclerosis or hypercholesterolemia, and then only "under the carefully controlled conditions of clinical investigation." Merrell's advertising campaign for MER/29 offered statements about efficacy that were tagged as "wholly unscientific" by New York physician Herbert Pollack and "offensive" by FDA medical officer Frank Talbot. Merrell advertisements soon became a sorry exemplar in the Bureau of Medicine's proposal for FDA control over advertising. As the reports on MER/29 complications continued to mount, the FDA secured Merrell's agreement to send a "Dear Doctor" warning letter on the drug. A market withdrawal was considered but was also held to be legally suspect, as other firms (including Norwich Pharmacal) were currently contesting the FDA's authority for market withdrawal, and as Merrell had indicated that it would legally challenge any market removal of its top-selling medication. The AMA Council on Drugs' November 1961 editorial suggesting controlled marketing of MER/29, moreover, had given the Bureau of Medicine some cover. And *Newsweek* had weighed in with a brief story entitled "Worth the Risk," stating general support among cardiologists for MER/29's continued but restricted distribution. Doubts within the agency about Merrell and MER/29 continued to mount, quite independently of the thalidomide case. Within the year, Associate Commissioner John Harvey would conclude that his agency's conditional approval of MER/29 in April 1960 was mistaken.[177]

1958; *ICDRR*, 824–5. Albert A. Brust, M.D., "Introduction to the Proceedings," February 1, 1960, *Progress in Cardiovascular Diseases*, Special Supplement 2 (6), part 1 (May 1960): 485. E. I. Goldenthal, Division of Pharmacology, memorandum to New Drug Branch, FDA, Attn: Dr. Talbot, "Triparanol Capsules, MER/29 (Wm. S. Merrell Co.), NDA 12-066," February 23, 1960; *ICDRR*, 840–42.

[177] "MER/29," *MLDT* 2 (21) (Oct. 14, 1960): 81–83. Mayo drug safety specialists had expressed their concerns within the hospital's Committee on the Safety of Therapeutic Agents (CSTA); see CSTA Minutes, November 9, 1961, and *Annual Report of the Committee on the Safety of Therapeutic Agents for the year 1961*; CSTA Records, MAYO. Mayo officials from the Section of Ophthalmology began to meet with John Nestor as early as October 1961; T. R. Kirby, "MER/29 Chronology," July 17, 1963; reprinted in *ICDRR*, 940–44. AMA-COD editorial in *JAMA*, November 11, 1961, p. 574. The potential affront to the FDA from the AMA-COD was recognized by trade journalists; *FDCR*, November 20, 1961; *ICDRR*, 893–5. Herbert Pollack, M.D. (New York) to O. L. Kline (FDA), November 9, 1960; Talbot to Pollack, December 1, 1960. Memorandum re "NDA 12-066, MER/29, The Wm. S. Merrell Co.," J Deutscheberger (BPPA), Frank J. Talbot, October 24, 1961. Pollack had alerted FDA officials

Kelsey's mistrust of Merrell Company officials, then, was organizationally embedded. She also cleaved tightly to a line of ambiguity about what
remained to be done. She avoided elaborating a set of conditions for approval, and instead preserved flexibility for later judgments. Her stance of
reluctance and ambiguity, was, moreover, explicitly and repeatedly legitimated by her superiors. While Ralph Smith allowed Murray and other Merrell officials to visit FDA headquarters and meet with Kelsey—it was common practice at the time, by no means unique to Larrick's tenure—he just as
often kept visitors at arm's length from his newest medical officer. Smith
refused to commit his organization to eventual approval of the Kevadon application, and he pushed for a wider consultation with central nervous system specialists. "I told [Merrell officials] that I could make no prediction as
to whether they would obtain an effective new drug application or when it
would be. I said that it was a matter for serious consideration and that possibly we might discuss the matter with some of our investigators or other
experts." When Murray later vented angrily that Kelsey was simply avoiding a decision on the application, Smith rebutted that "since she wanted to
investigate further," Murray was simply wrong.[178]

At the core of Kelsey's concern was a nagging hypothesis that peripheral
neuropathy might signal something much worse, perhaps irreversible central nervous system damage or perhaps harmful effects to the human fetus.
The sources of Kelsey's concerns about fetal effects of thalidomide ingestion
were multiple. As part of her work with Geiling in the 1940s at Chicago, she
had noted that the rabbit fetus differed markedly from its mother in tolerance of quinine. The lesson of this finding was of less importance for quinine and more importance for methodology. Kelsey was made "particularly
conscious of the fact that the fetus or newborn may be, pharmacologically,
an entirely different organism from the adult." Hence, studies involving
adult animal and human subjects were of little value in demonstrating safety
and efficacy for the fetus. Kelsey made this point repeatedly in her memoranda to Merrell and to Smith, and she was concerned about fetal effects of
thalidomide long before reports came in from Europe. Yet her pharmacological doubts were echoed by her husband, by Francis Tower, and by Ralph
Smith. And in an oral history in 1974, she acknowledged the influence of
John Nestor, Irvin Kerlan, and Irwin Siegel, all of whom were interested in

to other issues surrounding Merrell drugs; Kline memorandum to Ralph G. Smith, November
3, 1960; all in *ICDRR*, 877–89. "Adverse Side Effects Increasing as More New Drugs Hit
Market," *WSJ*, December 7, 1961, 2. "Merrell-FDA Discussions on Future of MER/29 Result
in Sending "Dear Doctor" Letter to All MDs Warning Against Side Effects," *FDCR*, December
4, 1961, 24–25. "Worth the Risk," *Newsweek*, December 23, 1961, 53.
[178]Smith, "Memo of Interview" and "Summary of Substance of Contact," NDA 12-611,
March 30, 1961; *ICDRR*, 88–9. On criticism of Smith for allowing Murray and Jones access
to Kelsey during the review, see "Shake-Up in FDA Seen as Thalidomide Result," *Washington
Evening Star*, September 18, 1962. Other evidence suggests that Smith was much more protective of Kelsey and had some of the more difficult discussions with Merrell officials; Hilts, *Protecting America's Health*, 153–4.

teratogenic effects of drugs. In many respects, Kelsey's questions regarding Kevadon were reinforced and deepened by her participation in the regulatory network of the FDA and her consultation with other officials.[179]

Kelsey's doubts mounted, and in the frustrated words of Merrell officials, the Kevadon application experienced "delay after delay after delay." She asked for more animal studies, including those with potential effects on the fetus, and she asked for long-term studies (following users for more than one year) monitoring the possibility of peripheral neuropathy and its reversibility among thalidomide patients. After an exasperated Murray wondered why the easygoing experience with Contergan in Germany did not constitute basis for approval, Kelsey told him that European experience with thalidomide was only of informational value and had no significance as precedent. Then, in a note to Murray, she set straight the legal and political terms on which Murray's company approached her.

> We have taken appropriate note of your contention that it has not been proved that Kevadon tablets actually cause peripheral neuritis, and the fact that the labelling of the drug proposed in your letter of March 29, 1961, fails to make a frank disclosure that the drug has been found to cause peripheral neuritis. In the consideration of an application for a new drug, the burden of proof that the drug causes side effects does not lie with this Administration. The burden of proof that the drug is safe—which must include adequate studies of all the manifestations of toxicity which medical or clinical experience suggest—lies with the applicant. In this connection we are much concerned that apparently evidence with respect to the occurrence of peripheral neuritis in England was known to you but not forthrightly disclosed in the application.[180]

Murray considered this letter "somewhat libelous" and immediately started pressing higher authorities at the FDA for a resolution. In a subtle but profound challenge to Kelsey's organizational membership and to the identity of Smith's Bureau, Murray asked Ralph Smith "whether the firm was dealing personally with Dr. Kelsey" or whether Kelsey's letter represented the

[179]The research on quinine was part of a larger pattern of cooperation between Geiling and his staff and military agencies during the war years. See Geiling to General J. I. Bonesteel (Commanding General, 6th Corp Area, U.S. Army, Chicago, IL), March 11, 1941; Box 12, Folder 7 (Pharmacology), Presidents' Papers, 1940–1946, University of Chicago Special Collections. Taussig, "The Thalidomide Syndrome," *Scientific American* 207 (2): 29–35. See Oldham, Geiling, and Kelsey, *Essentials of Pharmacology* (New York: Lippincott, 1947), 9–13 (on absorption, metabolism, and toxicity), 360–363 (on quinine). Oldham's was the first name on the book, and correspondence from the Geiling papers (Johns Hopkins) indicates that she was the principal author of the book. Walter Kahoe (Director, Medical Publications Division, Lippincott) to Geiling, July 14, 1964; Geiling to Kahoe, October 30, 1957; Box 503520, Folder "K I," EMKG. See also FOK Oral History, NLM, pp. 10–11; cited in McFadyen, "Thalidomide in America," 82. For memoranda on fetal effects and human absorption, see Kelsey, "Memo of Telephone Interview," July 27, 1961, and "Memo of Interview" (with Murray, Jones, and Louis Lasagna), Conference of September 7, 1961 (typed October 30, 1961); Smith, "Memo of Telephone Interview" (with Murray and Kelsey), September 26, 1961 (typed October 13, 1961).

[180]*Suffer the Children*, 78–9.

views of "this Administration." While acknowledging that any letter from any FDA officer could be reconsidered, Smith told Murray that Kelsey's handwritten letter "should be considered as from the FDA." Then in May 1961, Murray and a Merrell colleague visited William Kessenich, then FDA Medical Director. They complained that the Bureau of Medicine had not expressed clearly the problems with the Kevadon application, "a view I am not sure is justified," Kessenich noted. After a lengthy discussion of the requirements for a new drug application, Kessenich was puzzled: "This discussion should not have come as anything new to these men who regularly have such matters before us." Finally, as if non-committal ambiguity were the organization line, Kessenich "gave these visitors no specific remedy for the problems of their NDA."[181]

Well before the reports began to arrive from Germany and Australia tying thalidomide to birth defects, then, Frances Kelsey's chilly reception for thalidomide was legitimized within her Bureau as standard practice. Smith and Kessenich saw Kelsey's approach to the Kevadon application as customary, and they could only express puzzlement as to why Merrell had neither grasped the requirements for a new drug application nor taken seriously the peripheral neuropathy reports.

.   .   .

It is possible and worthwhile to pause the narrative here, in the spring of 1961—before thalidomide was withdrawn from global markets later that autumn, before Morton Mintz and the *Washington Post* made Frances Kelsey a household name, and just as Estes Kefauver was launching his ethical drug hearings and well before he took direct aim at issues of pharmaceutical safety. At this juncture, we can pose some counterfactuals to characterize more tightly the trajectory of organizational development—what had actually happened and what had been foreclosed.

Consider first the story of U.S. pharmaceutical regulation in the absence of its star heroine. What if Frances Kelsey and her husband had stayed in South Dakota, or she had joined the National Institutes of Health? What if she had never arrived to the agency? Would thalidomide have received the scrutiny it did? Would the FDA have been empowered to regulate efficacy and the investigational stage of drugs? Here the answer to the first question is "quite likely" and the answer to the second is clearly affirmative. The pivotal "aura" of Kelsey is not merely that she made the decision, but that she was a highly effective symbol. Thalidomide itself likely would have led to stronger regulation of investigational new drugs, though the fact that Kelsey ran the IND branch in the 1960s eventually made these regulations stronger. On the other hand, Kelsey's recruitment was endogenous to the story; she came as part of a preexisting network, and it is easily conceivable

---

[181] "Memorandum of Interview" between "F. Jos. Murray, M.D., Robert H. Woodward, Wm. S. Merrell Co., and William Kessenich," May 10, 1961; *ICDRR*, 94.

that had she not come, another doctor hired by Ralph Smith (John Nestor, for instance) would have resisted Kevadon's approval. Moreover, in the absence of either Kelsey or thalidomide, the United States would still have witnessed the rise of modern pharmaceutical regulation because its central precepts and institutions—efficacy, therapeutic value, clinical pharmacology's dominance, investigational-stage constraints, and the new drug application—were in place by 1959 at latest.

Second, consider the trajectory of pharmaceutical development in the absence of its congressional sponsor, Estes Kefauver. What if Kefauver had focused his attention elsewhere, or had not ascended to the chair of the Antitrust and Monopoly Subcommittee in the first place? Here the counterfactuals are easier to postulate. In the absence of Kefauver, the United States would have developed efficacy-based pharmaceutical regulation characterized by the pursuit and protection of reputation. Again, the United States had already developed efficacy standards, the new drug application as the pivot of the regulatory process, and standard of pharmacological evaluation (placebo controls, randomization, individualized case reports) before Kefauver ever turned his attention to drugs, and almost all of the pivotal development occurred under a Republican presidential administration.

Third, consider the trajectory of pharmaceutical regulation under alternative political scenarios. What if the Democrats had not made substantial midterm gains in the elections of 1958? What if Richard Nixon had won the election of 1960? The 1958 midterm counterfactual is more interesting, as perhaps Kefauver would not have pursued the pharmaceutical industry with as much vigor had the midterms not given his party renewed energy. Yet all of the officials who impelled and symbolized the transformation in U.S. pharmaceutical regulation were in place by the summer of 1958, and the impetus for greater FDA funding and for discretion was coming from the Eisenhower administration and the recommendations of its Citizens' Advisory Committee three years before.[182]

The interlacing of reputation and regulatory power would decisively shape the politics of pharmaceutical regulation in the late twentieth century. That interlacing arrived not merely through public cataclysm of thalidomide but years before, through ambiguous emergence. The institutional development of American drug regulation came in the procedural congealing of regulatory practice and concepts. The drama of thalidomide would reshape them again, on stages both national and global.

---

[182]Some of the Nixon counterfactuals can be addressed by examining the FDA under the Nixon administration, as headed by Commissioner Charles Edwards, as I do in chapter 5. It is worth noting that whereas food manufacturers received Edwards and the Nixon FDA warmly, pharmaceutical manufacturers and libertarians did not.

CHAPTER FOUR

Reputation and Power Crystallized: Thalidomide, Frances Kelsey, and Phased Experiment, 1961–1966

The thalidomide incident was a major factor leading to the enactment of the Kefauver-Harris Amendments of 1962. This has led to the conclusion by some that the law, and our investigational drug regulations, were hastily drawn and thus must have been poorly drawn. This is not correct. The Department's proposed legislation, which served as the basis for most of the provisions in the law as enacted which relate to drug testing, was very carefully drafted by experts and widely studied within the Executive Branch of the Government before it was sent to the Congress by our Secretary. Similarly the proposed investigational drug regulations were carefully prepared on the basis of many years of experience with the new drug law before the thalidomide situation came to public attention. Rapid developments in drug research and in promotional methods for drugs necessitated evaluation of the effectiveness of new drugs as well as their safety. Furthermore, the need for greater control and surveillance over the distribution and clinical testing of investigational drugs became apparent as abuses began to appear.

—Frances O. Kelsey, 1963

There is a certain concern and a feeling of uncertainty regarding the fact that all decision making authority rests solely and finally with the personnel of the Food and Drug Administration.

—Summary of Pharmaceutical Manufacturers' Association officials' complaints to the Modell Advisory Committee on Investigational New Drugs, 1963

The tame submission of the pharmaceutical industry to any and every regulatory suggestion or directive—regardless of the medical and scientific facts involved—is unsettling.

—James Z. Appel (President, American Medical Association), 1966[1]

IMAGE AND POWER in American pharmaceutical regulation took new shape in the early 1960s. In a series of events at the crossroads of legislative politics, national media attention, scattered personal tragedies and triumphs, scientific debate, and administrative interpretation and rulemaking, a new combination of reputation and power came into being. These changes were vast. In the policy tragedy of thalidomide, a new image of the Administration crystallized in the public and legislative imagination. Frances Kelsey came to national limelight and public commemoration as a new icon for the government physician and regulatory reviewer. A new statute—the Drug Amendments of 1962—codified the burgeoning powers and expansive practices of the 1950s, and it supplied the agency with commanding new authorities. The process of regulatory clearance for new drugs shifted subtly but durably, as the process of "pre-market notification" gave way to mandatory drug "approval" by the FDA. Standards of evidence changed, from "safety in use" (and implied judgments of "efficacy") to the formal "effectiveness" criterion. The governance of experiment became a central activity in pharmaceutical regulation, as the Administration seized upon the "adequate and well-controlled studies" clause in the new law to stipulate a model of three-phased experiment, to make incursions into the regulation of clinical trials and human subjects protections, and to shape the requirements for professional activity in pharmaceutical research.

These changes crystallized the emerging tools of directive, gatekeeping, and conceptual power. And they crystallized a set of organizational images—benevolent protector, fierce gatekeeper, arbiter of medical inquiry—that, with others, would hold sway in American politics for two generations.[2]

[1]Kelsey, "Problems Raised for the FDA by the Occurrence of Thalidomide Embryopathy in Germany, 1960–1961." Presented at the 91st Annual Meeting of the American Public Health Association, Kansas City, MO, November 14, 1963; FOK. Sidney Merlis, Untitled summary of PMA officials' complaints to the Modell committee, October 30, 1963; FOK. Appel, "New Drugs: The AMA and FDA Roles," speech delivered to the annual meeting of the American College of Allergists, Chicago, IL, April 29, 1966; AAMA.

[2]I consciously adopt the term "crystallization" as a metaphor in this chapter. The notion of crystallization—of a liquid solution reaching a state of "supersaturation" (an abundance of competing identities), followed by processes of primary and secondary nucleation that issue in solid crystals of varying size and shape (the solidified identity forms are subject to varying

The Kefauver Reform Initiative

For at least a century, American legislative politics has been marked by stasis and incremental change. The textbook norm of policy stability, marked by bargaining among numerous groups and factions that inhabited and spanned the major parties, was the basis for classic twentieth-century accounts of national policymaking in the United States, ranging from David Truman's *The Governmental Process* to John Kingdon's *Agendas, Alternatives and Public Policies*. Even the textbook models recognize an exception to their generalizations, however. There are moments even in American politics when heaven and earth seem to align, when the felt pressure for legislation produces quick, consensual action that subsumes and elides persistent disagreements.

Thalidomide created one of those moments. As the elixir sulfanilamide tragedy did for the 1938 Act, the thalidomide crisis busted a stalemate over proposed regulatory legislation. And like the 1937–38 episode, thalidomide helped to produce a regulatory regime—the Kefauver-Harris Amendments of 1962 and the Investigational New Drug Regulations of 1963—with stronger regulatory properties than any of the bills previously under discussion in Congress.[3]

The apparent coupling of tragedy to legislation—the pairing of sulfanilamide with the 1938 Act and the pairing of thalidomide with a new statute in 1962—has led many an observer to conclude that catastrophe itself is the mother of U.S. pharmaceutical policy. In fact, regulatory change has been far more measured and contingent upon shifts in interpretation and practice. Even at the level of formal authority, the transformation effected in 1962 and 1963 differs materially from that of the 1938 Act. The changes of the 1960s were wrought by different sorts of groups and organizations, most notably a Senate committee whose staff helped to organize the central hearings, helped connect crucial informants, journalists, and academics, and helped to advance the legislation. The writers of new policy at the Administration were not so much party elites like Henry Wallace but more like career civil servants such as Ralph Smith, Frances Kelsey, Julius Hauser, and

---

interpretations)—helps to express some of the properties of reputation building that I observe in the FDA in the late twentieth century. Crystallization solidifies one of many possible representations and the continuity of re-crystallization means that no reputation (or a particular solid form) is ever permanent. The continuity of a representation and its re-expression and contestation in political networks and discourse can be considered a form of "continuous crystallization." As with any model, there are weaknesses to this metaphor, among them its supposition of a homogeneous liquid in which nucleation occurs (political and historical environments are much more "heterogeneous," it would seem).

[3]The combination of incremental change and punctuated bursts of innovation has become a central subject of study in mathematical models. For the classic model in budgeting, see John F. Padgett, "Bounded Rationality in Budgetary Research," *APSR* 74 (June 1980): 354–72. For a more recent treatment, see Bryan Jones and Frank Baumgartner, *The Politics of Attention: How Government Prioritizes Problems* (Chicago: University of Chicago Press, 2006).

Irvin Kerlan, teamed with upper-echelon agents like William Goodrich. Perhaps most important, the 1962 Amendments to the Food, Drug and Cosmetic Act were both preceded and followed by extensive FDA rulemaking and transformation of administrative practice. The 1962 Amendments bespoke policy movement even as they authored it.[4]

In Congress, a mid-century reform initiative in ethical drug regulation started not with health and safety issues, but with Estes Kefauver's windmill tilt against industrial concentration in the American economy. Kefauver took the chair of the House's new Subcommittee on Monopoly in 1946. He quickly commenced general hearings on the problem of economic monopoly in the United States, inquiries that would continue with his election to the Senate in 1948. Kefauver's proceedings were interrupted by the Republican-controlled 83rd Congress (1953–54) and by the Senator's own campaign for the Democratic presidential nomination and the vice presidency in 1955 and 1956. In 1957, Kefauver became Chair of the Senate's Subcommittee on Antitrust and Monopoly. The Tennessee Democrat's interest in industrial organization dovetailed with two related worries among American citizens—the economic and political threats posed by monopoly and the persistence of price inflation. It was a mark of mid-twentieth century politics that Kefauver could credibly participate in the anti-communist legacy of Roosevelt and Truman and continually favor stronger regulation of American corporations. At the core of the hearings—whose early years were marked by daily television coverage—lay a regulatory defense of free enterprise. In a tradition of political economy that expressed the views of Louis Brandeis and earlier thinkers, Kefauver argued that capitalism, democracy, and the fabric of American society were equally threatened by economic concentration. It was significant, in this respect, that Kefauver's first hearings were an investigation of crime and racketeering. The tone of the early hearings identified antitrust and (later) pharmaceutical regulation as endeavors with moral and symbolic heft that transcended their economic significance.[5]

---

[4]Hilts, *Protecting America's Health*; Stephen J. Ceccoli, *Pill Politics: Drugs and the FDA* (Boulder, CO: Lynne Rienner, 2004); Daemmrich, *Pharmacopolitics*. For one narrative of more continual change in regulatory policy, see chapter 3 and the discussion of the emergence of pharmaceutical "efficacy" concepts; see also the narrative of nuclear energy regulation in Balogh, *Chain Reaction*.

[5]Richard E. McFadyen, *Estes Kefauver and the Drug Industry* (Ph.D. diss., History, Emory University, 1973), 6–16. Along with Richard Harris, *The Real Voice*, McFadyen's dissertation offers the most detailed account of the 1962 Amendments. On Kefauver's antitrust interests and philosophy, see Jack Anderson and Fred Blumenthal, *The Kefauver Story* (New York: Dial Press, 1956) and Joseph Bruce Gorman, *Estes Kefauver: A Political Biography* (New York: Oxford University Press, 1971).

Kefauver was appointed by Texas Democrat Wright Patman to his House chairmanship position. The Senate Subcommittee on Antitrust was created as a subsidiary to the Judiciary Committee during the 83rd Congress. Kefauver was in line to take control of the subcommittee when Democrats regained control of the Senate in 1955, but intra-party squabbles put fellow Democrat Harvey Kilgore at the head. Kefauver ascended to chair in 1957 with the dawn of the 85th Congress.

More than anything else, Kefauver's hearings placed the regulation of pharmaceuticals on the agendas of U.S. national politics and journalism. Part of the reason was the celebrity and expectations that the Tennessee senator's presence imparted to the cause. By 1960, Kefauver's was among the most recognized names in American society and electoral politics. He joined the Senate in 1948 and quickly made headlines with his nationally televised hearings on organized crime in 1950. Nearly 30 million Americans tuned in to see Kefauver's hearings, and his 1951 book *Crime in America* was a national bestseller. Re-elected easily in 1954, Kefauver was one of the lone Democratic senators who refused to sign the Southern Manifesto of 1956. After he and Adlai Stevenson lost resoundingly to Eisenhower in the 1956 general election, Kefauver began to target what he saw as a pattern of anti-competitive and inflationary behavior in the steel and automobile industries. Numerous industries made efforts to target Kefauver in 1960, but he prevailed again in a close election.[6]

In what was perhaps their most silent but persistent legacy, the Kefauver hearings associated the business of pharmaceuticals to that of other, more familiar "industries." In his inquiries into the concentration and pricing in the steel and automobile markets, Kefauver had begun his exploration with prototypical manufacturing sectors of the American economy. When he turned congressional and journalistic attention to ethical drugs, the makers of pharmaceuticals were presented to the American public as if they were much like other industrial giants: large corporations capable of manipulating prices, consumers, and politics. Combined with budding concerns about inflation in drug prices, the Kefauver hearings directed national attention to the details of ethical drug development and manufacture as perhaps never before.[7]

In the late 1950s and early 1960s, Estes Kefauver's intentions were the subject of weekly monitoring, scrutiny, and fantasy. To American business, the Senator from Tennessee appeared as a specter of haunting proportions. In part this was because of Kefauver's previous scrutiny of American manufac-

---

[6]Kefauver also graced *Time* magazine's cover in March 1951; "It Pays to Organize," *Time*, March 12, 1951. On Kefauver's activities in the House and Senate, see Gorman, *Estes Kefauver: A Political Biography*, and Julian Zelizer, *On Capitol Hill: The Struggle to Reform Congress and Its Consequences, 1948–2000* (New York: Cambridge University Press, 2004), 30, 40–41, 71.

[7]Harris (*The Real Voice*, 8–11) discusses Kefauver's notoriety. For publications from Kefauver's earlier hearings and inquiries, see U.S. Congress, House Committee on Small Business, Monopoly Subcommittee, *United States versus Economic Concentration and Monopoly*, Report, 79th Congress, December 27, 1946 (Washington, DC: GPO, 1949). See also Dominique Tobbell, "Pharmaceutical Networks: The Political Economy of Drug Development in the United States, 1945–1980," (Ph.D. diss., University of Pennsylvania, 2008). As a comparison, neither in 1905–1906 nor in 1937–38 had there been extensive national or congressional discussion about the process of pharmaceutical research and development or manufacturing. In part this is because congressional hearings accompanying this legislation were fewer in number, and because such hearings were not nearly as publicized as Kefauver's hearings were. Moreover, issues of food regulation played a much greater role in the 1906 and 1938 episodes.

turers and his rumored interest in health-care inflation. In part it was due to recent activities by the Department of Justice and the Federal Trade Commission targeting drug firms for price-fixing. Seeing the Salk vaccine prosecutions in 1958, the *Oil, Paint and Drug Reporter* predicted "heavy weather ahead for the drug business." Quoting "veteran observers of the Washington scene," the *Reporter* feared that the federal government "may have been only warming up for a long series of harassments to the pharmaceutical industry." The 1958 midterm elections and the 1960 general election contest—both largely dominated by national Democrats—worsened the industry's prognosis, and the pharmaceutical industry soon found itself facing scrutiny from the Fountain committee in the House as well as the Kefauver committee in the Senate.[8]

Kefauver's hearings into pharmaceutical production and pricing began in December 1959. The discussion was dominated by issues of "profit margin" and "markup." When accounting profits were calculated and compared across twenty-five industrial sectors by Kefauver's staff, it was reported that "the drug industry" had by far the highest profit rate. When the manufacturing cost of common medications was compared to the retail price, congressional investigators discovered markups of 1,000 percent or more—the per-tablet manufacturing cost of new drugs was often one-tenth or one-twentieth of the retail cost to consumers. These statistics and their propagation by the Kefauver committee occluded some important issues while keeping others from view. As in the early twenty-first century, industry representatives argued in 1959 and 1960 that drug prices needed to cover all costs of the production process, not just the marginal cost of synthesizing, tabletting, and packaging a finished product. Most notably, they maintained, drug prices needed to recoup the costs of research and development for drugs marketed as well as those developed but not marketed. Other company executives fairly complained that the costs of distribution, overhead, and taxation had been excluded from the committee's figures.[9]

Despite these protests and the genuine issues they raised—and in part because Kefauver had so bluntly and effectively simplified the process of

[8]A series of fearful articles in trade reporters of the time provides a helpful catalog of the industry's anxiety about Kefauver and other government actors. "'Wonder Drug' Output Figures Are Being Sought by the FTC," *OP&DR*, May 27, 1957, 4. "Gov't Vaccine Pricing Case Seen as a Warm-Up for Attack On Other Producers of Drugs," *OP&DR*, May 19, 1958, 5. "Drug Firms Shocked at Salk Pricing Case," *OP&DR*, May 19, 1958, 5. "Chemical Industry Sees Itself a Loser in 1958 Elections," *OP&DR*, November 10, 1958, 3. "Kefauver Prepares to Scatter Buckshot at the Drug Industry As It Reels From Gov't Blows," *OP&DR*, November 17, 1958, 5. On the Fountain committee, see "House Probers Turn Cold Stare On Drug Men," *OP&DR*, December 15, 1958, 3. "Drug Industry PR Outlook: Worse Before It Gets Better," *OP&DR*, April 11, 1960, 51. "Drug Industry Seen Target for Politicians," *OP&DR*, April 11, 1960, 51, 60.

[9]For an interesting account of how Kefauver's staff became interested in pharmaceutical issues, see Harris, *The Real Voice*, 1–7, 14–16. Kefauver Hearings, Part 14, 7860; Part 16, 8887–90; quoted in McFadyen, *Estes Kefauver and the Drug Industry*, chap. 2. See McFadyen's second chapter for an in-depth discussion of the complexities of the pricing and profits data.

drug development and manufacture—public doubts about the industry began to crystallize in a way that deeply worried its officials. A public opinion poll in spring 1960 told American respondents that "Recent congressional hearings have revealed that the mark-up on prescription drugs is extremely high." It then asked, "Do you think the government should take action to control prescription drug prices?" Over 65 percent of respondents said yes. Voices allied with the industry echoed and amplified these fears. Though their compassion for pharmaceutical manufacturers was overwrought, drug trade reporters properly described the Kefauver hearings as the latest in a durable wave of negative publicity buffeting the industry. Kefauver's ceremonies, one reporter stated, were "the feature attraction growing out of the rash of recent finger-pointing that has thrown the drug business off balance, forced its legal brains into overtime activities and is causing a reassessment by the industry of its public relations." One month before the hearings started, the Pharmaceutical Manufacturers' Association took the bold, unprecedented, and highly publicized step of hiring the public relations firm Hill & Knowlton. As an *Oil, Paint and Drug Reporter* editorial of December 1959 concluded, no issue facing the pharmaceutical industry was as daunting as the public relations challenge symbolized by the Kefauver investigation: "The drug trade has a most important and very big job in public relations before it—and it is in a pillory."[10]

Having identified and amplified a national problem, Kefauver's committee advanced several policy solutions. By the spring of 1961, these had been bundled into an omnibus bill, S.1552. The easiest of these, it appeared, was to amend the 1938 Food, Drug and Cosmetic Act to require the FDA to pass on the effectiveness as well as the safety of medicines before their marketing. Kefauver felt this would simply codify much of existing practice and prevent wasted consumer expenditure upon worthless pharmaceuticals. A second tactic was to allow the Department of Health, Education and Welfare to license drug producers under standards promulgated by the FDA. The third option was to require approval of advertising and inserts by FDA at the same time as the molecule itself was being reviewed. This plank was less worrisome to industry interests because it substituted for FTC regulation of advertising and because it mimicked existing FDA regulatory practices.[11]

---

[10] "Kefauver's Drug Industry Show Due to Take Road November 30 For What May Be a Long Run," *OP&DR*, September 28, 1959, 5; "Drug Men Find Kefauver Is Casting a Bigger Net," *OP&DR*, October 26, 1959, 3; "PMA Public Relations Job Goes to Hill & Knowlton," *OP&DR*, November 2, 1959, 7; "Drug Trade Pilloried," *OP&DR* (Editorial), December 21, 1959, 32.

On the public opinion poll, see Ralph L. Cherry, "Drug Industry, Already in a Burn Over the Antics of Sen. Kefauver, Finds a Newspaper Poll Now Adding Fuel to the Fire With Some Suspect Opinions About Government Control of Medicine Prices," *OP&DR*, February 8, 1960, 30. The *Washington Star* poll that formed the basis for Cherry's article suffered from loaded questions and from other methodological problems, but its effect upon industry perceptions of the threat from Kefauver's legislation was no less real for that fact.

[11] This narrative skips some of the developments in 1960, including Kefauver's bill S.3677,

To pharmaceutical manufacturers, the most controversial and worrisome provisions of the law were its patent provisions. Kefauver first proposed that qualified drug makers, by paying a small royalty fee to the pioneer firm, could receive a license to produce any patented drug within three years of the patent's effectuation (the statutory patent life was then seventeen years). This proposal would have the effect of maintaining the patent system in formality while requiring the pioneer company to relinquish its exclusive rights to companies willing to pay the cost. Second, Kefauver proposed eliminating patent protection for "me-too" drugs, which were defined as molecular alterations that did not show evidence of therapeutic superiority over the pioneer or, in the case of fixed-combination drugs, over the component drugs used alone. Third, Kefauver wanted to increase physician incentives for generic prescribing by enabling FDA inspectors to assess complaint files and the qualifications of technical staff. These authorities would give the Administration the capacity to declare generic drugs to be of equivalent quality and purity as trade name drugs. As if to give the Kefauver initiative greater credibility and heft, other voices in national politics were calling for even more drastic measures. Eisenhower HEW Secretary Arthur Flemming proposed automatic inspection of all drug products before their shipment in interstate commerce, a scheme tarred as "stronger than the Kefauver idea" by industry allies, who met Flemming's idea with cries of dictatorship. And by the fall of 1960, the Democratic Party had convened a twenty-one-member Advisory Committee on Health Policy of the Democratic Advisory Council, headed by medical celebrity Michael E. DeBakey, that issued an open call for federal licensing of drug firms and for strengthening of the FDA.[12]

---

introduced in June 1960, which empowered the Administration to assess efficacy and to assist in firm licensing but which did not include the patent reforms discussed in the next paragraph. Like other reform bills in the 86th Congress, it was stopped by industry lobbyists; "Chemical Men Like the Work Of a Now-Suspended Congress: It Ditched Troublesome Bills," *OP&DR*, July 11, 1960, 3. See McFadyen, *Estes Kefauver and the Drug Industry*, 213–14, for a synopsis of this interim legislation.

As the hearings were beginning in December 1959, the *OP&DR* observed that for the first time, Kefauver was also looking at industry expenditures on advertising. In addition, Kefauver had been rumored to have interest in regulatory checks on advertising claims for new drugs, in regulation of generic names and nomenclature, and in the general issue of "quack drugs"; "Kefauver's Head Now Buzzing With Master Plan for Reforming Practices in the Drug Industry," *OP&DR*, December 21, 1959, 3. "The proposal that new drug applicants submit their advertising matter simultaneously with their new drug application," the *OP&DR* reported, "was not new with FDA officials. To a certain degree this is done now. Manufacturers are required to submit their brochures and package materials to FDA along with the application" (37). The *OP&DR* story shows that FDA officials, who served as a source for the December 21 article and this attribution, perceived that they had already possessed many of the powers that S.1552 would grant to them.

[12] On other proposals, consult "Kefauver's Drug Licensing Plan Is Coming Out of the Shadows to Show Its Political Nature," *OP&DR*, June 27, 1960, 3; "Flemming Seeks Dictator's Control Over Drug Trade," *OP&DR*, July 4, 1960, 3. In Kefauver's proposal, authority for licensing would rest in the hands of the HEW Secretary, not the FDA. See also McFadyen, *Estes Kefauver and the Drug Industry*, 214–19 (proposed patent changes), 256–57 (Flemming proposal).

Through 1961 and the spring of 1962, Kefauver continued his hearings, and an influential series of articles by Jonathan Lear in the *Saturday Review* fueled wider concern among professionals and policymakers about the promotion, misuse, and regulation of antibiotics. Yet while Kefauver had succeeded in the task of problem definition, he had so far failed in the task of statutory change. There were numerous reasons for the stoppage of S.1552, not least the concerted opposition of the American Medical Association (to the new efficacy requirement) and the Pharmaceutical Manufacturers' Association (mainly to the patent system changes). In the Senate, the AMA-PMA alliance was personified by Republicans Everett Dirksen of Illinois and Roman Hruska of Nebraska, who skillfully induced the larger Judiciary Committee to disembowel Kefauver's legislation when it came out of subcommittee. S.1552 would never emerge from the Committee. Kefauver had, moreover, created numerous enemies with his idiosyncratic style and his flair for independence. Yet as much as anything else, it was the silence and diffidence of the new and popular President Kennedy and his White House staff that deflated Kefauver's initiative. Kennedy's policy advisers viewed Kefauver and anything he proposed as radical, and they were motivated to focus on those policy reforms for which the White House could claim credit. Presidential records suggest that in June 1962, when S.1552 was being emasculated in the Senate, Kennedy was focused upon four measures: trade expansion, tax reform, farm legislation, and his "Healthcare for the Aged" plan. In contrast with these priorities, all of them central to the Kennedy strategy and to his projected legacy, the safety, development, and marketing of medicines were near invisible issues. There was, finally, little citizen interest in pharmaceutical reform in June 1962. As Morton Mintz summarized matters, "a tranquilized, sedated public raised little outcry when the Senate Judiciary Committee gutted Senator Estes Kefauver's bill to strengthen the drug laws."[13]

FDA officials, particularly in the Bureau of Medicine, did not reflexively observe the legislative process but actively wrote drafts of new drug reform

---

[13] Lear was science editor of the *Review*; "Taking the Miracle Out of Miracle Drugs," *Saturday Review*, January 23, 1959. Lear's investigation also revealed the payments that FDA Antibiotics Division Chief Henry Welch had received from drug makers for his editorship of a serial. The activity of industry spokesmen in the 86th Congress (1959–60) was primarily one of obstruction; "Chemical Men Like the Work Of a Now-Suspended Congress: It Ditched Troublesome Bills," 3. Telling and specific narratives of legislative action in the 86th and 87th Congresses include Hilts (*Protecting America's Health*, 132–43), McFadyen (*Estes Kefauver and the Drug Industry*, 214–50, 295–99, 305, 309–17), and Harris (*The Real Voice*). Kennedy's attention was focused on the Trade Expansion Act (H.R. 11970), Health Care for the Aged (S.909, H.R. 4222), Tax Reform (H.R. 10650) and the Farm Bill (S.2786). "Legislative Items Recommended by the President," June 8, 1962, The White House; B 51, F 1 ("Legislative Files"), Papers of President Kennedy, John F. Kennedy Library, Boston, MA. See also McFadyen, 291–4.

The emasculation of Kefauver's measure by the Senate Judiciary Committee comprises a larger and more detailed story than can be conveyed here. See McFadyen, 303–15; Mintz, "Drug Tragedy Revives Hope for Cure," *WP*, August 19, 1962.

bills and directly lobbied Cabinet officials and House and Senate legislators. Such patterns of active bureaucratic participation in the legislative process were evident in President Eisenhower's second term (1957–60), and they were fueled by long-standing dissatisfaction among FDA officials with the weaknesses in their enabling statute. Congressional debate over legislation in 1953 had been interpreted by the courts as an authoritative "legislative history" so conservative as to sharply restrict the Administration's inspection powers. The agency had requested full certification authority over all antibiotics in 1950, but the demands fell silent on Capitol Hill. The Bureau of Medicine, even with the 1956 rules and the conceptual apparatus of efficacy at its disposal, was still shackled by the sixty-day review time limit. Sensing new opportunities and emboldened by Bureau of Medicine leadership, agency officials introduced reform bills to the House in 1960 and 1961. These bills were the products of drafting and research from numerous agency officials spread across and through its hierarchy, including General Counsel William "Billy" Goodrich and Bureau of Medicine officials Julius Hauser and Frances Kelsey who in the fall of 1960 studied the drug statutes and agencies of European nations.[14]

Besides changes to administrative practice and new legislation, FDA officials also changed policy in 1961 and the spring of 1962 by means of rule-making. Here the pivotal actors were Goodrich, Hauser, Bureau of Medicine physician Robert McCleery, Food and Drug officer Harold Chadduck, and advertising specialist Morris Yakowitz. In 1961, as part of the self-styled "full disclosure movement," Bureau officials proposed regulations requiring that all prescription drugs be accompanied by full instructions pertaining to uses, dosage, and possible side effects. The existing rules compelled companies to disclose this information only indirectly, by making relevant "literature available upon request." A second proposal, pushed by Yakowitz in particular, required any advertising circular distributed among physicians to include a balanced portrait of the drug's side effects. Both of these proposals had their roots in aspirations of Bureau of Medicine officials in the early 1950s, including Ernest Q. King and Ralph G. Smith. And both would eventually become embedded within American food and drug regulation, though not until after 1962.[15]

[14]McFadyen, *Estes Kefauver and the Drug Industry*, 252–4 (weak authority pre-1960), 257–60 (1960 bill), 286 (1961 bill), 261–66 (new regulations). Nate Haseltine, "Tough FDA Promises to Get Tougher in Future," *WP*, December 26, 1961. Kelsey corresponded with Geiling in 1960 about the Medical Research Council of the UK, as well as British statutes for food and drugs. She was specifically interested in the Therapeutic Substances Act of 1956; Geiling to Kelsey, May 16, 1960; F "Correspondence, K II," EMKG. The FDA's bills were "Factory Inspection and Drug Amendments of 1960" (S. 3815, H.R. 12949) and the "Factory Inspection and Drug Amendments Bill of 1961," which updated the 1960 measure in the 87th Congress (1961–62). Hauser had been active in the "full disclosure" regulations, the good manufacturing practice regulations, and the investigational drug regulations; Hauser, "Biography," attachment to Marsha J. MacIntosh to C. J. Cavallito, September 12, 1969; JHPP.

[15]On the drug advertising regulations and the full disclosure movement see "Julius Hauser,

Administration officials did not simply mind their own business by keeping track of FDA-sponsored legislation. They also offered commentary on other measures, including the committee markups of the Kefauver bill. When in June 1962 the Senate Judiciary Committee reported S.1552 and gutted Kefauver's favored provisions, three FDA administrators filed an angry brief with Commissioner Larrick and HEW Assistant Secretary Wilbur Cohen. Their laments were, eventually, communicated to Emanuel Celler, Chair of the House Judiciary Committee (and a friend and longtime ally of Kefauver's). "This is regressive legislation and should be defeated," the officials wrote. The Senate draft, they said, encumbered the work of FDA inspectors, failed to provide the Administration with robust withdrawal authority, and left the concept of "efficacy" so vaguely defined as to reduce the discretion of the Bureau of Medicine in new drug reviews. The FDA-sponsored bills of 1960 and 1961 differed in every manner conceivable from the Senate's markup. They elaborated upon the meaning of efficacy, gave factory inspectors new authorities, and compelled the federal government to refuse drug clearance in those cases where efficacy had not been shown.[16]

THALIDOMIDE AND THE PUBLIC TRIUMPH OF FRANCES KELSEY

As FDA and Merrell officials battled over the Kevadon application, reports were emerging of an outbreak of congenital birth abnormalities in West Germany, Britain, and Australia. Called "phocomelia" (from the Greek, for "seal extremities") because many of the victims were born without intermediate limb structures such as elbows, the syndrome produced macabre objects for public horror (figure 4.1). Television viewers and newspaper readers saw feet protruding from hips and "Knuckles at shoulder-blades," as Sylvia Plath would hauntingly mark the deformity in her poem *Thalidomide* (1962). Well beyond the visible carnage, the thalidomide epidemic included hundreds and perhaps thousands of cases of internal organ damage, brain impairment, and death; the number of children stillborn or aborted has never been accurately counted. The initial investigations into the phocomelia epidemic were conducted not by pharmacologists, but by epidemiologists and pediatricians. By the time that highly decentralized physicians' clinics in West Germany began to pool their observations in the summer of 1960, German authorities realized that they had an epidemic on their hands, one that added fifty to one hundred infants per day to the ranks of victimhood.[17]

Memoirs" (typescript, composed 1991–94, JHPP; in possession of the author), 125–29. Haseltine, "Tough FDA Promises to Get Tougher in Future."

[16] M. D. Kinslow, Winton Rankin, and "JHS" (probably Joseph Sadusk, then Medical Director), to Cohen and Larrick, July 18, 1962; Abraham Ribicoff (Secretary of Health Education and Welfare) to Emanuel Celler, May 17, 1962; B 3182—1962, DF 505, RG 88, NA.

[17] One version of this malady was known as "tetra-phocomelia," or "four seal's limbs." Such deformities were known to be rare and possibly congenital. A Danish study published in 1949

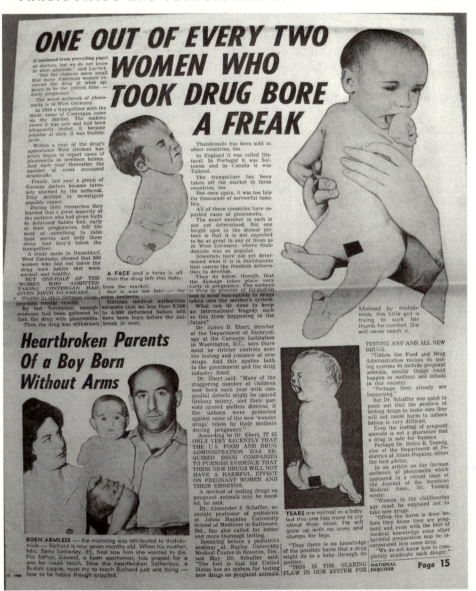

Figure 4.1. Thalidomide images from the *National Enquirer*, 1962.

Finally, in late 1961 two physicians—Widukind Lenz of West Germany and William G. McBride of Australia—each independently announced their conclusions that thalidomide was responsible for the birth defects. Lenz and McBride inferred from available data that, when taken in the first trimester of pregnancy, thalidomide would induce birth deformities. Tragically, thousands of pregnant women had taken thalidomide during this window of pregnancy because of its utility as an anti-nausea drug. Upon Lenz and McBride's announcements, Chemie-Grunenthal officials withdrew the drug from the European market, but Merrell continued to claim in its letters to FDA medical officer Frances Kelsey that there was no proven relationship between their compound and the abnormalities. Kelsey rejected this assertion and again imposed the burden of proof upon Merrell. As the stories became more numerous and as the link between drug and defects became clearer, Merrell quietly withdrew the NDA for Kevadon in March 1962.[18]

The thalidomide tragedy eventually assumed global proportions, becoming a worldwide crisis of science, politics, and capitalism. Yet its early public history was largely constrained to debate within and across particular medical communities—general practitioners and pediatricians in West Germany, Great Britain, Australia, and the United States. Numerically, the phocomelia epidemic emerged most rapidly in West Germany, where thalidomide was marketed under the trade name Contergan and where phocomelia victims would eventually be known as "Contergan babies." By 1960, according to a casual estimate, West Germans were ingesting over one million doses of

estimated that phocomelia occurred in one out of 4 million births. The *Sunday Times* Insight Team, *Suffer the Children: The Story of Thalidomide* (London: Viking, 1979); Rock Brynner and Trent Stephens, *A Dark Remedy: The Impact of Thalidomide and Its Revival as a Vital Medicine* (New York: Basic Books, 2001), chap. 2; Helen B. Taussig, "A Study of the German Outbreak of Phocomelia," *JAMA* 180 (June 30, 1962): 1106–24; "The Thalidomide Syndrome," *Scientific American* (Aug. 1962)–29.

While the primary focus of medical and historical analysis of the thalidomide tragedy has been placed upon the living victims, many fetuses and infants were in fact aborted (either electively or spontaneously). There were also abnormalities that quickly proved fatal, such as was witnessed among the three Australian infants born in 1961 with bowel atresia (no bowel opening), all three of whom died shortly after birth; *Suffer the Children*, 2–4. Separately, Brynner and Stephens estimate that "8,000 to 12,000 infants were deformed by thalidomide, of whom 5,000 survived past childhood" (*A Dark Remedy*, 37). For a study showing thalidomide's abortive effects in rhesus monkeys, see J. F. Lucey and R. E. Behrman, "The Effect of Thalidomide upon Pregnancy in the Rhesus Monkey," *Science* 139 (1963): 1295.

[18] Widukind Lenz, "Kindliche Missbildungen nach Mediakment wahrend der Graviditat," *Deutsche Medizinische Wochenschrift* 86 (1961): 2555–6; William G. McBride, "Thalidomide and Congenital Abnormalities," *Lancet* 2 (1961): 1358. See Arthur Daemmrich's insightful study comparing Lenz and Kelsey and their public profiles; "A Tale of Two Experts: Thalidomide and Political Engagement in West Germany and the United States," *Social History of Medicine* 15 (2002): 137–58. Other authors claimed to have found a relationship between the precise timing of thalidomide utilization (in the interval encompassing the twentieth and fiftieth days of gestation) and the particular deformity; "Drugs in Pregnancy: Are They Safe?" *Consumer Reports* (August 1967): 434.

the drug per day, giving it to their children so often as to endow Contergan with the epithet of "West Germany's baby sitter."[19]

In the United States of 1960 and 1961, however, there were few if any premonitions of impending disaster. Despite widespread popular attention to issues of birth defects, it would appear—judging from major city newspapers at the time—that American readers were little if at all exposed to the news that thousands of previously rare birth deformities were being observed in Europe and Australia. A survey of the *Chicago Tribune*, *Los Angeles Times*, *New York Times*, *Washington Post*, and *Wall Street Journal* reveals not a single article mentioning "phocomelia" or describing a new epidemic of "birth defects" or "deformed babies" in Europe until April 1962. On April 11, Dr. Helen B. Taussig presented her findings on the German thalidomide epidemic to the annual meeting of the American College of Physicians in Philadelphia. The following day, her appeal for stronger U.S. controls on foreign drugs was carried by the *Chicago Tribune* and the *New York Times*, followed by a *Washington Post* story and a *Times* editorial ("Control of Pharmaceuticals") on April 13.[20]

In the months following Taussig's presentation, thalidomide received little news coverage, even as medical journals in Europe and the United States continued to publish new reports of phocomelia. This dearth of public knowledge in the United States, combined with Merrell's quiet withdrawal of the drug, meant that there was essentially no public knowledge of Frances Kelsey's quiet regulatory struggle. No one asked or documented why the drug had been kept from official approval in the United States. Indeed, American citizens assumed that the drug had never made its way onto U.S. soil.

[19] An adequate global history of the thalidomide tragedy—the palpable fear that its withdrawal and subsequent publicity induced among expectant mothers, physicians, and regulators in dozens of countries—has yet to be written. For an exemplary transnational study of a similarly jarring event, see Lisa McGirr, "The Passion of Sacco and Vanzetti: A Global History," *Journal of American History* 93 (4) (March 2007): 1085–1113. The estimate of 1 million consumers per day comes from Contergan's maker, Chemie-Grunenthal; see Insight Team, *Suffer the Children*, 36. From West German archival records, Arthur Daemmrich has adduced a smaller estimate of approximately 700,000; Daemmrich, *Pharmacopolitics: Drug Regulation in the United States and Germany* (Chapel Hill: University of North Carolina Press, 2004), 61. Brynner and Stewart, *A Dark Remedy*, chap. 2.

[20] These statements are supported by a search of major city newspapers in the ProQuest™ historical newspapers database for the years 1960 to 1964, using the search terms "deformed babies," "malformed babies," "birth defects," and "thalidomide" sequentially and separately. Robert K. Plumb, "Deformed Babies Traced to a Drug," *New York Times*, April 12, 1962, 37; "Finds Sleeping Pill Deforms Unborn Child," *Chicago Tribune*, April 12, 1962, B6.

More generally, global political and media reaction to the thalidomide-phocomelia tragedy seems to have been largely contained within West Germany and Great Britain. Japan left the drug on the non-prescription market for more than a year after it had been removed from European markets, during which time several hundred deformed babies were born. In Italy, thalidomide pills were on sale a full ten months after the German market withdrawal (*Suffer the Children*, 2).

The decisive event linking thalidomide and the FDA was the front-page publication by Morton Mintz of an article describing Kelsey's heroism in the Sunday morning *Washington Post* of July 15, 1962 (see figure 4.2). Mintz was clearly moved and persuaded by the protagonist of his story, and he opened his narrative with a stunning counterfactual: were it not for Kelsey's resistance to the Merrell overtures, thousands of American families may well have experienced the fate of thalidomide victims in Europe and Australia and other countries. Mintz's opening lines praised obstinacy and championed Kelsey as an officer of the American state.

> This is the story of how the skepticism and stubbornness of a Government physician prevented what could have been an appalling American tragedy, the birth of hundreds or indeed thousands of armless and legless children.[21]

Just as Mintz's words and the accompanying photo introduced Kelsey to the nation, his story also equated her identity with that of the national state. Hers was not merely an individual act but the success of a "Government physician" whose "high standards" were inseparable from her "skepticism and stubbornness." Mintz essentially re-interpreted "bureaucratic nitpicking" and deliberation—core features of the regime of protocol that had predated Kelsey's arrival—as modern-day, scientific virtues that upheld protection of American families and infants.

Perhaps the crucial feature of Mintz's thalidomide article is that the discovery owed little to the story's author. It was Tennessee Senator Estes Kefauver's antitrust subcommittee that leaked the details to Mintz, encouraged Mintz to contact Kelsey, and apparently provided some of the data and documentation that Mintz relied upon in writing his classic. Frances Kelsey's story of quiet resistance and sober judgment was no less true for this fact, but the source of the narrative highlights the pivotal role that Congress and its committee system played in the production of the FDA's national reputation in the late twentieth century. Frances Kelsey's public triumph was not a newspaper scoop—as were the Watergate stories that would vault the *Post* to the top ranks of American newspaper journalism a decade later—but instead a carefully timed leak designed to influence the passage of impending legislation, in this case Kefauver's drug regulation bill (S.1552).[22]

The Mintz story of July 15, 1962, started an avalanche of publicity both about thalidomide and about Kelsey. In the two months before Mintz's article, not a single piece had appeared in the *Post*, the *New York Times*, the *Wall Street Journal*, the *Chicago Tribune*, or the *Los Angeles Times* that contained the word "thalidomide" (figure 4.3). Even the linking of thalidomide to birth defects in published research had failed to engender media

[21] Morton Mintz, "Heroine of FDA Keeps Bad Drug Off Markets—Linked to Malformed Babies," *Washington Post*, July 15, 1962, A1.
[22] For evidence that Kefauver's committee supplied Mintz with raw material for the Kelsey story, see James McCartney, "Kefauver's Publicity Bomb Kills Huge Lobbying Buildup," *Commercial Appeal* (Memphis, TN), November 8, 1962; Richard Harris, *The Real Voice*, 183–7.

Linked to Malformed Babies

'Heroine' of FDA Keeps Bad Drug Off of Market

By Morton Mintz
Staff Reporter

This is the story of how the skepticism and stubbornness of a Government physician prevented what could have been an appalling American tragedy, the birth of hundreds or indeed thousands of armless and legless children.

The story of Dr. Frances Oldham Kelsey, a Food and Drug Administration medical officer, is not one of inspired prophesies nor of dramatic research breakthroughs.

She saw her duty in sternly simple terms, and she carried it out, living the while with insinuations that she was a bureaucratic nitpicker, unreasonable — even, she said, stupid. That such attributes could have been ascribed to her is, by her own acknowledgement, not surprising, considering all of the circumstances.

What she did was refuse to be hurried into approving an application for marketing a new drug. She regarded its safety as unproved, despite considerable data arguing that it was ultra safe.

It was not until last April, 19 months after the application was filed with the FDA,

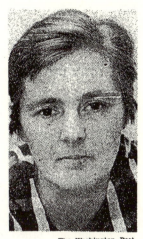

The Washington Post

DR. FRANCES O. KELSEY
. . . skepticism wins

that the terrible effects of the drug abroad were widely reported in this country. What remains to be told is how and why Dr. Kelsey blocked the introduction of the drug before those effects were suspected by anyone.

Dr. Kelsey invoked her high

standards and her belief that the drug was "peculiar" against these facts:

The drug had come into widespread use in other countries. In West Germany, where it was used primarily as a sedative, huge quantities of it were sold over the counter before it was put on a prescription basis. It gave a prompt, deep, natural sleep that was not followed by a hangover. It was cheap. It failed to kill even the would-be suicides who swallowed massive doses.

And there were the reports on experiments with animals. Only a few weeks ago the American licensee told of giving the drug to rats in doses 6 to 60 times greater than the comparable human dosage. Of 1510 offspring, none was delivered with "evidence of malformation."

In a separate study, one rat did deliver a malformed offspring, but the dosage had been 1200 times the usual one. Rabbits that were injected with six times the comparable human dose also were reported to have produced no malformed births.

Recently, the FDA publicly

See DRUG, A8, Col. 1

Figure 4.2. The *Washington Post* Thalidomide Story of July 15, 1962

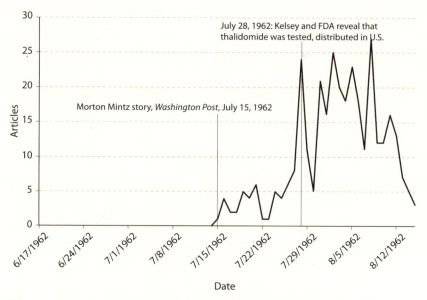

Figure 4.3. Major Newspaper Articles Mentioning "Thalidomide"

coverage in the United States. Helen Taussig's testimony linking thalidomide to birth defects before the Senate had also failed to generate news coverage, in part because the relevant House subcommittee had failed to notify the press that something big was about to occur. "I don't know what's wrong with those guys over there," complained one wire-service reporter of the committee's failure to alert the press about Taussig's May 17 testimony. "Biggest story of the year, and they just sat on it."[23]

Yet in the Monday papers following Mintz's report, stories appeared in the *Los Angeles Times*, the *New York Times*, and the *Chicago Tribune*, some of these syndicated directly from Mintz's *Post* article. The next uptick of coverage about thalidomide came on July 29, the day after Administration officials announced that thalidomide had entered the United States on an experimental basis. A scare whose confines had previously excluded the United States had now touched its domestic soil. In the wake of the stunning revelation of thalidomide's availability in the United States, President Kennedy held a press conference from the State Department auditorium on August 1. Even as diplomacy and espionage over nuclear weapons remained the central issues of the day, the President opened his remarks with a frank discussion of thalidomide's hazards and a note of reassurance to the American public.

[23]Harris, *The Real Voice*, 161. Richard McFadyen also concludes that America's "brush with tragedy" received sparse attention in U.S. media reporting, even as Taussig spread her findings in the medical community; "Thalidomide in America: A Brush with Tragedy," *Clio Medica* 11 (1976): 84.

Recent events in this country and abroad concerning the effects of a new sedative called thalidomide.emphasize again the urgency of providing additional protection to American consumers from harmful or worthless drug products. The United States has the best and the most effective food and drug law of any country in the world, and the alert work of our Food and Drug Administration, and particularly Dr. Frances Kelsey, prevented this particular drug from being distributed commercially in this country. Nevertheless, the drug was given to many patients on an investigational basis.[24]

From the *Washington Post* and other newspapers, the venue for regulatory triumph turned to Congress and the White House. Kefauver, whose staff had pushed the Kelsey story upon Mintz, immediately took legislative advantage of the news, calling for fresh action on his stalled bill. The Senator introduced Kelsey in Congress on July 18, 1962, along with Larrick and other leading FDA officials. He called upon President Kennedy to award Kelsey a national medal of service. On August 3, Congressman Harris McDowell (D-Delaware) introduced a House Joint Resolution that a gold medal be coined and given to Kelsey by the president. Then, in a highly publicized White House ceremony on August 7, Kennedy presented the Distinguished Federal Civilian Service Medal to Kelsey (figure 4.4). No such distinction had been awarded to a federal civilian employee since 1955, when President Eisenhower presented an identical medal to Jonas Salk for his discovery of the poliomyelitis ("polio") vaccine.[25]

Refractions and Complications of Gender

Kelsey's White House ceremony in August 1962 created images that were to appear for decades afterward, in the nation's newspapers, in television newscasts, in historical documentaries, and in continuing public commemoration. In the most commonly reproduced photograph, still used in Administration communications today and hanging in the FDA's library, the doctor wears her newly awarded medallion around her neck. Standing to the president's left, she clearly appears older than the handsome young president, as she was. On an August day, Kelsey is dressed modestly and darkly (perhaps in black) while Kennedy wears a lightly colored suit. Kennedy looks at Kelsey with a broad smile, but she does not return the gaze, instead looking downward and to the president's right. She holds a white purse and wears white gloves, one of which remains on her left hand while the right glove has

---

[24] "The President's Press Conference of August 1, 1962," in *Public Papers of the Presidents of the United States: John F. Kennedy, Containing the Public Messages, Speeches, and Statements of the President, 1961–1963* (Washington, DC: GPO, 1962–64), Title 321.

[25] At the time, Kefauver could not get the bill voted out of the very Committee he chaired. Mintz, "Great Tragedy Averted by Woman's Skepticism—Dr. Frances Kelsey Barred Drug Later Shown to Cause Deformities in Babies," *Los Angeles Times*, July 16, 1962, 16. Kefauver's remarks at *CR*, July 18, 1962, 12973. News release, Office of Congressman Harris B. McDowell, Jr., Friday, August 3, 1962; FOK.

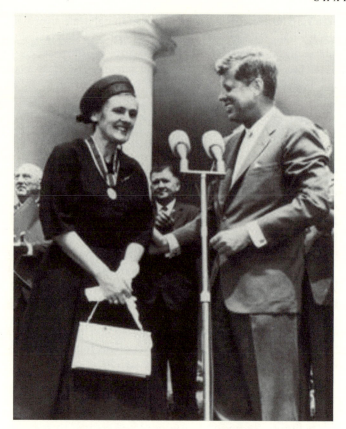

Figure 4.4. Kennedy Awards the Distinguished Civilian
Service Medal to Frances O. Kelsey, 1962 (National
Library of Medicine)

been removed, presumably for the presidential handshake. Kelsey's presence in the photo expressed features of Cold War urbane consumerism (white gloves, a white purse) while at the same time projecting professional gravity (a dark dress, an older stature). She was, in this shot, able to embody mature femininity while demonstrating circumspection and acumen.[26]

Frances Kelsey's limelight was perhaps the most intensive and positive experienced by any female federal official in the history of the United States. Throughout the story's telling and retelling at the hands of journalists, home-makers' journals, regulatory and scientific networks, congressional hearings and others, at least three facets of Kelsey's gender emerged. To the mass public, Kelsey appeared as a cerebral and maternal protector of sorts—quiet, unassuming, brilliant but circumspect. The *New York Times* cast her as "Guardian of the Drug Market," while the *Saturday Review* found in Kelsey the "Feminine Conscience of the F.D.A." Administration officials and Ke-fauver Committee staff gleefully shopped her image to homemakers' maga-zines and syndicated digests of the early 1960s. And along with newspapers, these venues drew moral lessons from the thalidomide case, obliging their readers to Kelsey and her organization. *Parents* magazine honored her for "Outstanding Service to Family Health." "Every American family stands in debt to Frances Kelsey," declared the *New York Herald Tribune*.[27]

In the public persona of Kelsey, the FDA's public and journalistic reputa-tion was for a time concrete, visually tangible, and widespread. Every time her story was told, reporters and editorialists sheepishly reminded their readers that they were, undoubtedly, already familiar with Kelsey, her orga-nization, and her accomplishment. "As everyone who can read or hear surely knows by now," prefaced the *Saturday Review* of September 1962 to

[26]It would push matters to infer that these features of Kelsey's appearance were inten-tional—that would be difficult and perhaps irrelevant to know—yet the way that the August 1962 photo of Kelsey with President Kennedy reinforces other portraits of Kelsey (both photo-graphic and textual) is important to highlight. Kelsey's White House appearance came in the midst of a pivotal transition in the history of American consumer culture, a moment in which mass marketing thoroughly segmented the American consumer market by gender. Lizabeth Cohen, "Reconversion: The Emergence of the Consumers' Republic" (chap. 3) and "Culture: Segmenting the Mass" (chap. 7) in *A Consumers' Republic: The Politics of Mass Consumption in Postwar America* (New York: Knopf, 2003). On the continuation of these trends in contem-porary audiences, see Joseph Turow, *Breaking Up America* (Chicago: University of Chicago Press, 1997).

At a 1997 public session on the re-introduction of thalidomide for erythema nodosum lep-rosum (ENL), Louis A. Morris described the importance of the Kelsey-Kennedy photo: "Tha-lidomide has special meaning for lots of people, and for someone who has worked at FDA, this is one piece of the meaning for thalidomide that I think FDA staff has. In the library in the Center for Drugs, there's a picture of Dr. Frances Kelsey receiving an award from President Kennedy. That picture, I think every time we go into the library, communicates to people at FDA in a very special way." Remarks of Louis A. Morris in FDA, "Thalidomide, Potential Benefits and Risks: An Open Public Scientific Workshop," Bethesda, MD, September 9–10, 1997; Natcher Conference Center, NIH, Bethesda.

[27]"Take Warning from Thalidomide," *New York Herald Tribune*, July 31, 1962.

its readers, "Dr. Kelsey is the Canadian-born medical officer of the U.S. Food and Drug Administration who refused to approve American marketing of thalidomide." In December 1962, on the basis of a national survey, George Gallup's National American Institute for Public Opinion named Kelsey as one of the ten "Most Admired Women of the World" among the American public, behind Jacqueline Kennedy and Queen Elizabeth II but ahead of Patricia Nixon, Princess Grace of Monaco, Lady Bird Johnson, Helen Hayes, and Bette Davis.[28]

The image of the vigilant and stubborn "heroine" shot through media coverage of the thalidomide tragedy. The titles of contemporary magazine articles are noteworthy for their blunt lionization of the doctor, and for the way they echoed facets of Kelsey's public portrait.[29]

- "Dr. Kelsey's Stubborn Triumph" (*Good Housekeeping*)
- "Dr. Kelsey, Heroine" (*Catholic Standard*)
- "Doctor and the Drug" (*Newsweek*)
- "Thalidomide Disaster" (*Time*)
- "Drug Market Guardian: Frances Oldham Kelsey" (*New York Times*)
- "Woman Doctor Who Would Not Be Hurried" (*Life*)
- "Inside Story of a Medical Tragedy: Interview" (*U.S. News*)
- "Thalidomide Lesson" (*Science*)
- "Vigilant Doctor Gets a Medal" (*U.S. News*)
- "Feminine Conscience of FDA: Dr. Frances Oldham Kelsey" (*Saturday Review*)
- "*Parents Magazine* Honors Dr. Frances Oldham Kelsey for Outstanding Service to Family Health" (*Parents Magazine*)
- "Doctor Kelsey Said No" (*Reader's Digest*)
- "Reward" (Saturday Review)
- "Thalidomide Heroine Seeks New Culprits" (*Scientific Digest*)
- "Lady Cop" (*Newsweek*)

[28] *Saturday Review*, September 1, 1962; George Gallup, "Mrs. Kennedy Is Most Admired Woman," *Washington Post—Tribune Herald*, December 26, 1962, B7.

[29] "Dr. Kelsey's Stubborn Triumph," *Good Housekeeping*, November 1962; "Dr. Kelsey, Heroine," *Catholic Standard*, August 10, 1962; "Doctor and the Drug," *Newsweek* 60 (July 30, 1962): 70; "Thalidomide Disaster," *Time* 80 (August 10, 1962): 32; "Drug Market Guardian: Frances Oldham Kelsey," *NYT*, August 2, 1962, A1; J. Mulliken, "Woman Doctor Who Would Not Be Hurried," *Life* 53 (Aug. 10, 1962): L28-29; "Inside Story of a Medical Tragedy: Interview," *U.S. News* 53 (Aug. 13, 1962): 54–55; D. Wolfle, "Thalidomide Lesson," *Science* 137 (Aug. 17, 1962): 497; "Vigilant Doctor Gets a Medal," *U.S. News* 53 (Aug. 20, 1962): 13; W. Jonathan, "Feminine Conscience of FDA: Dr. Frances Oldham Kelsey," *Saturday Review* 45 (Sept. 1, 1962): 41–43; "*Parents Magazine* Honors Dr. Frances Oldham Kelsey for Outstanding Service to Family Health," *Parents Magazine* 37 (Oct. 1962): 64; Morton Mintz, "Doctor Kelsey Said No," *Reader's Digest* 81 (Oct. 1962): 86–9; "Toward Safer Drugs," *Consumer Reports* 27 (Oct. 1962): 509–11; Jonathan Lear, "Reward," *Saturday Review* 46 (Feb. 2, 1963): 47; "Thalidomide Heroine Seeks New Culprits," *Scientific Digest* 53 (May 1963): 32; "Lady Cop," *Newsweek* 61 (June 24, 1963): 100.

Beyond this, journalistic coverage of Kelsey constructed and praised several facets of her personality. She was, first and foremost, exalted for her scientific judgment. The Mintz article itself had concluded by emphasizing her training in pharmacology. "For 20 years she taught pharmacology. She knows the dangers, and she has not the slightest intention of forgetting them." Kelsey was an eagerly sought speaker on the academic and medical lecture circuit. With the blessing of her superiors Ralph Smith and William Kessenich, Kelsey was invited to speak at numerous scientific conferences and meetings, including proceedings at the Mayo Clinic, the University of Pennsylvania, and European meetings on drug safety. She lectured to hundreds of alumni at the M.I.T. Club of Washington on "The Investigation of New Drugs."[30]

Two other facets of Kelsey's public image concerned ethical behavior. Quite apart from her scientific prowess and her "stubbornness," Kelsey was first praised for her evident reputation for wisdom and good judgment. "Her manner is pleasant but unhurried," the *Catholic Standard* observed, "and one senses that her responsibilities are not taken lightly." Kelsey's "common sense and knowledgeability come through like a great white light." A *Modern Medicine* report quoted Kelsey as saying that "My job is to pick these new-drug applications to pieces" and emphasized the "scrutiny" with which new drug applications were received and reviewed. An editorial in *Science* offered a quick causal suggestion, such that the thalidomide tragedy had been averted by means of personal virtue whose principles could be more broadly applied: "Dr. Kelsey's caution has prevented much heartache, and it appears that the thalidomide case may be useful in improving the procedures used in evaluating and appraising new drugs."[31]

A second ethical facet of the reputation that Kelsey had earned for herself and for her organization was a credit for dispassion, neutrality, and objectivity in the pursuit of "duty." As Mintz put it in his original *Washington Post* story, "She saw her duty in sternly simple terms, and she carried it out, living the while with insinuations that she was a bureaucratic nitpicker, unreasonable—even, she said, timid." Kelsey herself represented the decision in subtle, moral terms, not just as a matter of science, but a matter of ethics. As she told a *Catholic Standard* reporter in August 1962, "I only did what I thought was right." While the hypothesis has not received research, it is plausible that Kelsey's persona might have borne specific appeal to traditional Catholics and conservative Protestants who placed particular moral emphasis upon the developing fetus and who saw human life as preceding birth. Among this audience, Kelsey's moral stature was more impressive than her scientific or consumer protection esteem. "I thank God because

[30]Mintz, "Heroine of FDA Keeps Bad Drug Off Market." Announcement, February 8, 1963, M.I.T. Club of Washington; FOK. Mayo Clinic officials discussed plans for a visit from Kelsey in December 1963; Minutes, CSTA, November 21, 1963; MAYO.

[31]Mary Tinley Daly, "Dr. Kelsey, Heroine," *Catholic Standard*, August 10, 1962, p. 10.

intuitively I respect your integrity above almost all others," wrote Philadel-
phian Bernie Gold to Kelsey. "I know you won't be influenced by any
group—I've prayed all along that you, personally, will be in charge of [Kre-
biozen's] destiny." So seared into public consciousness were Kelsey and the
thalidomide tragedy that a career federal official was the subject of continuing private prayer, and her triumph an occasion for divine gratitude.[32]

Kelsey's award ceremony was one of many public appearances—all of
them occurring after the Mintz story was published—in which President
Kennedy spoke openly and plainly for stronger FDA authority and controls
on new drugs. In some respects, this advocacy echoed an existing rhetoric of
consumer representation in the Kennedy administration. In March 1962,
the president had delivered a special message to Congress calling for "a
Consumer Bill of Rights—the right to safety, to be informed, to choose, and
to be heard." As historian Lizabeth Cohen has characterized it, Kennedy's
rhetoric launched the "third wave" of the consumer movement in the
twentieth-century United States, a movement whose symbolic agent was
male. As Kennedy had intoned in his 1960 campaign, "The consumer is the
only man in our economy without a high-powered lobbyist. I intend to be
that lobbyist." Yet whereas Kennedy's generic consumer was a man, and
whereas his portrait of the protector was general—terms of the "federal
government"—the President's language changed subtly but significantly in
discussing drug law. In an August press conference, after a reporter asked
Kennedy whether the government was tracking down the supply of thalidomide, Kennedy responded that "The Food and Drug Administration have
had nearly two hundred people working on this, and every doctor, every
hospital, every nurse has been notified." His praise was organizationally
specific, and his warning was gendered. "Every woman in this country, I
think, must be aware that it is most important that they check their medicine cabinet and that they do not take this drug and that they turn it in."[33]

As the images and lessons of the thalidomide tragedy slowly cemented
into public and private commemoration, the person of Frances Kelsey became obscured and the role of her organization became exalted. When in
1989 the editors of the Washington Post recounted the thalidomide tragedy,
they mentioned not Kelsey but the agency. A generation after 1962, few
would remember the woman who stopped thalidomide in its regulatory
tracks, but a healthy majority of Americans could identify "thalidomide."
The initial merging of individual and organizational praise was due in part

[32] Morton Mintz, "Heroine of FDA Keeps Bad Drug Off Market." Bernie Gold, 5057 N.
Ninth Street, Philadelphia, to FOK, June 8, 1963; FOK, B1, F2. Mary Tinley Daly, "Dr. Kelsey,
Heroine," 10.

[33] "Kennedy Submits a Broad Program to Aid Consumer," and "Text of Kennedy's Message
on Protections for Consumers," NYT, March 16, 1962. Kennedy's attribution of male sexual-
ity to the consumer is noted in Cohen, A Consumer's Republic, 513; see also 146–7, 345. "The
President's News Conference of August 1st, 1962," in Public Papers of the Presidents of the
United States: John F. Kennedy, Containing the Public Messages, Speeches, and Statements of
the President, 1961–1963, Title 316.

to Kelsey's rather humble accreditation of her organization and her superiors. Kelsey transferred recognition to her organization and said that the tribute must be shared. "Many people must be nominated for this award," she reminded reporters in August. And it was not only Kelsey who widened the ambit of praise and ascription. Morton Mintz's original *Washington Post* article projected her virtues of stubbornness and skepticism onto her wider organization, emphasizing that "Dr. Kelsey's tenacity... was upheld by her superiors, all the way." When Kelsey appeared on the floor of Congress, Commissioner George Larrick and other FDA officials accompanied their star medical officer, and all were warmly noted and praised by Kefauver in his speech.[34]

In light of the Administration's transformation in the 1950s, along with the conflicts that attended those changes, this universality of praise was neither trivial nor foreordained. At the time of the thalidomide tragedy and for years afterward, there were enduring suspicions about the zeal of some of Kelsey's superiors, not least Commissioner Larrick and Kelsey's very recruiter and superior, Ralph Smith. Doubters complained that FDA superiors had supported a culture in which the pressure applied by Merrell company officials to Kelsey was all too common. Mintz himself would later write—in his book *By Prescription Only*—that Larrick would later retire into "well-earned obscurity." Yet the lesson that the American public drew during the glaring regulatory lights of 1962 was that Administration officials generally, even those not involved with the case—had supported Kelsey in her stringency with thalidomide. Credit was bestowed not merely upon an individual but upon the organization she inhabited. In the public imagery of the FDA, the lessons of Frances Kelsey's public achievement were extensible to other Administration officials. This equation was a powerful one, to be repeated in public, media, congressional, medical, and scientific dialogue thousands of times over the ensuing decades: If given the discretion and the resources, FDA medical officers will make the right decision, most of the time.[35]

It is today difficult to imagine or recreate the simultaneous sense of fear of thalidomide, the general worry about the capacity of national institutions to prevent another occurrence of a like disaster, and the widespread admiration for Frances Kelsey. Mothers throughout the nation held Kelsey personally responsible for the good health of their infant children. As a Dubuque, Iowa, mother wrote to Senator Hubert Humphrey in March 1963, "Our [child] was born shortly after the thalidomide scare and we have been so thankful that she is a normal, healthy 6-month old baby. Due to difficulties in pregnancy I was given different preparation but, thanks to Dr. Frances Kelsey, no thalidomide." Newspapers and local television syndicates typically took separate time and space to address the thalidomide issue. John

---

[34]Mary Tinley Daly, "Dr. Kelsey, Heroine," 10. Mintz, "Heroine of FDA Keeps Bad Drug Off Market."

[35]Mintz, *By Prescription Only* [originally published as *The Therapeutic Nightmare*] (Boston: Beacon, 1967), Preface, xxi; see also 131.

Madigan, editorial anchor for WBBM-TV, a CBS affiliate in Chicago, delivered the station's perspective in their "Standpoint" program, a program devoted to the thalidomide scare. He began by noting the tangible apprehension in the Chicago area.[36]

> Standpoint senses a note of hysteria seeping into some of the local reaction [to
> thalidomide]. We believe that every channel of proper investigation should be pur-
> sued. But this should be done in light of considerable reassurance.

The source of this reassurance, Madigan thought, should flow from the
FDA's regulatory system, and he described the FDA as the safety net for the
pharmaceutical market, reminding them of Kelsey's singular role, though
without naming her.

> It serves no purpose . . . to score the Food and Drug Administration, as some have
> done here, for not sounding a general alarm seven months ago. They forget that
> the drug manufacturer notified FDA the moment word was received of the Euro-
> pean birth tragedies. . . . These scolders forget, too, that it was a woman doctor
> in the FDA who kept the drug off the American market almost single-handedly.

Madigan concluded with a reminder that FDA regulators had been very
active in recent years, and that those agents should be endowed with even
more power.

> WBBM-TV feels there are constructive suggestions which can be made in this
> case. And from the fact that since 1958, 21 drugs have been forced from the mar-
> ket because they were proved to be dangerous. Medical science should not be
> impeded and after proper testing with animals there must be some human experi-
> mentation. But, obviously, federal controls over testing of new drugs on humans
> must be tightened. There should be more complete records of what doctors get what
> drugs and what they are doing with them. And, if Americans are wise, they'll use no
> drugs bought overseas without consulting their physicians at home, and the doc-
> tors should check with the Drug Administration.
>   To date, there are no known tragedies resulting from the Thalidomide pro-
> cured in the U.S. The next time we may not be so fortunate.
>   I'm John Madigan.

While Madigan credits the unnamed heroine, he esteems her organization
even more, shunning his viewers from foreign markets where the FDA's authority did not reach, and telling his viewers that their family doctors should
be in contact with the agency. His editorial serves as an historical reminder
that widespread criticism of the FDA did in fact accompany the thalidomide
scare. The cumulative effect of reports such as Madigan's and Mintz's, however, was essentially to rewrite the thalidomide story not as regulatory collapse (or even a narrowly averted disaster), but as a bureaucratic triumph

---

[36]"Editorial, Program: Standpoint," WBBM-TV 2, Chicago. Enclosure in John Madigan,
Editorial Assistant of the General Manager, WBBM-TV, Chicago, IL, to Larrick, July 31, 1962.
Corrected for orthography. FOK, B1, F2. Unnamed correspondent (Dubuque, IA), to Sen.
Hubert Humphrey, March 19, 1963; *ICDRR*, 1239–40.

that pointed clearly toward the need for new statutory powers for the Administration.[37]

In these and other projections, national news organizations and their syndicates exercised pivotal influence in shaping public facets of the FDA's reputation. In the end, Morton Mintz's reportage would become the dominant narrative of thalidomide. A half-century later it is worth asking why. Why were there no other narratives—including narratives of failure that would later surface in Congress—reproduced widely among the American reading and viewing public? One answer lies in the power of first impressions, the agenda-setting and framing effect of the Mintz story. By casting thalidomide as a tale of regulatory success, replete with a protagonist (Kelsey) and an antagonist (the drug, or its manufacturer Merrell), the Mintz story personified world news and made bureaucracy more human, more intimate, and more tangible. Many of the newspaper accounts, magazine summaries, and television broadcasts of 1962 and 1963 would rehearse the thalidomide episode in nearly identical terms. A second answer lies in the utility of the news that American citizens were receiving. The Mintz story and the Madigan editorial offered explicit warnings about thalidomide, as well as implicit warnings about the dangers of using drugs that had not received U.S. approval, and about the importance of Americans' and physicians' deference to their federal government in these matters. Long before the morals of thalidomide were cemented in public understanding, Mintz, Madigan, and other journalists at the national and local levels were actively describing and shaping those lessons for their readers and viewers.[38]

In public and legislative debates over the Kefauver bill, senators and representatives and White House officials repeatedly employed caricatures of Kelsey and images of the Administration and its officers. In part for this reason, the 1962 amendments went well beyond changes to the formal power of the Administration (changes discussed in the ensuing chapter). The legislative process and its statutory product also bore an ideational residue, a reputation in stone and rhetoric to which federal courts, Congresses, and scientific and public organizations would show deference.

·   ·   ·

[37]In this respect, it is interesting that Madigan would send a copy of his editorial remarks to Commissioner George Larrick; Madigan to Larrick, July 31, 1962; FOK, B1, F2.

[38]On the instrumental utility of narratives as an essential element of their newsworthiness, see W. Lance Bennett, *News: The Politics of Illusion*, 3rd ed. (New York: Longman, 1995). The thalidomide case functions as a partial example of "event-driven problem definition" as the concept is framed by Regina Lawrence, *The Politics of Force: Media and the Construction of Police Brutality* (Berkeley: University of California Press, 2000). Lawrence contrasts her "event-driven" account with a standard "institutionally determined" model. Yet the case of thalidomide points to dependencies across Lawrence's binary divide, as the regulatory and policy context for understanding the tragedy was created by Administration officials and by Kefauver and his committee staff. It was the *meeting* of event and institutions, not thalidomide alone, which transformed the policy agenda. I thank Thomas Birkman, a political scientist and communications specialist at SUNY-Albany, for these references and for other helpful remarks on the thalidomide case.

In July 1962, FDA officials including Larrick (now on board the reform train) aggressively pressed for an expansion of regulatory authority. The initial target of Kefauver, FDA officials, and White House policymakers was the automatic approval provision in the current Food, Drug and Cosmetic Act. Kefauver's principal argument against the automatic approval clause was that Administration officials opposed the deadline. "Commissioner Larrick, and other officials of the Food and Drug Administration are strongly of the opinion that they should not have to approve a new drug application until they are satisfied beyond any reasonable doubt as to the safety and efficacy of the drug."[39] Kefauver capitalized upon the Kelsey triumph to push for new administrative discretion. If "the physicians of the FDA" wished to wait on the approval of a drug, then federal statute should explicitly and clearly provide for an opportunity to deliberate.

> The thalidomide episode dramatically illustrates the necessity of incorporating strong and fair provisions to protect the public against drugs with adverse side effects. . . . At the present time, a new drug application is approved automatically in 60 days unless the Commissioner of the FDA acts to prevent its sale. This, of course, places great strain upon the physicians of the FDA who are trying to protect the American people from drugs with dangerous side effects, such as thalidomide. They should have an adequate time to assure themselves that the drug is safe, and applications should not become effective automatically during any time period.[40]

One irony of these claims is that their reverberation was fueled by interpersonal competition. Kennedy, Kefauver, and Larrick fought over the implicit title of consumer protection advocate in the area of ethical drugs. In so doing, they all publicly but implicitly underscored the assumption that FDA officials were deserving of the discretion, that additional time in review was time spent deliberating, appraising, reassuring. President Kennedy's early August remarks celebrated the 1938 statute as "the best and the most effective food and drug law of any country in the world," and he immediately credited "the alert work of our Food and Drug Administration" and Kelsey especially for keeping thalidomide from commercial distribution. Two weeks after Kefauver intoned from the Senate floor on the need for administrative discretion in new drug review, Kennedy issued a letter to Senator James O. Eastland, chairman of his chamber's Judiciary Committee, accompanied by recommended amendments to Kefauver's bill. The most noticeable amendment eliminated automatic approval of drugs after sixty days of review; another gave the Administration (through the Department of Health, Education and Welfare) nearly unilateral power to remove a previously approved drug from the market. Kennedy's letter called upon Eastland to recall Kefauver's bill (S.1552) from the Senate floor and add the president's amendments. As reporter Richard Harris would summarize it, Kennedy's letter and amend-

[39]Kefauver, CR, July 18, 1962, 12973.
[40]Kefauver remarks at CR, July 18, 1962, 12973.

ments converted Kefauver's policy into "the President's bill." Presidents, senators, and House members pushed one another aside to shower ever more praise and ever more discretion upon the officers of the Food and Drug Administration.[41]

Even as politicians observed and reiterated the policy lessons of thalidomide, other voices, not as pivotal to the bill's passage, saw less obvious implications from the thalidomide experience. New York Republican Jacob Javits followed Kefauver's July 18 speech with a cautionary note, saying "It may not be necessary to pass such legislation... Indeed, the Kelsey case may show that the present system is working pretty well and that legislation may not be needed." Arthur Rankin himself told Mintz that "the significant thing about the law is that it gave Dr. Kelsey the weapon she needed to block the marketing of thalidomide in the United States." Yet these were claims from July, in the immediate wake of the Mintz story and the Kelsey award ceremony; by August and September, they were scarcely heard.[42]

Few if any FDA officials had wanted this publicity. Yet the visible and evocative horror of the thalidomide tragedy—babies born limbless, their pictures scattered across the front pages of newspapers and magazines, their horrific deformities and stories of agony repeatedly narrated on television and over radio—created the substrate for a powerful historical lesson. Drugs were inherently dangerous, and the Administration could protect the unaware American family from them, not merely through police-like enforcement but through regulatory gatekeeping. Although data are sparse, this lesson was probably learned (albeit implicitly and ambiguously) by tens of millions of U.S. citizens. Though the 1960s and through the ensuing decades, thalidomide remained a household word in the United States, Europe, Australia, and Canada. At a 1997 meeting at the NIH in which the return of thalidomide for erythema nodosum leprosum (ENL) was discussed in front of a large audience, FDA official Louis Morris presented the results of a small opinion survey. His data showed that over two-thirds of survey respondents over the age of forty-five could correctly define "thalidomide," whereas approximately one-third of respondents under the age of forty-five

---

[41]Kennedy, "Letter to the Chairman, Senate Committee on the Judiciary, on the Need for Safer Drugs," *Public Papers of the Presidents of the United States: John F. Kennedy, Containing the Public Messages, Speeches, and Statements of the President, 1961–1963*, Title 321. Despite being released on August 5, Kennedy's letter was dated August 3. Harris offers an apt summary of the Kennedy announcement of August 5: "the quest for public credit gave birth to a unique parliamentary tactic" (Harris, *The Real Voice*, 197–8). The Senate would make many of these changes—some of them favored by Administration officials and Kefauver well before Kennedy's advocacy. At a press conference less than three weeks after the letter's release, Kennedy would claim credit for the late-summer revisions to S.1552: "the drug bill, which has been tightened in the Senate Judiciary Committee, much along the lines that I requested, will give us every safeguard to protect our American citizens"; "The President's News Conference of August 22nd, 1962," *Public Papers*, Title 340. George McGovern would also congratulate Kelsey publicly; Kelsey to Hon. George McGovern, January 29, 1963; FOK, B1, F2.

[42]Javits in *CR*, July 18, 1962, 12973; Mintz, "Heroine of FDA Keeps Bad Drug Off Market."

were able to do so. Interestingly, Morris and his colleagues found no effect of gender on the recall rate; men were just as likely as women in his sample to correctly identify thalidomide. The crucial variable was the "cohort effect." The generation of people who had been eight or more years of age during the thalidomide tragedy simply could not forget its imagery and its lessons.[43]

As for the humble protagonist of the thalidomide tragedy, Frances Kelsey, her identities would soon refract among different audiences. Kelsey faded from the immediate spotlight, but her deeds in the Kevadon review became the material of legend. She was cast as an ordinary citizen doing extraordinary things in Ray and Beryl Epstein's *Who Says You Can't?* (1969), and profiled and lionized in Margaret Truman's 1976 volume *Women of Courage*. As a reticent heroine who became less recognizable to the American mass public, she became agonizingly familiar to American pharmaceutical companies and clinical researchers. In her accession to the head of the new Investigational Drug Branch of the Bureau of Medicine, Kelsey would become responsible for the interpretation, construction, and enforcement of federal regulations governing clinical trials. It was in this position, and less in the thalidomide tragedy, where Kelsey's legacy was most tangible, most concrete and, perhaps, most far-reaching.[44]

The Rebirth of Regulatory Reform

In the weeks following Morton Mintz's Sunday morning, July 15, 1962 story on thalidomide and Frances Kelsey, the agenda, content, and emotion of pharmaceutical politics changed. It is tempting to conclude or assume, as many writers have, that the thalidomide crisis transformed everything and paved the way for the new legislation signed by President Kennedy on October 10, 1962. For all of its emotional and political weight, however, the thalidomide episode left some hefty questions awaiting resolution and some vital battles to be waged. The crisis ensured only that some version of reform would pass, not that anything Kefauver or the Bureau of Medicine wanted would materialize.[45]

Perhaps the most immediate result of the crisis was that the Kennedy White House took on a new and more aggressive posture in the proceedings.

[43]Remarks of Louis A. Morris in FDA, "Thalidomide, Potential Benefits and Risks: An Open Public Scientific Workshop," Bethesda, MD, September 9–10, 1997; Natcher Conference Center, NIH, Bethesda. As Morris summarized his data to the assembly, "I think my explanation for it is, again, if you ask people over 45 about thalidomide, they just see these very vivid images. They retrieve it. Under 45, they just don't have those memories." I thank Susanne White-Junod for bringing Morris's presentation to my attention.

[44]Margaret Truman was the daughter of the deceased president; *Women of Courage* (New York: Morrow, 1976); Beryl and Samuel Epstein, *Who Says You Can't?* (New York: Coward-McCann, 1969).

[45]Daemmrich, for example, states that "attention to [thalidomide] breathed new life into Kefauver's bill" but ignores the role played by FDA and HEW officials in the drafting of new legislation (*Pharmacopolitics*, 26–7).

After the second round of thalidomide reporting on July 28 and 29—most of which revealed the widespread distribution of the drug in the United States—Kennedy gave a nationally televised press conference and demanded quick legislative action. Kefauver's bill had been emasculated, so it was not the template with which to start. Instead, the Kennedy administration drafted a new bill based in part upon legislation introduced by Arkansas Representative Oren Harris. The drafting was led by HEW functionaries Jerome Sonosky and Theodore Ellenbogen. Sonosky and Ellenbogen's draft began to look more and more like the original Kefauver bill, but it lacked the crucial ingredient of the Senator's plan: patent law revision.[46]

The demise of patent law reform was one legacy of thalidomide. Fights over definition of concepts were next. If the Bureau of Medicine was to achieve its vision—if pharmacological drug development and efficacy regulation were to become the standard of the land—then terms such as "efficacy" and "investigation" would require stable definition in terms sufficiently favorable as to permit stringent approaches to clinical trials and new drug submissions. In their negotiations with House and Senate committees and with the Department of Health, Education and Welfare, Administration officials repeatedly and thoroughly targeted the definition of efficacy and the language of experiment as the major aims of reform. Allies of the organized industry and organized medicine fought back on both fronts. It was in these late-summer struggles over concept and phrasing that political contingency would reappear in the wake of thalidomide. In the bill that emerged from these deliberations, neither the Bureau of Medicine nor Kefauver received what they first desired. Yet the resulting terminology was sufficiently flexible as to hand broad interpretive license to FDA officials.[47]

With the Kennedy White House pushing for quick congressional action, and Kefauver and his allies emboldened by the president's support and by new press coverage, reform opponents suspected that some statutory revision was imminent. Lobbyists for the Pharmaceutical Manufacturers' Association began to press for restricted FDA authority and limited and favorable statutory terms. The Kennedy administration's bill called for drug

[46]Hilts, *Protecting America's Health*, 158–9. The Harris bill was in part a Kennedy administration bill.

[47]The battle over definition of terms in the law was one that attracted the energies of agents throughout the FDA hierarchy. Ralph Weilerstein (now Associate Medical Director of the San Francisco District) wrote a long memorandum asking for numerous changes, and his suggested amendments to the definition of "new drug" under the law were influential; Weilerstein to Director, San Francisco District, re "Commissioner's letter of May 1, 1962 re legislative proposals," May 22, 1962; Ellenbogen to Winton Rankin, February 16, 1962; FDA, "Comments on Testimony, H.R. 11581"; FDA General Correspondence, DF 062.1, RG 88, NA. Because different bills used different terms for "effect" ("effectiveness," "efficaciousness," and "efficacy"), FDA General Counsel Goodrich tied these disparate words to the term "efficacy" that had been in use in FDA practice of the 1950s; Goodrich to Sam Spal (Counsel, House Committee on Interstate and Foreign Commerce), August 18, 1962; General Correspondence, DF 062.1, B 3183, RG 88, NA.

applications to present a "preponderance" of evidence for safety and efficacy, while Lloyd Cutler and drug company lobbyists wanted a requirement of "substantial" evidence. Kefauver committee staffer John Blair agreed to the term "substantial" as long as Cutler would agree that "substantial" would be accompanied by a requirement of "adequate and well-controlled investigations" conducted by "experts qualified by scientific training and experience." These were terms that had already received substantial elaboration in FDA rulemaking and administrative practice, most notably in Ralph Smith's New Drug Application form first published in the September 1955 *Federal Register*. Cutler and his coterie accepted this compromise, which implied a partial victory in the sense that preponderance would have required a majority of a company's studies to have demonstrated positive results. Yet the terms "adequate," "well-controlled," and "qualified by scientific training and experience" also meant that FDA officials would be able to define the minimal standards of research for drug approval.[48]

Another crucial amendment to the June 1962 bill—a full enabling of the Administration's capacity to deny market entry to new drugs—was the subject of only rhetorical contestation. Spurred by FDA officials, Kefauver seized upon the Kelsey triumph to target the automatic approval clause of current federal law. "The thalidomide episode," Kefauver intoned, "dramatically illustrates the necessity of incorporating strong and fair provisions to protect the public against drugs with adverse side effects.... At the present time, a new drug application is approved automatically in 60 days unless the Commissioner of the FDA acts to prevent its sale. This, of course, places great strain upon the physicians of the FDA who are trying to protect the

[48]The narrative of the compromise here generally follows Harris (*The Real Voice*, 204–5) and Hilts (*Protecting America's Health*, 160), whose evidence and interviews are instructive; see also McFadyen, *Estes Kefauver and the Drug Industry*, 359–60. Harris and Hilts tell the story as if John Blair inserted the terms "adequate and well-controlled investigations" and "qualified by scientific training and experience" on his own; Hilts quotes Sonosky as saying, "I just couldn't believe it when Blair pulled that off." Yet the terms that Blair proposed as part of the compromise were terms synthesized by FDA officials; consult Part 1(a) of FDA "Form FD 356—Rev. 1956," published in *FR* 20:175 (Sept. 8, 1955): 6586; *FR* 21:143 (July 25, 1956): 5578; see also chapter 3.

FDA officials seized on their perceived victory in the Senate to push for favorable terms in the House bill (H.R. 11581); Goodrich to Sam Spal (Counsel, House Committee on Interstate and Foreign Commerce), August 18, 1962; John L. Harvey (Deputy Commissioner), "The Omnibus Bill," presented to the Division of Food, Drug and Cosmetic Law of the Section of Corporation, Banking and Business Law of the American Bar Association, August 8, 1962; General Correspondence, DF 062.1, B 3183, RG 88, NA.

This episode points to a different interpretation of the Kefauver committee staff in the history of U.S. pharmaceutical regulation. Blair had been in regular contact with Kelsey and Bureau of Medicine officials throughout the Kefauver hearings and the summer of 1962, and it was Blair who leaked the thalidomide story to Mintz's superiors at the *Washington Post* (Hilts, 156–7). In this respect, Blair was pivotal in part because he was a broker of information and advice between Frances Kelsey and Ralph Smith, on one hand, and the *Washington Post* and the national legislative process, on the other.

American people from drugs with dangerous side effects, such as thalido-mide. They should have an adequate time to assure themselves that the drug is safe, and applications should not become effective automatically during any time period." Senator Javits took less obvious policy lessons from the thalidomide experience; to him, Frances Kelsey's triumph was a living and tangible endorsement of the present system of drug review and its proce-dural safeguards. What was needed, in Javits' view, was not "legislation" but continued deference to the Administration's medical reviewers."[49]

In debating the meaning of "the Kelsey case" and whether or not it called for new legislation, Kefauver and Javits were negotiating the meaning of the Administration's organizational legitimacy. Kefauver's exemplar of regula-tory protection was the Administration medical officer, not just Kelsey her-self, but the "physicians of the FDA who are trying to protect the American people from drugs with dangerous side effects." Javits disagreed only in his perception that existing law allowed the FDA's protectors to fulfill their charge. As it turns out, the fate of the sixty-day clause and the automatic approval provision would be sealed not in Senate debate, but by the presi-dent's August 3 letter to Senate Judiciary Chair James Eastland containing seven amendments that Kennedy said must be attached to any legislation. This third of these amendments required an affirmative FDA approval of a drug application before interstate marketing or distribution. Another Ken-nedy amendment strengthened the Commissioner's authority to withdraw drugs from the market.[50]

Despite elite disagreement about thalidomide's implications, public opin-ion appeared to congeal in favor of stronger federal controls. In early Au-gust 1962, the "What America Thinks" poll posed the following question to hundreds of American respondents: "Do you think that Government con-trol over drugs should be more strict, less strict, or about the same as it is now?" Over three-quarters of respondents (76.3 percent) answered "more strict." The poll demonstrated the fluidity of public opinion and its con-struction by events and, indeed, by survey questions themselves. It also dem-onstrated that, in the shadow of an impending midterm election and the fact

[49]Kefauver and Javits remarks at *CR*, July 18, 1962, 12973. Kefauver had been lobbied di-rectly on this provision by Larrick (now on board the reform train) and other FDA officials: "Commissioner Larrick, and other officials of the Food and Drug Administration are strongly of the opinion that they should not have to approve a new drug application until they are satis-fied beyond any reasonable doubt as to the safety and efficacy of the drug" (ibid.). Javits's point had been made by others, including the Administration's own Winton Rankin when he told Mintz that "the significant thing about the law is that it gave Dr. Kelsey the weapon she needed to block the marketing of thalidomide in the United States"; Mintz, "Heroine of FDA Keeps Bad Drug Off Market."

[50]Kennedy's amendment was significant because the Senate version of the drug reform bill had simply extended the time limit from 60 days to 90, without eviscerating compulsory ap-proval; Kennedy to Eastland, August 3, 1962; *ICDRR*, 241–4; McFadyen, *Estes Kefauver and the Drug Industry*, 353–5.

that final passage votes would be held in the fall, President Kennedy's repeated public call for prompt legislative action was not a losing wager.[51]

By late August, a sense of inevitability had set in among journalists and other observers of drug reform. Pharmacist Robert P. Fischelis tied the impending passage of legislation directly to issues of new drug review. "It is quite apparent," he wrote in *The American Druggist*, "that a crisis in the evaluation of new drugs is upon us and it looks now as though food and drug legislation will be passed at this session of Congress after all." Thalidomide "is quite apt to be the determining factor in the enactment of the emasculated Kefauver bill (S.1552) with some of its strong original provisions restored." The Pharmaceutical Manufacturers' Association decided to agree to the Kefauver bill because, according to a *Wall Street Journal* reporter, "the companies don't think they have any choice." "Ruefully, the industry admits it could do little to block new controls, even if it tried. 'In the past month or so, our political situation has changed, and we can't get anyone's ear in Washington,' laments one company official." Concluded the *New York Post*, "It is almost certain that new drug controls will emerge before Congress adjourns this fall. The reason is simple—thalidomide."[52]

President Kennedy signed Public Law 87-781, the "Drug Amendments of 1962," into law on October 10, with Frances Kelsey standing behind him. Estes Kefauver would receive the resident's signatory pen. The Administration's Bureau of Medicine would receive presumptive authority over much of the global pharmaceutical industry.

Thalidomide Revisited: A Reading in Comparative
Context and through the Lens of Reputation

The 1962 Amendments both expressed and commenced a series of vast changes to the sphere of pharmaceuticals, and the particulars of the statute have been extensively interpreted in the American legal disciplines of food and drug law and administrative law. At their core, the Amendments contained three provisions governing pharmaceutical regulation (table 4.1). They first required affirmative evidence of "effectiveness" and "safety," evidence in the form of "adequate and well-controlled investigations," before any "new drug" could enter into interstate commerce. Second, they required

[51] The percentages were 76.3 percent for "More strict," 16.9 percent for "About the same," 1.9 percent for "more or less" or "depending," 1.2 percent for "Less strict," and 3.7 percent reporting "No opinion." Jack Boyle (Director, "What America Thinks" polls), "What America Thinks: Stricter Drug Controls Needed, Poll Reveals," *Washington* (Sunday) *Star*, August 13, 1962; *ICDRR*, 606–7.

[52] Fischelis, "Coming: Supreme Court of Drug Evaluation," *The American Druggist*, August 20, 1962; Herbert G. Lawson, "Regulating Drugs—New Federal Rules No Cure-All for Safety Complications," *WSJ*, August 27, 1962; Barbara Yuncker, "Pills and You—Is the Kefauver Bill Enough?" *New York Post*, September 16, 1962; Mintz, "Drug Tragedy Revives Hope for Cure," *WP*, August 19, 1962; *ICDRR*, 608–10, 614, 621, 624–5.

designation of a medicine as an Investigational New Drug during its period of experimentation (and submission of the IND to the agency), and empowered the Administration to nullify this status (and hence development of the drug) if research protections for patients were not being observed, if the clinical trial protocol was not sufficiently rigorous, if pregnant women were being exposed to teratogens, or if any evidence of research as commercialization emerged. Third, they required the Administration to lay out and enforce new procedures to protect the interests and rights of patients in medical research.[53]

Frances Kelsey's contribution to the Administration's public image—the variable faces seen by industry, by Congress, and by the public—allows us to ask anew about her role in creating the modern pharmaceutical regime. What if Kelsey and her husband had stayed in South Dakota, or she had joined the National Institutes of Health instead of going to the FDA? It is difficult to address such counterfactual queries. The legal, procedural, and structural residue of the thalidomide tragedy receives treatment in the following chapter. For now, it merits remark that Kelsey's pivotal legacy is not merely that she made a crucial decision, but that she and her choices formed highly memorable and effective symbols that attached to an organizational image for decades to come.

Under this symbolic reading of thalidomide and Kelsey, what happened in 1962 and 1963 is not that the regulatory world changed abruptly, but that one among a set of competing and emerging organizational identities crystallized in public, professional, business, and government belief. The Administration's reputation took shape in new form, a fusion of its cop, gatekeeper, and protector identities. Yet the process was far more continuous than public commemoration of the thalidomide affair would suggest. The FDA's reputation was symbolically multiplied, and the process of reputation making owed its energy to numerous political and social processes—to the Kefauver hearings and the follow-on hearings in the House, to the new law and its codification of Administration power, to the affirmation and legitimization of the new pharmacology-based regulation by the thalidomide

---

[53]This three-part summary excludes many important provisions in order to focus on those most relevant to FDA regulatory power. For a synopsis of the measure, see *ICDRR*, 409ff. The most comprehensive and accessible review appears in Merrill, "Architecture"; esp. 1764–8. Merrill argues that the 1962 amendments converted what was a "premarket notification system" into a genuine "premarket approval system," by doing away with presumptive approval after 180 days of review ("Architecture," 1764–5). Yet in this respect, much of what the Amendments accomplished had already been achieved by the Administration in its administrative practices; see chapter 3.

For other summaries of the amendments, consult "Note: Drug Efficacy and the 1962 Drug Amendments, *Georgetown Law Journal* 60 (1971): 185; David F. Cavers, "The Legal Control of Clinical Investigation of Drugs: Some Political, Economic and Social Questions," *Daedalus* 98 (1969): 427; Peter Barton Hutt and Merrill, *Food and Drug Law: Cases and Materials*, 2nd ed. New York: Foundation Press, 1991).

TABLE 4.1
Partial Summary of Changes Effected by Kefauver-Harris Amendments of 1962

	Criteria of Marketability for "New Drugs"	Burden of Proof for New Drug Applications
1938 Food, Drug and Cosmetic Act	Safety [Section 505(b), (c)]	Upon FDA, after 60 days review
Modifications from 1939–1961, incl. FDA proposals-and new interpretations of the 1938 Act	"Safety in use" considerations, from 1939 onward "Efficacy" as inseparable from "safety"	Upon sponsor, informally, after 1956 new drug rules and regular reliance on-"incomplete" rulings
1962 Amendments	"Effective" and/or "the drug will have the effect it purpurports or is represented to have" [Section 505 (b), (c), (d)]	Upon sponsor, formally [Section 505 (b), (c), (d)]

Note: This is summary and partial. See text of the chapter for more detailed and nuanced discussion.

*Section 505(i) of the Federal Food, Drug and Cosmetic Act, as amended by the 1997 FDA Modernization Act, verifies the agency's authority to issue a clinical hold.

experience. Thalidomide was, in this view, important less for inaugurating a new era, and much more for legitimizing one among a competing complex of orders and images that had emerged in the previous decade. Competition and indeed confusion about the essential nature of drug regulation persisted through the 1960s, but both were restricted considerably by the late days of the Eisenhower administration. Thalidomide and the Kefauver hearings allowed for the triumph of a new regulatory order, a triumph over a set of competing regimes that had been substantially narrowed during the preceding decade.

The force and spillover of organizational image emerges clearly when the U.S. thalidomide experience is compared with that of other nations touched by the drug, notably West Germany, Britain, and Australia. The most vivid contrast emerges in the German reaction to the episode. At the time of Contergan's distribution, drug development in Germany was governed by (and expressed in) a federal statute passed in 1961. The statute prohibited dan-

Investigational Drugs	Human Subjects Protections	Inspection Powers of FDA
Small, insignificant regulation	No government regulation	Enhanced powers
FDA officials propose stronger regulation of drugs in late 1950s	No FDA modification before 1962; Considerable development of standards in medicine- and medical ethics (Helsinki Declaration).	*U.S. v. Cardiff* (1952) Supreme Court decision vacates criminal application of 1938 law following FDA inspection Factory Inspection Amendments of 1953 restore and clarify criminal application of factory inspection provisions; FDA must notify company as to conditions observed and sample taken
Rulemaking authority over "Investigational New Drugs" handed to FDA FDA given power to halt clinical trials by placing "clinical hold" upon INDs*	Expansive rulemaking authority over clinical trials.	FDA inspectors receive authority to inspect company records regarding development, clinical testing, and production in addition to samples and observations of behavior.

gerous medicines but did not give any agency of the federal government the power to conduct pre-market review, nor the power to regulate medical research or other pre-marketing aspects of drug development. The 1961 law preserved important features of West Germany's federalist structure and left discretion over drug adoption in the hands of state governments (Länder) and German physicians, keeping authority away from the central state.[54]

In the immediate wake of the "Contergan baby" epidemic, the German difference did not wane but persisted. *Washington Star* correspondent Crosby Noyes would report in August 1962 that German politics offered a "curious contrast" to legal and regulatory developments in the United States,

[54]The most direct treatment of the 1961 law appears in Ute Stapel (with a Foreword by Rudolf Schmitz), *Die Arzneimittelgesetze 1961 und 1976 Quellen und Studien zur Geschichte der Pharmazie* 43 (Stuttgart: In Kommission Deutscher Apotheker Verlag, 1988). An excellent comparison of these laws with those of the United States appears in Arthur Daemmrich, *Pharmacopolitics: Drug Regulation in the United States and Germany* (Chapel Hill: University of North Carolina Press, 2004). I have relied upon Daemmrich's book and on characterizations from conversations with him. I assume all responsibility for any errors, omissions, or characterizations.

Britain, and France. Almost everywhere else that a debate on drug regulation was happening, Noyes observed, the call for more stringent government regulation of drugs was being heeded. Yet in Germany, Noyes located a cultural resistance to government pharmaceutical regulation, a "general attitude" attributable to "Germany's peculiar federal structure and to what amounts to a genuine horror of centralized control in a large number of fields." At its core, this attitude expressed a distrust of state mechanisms; "the one point on which everyone involved—including doctors, public health officials, politicians and drug manufacturers—appears to be in close agreement is that no amount of Government control could have prevented the thalidomide tragedy." Unlike the United States, where legislators, scientists and consumer advocates saw abiding flaws in pharmaceutical industry practices and vested greater hope in the science and procedures of the Food and Drug Administration, Germans were inclined to defer to the capacity of their pharmaceutical companies. "So far as the testing of drugs is concerned," Noyes observed, "it is pointed out that the Government itself could never duplicate the great variety of facilities available to the industry. And it is argued that the improvement of testing procedures should be left to the industry which has itself the liveliest and most direct interest in insuring the safety and effectiveness of its profits." In addition to relative trust of industry over central state agencies, German politics in the wake of thalidomide witnessed other legitimized organizations lobbying for more power over drug development. The most important of these were medical and scientific organizations—the Federal Chamber of Physicians (Bundesärztekammer, or BÄK) and Germany's principal pharmacology society. In the absence of a central state agency with drug evaluation capacity—an institutional and reputational niche filled by industry and the organized medical profession— German politicians' instinctual response to thalidomide was seemingly to consider every solution *except* for government pre-market review.[55]

In other nations—in their legislatures, in their public discourse, and in their networks of medical research and dialogue—the Administration was widely considered a model for emulation in the design of pharmaceutical policy. In France and Great Britain there were immediate, sonorous calls for the empowerment of the federal government in regulating the development and marketing of new medicines. There was, to be sure, a different system of federalism in Germany, but in other nations with federalist systems that erected new institutions of governance for pharmaceuticals, open emulation

[55]Crosby S. Noyes (foreign correspondent, *Washington Star*), "Thalidomide's Shadow: Germany Shuns Controls," *Washington Star* (evening edition), August 28, 1962, p. 2; *ICDRR*, 452. Daemmrich also observes that proposals for greater government regulation by agents in Bonn "were widely discredited as too costly, inefficient and unlikely to guarantee product safety" (*Pharmacopolitics*, 39). The Deutsche Gesellschaft für Experimentelle und Klinische Pharmakologie und Toxikologie (DGPT) was founded in 1920 and, with members scattered throughout Germany's universities, was well poised to capitalize on the Federal Republic's federalist structure. See also chapter 11.

of the FDA was commonplace and celebrated. These included Australia and Canada, where the agency now known as Health Canada was modeled upon FDA structure and procedures and where Canadian medical authorities were to constantly lament that their agency did not measure up to its southern counterpart.

British medical experts and public health officials gestured to the FDA as an entity whose presence, strength, and accumulated judgment was sorely lacking in their country. With the use of oral contraceptives on the upswing in Britain, the editors of the *British Medical Journal* noted with suspicion an August 1962 circular letter sent by drug maker Searle (manufacturer of the contraceptive Enovid) to British physicians. Detecting the weight of the FDA in Searle's decision to issue a broad warning about thromboembolic risks associated with Enovid, the editors pointed to the multiple roles that the Administration could play in improving the quality, safety, and information available about medicines.

> It is of course impossible to know how much of the contents of the Searle letter is due to its consultations with the FDA. Certainly the fact that it was prepared in association with a Government agency lends it a weight and authority which it could hardly lay claim otherwise. This is perhaps a welcome reminder that the FDA has a wider function than merely registered drugs—it can also exercise a useful effect on the amount and quality of information which the pharmaceutical houses disseminate to the profession. It can insist, for instance, on the notification of side-effects in promotional and package literature. We have, by contrast, no official provision in this country for insuring that dangers and disadvantages of preparations are so notified—this is left entirely to the judgment of the industry.[56]

At the level of personality, cross-national differences in the politics of reputation are observed in the differing trajectories of the three national protagonists in the thalidomide tragedy—Kelsey, Widukind Lenz, and William McBride. Lenz would become involved in civil litigation against thalidomide manufacturers and, in the process, would have his claims discredited and his name tarnished through cross-examination and media reporting. William McBride's fame in Australia would persist, as he launched a research center with the substantial contributions given him after his role in the thalidomide revelations. Still, his profile slowly faded into one of cultural and international obscurity, and he would resurface a generation later only to experience humiliation. In a stunning 1982 article, McBride would allege that one of the ingredients of Debendox—a morning sickness compound marketed as Bendectin in the United States—was the cause of birth

---

[56] "Today's Drugs: Oral Contraceptives and Thrombophlebitis," *BMJ* (Sept. 15, 1962): 727. The *BMJ* statement ends with a request that any cases of thrombophlebitis, stroke, or other cardiovascular adverse events should be referred to the FDA. In the United States, Searle and FDA apparently bargained and fought over the contents of the letter, and on whether Searle had properly complied with the FDA's request that it inform physicians (*Medical Tribune*, August 20, 1962, 23).

defects. Soon after McBride's warning, global sales of Debendox plummeted and by 1983, the drug was withdrawn by its American manufacturer, Merrell Dow. After a charge of research fraud was leveled against McBride by one of his researchers, the gynecologist's name plummeted, his research institute closed and, in 1993, he was convicted by a medical tribunal in the case and removed from medical practice. [57]

By the 1990s, of the three temporary heroes—Kelsey, Lenz, and McBride—only Frances Kelsey was left standing in name and in government service. In some respects, the falls from grace experienced by Lenz and McBride owed to fabricated claims and issues of individual judgment. Yet a key variable in the contrast remains the intimate connection of the American expert to her federal government organization. Neither Lenz nor McBride worked for a legitimate agency of state, and neither was endowed with formal regulatory power in the years following the global phocomelia epidemic. In this respect, the FDA assisted with Kelsey's longer-term reputation even as Kelsey lent her good name to the Administration. A contrast in individual reputations reproduced the gulf in the organizational reputations attached to national regulators. In the years following thalidomide, no global pharmaceutical regulatory agency carried a more prominent public profile than did the Food and Drug Administration. This profile would open the FDA to immense and enduring criticism, yet the alternating flow of contest and acclaim would only serve to cement certain images in public and local discourse and memory.

Despite the impermanence of failure narratives attached to thalidomide, the Administration and its officials did receive significant criticism. Some of the criticism flowed from the narrowness of the agency's success in thalidomide. If the drug came so close to getting approved, such that only one vigilant heroine stood in the way, national elites reasoned, then did not the thalidomide episode reveal the fragility of the American pharmaceutical regime as much as its vigor? Journalists and national politicians noted the razor-thin procedural margin by which thalidomide was kept from the market, and by August 1962, they knew that the drug had been tested in the United States without being formally approved here. Lawrence Fountain, North Carolina Democrat and Chair of the House Intergovernmental Sub-

---

[57] As Arthur Daemmrich reads these individual reputations, Kelsey's embedment in a legitimized organization contributed to her surfeit of cultural and professional authority: "Whereas Kelsey retained her credibility as an FDA regulator, Lenz became isolated and failed to carry his credibility through legal-cross examination and courtroom demonstration of his biased stance." Daemmrich, "A Tale of Two Experts: Thalidomide and Political Engagement in the United States and West Germany," *Social History of Medicine* 15 (2002): 137–58.

McBride's 1982 publication was "Effects of Scopolamine Hydrobromide on the Development of the Chick and Rabbit Embryo," *Australian Journal of Biological Sciences* 35 (2) (1982): 173–8. In 1993, the Medical Tribunal of New South Wales convicted McBride of research fraud and removed him from the Register of Medical Practitioners there. See Daniel John, "Medical Hero Guilty of Research Fraud: Australian scientist faces end to career of acclaim," *The Guardian* (London), March 20, 1993, 11; Brynner and Stephens, *Dark Remedy*, 198–9.

committee, prepared in October 1962 to hold a set of hearings on the FDA's "inadequacies." And even as Congress prepared to endow the Administration with vast new formal authority, major voices such as Hubert Humphrey openly accused the agency of gross shortcomings in its application of existing federal statute. The Bureau of Medicine had, in Humphrey's expressed fears, become "a scientific backwater," despite the presence of "a small nucleus of dedicated FDA scientists." So rutted was the agency in its past as "police department"—Larrick continued to defend his organization as "essentially an enforcement agency"—that it had failed to develop the necessary scientific capacity to administer the 1962 law. The Administration would need abiding and enduring assistance from federal advisory committees.[58]

For some audiences, George Larrick would come to personify these failures. The commissioner was a convenient and plausible target of scorn and a scapegoat to whom the agency's critics could ascribe its shortcomings. The *Drug Trade News* saw potential in the Administration, but potential that was being hindered by Larrick's presence and by structural flaws imposed from without. "There is a good basis for feeling that FDA is not set up to do today's job as efficiently as it could. Mr. Larrick will have to bear the responsibility for this." Other observers attributed less good will to Larrick and argued that it was long past time for his departure. "The implication is clear," concluded a *Washington Post* editorial, "that Commissioner George P. Larrick has been an indifferent steward of an important post." Larrick's poor personal reputation was, in some sense, a catharsis for the FDA's organizational failings. A failure of leadership and a stunting of potential were, at the same time, the basis for an exoneration of the agency corps of career civil servants.[59]

Other faces in the FDA, including some personalities central to the reform movement, were perceived in tones quite different from the warm light cast upon Kelsey. Kenneth Milstead, deputy director of the Bureau of Enforcement, warned of an impending shake-up in the agency as a result of thalidomide. Critics of the agency faulted Larrick for supporting an open-door policy—one in which aggressive industry representatives were free to roam the halls of the Administration and hound medical reviewers—though Larrick would deny in his testimony to Congress that any such environment existed. A further irony of the thalidomide episode was that some of the very architects of the new pharmacological regime in federal regulation, not least Ralph Smith (who was at that time Kelsey's immediate superior), were accused of hindering Kelsey and allowing company officials unfettered access to the new drug reviewer.[60]

[58]Humphrey's October 3, 1962, remarks from the Senate floor appear in Exhibit 94, *ICDRR*, 579–83. Stephens Rippey, "FDA's Leadership Is Having Trouble," *DTN*, September 17, 1962, 2; *ICDRR*, 627–8. Larrick's defensive remarks appear in "FDA: A Time of Crisis—Growth Patterns Cause Problems, Larrick Believes," *Medical Tribune* 4 (65) (Aug. 16, 1963): 16.

[59]Rippey, "FDA's Leadership Is Having Trouble," 2; "Energizing FDA," *WP*, October 28, 1962, E6; *ICDRR*, 627–32.

[60]"Shake-Up in FDA Seen as Thalidomide Result," *Washington Evening Star*, September 18,

When it came time to assign organizational blame, the Administration again dodged and deflected much of the harshest criticism. In their public agonizing over the drug safety crisis of the early 1960s, politicians, scientists, and journalists echoed the Citizens' Committee of 1955: the most systematic failures of the agency were failures of Congress. The Administration was ill-equipped due to legislative thrift. This assignment of regulatory failure to Congress was widespread, including within the national legislature itself. Cornell pharmacologist Walter Modell—a leading voice in therapeutic reform in the mid-twentieth century—thought that Congress had so under-equipped the FDA that the Kefauver bill was doomed. "It just doubles an impossible burden unless we also give them lots more money and much more vigorous leadership," Modell worried. "I see no disposition on the part of Congress to give FDA the support it needs." "Penury is the lot of this key agency," summarized Johns Hopkins pharmacologist Frederick Wolff, who framed the Administration in mythic terms.

> The Food and Drug Administration is generally known as the Cinderella of the health agencies. It is exposed to such continuous pressures from the people's representatives, industry and others, is so underpaid, understaffed, overworked and neglected that it is constantly losing its best people to industry and the intellectually more stimulating atmosphere of the universities.

This verbal portrait of indigence resounded continually in Washington politics. "Though the FDA has a solid record of accomplishment," the *Washington Post* concurred, "the agency has simply not grown with the times and is in urgent need of reinvigoration." Hubert Humphrey himself, in introducing his 1963 hearings at which the Administration would be excoriated, took time to blame his resident institution for many of the FDA's shortcomings. "FDA has been seriously handicapped for many years by acute shortages of men, money, manpower, material," the senator admitted. "The Congress has its responsibilities for this shortage and for this limitation. FDA, I think, has never been given the public support that is justified."[61]

1962. One national magazine reported that Smith, who was Kelsey's immediate superior at the time of the Kevadon NDA, had allowed thalidomide producers repeated access to her while she was processing their application. As numerous observers of the thalidomide review have noted, Smith actually backed Kelsey against the accusations and ire of Merrell officials and often delivered the bad news of another delay to Merrell executives (Hilts, *Protecting America's Health*, 153–4). For more detailed claims of Merrell executives working the halls of the Administration's offices, see also Miriam Ottenberg, "The Story of MER/29—Was the Public Protected?" *Washington* (Sunday) *Star*, August 26, 1962.

[61] Humphrey remark at *ICDRR*, 779; Barbara Yuncker, "Pills and You—Is the Kefauver Bill Enough?" *New York Post*, September 16, 1962; *ICDRR*, 624. In an October 1962 letter to Senator Humphrey, L. T. Coggeshall, Chairman of the Commission and Drug Safety and then a Vice President at the University of Chicago, would describe his 1950s experience with the FDA in terms that echoed Modell's portrait: "As a former assistant to Secretary Folsom in 1956, I had the responsibility of guiding the [FDA's] program and became familiar with its strengths and weaknesses. At that time it was not adequate to meet its tasks, housed in inade-

The timing and form of the Drug Amendments of 1962 point to organizational reputation as the primary force advancing and shaping regulatory change. The dynamic of industry capture—of large firms using the political process to erect new entry barriers for their smaller and less mature competitors—was never a possibility. The Pharmaceutical Manufacturers' Association, whose lobbyists served as the mouthpiece for large pharmaceutical firms, steadfastly resisted any provision that strengthened the Administration's gatekeeping authority. Industry influence over regulatory legislation was evident in the spring of 1962 but was nullified by the thalidomide crisis and its distillation in national politics. Perhaps the best evidence that reputational politics carried the day is that the final measure could have been quite different, and much stronger. The patent provisions of Kefauver's original legislation were dropped, as was the proposal to endow the Department of Health, Education and Welfare with authority to license drug companies. What survived in the legislative rush of August and September 1962 were the efficacy standard and the investigational new drug provisions, in other words, those provisions that expressed the wishes of the FDA's Bureau of Medicine and that deferred to its emergent vision and practices.

The other legacy of organizational reputation comes not in the Amendments' language, but in its many spaces of silence and brevity. While champions and critics of the Kefauver-Harris Amendments have devoted most of the attention to the addition of an "efficacy requirement," they have largely ignored the ambiguity with which the Amendments elaborated a new pharmaceutical regime. Mindful and generally trustful of the Bureau of Medicine's capacity and legitimacy, the 87th Congress and President Kennedy willfully left many questions and concepts undefined. Among these were "new drug," "efficacy," "adequate," "well-controlled," "investigations," and "scientific training and experience." In the Drug Amendments of 1962, national politicians handed to the Administration the power of interpretation and concept definition, all but ensuring that the key developments in American pharmaceutical policy would come not from statute but from administrative rulemaking and regulatory practice.

Conceptual Power Elaborated: The Administrative Construction of Effectiveness and Experiment

From 1963 onward, the basic terms of the Federal Food, Drug and Cosmetic Act—and hence some of the central concepts of the modern pharmaceutical world—were elaborated in rhetoric, in rulemaking, and in rote application of the new law. The Administration's officers did not invent all of

---

quate quarters, and understaffed; and at best, it received only indifferent support from the Congress. The new Federal drug law and regulations spell out ways and means of correcting some of the faults, but at the same time will result in throwing upon the [FDA] a greater load than they can possibly cope with"; Coggeshall to Humphrey, October 16, 1962; *ICDRR*, 727. Wolff to Editor, *New York Times*, August 14, 1962; *ICDRR*, 541–2.

these terms from scratch. Many terms were the co-creation of pharmacologists, industry-based clinicians, academic physicians, and others in a process of therapeutic reform that extended through the twentieth century. The notion of efficacy had a European past and was inscribed in Swedish statutes before its incorporation in American law. The idea of a randomized controlled trial—an experiment where chance alone assigned a patient to the population receiving the medical treatment in question or to an "arm" of experimental "control" subjects who did not receive the treatment—possessed a decades-old history in statistics, in agronomy, and in the evaluation of antibiotics before general pharmacologists and the FDA's Bureau of Medicine seized upon it in the late 1940s and 1950s. Normative constructs of informed consent and patient protection had evolved from global reaction to wartime medical atrocities and developments in bioethics. In these cases and many others, the FDA officials who were opening the uncertain spaces of late twentieth-century drug development were mere participants in a much grander dialogue.[62]

What happened in the pharmaceutical politics of the 1960s and 1970s was not invention but reinvention. In their active and passive construal of the law and in the elaboration and extension of their formal power, FDA officials became more than participants or referees. They became founders. The task of the Administration's officers was to formalize and give concrete meaning to a new regime of drug development and approval. In doing so, they drew in part from the conceptual apparatus that had been developed in European and American medicine and science, in part from the habits of notable companies and medical centers, and not least from their own patterns of regulation, most of which had been developed in the decade and a half before 1962. These decisions were only partially coordinated, and they were guided as much by trial-and-error learning and by political considerations as by directed plan. Yet because the Administration alone stood sentry at the crossing from medical science to the therapeutic marketplace, its administrative decisions and actions transformed science and therapy outright. When three phases of experiment were delineated as the legitimated schedule of drug development, the basic notion of experiment itself changed. When new drugs were rejected, delayed, or withdrawn based upon insufficient demonstration of efficacy, these sometimes alarming precedents altered the very concept of efficacy. When drug companies worldwide boosted their ranks of pharmacologists and statisticians by the dozens and hundreds—because the Administration had told them to do so and would accept no other form of oversight for sponsored new drugs—the very understanding of scientific expertise had changed. In the particular administration of a legal regime, the generalities of science and statute were shaped again. The applied reordered the pure.

[62]Harry Marks, *The Progress of Experiment: Science and Therapeutic Reform, 1900–1990* (New York: Cambridge University Press, 1997). Beauchamp, *A History and Theory of Informed Consent* New York: Oxford University Press, 1986).

Two remarks are in order. First, the ability to define basic terms of legislation and statute through particular decisions does not imply any sort of constitutional or legal violation. At no point in the elaboration of formal authority did FDA officials engage in unconstitutional interpretations or illegal behavior. The organizational legitimacy of the Administration was such that courts and national politicians deferred consistently to its interpretations, actions, and decisions. If the aggregation of particular decisions into general principles were an illegitimate course of legal construction or policymaking, then much of American case law and British common law would be invalidated as well.[63]

A second point concerns the facets of regulatory power. The Administration's pronouncements and actions stuck because its gatekeeping authority compelled any sponsor of a new medication to satisfy its terms and interpretations. In this sense, directive regulatory power (formal authority) and gatekeeping power supported the conceptual facet of regulatory power. Yet in another way, the Administration's attempts to compel or induce particular behavior by regulated entities (gatekeeping and directive power) relied continually upon its ability to secure acceptance of the meanings it had attached to basic concepts and phrases. In this way, the conceptual face of regulatory power gave necessary weight and cement to the other faces.

More than other interpreters of the 1962 law, Bureau of Medicine officials sought to tie the statute's various terms together into a regulatory equilibrium of concepts and powers. At the core of this equilibrium was the power of the Administration to refuse. When Administration Medical Director Joseph Sadusk spoke of the definition of drug "efficacy" under federal law in an October 1964 speech to the American College of Physicians in Los Angeles, he did not begin his speech with an examination of the word, but rather described the authorities of his agency in terms of negation.

> As a result of these Amendments, a new drug application can now be rejected not only when there is insufficient evidence to establish its safety, but also if there is a lack of substantial evidence to show that the drug will have the effect it purports or is represented to have under conditions of use recommended in the proposed labeling.[64]

In casting the Administration's veto power in broad terms, Sadusk was leading his audience (and his agency) away from other meanings and interpretations of the Act. Industry officials and attorneys saw in the "substantial evidence" standard a much lighter burden for new drug approval, including

---

[63] This point is all the more relevant because in one crucial area of economic regulation—the constraint of trusts—the United States was governed by the British common law case *Horner v. Graves* for much of the nineteenth century; Martin J. Sklar, *The Corporate Reconstruction of American Capitalism, 1890–1916: The Market, the Law and Politics* (New York: Cambridge University Press, 1988).

[64] Sadusk, "The Definition of the Efficacy of a Drug Under the Law," presented in a Symposium on Drug Investigation and Therapy, at the Second Fall Meeting of the American College of Physicians, Los Angeles, October 8, 1964, p. 1; DF 505, RG 88, NA.

the possibility of "reasonably substantiated efficacy claims" that could obtain even if equal or preponderant evidence against efficacy had emerged during clinical trials.[65]

The other innovation of Sadusk's Los Angeles address was one of ideation. Sadusk presented the concept of efficacy as significant not in and of itself, nor in its legacies of therapeutic reform, but in its provision of a new rationale for FDA rejection of new drug applications. Since the concept of efficacy served to empower regulatory rejection, the term would be identified as much by administrative practice as by science. In the remainder of his speech, Sadusk defined labeling and then offered an exegesis of sorts on the term "substantial evidence." The "definition of efficacy as expressed in the law," Sadusk remarked, came down to three clauses associated with the substantial evidence requirement of the Amendments.

   1. Adequate and Well-Controlled Investigations.
   2. Experts Qualified by Scientific Training and Experience.
   3. On the Basis of Which It Can Fairly and Responsibly be Concluded That the Drug Will Have Its Claimed Effect.

On the first clause, Sadusk repeated the well-worn insistence of Administration functionaries that efficacy demonstrations required "placebo comparisons in well-designed double-blind clinical studies." He then quickly acknowledged that in many cases, randomized and controlled trials with a placebo arm were neither feasible nor ethically appropriate. Yet his instruction to the assembled physicians in Los Angeles in these cases was not that any method could then be applied, but that the Administration itself would employ other criteria to assess the evidentiary value of the experiment.

> Here the design of the study, the competence and experience of the investigators, the adequacy of the observations and laboratory and other test procedures that are employed to record and weigh the clinical effects of the drug take on paramount importance. With some drugs intended for use in disease states, the natural histories of which are reasonably well understood and in which the pharmacological behavior of the drug can be observed by objective measurements, the blind

---

[65]These interests seized upon the Senate Judiciary Committee's rejection of the "preponderant" evidence standard; see Senate Report 1744, 16, n.116; reprinted in FDA, *A Legislative History of the Federal Food, Drug and Cosmetic Act and Its Amendments*, 22: 109. Joel E. Hoffman, "Administrative Procedures of the Food and Drug Administration," in David G. Adams, Richard M. Cooper, and Jonathan S. Kahan, eds., *Fundamentals of Law and Regulation, Volume II, An In-Depth Look at Therapeutic Products* (Washington, DC: Food and Drug Law Institute, 1997), 29. Hoffman's reading of the legislative history is a revisionist one; neither the Senate report nor the statute ever counseled approval based upon "reasonably substantiated efficacy claims," and even as legal constructs of "reasonable" plans of experiment, "reasonable variations" from plan and "reasonable promptness" suffused the law, the committee deliberations and the subsequent rules, language of reasonable *evidence* was strikingly absent from all of these venues. See also the decision of the Third U.S. Circuit Court in *Warner-Lambert v. Heckler*, 787 F.2d 147, 157 (1986).

and double-blind studies take on less significance. And even in states where there are little or no objective measures of patient response, careful planning coupled with systematic observation and accurate recording of the patient's course may qualify as a well-controlled study. The use of other disciplines such as statistics may provide the extra support to make the study an acceptable and convincing one.[66]

Whether or not Sadusk meant them to, these remarks struck a revolutionary posture. For a wide variety of drugs, the quality of investigation would be defined not simply by its observable procedures, but by the status of the people carrying it out, the perceived quality of its facilities, and by an array of terms that described a morality of clinical experiment and research conduct. How "careful," how "systematic," how "accurate," how "acceptable," how "convincing" would a study be? These were the questions that Sadusk's colleagues at the FDA would answer. What the director's speech implied was that the meaning of "adequate and well-controlled" lay in the eye of the gatekeeper.

Sadusk endowed the phrase "experts qualified by scientific training and experience" with similar ambiguity. Since "the scientific community" had nowhere nailed down explicit criteria to define the competency of an investigator, "it does not seem likely that a Governmental agency will ever be able to establish such standards." The FDA, then, would approach qualification judgments on a case-by-case basis, considering each investigator "on the merits of his curriculum vitae, his past record of accomplishment, the scientific environment in which he is doing the investigation, and the nature and quality of the recorded observations." Whereas Sadusk had already defined the quality of experiments in part by the competence of the experimenter, he now defined the competence of experimenters in part by the observable quality of their experiments. In a revealing addendum to this discussion, Sadusk pronounced that his agency would probably never produce a list of qualified investigators. As he was speaking, his resource-constrained Bureau of Medicine was doing the inverse by sketching out procedures for the disqualification of researchers.[67]

On the third clause regarding the drug's "claimed effect," Sadusk once again pointed to the absence of consensual standards for evaluating efficacy claims. He began by outlining those implications excluded from the meanings of the statute. "Neither legally nor medically is there any requirement that all investigators show effectiveness," he said. Furthermore, the law specified neither a fixed number of studies nor a fixed number of experimenters. In a bow to industry critics of the law and the agency who worried about the possibility of comparative efficacy judgments, he saw no requirement that a drug "be found more effective than other drugs for the same purpose." Beyond this, scientific considerations could not pin down the criteria of efficacy, so the job was left to the gatekeeper.

[66]Sadusk, "The Definition of the Efficacy of a Drug Under the Law," 3.
[67]Ibid., 3–4. On disqualification, see chapter 8.

Since medical investigation cannot always be an exact science, the law does not require that the evidence demonstrate effectiveness beyond peradventure.

What is required is a body of scientific data drawn from the investigations that will be convincing to those responsible for the decision to approve or not to approve the marketing of the drug.[68]

Joseph Sadusk's Los Angeles address about efficacy was in fact a speech about power. It was one of many addresses that he and other mid-level officials—Ralph Smith, Frances Kelsey, John Harvey, William Goodrich—would make in the early 1960s. Most of these were circulated extensively within the Administration and particularly among the staff of the Bureau of Medicine. Most of them were officially approved and edited for delivery. In all of these addresses, the basic terms of the 1962 Amendments received little elaboration, and the audiences (physicians, business executives, lawyers, advertisers) were told that the terms of the modern pharmaceutical world meant what the Administration would make of them. The agents of power were those entrusted with "the decision to approve or not to approve the marketing of the drug." The power to refuse was, moreover, premised upon the particular standards by which the agency evaluated drugs, and the particular methods and hurdles that the agency could demand of drug sponsors. The power of veto would rest upon definition of the terms in which vetoes were justified, and these definitions in turn received their meaning from regulatory considerations. The result was not circularity but an ambiguous equilibrium of practice and meaning, an equilibrium sketched out slowly in regulatory experience. As with the ambiguity that characterized the elaboration of standards of efficacy and new drug review in the 1950s, the ambiguity that emerges from official FDA communications of the early 1960s was strategic in part, but also normative. Ambiguity preserved space for discretion. It also obviated the need for rulemaking and copious delineation of terms. And ambiguity meant that any single official could partially clarify the terms of the new pharmaceutical regime while not speaking inappropriately for the larger entity or constraining the action of others. The resulting equilibrium was not one of rational action but of ideation, a nexus of concepts tied to one another.[69]

---

[68]Ibid., 4. Matters would become more specific in the coming years, as the Administration interpreted the statute's words "experiments" to call for at least two studies demonstrating efficacy; for an acknowledgment and rationale, see *FR* 60 (Aug. 1, 1995): 39180–81. Sadusk's denial that a new drug had to show superiority to others for the same disease did not, moreover, rule out all comparative efficacy considerations. FDA officials would still consider whether new drugs (1) treated a target disease as well as existing treatments or (2) treated those who fared poorly under medicines previously approved for the condition. See chapter 7 for a more extended discussion.

[69]For similar addresses, see Sadusk, "The Relationship of the Food and Drug Administration to the Practice of Medicine and the Aminopyrine-Dipyrone Problem"; Kelsey, "Use of Investigational New Drugs in Hospitals under the New FDA Amendments," June 24, 1964; Kelsey, "The Control of Investigational Drugs," December 4, 1963; "Chicago and New Drug Legislation," June 6, 1963; in DF 505, RG 88, NA. Having read the Sadusk address, former

The Idea of Phased Experimentation. With terms such as "new drug" and "efficacy" defined in terms of evidence, the architecture of the 1962 law became increasingly dependent upon the rules governing medical experiment and drug development. The 1962 Amendments compelled the FDA to issue regulations governing clinical experimentation, and FDA leadership responded quickly with a wider set of draft rules issued in January 1963. The "Investigational Drug Regulations" were finalized in August 1963 and distributed widely, and FDA leadership set in motion a variety of mechanisms to enforce and clarify their meanings. The 1963 IND rules expressed core features of the new pharmaceutical world, including many features that had been crafted partially or wholly outside of the Administration such as notions of informed consent, controlled experiments, and study protocols. Yet in one particular innovation whose roots lay squarely within the FDA, the 1963 rules forever changed the realm of clinical experiment by imposing a structure of "phases" upon clinical trials.[70]

Along with the 1956 new drug application rules, the 1963 investigational new drug rules compose some of the most important federal regulations ever to be issued by the Administration. Indeed, along with the National Ambient Air Quality Standards (NAAQS) issued by the Environmental Protection Agency in 1977 and perhaps the "Part 68" rules issued in 1975 by the Federal Communications Commission (FCC) governing connections to the public telephone network, the 1956 and 1963 rules arguably represent some of the most consequential regulations issued by any agency in American

FDA general counsel Peter Barton Hutt (private correspondence, November 14, 2008) informs me that "I made the same speeches, as does the FDA today." This points to the durability of Sadusk's interpretations.

On the logic of ambiguity in pharmaceutical regulation, consult Daniel Carpenter and Colin D. Moore, "Robust Action and the Strategic Use of Ambiguity in a Bureaucratic Cohort: The Investigational New Drug Rules of 1963," in Stephen Skowronek and Matt Glassman, eds., *Formative Acts: American Politics in the Making* (Philadelphia: University of Pennsylvania Press, 2007). For mathematical models that express some of this logic but also strip away much of the necessary complexity and nuance, see Stephen Callendar and Daniel Carpenter, "Ambiguity and Commitment in Approval Regulation," manuscript, Northwestern University; B. Douglas Bernheim and Michael Whinston, "Incomplete Contracts and Strategic Ambiguity," *American Economic Review* 88 (4) (Sept. 1998): 902–32. Several FDA officials and drug company attorneys were consciously aware that the Administration's informal statements and policy decisions were not being aggregated in a way that would allow for greater clarity. At the suggestion of attorneys for Mallinckrodt Chemical Works in St. Louis, FDA officials considered adopting practices from the Internal Revenue Service, which was in the habit of compiling and annotating its rulings. See M. R. Stephens (Director, Bureau of Enforcement) to Commissioner, "Issuing of Informal Policy Statements," September 23, 1963; Leo L. Miller (Assistant Commissioner for Administration) to Rankin, "Issuing of Informal Policy Statements," December 5, 1963; FDA General Correspondence, 1963—051.155, B 3422-23, RG 88, NA. In lieu of a new publication, FDA officials of the early 1960s preferred to use the *Federal Register* for these statements.

[70]See William W. Goodrich Oral History, FDA Oral History Collection, NLM; published electronically at http://www.fda.gov/oc/history/oralhistories/goodrich/part3.html (accessed Feb. 20, 2007), 12–13.

history. Like the 1956 rules—which had refined and publicized the New Drug Application form—the 1963 regulations had their primary effect by institutionalizing a new government document, "Form FD 1571: Notice of Claimed Investigational Exemption for a New Drug." Without having filed a completed "IND form" with the FDA, no sponsor could begin clinical trials with any new drug.[71]

The Administration had already issued new proposed rules governing investigational drugs in August 1962, two months before Kennedy had signed the Drug Amendments of 1962 into law. These rules were based on draft regulations authored by Julius Hauser—serving as assistant to the Medical Director in the Bureau of Medicine—earlier that year. When Mintz's thalidomide story hit, general counsel William Goodrich and associate commissioner Winton Rankin revised Hauser's draft rules. It was in these proposed rules—published in the *Federal Register* of August 10, 1962—that Form FD 1571 made its first public appearance. The proposals, particularly their requirements for extensive record keeping, were assailed with charges of government paternalism, but Goodrich and other top regulators did not budge from imposing the obligations. The tenth item of the new form directed the sponsors of new drugs to provide "an outline of the planned clinical investigations of the new drug," including any "planned stages of investigation." Yet in the summer of 1962 there was little hint of a favored or established sequence of experiments, one before the other, progressing toward a randomized, controlled clinical trial.[72]

---

[71]To compare the significance of federal rules across history is a difficult undertaking. My point is that, aside from the particulate standards in the EPA's NAAQS rules, it is difficult to find federal rules that, like the 1956 and 1963 FDA rules, established the organizational structure of science and industry. There are many examples of highly consequential federal rules— the cotton dust standard or the 1983 hazard communication rules of the Occupational Safety and Health Administration, the concentrated animal feeding operations (CAFO) rules of the EPA, even FCC's Part 68 rules—that were enormously consequential economically but did not generate new concepts that governed a generation of subsequent science and generate a new industry founded on these concepts, both in the United States and other nations.

[72]Hauser, "Proposed Revision of Regulation 130.3, first draft," May 24, 1962; Hauser to FDA Division Directors, "Proposed Revision of Investigational Drug Regulations," June 5, 1962; Hauser to Commissioner's Office, July 23, 1962, summary memo re "Draft Revision— Investigational Drug Regulations"; *Julius Hauser Memoirs*, 130–31; all in JHPP. See also Hauser's first draft of May 24, where he apparently penciled "2 3 stages" next to the section discussing the "outline of the planned clinical investigations" (p. 3); however, these terms did not enter subsequent drafts or the August 10 proposed rules.

Larrick, "New Drugs for Investigational Use: Proposed Exemptions," *FR* 27 (Aug. 10, 1962): 7991. On the opposition, Goodrich would later remark that "We got tremendous opposition on the thing. Every organized piece of medicine came here arguing that they were responsible people, that they didn't need any government supervision, and that the record keeping and reporting was onerous and would cut down the development of new drugs. We had a deaf ear to all that" (Goodrich Oral History, NLM). Pharmacologist Carl Pfeiffer would also remark that the IND rules "were presented and passed as a fait accompli in spite of protests by scientists and scientific societies." "Problems in Drug Development as they Relate to the Clinical Investigator," *Journal of New Drugs* (Nov.–Dec. 1964): 299.

The notion of experimental phases emerged in the Administration's Bureau of Pharmacology and Bureau of Medicine and a small network of clinical oncologists centered in the National Cancer Institute. Among pharmacologists in the late 1950s, a "Phase 1 study" referred to the first experiments in humans for assessing toxicity, dosage, and preferred route of administration. The idea of a "first phase" human trial stemmed from a methodology for animal studies developed by FDA pharmacologists A. J. Lehman and O. Garth Fitzhugh. Lehman and Fitzhugh made two contributions. First, they wanted to order the study of safety and effectiveness so that experiments moved systematically from the former question to the latter. In this way, the architecture of the 1938 Food, Drug and Cosmetic Act placed safety studies at the start of research on any drug. The second contribution was to create a sequence of toxicity studies that reflected rational, orderly transitions from one kind of experiment to the next. In Lehman and Fitzhugh's design, studies would move from questions of safety in short-term drug utilization to questions about longer-term use.[73]

Lehman and Fitzhugh's approaches were picked up in the Bureau of Medicine and in human trials for the first time in cancer chemotherapy research. In 1955, the National Cancer Institute began to establish a handful of regional oncology research networks, in part to facilitate multicenter clinical trials. The most prominent of these networks were the Eastern Cooperative Group on Solid Tumor Chemotherapy, the Midwest Cooperative Chemotherapy Group, and the Southwest Cooperative Oncology Group (centered at M. D. Anderson). The officials leading this effort—chiefly Charles G. Zubrod, head of the National Cancer Institute—were interested in controlled clinical trials for comparative efficacy. At the organizational and procedural level, however, these groups quickly confronted the question of when a drug was sufficiently nontoxic to qualify for tests of its anti-tumor activity. The methods by which this question would be answered were imported from pharmacology circles, chiefly the Lehman-Fitzhugh group at the FDA. A crucial lesson drawn from the Lehman and Fitzhugh studies was that of using the results of toxicity studies in the design of effectiveness studies. The cooperative oncology groups soon began drawing up plans for Phase 2 studies, including randomized studies, which started with dosage schedules derived from the Phase 1 trials.[74]

[73]On Lehman and Fitzhugh's development of standards in chronic toxicity, see chapter 3, and J. M. Barnes and F. A. Denz, "Experimental Methods Used in Determining Chronic Toxicity," *Pharmacological Review* 6 (1954): 191–242. Referring to Lehman's 1949 paper, Barnes and Denz wrote that "The standard publication on the toxicity test is that of Lehman and his colleagues." The four-stage sequence of toxicity studies developed by Lehman and Fitzhugh started with examination of the drug's chemical and physical characteristics, and then proceeded to acute toxicity studies (where for instance LD 50 levels were determined), to sub-acute toxicity studies, then finally to chronic toxicity studies. Late 1950s textbooks in pharmacology then began to incorporate discussions of sequenced experiment; Torrald Sollman, *A Manual of Pharmacology and Its Applications to Therapeutics and Toxicology*, 8th ed. (Philadelphia: Saunders, 1957).

[74]In the electronic databases of medical journals of the National Library of Medicine known

The idea of applying three sequentially ordered phases of experiment to all drug research was hatched in discussions between FDA attorneys and the Bureau of Medicine in the fall of 1962. The web of officials in which these concepts took shape appears to have included Frances Kelsey, William Goodrich, Julius Hauser, J. Kenneth Kirk, Joseph Sadusk, and Ralph Smith. Hauser was probably the most actively involved author, having circulated earlier rules governing investigational new drugs to Goodrich, Smith, Kessenich, and even Ralph Weilerstein. Crucially, the concept was synthesized and sounded out by FDA administrative and legal officials as well as by medical staff. Bureau of Medicine leaders such as Kelsey and Smith wanted compulsory phases in order to establish prospective research design. Regulatory personalities like Goodrich, Hauser, and Kirk were particularly keen to quash the growing pattern of companies using experimentation to market their product to physicians before FDA approval. All of these officials wanted to endow drug development with "rational," "orderly," and "comprehensive" characteristics. Kelsey's hope, in particular, was that lessons learned in the earlier experiments would be systematically incorporated into later, more thorough trials.[75]

as PubMed, the first reference in an article title to a clinical trial with a numbered phase appears in F. H. Bethell, et al., "Phase II evaluation of cyclophosphamide," *Cancer Chemotherapy Reports* 8 (July 1960):112–15. For some insight into practices of phased experimentation in their infancy, see Bruce I. Shnider, "Early clinical trials with anticancer agents; phase I and phase II studies. A. Dosage schedules and routes of administration," *Cancer Chemotherapy Reports* 16 (Feb. 1962): 61–7; John Louis, "Coordinated Phase I Studies for Cooperative Chemotherapy Groups," *Journal of Chronic Diseases* 15 (1962): 273–81. Perhaps the most influential early comparative clinical trial in anti-tumor research appears in Charles G. Zubrod, et al., "Appraisal of Methods for the Study of Chemotherapy of Cancer in Man: Comparative Therapeutic Trial of Nitrogen Mustard and Triethylene Thiophosphoramide," *Journal of Chronic Diseases* 11 (1) (Jan. 1960): 7–33. Most Phase 2 trials in the cooperative oncology groups were incredibly exploratory, testing a drug upon numerous different forms of tumor. Some insightful work on the idea of protocol in cancer clinical trials has been conducted by Peter Keating and Alberto Cambrosio; "From Screening to Clinical Research: The Cure of Leukemia and the Early Development of the Cooperative Oncology Groups, 1955–1966," *BullHistMed* 76 (2002): 299–334; "Cancer Clinical Trials: The Emergence and Development of a New Style of Practice," *BullHistMed* 81 (2007): 197–223.

The development of phased experimentation was part of a larger conversation about the design of clinical experiment, and participants from drug companies, university medical centers, and research hospitals also occupied important places in this conversation. See generally Marks, *The Progress of Experiment*. Industry leaders included Karl Beyer at Merck, Sharp and Dohme, and C. H. Ellis at Wellcome Laboratories. Among medical centers, Louis Katz at the Michael Reese Hospital in Chicago, and P. J. Huntingford at St. Thomas Hospital in London were active. Academic leaders included Thomas Chalmers and Louis Lasagna (then at Massachusetts General Hospital). None of these authors was explicit in conceptualizing phased experimentation, however.

[75]Some sense of the network comes from the circulation ("cc") lists in Hauser's May and June 1962 memoranda; Hauser, Hauser, "Proposed Revision of Regulation 130.3, first draft," May 24, 1962; Hauser to FDA Division Directors, "Proposed Revision of Investigational Drug Regulations," June 5, 1962; JHPP. The terms "rational," "orderly," and "comprehensive" are taken retrospectively from 1963 speeches that Kelsey and Sadusk gave to medical audiences.

The new vision of ordered medical experiment would surface in the draft IND rules of January 1963, where a new Form FD 1571 was presented. The tenth item of the form compelled a drug sponsor to convey "an outline of any phase or phases of the planned investigations." The form then listed three phases of trials.

> a. Clinical pharmacology. This is ordinarily divided into two phases: **Phase 1** starts when the new drug is first introduced into man—only animal and in vitro data are available—with the purpose of determining human toxicity, metabolism, absorption, elimination, and other pharmacological action, preferred route of administration and safe dosage range; **phase 2** covers the initial trials on a limited number of patients for specific disease control or prophylaxis purposes. A general outline of these phases shall be submitted, identifying the investigator or investigators, the hospitals or research facilities where the clinical pharmacology will be undertaken, any expert committees or panels to be utilized, the maximum number of subjects to be involved, and the estimated duration of these early phases of investigation....
>
> b. *Clinical trial*. This **phase 3** provides the assessment of the drug's safety and effectiveness and optimum dosage schedules in the diagnosis, treatment, or prophylaxis of groups of subjects involving a given disease or condition. A reasonable protocol is developed on the basis of the facts accumulated in the earlier phases, including completed and submitted animal studies. This phase is conducted by separate groups following the same protocol (with reasonable variations and alternatives permitted by the plan) to produce well-controlled clinical data.[76]

See Kelsey, "The Control of Investigational Drugs," presented to a meeting of the Mayo Clinic staff, December 4, 1963 (pp. 3–4 of this speech present the idea of learning within and between trials); "Use of Investigational Drugs in Hospitals under the New FDA Amendments," presented at the Catholic Hospital Association's 49th Annual Convention, June 24, 1964, New York City; Sadusk, "The Relationship of the Food and Drug Administration to the Practice of Medicine and the Aminopyrine-Dipyrone Problem," presented in a Symposium on Drug Therapy at the meetings of the Southern Medical Association, November 16, 1964, Memphis, TN; DF 505, RG 88, NA. In Sadusk's Memphis address he asserted FDA authorship of the phase definitions (p. 2). See also the William W. Goodrich Oral History, FDA Oral History Collection, NLM.

[76]FDA, "Investigational New Drug Regulations under the Kefauver-Harris Amendments of 1963," reprint from CFR—Part 130, Section 130.3, August 1963, 4. Emphasis added. The draft rules of January 1963 contain the first mention of phase 1, 2, and 3 trials in the history of federal regulation. Goodrich and the Bureau of Medicine rejected internal proposals for mandatory "phase IV" trials which would have accompanied the first marketing of the drug; Goodrich Oral History, NLM.

I have not been able to locate any document in which the three phases were clearly proposed by a single individual, though Hauser's draft legislation and notes come close. The authorship of phased experimentation appears to have been collaborative, with Hauser and Kelsey assuming crucial leadership roles. After the passage of the Kefauver-Harris Amendments, the final IND rules were edited and written by Goodrich, Assistant Commissioner J. Kenneth Kirk, and O. M. Kline. Kirk appears to have taken the lead, and in October 1962 he drafted "a memo to BM [Bureau of Medicine] requesting them to propose a set-up to review clinical investigation plans." M. D. Kinslow, "Memorandum of Meeting: Drug Amendments of 1962—Steps Needed

Nowhere in the Administration's regulations had any phase of experiment been designated as mandatory. Yet by establishing the IND form as the template for the normal and expected structure of pharmaceutical research—by describing what was stark and novel as "ordinary"—FDA officials had essentially compelled all firms and researchers to arrange their investigations according to sequential phases. Beyond this, mandatory completion of the IND form before clinical research would force sponsors to design their studies prospectively and to disclose the plan of experiment to the Administration, in particular Frances Kelsey and her Investigational New Drug Branch.

Projection of Conceptual Power: The 1963 Conference on New Regulations

In February 1963, the FDA convened an open public hearing on the draft IND rules. Here more than anywhere else, the internal identity and external presentation of pharmaceutical regulation were symbolically fused. Virtually every audience involved with the Administration—in Congress, in the pharmaceutical industry, in regulatory agencies around the globe, in academic medical centers, in general and specialty medical organizations, and in the press—was waiting for the rules. And here they would get their first public discussion of the terms of the new pharmaceutical world.

Over 1,000 people were in attendance, and the ballroom of a Washington hotel was packed. The meeting was billed by New Drug Branch Director Arthur Ruskin as an "open public forum to discuss how you and we can best operate" under the new amendments. Ruskin projected a common identity for the audience as "citizens in a democracy." Yet Ruskin's meeting had a decidedly undemocratic feel. The March 1963 meeting was not a roundtable, not a "discussion" or a "forum," but a question-and-answer period where FDA officials answered queries with authority and where the regulations on the table had the feeling of inevitability.

If 1950s observers and clients of the FDA doubted whether the agency's inspection and field arms of the FDA were projections of a unified regulatory ideology, they could no longer doubt it now. Yakowitz from the Bureau of Enforcement was there; Evans from manufacturing control was there; Kelsey was there, now heading the Investigational New Drug Branch of the Administration. The meeting was called to order by Arthur Ruskin, Acting Director of the Division of New Drugs in the Bureau of Medicine. Ruskin explained the new organization of the New Drug Division and the Bureau

for Implementation," October 11, 1962; FDA General Correspondence, 1963—051.155, B 3422-23, RG 88, NA. The three phases of experimentation surfaced in the Bureau of Medicine in the fall of 1962. See also Smith to Kirk, "Proposed Revision of Regulation 130.3(e)," February 25, 1963; FDA General Correspondence, 1963—051.155, B3422-23, RG 88, NA. Kelsey and Hauser were copied on this communication.

of Medicine; how enforcement, inspection, drug review, pharmacology, manufacturing controls evaluation, would all be pressed into the unified service of regulation premised upon the New Drug Application. Even as the projection of identity ran ahead of the administrative reality, it was formidable: the different divisions were projected as "on the same page," perhaps literally in the sense that "the various offices collaborated closely (under the leadership of the Bureau of Medicine) in writing the new regulations." Kelsey's appearance conveyed startling news to company officials—many of whom did not then know that she would be the primary federal regulator of clinical trials in the late 1960s. Yet it also projected a face of regulatory defiance. Was any company official or lawyer, however upset over the new rules, going to argue with Frances Oldham Kelsey on the propriety of regulations governing clinical experiment?[77]

This theme of procedural unification of state, science, and management was one rehearsed throughout the early 1960s by FDA officials—in Ruskin's 1963 address to the Pharmaceutical Manufacturers Association; in a Bureau of Medicine Program circular describing the orchestration of enforcement activities during a drug's investigational stage; in FDA communications with the Mayo Clinic and other medical research centers. Every dimension of government drug regulation—enforcement, manufacturing control, medical evaluation, the governance of investigational drugs, and new drug status branch—would now revolve about the IND-NDA process. The process of modern drug development was now established and demarcated administratively. It was segmented in a form that evinced vast and intricate procedural control of every feature of drug development, control housed institutionally and symbolically within the Division of New Drugs.[78]

In the February 1963 conference where this new vision was elaborated, George Larrick found himself in the odd and uncomfortable position of interlocutor. He quietly and perfunctorily took written questions from the audience and vocalized them to his Bureau and Division chiefs. It was clear that, in matters of pharmaceutical regulation at least, the Commissioner of Food and Drugs was no longer running or representing the Food and Drug Administration.

Arthur Ruskin promoted a different gatekeeper image, one more daunt-

[77]*Proceedings: FDA Conference on the Kefauver-Harris Drug Amendments and Proposed Regulations, February 15, 1963* (U.S. Department of Health Education and Welfare, Food and Drug Administration, Washington, DC, 1963. Hereafter cited as *Proceedings: FDA Conference*. It was evident from his prepared remarks that Ruskin in fact planned to describe a new division of regulatory labor. Ruskin, "New Drug Procedures," prepared for delivery, FDA Conference on Kefauver-Harris Amendments and Related Regulations, February 15, 1963; copy in DF 505, RG 88, NA.

[78]Ruskin, "The Current Reorganization and Functions of the Division of New Drugs," presented at the annual meeting of the American Pharmaceutical Manufacturers Association, March 21, 1963, Clearwater, FL; FDA, Program Circular 47A-9, Subject "Investigational New Drugs and Antibiotics," June 4, 1963; DF 505, RG 88, NA; John G. Mayne (CSTA), "Annual Report of the Committee on the Safety of Therapeutic Agents for the Year 1963," February 8, 1964, CSTA Records, MAYO.

ing than industry executives had seen even as recently as the late 1950s. He plainly stated the FDA's veto power over pharmaceutical development, and implicitly, over careers. "Experience and training of key personnel in charge of manufacturing and controls," he stated, "are to be included in the new drug applications." The Administration would simply reserve "the right to withhold approval of applications in which clearly unqualified people play important roles." The governance of new drug development had been leveraged into the regulation of scientific expertise.[79]

Firms, too, received a new identity in the regulations. Companies were no longer "manufacturers" but "sponsors"; the "sponsor" concept implied that a company was not a manufacturer of medicines until the FDA approved a new drug application for the product. The primary identity of the firm in this lens, moreover, was neither maker nor discoverer, but rather rhetorician. Ruskin and Kelsey voiced their implicit belief that the two processes of research and commercialization should be separated, with the science of drug development divorced thoroughly from the "business" of drug promotion. For many representatives of the industry, these were inseparable functions.

And finally, a vivid contrast arose between Frances Kelsey's general public image and her image as projected to industry and clinical researchers. In the projection of national journalists and homemakers' magazines, Kelsey was skeptical but quiet, sweet, a maternal protector. In her remarks to academic clinical investigators and industry officials—an audience-specific image projected sparingly but formidably to organized industry—she was dismissive, micromanaging, distrustful, a maternal disciplinarian. She regarded much of the industries' criticism of the law as unnecessary, groundless, and beyond this, even morally illegitimate.

> It is difficult to understand why any conscientious and experienced clinical investigator would object to supplying detailed reports of his work. It is to be presumed that he would keep such reports for the protection of his patient, and, it is assumed that as a scientist he would want the optimum benefits to come from his work.
>
> It is also somewhat surprising that objections should have been made to the provision that patients or persons used as controls, or their representatives be informed that investigational drugs are being used and that their consent be obtained before they serve as experimental or control subjects. These provisions are embodied in the Code of Ethics of the American Medical Association and have been upheld in civil courts.[80]

Kelsey concluded her remarks by saying that the pharmaceutical industry could use a broad lesson in clinical pharmacology and scientific drug evaluation. "Improved procedures" would come not from industry learning or adaptation, but from new federal statute and FDA-issued regulations. Before lamenting the added burden of the new rules, she cautioned, clinical

---

[79] *Proceedings: FDA Conference*, 5.
[80] Ibid., 11.

researchers and companies should revisit their own practices of drug development and appraisal, both of which lay in disrepair.

> Fears have been expressed that the additional requirements will discourage clinicians from testing drugs. However, it is acknowledged that the current status of drug evaluation leaves much to be desired. Much of this is due to the lack of adequately trained and experienced clinical investigators. It is hoped that the new requirements for improved testing procedures will give added stature to the field of drug testing and that recent steps taken to provide fellowships and training programs in clinical pharmacology will be accelerated.[81]

Among those in attendance at the February 1963 forum was Harold Upjohn, Clinical Director of the research arm of the Upjohn Company. Upjohn lamented the dearth of information presented, especially the noncommittal character of the agency's answers to questions about the regulations. And he came away with abiding fears about the regime to come. "What was said at the meeting was nothing new," Upjohn would write to Harvard pharmacologist Maxwell Finland later that month. "For the most part, the speaker simply said what the regulations were." Upjohn's notes portray not the "good cop" face of the Administration witnessed by the general public, but the "bad cop" face that alarmed pharmaceutical companies and clinical researchers. He saw "extremely bad" features of the regulations, whose "emphasis is far too great on safety" and whose provisions contained "a very real possibility of stifling clinical research in this country." And he envisaged the specter of asymmetric power possessed by the Administration, not only in authority but also in information. "I think it is intolerable that the FDA can force a drug company to stop testing a drug or for that matter remove a drug from market based on data they refuse to show the drug house."[82]

The conference of February 1963 and Harold Upjohn's worried reaction to it mark a transitional moment in the American and global history of pharmaceuticals. In a partial way, and for a time, the procedural and theoretical architecture of the Eisenhower-era Bureau of Medicine had come to political, legal, and scientific domination. The symbols and principles expressed in February 1963 would become sewn into the fabric of late-twentieth century medicine and pharmaceutical development: concepts of therapeutic efficacy as inseparable from safety; government oversight of clinical trials in every phase and moment (supervised by Kelsey herself); an insistence upon prospectively designed, randomized clinical trials with placebo arms; and, not least, the inevitability of the federal government's moral

---

[81] Ibid., 12.

[82] Harold L. Upjohn, M.D. (Clinical Director, Research, The Upjohn Company), to Finland, February 22, 1963; Box 2, F 24, MIF. It was a measure of Upjohn's frustration and of the political status of clinical pharmacology in 1963 when Upjohn concluded his letter by expressing his wish "that we can get together sometime to visit about the regulations and particularly these points. I personally am going to do everything I can to see that changes are made in these areas."

and social evaluation of clinical researchers and of drug sponsors. And just as new procedures and institutions became a cemented and familiar feature of the American economic, political, and scientific landscape, so too did the emotions accompanying them, emotions expressed at the conference of February 1963: conscious deference to the Administration and its top functionaries, anxiety of an all-powerful regulator, fearful anticipation of the government's next moves, private anger.

For the officials of a previous era—Ralph Smith, Jerry Holland, Barbara Moulton, Irvin Kerlan, Ralph Weilerstein, Arnold Lehman, Julius Hauser— their labor had come to an odd, ironic, and mostly anonymous fruition. For George Larrick, the 1963 hearing demonstrated an organizational momentum that had left him behind. For Frances Kelsey and her coterie, a regime was just beginning.

Digesting the New Regime

As the Investigational New Drug rules made their way to final print, clinical investigators and drug companies across the United States clearly perceived that the structure of drug development had been changed, and they identified the origin of these changes in the FDA. The IND rules effected many revisions of practice and procedure within clinical research centers, revisions that began before the Administration's rules were finalized. At the Mayo Clinic, the Board of Governors asked its staff to classify all ongoing drug trials into one of the three phases that had been defined by the FDA rules. Mayo officials then required any new trial to be classified as Phase 1, 2, or 3 and to be cleared by the Clinic's Committee on the Safety of Therapeutic Agents. Cancer researchers at Roswell Park Memorial Hospital in Buffalo adopted procedures for handling new chemotherapy drugs, and the Mayo Clinic followed them. The Clinic also began to centralize reporting from all of its research in a single Central Distributing Unit ("under supervision of Miss Nystrom at Desk R") that would store all drugs and keep all records relating to their storage, use, and administration.[83]

[83]Excerpt from Board of Governors meeting of January 21, 1965: "Doctor Faulconer reviewed the recommendations of the Committee on the Safety of Therapeutic Agents concerning receipt, custody, records and reporting related to investigational drugs. These recommendations have resulted from study of recently adopted Federal Drug Administration [sic] Regulations pertaining to investigational drug usage in hospitals. These Regulations divide such uses into phases as follows: Phase 1—First use of a drug in humans in this country; Phase 2—Clinical trial in a single series of patients; Phase 3—Clinical trial in multiple series of patients"; Minutes, CSTA, February 18, 1965; MAYO. Richard W. Hill, M.D., Chairman, CSTA, to Heads of Sections, Re "Procedure for New Drug Investigations," September 23, 1965. "Proposals for all drug investigation will be forwarded to the Committee on Safety of Therapeutic Agents in investigative studies involving Phase 1, Phase 2, and Phase 3 programs as defined by the Food and Drug Administration." John G. Mayne (CSTA), "Annual Report of the Committee on the Safety of Therapeutic Agents for the Year 1963," CSTA records, MAYO. "Similar procedures used for the control of investigational drugs at the Roswell Park Memorial Hospital

By late 1964, Frances Kelsey's office had created a separate trial registration form for each of the three phases. One version of Form FD 1571 was now required for Phase 1 trials, while different versions were necessary for Phase 2 and 3 trials, respectively. In addition, a new Form FD 1572 was created for qualification of investigators, while a Form FD 1573 was created for qualification of Phase 3 researchers. Research-oriented medical centers began to create their own trial registration forms to facilitate its compliance with federal regulations.[84] All the while that the AMA and pharmaceutical industry associations were disparaging the new rules and demanding revisions, the deference of top hospitals such as the Mayo Clinic and Roswell Park was blunting medical conservatives' criticism. Mayo leaders were especially anxious to please Kelsey, inviting her to visit the hospital in 1963 and preparing an elaborate plan for her visit. They would continue corresponding with her and courting her favor through the entire decade. When in July 1965 PMA President Austin Smith circulated a statement detailing the Association's reaction to the new rules, accompanied by a questionnaire, Mayo leadership tabled the documents and restricted their physicians from sending official protests to the FDA.[85]

The process of elaborating the three phases of experimentation and the FDA forms accompanying them was one taken up by Kelsey and Sadusk. They detailed their expectations in speeches and in a new circular issued by Kelsey's office. In her December 1963 speech to the Mayo Clinic staff, Kelsey assured her audience that medical researchers would have "considerable leeway" in the first two phases, including the ability to change route of administration so that, for instance, a drug that began Phase 1 trials as an oral agent could be tested by being given intravenously. In Phase 3, too, the agency would allow "reasonable variations" from protocol. Whatever flexibility lay in the new rules, however, could add to a sponsor's burden as well as subtract from it. Kelsey and Sadusk both remarked that animal studies

---

are under study by Dr. Moertel." The document appears at "Procedure for Handling of Cancer Chemotherapeutic Investigational Drugs," January 7, 1963, CSTA Records, MAYO.

[84] Kelsey, "Investigational Drug Branch: Intra-FDA Relationships," *FDLJ* 12 (Feb. 1966): 102–5. CSTA memorandum to Board of Governors, Mayo Clinic, December 17, 1964; MAYO. John G. Mayne (CSTA), "Annual Report of the Committee on the Safety of Therapeutic Agents for the Year 1963," February 8, 1964. "Kelsey... informed us by letter on December 30, 1963, that her office is now giving serious attention to preparing standard forms 1572 and 1573. Final modification of our own registration form will await development of the FDA forms 1572 and 1573 so that we can use a similar or identical form thereby considerably simplifying work of our own investigators."

[85] For invitations to Kelsey and plans, see Minutes, CSTA, July 25, 1963; September 26, 1963; October 10, 1963. The CSTA announced Kelsey's planned visit in November: "The Committee, most anxious to make Dr. Kelsey's two-day visit pleasant and memorable, discussed how best to acquaint her with the Clinic and also arrange for as many opportunities for members of the staff to discuss with her their problems in compliance with the new drug regulations"; Minutes, CSTA, November 21, 1963. For tabling of Austin Smith communication and restrictions on protest, see Minutes, CSTA, October 10, 1962, and July 29, 1965; MAYO.

would be expected to accompany Phase 2 human trials and would extend into Phase 3. The Bureau of Medicine's vision of experiment was that the first two phases would reveal clearly unsafe and inefficacious drugs and exclude them from further testing and the possibility of being marketed. In addition, the first two phases would set up the third, where "the route of administration and the formulation of the drug would be more or less standardized." This phase of "critical assessment" might, in the Bureau's vision, include thousands of patients as subjects. Holding the route of administration and formulation equal across trials would allow investigators and the agency to examine optimal dosage schedules. At the center of the Administration's vision of phased experiment was the idea that the eventual utilization of the drug would be honed through the scrutiny of Phase 3.[86]

Backing the Administration's power to define these trials and their sequence was the agency's formal authority to place a "clinical hold" upon experiments. The IND was important because it created a temporary exemption from the prohibition on interstate distribution of non-approved drugs. By revoking an IND exemption, the Bureau of Medicine ended the legality of testing. The operation of this authority was passive rather than active. There was no requirement for FDA approval of clinical trials before they could begin, but agency could intervene (in the person of the Commissioner) to place a "hold" on all studies. The reasons justifying such clinical holds were varied and functioned as a message for what the Administration expected of the investigational stage of drug development.

- Insufficient clinical data, including control data to evaluate the study's safety
- Information showing lack of safety or efficacy
- Inadequacy of the proposed plan of investigation
- Evidence of commercialization
- Inadequate presentation of animal safety data to the clinical researchers
- Failure to submit proper reports to the FDA
- Failure to report "serious side reactions or contraindications" to the FDA

By July 1964, nine INDs had been terminated by the Administration, of about 1,800 submitted. The fact that so few drug investigations were stopped was due in part to the small staff that Kelsey had for policing clinical trials, but it also gestured to the wide adherence to new rules by the vast majority of companies and researchers.[87]

---

[86]Bureau of Medicine, FDA, *Investigational Drug Circular* 1 (Feb. 20, 1964) (Washington, DC: FDA, 1964). Two other circulars were published in 1964. Kelsey, "The Control of Investigational Drugs," presented to a meeting of the Mayo Clinic staff, December 4, 1963 (pp. 3–4 of typescript); "Use of Investigational Drugs in Hospitals under the New FDA Amendments," presented at the Catholic Hospital Association's 49th Annual Convention, June 24, 1964, New York City; Sadusk, "The Relationship of the Food and Drug Administration to the Practice of Medicine and the Aminopyrine-Dipyrone Problem" (pp. 2–3 of typescript), presented in a Symposium on Drug Therapy at the meetings of the Southern Medical Association, November 16, 1964, Memphis, TN; DF 505, RG 88, NA.

[87]Kelsey, "Use of Investigational Drugs in Hospitals under the New FDA Amendments," 3.

An expanded regimen of clinical testing also allowed the Bureau of Medicine, especially Kelsey, to rein in investigators who lacked credibility. Kelsey's early decisions to terminate INDs were often contested, but they sent powerful signals to the research community about which practices and which *practitioners* would be regarded as substandard. The two most salient precedents were established in Kelsey's refusal to permit continued experimentation with the acronym-known drugs DMSO (dimethyl sulfoxide) and LSD (lysergic acid diethylamide). DMSO was the pet project of University of Oregon researcher Stanley Jacob. Jacob had teamed with the Crown Zellerbach Corporation in 1964 to begin clinical tests for DMSO for the treatment of arthritis. Kelsey and her colleagues greeted Jacob's IND with skepticism from the start. They saw no plausible pharmacological mechanism that would have supported DMSO's supposed curative properties. There were also safety problems. Animal studies demonstrated abnormal changes in vision, and over twenty cases of adverse vision experience associated with DMSO use had been reported to the agency. Perhaps most jarring, a woman in Ireland had recently died after three days of DMSO treatments for her sprained wrist. Jacob had also allegedly violated the 1963 rules on clinical experimentation and patient protection.[88]

Kelsey terminated Jacob's IND in November 1965, citing lack of basic evidence for the drug's safety and efficacy; she and other officials saw no basis for attributing any plausible clinical value to the drug. At the core of Kelsey's doubts about DMSO, moreover, lay the same sort of concerns that animated her skepticism of the Merrell Company's application for thalidomide in 1960. She questioned Jacob's credibility and his training, and she worried about Jacob's status as a patent holder for DMSO. Hence, she not only revoked approval of the drug's experimental status (Form FD 1571), she also revoked Jacob's status as an approved investigator (Form FD 1572). Commissioner George Larrick then terminated all human testing of DMSO by an administrative order.[89]

Jacob and his supporters fought back by attracting publicity to Kelsey's decision and securing congressional pressure for permission for continued testing and outright approval. Members of Congress began to demand action on the drug. At a New York Academy of Sciences symposium in March 1966, the evidence on eye damage from DMSO was questioned. Even as Kelsey and her outfit were cracking down on Jacob, newspapers and popular magazines had begun to warm to his therapy; in an April 1965 editorial, the *New York Times* called DMSO "the closest thing to a wonder drug

---

For Kelsey's understanding of the IND activation process as passive rather than one in which permitting was involved, see Kelsey to William A. Kaloss, M.D., Red Bank, NJ, January 21, 1966; F4, B1, FOK.

[88] Kelsey to Sadusk and Ralph G. Smith, January 27, 1966; F3, B1, FOK. Phillip W. Davis, "An Incipient 'Wonder Drug' Movement: DMSO and the Food and Drug Administration," *Social Problems* 32 (2) (Dec. 1984): 197–212. On the lack of mechanism, see "Controversial DMSO Drug 'Seems Useful' In Treating Psychoses, 2 Researchers Say," *WSJ*, March 17, 1966, 10.

[89] Larrick's order appears at *FR* 30 (228) (Nov. 19, 1965): 14639.

produced in the 1960s." These doubts and pressures eventually persuaded Kelsey's superiors. In 1966, Joseph Sadusk and Ralph Smith agreed to allow Jacob to participate in DMSO testing as long as he could find a reputable company to give him supplies for his studies. There was no proof that he had violated the 1938 Act, Sadusk and Smith reasoned, and Jacob was still a licensed physician with good standing in his state. In December 1966, the agency's administrative order was reversed. Long before the reversal became public, Kelsey shot off a long, sober memorandum to Sadusk and Smith. Their action would "violate the spirit of the Investigational Drug Regulations," she said, and would undermine the agency's reputation in several ways.

> I do not feel that the exclusion of Dr. Jacob as an investigator should require that he be first indicted and found guilty of having violated any of the regulations pertaining to the use of investigational drugs. The judgment that we can offer in the Investigational Drug Branch is that of a man's suitability, on the basis of training, experience, and demonstrated accomplishments, as an acceptable investigator. In this, of course, we are partly guided by recommendations furnished by the drug firms. We have plenty of information that suggests that many of these were not particularly impressed by Dr. Jacob's objectivity as a clinical investigator. I feel we have weakened our position with the sponsors by reaching an agreement with Dr. Jacob whereby we would approve his [status] as an investigator if he could find a sponsor willing to supply him with the drug.[90]

[90]For an example of congressional pressure, see the Administration's correspondence with Rep. Al Cederburg (R-MI); Cederburg to Larrick, September 28, 1965; Unnamed official [David] to Cederburg, October 6, 1965; Rankin to Cederburg, "Rough Draft," September 30, 1965; FOK, B1, F3. Other IND sponsors also pursued this channel of influence. In 1963, transplant researcher Thomas E. Starzl asked Kelsey for relief from the regulations for studies of antinomycin C, for reversal of transplant (homograph) rejection, but he simultaneously lobbied the Senate; Starzl to Senator Gordon Allott, June 26, 1963. Starzl's letter to Allott copied Kelsey and Donald Whitfield of the Harvard Medical School; Dr. Joseph Murray, head of the transplant team at Harvard Medical School, also personally appealed to Kelsey; FOK, B1, F2.

For the reversal, see FR 31 (248) (December 23, 1966): 16403-04. "DMSO— Promise and Danger," NYT, April 3, 1965, 28. "A Limited Wonder," Time, September 17, 1965; "Controversial DMSO Drug 'Seems Useful' in Treating Psychoses, 2 Researchers Say," WSJ, March 17, 1966, 10. Sadusk was adhering in part to a practice that he had established in the agency, namely, that physician licensure was a necessary and significant component of qualification for clinical investigation; Sadusk to Seymour Fisher (Division of Psychiatry, Boston University School of Medicine, Boston), January 21, 1966; FOK, B1, F4. The sufficiency of licensure for clinical investigation was never conclusively discussed or established in the 1960s. Kelsey and others wanted any physician to be accompanied by a trained clinical pharmacologist. Sadusk disagreed. The possible equivalence of physician license and investigator qualification would be discussed by the Modell Committee as well; Advisory Committee on Investigational Drugs, Summary of Proceedings, 13th Meeting, December 3, 1964, Washington; John Adriani Papers, NLM. At these meetings, Julius Hauser also saw an important reputational politics at work, but one that favored the FDA. "If the industry sponsor knows that its NDA's won't be approved if poor investigators are employed, the situation may solve itself," he reasoned. Administration officials sent precisely this message in numerous communications, implied and explicit. As the decade wore on, Sadusk would drift further away from the reform cohort of the Administration, and closer to the viewpoint of the organized pharmaceutical industry. He

Kelsey's lament reveals much of her thinking about the function and capacity of the Administration in overseeing pharmaceutical experiment. At first, it is clear that she intended her Investigational Drug Branch to serve as something of a moral and professional arbiter, to determine who was "suitable" and "acceptable" for drug research and who was not. This capacity, she felt, lay squarely within her talents and training as a lifelong pharmacologist with extensive experience in both animal and clinical settings. In addition, Kelsey's worry about "position" with respect to sponsors displayed her concern for two faces of her Bureau's reputation. The Bureau's professional judgments would be seen as superfluous by reputable companies, she felt, if someone so ill-equipped as Jacob were allowed to conduct drug studies. Furthermore, permission for Jacob could well establish a debilitating precedent. Other companies might more eagerly challenge FDA skepticism about their clinical investigators if they could point to Jacob as someone whom the agency had qualified. In Kelsey's ultimate worry, the Bureau of Medicine would command neither esteem nor fear.[91]

Among the few other drugs whose IND exemptions were terminated or withdrawn under pressure, there were some remarkable features. Like DMSO, the Bureau's termination of clinical studies with Krebiozen received tremendous publicity but also sent a signal to American markets and research communities that the days of quack medicine for prescription drug development were over. Yet outside of DMSO and Krebiozen, most of the other terminations did not include "easy targets." Instead, some of the world's most reputable drug firms saw their experiments halted. European megalith Geigy had developed a new tranquilizer and antidepressant in the early 1960s, but its early clinical trials were halted when Kelsey perceived too little protection for pregnant women and the unborn fetus. Upjohn had been developing an ophthalmic ointment but stopped clinical trials when severe eye irritation developed in dogs treated with the product, killing one of them, in an ongoing animal study. The company reapplied for an IND for smaller doses, but Kelsey and her colleagues held it from approval. Other companies whose INDs were targeted for termination included Ortho and Johnson and Johnson.[92]

---

would be invited to resign his position by Commissioner James Goddard in 1966. Kelsey's response appears in Kelsey to Sadusk and Ralph G. Smith, January 27, 1966; F3, B1, FOK.

[91]Permitting Jacob to test DMSO on a single patient, Kelsey worried, would eventually "permit any person, with a license in the healing arts in the State in which he resides, to use a drug, such as Krebiozen, for which we think any evidence of safety or effectiveness has been gained fraudulently." Kelsey to Sadusk and Smith, January 27, 1966; F3, B1, FOK. For a detailed review of the DMSO controversy, see Davis, "An Incipient 'Wonder Drug' Movement."

[92]On Geigy's tranquilizer G-38072 (IND 054), see W. D'Aguanno (Division of Pharmacology) to Kelsey, July 9, 1963. D'Aguanno summarized that "The reports of animal investigations consist of a poorly prepared summary. The acute studies should be expanded to include non-rodent species." Yet chief among the reasons for termination was "the fact that the protocol for clinical studies states that only females between the ages of 17–59 will be used in the study and that no reproduction studies have been performed"; F "Fountain Hearings," B11, FOK. On Upjohn's ophthalmic ointment (IND 227), see Alan B. Varley (Upjohn Company), to

Kelsey's management of the Investigational Drug Branch expressed a subtle politics of reputation. Her concerns for the status and prominence of her Branch, and the larger Bureau of Medicine, were shared by Smith, Julius Hauser, and Goodrich. In part to assuage the concerns of congressional audiences, particularly Lawrence Fountain's House Committee, and in part to give scientific prominence to her group, Kelsey elevated the status of pharmacologists and chemists in the Investigational New Drug Branch. Her May 1965 rules stipulated that, in reviewing an IND, any licensed physician in the Branch would have to take account of any recommendations made by pharmacologists or chemists and would have to justify any disagreements with these assessments in a written memo to Kelsey herself. She also commenced a series of investigations and inspections of different companies and clinical research centers, a series of inquiries overseen by her Branch. Kelsey often enlisted the services of esteemed academic physicians (including members of the Modell Committee on Investigational Drugs) in these inspections. Along with Goodrich and Julius Hauser, she wanted to project the presence and authority of the Investigational New Drug Branch while avoiding a heavy-handed stance that might provoke complaints of interference from otherwise supportive research communities.[93]

When it came to the exercise of its ultimate authority, Kelsey's group terminated few INDs but raised concerns about many, prompting numerous complaints from industry but also sprints toward compliance. By February 1965, the Branch had received about 2,200 Notices of Claimed Investigational Exemptions for a New Drug. Only twelve of these had been revoked. Yet the reach of the Investigational New Drug Branch was far greater than

---

Kelsey, September 11, 1963; F. N. Narzulli (Division of Pharmacology) to Kelsey, July 17, 1963; Amos E. Light (Division of Toxicological Evaluation) to Kelsey, Subject: "IND 227 – Supplemental Data dated May 22, 1964," September 3, 1964; F "Fountain Hearings, B11, FOK. For a list and discussion of INDs targeted for termination, see Memorandum from E. I. Goldenthal (Division of Toxicological Evaluation/Drug Review Branch) to Kelsey, "Adverse Comments—INDs," September 28, 1964; F "Fountain Hearings," B11, FOK.

[93]In a 1965 memorandum Kelsey stated that "It is important that for every IND the recommendations of the reviewing chemist and pharmacologist be taken into consideration by the medical officer." In the officer's "summary he can indicate whether he has followed the suggestions offered and if he does not propose to do so, he should indicate the reasons for his decision." Kelsey, "Memorandum to Medical Officers and Chemists, Investigational Drug Branch," "Subject: IND Review Guidelines," May 25, 1965; F "Fountain Hearings," B11, FOK. Kelsey's missive was a response to Memorandum from W. B. Rankin (Assistant Commissioner for Planning), to Bureau of Medicine, "Subject: Hearings on Drug Safety before the Fountain Subcommittee, May 4, 1965," May 13, 1965; F "Fountain Hearings," B11, FOK.

The involvement of the Modell Committee in Investigational Drug Branch inspections worried Modell himself. He expressed concern that its "members may be regarded as 'hatchet men' by disgruntled sponsors." Julius Hauser (also a member of the Modell Committee) responded with the idea that inspections include "a specific outside expert," as "a sort of ad hoc committee" for each inspection. "That way," Hauser reasoned, "no particular group would receive a bad reputation." Advisory Committee on Investigational Drugs, Summary of Proceedings, 14th Meeting, January 14, 1965; John Adriani Papers, NLM.

the small number of revocations might suggest. Merely by pointing to possible problems with a study, Kelsey's unit induced the abandonment of hundreds of questionable drug projects. Somewhat over 10 percent of INDs—at least 250, in the first two years after the IND rules—had been discontinued by sponsors, usually after Kelsey's group had notified the sponsor that preclinical data were inadequate to assess the safety of the proposed human studies. Hundreds of others had been substantially modified for compliance. Here the second face of power and the agency's fearsome reputation worked hand in hand. If Kelsey was raising doubts about the project as Phase 1 trials were just beginning, firms would reason, it was unlikely that the drug would ever gain approval even if she did not revoke the IND. In addition, Kelsey was making the job of the Bureau of Medicine easier, as these dubious projects never saw the light of a new drug application.[94]

For their part, drug company officials assumed an indistinct political carriage toward the IND regulations and toward Kelsey herself. Privately, they were often infuriated by the ambiguity that connected Kelsey's public statements and her individual decisions and communications to specific companies. Yet companies rarely challenged Kelsey openly. Instead, they chose to direct their complaints anonymously through safe channels such as the Modell Committee or the Pharmaceutical Manufacturers Association. Company officials exhibited what J. K. Weston of Burroughs-Wellcome called "a general reluctance in industry to argue with FDA because of 'fear of reprisals and arbitrary delays.' There is a feeling of mutual distrust and little has been done to dispel this." The relationship between the Bureau of Medicine and pharmaceutical companies was one of mutual fear. Kelsey, Hauser, and Goodich, like many FDA officials, feared that overactive application of the new law and regulations would infuriate companies and general practitioners and undermine the very political legitimacy that lay beneath the agency's powers. Firms feared that too much protest about the FDA's decisions on a particular drug would convey a lack of organizational credibility and possibly an underlying problem in the drug they were sponsoring. This equilibrium of fear produced currents of ambiguous communication. Whereas Kelsey's organization wanted specificity and sponsors wanted particular guidance, communication tended toward generalities.[95]

[94]Kelsey, "Comments," *FDLJ* 20 (Feb. 1965): 86. The pattern whereby Kelsey's group could induce termination of clinical studies by the sponsor appears to have been a common one. In February 1964, Kelsey would remark that whereas only five or six INDs had been "subject to outright termination proceedings... a great number of letters and calls have gone out objecting to parts of investigations." Advisory Committee on Investigational Drugs, Summary of Proceedings, 7th Meeting, February 27, 1964; John Adriani Papers, NLM. For a simplified mathematical treatment of how regulators such as the FDA can induce product abandonment well before submission and thereby establish a more favorable "agenda" of drugs that are later reviewed, see Carpenter and Ting, "Regulatory Errors with Endogenous Agendas."

[95]Advisory Committee on Investigational Drugs, Summary of Proceedings, 7th Meeting, February 27, 1964; John Adriani Papers, NLM.

For the more strident drug researchers of the time, these patterns of ambiguity were intolerable. Pharmacologist Carl Pfeiffer directly expressed some of the frustrations experienced by pharmaceutical sponsors at the inaugural meeting of the American College of Clinical Pharmacology and Chemotherapy in October 1964. "At the very least," Pfeiffer intoned, the FDA "has been remiss in not clarifying the interpretation it will choose to place on the law.... Until now, its flabby practice has been to avoid committing itself to any stand while always maintaining the possibility of saying 'nay.' This refusal often comes in serial form, so that an IND may have to be submitted in as many as five revisions only to be rejected each time by a new reviewer. These dilatory tactics may safeguard them from criticism by anyone who is interested only in status quo, as is typically true of bureaucrats."[96]

The Legacy of Regulated and Phased Experiment

In a way that has eluded perception, the FDA's 1963 rules and their implementation by Frances Kelsey's outfit would establish the accepted structure of medical experiment in the late twentieth century. Before 1960, there are no references to phased trials in the American and European medical literature, and there is no reference to a "Phase 3" study in Western medical literature before 1964. In the early 1960s, reports of "Phase 1" and "Phase 2" experiments appear haltingly, then rapidly near the end of the decade (table 4.2). What is more, American researchers and doctors began to reflect systematically on the relationship between earlier phases and later phases. They published theoretical reflections and surveys of practice, articles that conveyed the normal, appropriate, and efficient design of trial phases as well as transitions from one phase to another. The three-phased system of experiments begun in the 1970s appears as a normal course in the introductions to American pharmacology textbooks. In the 1960s and 1970s, firms and hospitals hired clinical pharmacologists by the hundreds in order to oversee these sequences of experiments, or to consult for them. In the 1980s and 1990s, statisticians and engineers began to design computer software to inform decisions about when to end one phase of trials and commence another.[97]

---

[96]Carl C. Pfeiffer, "Problems in Drug Development as they Relate to the Clinical Investigator," *Journal of New Drugs* (Nov.–Dec. 1964): 299–305. Presented at a symposium on "Problems in the Development of New Drugs" at the First Annual Meeting of the American College of Clinical Pharmacology and Chemotherapy, New York City, October 29–30, 1964.

[97]Kenneth L. Melmon and Howard F. Morelli, eds., *Clinical Pharmacology: Basic Principles in Therapeutics*, 2nd ed. (New York: Macmillan, 1978), chap. 1. John Whitehead, *The Design and Analysis of Sequential Clinical Trials* (Chichester, Horwood, NY: Halsted Press, 1983); P. C. O'Brien and T. R. Fleming, "A Multiple Testing Procedure for Clinical Trials," *Biometrics* 35 (1979): 549–56. For a summary review, see Whitehead, "Stopping Clinical Trials by Design," *NRDD* 3 (Nov. 2004): 973–7. In recent years, two of the representative statistics packages for clinical trial design are Cytel's EaSt software and the SeqTrial module in the S-Plus programming language. For representative statistical software, see Cytel Software Corporation, *EaSt: A Software Package for the Design and Interim Monitoring of Group Sequential Clinical Trials* (Cambridge, MA: Cytel, 2000); Mathsoft, Incorporated, *S-Plus SeqTrial* (Seattle: Mathsoft, 2000); both of these programs have been succeeded by more advanced versions.

TABLE 4.2.
References to Phased Clinical Studies in Western Medical Literature,
1950–1980

Year	Phase I	Phase II	Phase III	Total
1950–1954	0	0	0	0
1955–1959	0	0	0	0
1960	0	1	0	1
1961	0	0	0	0
1962	5	2	0	7
1963	3	0	0	3
1964	6	8	0	14
1965	7	0	1	8
1966	0	0	0	0
1967	3	0	0	3
1968	4	2	1	7
1969	2	2	0	4
1970	4	4	0	8
1971	7	2	0	9
1972	11	11	0	22
1973	17	6	1	24
1974	12	11	2	25
1975	25	30	6	61
1980	82	120	13	215

Searches conducted in PubMed [http://www.ncbi.nlm.nih.gov/sites/entrez] under Arabic and Roman numerals for the three different phases. For example, for phase I trials between 1971 and 1975, the following two searches were conducted:

(1) phase 1 [Title/Abstract] AND ("1971"[PDAT] : "1975"[PDAT]) and
(2) phase I [Title/Abstract] AND ("1971"[PDAT] : "1975"[PDAT]).

From the list of articles returned by these searches, articles referring to animal trials or articles with primary reference to phasic concepts in bacteriology, immunology and cardiology were all dropped from the count. Counts were then checked for duplicates, such that each title was counted only once. Note that this aggregation (1) is not an enumeration of trials completed or ongoing in a given year, and (2) provides only those articles where phasic concepts were cited in the title or abstract.

The number of drugs, clinical trials, hospitals, companies, and employees affected by this transformation is immense and probably beyond reliable calculation. In the early 1960s, even as the pace of clinical development was slowing, Kelsey's IND Branch received over 1,000 notices of claimed investigational exemption per year. Each of these documents included a detailed plan for phased studies. Each of these plans, in turn, implemented the

Administration's definition of experiment. Each of the forms represented, moreover, at least one clinical trial (often a dozen or more) ordered upon concepts, assumptions, and premises that had been thoroughly shaped by the FDA. Since the 1960s, with the expansion of the global pharmaceutical economy, the activity of commencing experiments through IND forms has taken on immense proportions; from 1986 to 2006, the Administration's drug reviewing division received 35,700 separate exemption claims.[98]

The enormity of pharmaceutical experiment in the late twentieth century implies that miniature patterns of adaptation and deference to the Administration were played out on a vast, global scale. The ambiguity that motivated Carl Pfeiffer's lament, the fear of the agency expressed by Burroughs-Wellcome official J. K. Weston (and the many other fears unspoken), the worried compliance that clinical researchers and company employees displayed toward the FDA—these emotions and interactions were probably repeated tens of thousands of times in the United States alone over the past half-century.

In American and global financial markets, phased experimentation now organizes the disclosure of information used in pharmaceutical company valuations. The beginning and ending of a clinical trial phase has become a temporal pivot for movements in financial asset prices. The long saga of drug development is partitioned by FDA concepts into distinct phases, and the transitions between these phases mark the largest movements in stock values. This pattern is heightened in the United States by virtue of a twin institutional combination: the patent expiration system and the lack of government price controls on pharmaceutical products. Since drug companies gain far greater revenue from patented drugs than from drugs whose patents have expired—and the revenue is much greater in the United States where drug prices are not constrained—the valuation of a publicly traded drug company depends heavily upon its pipeline of patented but yet-to-be-marketed treatments. Unexpected changes in clinical trial results can induce tremendous swings in company-wide stock prices. When the findings are surprisingly bad ones, their announcement can erase individual and organizational fortunes within minutes. So heavily do investors cling to the structure of phased experimentation for their news that it has become customary for companies to publicize results from each phase of experiment well before they are published in a medical or scientific journal. In the past twenty years, the *Wall Street Journal* has published over 1,300 original stories covering phased trial results. Financial papers, wire services, cable news television channels, and other media organizations have likely published tens of thousands more.[99]

---

[98]Kelsey, "Comments," *FDLJ* 20 (Feb. 1965) 86. FDA/CDER, "INDs Received, Calendar Years 1986–2006" (Rockville: FDA, 2006).

[99]In the 1980s, the *Wall Street Journal* and other financially oriented newspapers began running front-page stories for Phase 1 clinical trials. An early story on tumor necrosis factor (TNF) appears in Marilyn Chase, "Biotech Battle: Newest Cancer Drug Gets Favorable Results in

Pharmaceutical and biotechnology companies also rely upon venture capital financing for their early existence, and a three-phase system of experiment has come to define the basic structure of companies' legal contracts with equity firms and other investors. Early biotechnology companies such as Genentech were crucial in establishing these patterns, for they were experimenting with technologies to which stable expectations about efficacy and profitability were nearly impossible to assign. Struggling to secure funding, Genentech and its investors struck upon contractual "benchmarks." By reaching intermediate goals in the development and approval process, Genentech would trigger the flow of cash from its investors. A high fraction of these benchmarks were premised upon successful initiation or completion of a clinical phase—usually the initiation and completion of Phases 2 and 3— or regulatory events such as NDA filing or approval. For investors, the benchmarks allowed for the incremental and evidence-based bearing of risk. For company scientists, these benchmarks defined their living. As one Genentech scientist later recalled, "Each time we reached a benchmark, we would get more money. Of course, that was our salaries."[100]

The three-phase system of human experiment has also diffused to other nations. National regulators in Europe adopted a three-phase system with few changes from its legacy in the United States. In the 1990s, the European Union began to harmonize clinical development across European member nations, the effect being to cement phased experimentation throughout the continent. The Union's Directive on Good Clinical Practice (Directive 65/65/EEC) prescribes "phase 1 trials in normal healthy subjects, phase 2 dose ranging efficacy trials in subjects expected to derive medicinal benefit through

---

Early Tests in Japan—Three U.S. Firms Plan Trials With TNF, and the Race To Market It Has Begun—A New Ally for Interferon?" *WSJ*, June 19, 1985, A1. By contrast, *Journal* reporters habitually explained phased trials in very simple terms in the 1960s, if they referred to them at all; "Merck May Face Charges on Time It Took To Say Birth Drug Caused Cancer in Dogs," *WSJ*, March 11, 1966, 6. For an example where a single clinical trial result induced a 42 percent single-day drop in a company's share price, see Geeta Anand, "Burden of Proof: Cancer Drug Fails, So Maker Tries New Pitch; Biotechs Challenge FDA Approval Process; Mr. Creel's Tumor," *WSJ*, August 2, 2007, A1. SEC rules now require disclosure of clinical trial results for publicly traded companies.

[100]As former Genentech chief financial officer Fred A. Middleton would later describe the contracts, "Typically, there are some research benchmarks: product yield, the amount of protein per milliliter of fermentation broth, percentages of the cell that has the protein you want, making the first gram or first ten milligrams of a pure product, delivering to them the protocol for manufacturing a batch of this material, filing an IND, getting permission from the FDA to start a Phase II clinical trial, getting human results from a Phase II clinical trial that are positive, starting a Phase III clinical trial, getting data from the Phase III trial that's statistically significant, filing an NDA, getting FDA approval. Everything I told you there is a basis for a benchmark, and all of those benchmarks were used by Genentech in various of its contracts. The partner will argue for making the benchmark payments bigger and bigger in the later years when there's more certainty and less risk on their part." Sally Hughes, interview with Fred A. Middleton. On salaries, see Hughes, Interview with Daniel G. Yansura. In Genentech Oral History Series (October 2002), Regional Oral History Office, The Bancroft Library, University of California, Berkeley.

large efficacy and safety phase 3 trials." At the end of these trials there stands an administrative culmination quite similar to the New Drug Application of the United States—the Marketing Authorization Application (MAA).[101]

In Japan, national pharmaceutical regulators in the Ministry for Health and Welfare have both resisted and copied the conceptual structure established by the FDA. Whereas the FDA and European agencies have usually required two Phase 3 clinical trials showing efficacy for drug approval, Japanese authorities have usually required only one "pivotal" trial of the randomized, controlled sort in the third phase. In other ways, regulators in Japan have imposed more stringent requirements upon the phases. Whereas American and European authorities require sponsors to demonstrate superiority of their drug to placebo in the third phase, Japanese regulators have often demanded that the control arm contain not a placebo but an actively used therapy. Hence, in Japan efficacy judgments are explicitly comparative across drugs. While Japanese requirements placed upon the third phase are different, however, the structure and meaning of the phases displays enduring similarities to that of the 1963 FDA model. In governing clinical trials, the Ministry of Health has implemented "Good Clinical Practices" whose title and content match the guidance issued by the FDA in the 1970s and 1980s.[102]

In the arrival of partitioned experiment, the different facets of regulatory power have overlapped and interacted. Gatekeeping and conceptual power are demonstrated in the Administration's capacity to fashion the precise structure and content of the submissions it receives. Gatekeeping power also shows in the agency's ability to prevent many submissions from appearing in the first place, mainly by sponsors' abandonment of drugs. These abandonment decisions are less visible, in part because they are induced through the Administration's powers. Supporting this gatekeeping power are the formal authorities of directive power that the Administration retained from the 1962 Amendments (and which were extended and legitimated in rulemak-

---

[101] "Directive of the European Parliament and the Council on the approximation of the laws, regulations and administrative provisions of the Member States relating to implementation of good clinical practice in the conduct of clinical trials on medicinal products for human use," *Official Journal of the European Communities*, May 1, 2001 (Brussels: European Commission, 2001). P. Mermet-Bouvier and F. de Cremers, "Clinical Trial Initiation in Europe: Current Status," *Regulatory Affairs Journal* (July 2002): 571–8. International Committee on Harmonization "Tripartite Guideline for Good Clinical Practice," ICH E6 CPMP/ICH/135/95/ Step 5, July 1996. K. Hill, "The European Union Directive on Good Clinical Practice in Clinical Trials: Implications for Future Research," in Richard A. Guarino, ed., *New Drug Approval Process: Accelerating Global Registrations* (New York: Marcel Dekker, 2004).

[102] A. Kouseishou, *A Guideline for the Statistical Analysis of Clinical Trials* (Tokyo: Japanese Ministry of Public Health, 1992) [in Japanese]; Chihiro Hirotsu and Ludwig A. Hothorn, "Impact of the ICH E9 Guideline Statistical Principles for Clinical Trials on the Conduct of Clinical Trials in Japan," *Drug Information Journal* (2003); "FDA-Style Agency for Japan," *Nature Biotechnology* 17 (Jan. 1999): 7. Ministry of Health and Welfare, "Approval and Licensing System for Drugs, Quasi-Drugs and Cosmetics," *Annual Report on Health and Welfare* 1999 (Tokyo, Ministry of Health and Welfare, 1999). The 1997 Food and Drug Administration Modernization Act (FDAMA) changed the federal requirement to one Phase 3 trial.

ing and court decisions), and the conceptual power that engendered the consensual and often automatic adoption of terms and procedures that were initially sketched and elaborated by the Administration itself. As the directive, gatekeeping and conceptual facets of regulatory power sustain one another, they are in turn shaped and supported by organizational image. The three-phase structure of research has endured as a "natural" and "rational" mode of drug development in great measure because Frances Kelsey, Ralph Smith, and other Administration officials spoke with esteem and authority on the subject. The collective decisions of firms to cleave tightly to FDA regulations, and to abandon thousands of their drug projects at the slightest hint of skepticism from the agency, flows from the fearsome side of the agency's reputation. The stability of pharmaceutical gatekeeping in federal law—despite continued attacks from industry, organized medicine, and libertarians—rests upon the robustness of the agency's image as protector of a citizenry.

. . .

The evolution of regulatory power at the Food and Drug Administration is marked by contingency, by dispute, and by limits. The basic authority of veto—the Administration's pre-market review procedure—was created in the 1938 Food, Drug and Cosmetic Act, but its expanse was limited. In most respects the burden of action remained upon the FDA and not with applicants for drug approval. A default clause in the 1938 law permitted marketing for any drug that the FDA had not reviewed within sixty days of receiving the company's application. Only the pharmacologic revolution of the 1950s FDA—led by officials like Ralph Smith, Albert "Jerry" Holland, William Kessenich, Barbara Moulton, Irvin Kerlan, William Goodrich, and Julius Hauser—would bring weight and meaning to the formal capacity of the 1938 Act. And as Frances Kelsey remarked to her Kansas City audience in 1963, many of the ideals and practices of the Ralph Smith era lacked textual and legal expression until the 1962 Kefauver-Harris Amendments and the 1963 Investigational New Drug rules.

From the time of Kelsey's speech to the American Public Health Association in 1963, it would take another two decades for her agency's powers to stabilize. No part of this process was foreordained, and contestation suffused every part of it. In the 1962 statute, the 1963 rules and other regulations, and in the legitimation of FDA procedures in the 1960s and 1970s, the fortification of American regulatory power over pharmaceuticals depended upon the assent of pivotal cultural and political actors in the United States and the world. It depended upon the continued deference of the American federal judiciary to the Administration, and it depended upon bipartisan agreement within Congress on the agency's basic legitimacy and authority. It depended upon particular FDA actions, not only those aimed at expanding powers but those cognizant of battles better left unfought and of administrative expressions of grace and good will. Most important, the cementing of power depended crucially upon organizational legitimacy.

Reputation and Power Institutionalized: Scientific Networks, Congressional Hearings, and Judicial Affirmation, 1963–1986

> The women in this country, and the women in Great Britain,
> and in Scandinavia, and in Australia, and in South America,
> are consuming oral contraceptive medications in the belief
> that they are considered safe by the American Food and Drug
> Administration and for no other reason, because they have
> no other way to assess the safety of this medication.
>
> —Dr. Victor Wynn, on NBC News, 1970

> There are no villains in the FDA, only victims
> of inadequate public support.
>
> —Cornell pharmacologist Walter Modell, 1967[1]

IN THE quarter-century following the thalidomide crisis, reputation and power in American pharmaceutical regulation slowly became institutionalized. By the 1980s, the politics of reputation and the patterns of government power had become somewhat predictable, though not entirely so. For nearly every debate about drug regulation, a set of audiences arose and aligned upon the theme of safety and consumer protection, while another set of audiences emerged on the theme of research, innovation, and the "drug lag." The politics of reputation became predictable in the minimal sense that voices surfaced that would stably characterize and inform much of the debate. These voices included Sidney Wolfe, Morton Mintz, and Democratic congressional committee chairmen in one nexus, and William Wardell, Louis Lasagna, and the *Wall Street Journal* editorial page in another. In part, institutionalization occurred because different audiences and voices were slowly

---

[1] Wynn statement in Elizabeth Siegel Watkins, *On the Pill: A Social History of Oral Contraceptives, 1950–1970* (Baltimore: Johns Hopkins University Press, 1998), 112. Modell, "Editorial: An End to the Means; FDA papers III," *CP&T* 9 (6) (Nov.–Dec. 1968): 710.

embedded into organizational homes—House and Senate committees, pharmacology journals, the American Enterprise Institute, Ralph Nader's Public Citizen group, the Center for the Study of Drug Development (first at the University of Rochester), and major national newspapers.

Institutionalization brought relative stability and predictability, but not the absence of contest. The Administration's activity in drug regulation came under attack from numerous quarters. Moreover, reputation evolved not only as public spectacle but also as a networked phenomenon, with various debates raging in correspondence networks among physicians and pharmacologists, in medical publications, in financial and trade journals, and in the reports and discussions of congressional committees and watchdog agencies and groups. The powerful symbols of thalidomide and Frances Kelsey were distilled and embedded in common memory even as Kelsey herself faded into public obscurity. The criticisms reminded the different audiences of the Administration's possibilities. Every expression of censure rehearsed something that was known or widely believed about the FDA—that it could protect public health, but was not doing so, or that its keen scientific scrutiny was being carried too far, overburdening clinical researchers and drug companies—and in so doing, every lament reproduced and reinforced those facts. For this reason, among others, criticism of the FDA more than coincided with a period of high visibility and public trust. A surfeit of criticism may have strengthened an organizational image.

Regulatory power was also transformed and institutionalized. Directive, gatekeeping, and conceptual powers were challenged by political organizations and by new alliances between American business and American medicine. Yet the relative quietude of activity betrays some vast transformations, not least the elaboration of standards of experiment ("adequate and well-controlled investigations") and the massive social intervention undertaken in the Drug Efficacy Study Initiative, both legitimated in the Supreme Court's *Hynson* decision of 1973. Corporate challenges to all three facets of regulatory power failed in the courts, in Congress, and in public opinion. When the Administration was observed to fail, the most common explanation (one popular among its supporters and detractors, both Sidney Wolfe and Walter Modell) was that it was underequipped. In a period of challenge, much was cemented. The expansion of reputation and power in the early 1960s became normal, as authority was converted into patterns of protocol, expectation, and practice, and as everyday life in the modern pharmaceutical world was restructured.

THE CONTOURS OF A REPUTATION

The reputation of the U.S. Food and Drug Administration in the late twentieth century was manifold. The agency was known, admired, and despised for many different properties: expertise, puffery, vigilance, caution and "overcaution," deliberation, plodding. There were hundreds, perhaps thousands of competing claims made by and about the organization, by different members of the Administration, by different clients of the agency, and by different tribunals in the U.S. Congress, in medical and scientific associations, and in mass media outlets. Each of these claims carried a partial or potential truth. Occasionally, the various potentialities came together and solidified into a common understanding, if only for a time. One claim about the FDA would concatenate with another, would be echoed by a third, contested by a fourth, appropriated by a fifth, and so on, until the train of repetition rendered an image or concept so familiar as to elude conscious notice. In such a pattern of political echo and social reverberation did the public myth of Frances Kelsey and terms like "gold standard" and "guardian of health" take shape. One crystallization often re-expressed features of an earlier form, as when libertarian critics of the Administration reoriented its reputation for caution and deliberation, combined it with resurgent anti-government ideology, and created a new discourse centered upon "the drug lag." In its embedded assumption that the Administration displayed patterns of caution and stringency, the "drug lag" debate actually cemented some positive features of the FDA's reputation even as it reframed them in a negative light.

In retrospect, it is possible to detect a deep irony in the FDA's reputation of the late twentieth century. The Administration stood as one of the world's most admired public organizations—with surprisingly high name recognition and approval in national surveys, admiration and emulation from dozens of foreign governments and hundreds of scientific communities, and deference from pharmaceutical and biomedical companies. Yet, along with this aggregate pattern of acclaim came consistent lament from scientific, business and, most powerfully, congressional audiences. In these and other venues, America's pharmaceutical regulator was just as often assailed as praised. Notable committees in Congress—particularly in the Senate, chaired by luminaries like Nelson, Kennedy, Fountain, even Kefauver himself—repeatedly held excoriating hearings during the very decades that the FDA's power and reputation were at their zenith, in 1962, 1963, 1967, 1970, 1972, 1974, 1975, 1976, 1977, 1978, and 1979. The American Medical Association and other professional societies loudly rehearsed their opposition to federal efficacy standards, while business and libertarian groups located fresh ammunition and allies with which to wage new battles against the federal government's most powerful regulatory agency. In medical and pharmacological circles, the Administration had by the early 1970s alienated some of its earlier champions, most notably pharmacologists Walter Modell and Louis Lasagna.

How, then, did the Administration's image weather this acrimony? In part it was the vividness of the original images and memories from the thalidomide tragedy, and the way that they evoked core fears of American and world citizens confronting the risks of new technologies. The legacy of thalidomide was a powerful one, and every time a new drug safety issue arose, the memory of the drug and its disfigured victims was evoked. These fears often left citizens in a state of governmental embrace, one that metaphorically echoed the world described by English political theorist Thomas Hobbes in his *Leviathan*, the state whose citizens' allegiance was founded in part upon their horrified flight from a brutal and atomistic "state of Nature."[2]

In part, however, the Administration's reputation persisted because of the acrimony itself. The ceaseless contestation of the organization's power and its image yielded not an abiding uncertainty about the Administration, but instead a persistence of the metaphors representing it. The prospect of a vigorous and independent "protectorate" was made possible, in part, because politicians, consumer safety advocates, and even some insiders nagged the FDA incessantly and complained publicly of "industry bias" commingled with regulatory negligence. The political reality of a scientifically deliberate body of medical specialists was constructed in part through the laments of pharmaceutical firms and libertarians despairing of "overcaution" and the wrong kind of "conservatism." The toughness of the agency's police functions and the stringency of its review practices was amplified, perhaps unintentionally, by physicians and specialists who complained weekly of interference in the holy and autonomous practice of medicine. Every criticism embedded a portrait. And every portrait displayed an organizational capacity that someone in the pluralistic soup of American national politics could admire.

The images constituting this reputation were many, but certain forms continually reappeared and remain with us today. They include the notion of the agency as a "guardian" and protector, the idea of the agency's practices as a global "gold standard," the person of Frances Kelsey and her public triumph in the thalidomide tragedy, the controversial politics of different commissioners (most notably James Goddard, Donald Kennedy, and David Kessler), the growing scientific status and influence of FDA medical official Robert Temple, and the emergence of debate about the "drug lag."

These images were suspended in a system of audiences and networks that, while ever changing in the late twentieth century, retained a degree of stability. One set of audiences was created by the unique congeries of institutions and organizations that ferried "news" to the Cold War American household. In some respects the reputation was made possible by the centralization of national media outlets—the dominance of large newspapers with capable Washington staff writers, and the preeminence of broadcast television syndicates such as the Columbia Broadcasting System (CBS) before the era of cable television networks. Another set of audiences lay in the burgeoning and rapidly fractionating societies of scientists and professionals in the United States.

[2]Thomas Hobbes, *Leviathan: Or the Matter, Forme and Power of a Commonwealth Ecclesiastical and Civil* (1651); The First Part, chapter 11, "Of the Difference of Manners," and chapter 13, "Of the Natural Condition of Mankind as concerning their Felicity and Misery."

Perhaps the most important of these audience structures lay in America's national legislature and its committee systems. It was in Congress where the various images and terms of debate were presented before national audiences, where discourse took shape, and where the pitch of contestation was so high. And in this making and remaking of an agency reputation, the political and historical contingency of Congress in the Cold War era was significant. The U.S. Congress of the late twentieth century was a propitious place for the production and reproduction of the FDA's image. American national politics from the 1950s through the 1980s bespoke the pluralism of numerous interests competing for access and advantage in manifold venues. In both chambers of the national legislature, the decades of the 1960s, 1970s, and 1980s witnessed the zenith of committee decentralization and subcommittee autonomy. Each committee and subcommittee chair—parochially lording over his yard of turf—could call and orchestrate a hearing that exposed a different side of the agency. Congress became for the Food and Drug Administration an arena for simultaneous criticism and praise, an amphitheater for projections onto the agency, for the mapping of images as metaphors onto the organization. Congress became, in the language of cultural anthropology, the preeminent "site" where the FDA's image and reputation were produced and reproduced. And of course, Congress and its committees were anything but passive listeners. Strategic committee chairs would call witnesses to influence the content of news. Senators would hold hearings to persuade their colleagues in the House of Representatives, and vice versa. And legislators would call hearings to praise, tarnish, and influence the FDA itself.[3]

Audiences in Science and Medicine

The Administration's reputation among the American mass public, supported by public relations and reproduced in national journalism, was a source of constant notoriety, occasional pity, and general prestige in the Cold War United States. Yet there were other facets to the FDA's organizational image, facets visible to other audiences where other understandings prevailed, where other languages were spoken. As important as any other venue was the scientific-medical audience composed of the various burgeoning and refracting professions of medicine and allied sciences related to drug development. At the symbolic level, the Administration's image among scientific audiences consisted of a simplex of concepts, texts, and images—

[3] For anthropological research on "sites" of reproduction of social and cultural structures, see June Starr and Jane Fishburne Collier, *History and Power in the Study of Law: New Directions in Legal Anthropology* (Ithaca: Cornell University Press, 1989); Geoffrey White, *Identity through History: Living Stories in a Solomon Islands Society* (New York: Cambridge University Press, 2002). For a more historical treatment of how legislative and institutional politics can perpetuate myths and fictions necessary for political order, see Edmund S. Morgan, *Inventing the People: The Rise of Popular Sovereignty in England and America* (New York: Norton, 1988), introduction to part 1, and chapters 6 and 9.

ranging from orthodox but influential accounts of the FDA in classic pharmacology textbooks (such as Goodman and Gilman's *The Pharmacological Basis of Therapeutics*), to public praise and scorn heaped upon the agency in the pages of medical journals and at scientific and industry conferences, to musings and frustrations about the FDA expressed in correspondence among top scientists.

At the structural level, the Administration's scientific reputation was grounded in extensive networks of association, information flow, and resource exchange between the agency, its committee system, universities and clinical researchers, pharmaceutical firms, and specialized medical and scientific societies and their members. The full set of scientific networks and liaisons connecting the Administration to American and international scientific audiences is too exhaustive (and its links too little observed) to be portrayed accurately in total. Yet one vital web connecting the FDA to this audience structure lies in the agency's committee structure and organizational memberships. Like many of the symbols that later constituted the FDA's organizational identity, these webs of professional and scientific association were an historical residue from the Ralph Smith era. Embodied in networks of committee memberships, the structural nexus undergirding the FDA's Cold War reputation predated the thalidomide tragedy and in fact evolved rather independently from that event.

From the beginnings of the Eisenhower administration and probably earlier, FDA officials acted intentionally, strategically, and with foresight to establish numerous committees of liaison to the professions. Agency officials established not just medically specialized "advisory committees" of the sort that became institutionalized in the late twentieth and twenty-first centuries, but also more temporary committees that helped the FDA recruit and retain allies and consultants. In cases where the official initiative in establishing these committees came from the White House or Congress, FDA officials were usually pivotal in deciding upon relevant appointments and leadership.

Among the most important panels in terms of precedent and reputation building were the Advisory Committee to the Secretary of Health, Education and Welfare of 1960, the Advisory Committee on Investigational Drugs, and the Medical Advisory Board. The first committee—also known as "the Miller Committee" for its chairman Philip Miller of the University of Chicago—served to link the pharmacological and medical luminaries of the 1950s with the Administration's emerging leadership (table 5.1). It was appointed in the wake of a scandal involving Division of Antibiotics Director Henry Welch, who among other things had been discovered to receive tens of thousands of dollars for steering FDA publishing contracts to a press that he owned. The second of these groups, commonly known as "the Modell Committee" after its chairman, pharmacologist Walter Modell of Cornell Medical School, was established in 1963 to assist and legitimate Frances Kelsey's Investigational New Drug Branch (see table 5.2). Of its members, several of the most distinguished (Modell, Gordon Zubrod) were already

TABLE 5.1.
Membership of the HEW Advisory Committee on the FDA, September 1960

Philip Miller [Chairman], University of Chicago School of Medicine

John Holmes Dingle, former director, Commission on Acute Respiratory Diseases

Maxwell Finland, Harvard Medical School

Colin MacLeod, Professor of Medicine, New York University

Karl Meyer, Professor of Biochemistry, Columbia University; Lasker Award winner (1957)

Carl Schmidt, Professor of Pharmacology, University of Pennsylvania; editor, *Circulation Research* (1958–62)

Wesley Spink, University of Minnesota; President, American College of Physicians

Allen Pond, Staff Assistant to Secretary of Health, Education, and Welfare

Franklin Clark, Bureau of Field Administration, FDA

Paul Cay, Office of the Commissioner, FDA

Donald Grove, Acting Director, Division of Antibiotics, FDA

George Larrick, Commissioner, FDA

William Kessenich, Bureau of Medicine, FDA

Winton Rankin, Office of the Commissioner, FDA

Robert Roe, Bureau of Biological and Physical Sciences, FDA

Ralph Smith, Head, New Drug Branch, Division of Medicine, FDA

Saul D. Cornell, Executive Officer, NAS / NRC

R. Keith Cannan, Chairman, Division of Medical Sciences, NAS / NRC

Herbert Gardner, Professional Associate, Division of Medical Sciences, NAS / NRC

Source: "Committee," September 8, 1960; B 2, F 24 ("FDA"), MIF.

well known to members of the Bureau of Medicine. The committee did not include a single industry representative.[4]

As the Modell Committee began its work of facilitating and easing relations between clinical investigators at the FDA, its members began to elaborate plans for an expanded network of ties to American science and medi-

[4]The official title of the Miller Committee was "Special Advisory Committee to the Secretary of Health, Education, and Welfare to review the Policies, Procedures, and Decisions of the Division of Antibiotics and the New Drug Branch of the Food and Drug Administration"; B2, F 24, MIF. Advisory Committee on Investigational Drugs, Ninth Meeting, April 30, 1964, "Summary of Proceedings," 2; B 13, F 1, FOK.

TABLE 5.2.
Membership of the Advisory Committee on Investigational Drugs, January 1965

Walter Modell (Chairman), Cornell University Medical School, New York

Dr. John Adriani

Sidney Merlis, Director of Psychiatric Research, Central Islip State Hospital, New York

Dr. Joseph Volker

Dr. John A. D. Cooper

Dr. C. Gordon Zubrod

Dr. Harold Hodge

Dr. Joseph F. Sadusk, Jr.

Dr. Joseph M. Pisani

Dr. Ralph G. Smith

Frances O. Kelsey, Chief, Investigational New Drug Branch, FDA

Dr. Clem O. Miller

Dr. Merle Gibson

Mr. Winton Rankin

Mr. Julius Hauser

Dr. Paul Palmisano, Executive Secretary

Source: Summary of Proceedings, 14th Meeting, January 14, 1965; Adriani Papers, NLM.

cine. Behind these plans was a keen and shared recognition of the need to build scientific capacity and to "improve FDA's image" and its "stature," not among the mass public but among scientists and medical academics. Frances Kelsey reminded her committee colleagues that her newly established branch was "forty years behind the times" in pharmacology. Boisfeuillet Jones, assistant to the Secretary of Health, Education and Welfare, outlined a vision for "the FDA's Scientific Future." National Academy of Sciences officials called for an expanded and regularized FDA advisory system, lamenting the Administration's "habit of seeking advice only on an ad hoc basis when in a sticky situation." The Administration needed "medical competence beyond its ability up to that time," Jones argued, competence that could support "recognition and an improved image."[5]

[5]Advisory Committee on Investigational Drugs, Ninth Meeting, April 30, 1964, "Summary of Proceedings," 2; B 13, F 1, FOK. On NAS complaints of FDA advice-seeking behavior, see R. Keith Cannan (Director, Division of Medical Sciences, NAS) to Maxwell Finland, February 22, 1963; B 4, F 3 ("National Research Council, 1931–1978"), MIF.

As Boisfeuillet Jones recognized, Administration officials had already taken concrete steps to address these concerns. Sadusk had been appointed as Medical Director in 1964. Then in 1965, Sadusk announced his intention to appoint a Medical Advisory Board and as many as twelve other special committees, some of which might absorb the Modell Committee itself. The agency had been reorganized to "put the scientific areas on a higher level," and to augment the medical staff. The assignment of Frances Kelsey to lead the Investigational New Drug Branch was the most notable example of taking an individual with broad scientific (and now, mass public) recognition and delegating important official responsibilities to them. Other luminaries of American pharmacology—Harry Dowling, Maxwell Finland, Eugene M. K. Geiling—were brought within the agency's regulatory orbit as consultants or, for a time, as fully employed staff. Yet the members of the Modell Committee were in unanimous agreement that internal appointments were of limited value in enhancing the FDA's scientific image. At least two other mechanisms were needed, one of dialogue and one of association.[6]

At the level of dialogue, Jones spoke of a "'forum' through which all interested parties could come together to discuss their mutual problems." Lowell Coggeshall's Drug Safety Commission was one such venue, committee members noted, but it was "not entirely satisfactory since it was sponsored by the regulated industry." The primary problem with "regulated industry" was not one of ethics but of scientific politics. Put simply, much of the American pharmaceutical industry carried poor scientific esteem. Episodes associated with chloramphenicol, MER/29, and thalidomide had combined with increasing alarm expressed in scientific and medical journals about the analytic and procedural rigor of drug development. This is not to deny that particular companies and their laboratories—Merck, Sharp and Dohme, and Hoffmann-La Roche, in particular—garnered broad respect. Yet when American scientists and medical academicians spoke of "the industry," they thought less frequently of these companies and their prized scientists and more commonly of a leviathan personified by the Pharmaceutical Manufacturers Association or the William S. Merrell Company.[7]

[6]Advisory Committee on Investigational Drugs, Ninth Meeting, April 30, 1964, "Summary of Proceedings," 2, 4; B 13, F 1, FOK. Finland had assisted the Bureau of Medicine in its investigation and withdrawal of Eaton Laboratories' Altafur; David Davis; Medical Officer, New Drug Branch, Bureau of Medicine, to Finland, September 22, 1960; B2, F 24 (FDA"), MIF. Geiling joined the Administration from 1959 to 1961 (HEW Press Release. Friday, August 28, 1959; Robert Roe (Director, Bureau of Biological and Physical Sciences) to Geiling, May 21, 1959; B 503517, F "Personal Materials," EMKG). Before his 1959 appointment, he had consulted formally with the Bureau of Medicine and maintained frequent contact with Irving Kerlan and Albert "Jerry" Holland on numerous issues ranging from regulatory toxicology to staff recruitment; Geiling to Kerlan, March 29, 1957; Kerlan [handwritten] to Geiling, March 27, 1957; Folder "Correspondence, K II," EMKG. After 1961, Geiling continued to serve as a consultant; Geiling to Harvey, June 20, 1961; B 503517, F "Personal Materials," EMKG. Dowling to Boisfeuillet Jones, July 11, 1963; HFD, NLM.

[7]On the reputational fallout of the MER/29 and thalidomide tragedies, see Jeremy Greene, *Prescribing by Numbers*, 161–3.

At the level of association, Sadusk spoke of "plans to develop close liaison between the Bureau of Medicine and the general scientific community." Sadusk's designs included a scheme of rotation where FDA physicians would spend up to one day per week in a university setting; he wanted his new recruits not to become internalized within the Bureau of Medicine but to form relationships with scholars outside. The Bureau would support new symposia and would encourage additional research by means of contract financing through medical schools. Sadusk's Medical Advisory Board was established in 1965. In 1969, its membership included names and faces familiar to FDA officials: Harry Dowling, William Kirby, Wesley Spink (see table 5.3). The legitimizing function of the Medical Advisory Board was all the more important after FDA Commissioner James Goddard and General Counsel William Goodrich became involved in a public spat over patient package inserts and medical journal advertising in the late 1960s. As Modell himself became a caustic critic of the Administration, the Modell Committee became of less reputational use.[8]

As early as 1967, when James Goddard was beginning just his second year as Commissioner of Food and Drugs, the FDA's system of committee memberships could plausibly be described as vast. FDA personnel sat on nearly sixty committees in prestigious and influential scientific organizations ranging from the American Cancer Society and the International Union of Pure and Applied Chemistry to the National Academy of Sciences (NAS) and the World Health Organization (WHO) (see table 5.4). Most of the FDA personnel sitting on these committees were from the Bureaus of Medicine or Pharmacology (or related scientific bureaus and divisions), and in nearly every case the committee members were careerists who represented the pre-thalidomide regime of protocol—Ralph Smith, A. J. Lehman, O. Garth Fitzhugh, Edwin Goldenthal, even Frances Kelsey.

Another crucial pattern of scientific and professional liaison was the recruitment of top medical scientists to serve on public advisory committees. The advisory committee system was launched in the mid-1960s, although the FDA had employed some committees since the early twentieth century. In a pattern that was established quickly and would become pivotal in regulatory politics in the late twentieth century, the Director of the Administration's drug regulation division was given primary responsibility for appointments to these committees and for their meetings. In the late 1960s, the Director of the Bureau of Medicine was the primary officer responsible for fully nineteen (73 percent) of the entire agency's twenty-six advisory committees. This pattern not only reflected not the creation of advisory committees for drug review assistance, but also held for connections to basic science advisory committees, such as those representing expertise in the biological and physical sciences and toxicology (see table 5.5). The centrality of the

[8] Advisory Committee on Investigational Drugs, Ninth Meeting, April 30, 1964, "Summary of Proceedings," 6; B 13, F 1, FOK. The dispute between Modell and Lasagna, on the one hand, and Goddard and Goodrich on the FDA side, is discussed below.

TABLE 5.3.
Membership of the Medical Advisory Board (FDA Bureau of Medicine), 1969

Mark W. Allam

Allan D. Bass

Harry Dowling, University of Illinois

William M. M. Kirby, University of Washington Medical Center, Seattle

William R. Mann

John G. Morrison

Arthur P. Richardson

Wesley W. Spink, University of Minnesota; President, American College of
    Physicians

From FDA (Bureau of Medicine unless noted):

B. Harvey Minchew

John J. Schrogie

Jean D. Lockhart

William J. Murray

William Gyarfas

Paul Bryan

C. D. Van Houweling (Bureau of Veterinary Medicine)

J. Giel (Research and Development Office, CPEHS)

Source: FDA Bureau of Medicine, Medical Advisory Board, Eighteenth Meeting, March 27
and 28, 1969, Minutes; HFD, NLM.

Bureau of Medicine prevailed despite the long-term presence of a Bureau of
Pharmacology and a Bureau of Physical and Biological Sciences (later the
Bureau of Science).

   In aggregate, the Administration's network of scientific relationships was
less organic than sponsored. Whereas earlier advisory committees had sketched
a vision for the systematic webbing of FDA personnel to scientific organizations, the agency now began to bureaucratize this function. The FDA Commissioner's Office included a Committee Management Office with a full-
time staff. In their committee appointments, FDA officials were directed by
a guidance document ("issuance") for internal use entitled *Food and Drug
Administration Committee Management*. These formalized patterns of liaison were accompanied by less formal efforts that were themselves coordinated through the FDA network of external advisers. At meetings of the

TABLE 5.4
Committee Memberships Formally Managed by the FDA, 1967

Name of Association or Organization	Name of Committee	FDA Representative
Advisory Council	Educational Seminar on Birth Defects	Frances O. Kelsey
American Academy of Pediatrics	Committee on Nutrition	not named
American Association of Avian Pathology	Committee on Nomenclature	2 members of the Bureau of Veterinary Medicine
American Cancer Society	Committee on New and Unproved Methods	William Evans
American Chemical Society	Committee on Analytical Reagents	W. D. Hubbard
American Chemical Society	Division of Agriculture and Food Chemistry Nominating Committee	Leonard Stoloff
American College of Clinical Pharmacology and Chemotherapy	Long-Range Planning Committee	A. J. Lehman
American Industrial Hygiene Association	Toxicology Committee	Keith Jacobsen
American Medical Association	Analytical Microbiology Section	A. Kirshbaum
American Medical Association	Evaluation of Drugs for Microbial Contamination	Frances Bowman
American Public Health Association	Standard Methods Committee	L. R. Shelton
American Society for Pharmacology and Experimental Therapeutics	Committee on Toxic Reactions to Drugs	A. J. Lehman

TABLE 5.4
cont.

Name of Association or Organization	Name of Committee	FDA Representative
American Society for Testing and Materials		Dr. Joseph Davis
American Veterinary Medical Association	Council on Biological and Therapeutic Agents	Fred J. Kingman
Army Scientific Advisory Panel		Herbert L. Ley
Association of American Feed Control Officials	Pet Food Committee	William McFarland
Association of American Feed Control Officials	States Relations Committee	William McFarland
Association of Food and Drug Officials of the United States		not named
Chemical Society of Washington	Analytical Topical Group	Edward Haenni
Coordinating Conference on Health Information		William Evans, Wallace Janssen
Food and Agriculture Organization (FAO) (United Nations)	FAO Working Party of Experts on Pesticide Residues	J. W. Cook
World Health Organization (WHO) (United Nations)	WHO Committee on Quality Control	J. J. DiLorenzo
FAO-WHO	4th Codex Alimentarius Committee on Food Additives	O. Garth Fitzhugh, H. Blumenthal
FAO-WHO	Alimentarius Commission on Labeling Committee	J. Kenneth Kirk

TABLE 5.4
cont.

Name of Association or Organization	Name of Committee	FDA Representative
FAO-WHO	Codex Alimentarius Commission	J. Kenneth Kirk
FAO-WHO	Codex Alimentarius Expert Group on Cocoa and Chocolate Products	L. M. Beacham
FAO-WHO	Codex Alimentarius Expert Group on Frozen Foods	L. M. Beacham
FAO-WHO	Codex Committee on Fish and Fishery Products	L. M. Beacham
FAO-WHO	Codex Committee on Methods of Analysis and Sampling	W. Horwitz
FAO-WHO	Codex Committee on Pesticide Residues	O. Garth Fitzhugh
FAO-WHO	Committee on Microbiological Specifications for Foods	M. T. Bartram
FAO-WHO	ECE/Codex Alimentarius on Standardization of Fruit Juices	L. M. Beacham
FAO-WHO	Expert Committee on Biological Standardization	W. W. Wright
FAO-WHO	Government Experts on the Code of Principles for Milk and Milk Products	R. W. Weik
Institute of Food Technology		not named
International Society of Chemotherapy		R. E. Barziliai
International Union of Pure and Applied Chemistry	Trace Substances Division	H. Fischbach

TABLE 5.4
cont.

Name of Association or Organization	Name of Committee	FDA Representative
National Academy of Sciences/ National Research Council	Advisory Board, Office of Biochemical Nomenclature	Daniel Banes
National Academy of Sciences/ National Research Council	Advisory Panel on the Food Chemicals Codex	H. Fischbach
National Academy of Sciences/ National Research Council	Agricultural Research Institute	J. Fritz and Dr. Van Houweling
National Academy of Sciences/ National Research Council	Committee in Toxicology	A. J. Lehman
National Academy of Sciences/ National Research Council	Committee on Applications of Biochemical Studies in Evaluating Drug Toxicity	Edwin Goldenthal
National Academy of Sciences/ National Research Council	Committee on Problems of Drug Dependence	Ralph Smith
National Academy of Sciences/ National Research Council	Drug Research Board	not named
National Academy of Sciences/ National Research Council	Food and Nutrition Board, Recommended Dietary Allowances Revision Committee	Philip Harris
National Academy of Sciences/ National Research Council	Institute of Laboratory Animal Resources Advisory Council	Charles Durbin
National Academy of Sciences/ National Research Council	Subcommittee on Carcinogenesis, Food Protection Committee	A. A. Nelson

TABLE 5.4
cont.

Name of Association or Organization	Name of Committee	FDA Representative
National Academy of Sciences/ National Research Council	Subcommittee on Reference Materials of the Committee on Analytical Chemistry	H. Fischbach
National Better Business Bureau		Theodore Byers
National Health Council		not named
Research and Development Associates. Inc.		J. William Boehne
Second International Workshop in Teratology		Frances O. Kelsey
Society of Toxicology	Technical Committee	Stephen Krop, Kent J. Davis
United States Livestock Association		not named
United States Pharmacopeia/ National Formulary	Joint Panel on General Notices	James B. Kottemann
United States Pharmacopeia/ National Formulary	NF Advisory Panel	Jonas Carol
United States Pharmacopeia/ National Formulary	USP Advisory Panel on Radioactive Pharmaceuticals	Carl E. Myers
United States Pharmacopeia/ National Formulary	USP Advisory Panel on Sterilization Procedures	Frances Bowman
US-Japan Cooperation on Development of Natural Resources	Panel on Mycoplasmosis of Domestic Animals	C. Durbin

TABLE 5.5.
FDA Public Advisory Committees, 1967

Name of Committee	Year Authorized	FDA Officer with Responsibility
National Advisory Food and Drug Council	1964	Commissioner
Anti-Infective Agents Advisory Committee	1967	BOM Director
Board of Tea Experts	1897	Board Secretary (appointed)
Cardiovascular and Renal Disorders Advisory Committee	1967	BOM Director
Advisory Committee on Clinical Research Contracts	1965	BOM Director
Advisory Committee on Abuse and Depressant and Stimulant Drugs	89th Congress	Director, Bureau of Drug Abuse Control
Dental Advisory Committee	1967	BOM Director
Dermatology Advisory Committee	1967	BOM Director
Drug Experience Advisory Committee	1967	BOM Director
Drug Nomenclature Advisory Committee	1967	Commissioner
Endocrinology and Metabolism Advisory Committee	1967	BOM Director
Food Standards Committee	1964	Office of Legislative and Governmental Services
Hematology Advisory Committee	1967	BOM Director
Medical Advisory Board	1964	BOM Director
Neuropharmacology Advisory Committee	1967	BOM Director
Oncology Advisory Committee	1967	BOM Director
Ophthalmology and Otorhinolaryngology Advisory Committee	1967	BOM Director
Advisory Committee on Protocol for Safety Evaluations	1965	BOM Director
Psychomimetic Agents Joint FDA-PHS Advisory Committee	1967	BOM Director
Advisory Committee on Obstetrics and Gynecology	1965	BOM Director
Radioactive Pharmaceuticals Advisory Committee	1967	BOM Director
Advisory Committee on Research in the Biological and Physical Sciences	1964	BOM Director
Respiratory and Anesthetic Drugs Advisory Committee	1966	BOM Director
Advisory Committee on Veterinary Medicine	1964	Director, Bureau of Veterinary Medicine
Advisory Committee on the Teratogenic Effect of Certain Drugs	1965	BOM Director
Advisory Committee on Safety of Pesticide Residues in Foods	1965	Director, Bureau of Science

Medical Advisory Board, members regularly talked through strategies of connecting the Bureau of Medicine to external scientific organizations by means of appointments, "representation," and symposia. Through formal and informal committee management, a significant portion of the Administration's liaison with scientific audiences had taken shape in an official, publicized, and hardened form. By the late 1960s, the FDA's committee management system—which would persist and grow for the remainder of the century—was a structure not simply of networks, but of publicly established associations that served to legitimate both the committee members and the FDA.[9]

The existence of these relations should not be taken as evidence of their temperature. The networks linking the Administration to scientific and medical organizations were not always couriers of support and praise. Often enough criticism and doubt streamed through them. Far more than creating an echo chamber of glorification, the networks helped to hone and stabilize expectations about the roles and capacities of the Administration. With repeated interaction—even of the sort that embedded sustained disagreement and criticism—these scientific and medical networks also bred familiarity and trust.

At crucial times, these scientific ties would pay immediate political dividends. When following the Kefauver-Harris Amendments, the Administration began to conduct a review of all drugs approved between 1938 and 1962 as part of the Drug Efficacy Study, FDA Commissioner James Goddard enlisted the assistance of the National Academy of Sciences and the National Research Council (NAS/NRC). The Drug Efficacy Study entailed the creation of dozens of panels to review drugs in different therapeutic categories, a nexus headed by a Policy Advisory Committee. In the constitution of these panels, it was clear that friends of the FDA would largely direct the Drug Efficacy Study. The chairman of the Policy Advisory Committee was Alfred Gilman, and its other star member was Maxwell Finland. The Policy Advisory Committee orchestrated the entire study. Medical Advisory Board member William M. M. Kirby chaired a panel on anti-infective drugs and another Board member, Sidney Merlis, was on the psychiatric drugs panel. Goodman student Mark Nickerson was on the cardiovascular drug panel. When the Administration began to withdraw hundreds of drugs—including widely used fixed-combination therapies—from the market beginning in 1969, its allies on the NAS/NRC helped to cement the FDA's position and secure its decisions.[10]

[9]Source: Memo from E. R. Lannon (Asst Commissioner for Administration) to "Associate Commissioners, Assistant Commissioners, Bureau, Office and Division Directors," Subject "FDA Committee Management," November 24, 1967; HFD, NLM. See the suggestions of Harry Dowling and William Kirby at the Medical Advisory Board, Eighteenth Meeting, March 27 and 28, 1969, Minutes; HFD, NLM. By 1970, many of these committees had been disbanded, only to re-emerge under the direction of Charles Edwards; Peter Barton Hutt, personal communication, September 2008.

[10]Division of Medical Sciences, National Research Council, *Drug Efficacy Study: Final Re-*

Along with the general legitimacy bestowed upon the Administration by its nexus of contacts and affiliations with American medicine and science, there were also persistent strains of disapproval. The pharmacological revolution of the 1950s, the 1962 Kefauver-Harris Amendments, and the 1963 Investigational New Drug rules had all made drug development more scientific. Yet they had also made drug development more costly, at least in the nominal sense of additional time and money spent in compliance with the regulations. This fact was a surprise to no one. The major point of contention was just how much burden the regulations had added and whether the new and official commitment to scientific drug development justified the hindrance. On these points, some notable voices in American medicine were as sour on the new regulations as they were respectful of the agency.

One Carl Pfeiffer would provide a prescient example in his address to the newly assembled American College of Clinical Pharmacology and Chemotherapy in 1964. Pfeiffer was a clinical pharmacologist who specialized in issues relating to nutrition and psychiatric drugs. His primary concern with the new regulations was their encumbrance of therapeutic freedom. The federal government's "restriction of drugs to their licensed use alone," Pfeiffer intoned, "is a travesty on the physician's free choice in the practice of medicine." This was as much a criticism of the Durham-Humphrey Amendments of 1952, which recommended regulations for the prescribing of ethical drugs, as it was of the changes of 1962 and 1963. Pfeiffer also believed that the governance of clinical investigation was not core to the efficacy concerns of the 1962 law but instead constituted "fringe aspects of the regulations." They "interfere with, and will continue to obstruct, advances in the field of basic clinical pharmacology." Pfeiffer reserved his most pointed language for the application of the rules and for the FDA, scoring the agency's "flabby practice" of ambiguity and its "dilatory tactics" and behavior that were "typically true of bureaucrats."

Carl Pfeiffer's imagery of the FDA was manifold, influential, and partially inaccurate. It would be reproduced continually in the coming years, often enough by clinical pharmacologists who had heard similar rhetoric reverberating through the conferences and networks of their discipline. At its core, the Administration in this portraiture was an agent with the power of negation. Only once its assent to proceed with clinical trials had been granted could a scientist move forward with human research. Armed with scientific veto power, the Administration's behavior displayed two "bureaucratic" facets: delay and ambiguity. The Administration's refusals to permit new clinical studies were based not upon legitimate scientific rationales, Pfeiffer intimated, but were "dilatory tactics." The justifications for these decisions, moreover, were never clear but were accompanied by noncommittal explanations that always left the FDA with discretion to negate

port to the Commissioner of Food and Drugs, FDA (Washington, DC: National Academy of Sciences, 1969), 2, appendixes A-1 A-2.

once again. In fact, the Administration's powers under the 1962 law and the 1963 rules were considerably more restricted than Pfeiffer's rhetoric implies. Clinical investigators did not need to secure FDA approval of every single Investigational New Drug application. Instead, once an application had been submitted, it was the sponsor's presumptive right to commence research thirty days later. The FDA could halt the study only by issuing (within 30 days of the IND's receipt) a "clinical hold" delaying the initiation of the trial. Unlike the new drug application process in which active assent from the Administration is required, the IND process required active intervention by the FDA if a study was to be stopped or delayed.

Despite their brute depiction of what were more complex regulatory realities, images like Pfeiffer's endured through the 1960s and 1970s. They were already on display in the summer of 1963, when approximately 200 clinical pharmacologists and academic physicians from around the globe had convened for a two-day conference in Chicago. The meeting was sponsored by Lowell Coggeshall's Commission on Drug Safety. The specter of bureaucratic power, exercised over medical practice and clinical research, was the most common fear expressed. The Administration now possessed "awesome powers, not subject to effective judicial review," said Dr. Theodore G. Klumpp, president of Winthrop Laboratories in New York City. Winthrop attorney James H. Luther, Jr., argued that the broad discretion embedded in such terms as "substantial doubt" of safety or the "reasonableness" of an investigation rendered the FDA, in all effect, "the arbiter of medical opinion." Another panelist warned that "The regulatory agencies, by a literal interpretation of the regulations, have the power to snuff out the life of clinical pharmacology." William M. M. Kirby of University of Washington Medical Center in Seattle presented results from a survey of 640 investigators from seventy-five medical schools. Fully 57 percent of Kirby's respondents said that the 1963 regulations hindered their research or that of their colleagues, and nearly three-quarters agreed with the statement that the increased paperwork had induced a "reluctance to carry on old projects or to initiate new ones."[11]

Coggeshall's conference of July 1963 demonstrated widespread concern with the new FDA-centered regime of drug development, but also what one medical reporter described as a "spirit of cooperation" with the Administration. "The consensus appeared to be that better standards in drug testing have been needed and that the regulations, at the least, will discourage incompetent investigators." FDA ally Wesley W. Spink of the University of

[11] *Modern Medicine*, July 22, 1963, 32. Coggeshall's full-time position was at the University of Chicago, and Chicago was also home to the headquarters of the AMA, which had opposed the efficacy requirements of the 1962 Kefauver-Harris Amendments. Kirby's percentages were derived from "adequate" responses to his survey, and the definition of "adequate" is not clear from the *Modern Medicine* article. Klumpp would rehearse some of the same arguments at a October 1963 conference at the University of Pennsylvania, where he attributed the 1962 law to "hysteria"; "Scientists Explore News Problems," *Philadelphia Inquirer*, October 18, 1962, 1.

Minnesota, Minneapolis, president of the American College of Physicians, considered much of the criticism rather frivolous. "I find it very difficult to find anything highly specific and significant except that they do not like the increased amount of paper work, and they do not like to feel that their clinical investigation is being regulated," he said. Other panelists placed the blame for the disruption of research upon medicine itself, and particularly upon "the medical schools." American academic medicine had failed to train enough clinical pharmacologists who could bring the methods of modern therapeutics to the process of drug development, and many pharmaceutical companies had failed to hire them.[12]

Administration officials were not passive listeners at the Coggeshall conference. Frances Kelsey attended the proceedings with HEW official Boisfeuillet Jones and tried to allay the fears of clinical researchers. If the rules "do, in fact, become a bottleneck to the development of new drugs beneficial to mankind, they can and will be modified," said Jones. Kelsey concurred, stating that "a reasonable degree of freedom is essential if the full potentialities of a drug are to be developed." Kelsey's attendance at the Chicago conference was part of a larger nationwide tour in which she visited some of the nation's most distinguished research hospitals, including the Mayo Clinic in Rochester, Minnesota. Kelsey was hosted as a medical celebrity, with a guided tour of the Clinic, a dinner at the Mayo Foundation house, and numerous one-on-one meetings with the Clinic's top investigators. Mayo leadership urged their research staff to attend these meetings. Companies and patient organizations also hosted Kelsey in this manner, and in many cases she was honored with an award or some form of recognition.[13]

Kelsey's political and scientific tourism notwithstanding, there remained considerable ambiguity about how the Administration would interpret and apply the 1962 law. As the FDA officials began in 1963 to discuss the patient consent provisions of the Kefauver-Harris Amendments, officials sought to assuage the worries of clinical investigators that the patient consent rules were stifling research and patient relationships. Yet there was another audience that needed pacification, namely members of Congress and medical ethicists who were concerned that the future of patient protection rested in the hands of a potentially unstable agency. The Administration's earliest statements on patient consent resulted from conscious but uncoordinated

[12] *Modern Medicine*, July 22, 1963, 32.
[13] Ibid. On Kelsey's Mayo visit, see Minutes, CSTA, November 21, 1963; MAYO. "It is hoped that as many as possible who are carrying out clinical investigation and who will have to work with the FDA will meet Dr. Kelsey. To this end special notices and invitations to attend the Staff Meeting will be sent to representative staff investigators." For an example of one of many companies to invite Kelsey to its premises, see Arthur J. Palliota (Director of Research, Bionetics Research Laboratories, Inc.), to FOK, March 16, 1967; B1, F "1967, Jan–May," FOK. The Washington, DC, Area Chapter of the National Multiple Sclerosis Society also invited Kelsey to its "MS Fashion Show and Luncheon" in 1967, recognizing her as an "Outstanding Woman of Achievement"; Edwards W. Alfriend, IV, Chairman, Board of Trustees, National Multiple Sclerosis Society, to FOK, March 16, 1967; B1, F "1967, Jan–May," FOK.

navigation between these critical audiences. The only federal statute particular to patient consent was the Kefauver-Harris Amendments, and they
spoke briefly and vaguely on the subject. The Amendments required that
consent be obtained "except where they [the doctors] deem it not feasible or,
in their professional judgment, contrary to the best interests of such human
beings." One reporter continued that

> The words, "not feasible," look like a wide open hatch. However, Dr. Frances O.
> Kelsey, who polices this part of the law for the Food and Drug Administration,
> says the legislative intent was only to cover emergencies when consent could not
> be gotten in time. "There is," she says, "no basis for concluding that such excep-
> tions would include circumstances in which the investigator feels that informed
> consent would interfere with the design of the experiment or would disturb the
> 'doctor-patient' relationship."

When Kelsey's reading of the law was published in 1964, her lines alarmed
one of the nation's preeminent clinical researchers, Henry K. Beecher of
Harvard Medical School and the Massachusetts General Hospital. In Beecher's work on subjective drug response and its statistical measurement, he
often did not inform patients that they might be receiving a placebo. Strictly
construed, informed consent requirements would interfere with the design
and conduct of these trials. Beecher wrote Commissioner George Larrick to
report that he found Kelsey's interpretation "disturbing."[14] As he asked Larrick:

> May I inquire just how it is possible for Dr. Kelsey to issue single-handed such a
> ruling [?] Those of us who carry on experimentation of this type have been as-
> sured repeatedly that the opposite of Dr. Kelsey's conclusion is possible. Are the
> officials of the Food and Drug Administration free to interpret the law as they see
> fit? If not, what restraints are put on personal and individual interpretation?

Henry Beecher's simple inquiry was a bold challenge, not merely to the Administration's interpretation of the law, but to its organizational identity
and authority. Who represents the agency, Beecher wondered, and for whom
does Kelsey speak? At some level, Beecher was contesting Frances Kelsey's
authority within the Administration, and the relationship of her authority to
federal statute. Beecher's letter sent FDA leadership scurrying to find the
source of Kelsey's remarks and to consult with their in-house attorneys on
what statutory basis underlay their heroine's interpretation. Larrick and
Medical Director Joseph Sadusk would remind Beecher that the Administra-

[14]Kelsey's statement was published in *Hearings before the Subcommittee on Reorganization
and International Organizations of the Committee on Government Operations of the United
States Senate*, Part V, June 19, 1963 (Washington, DC: GPO, 1964), 2454. The original statement appeared in her chapter "Patient Consent Provisions of the Federal Food, Drug and Cosmetic Act," in Irving Ladimar and Roger W. Newman, eds., *Clinical Investigation in Medicine:
Legal, Ethical and Moral Aspects* (Boston: Boston University Law-Medicine Research Institute,
1963), 336–40. Beecher (from Massachusetts General Hospital) to Larrick, December 22, 1964;
Beecher to Larrick, September 8, 1965; DF 505.51 (Patient Consent), RG 88, NA.

tion had not yet issued any regulations, and that the only legal source of American "patient consent" policy lay in the terse provisions of the 1962 law. Beyond this, Sadusk replied that Kelsey was no cop but rather a scientist, and that her remarks must be interpreted as issuing from a scientific role that was shared by the members of her Bureau. "I would take issue," he wrote Beecher, "with the reporter who stated that Dr. Kelsey 'polices' this part of the law.... [T]hose of us in the Bureau of Medicine are responsible to the Commissioner for scientific recommendation and not for 'police' or 'enforcement' activities." Sadusk's response both undermined the police metaphor used by trade reporters (and taken up by Beecher) and gave added weight to Kelsey's interpretation as being based not simply upon the 1962 statute but upon technical considerations.[15]

Two years after the Beecher-Kelsey tension died down, the FDA's application of its new pharmaceutical regulations would create another public conflict involving another medical luminary. Speaking at a medical conference in 1967, General Counsel William Goodrich announced that publishers, authors, and editors who had written, approved, and published drug dosages different from those approved by the Administration were liable for damages to the patient and the manufacturer. And in another speech he intimated that medical journals might be legally liable for publishing misleading advertisements. This pronouncement met with a harsh reply from Cornell pharmacologist Walter Modell, editor of *Clinical Pharmacology and Therapeutics* and previously a reliable ally for the Administration's procedural reform cohort. "The FDA," Modell complained, "has now taken the stand that in this country it is the sole arbiter of drug dosage and that its pronouncements on this subject in drug package stuffers are inviolate." From the implied threat of legal vulnerability, Modell inferred a direct threat to free scientific and medical expression. "The implications of this unprecedented FDA program are shattering. Absolute freedom of dialogue and communication has long been accepted as essential to all scientific progress and to medical progress as well." Medical journals and academic symposia were critical fora in which this dialogue coursed, but now "the FDA has begun to discourage, to hobble, to stifle, to castrate such publications." Modell concluded that the public and the medical community in the United States needed safeguarding from the Administration. "The public is protected by existing legislation against irresponsible errors by publishers, editors, and authors. Who will protect the public against the FDA?"[16]

Walter Modell had inverted the metaphor of protection that lay at the foundation of the FDA's image. In other ways, he belittled some of the in-

[15] Joseph F. Sadusk (Medical Director) to Beecher, January 27, 1965; Memo from William W. Goodrich (Assistant General Counsel) to Sadusk, April 13, 1965; Beecher to Larrick, September 8, 1965; Larrick to Beecher, September 24, 1965; DF 505.51 (Patient Consent), RG 88, NA.
[16] "Editors Assail Punitive View of Liability for Advertising," *Medical Tribune*, January 25, 1967, 1; Modell, "Editorial: FDA Censorship," *Clinical Pharmacology and Therapeutics* 8 (3) (May–June 1967): 359.

struments and signs of the Administration's power. In rendering the package insert as a "drug package stuffer," he mocked one of the Administration's central regulatory tools, dismissing it as too costly and perhaps altogether unnecessary. "The stuffer," Modell later carped, "is not a legal directive to the physician. It is a label, a label!" Other editorial celebrities—including *New England Journal of Medicine* editor Joseph Garland and *Journal of Pediatrics* editor Waldo E. Nelson—expressed concern, but in more measured tones. Goodrich's view of advertising was supported by Philadelphia doctor S. Leon Israel, editor of *Obstetrics and Gynecology*, who remarked that "we do not think it a threat when the FDA issues a warning concerning pharmaceutical advertisements that may be in error." Yet Modell's thrust and parry had established a troubling precedent. Some of the same networks and organizations of clinical pharmacology that had supported the Administration's stringent standards of evaluation could quickly become chambers in which laments of "censorship" and "bureaucratic malfeasance" could amplify through reverberation and feedback. FDA officials took notice.[17]

Julius Hauser and General Counsel William Goodrich would later collaborate on a statement that disavowed any intention to regulate the communications of medical societies. The FDA, Hauser declared to the American Medical Writers Association meeting in New York City, "has no intention of attempting the censorship of the *Journal of the American Medical Association*, the medical journals published by State medical societies, medical textbooks, or any other private medical publications." Modell immediately claimed "a sense of victory" and noted that the episode was one in which the politics of reputation and criticism would constrain even the FDA with its vast new armature of legal authority: "The small voice, if insistent and reasonable, will be heard by the FDA," he reasoned, and "the FDA may even bend to the pressures it exerts."[18]

Modell's voice was soon echoed by Louis Lasagna, the Johns Hopkins pharmacologist who had notably supported the Administration's efficacy regulation in the Kefauver hearings of 1960 and 1961. As with Modell, Lasagna's earlier support of the FDA pharmacological regime helped to legitimate his subsequent criticism. An FDA "champion" had turned into a strident critic. When James Goddard took over the post of Commissioner in 1966, he floated the idea that mandatory package inserts could perhaps be replaced by a single drug compendium, approved by the Administration but funded by a tax upon the industry. Modell worried that a compendium

---

[17] Modell, "Editorial: An End to the Means; FDA papers III," *CP&T* 9 (6) (November–December 1968): 705–11; "Editors Assail Punitive View of Liability for Advertising," *Medical Tribune*, January 25, 1967, 16–17.

[18] Modell, "Editorial: FDA Censorship," *CP&T* 8 (3) (May–June 1967): 359; "How to Stuff a Stuffer and Cook a Wolf," *CP&T* 8 (1967): 775–81; "On Speech and Silence and the FDA," *CP&T* 9 (1968): 139–41; "How to HEW the FDA into Shape," *CP&T* 9 (1968): 285–89; "To Protect the American Patient," *CP&T* 9 (1968): 413–20. Hauser's statement appears in "FDA Papers II," *CP&T* 9 (1968): 711–17.

would amount to "stuffers bound instead of stuffed" and compared the idea to "a modern '5-foot shelf' of package inserts." The Pharmaceutical Manufacturers Association (PMA) reacted coolly to Goddard's proposal, and pharmacy societies also expressed their disapproval. Surveys of practicing physicians by the PMA and the Opinion Research Corporation found that two-thirds of respondents felt that current options—mainly the *Physicians' Desk Reference*—were adequate. When Goddard, in a speech to the American College of Legal Medicine in June 1968, referred to the compendium imbroglio as "one pathetic little fire" and a "manufactured controversy," the acrimony became increasingly hard-edged, and much more serious accusations were leveled. "When the nonexpert group of the FDA threatens to become the dictator of American medicine," Modell warned, the inevitable outcome would be "Therapeutic Nihilism." Lasagna thought Goddard's compendium proposal a "cavalier suggestion" and an act of "arrogance." It was the equivalent, he wrote, "of passing a bill commanding Hugh Hefner to buy solid gold falsies for Elizabeth Taylor and Sophia Loren and every Bunny in each of Mr. Hefner's Playboy Clubs."[19]

The Walter Modell imbroglio stands as a reminder that, in the aftermath of the 1962 law and the 1963 rules, the Administration's audiences were composed of numerous voices and cross-cutting pressures. Laments flowed in from clinical researchers about the disruption of drug development, while general practitioners complained of interference in their patient-physician relationships. All the while, members of Congress were pressuring the Administration to take a more aggressive stance toward Upjohn, which housed the most strident and aggressive of the agency's critics. So direct and public was the pressure from Congress that some clinical pharmacologists smelled political interference with science. North Carolina Democrat Lawrence Fountain had contacted the FDA to say that the agency should have "moved more quickly" to remove Upjohn's combination antibiotic Panalba from the market, and "not allowed 120 days grace." He also held hearings in 1969. Fountain's rhetoric had incensed some of the Administration's academic advisers, including Harry Dowling, who questioned "the propriety of a Congressional Committee holding a hearing on a drug while this drug is being considered by the regulating agency." FDA general counsel William Goodrich replied that hearings were "good for the country regardless of how painful they may be for the FDA." Yet Goodrich probably knew as he spoke that the hearings were in fact beneficial for his agency's authority. The fact that a powerful subcommittee chair was lobbying the Administration to act more stringently meant that the agency's powers over post-

[19]Goddard, "To the fullest extent," presented to the American College of Legal Medicine, AMA, San Francisco, June 16, 1968; reprinted in *CP&T* 9 (6) (Nov.–Dec. 1968): 711–17; Lasagna, "Setting the Record Straight on 'To the fullest extent,'" *CP&T* 9 (6) (Nov.–Dec. 1968): 719. "FDA and Doctors Clash on Compendium," print in Dowling Papers; NLM. "Only 15% of MD's Want All-New Compendium," *DTN*, July 29, 1968, 1, 7.

market withdrawal for efficacy rationales would not be weakened in the near future.[20]

As the rhetoric continued to escalate, the critique focused less and less upon the Administration as organization and more and more on the FDA's leadership. In concluding one of his most acerbic essays, Modell felt compelled to proclaim that he meant no ill will toward the agency's "staff" or permanent structure, but that his laments were directed at Goddard and Goodrich.

> I have never disparaged the hopes and aspirations or the benevolent intentions of the Food and Drug Administration, nor do I do so now. I have never suggested that they were not devoted public servants. There are no villains in the FDA, only victims of inadequate public support. I have suggested that actions unacceptable to me were the result of frustrations of incompetence due to insufficient funds and that deviousness was a compensatory device for inadequacy. I have written that the FDA is understaffed and underbudgeted and that the job of the Commissioner as well as that of the FDA as a whole is impossible. I have made serious and detailed recommendations for the alleviation of some of its burdens and for the modernization and increase of efficiency of its operation, which I consider vital to the health of the nation.[21]

Modell couched and conditioned his laments within a blanket of general praise and pity for the Administration. In doing so, he echoed within pharmacology circles the refrain of "FDA as victim of public neglect." The failures of the agency were legion and threatening, but like other critics Modell blamed them either on poor leadership or on lack of funding. While some critiques from academic medical researchers did in fact target the organization as a whole, a material fraction of the criticism absolved the Administration's structure and career officials.

Whereas Administration leadership disgruntled therapeutic luminaries like Lasagna and Modell, most pharmacologists and medical researchers appear to have viewed the 1960s FDA in warmer and more benign terms. The Administration's posture and its powers were, after all, a favorable projection of the discipline of clinical pharmacology over the world of ethical drugs. Statistical and methodological purists might have worried about the FDA's new stances and pronouncements, but if they did, they rarely voiced these concerns. More often than not they publicly and privately defended the Administration against its critics.

No two twentieth-century academic physicians better represented this genial consensus than Utah's Louis Goodman and Harvard's Maxwell Finland. Here the Administration's networks of medical communication and academic familiarity redounded to its advantage. Ralph Smith had known

[20]FDA-BOM, Medical Advisory Board Minutes, Nineteenth Meeting, June 26 and 27, 1969, pp. 9–10; Harry F. Dowling Papers, NLM.
[21]Modell, "Editorial: An End to the Means; FDA papers III," 710.

Goodman for years and remained on a first-name basis with him. Well into the 1960s, the two corresponded and kept tabs on each others' careers. Goodman's support was pivotal for FDA career officials; by 1965, he was already a celebrity in the world of pharmacology. His perch in academic medicine was not necessarily higher in status than Louis Lasagna's or Walter Modell's, but Goodman was probably more influential. Much of Goodman's authority lay in his authoritative textbook with Alfred Gilman, *The Pharmacological Basis of Therapeutics*, which issued in its third edition in 1965 and was in the late 1960s (and for at least two decades thereafter) the most oft-assigned pharmacology text in U.S. medical schools. Goodman had also mentored some of the nation's top pharmacologists in his research hub at Utah, including George Sayers, Mark Nickerson, Herbert L. Borison, Dixon Woodbury, and Don W. Esplin, all winners of the John Jacob Abel Prize. Beyond his academic notoriety, Goodman also carried enduring ties to pivotal pharmaceutical companies and the most heralded scientists working in them—including Harold Clymer and Bryce Douglas at Smith Kline and French, William Creasy at Burroughs-Wellcome, and Barney Pisha at Hoffmann-La Roche. Gilman went on to win the Nobel Prize in Medicine, but in the 1960s and 1970s, he connected less with the academic and industry pharmacology community, while his co-author Goodman engaged more and more. Finally, and as significant as any other reason, Goodman's papers were widely read in congressional committees investigating the ethical drug industry and the FDA. As Hubert Humphrey (then U.S. vice president but formerly a pharmacist and a senator on one of the FDA's oversight committees) would remind Goodman in a 1965 letter, "excerpts from your papers proved to be our best source of guidance as laymen."[22]

In the 1960s and 1970s, Goodman kept an ongoing series of notes for revision of the *Pharmacological Basis of Therapeutics*, for deployment in his medical school lectures, for communications with his longtime friend Gilman, and for occasional essays in medical and scientific journals. In these sketches of academic thought and clinical practice, he often discussed what he perceived to be the "role," "function," "position," and "job" of the Administration. The tasks that Goodman assigned to the FDA derived not so

[22]Smith to Goodman, May 10, 1965; Goodman to Smith, May 24, 1965; Vice President Hubert Humphrey to Goodman, April 29, 1965; Hallowell Davis (Section of Physiology, National Academy of Sciences) to Goodman, April 29, 1965; LSG. *The Pharmacological Basis of Therapeutics*, also known as "Goodman and Gilman" among pharmacologists and thousands of medical students, is often referred to as "the bible of pharmacology" within academic and medical circles. Goodman also served on the AMA Committee on Drugs and was elected in 1965 to the National Academy of Sciences. On his mentorship of top pharmacologists, see Goodman to Ellsworth B. Book (Executive Officer, ASPET), October 15, 1974; LSG. On ties to industry officials and scientists, see B. V. Pisha (Roche Laboratories) to Goodman, August 31, 1972; Goodman to Pisha, September 15, 1972; Douglas (Vice President, Smith, Kline and French) to Goodman, July 27, 1979; Clymer (Vice President, Research and Development, Smith, Kline and French) to Goodman, January 25, 1971; Goodman to Clymer, January 27, 1971; Creasy (President, Burroughs Wellcome) to Goodman, May 14, 1965; LSG.

much from law as from an ethics of pharmacology and sound medical practice. The world of pharmaceuticals, in this view, was less Morton Mintz's "Therapeutic Nightmare" and more a "Therapeutic Jungle," a chaotic state of national over-medication and mismatch of therapy to disease, a condition whose faults lay with government, the medical profession, and American business.[23]

Goodman's ethical worldview of medicine and drugs was one widely shared among scientists, academic physicians, journalists, and social critics. The notion that the United States was chronically "over-medicated" was commonly acknowledged in scientific and medical journals, intellectual outlets and newspapers. Pharmaceutical companies were widely seen as selfish and politically powerful corporate entities, a part of the "drug establishment" that Commissioner James Goddard decried in an *Esquire* article in 1969. Popular notions of physicians were bound up with distrust of the American Medical Association, still widely seen as a quasi-corporate trust. Patients and "the public" were fused in this view as needing institutional protection. They were perceived as subject to the whims of physicians who knew not what they were prescribing, and to companies marketing drugs to them directly and to their physicians.[24]

Goodman saw a protective role for the FDA in part because he observed a lack of ethical business practices among pharmaceutical manufacturers and, in particular, their marketing divisions. With other academic physicians and pharmacologists of his day, Goodman harbored enduring concerns about the mixture of profit-maximizing development and clinical research. And his distrust of many pharmaceutical companies came not from his knowledge of the persons who labored for them but from his perceptions about what happened when they took on the identities of their firms. "Many of the pharmaceutical co. people—both business & scientific personnel—are high-minded and capable as individuals," he penned in his notes. "I have trained some of them, I know many of them, and some contributed $ to our dept. and our Med. Center Bldg. Yet their activities as corporate entities often go far beyond the bounds of reasonableness and legitimacy." Pharmaceutical marketing was essentially untrustworthy. In teaching his medical students how to "keep abreast of new drug developments," his central point was "Don't read the ads." In this "jungle"-like world where patients and physicians could be so easily misled, the rationale for FDA regulation was

[23]Goodman handwritten notes for *Pharmacological Basis of Therapeutics*, undated, pp. 6, 8; Goodman, "A Global View of Drugs and Society," lecture notes, University of Utah, 1969, 1970, 1971; F 6, B50, LSG.

[24]David Cowen, "Ethical Drugs and Medical Ethics," *The Nation* 189 (22) (Dec. 26, 1959): 479–82; "The A.M.A. and the U.S.A.," *Time*, July 7, 1961, 56; Charlotte Muller, "The Overmedicated Society: Forces in the Marketplace for Medical Care," *Science* 176 (1972): 488–92; Goddard, "The Drug Establishment," *Esquire*, March 1969, 120–21; Mintz, *The Therapeutic Nightmare*; Jesse D. Rising, "The Practicing Physician's Approach to the Evaluation of New Drugs," *Canadian Medical Association Journal* 19 (Nov. 16, 1964): 1046–50. Goodman kept a folder of papers on "Medical Ethics" in which he had placed the Cowen article.

not a matter of efficiency, aggregate welfare, or even patient benefit. It was a matter of ethics. As he would underscore in his notes, the

> MORALITY of drug industry must be diff. than that of other industries because it affects public health and welfare. Federal regulation & self regulation are essential, & if the latter fails there must be more of the former.[25]

These portraits eventually surfaced in *The Pharmacological Basis of Therapeutics*. In the third edition of their text, first published in 1965 and reprinted continually through the late 1960s and early 1970s, Goodman and Gilman described American pharmaceutical regulation in generic and favorable terms. They ascribed pure motives to federal regulation and its originators. The penumbra of statutes and rules were "designed for the protection of the public health and for the protection of the physician from unethical practices of irresponsible manufacturers." Thanks to federal statute and its administrative enforcement, they stated, "physicians in practice today can prescribe drugs with the knowledge and confidence that they are essentially as represented by the manufacturers." So indebted were modern physicians to federal law and the Administration that Goodman and Gilman counseled their readers to lend a hand to the agency in realizing the goals of the law: "The physician should be familiar with the major provisions of the act and assist in every way with its enforcement." Beyond this, the general positive regard for the Administration went so far as to affect guidance for prescribing. Whereas an earlier generation of physicians and pharmacists had been counseled to prescribe by brand name, Goodman and Gilman explicitly rejected this view, maintaining that the FDA's regulation of drug equivalence was sufficiently trustworthy as to obviate this practice.

> It is often argued that prescribing by nonproprietary name permits the pharmacist to dispense preparations of inferior quality, and that this can be prevented by prescribing the proprietary name of a reputable manufacturer. However, this argument ignores the role of the FDA in assuring uniformity and quality of medicines.[26]

Harvard's Maxwell Finland was another advocate of pharmaceutical reform and also influential in medical, scientific, and regulatory circles. He

---

[25] Goodman handwritten notes for *PBOT*, undated, pp. 6, 8; "Advice to Students & M.D.s: How to Keep Abreast of New Drug Developments," Lecture Notes; F 6,.B50, LSG. I have not corrected these notes for orthography; underlining in original. In the late 1950s and 1960s, academic physicians worried continually about how their medical students approached drug advertising and "detail men"; Solomon Garb, "Teaching Medical Students to Evaluate Drug Advertising," *Journal of Medical Education*, 35 (8) (Aug. 1960): 729–39.

[26] Louis S. Goodman and Alfred Gilman, *The Pharmacological Basis of Therapeutics*, 3rd ed. (5th printing) (New York: Macmillan, 1968), 31, 33. The argument against which Goodman and Gilman were counseling had been characterized by Rutgers historian David Cowen in 1959. Presaging Goodman and Gilman's claim that brand names carried no special value because of the uniformity induced by FDA regulation, Cowen argued that "increased governmental supervision, through the FDA, would be needed to guarantee the integrity of the 'USP' legend" ("Ethical Drugs and Medical Ethics," 481–2).

had consulted with the Administration's Antibiotics Division in the early 1950s, had defended the agency's rejection of the drug Altafur in 1961, had championed efficacy standards at the 1960 and 1961 Kefauver hearings (corresponding with Kefauver himself about the content of the legislation), and would assist the Administration regularly in the 1960s. Finland surveyed the state of American medicine in 1957 and saw a vacuum of responsible drug regulation; no authority was carefully and vigorously keeping tabs upon drug promotion and development, especially for the newest molecules. The U.S. Pharmacopeia, "while still the bulwark of American Medicine," was too little used and was of poor guidance for new drugs. The AMA's Council on Drugs had surrendered its approval process and "now merely serves to collect data for the publication of the so-called 'monographs' on new drugs usually appearing sometime after they have been pretty well 'sold' to the public by the manufacturer." The FDA, for its part, "has failed to exercise the restraining influence which the people and the medical profession have a right to expect from their representatives." Alone among the institutions he blamed in 1957 for the drug malaise, the Administration served as a representative of "the people" and the American medical profession. The limitations he perceived in the agency were attributable to its lack of legal authority and the need for independent, external advice. He strongly favored additional FDA control over the "quality and effectiveness of products before and after their release for sale." And like other clinical pharmacologists, Finland favored a more expansive FDA role in the postmarketing regulation of new drugs.[27]

Along with celebrity academicians like Goodman and Finland, the clinical pharmacology audience was represented in new publications emerging in the area of "therapeutics." Most notable among these was the *Medical Letter on Drugs and Therapeutics*, launched in January 1959 and published by Drug and Therapeutic Information, Incorporated of New York. Along with Modell's *Clinical Pharmacology and Therapeutics*, the *Medical Letter* served to create a subprofessional audience outside of the mainline medical journals—the *Journal of the American Medical Association*, the *New England Journal of Medicine*, the *Annals of Internal Medicine*, and the like. The letter's executive director was Arthur Kallet of the Consumers' Union, and Manhattan physician Harold Aaron served as chairman of its editorial board.

[27]Kefauver to Finland, September 22, 1960; Finland to Kefauver, October 10, 1960. B 2, F 24 ("FDA"); MF. Finland began consulting the Division of Antibiotics as early as August 1952, when his expertise was requested by the FDA on chloramphenicol and its association with blood dyscrasias; R. Keith Cannan (Director, Division of Medical Sciences, NAS-NRC) to Finland, December 8, 1960, F 3, B 2 ("National Research Council, 1931–1978"); MF. On his assistance to the FDA in the Altafur case, see Finland to Joseph Garland (Editor, *NEJM*), January 12, 1961; Finland to Paul F. MacLeod (Eaton Laboratories), January 12, 1961; B 3, F 36 ("Miscellaneous, Pubs and Reprints"), MF. Finland to Thomas Bradley (professional associate, National Academy of Sciences), April 16, 1957; F 3, B 4 ("National Research Council, 1931–1978"), MF. For advocacy of efficacy standards, see Finland to K. F. Meyer (UCSF Medical Center), February 13, 1961; B2, F24 ("FDA"), MF.

The *Medical Letter* billed itself as "a non-profit publication," though its industry-aligned detractors would argue that Kallet, Aaron, and others profited indirectly and materially from its success. It served as a voice of consumer protection and conservative therapeutics—so much so that Aaron and Kallet were attacked as Communists and therapeutic "nihilists." Linus Pauling accused the editors of "bias and malice" after the *Letter* published a negative review of the Stanford chemist's *Vitamin C and the Common Cold* (1976). Yet none of these controversies slowed the *Medical Letter*'s popularity—by 1977 its editors could count over 100,000 subscribers in the United States and Canada and another 20,000 in Latin America who received the Spanish edition. Just as the *Medical Letter* backed the new pharmacological regime centered in the FDA, its editors would continually scrutinize and lament many of the FDA's drug approval decisions. Administration decisions to approve new drugs such as the antibiotics cephapirin and cephradine were blasted in the *Medical Letter*, to the extent that Goodman and Gilman saw fit to exclude these drugs from their textbook.[28]

The Administration's good favor with top academic pharmacologists would help to buffet it against criticism in the wake of some of its more controversial regulatory moves. One of these came in 1969 when the FDA acted to remove the Upjohn Company's combination antibiotic Panalba from the American market. Panalba was a combination of novobiocin and tetracycline that was found "ineffective as a fixed combination" by a NAS/NRC review panel. The regulation of fixed-combination antibiotics brought up some of the stickiest issues in pharmaceutical regulation. Both novobiocin and tetracycline had long been certified as effective antibiotics; either of the compounds could be marketed, prescribed, and utilized alone. The question was whether the combination of novobiocin and tetracycline possessed a broader spectrum of antibacterial activity than either molecule used by itself. Once this question was asked, however, it immediately raised politically contentious issues of "comparative efficacy." In the Kefauver hearings and in legislative debates over the 1962 law, opponents of reform (who begrudgingly supported the bill in the wake of Frances Kelsey's public triumph) stated consistently that the new law would give the FDA power to judge a drug's effectiveness as against a baseline, but would not judge one drug's efficacy as against another. Beyond its political ramifications, the evaluation of combination antibiotics also raised difficult and novel issues of scientific and statistical inference. Regulatory practice and statute had generally required efficacy to be tested against a null hypothesis; the prospect that

[28] *The Medical Letter on Drugs and Therapeutics* (New York, New York; 1959–); Harold Aaron to Goodman, October 30, 1968; Louis Lasagna to Kallet, September 2, 1971; LSG. Linus Pauling, *Vitamin C and the Common Cold* (San Francisco: W. H. Freeman, 1970); "Vitamin C and the Common Cold," *MLDT*, 12 (26) (312) (Dec. 25, 1970); Pauling to Aaron, February 16, 1971; LSG. On subscription totals, see Aaron to Goodman, September 11, 1975; Aaron to Goodman, December 27, 1976; LSG. Goodman would attach the moniker "junkapirin" to cephapirin; Goodman to Gilman November 4, 1974; LSG.

a medicine had "some" efficacy would be assessed against the baseline of "zero" efficacy. If the "null hypothesis" of zero efficacy could be rejected, then the alternative hypothesis of efficacy could be accepted. Yet combination antibiotics clouded this neat and tidy statistical framework in at least two ways. First, the baseline had disappeared. No longer was a drug's efficacy being compared against zero; it was being compared against the efficacy of another drug, which was itself a random variable. Second, the combination antibiotic was being assessed not just against any other drug, but against two or more of its own components, each of them acting alone. There was no randomized, controlled trial pitting Panalba against novobiocin or tetracycline alone, and on this basis, the NAS/NRC panels did not find adequate evidence of efficacy. Accordingly, the Administration removed certification from all novobiocin-tetracycline combinations in May 1969, a rule that essentially banned Panalba's marketing. The Upjohn Company sued the agency a month later, arguing that it had been denied a full judicial hearing and asking the U.S. Sixth Circuit Court of Appeals to revoke the decertification order.[29]

Perhaps the most notable feature of the case came when Louis Lasagna filed a signed affidavit accompanying the Upjohn lawsuit with the Sixth Circuit. In the affidavit, Lasagna not only vouchsafed for Panalba's efficacy, he also defended all combination antibiotics and, more stridently, trashed the NAS/NRC review panels that had cast doubt upon them. The review committees had been driven by "personal opinion and experience (including 'uncontrolled' and unpublished trials)," he wrote, and the NAS/NRC findings on combination antibiotics "should not be regarded as final, conclusive, or irrevocable scientific determinations, decisions or recommendations."[30]

At the core of Lasagna's apologia for Panalba was an emergent libertarian argument with two strains. First, echoing Upjohn's legal defense, Lasagna argued that the Administration's procedures were by definition a denial of due process. Once a product of any sort had been marketed, any governmental decision to remove it from the market, Lasagna felt, should be subject to full judicial proceedings. "It seemed to me important," he would later write to Goodman, "for the company to have their day in court." In this sense Lasagna's frustration stemmed with the administrative character of the regulation. As he would later confide to the editors and advisers of the *Medical Letter,*

I have never prescribed Panalba in my life, and probably never would have. My main objection to the way this problem was handled was that it did not represent

---

[29]William M. M. Kirby (Professor of Medicine, University of Washington School of Medicine, Seattle), "Fixed Combinations of Antibiotics," testimony before the Monopoly Subcommittee of the Senate Small Business Committee, May 6, 1969.

[30]"Lasagna Says Panalba Is Effective," *FD&CR*, November 17, 1969, 10; "Combination's Efficacy Backed, Hearing Urged: Dr. Lasagna Disputes FDA on Panalba Ruling," *Medical Tribune*, December 15, 1969, 1, 18.

due process. I have always believed that one should back liberty no matter who was involved.[31]

Lasagna's second argument for Panalba was a novel defense of the therapeutic marketplace. If so many physicians were prescribing Panalba in their clinical practice, Lasagna argued, then their aggregated judgment created a scientific rationale for Panalba's continued marketing. The FDA's regulations on fixed-combination therapies were "scientifically unreasonable" under this logic, mainly due to their insistence upon randomized, blinded, and controlled trials as the basis of efficacy demonstrations. The Administration failed to "accord any weight to clinical studies that do not meet requirements of the regulation or to extensive, well-documented clinical experience with drug products." The symbolic battle of "rigor versus testimony" had commenced again, but testimony now included informally accumulated medical observations that were "well-documented," a criterion that Lasagna never defined. Later, in April 1971, Lasagna penned a *Wall Street Journal* editorial in which he argued that aggregated medical opinion could effectively serve as a legal basis for drug marketing even in the wake of the 1962 Kefauver-Harris Amendments. A "respectable minority opinion" favorable to a drug's efficacy should be regarded as sufficient for FDA approval. To make his point emotive and tangible, he again took space to score the NAS/NRC review panels and their recommendations: "I'm not sure which metaphor is apt, Pandora's box or Frankenstein's monster, but the results are frightening to view."[32]

Lasagna's advocacy for Panalba was risky and vocal, and it marked the beginning of a steady decline in his status among medical academicians. Lasagna's name was golden in the 1950s, when he had authored pathbreaking papers on the placebo response and clinical trial design, when he had founded the nation's first clinical pharmacology department at Johns Hopkins, and when he had testified in support of efficacy standards at the Kefauver hearings in 1960. In siding with Upjohn, Lasagna had aligned himself with one of America's oldest and most notable pharmaceutical companies, but in the process he had reversed his own judgment on combination antibiotics. FDA General Counsel William Goodrich stated flatly that Lasagna's rhetoric "stands in bold contradiction to every scientific precept he has advocated publicly and to his profession." Indeed, as late as February 1969, just nine months before the Upjohn affidavit was filed, Lasagna had signed a statement holding that promotion of pain relief combinations encouraged

[31]Lasagna to Arthur Kallet, September 2, 1971; LSG. See also Lasagna to Goodman, October 25, 1971; LSG. Lasagna also called for an "evidentiary hearing" and rehearsed the due process claim in an April 1971 *Wall Street Journal* editorial; "FDA 'Efficacy' Rule: Does It Work?" *WSJ*, April 8, 1971, 12.

[32]"Lasagna Says Panalba Is Effective"; "Combination's Efficacy Backed, Hearing Urged,"; Lasagna, "FDA 'Efficacy' Rule: Does It Work?" *WSJ*, April 8, 1971, 12; "Drug Efficacy Study: FDA Yields on Fixed Combinations," *Science* 172 (June 4, 1971): 1013.

"bad therapeutics." FDA officials quickly reproduced other statements that Lasagna had published just years earlier, some disparaging the therapeutic marketplace's ability to aggregate valid information on efficacy, some doubting the capacity of individual physicians to make general therapeutic judgments. "It is a sad fact," Lasagna concluded in one of these refrains, "that the individual physician cannot really gauge the true worth of many remedies." Elsewhere, Lasagna's stance infuriated NAS/NRC panel chairmen, some of whom were "outright perturbed" with his rhetoric and its open publicity. At the *Medical Letter*, Lasagna's public stances became the subject of so much embarrassment and fretting that Arthur Kallet asked for his resignation from the journal's advisory board.[33]

Lasagna was stunned and apparently hurt by his dismissal from the *Medical Letter*, which he regarded as "one of the most depressing communications I have received." The Rochester pharmacologist responded with an angry three-page letter decrying Kallet's "disgraceful" action, which represented a "party-line approach" to therapeutics. Then, as he turned from the offensive to the defensive, Lasagna began to account for his odd and vocal stance on Panalba and to make his case that his stance on combination drugs was legitimate and respected, even if dissident. It was none other than the officials of the Administration itself who had retained their respect for Lasagna and his writings.

> At the same time that you were writing me your letter of dismissal, Dr. Henry Simmons, of the Food and Drug Administration, was in Vermont quoting my own published requirements for combination drugs as the basis upon which the FDA would move in the future. I am on Commissioner Edward's [sic] policy committee, and on the FDA Neuropharmacology Review Committee. In February I am going down to spend two weeks with the Food and Drug Administration to help them out in regard to their review procedures. Are these acts one of which the Medical Letter Editorial and Advisory Board members are ashamed?

To Kallet and his boards, Lasagna's message was a simple one: the FDA still relies upon me, and still retains my services as a consultant and official adviser. Why then does the *Medical Letter* alone "throw me off the Advisory Board"? Lasagna's plea marked an ironic but resounding affirmation of the Administration. Having attacked the FDA over its Panalba decision and its regulatory framework for efficacy review of marketed compounds, Lasagna turned around and relied upon his links to the agency—including Nixon appointee Charles Edwards—as a defense of his public and professional legitimacy.[34]

[33] "Combination's Efficacy Backed, Hearing Urged; "Drug Efficacy Study: FDA Yields on Fixed Combinations." Kallet to Lasagna, August 23, 1971; Lasagna to Kallet, September 2, 1971; Kallet memo to Members of the Medical Letter Editorial and Advisory Boards, September 15, 1971; Mark H. Lepper to Kallet, September 16, 1971; Lasagna to Goodman, October 12, 1971; Goodman to Lasagna, October 20, 1971; Lasagna to Goodman, October 25, 1971; LSG.

[34] Lasagna to Kallet, September 2, 1971; LSG.

Lasagna pleaded with Louis Goodman for a favorable response and an intervention with the *Medical Letter*'s boards, but Goodman politely and firmly declined. Goodman worried that Aaron and Kallet had erred in "dropping you," he wrote Lasagna, but "in view of the great service of the *Medical Letter* to the medical profession, it would be wrong for members of the Advisory Board to withdraw their services." Beyond this, Goodman's letter intimated a subtle but genuine decline of respect for Lasagna. He chided Lasagna for his written outbursts and confided that "I must tell you in all frankness that your support of Panalba came as a surprise to me."[35]

The diverging paths of Louis Goodman and Louis Lasagna marked the splintering audiences of the Food and Drug Administration as well as the agency's enduring scientific legitimacy. In the status-conscious world of academic medicine, Louis Lasagna never fully recovered from the Panalba battle. By 1970, Lasagna had left the heights of Johns Hopkins pharmacol-ogy—the home of John Jacob Abel and Eugene M. K. Geiling—for the University of Rochester, where he founded the industry-funded Center for the Study of Drug Development whose researchers would contribute to public and congressional perceptions of "the drug lag." His correspon-dence with star academicians such as Goodman, Maxwell Finland, Alfred Gilman, Henry Beecher, and others all but vanished. Lasagna's status had not disappeared, but his currency among academic pharmacologists had declined appreciably. He would publish more in opinion outlets than in top medical journals, and he would not receive the sort of career recognition enjoyed by Finland, Goodman, and Gilman. Later in his career Lasagna would move his Center for the Study of Drug Development to Tufts University in Massachusetts, where he became Dean of the Tufts Medical School.[36]

Goodman would remain aligned with the *Medical Letter*, would continue publishing the world's most authoritative pharmacology text, and would maintain his esteem for the Administration and its Bureau of Drugs. Gilman and Finland would serve on the governing committee of the NAS/NRC Drug Efficacy Review Study and would continually support the FDA's most aggressive regulatory actions. Other luminaries such as Wesley Spink and William M. M. Kirby would continue to question the agency's doubters. And the disciples of these luminaries—the award-winning students of Good-man, Gilman, Finland, Spink, Kirby, and others—would generally reaffirm their mentors' respect for American pharmaceutical regulation. In the world of clinical pharmacology and academic medicine, debate over the FDA—its powers, its officials, its practices—would persist and flourish. Yet suffusing this discourse was a general deference to the Administration that, by the early 1970s, had become a fact of the medical academy.

[35]Goodman to Lasagna, October 20, 1971; LSG.

[36]Characterizations of Lasagna correspondence are based upon registers of letters received and sent in the Louis C. Lasagna Papers, University of Rochester.

AUDIENCES WITHIN THE OVERSEER: THE PRODUCTION
OF REPUTATION IN CONGRESSIONAL HEARINGS

What an agency's audiences see in the organization depends directly upon what is shown to them, and who presents it. To be sure, organizational reputations cannot be manipulated endlessly. Nor is an organizational reputation the kind of thing that can be perfectly controlled by the organization itself, its friends, or its enemies. Yet the purposeful depiction of an administrative agency—in terms favorable or unkind, or both—is a constant feature of American national politics since the early twentieth century. In the continuous crystallization of the FDA's organizational reputation, no structural interface has been more consequential than the committees of the U.S. Congress. The properties and ascriptions various audiences saw in the FDA were most often those that had been presented—explicitly or inadvertently, but always with some set of intentions and emotions—in congressional hearings.[37]

The relationship between a national legislature and administrative agencies is usually conceived as a hierarchical one, and for good reason. In republican democracies founded upon popular sovereignty, electoral representation, and the rule of law, acts of the legislature create, enable, constrain, and even terminate agencies. The committee systems of many legislatures, including the U.S. Congress, allow a busy, multifaceted council to effectively monitor and instruct the organizations that transform its statutes into policy. Hearings are the most familiar and publicized mechanism of agency monitoring. Yet even as they function as instruments of constraint and revelation, legislative hearings have two juridical features that allow for the production of agency reputations. First, hearings are formally adversarial and they embed political conflict. The committee in question—particularly its chair—establishes the agenda for a hearing, including the list of witnesses and the questions that will be posed. Yet if an agency is the target of inquiry, its officials will almost always have the opportunity to speak and defend their organization. Beyond this, for every majority party member scheduling a hearing to expose problems with a given agency, there is likely a minority member or a renegade legislator who insists upon revealing a different story. The second relevant feature of hearings is that they rely not upon speeches but upon testimony. Whether prepared or in response to questions from legislators, testimony often takes directions that were not anticipated, and observers can and usually do take note of the surprises and tangents. More commonly,

[37]To be sure, there were purposeful depictions of executive agencies in nineteenth-century congressional hearings as well, but the twentieth century has witnessed a stark rise in a particular kind of hearing and a particular kind of committee (or committee function): oversight. As a generalization, oversight hearings involving extensive testimony and demonstration of evidence from administrative agencies are a feature of the twentieth century much more so than the nineteenth. See John Mark Hansen, *Gaining Access: Congress and the Farm Lobby, 1919–1981* (Chicago: University of Chicago Press, 1991); also Carpenter, *The Forging of Bureaucratic Autonomy.*

congressional testimony includes many symbols that carry multiple and ambiguous meanings. These symbols appear as statements and images that quietly affirm one representation even as they openly negate another.[38]

The late twentieth century provided a lush context for the elaboration of
organizational reputations through congressional hearings. Numerous administrative agencies in the federal government—among them the Departments of Defense and Agriculture, the Interstate Commerce Commission and
the Federal Trade Commission, and the Environmental Protection Agency
and the Food and Drug Administration—were the subject of well-publicized
investigations. In part, the growth in number and breadth of congressional
hearings was dependent upon changes in the House and Senate committee
systems. As committees acquired greater autonomy in the twentieth century,
as linkages with national press organizations became more routine, and as
delegation to congressional subcommittees peaked in the 1970s and 1980s,
hearings more often reflected the interests of committee chairs who served
less at the preference of their party leaders and more by virtue of their accumulated tenure under the seniority systems of their chambers. While every
bit as strategic as before 1947, postwar congressional hearings embedded a
further element of randomness and the personal agenda.[39]

The double-edged implications of congressional hearings were evident
even during the height of the Administration's post-thalidomide glow. At the
same time that the Kefauver Committee praised Administration officials for
withholding Kevadon, new questions were arising about the anti-cholesterol

[38]These properties of congressional hearings have long been recognized by legislative scholars in political science. For exemplary studies of the political construction of congressional
hearings, see Hansen, *Gaining Access*; Richard L. Hall, *Participation in Congress* (New Haven:
Yale University Press, 1996); Kevin Esterling, *The Political Economy of Expertise: Information
and Efficiency in American National Politics* (Ann Arbor: University of Michigan Press, 2004);
Frank Baumgartner and Bryan Jones, *Agendas and Instability in American Politics* (Chicago:
University of Chicago Press, 1992).

[39]A pivotal institutional development in this era was the "Subcommittee Bill of Rights" of
1973, adopted by resolution of the House Democratic Caucus, which defined the rights and
powers of the subcommittees. As political scientists then and now have noted, the early 1970s
reforms in the House empowered the House leadership at the expense of committee chairs;
David W. Rohde, "Committee Reform in the House of Representatives and the Subcommittee
Bill of Rights," *Annals of the American Academy of Political and Social Science*, 411 (*Changing Congress: The Committee System*) (Jan. 1974), 39–47. Julian Zelizer, *On Capitol Hill: The
Struggle to Reform Congress and Its Consequences* (New York: Cambridge University Press,
2004). Eric Schickler, *Disjointed Pluralism* (Princeton: Princeton University Press, 2001).
    As political scientists have argued, delegation to committees is not necessarily abdication of
policy responsibility and is often consistent with centralized partisan objectives; Roderick
Kiewiet and Mathew McCubbins, *The Logic of Delegation* (Chicago: University of Chicago
Press, 1991); Gary Cox and McCubbins, *Legislative Leviathan*, 2nd ed. (New York: Cambridge University Press, 2006). Yet this portrait of "control despite delegation" holds more
readily for committee functions such as markup and bill reporting than it does for hearings.
The content of markup must eventually be affirmed by vote of the entire legislature in order to
have effect. Hearings as such are not subject to veto or modification by the larger chamber or
"floor" of the legislature.

drug MER/29 marketed by Kevadon's sponsor, the William Merrell Company. MER/29 was known chemically as triparanol and had been approved for its anti-cholesterol activity in June 1960. There were early questions about the strength of the evidence for its efficacy, and in the months after it was marketed, reports began to flow into the Bureau of Medicine about cataract formation in patients taking MER/29. For several months, these doubts were entertained mildly. But with the arrival of John Nestor to the Bureau in 1960, new data were demanded of Merrell. Merrell supplied data with such rapidity, data that all-too-perfectly refuted Nestor's concerns, that the agency decided to investigate. Echoing the confrontation of seven years earlier, FDA inspectors descended on the Cincinnati manufacturing facility of Richardson-Merrell in April 1962 in an unprecedented regulatory strike. Inspectors found evidence of falsified research reports involving chronic toxicity of MER/29 in monkeys. Monkeys that had died or fared poorly in the trials disappeared from the labs but were listed as having fared well in the clinical trial summaries. Merrell also withheld information on weight loss and liver and gall bladder damage that had been observed in monkeys taking MER/29. The inspectional investigations led to criminal charges against Merrell and its officials.[40]

National media outlets reported the MER/29 experience not as one of regulatory success but as one of system failure. *Washington Star* reporter Miriam Ottenberg wrote that the MER/29 story "illustrates what can happen with too little law, too much pressure, and too much responsibility resting on a single doctor." In March 1963, as the shock from the Administration's proposed rules on investigational new drugs began to settle in, and as something of a soul searching over thalidomide and MER/29 continued in clinical research communities, pharmaceutical firms, and at the FDA, Senator Hubert H. Humphrey announced a second set of hearings on drug regulation.[41]

Humphrey's star witness was Nestor, who had been with the Bureau of Medicine for less than two years, yet enough time to compile a battery of complaints about his organization. His testimony was withering. Nestor provided a laundry list of problems in new drug approval and post-marketing surveillance at the Bureau of Medicine. In some cases, data for approved new drugs did not substantiate safety, an allegation which if true revealed an

---

[40]The narrative here relies upon Greene, *Prescribing by Numbers* (159–64) and Hilts, *Protecting America's Health* (144–6); Hilts states that MER/29 was on the market by April 1960, whereas Greene remarks that the drug was approved by the FDA in June. Nestor's remarks on MER/29 appear in *ICDRR*, 785, 822. On the March 1954 inspection, see chapter 3 of this study. The criminal charges were leveled against Richardson-Merrell and associated companies, their pharmacologist E. F. van Maanen; laboratory chief William King; and VP Harold Werner. All three officials were indicted on charges of making false, fictitious, and fraudulent statements to the FDA about MER/29, and all three defendants entered a nolo contendere plea in March 1964. Insight Team of the Sunday Times of London, *Suffer the Children*, 67; Greene, *Prescribing by Numbers*, 161–3.

[41]Miriam Ottenberg, "The Story of MER/29—Was the Public Protected?" *Washington (Sunday) Star*, August 26, 1962.

open violation of not just the 1962 Amendments but also the 1938 law. Basic records were not kept, leaving the Administration ignorant of fundamental questions such as the status of therapies as "new drugs," as well as broader issues like the trustworthiness and behavior of a clinical investigator. Agreements with companies and clinical researchers were more likely to be made informally by telephone than fixed in writing. Alaska Senator Ernest Gruening called Nestor's statements "a shocking indictment of the administration of the Food and Drug Administration."[42]

Despite its caustic tone, Nestor's testimony reaffirmed the increasing trust the medical communities and Congress could place in FDA procedures. Nestor spoke of the centrality of the new drug application, and of how American society and American physicians could not trust any drug that had been put on the market "without the benefit of a New Drug Application." In other ways, Nestor's testimony showed evidence of vigorous and open disagreement within the Bureau of Medicine. Smith and Kessenich had given the conditional okay to MER/29 and the Division of Pharmacology had opposed approval. And Administration inspectors and medical officers had discovered Merrell's wrongdoing and had prosecuted the case aggressively.[43]

As Nestor's testimony suggests, MER/29's withdrawal and thalidomide might have spelled significant reputational trouble for the FDA and its regime of drug evaluation. The Bureau of Medicine had approved a drug that later had to be withdrawn, and for which the FDA's own Division of Pharmacology had opposed approval. Yet the financial press and medical publications alike tended to attribute the conditionality of the FDA's response to Merrell to the weakness of its formal powers, not the weakness of its resolve. The *Wall Street Journal* seemed to suggest that the agency's hunches were right all along. "The FDA, for some time," it noted, "has taken a dim view of the side effects of the drug."[44]

While national media outlets aggressively and thoroughly covered FDA oversight hearings, much of the relationship between Administration officials and congressional committees occurred out of public view. Long meetings between Bureau of Medicine administrators and committee staff were commonplace, both before and after hearings and as part of ongoing oversight of Administration activities. These meetings concerned everything from the major issues of the day to regulatory minutiae and internal FDA organization. At a three-hour meeting between officials from the Division of New Drugs and Fountain Committee staff in 1965, parties discussed the reorganization of the Bureau of Medicine (including patterns of mail flow), the role of pharmacologists in the Bureau, the workflow of new drug applications, coordination between offices of the Division of New Drugs, the

[42] *ICDRR* 777–807 (Nestor's remarks), 807 (Gruening).

[43] *ICDRR*, 797. The case pharmacologist was E. I. Goldenthal, and the medical officer in charge of the triparanol NDA was Frank J. Talbot; Hilts, *Protecting America's Health*, 144–5.

[44] "Richardson-Merrell Is Withdrawing Drug Used on Heart Patients; Side Effects Cited," *WSJ*, April 17, 1962. *ICDRR*, 902–4; Hilts, *Protecting America's Health*, 144–5.

method of informing firms about problems in an application, and research practices of FDA medical officers.[45]

With the consumer protection movement in full swing and the pace and number of hearings accelerating rapidly in the 1970s, the FDA would come in for regular and extensive scrutiny at the hands of different House and Senate committees. Commissioner Alexander M. Schmidt stated that in the three years of his tenure (1973–76), the agency had "averaged between 35 and 40 formal Congressional hearings a year, before 20 to 25 different Congressional subcommittees." Some of these hearings were perfunctory and reflected the odd amalgamation that had created the modern FDA, which combined elements from the USDA, the Federal Security Agency, and several public health agencies. Yet many of the hearings were discretionary and occupied days and weeks of the Administration's scarce time. Schmidt also stated in 1974 that, as an historical fact, the scrutiny from Congress was not only frequent but also fairly one-sided. "In all of the FDA's history," he told a panel, "I am unable to find a single instance where a Congressional committee investigated the failure of FDA to approve a new drug." Schmidt's statement has been repeated many times since in scholarship, in policy reports, and in drug lag rhetoric. In fact, the reality of congressional-FDA liaison in the 1970s is far more complicated than the Commissioner's portrait suggests. While many hearings did examine safety and procedural issues with approved drugs, there were hearings in which the Administration was criticized for slowing drug approval, including the review of thalidomide itself. And in the years immediately following Schmidt's tenure, the Senate would hold high-profile hearings in 1976, 1977, and 1978 that publicized the drug lag and investigated the Administration's effects upon pharmaceutical development (see table 5.6). Beyond these visible interventions, there were numerous cases in which legislators applied pressure behind the scenes and lobbied for approval of a particular drug. Yet like other brute characterizations of American pharmaceutical regulation, Schmidt's 1974 portrait persisted years afterward, not despite its simplified inaccuracy, but because of it.[46]

[45]Ralph Smith described the conversation as "cordial and informal." FDA officials at the meeting included Howard Cohn, Earl Meyers, and Ralph Smith; committee staff included W. Donald Gray (Senior Investigator) and Delphis Goldberg (Professional Staff Member) of the Intergovernmental Relations Subcommittee of the House Committee on Government Operations. Ralph G. Smith, "Memorandum of Interview," Subject "Handling of New Drug Applications," January 14, 1965; DF 505.5, RG 88, NA.

[46]Alexander M. Schmidt, "Great Expectations or Giving the FDA the Dickens," paper presented at the Health Industry Manufacturers' Association meeting, Scottsdale, Arizona, February 1976; quoted in Jeanne Herzog, *Recurrent Criticisms: A History of Investigations of the FDA*, (Rochester, NY: Center for the Study of Drug Development, University of Rochester Medical Center, March 1977). Peter Barton Hutt, "Investigations and Reports Respecting FDA Regulation of New Drugs (Part I)," *CP&T* 33 (1983): 537–48; "Investigations and Reports Respecting FDA Regulation of New Drugs (Part I)," *CP&T* 33 (1983): 537–48. Hutt estimates that in his four-year tenure (1971–75), he appeared before Congress "on about 80 occasions in 4 years"; personal communication, September 2008. Arthur Daemmrich, in reviewing the drug lag debate, interprets Hutt's summary as describing "a nearly unbroken series of Congressional

TABLE 5.6.
List of Congressional Hearings on Pharmaceutical Regulation at FDA, 1960–1980

Year	Chamber, Committee	Title
1961*	Senate, Judiciary (Subcommittee on Antitrust and Monopoly)	Drug Antitrust Act of 1961
1962	Senate, Judiciary (Subcommittee on Antitrust and Monopoly)	Drug Regulation Act of 1962
1963	Senate, Government Operations	Interagency Coordination in Drug Research and Regulation
1963		Regulatory Policies of the Food and Drug Administration
1967–	Senate, Small Business [Select]	Competitive Problems in the Drug Industry
1969, 1970	House, Commerce	FDA Consumer Protection Activities—FDA Reorganization
1971	House, Government Operations	Recall Procedures of the Food and Drug Administration
1971	House, Government Operations	Safety and Effectiveness of New Drugs [four sets of hearings]
1971	House, Government Operations	FDA Regulation of Oral Contraceptives
1972	House, Commerce	Food and Drug Administration Act
1972	House, Government Operations	FDA Regulation of the New Drug "Serc."
1972	House, Commerce	Review of Transitional Issues in Drug Amendments of 1962
1973	House, Government Operations	Safety of a New Combination Drug, Innovar
1974	Senate, Committee on Science, Commerce and Transportation	Food, Drug, and Cosmetic Amendments of 1974
1974*	Senate, Labor and Public Welfare	Regulation of New Drug R&D for the Food and Drug Administration
1974	Senate, Judiciary and Senate, Labor and Public Welfare	The Commissioner's Report of Investigation of Charges from Joint Hearings

TABLE 5.6.
cont.

Year	Chamber, Committee	Title
1975	House, Government Operations	Use of Advisory Committees by the Food and Drug Administration, Part 3
1975	House, Commerce	Regulatory Reform. Vol. 2: Federal Power Commission, Food and Drug Administration
1976	House, Government Operations	FDA's Regulation of the Drug "Triazure"
1976*	Senate, Judiciary and Senate, Labor and Public Welfare	Food and Drug Administration Practice and Procedure, 1976
1976	House, Commerce	Drug Safety Amendments of 1976
1977	House, Commerce	Prescription Drug Labeling and Price Advertising
1977	House, Commerce	Conflict of Interest in Regulatory Agencies
1977*	Senate, Human Resources	Banning of the Drug Laetrile from Interstate Commerce by FDA
1978*	Senate Human Resources [two hearings] House, Commerce	Drug Regulation Reform Act of 1978
1978	House, Commerce	"Man-in-the-Plant": FDA's Failure To Regulate Deceptive Drug Labeling
1979*	Senate, Labor and Human Resources	Drug Regulation Reform Act of 1979
1980	House, Commerce	"Man-in-the-Plant" Revisited— A Deceptive Drug Labeling Practice Continues
1980*	House, Commerce	Drug Regulation Reform—Oversight; New Drug Approval Process

*These rows reflect hearings at which concerns about slow drug approval or reduced innovation were voiced.

A more accurate portrait of congressional hearings in the 1960s and 1970s is that the Administration was continually appraised on numerous dimensions of evaluation and was criticized from many sides. For example, three different congressional committees publicly investigated the Administration's regulation of lysergic acid diethylamide (LSD) in the mid-1960s. As the Drug Abuse Control Amendments of 1965 had just been passed, these were issues high on the national legislative agenda. The FDA's partial but real responsibility for enforcement of illicit drug controls following the 1965 Amendments—anyone not holding an IND for the drug was required by the 1965 statute to turn over their supplies to the Administration—conflicted with its duty to regulate possible commercial development of the same substance. The second responsibility was triggered by Sandoz Pharmaceuticals' submission of a notice of claimed investigational exemption for LSD in 1963. In 1966, at least three different congressional subcommittees, each observing a different dimension of FDA behavior, used different criteria to praise and castigate the Administration. The Special Subcommittee on Juvenile Delinquency of the Senate Committee on the Judiciary, chaired by Connecticut Senator Thomas J. Dodd, expressed concern as to "why FDA allowed any kind of use of so dangerous a drug as LSD." The Subcommittee on Executive Reorganization of the Senate Committee on Government Operations, chaired by Massachusetts Senator Robert Kennedy, bespoke a different worry. Kennedy, whose wife Ethel had reportedly benefited from LSD treatment, argued that "we have given too much emphasis and so much attention to the fact that [LSD] can be dangerous," so much so that "we have lost sight of the fact that it can be very, very helpful in our society if used properly." As Administration officials privately interpreted Kennedy's remarks, the Senator was worried about "FDA interference with the scientific investigation of so promising a drug as LSD." Meanwhile the Subcommittee

---

hearings led by Estes Kefauver, Hubert Humphrey, Gaylord Nelson, Lawrence Fountain, and Edward Kennedy between 1959 and the mid-1980s"; "Invisible Monuments and the Costs of Pharmaceutical Regulation," 16, n.32.

On the character of congressional criticism, see Schmidt's testimony at *Regulation of New Drug R&D by the Food and Drug Administration*, Hearings before the Committee on Labor and Public Welfare, U.S. Senate, 93rd Congress, Second Session (Washington, DC: GPO, 1974), 207. Schmidt's statement would appear in Grabowski, *Drug Regulation and Innovation*, 76, and frequently thereafter in other venues. In a 2004 article in *Health Affairs*, I also quoted the statement without appreciation for the more complicated reality that it betrays; "The Political Economy of FDA Drug Approval: Processing, Politics, and Lessons for Policy," *Health Affairs* 23 (1) (Jan./Feb. 2004): 54. For a critique of the misuse of this statement, see Merrill, "Architecture." On the congressional investigation into the agency's non-approval of thalidomide, see Daemmrich, "Invisible Monuments," n.32. For one among many examples of congressional pressure for drug approval discussed at 1976 hearings, see the discussion of Mary Bruch, Merle Gibson, and Massachusetts Senator Edward Kennedy, *Food and Drug Administration Practice and Procedure, 1976,* Joint Hearing before the Subcommittee on Health of the Committee on Labor and Public Welfare and the Subcommittee on Administrative Practice and Procedure of the Committee on the Judiciary, U.S. Senate, 94th Congress, Second Session; hereafter cited as *FDAPP*, 81–2. See also discussion of the approval of cisplatin (Platinol) in chapter 7.

on Intergovernmental Relations of the House Committee on Government Operations, chaired by Lawrence Fountain, asked "whether FDA was effectively administering the law, regulations, and its own policies with respect to the control of LSD." In navigating among these shoals of committee audiences, Administration officials distinguished between "illegal distribution and use" and "legitimate use and investigation." The illegitimate modes of LSD were governed by the FDA's Bureau of Drug Abuse Control, while the legitimate modes of LSD were governed by Frances Kelsey and the Investigational New Drug Branch.[47]

The slew of hearings in the 1970s provides evidence of the feedback relationship between regulatory agencies, the burgeoning consumer protection movement, and the structure of Congress. The emergence of "consumer protection" as a theme and a rationale for federal legislation owed much to the transformation of American consumer culture more generally. The animating idea of new federal regulations in areas ranging from health and safety to antitrust was less to correct moral imbalances or to counter concentrated social and political power, but more to enhance the "interests" and "welfare" of consumers. The transformation of "citizen" to "consumer" as a primary identity for the American individual and family had been under way since the late 1800s, but it accelerated during the years following the Second World War. Yet the reverberation of this rhetoric in the chambers of Congress suggests that American consumerism was as much an institutional creation as a social movement. The consumer movement in the United States found much of its expression, embedment, and animation in the increasingly decentralized nature of the executive and legislative branches of American government.[48]

---

[47]Sandoz began experimentation with LSD in 1953, before an IND exemption was required. On the Administration's complicated stances toward LSD in the wake of the 1965 legislation, see "The Regulation of LSD Use," statement presented by Julius Hauser at the Medical Advisory Board, June 23, 1966; Minutes, FDA-BOM, Seventh Meeting of the Medical Advisory Board, June 23 and 24, 1966; Harry F. Dowling Papers, NLM. Commissioner Goddard and Assistant Commissioner Winton Rankin announced new controls in "Proposed Listing of Additional Drugs Subject to Control," FR 31 (11) (Jan. 18, 1966): 565; "Listing of Additional Drugs Subject to Control," FR 31 (54) (March 19, 1966): 4679–80. The Bureau of Drug Abuse control was headed by Administration official James Finlator. Kennedy's criticism of the agency's stance against LSD appears in Organization and Coordination of Federal Drug Research and Regulatory Programs: LSD, Hearings before the Subcommittee on Executive Reorganization of the Committee on Government Operations, U.S. Senate, May 24–26, 1966, (Washington: GPO, 1966), 72–5. Some useful if stridently written coverage of the FDA's regulation of LSD appears in Martin A. Lee and Bruce Shlain, Acid Dreams: The Complete Social History of LSD: The CIA, The Sixties, and Beyond (New York: Grove Press, 1985), esp. 79.

[48]For a survey of developments in antitrust that highlights its transformation from civic republican discourse to the "procedural republic" of neutrality, see Michael Sandel, Democracy's Discontent (Cambridge: Harvard University Press, 1998). On the evolution of consumer culture in the United States, see William Leach, Land of Desire (New York: Vintage, 1994); Cohen, A Consumer's Republic, esp. chap. 8; Jacobs, Pocketbook Politics. On the decentralization of the executive and legislative establishments in this period, see Hugh Heclo, "Issue Networks and the Executive Establishment," in Anthony King, ed., The New American Political

No episode better typified the new environment than the hearings on oral contraceptives held by Wisconsin Democrat Gaylord Nelson in 1970. Nelson chaired the Senate Committee on Small Business Practices and in 1968 commenced a long-running series of hearings under the theme "Competitive Problems in the Drug Industry." Nelson's sessions in 1968 echoed the themes that Estes Kefauver had identified a decade before: drug pricing, lack of competition within therapeutic classes, concern about the activities of pharmaceutical industry "detail men" and whether they were regulated with sufficient stringency. In evaluating the Administration, Nelson and his committee provided general support and praise for FDA drug safety efforts.[49]

In December 1969, however, after reading Barbara Seaman's critique of oral contraceptives, *The Doctor's Case Against the Pill* (1969), Senator Nelson announced a new set of inquiries into the safety of oral contraceptives. What followed were some of the most watched and influential hearings in the history of the U.S. Congress. In January 1970, as Nelson and his witnesses—not one of them a woman—discussed the safety risks associated with oral contraceptive use, women by the hundreds of thousands began to abandon oral contraceptives in favor of more traditional (and less effective) birth control methods. Requests for intrauterine devices (IUDs) and diaphragms at the nation's Planned Parenthood Clinics skyrocketed, diaphragm queries rising tenfold and IUD queries doubling in Detroit during the four weeks in which Nelson held hearings. *Business Week* estimated a fivefold increase in diaphragm sales nationwide. The hearings received daily, front-page coverage in the nation's major newspapers and headliner attention on the nightly news broadcasts of the major syndicates.[50]

The Nelson hearings followed the release of the *Second Report on the Oral Contraceptives*, issued by the Administration's Advisory Committee on Obstetrics and Gynecology. The Committee generally vouchsafed for the safety of the drugs but also presented evidence of cardiovascular risks associated with their use. As gynecologists, epidemiologists, and cardiovascu-

---

System (Washington, DC: American Enterprise Institute, 1978); Charles O. Jones and Randall Strahan, "The Effect of Energy Politics on Congressional and Executive Organization in the 1970s," *Legislative Studies Quarterly* (May 1985): 154–5; Roger H. Davidson and Walter J. Oleszek, *Congress Against Itself* (Bloomington: Indiana University Press, 1977); David C. King, *Turf Wars: How Congressional Committees Claim Jurisdiction* (Chicago: University of Chicago Press, 1997); Eric Schickler, *Disjointed Pluralism: Institutional Innovation and the Development of the U.S. Congress* (Princeton: Princeton University Press, 2001).

[49]In these hearings, Administration officials felt that "Senator Nelson strongly endorsed the FDA position"; FDA-BOM, Medical Advisory Board, Sixteenth Meeting, October 3, and 4, 1968; Harry F. Dowling Papers, NLM.

[50]The "Nelson hearings" appear as part of the goliath collection, *Competitive Problems in the Drug Industry*, Hearings before the Subcommittee on Monopoly, U.S. Senate, 14 volumes (Washington, DC: GPO, 1967–). My understanding of the Nelson hearings and the issues surrounding oral contraceptives has benefited greatly from reading Watkins, *On the Pill*, 107–20. See also Lara V. Marks, *Sexual Chemistry: A History of the Contraceptive Pill* (New Haven: Yale University Press, 2001), 150–51. Four women would testify at the second set of Nelson hearings in February 1970; Watkins, *On the Pill*, 118.

lar specialists, echoed by consumer safety advocates, subjectively enumerated the risks of oral contraceptive use, the Administration was immediately attacked from two angles. In Congress and in national media coverage, audiences began to doubt the basis on which the pills received FDA approval. How could these medicines have reached the market, critics wondered, without adequate tests for their long-term safety? Beyond the fact of approval, physicians testifying at the Nelson hearings berated the FDA for supplying so little information to women using the pill. "Never in history," declared Hugh Davis of Johns Hopkins in a widely televised statement, "have so many individuals taken such potent drugs with so little information as to actual and potential hazards."[51]

A second line of attack came from feminist organizations such as D.C. Women's Liberation who, for a time, identified oral contraceptives with the male-dominated medical profession and those with the FDA. Here the Administration was represented by Charles C. Edwards, President Nixon's first Commissioner of Food and Drugs, who repeated the decades-old refrain among FDA officials that patients should first consult their doctor about the pill but also insisted that American women "should continue to take it." It was Edwards who embodied the FDA to Congress, and Edwards who met with members of the D.C. Women's Liberation Group in March 1970 (before storming out after an hour with HEW Secretary Robert Finch, who called the meeting a "waste of time"). And it was Edwards who would set in motion the Administration's response to the hearings and, indirectly, to Hugh Davis's indictment, by announcing the creation of the first "patient-package insert" for an orally administered prescription drug in February 1970 (see chapter 9).[52]

At their core, the Nelson hearings both evinced and undermined the immense social, economic, and political trust that American citizens had placed in the Administration. The hearings and the intense, searching exposure they received in national media outlets opened new concerns about the Administration's procedures, capacities, and limitations. How could a government agency that churned through drug dossiers in two years or less and that required six to twelve months of testing on investigational drugs possibly uncover safety problems that would emerge only after years of use? The criticism reverberating from the Nelson hearings touched the very facets of the Administration that were embodied by Frances Kelsey's tenure—attention to drug safety and enforcement of patient consent. These themes comprised pillars of the 1962 Amendments and the 1963 IND rules, so both themes struck at the core of the Administration reputation and its power. Yet as the hearings were digested in national, local, private, and professional

---

[51]The *Second Report on the Oral Contraceptives* is discussed at greater length in chapter 9. Watkins, *On the Pill*, 111.

[52]The regulatory apparatus of the patient-package insert, and the discord it introduced between the Administration and the general practitioner community in the United States, are discussed in chapter 9.

debates about the safety of oral contraceptives, Americans learned just how much trust their culture, their institutions, their economy, and their bodies had placed in the FDA. In a statement broadcast by NBC News on January 22, 1970, physician Victor Wynn pointed to the Administration's endorsement of oral contraceptives as the fundamental truth shaping their use and the national and international debate over them.

> The women in this country, and the women in Great Britain, and in Scandinavia, and in Australia, and in South America, are consuming oral contraceptive medications in the belief that they are considered safe by the American Food and Drug Administration and for no other reason, because they have no other way to assess the safety of this medication.[53]

Victor Wynn's statement was one of worry, not of praise. Yet as part of a larger critique of drug safety policy in the United States, his characterization reminded NBC viewers of the FDA's charge and its capacity. Like so much of the concern expressed in the rhetoric of consumer protection and FDA oversight of the 1970s and 1980s, Wynn's anxiety magnified abiding beliefs about how Americans and citizens worldwide trusted the judgments of the Administration.

A similar pattern of symbolic reinforcement through public criticism would mark other hearings in the 1970s and 1980s. Seizing upon the power granted to subcommittees by his party's congressional reforms, Democratic Senator Edward Kennedy of Massachusetts began to hold hearings on FDA issues in 1974. The witnesses included Nestor (still at the Administration) as well as other reformists like William Gyarfas, Marvin Seife, Julia Apter, and Carol Kennedy. FDA careerists described numerous inversions of the 1962 Amendments and FDA rules—medical officers putting the burden of proof upon claims of the drug's toxicity rather than upon the drug's safety claims, extensive undocumented consultation with pharmaceutical companies, and drug reviewers being overridden in their decisions without documentation or justification. Beyond renewed claims of industry bias, FDA dissidents also voiced their hypotheses as to what explained the "drug lag." Kennedy's hearings would continue through the 1970s and would form the basis for his ill-fated reform bill, the Drug Regulation Reform Act of 1978. As drug safety concerns were tossed about with worries of "industry bias" and "drug lag" anxieties, Administration officials rightly perceived that they were taking a fusillade from "all sides." Perhaps most damning were the quotable laments of the agency's own employees. Marvin Seife likened his organization to "a toothless tiger," while an insider in the Cardio-Renal Division in the Bureau of Drugs announced that his unit "could qualify for federal disaster relief."[54]

The Administration's own personnel conveyed various information and

---

[53]NBC Huntley-Brinkley Report, January 22, 1970; VTNA; quoted in Watkins, *On the Pill*, 111.

[54]*FDAPP*. Subcommittee power enabled Kennedy to hold his hearings. In 1976, Kennedy was chair neither of Labor and Public Welfare nor of Judiciary. But he served as chair of both of the subcommittees that hosted the 1976 hearings. For FDA officers' claims, see *FDAPP*, 349

symbols in these public dramas. Lower-level functionaries criticized their superiors and the companies that sponsored new medicines. They also took advantage of the platform given them by the hearings and boldly offered new proposals for legislative reforms. Top officials alternately conditioned, accepted, and reinterpreted the statements of their subordinates. More than anything else, the Administration's leadership pointed to powers and resources that the agency lacked. The agency was constrained by congressional thrift and by the importance of respecting medical autonomy. "FDA shouldn't play the role of doctor," said Commissioner Charles Edwards repeatedly, even as he counseled American physicians to change their prescribing practices with oral contraceptives. Later in the decade, Edwards' successor, Donald Kennedy, conceded that his agency's timeworn insistence that it regulated "drugs, not doctors" had lost credibility. The claim had the resonance, he admitted, of the National Rifle Association's refrain that "guns don't kill people; people kill people." He straightforwardly dismissed the distinction: "If you regulate drugs, devices, vaccines, radiological products, diagnostic products, you surely regulate practice."[55]

THE EXTENSION AND AFFIRMATION OF AUTHORITY: DESI, PANALBA, AND RULEMAKING

One of the quieter but nonetheless crucial victories in the institutionalization of reputation and power came in an encounter of the "new" regime with "old" commodities. In the Drug Efficacy Study Initiative of the 1960s and 1970s, the Administration's directive power was asserted in its ability to haul drugs from the market with minimal procedural effort. Its conceptual power was asserted in its ability to define "adequate and well-controlled studies." Pivotal court decisions strengthened the agency's reputation of invincibility in judicial venues, while judges and other observers saw sufficient technical reputation in the FDA that legitimacy did not require an administrative hearing for each and every drug withdrawal.

The passage of the Kefauver-Harris Amendments solved many a regulatory problem for the Administration, but it also created some new ones.

(industry bias); 140, 189, 199, 211, 353 (drug lag), 364, 371–2 (undocumented contacts); 80 ("toothless tiger"), 126 ("disaster relief").

For another case where top Administration officials frankly admitted that their administrative practices violated federal statute, see Peter Barton Hutt's admissions before California Democrat John Moss's committee in 1978; U.S. House of Representatives, Committee on Interstate and Foreign Commerce, Subcommittee on Oversight and Investigations, *"Man-in-the-Plant—FDA's Failure to Regulate Deceptive Drug Labeling,"* Report, 95th Congress, Second Session (Washington, DC: GPO, December 1978), 9–10, 14.

[55] Many FDA officials —particular Bureau of Drugs director J. Richard Crout in his perceptive essay "The Nature of Regulatory Choices" (*FDCLJ* 33 (1978)) —realized that there were two stock narratives, one story (from consumer safety activists) of the Administration as captured by industry and another story (from industry and its allies) of the agency as too cautious. For Edwards' remark, see his "Address to the Institute of Medicine" in October 1977.

Perhaps the thorniest issue concerned how to regulate the thousands of drugs that had been cleared from 1938 to 1962, but that had not been officially reviewed for their effectiveness. This issue was not a merely academic query. The medicines reviewed in the two decades before 1962 now suffused therapeutic practice among generalist and specialist physicians alike.

The Amendments precluded any default policy of "grandfathering" the pre-1962 approvals. The statute exempted pre-1962 approvals from effectiveness requirements for two years (until October 10, 1964) to give their manufacturers time to gather "substantial evidence" of effectiveness for indications claimed in the labeling, unless such evidence was already published. Drug makers would in fact receive much more than two years because much of the available information was deemed "inadequate" by FDA officials, because the agency was slow to commence its review, and because scarce administrative resources in the Bureau of Medicine were being diverted to new drug review and investigational drug review.[56]

Accompanying the procedural questions were fundamental issues of legitimacy, reputation, politics, and power. Who would decide whether an already marketed drug was effective? FDA officials, including George Larrick and his successor, James K. Goddard, approached this issue with some trepidation. They knew intuitively that the regulation of pre-1962 approvals would signify the most raw extension of Administration power. When a new drug had yet to be introduced into interstate commerce, the FDA's judgments about its efficacy stuck in part because they were announced in a vacuum of previous assessments. Yet where patients and practitioners had already used these drugs on a massive scale, the evaluation of efficacy became a much more direct intervention into medical practice, a potentially open upheaval of thousands upon thousands of individualized therapeutic choices. A related political question was just how far to press the review. Some of the suspect drugs were popular therapies. They had enriched their manufacturers, so much so that the companies in question possessed deep pockets and enduring political connections. The Administration's leaders faced a tension between wishing not to antagonize larger companies and other powerful interests, and wishing to make sure that efficacy requirement meant something. Because decisions about how to apply efficacy to pre-1962 drugs would establish multidimensional precedents—precedents that were legal, regulatory, scientific, and political—the question of legitimacy was forefront.[57]

[56]The new authority was embedded in Section 505(e) of the Food, Drug and Cosmetic Act, 21 U.S.C. 355(e). For an accessible summary, see Paul A. Bryan and Lawrence H. Stern, "The Drug Efficacy Study, 1962–1970," *FDA Papers* (Oct. 1970): 14–15. As many as twenty drugs from 1938–62 period have not been reviewed under DESI.

[57]One facilitating factor was the definition of "new drug" as any drug not "generally recognized as safe for its intended uses," language that had been specified in the 1938 Food, Drug and Cosmetic Act. Hence, previously approved drugs could be regarded as "new ones" when there was a lack of general recognition as to safety and efficacy. Yet any application of this standard would have begged the questions of what "general recognition" meant and who would stand as the arbiter of this criterion.

A final question entailed procedural and political dimensions; it concerned how to go about the process of reviewing the drugs and, where necessary, removing them from the marketplace. This question put some difficult issues before the Adminstration's leaders, especially its General Counsels William Goodrich and (later) Peter Barton Hutt and Richard A. Merrill. Removal of an already marketed product from interstate commerce usually required a mechanism with judicial properties such as a formal adjudication hearing. This principle was embedded in longstanding federal law, not least the Federal Food, Drug and Cosmetic Act itself, and had been enshrined in the Administrative Procedure Act of 1946. Yet to conduct a separate hearing for each of the more than 4,000 drugs reviewed would have rendered the law null in its effect. Drugs that were questioned would have remained on the market for decades while the hearings and court battles wore on. The problem was that legislative rulemaking, or issuing "agency rules with the force of law," was not standard practice in American pharmaceutical regulation in the 1960s. The problem of pre-1962 drugs compelled the FDA to rethink its regulatory practices in a way that other federal agencies had done.[58]

The crucial decisions on pre-1962 drugs were undertaken by new Commissioner James L. Goddard. Goddard's appointment in January 1966 was greeted with a mixture of relief and unease. On the one hand, many audiences felt that George Larrick had been unable to shepherd the agency through implementation of the 1962 law and the 1963 rules. On the other hand, Goddard entered the Commissioner's office as something of an unknown personality to the industries regulated by the agency. He had not been mentioned as a front-runner for the post being vacated by Larrick, and his previous experience was in aviation medicine and public health. He came to the FDA from his post as chief of the federal Communicable Disease Center in Atlanta. In speech and in action, Goddard immediately struck a confrontational pose toward the organized pharmaceutical industry. Trade journals predicted the end of "gamesmanship" in FDA-industry relations. Within months of Goddard's appointment, many of the drug industry's worst fears had been confirmed. Goddard began his tenure by excoriating companies and their research practices. And to add action to the rhetoric, the Administration began a criminal prosecution of Merck for allegedly falsifying the results of animal trials in its development of its new anticancer drug, MK-665. Goddard was well-versed on the case and followed it closely.[59]

James Goddard would serve just two and a half years as Commissioner of Food and Drugs, but his choices on how to implement the review of pre-1962

[58] M. Elizabeth Magill, "Agency Choice of Policymaking Form," *University of Chicago Law Review* 71 (2004): 1383–1447. Peter Barton Hutt informs me that legislative rulemaking "was standard practice for promulgating food standards of identity" (personal correspondence, Nov. 14, 2008).

[59] "End of "Gamesmanship in FDA-Industry Regulatory Battles Among Major Changes from Appointment of PHS' Dr. James Goddard as FDA Head: Respect in Congress," *FDCR*, January 17, 1966, 3–8. The CDC is now known as the Centers for Disease Control and Prevention. Trade journals trained their attention on the Bureau of Medicine to see what changes

drugs established precedents as far-reaching as any in the Administration's history. In June 1966, Goddard announced a twin institutional strategy. First, the Administration would formally contract with the National Academy of Sciences (in particular its National Research Council) to review the full set of drugs for which an NDA became effective from 1938 to 1962. Goddard's tactic carried advantages for both reputation and resources. Review by the NAS/NRC would provide legitimacy for the agency's most difficult and contentious judgments and would allow Goddard to overcome the expected objection that his agency had insufficient staff resources (both in numbers and in training) to carry out the review. Goddard's second stratagem was to announce and effectuate the agency's decisions as much as possible by publication of orders in the *Federal Register*, thereby carrying out enforcement by acts of rulemaking.[60]

The Administration and the National Academy established thirty different committees to review pre-1962 drugs. The deadline for manufacturers to submit new evidence of effectiveness was reset at January 4, 1967 for antibiotics and at September 6, 1966 for all other drugs. By April 15, 1969, the NAS/NRC panels had issued 2,824 reports that offered efficacy assessments on 4,349 different drug products. Goddard and other FDA leaders agreed with Academy officials that these reports would remain confidential until the Administration published them in the *Federal Register*. The Bureau of Medicine would then digest the reports, examine other literature, and assign the reviewed drugs into one of five categories that bluntly summarized the evidence—"effective," "probably effective," "possibly effective," "ineffective," or "ineffective as a fixed combination." Manufacturers wanted to avoid the last two of these designations, as they implied that the drug in question was eligible for withdrawal from the therapeutic marketplace. Designation as "possibly effective" might compel revisions to a drug's labeling, but this was a far less costly outcome for manufacturers.[61]

Goddard would make there. For other reactions to the appointment, see "A Strong Man for FDA," *WP*, January 12, 1966, A22. Affected industries approached Goddard with tact and deference; see the congratulatory letters in B1, JLG, NLM. On the Merck prosecution, see Karl H. Beyer (Senior Vice President, Merck, Sharpe and Dohme) to Goddard, May 24, 1967; B2, JLG, NLM. On Goddard's public criticism of the drug companies, see Hilts, *Protecting America's Health*, 168–9.

[60]Bryan and Stern, "The Drug Efficacy Study, 1962–1970." Much of this publication strategy was effected by William Goodrich, whose activity followed a statutory requirement.

[61]My summary of the administrative procedure of the Drug Efficacy Study ignores the role of the DESI Policy Advisory Committee in choosing the panels, as well as the particular machinery of Bureau of Medicine (especially its DESI Task Force); see Bryan and Stern, "The Drug Efficacy Study, 1962–1970," 15. Temin's summary of the DESI panels—"it seems curious to replace reliance on the clinical experience of some doctors with reliance on the clinical experience of other doctors" (*Taking Your Medicine*, 130)—is particularly egregious. The panels relied on a vast array of medical literature, employed the two-trial standard that had been developed in the previous decade, and actively helped to flesh out logic that would appear in the "well-controlled studies" rule in the 1970s. Temin also slights the FDA for "definitively" excluding informal experience from drug evaluation in the 1970 rule (137–38), when in fact

In January 1968, the Administration began to publish notices of intent in the *Federal Register* to withdraw drugs. Some twenty-one drugs had been withdrawn from the market in the five years following the enactment of the Kefauver-Harris Amendments, but they were generally non-controversial, their removal did not follow from the NAS/NRC recommendations, and none of them had involved an entire class of therapies. With the *Federal Register* announcements of January 1968, the Drug Efficacy Study was immediately transformed from a problem of review to a problem of implementation. Drugs that were deemed ineffective would now be withdrawn from the market, and the FDA's initial offensives implied that the most popular medicines, sold by the most respected names in the drug business, would be targeted. The politics of efficacy quickly became more visible and more polarized.[62]

On January 23, Goddard announced in the *Federal Register* that a class of products known as bioflavonoids would be targeted for market withdrawal. Bioflavonoids were derived from citrus fruit skins, and manufacturers sold them for relief from hemorrhage to amelioration of skin conditions. The informal theory of their operation was that they improved circulation by dilating blood vessels, bringing greater nutrition to the extremities, the skin, and the developing fetus, and reducing the risk of hemorrhage and stroke. Bioflavonoids were sold by firms small and large, ranging from regional specialists such as Table Rock Labs of Greenville, South Carolina, to global giants like Abbott, Bristol-Myers, and Merck.[63]

The earliest complaints came from general practitioners and libertarians, and they were voiced in national media and directed through Congress. The reaction of many segments of society was expressed tidily by a writer for the *Saturday Evening Post* in an article entitled "Uncle Sam Coddles the Consumer." The writer attacked the bioflavonoids decision and pointed to the case as a metaphor for the intrusion into patient autonomy and consumer freedom.

> This same arrogant self-assurance is behind the FDA's simultaneous campaign this
> year against certain drugs it deems to be "ineffective." In January, the FDA set in

---

much of this work was accomplished in practice long before the 1970 rule, and academic pharmacologists had been strongly favoring statistical evidence (especially randomized controlled trials) at the same time; Marks, *The Progress of Experiment*, chapters 5 and 6.

[62] John F. Palmer (Assistant to the Director for Scientific Coordination, BOM) to William B. Deichmann (Miami, Florida), May 2, 1968. Deichmann was author of several well-known volumes on toxicology. Enforcement decisions were often the subject of extensive discussion among FDA leadership; J. Kenneth Kirk (Associate Commissioner for Compliance) to T. E. Byers (Director, Division of Case Guidance, Bureau of Regulatory Compliance), January 29, 1968; DF 505.6, RG 88, NA.

[63] FDA, "Drugs for Human Use Containing Rutin, Quercetin, Hesperidin, or any Bioflavonoids: Notice of Opportunity for Hearing on Proposal to Withdraw Approval of New Drug Applications," *FR* 33 (133) (July 10, 1968): 9908–9. For the original announcement, see *FR* 33 (15) (Jan. 23, 1968): 818.

motion legal machinery to bar a whole class of drugs, known as the bioflavonoids, from the market. Here again it is not suggested that these citrus derivatives are dangerous; it would be almost impossible for anyone to hurt himself from an overdose of rutin or hesperidin in the forms in which the drugs have been prescribed for more than 20 years. No. The finding of the FDA's experts is that the drugs are "ineffective for use in man in any condition."

Is it true? The FDA has said so, relying on its experts. Yet some reports in medical literature suggest that in certain cases, the bioflavonoids do indeed appear to inhibit hemorrhage, help skin diseases, and prevent miscarriage. But the FDA has spoken. If its preliminary order runs the course, the bioflavonoids will be withdrawn, and no doctor may prescribe them thereafter. Patients who have benefited from these drugs—or believe they have benefited from them—will be out of luck.[64]

Patients who had used bioflavonoids—and their doctors—began lobbying Congress for a reversal of the FDA's decision. G. W. Campbell of Phoenix, Arizona wrote to his state's conservative junior Senator, Paul Fannin, asking Fannin to prevent the removal of bioflavonoids from the market. Campbell's doctor had prescribed a bioflavonoid to him for a retinal hemorrhage in his right eye, and Campbell was convinced that the drug had prevented further eye damage. "It is frightening," Campbell wrote, "to discover that someone can countermand instructions of my personal physician of almost twenty years, who is totally familiar with my physical condition." Despite these complaints, and an increasing volley of criticism aimed at Goddard from congressional Republicans, the Drug Efficacy Study recommendations were often accepted as impending fact by medical authorities and citizens alike. Authors of pharmacology textbooks wrote to the Bureau of Medicine asking for quick updates on which drugs would be withdrawn and when. "I would like to delete all ineffective drugs" from "our book," wrote one author.[65]

A year later, with James Goddard having departed and former Bureau of Medicine director Herbert Ley in the Commissioner's seat, the Administration set its sights upon fixed-combination antibiotics. Fixed-combination antibiotics, as the name implies, were mixtures of antibiotic medicines that were also marketed individually. For two reasons, Bureau of Medicine skeptics and doubters in pharmacology circles like Maxwell Finland had long questioned the clinical value of these products. The combinations were no more effective than each antibiotic used separately, for one, and the prede-

[64]James J. Kilpatrick, "Uncle Sam Coddles the Consumer," *Saturday Evening Post,* July 13, 1968.

[65]G. W. Campbell to Paul Fannin, July 12, 1968; Campbell to Fannin, September 9, 1968; Fannin to Commissioner Herbert Ley, September 20, 1968; Paul Schuette (Deputy Assistant Commissioner for Education and Information) to Fannin, October 1, 1968; DF 505.6, RG 88, NA. Ruth D. Musser to Edwin I. Goldenthal (Acting Deputy Director, Office of New Drugs, BOM), December 31, 1967; Musser and John O'Neill, *Pharmacology and Therapeutics* (New York: Macmillan, 1961); Herbert Ley (Director, BOM) to Musser, January 12, 1968; DF 505.8, RG 88, NA.

termined fraction of each drug contribution meant that antibiotic therapy could not be "rationally" tailored to an individual's needs. In two series of *Federal Register* announcements—one in December 1968, the other in April and May 1969—Ley and FDA leaders proposed to withdraw a total of eighty-five separate combination products from the American marketplace. The new efficacy initiative targeted widely prescribed medicines and, moreover, the large companies that produced them. Two of the most powerful and well-organized agents of late twentieth-century politics—the general medical practitioner and the pharmaceutical company—would be directly antagonized, and FDA authorities and observers knew it.[66]

Yet another logic impelling the offensive against fixed-combination antibiotics involved not assertion but caution. Officials in the Commissioner's Office and the Bureau of Medicine chose to direct their energies at fixed-combination antibiotics in part because the case against them was more consensual and the evidence for that case was rather solid. The "prime target" of this offensive, as contemporaries observed, was Upjohn's drug Panalba, a widely prescribed antibiotic that contained a preset mixture of novobiocin and tetracycline. On December 24, 1968, the Administration announced its agreement with the NAS/NRC finding that Panalba was ineffective as a fixed-combination drug, and then notified Upjohn and the public of its intent to withdraw the drug's certification. The FDA's action was motivated in part by safety concerns, in particular the emergence of evidence that novobiocin carried severe risks.[67]

The Drug Efficacy Study took on new tones of political and legal controversy with Upjohn's May 1969 decision to contest the withdrawal of Panalba. The company challenged the Administration in several venues—some publicly visible, others not. Less perceptibly, Upjohn and other companies stoked protest through administrative procedures of notice and comment, as doctors and patients sent hundreds of testimonial letters to the Administration vouching for Panalba's safety and efficacy. In executive branch politics, Upjohn brought pressure through Nixon's Secretary of Health, Education and Welfare Robert Finch, who pressured the agency to hold off on the withdrawal and conduct a full hearing. The Administration fought off this parry by threatening to expose the pressure at upcoming hearings in Congress. Finally, in a federal lawsuit, Upjohn challenged the right of the Administration to remove its product without a hearing. Before Upjohn's suit, many firms had dealt deferentially with FDA proposals to withdraw their products. Where the withdrawal was premised on a clear lack of evidence, the firm often requested a hearing on the proposed withdrawal but later

[66]The April 2 order appears at *FR* 34 (62) (April 2, 1969): 6003–10. "Ban on 78 More Antibiotic Mixes Proposed by FDA; Firms to Fight," *WSJ*, April 2, 1969, 2; "FDA Crackdown: Government, Industry Clash Over Bid to Curb Combinations of Drugs," *WSJ*, May 6, 1969, 1.
[67]The proposed withdrawal was announced in *FR* 33 (Dec. 24, 1968): 19203; separate restrictions on novobiocin labeling appear in *FR* 34 (May 2, 1969): 7252.

backed off and either withdrew the product voluntarily or announced a revision of the product's labeling. Upjohn's legal strategy was different, and FDA officials and industry observers perceived that its success or failure would serve as a bellwether for other challenges to the Administration's authority. Upjohn ran the process of requesting a hearing and filed a federal lawsuit challenging the legality of the DESI process and the agency's use of summary judgment to circumvent adjudication. Upjohn president R. T. Parfet presented the basic issue as one of rights and due process, as a question of "whether a regulatory agency has the right to order a widely used product from the market summarily without a hearing." Pharmacology celebrity Louis Lasagna brought academic weight to Upjohn's cause when he filed an amicus curiae brief in support of the company's suit. He later penned a *Wall Street Journal* editorial assailing the NAS/NRC review panels as composed of too many academicians with too little clinical experience.[68]

Because it raised so many issues, the FDA-Upjohn tangle over Panalba was watched closely by the entire pharmaceutical industry, by the American Medical Association and thousands of generalist doctors, by regulatory agencies whose missions had nothing to do with food and drugs, and by legal scholars. The narrow issue in the case was whether the Administration could remove a drug by means of summary judgment, or whether each and every efficacy-based drug withdrawal required a formal proceeding with judicial features. Other suits whose purpose was to enjoin the FDA from enforcing the withdrawal were also filed. In their challenges to the DESI withdrawals, however, drug companies were addressing a broader issue— whether it was appropriate for an agency to withdraw a product that had the imprimatur of widespread medical use, use that in some cases endured over decades. The FDA's Medical Advisory Board noted that "the entire pharmaceutical industry is looking at this case with deep interest. The attack on the NAS/NRC panels was expected." For this reason, the Administration's top attorney anticipated the precedent-setting value of the Panalba case in its legal strategy. William Goodrich remarked that the agency "could not have picked a better example than Panalba to substantiate the excellent work and painstaking findings of the NAS/NRC panels."[69]

[68]Contemporaries saw "strong evidence" that the spring 1969 testimonials sent to the Administration "were inspired by the drug companies"; "Drug Efficacy and the 1962 Drug Amendments," *Georgetown Law Journal*, 214, n.186; *1969 Hearings on Drug Efficacy*, 223, 239. On the pressure from HEW superiors and Commissioner Herbert Ley's response, see Hilts, *Protecting America's Health*, 174–6; see also Morton Mintz, "FDA and Panalba: A Conflict of Commercial, Therapeutic Goals?" *Science* 165 (1969): 875–81. The Administration also proposed to decertify existing batches of Panalba that had not yet been sold (*FR* 34 (93) (May 15, 1969): 7687); this order came separately from the agency's larger listing of combination products on April 2. "Upjohn Seeks to Enjoin FDA From Removing Drug Prior to a Hearing," *WSJ*, May 28, 1969, 2. Upjohn's initial suit appears at *Upjohn Co. v. Finch*, 422 F. 2d 944 (6th Circuit, 1970). The Bureau of Medicine often tried to induce voluntary withdrawal of those drugs deemed ineffective in the NAS-NRC review; B. Harvey Minchew (Acting Director, BOM) to Goddard, Re: Withdrawal of NDA 7-875 ("Nurobloc"), June 27, 1968, DF 505.6, RG 88, NA.
[69]FDA-BOM, Medical Advisory Board Minutes, Nineteenth Meeting, June 26 and 27, 1969,

The Drug Efficacy Study was an initiative characterized by ambiguity as much as by assertion. The initiative was beset in its early years by delays and timidity that stemmed from the intertwined political logics of organization and reputation. On the basis of resources and procedure alone, it was well known from discussions in the Kennedy administration that a thorough review of previously approved NDAs would take two decades. Organizationally, the NAS/NRC drug review panels were composed almost entirely of academic physicians, and the problem of coordinating schedules was a substantial one. Further displays of reluctance stemmed from the agency's uncertainty about its authority and its wish to avoid too much provocation of established players in the pharmaceutical field. The Administration might have immediately withdrawn ineffective drugs under the "imminent hazard" clause of the Food, Drug and Cosmetic Act, but its officials refused this course of action. This brought criticism from consumer safety advocates who wanted the Administration to proceed more aggressively against poor quality therapies; one former FDA official lamented that "Apparently people have to be dropping like flies all over the country before the FDA will employ the imminent hazard procedure." Agents in the Bureau of Medicine, the general counsel's office, and the Office of the Commissioner also refused to publicize the recommendations of the NAS/NRC panels. This tight-lipped strategy brought a lawsuit from the American Public Health Association and the National Council of Senior Citizens, which sought to compel the release of the NAS/NRC findings. In federal court, the Administration argued that any release of the panel's advice before FDA action would be premature—since the Administration did not always accept the panel's recommendations—and would possibly cause panic. Nevertheless, and in part to address these consumer protection audiences, the Administration published a temporary list of the drugs withdrawn or under withdrawal order in the *New York Times* in 1970. The FDA's implementation of the study also began to take genuine effect at this time, with often jarring results. Of the first 900 rulings made by the Administration under DESI, 40 percent were declarations that drugs were "ineffective."[70]

pp. 9–10; FDA-BOM, Medical Advisory Board Minutes, Twenty-First Meeting, December 18 and 19, 1969, pp. 1–2; Harry F. Dowling Papers, NLM. "Two Upjohn Antibiotics Barred From Sale; FDA-Drug Company Confrontation Is Seen," *WSJ*, May 15, 1969, 38. The FDA's guidance appears in "Hearing Regulations and Regulations Describing Scientific Content of Adequate and Well-Controlled Clinical Investigations," *FR* 35 (90) (May 8, 1970): 7250–53. For earlier withdrawals without hearings, consult J. Kenneth Kirk, "S. E. Massengill Company, Gallogen Injectable: Notice of Withdrawal of New Drug Application," *FR* 33 (Jan. 20, 1968) 770; Kirk, "Abbott Laboratories, Stendin Tablets; Order Vacating Opportunity for a Hearing," and Kirk, "Chesebrough-Pond's, Inc., Measurin Tablets; Order Vacating Opportunity for Hearings," *FR* 33 (Jan. 18, 1968): 650. Ironically, the Administration lost the first Panalba case, which induced Goodrich to revise his legal strategy; I thank Peter Barton Hutt for pressing this point.

[70] On FDA leadership's judgment that a review of NDAs approved from 1938 to 1962 would have taken "about 20 years," see Theodore Ellenbogen to Winton Rankin, February 16, 1962; FDA General Correspondence, DF 062.1, RG 88, NA. The delays in DESI implementation also

In respects that were both legal and scientific, the Administration's work with pre-1962 drugs blended the regulation of the past with the governing of the future. The lawsuits from Upjohn and other parties compelled the agency to speak more clearly on the criteria it would use to assess pre-1962 drugs. Yet the initiative to define "effectiveness" standards in the Drug Efficacy Study was in part an articulation of what the efficacy criteria would be for drugs yet to come. As of the summer of 1969, the Administration had not yet codified its interpretation of the Food, Drug and Cosmetic Act's requirement for "substantial evidence" of effectiveness. The main criteria for effectiveness had instead been elaborated informally, often in speeches by Joseph Sadusk, Frances Kelsey, and Commissioner James Goddard in the early and mid-1960s. In this sense, one of the FDA's most important rules of the period—the final "well-controlled studies" rule of May 8, 1970—served legal and political as well as scientific purposes. The May 1970 rules were adopted partially from FDA official William Beaver's testimony in the Upjohn suit of 1969, but like Beaver's testimony, they also expressed previous opinion and practice within the Bureau of Medicine. The May 1970 rules defined "well controlled studies" in flexible but rigorous terms, explicitly excluding "isolated case reports, random experience, and reports lacking the details which permit scientific evaluation." This rule clarified the statute, of course, but it also answered congressional criticisms that the agency had moved too slowly to clarify and enforce the efficacy requirements of the 1962 Amendments. Beyond this, the minimum-of-two-controlled-trials standard created a hurdle that any drug sponsor would have to surpass in order to qualify for an evidentiary hearing on a drug withdrawal. Testimonial evidence of the form fomented by Upjohn for Panalba would be ignored, and even evidence from studies using non-randomized, historical controls would be deemed insufficient. The May 1970 rule thus addressed the legal needs raised by the Upjohn challenge, at the same time that it addressed concerns from Congress and medical academics eager for illumination of the agency's clinical trial requirements. And, like the 1963 IND rules, it shaped the content of legitimate science.[71]

---

brought a lawsuit by American Public Health Association in 1972; a district court decision agreed with the Association and ordered the FDA to conclude the DESI review within four years, focusing first on those drugs deemed "ineffective" by the NAS/NRC panels; *APHA v. Veneman*, 349 F. Supp. 1311 (D.D.C. 1972). Southwick, "Faster FDA Action Asked in Lawsuit," *Science* 168 (1970): 1560; Southwick, "FDA: Efficiency Drive Stumbles Over the Issue of Drug Efficacy," *Science* 169 (1970): 1188–9. "Drug Efficacy," *Georgetown Law Review* 60 (1971): 213. In 1971, the editors of the *Georgetown Law Journal* would write that the *Times* listing "was published in part at least to mollify critics complaining about the agency's failure to publish the NAS/NRC findings"; "Drug Efficacy," 212, n.175. Charles C. Edwards, "Positive and Rational Drug Therapeutics," presented at the Symposium on Drugs—Hospital Pharmacists, September 26, 1970, p. 243 in Speech 27, V 1, F 2, CCE.

[71] Charles C. Edwards, "Hearing Regulations and Regulations Describing Scientific Content of Adequate and Well-Controlled Clinical Investigations," *FR* 35 (90) (May 8, 1970): 7250–53. The proposed rulemaking occurred three months earlier; *FR* 35 (33) (Feb. 17, 1970): 3073–4. I

With the "well controlled studies" rule published in final form, and with a favorable decision from the federal courts in *Upjohn v. Finch*, the essential logic and sequence of efficacy-based drug withdrawals had been established. By virtue of the standards announced in its rulemaking, the Administration would adjudicate drugs on a case-by-case basis, but where the company could not produce two studies satisfying the FDA's "substantial evidence" standard, the drugs would be withdrawn without a formal hearing. This mode of regulation was challenged anew in several lawsuits filed in 1970 and 1971 by companies whose drugs were being withdrawn. The implications of the lawsuits were manifold, but at their core they concerned the ambit of regulatory power. One set of suits was premised upon the claim that Section 505(e) of the Food, Drug and Cosmetic Act entitled any sponsor of a withdrawn NDA to a formal hearing, namely a full judicial hearing with an administrative law judge, as opposed to an informal or "oral hearing." Another suit from the Pharmaceutical Manufacturers' Association contended that while the Administration possessed authority to review documentation and data relating to drug efficacy, the agency had "doubtful" authority to act on the reviews and recommendations of the NAS/NRC. Behind this dispute lay a deeper challenge to the concepts elaborated in the 1962 statute and the 1963 regulations. As FDA officials saw it, the companies' Association was in fact contesting the application of post-Kefauver standards of efficacy to drugs developed before 1962, as well as the "FDA-proposed essentials of a well-controlled trial." And to challenge the capacity of the Administration to remove drugs without a formal hearing was a proposition to render the efficacy requirement null and void for pre-1962 drugs.[72]

The judgment of the Supreme Court on this matter came in a group of cases headed by the decision *Weinberger v. Hynson, Westcott & Dunning, Inc.* (1973). The *Hynson* decision, as it is now known, was a near complete victory for Hutt and the Administration. Writing for the Court, Justice William O. Douglas agreed with Hynson (the sponsor of Lutrexin) that Section 505(e) of the Food, Drug and Cosmetic Act did indeed require a hearing on whether its submission met the threshold criterion of "substantial evidence." Yet the Court also ruled that the hearing right was conditional. Only if a company submitted "substantial evidence" of effectiveness—data of a particular kind (and quality), meeting the standards of the May 8, 1970 "well-

am grateful to Richard A. Merrill and M. Elizabeth Magill for discussions and suggestions on the points in this and subsequent paragraphs. For the Commissioner's assertive presentation of the May rule, as well as a claim that the rule codified established regulatory and scientific practices, see Edwards, "Positive and Rational Drug Therapeutics"; Speech 27, 236; V 1, F 2, CCE. Beaver's testimony appears at U.S. District Court for the District of Delaware: Pharmaceutical Manufacturers Association v. Robert H. Finch, Secretary of Health, Education and Welfare, and Herbert Lay, Commissioner of Foods and Drugs; Affidavit of William Thomas Beaver, M.D. (Civil Action no. 3797, 1969), 455; cited in Curtis L. Meinert and Susan Tonascia, *Clinical Trials: Design, Conduct, and Analysis* (New York: Oxford University Press, 1986), 8.

[72]FDA-BOM, Medical Advisory Board Minutes, Twenty-First Meeting, December 18 and 19, 1969, pp. 1–2; Harry F. Dowling Papers, NLM.

controlled studies" rule—would it be entitled to a formal hearing. Hence, the summary judgment procedure—the ability of the Administration to vacate the opportunity for a formal hearing—was affirmed. If sponsors could not produce at least two well-controlled studies (as defined by the Bureau itself three years before) in favor of the drug's efficacy claims, no elaborate administrative procedure would be required for a withdrawal. The Bureau of Drugs and the Commissioner could limit adjudication to the question of whether the sponsor had met the steep burden of the "well-controlled studies" rule. In a sister case decided the same day as Hynson—*USV Pharmaceutical Corp. v. Weinberger*—the Court also affirmed the Administration's withdrawal of bioflavonoids.[73]

In combination with its sister cases, the *Hynson* decision expressed an affirmation of the Administration's reputation for scientific competence and public protection. As a general matter, Douglas wrote that "The heart of the new procedures designed by Congress is the grant of primary jurisdiction to FDA, the expert agency it created." The principle undergirding the particular decision was the consensus that the 1962 Amendments and the Administration's rules "express well-established principles of scientific investigation, in their reduction of the 'substantial evidence' standard to detailed guidelines for the protection of the public." It was this legitimacy and the "strict and demanding standards" of the May 8, 1970 "well-controlled studies" rule that rendered the FDA's summary judgment procedure "appropriate." In the *USV* case, Justice Douglas noted that "the 1962 regulatory scheme proposes administrative control through an expert agency in lieu of more cumbersome 1938 devices." The Court also amplified the agency's claims about the limits of individual physician learning, stating boldly that "impressions or beliefs of physicians, no matter how fervently held, are treacherous." In sum, the *Hynson* decision affirmed the capacities of the Administration to make efficacy judgments, as it rejected the capacity of general practitioners to render those same evaluations.[74]

---

[73] *Weinberger v. Hynson, Westcott & Dunning* 412 U.S. 609 (1973). The *Hynson* decision was accompanied by three others—*Weinberger v. Bentex Pharmaceuticals, Inc.* (412 U.S. 645), *Ciba Corp. v. Weinberger* (412 U.S. 640), and *USV Pharmaceutical Corp v. Weinberger* (412 U.S. 455)—and the set of cases is variously known as the "*Hynson* quartet," or the "*Weinberger* trilogy," depending on which combination of cases is of reference. *Hynson* essentially upheld a ruling of the Fourth Circuit a year earlier; 461 F.2d 215 (Fourth Circuit, 1972). The Bureau of Medicine had been renamed the Bureau of Drugs in 1969 under the initiative of Commissioner Charles C. Edwards; see chapter 7 for a review. In the *Hynson* and *USV* cases, the Supreme Court took the step of ordering a hearing for Hynson and for Lutrexin.

[74] See Douglas's opinion at 412 U.S. 610–11, 618 (*Hynson*); 412 U.S. 655, 665 (*USV Pharmaceutical Corp. v. Weinberger*). Several other Justices, including Byron White, felt that Douglas had taken the case beyond what the FDA was asking for. Blackmun clerk Ralph I. Miller felt that "Justice Douglas has rewritten the statute," particularly in his assessment that the FDA could issue a "declaratory order" on the new drug status of a product (412 U.S. 626–27); Circulation Memo, 72-394, 414, 528, 555, 666 [FDA Drug Cases]," May 11, 1973; File 72-394, Harry A. Blackmun Papers, Library of Congress. Douglas, in turn, felt that "the result reached is necessary lest the Act be turned on its ear"; Douglas, Memorandum to the Conference, May 8, 1973; File 72-394, Thurgood Marshall Papers, Library of Congress.

The *Hynson* decision also facilitated the Administration's review and removal of over-the-counter (OTC) drugs, which had begun more than a year before the Supreme Court announced its verdicts. Fully 300 of the 400 OTC medications reviewed were found to be rankly ineffective for one or more of their intended uses. With the summary judgment procedure legitimated under *Hynson*, and with the well-controlled studies rule in place, it was relatively straightforward for the Bureau of Drugs to use rulemaking rather than adjudication, and thereby issue review and withdrawal decisions for the hundreds of ineffective candidates. Having followed the Drug Efficacy Study initiative and the *Hynson* decision, the OTC drug removals of the 1970s occasioned much less political controversy and judicial oversight than they would have if they had come a decade earlier.[75]

Rulemaking, Reputation, and Gatekeeping. As fights over pre-1962 drugs, over-the-counter medications, and the meaning of efficacy wore on, a subtle but durable shift was occurring in the Administration's practices of regulation. Like several other federal agencies, but with far greater assertiveness and success, the Administration began to use rulemaking as a mode of governing. The patterns of behavior noticeable in this shift had been under way since the 1950s, but beginning in 1973, FDA officials made their intentions clear. The agency began to issue federal rules "with the force of law," premised upon the Food, Drug and Cosmetic Act as an organic enabling act with the status of a miniature constitution.[76]

The Administration's rulemaking initiative of the 1970s and early 1980s was undertaken in a rather intricate setting of changes in federal rulemaking activity and their reception in the national courts. The changes affected the production and meaning of "substantive legislative rules," or those rules with policymaking content that also carry the force of law. In modern administrative law, "legislative" rules are those that have the effect of statute in the sense that they bind regulated parties much as an explicit act of Congress would. Rules of the "nonlegislative" sort do not carry this force and take the form of agency statements about intended actions in the future. In addition, administrative law distinguishes between "substantive" and "procedural" rules. Substantive rules govern the behavior of regulated parties—those entities outside the agency—while procedural rules govern matters

---

[75]John H. Moxley III, Gary L. Yingling, and Charles C. Edwards, "The Food and Drug Administration's over-the-counter drug review: why review OTC drugs?" *Proceedings of the Federation of Independent Scientists* 32 (4) (April 1973): 1435–7. Lars Noah, "Treat Yourself: Is Self-Medication the Prescription for What Ails American Health Care?" *Harvard Journal of Law and Technology* 19 (2) (Spring 2006): 359–92. The agency also proceeded with summary judgment and rulemaking in securing labeling revisions for OTC drugs; *FR* 44 (Aug.31, 1979): 51525. For more recent and comprehensive regulations, see "Over-the-Counter Human Drugs: Labeling Requirements," *FR* 64 (March 17, 1999): 13286.

[76]For the understanding of rulemaking and agency practice elaborated here, I have relied heavily upon Thomas W. Merrill and Kathryn Tongue Watts, "Agency Rules with the Force of Law: The Original Convention," *Harvard Law Review* 116 (2) (Dec. 2002): 467–592. See also Richard A. Merrill, "Architecture."

inside the agency. Substantive rules include binding legislative rules, but also include two sets of nonlegislative rules, "interpretive rules" (nonbinding information on how the agency reads its powers under a statute or legislative rule) and "policy statements" (nonbinding suggestions that announce the agency's intention to exercise discretion in a certain way).[77]

The rulemaking shift at the FDA mainly involved substantive legislative rules, namely those rules that govern regulated parties with the force of law. The initiative was not isolated to the Administration, and it developed at the intersection of agencies and federal appellate courts. In the 1960s and early 1970s, attorneys at two federal agencies—the Administration and the Federal Trade Commission (FTC)—began to interpret their organizations' authorities more expansively. At the FTC, attorneys and commissioners began to abandon case-by-case adjudication in favor of Trade Regulation Rules that governed economic activity broadly. When in the late 1960s and 1970s the Commission used legislative rulemaking to require the posting of octane levels on gasoline pumps, the National Petroleum Refiners Association brought suit in federal court, claiming that the Commission lacked statutory authority to issue Trade Regulation Rules. The ultimate judgment of the federal courts on this issue was given by Judge J. Skelly Wright of the D.C. Circuit Court in *National Petroleum Refiners Association v. FTC* (1973). Wright wrote for a unanimous three-judge panel, arguing not only that the Commission held legislative rulemaking power under the Federal Trade Commission Act, but also that Congress had in effect granted this power to a wide array of other administrative agencies and that the federal courts had in previous decisions assented to this implicit grant of rulemaking authority. The "Skelly Wright decision" of 1973, as it has come to be known, created a presumption in favor of agencies that claimed legislative rulemaking authority. Wright's decision was carefully studied by administrative lawyers and by attorneys at other agencies in the federal government, not least by shrewd attorneys at the FDA.[78]

---

[77]Richard J. Pierce, Jr., "Distinguishing Legislative Rules from Interpretive Rules," *Administrative Law Review* 52 (2000): 549–54. Merrill and Watts, "Agency Rules with the Force of Law," 476–7. U. S. Department of Justice, *Attorney General's Manual on the Administrative Procedure Act* (Washington, DC: GPO, 1947), 30, n.3. The Attorney General's Committee on Administrative Procedure, *Administrative Procedure in Government Agencies*, Senate Doc. 77-8 (Washington, DC: GPO, 1941), 100. For an accessible and nontechnical review of these concepts, see Cornelius Kerwin, *Rulemaking: How Government Agencies Write Law and Make Policy*, 3rd ed. (Washington, DC: CQ Press, 2003), 22–3, 43–5, and chapter 2, passim.

[78]*National Petroleum Refiners Association v. FTC*, 482 F.2d 672 (D.C. Circuit, 1973); the Circuit's decision reversed a district court judgment that overturned the Commission's rules. For the FDA's response, see the following paragraphs. The FDA had used 701(a) rulemaking authority before, in 1972, when dealing with nutrition labeling and the OTC drug review. For another act of scrutiny, see Robert H. Becker, "Thoughts for Food," *FDCLJ* 28 (1973): 679–85. Congress would expressly delegate legislative rulemaking capacity to the FTC in the Federal Trade Improvement Act of 1975, but Merrill and Watts argue that Wright's decision had a greater impact outside of federal trade law. "The importance of Judge Wright's opinion went

At the Administration, the most aggressive and ingenious steps were taken by General Counsel Peter Barton Hutt, who had arrived by appointment from Commissioner Charles Edwards in 1971. In 1972, Hutt seized upon a particular section of the agency's enabling act—Section 701(a) of the Federal Food, Drug and Cosmetic Act—and argued that it gave his agency "ample legal authority" to adopt general procedures for enforcement. This was an important shift from the agency's previous reliance on Section 701(e) of the Act for rulemaking; "701(e) rulemaking" compelled a public evidentiary hearing under formal rule-making procedures, whereas "701(a) rule-making" entailed a less cumbersome notice-and-comment process. Well beyond this, Hutt claimed that the Act held the status of a "constitution" that granted broad authority to the agency to achieve "a set of fundamental objectives." The 1938 law and its amendments, Hutt argued, gave the Administration the power to do anything that was not expressly prohibited or constrained by the Act itself. Attorneys allied with regulated industries decried Hutt's reading of the law, one echoing Justice Benjamin Cardozo's 1935 lament that it amounted to "delegation running riot," while correctly noting that Hutt had proposed to reverse the burden of proof in disputes over the FDA's rulemaking authority. If courts accepted Hutt's reading of the Act, the Administration would need only show that its rulemaking was not expressly prohibited by its enabling act, not that the Act clearly permitted the rulemaking.[79]

In the wake of the *Hynson* case and the "Skelly Wright" decision, Peter Barton Hutt's confidence in the FDA rulemaking process crested. Speaking in 1973 to an audience of food and drug lawyers, Hutt claimed that the Skelly Wright decision would permit the agency to use Section 701(a) of its enabling statute to engage in legislative rulemaking. Hutt boldly declared that the Administration would prevail in any legal challenge to legislative rulemaking based on Section 701(a), and two years later his prescience proved correct in a 1975 decision of the Second Circuit court. Modern courts had "learned from experience," wrote Judge Mansfield for the Circuit, "to accept a general delegation as sufficient in certain areas of expertise."[80]

---

far beyond its impact on the FTC's rulemaking powers. His self-confident tone and masterful blending of Supreme Court precedents provided the road map for a more general erasure of the [earlier rulemaking] convention and invited other agencies, including the FDA, to assert generalized legislative rulemaking powers that Congress had not expressly granted"; "Agency Rules with the Force of Law," 557.

[79]Hutt, "Philosophy of Regulation under the Federal Food, Drug and Cosmetic Act," *FDCLJ* 28 (1973): 177. This article was a publication of Hutt's prepared remarks to the Food and Drug Law Institute in 1972. Merrill and Watts, "Agency Rules with the Force of Law," 557–9. For responses, see H. Thomas Austern, "Philosophy of Regulation: A Reply to Mr. Hutt," *FDCLJ* 28 (1973): 189, 191; Merrill S. Thompson, "The FDA: They Mean Well, But...," *FDCLJ* 28 (1973): 205, 209.

[80]Hutt, "Impact of Recent Court Decisions on the Future of FDA Regulations: An Impromptu Response to the Remarks of the Speakers," *FDCLJ* 28 (1973): 707, 712. *National Nutritional Foods Association v. Weinberger* 512 F. 2d. 688 (Second Circuit 1975). Merrill and

With these critical victories in the early 1970s, rulemaking became a primary mode of policymaking and regulatory planning at the Administration. Legal observers pointed to the rulemaking process as a method for avoiding formal hearings and for infusing the efficacy review process with greater efficiency. The shift to rulemaking struck one writer in 1979 as a basic transformation of the agency's identity. "During the late 1960s and 1970s," James O'Reilly wrote, the FDA had grown "from a law enforcement agency which brought deterrent actions against violators, into a more paper-bound generator of rules and regulations." The shift from interpretive rulemaking to substantive rulemaking had been a gradual one, as the "in-house" rules of the 1950s had in many ways bound external parties by specifying what was necessary in a New Drug Application form. Yet the assertiveness and the judicial affirmation of rulemaking at the FDA in the early 1970s marked a watershed in the agency's powers and its growth. The Administration had been endowed with the capacity to issue "rules with the force of law" without necessarily holding an administrative hearing.[81]

While the shift to rulemaking as a mode of regulatory government received its force from judicial affirmation, what buttressed rulemaking as much as anything else was the agency's product veto authority. Because the Administration has the ultimate say over whether and when a new drug will be marketed, its mere suggestions and intimations induce compliance even where they are not backed by legal authority. The agency's use of *Federal Register* policy statements and "guidance documents" (nonbinding statements of policy that are not customarily published in the *Federal Register* but are published under the auspices of the FDA itself) permits its officials to avoid the more costly and elaborate process of formal rulemaking, while still gaining acquiescence with its regulatory wishes. There is no constitutional or legal violation here, and several federal court decisions have upheld the agency's authority as exercised in this way. Yet the effect of the Administration's move to suggestive regulation is undeniable. Over the past few decades, the agency has successfully used its veto authority, in combination with its gatekeeping authority, to impose numerous procedural requirements upon pharmaceutical sponsors without having to engage in the sort of notice-and-comment rulemaking in which such requirements might be moderated or substantially changed.[82]

Watts, "Agency Rules with the Force of Law," 560–61. Attorney Joel E. Hoffman, who filed an amicus curiae brief for Hynson in the 1973 case, has argued that the agency's assertive use of Section 701(a) began with the Supreme Court's 1967 decision in *Abbott Laboratories v. Gardner* (387 U.S. 136); Hoffman, "Administrative Procedures of the Food and Drug Administration," in David G. Adams, Richard M. Cooper, and Jonathan S. Kahan, *Fundamentals of Law and Regulation*, vol. 2 (Washington, DC: FDLI, 1997).

[81] James T. O'Reilly, *Food and Drug Administration* (St. Paul, MN: West Group, 1979), chap. 4; cited in Merrill and Watts, "Agency Rules with the Force of Law," 558, n.488. Virgil Wodicka, "The 1970s: The Decade of Regulations," *FDCLJ* 45 (1990): 59–61; Fred H. Degnan, *FDA's Creative Application of the Law* (Washington, DC: Food and Drug Law Institute, 2000), 40–43.

[82] The connection between gatekeeping authority and the compulsory force of agency pro-

In the realm of law, too, the Administration's power was bound up in and expressed through its reputation. In the slew of cases that were decided in the 1970s—*Upjohn Company v. Finch* (1970), *Pharmaceutical Manufacturers' Association v. Richardson* (1970), and *Weinberger v. Hynson, Westcott & Dunning, Inc.* (1973) and its companion cases—the federal judiciary was observed to confirm nearly every aspect of the Food and Drug Administration's implementation of efficacy regulation. It was a stunning string of legal victories for Peter Barton Hutt (and for William Goodrich before him), and it led to a characterization of the FDA as somehow unique in the realm of administrative law. Relatedly, legal scholars at the time noted that Department of Justice attorneys exhibited a high rate of deference to the Administration in accepting for prosecution those cases that the agency referred to it. Indeed, no agency in the federal government was less likely to have its case referrals rejected by the Department of Justice. As early as 1963, industry lawyer Thomas Austern uttered words that would become accepted as fact in legal circles in the late twentieth century:

> [E]very experienced food and drug lawyer will tell you that in 999 out of 1,000 cases, even the most sanguine counsel knows that he hasn't a prayer of persuading an appellate court to second guess the FDA.
>
> Every finding is dressed up as a scientific determination... Colorful phrases of remote bearing—such as "poisoning the public," "prevention of cancer," "deleterious food injuring the public"—are regularly trotted out.
>
> It is indeed a sturdy appellate judge who is not tempted to clutch his stomach, to recall every episode of family illness, and to react in favor of those who march under the banner of protecting the aged, lactating mothers and infant children.[83]

It was not the first time that Austern had written hyperbolically about the Administration's powers. In 1963, Austern declared that "the FDA rulemaking process, by and large, has virtual immunity from judicial intervention or correction." Revisiting Austern's judgment a decade later, two scholars would argue that other agencies might pay heed to the FDA example and build rulemaking power on the basis of "broadly applicable principles of

---

posals, advice, and guidances is beautifully rendered in Merrill, "Architecture." For examples of the FDA's use of its "arm-twisting" power in regulatory negotiations, especially with respect to accelerated approval procedures for new drugs and corrective advertising campaigns, see Lars Noah, "Administrative Arm-Twisting in the Shadow of Congressional Delegations of Authority," *Wisconsin Law Review* 1997 (5): 874–941. The courts have, on occasion, invalidated an informal agreement between the FDA and a drug sponsor; *American Pharmaceutical Association v. Weinberger* 377 F. Supp. 824, 831 (D.D.C. 1974).

[83] The Panalba case was decided in *Upjohn Company v. Finch* (422 F.2d 944) (Sixth Circuit, 1970), a case that the Supreme Court declined to review. See also *Pharmaceutical Manufacturers Association v. Richardson* (318 F. Supp 301) (D. Del. 1970). Austern, "Sanctions in Silhouette: An Inquiry into the Enforcement of the Federal Food, Drug and Cosmetic Act," *California Law Review* 51 (1) (Jan. 1963): 45. Austern was an adjunct at New York University Law School at the time he wrote the decision, but was well known as legal counsel for many drug companies, including Upjohn. I thank M. Elizabeth Magill for this information. On case referrals, see Robert L. Rabin, "Agency Criminal Referrals in the Federal System: An Empirical Study of Prosecutorial Discretion," *Stanford Law Review* 24 (6) (June 1972): 1036–91.

administrative law." The truth of Austern's characterization is only partially relevant. In creating and replicating a social fact—that the Administration and especially its rulemaking process could not be beaten in court—Austern and a generation of administrative lawyers created another facet of the Administration's reputation, and a new font of regulatory power. The number and severity of legal challenges foregone or abandoned early on in recognition of the FDA's legal reputation is impossible to calculate, but it is plausibly substantial. And the string of conquests also influenced the judgment of later jurists. Judge Henry Friendly, in affirming the Administration's power to regulate over-the-counter (OTC) drugs in *National Association of Pharmaceutical Manufacturers v. FDA* (1981), interpreted expansive FDA powers in part from the string of legal victories that the agency had won in the previous decade. Along with other federal judges, Friendly was recognizing a different form of legal precedent, deferring not to the explicit language of other rulings (as in *stare decisis*), but to the flavor or temperature of those rulings and the implied portraits of administrative agencies they embedded.[84]

"Tame Submission" and Lament: The Response of Medical Associations, Organized Business, and Economic Conservatives

With its arsenal of new authorities and the powers that flowed from them, the Administration began in the 1960s and 1970s to exercise vast sway over the medical marketplace. Familiar over-the-counter remedies and doctor-prescribed pills vanished. The place of the general practitioner in drug development waned to the point of disappearance, as companies could no longer rely upon doctors' casual observations or observations of patient histories to buttress claims of safety and effectiveness. FDA rules compelled sea changes in the structure and composition of pharmaceutical manufacturers, whose development costs increased and whose ranks were quickly filled with more pharmacologists, statisticians, and medical specialists.

Some measure of the Administration's power, as well as insight into how that power endured political and cultural challenges, can be gleaned from the reactions and expressions of two major associations whose members were most influenced by the post-thalidomide world of drugs: the American Medical Association and the Pharmaceutical Manufacturers Association. The AMA leadership had opposed efficacy standards in the Kefauver bill throughout the late 1950s and early 1960s. Even as Frances Kelsey and Ralph Smith were rolling out the investigational new drug rules, AMA Gen-

---

[84]Charles C. Ames and Steven C. McCracken, "Framing Regulatory Standards to Avoid Formal Adjudication: The FDA as a Case Study," *California Law Review* 64 (1) (Jan. 1976): 16. Ames and McCracken were students of Virginia law professor Richard A. Merrill, who originally wrote the article with them but dropped his name from authorship when he became FDA General Counsel in 1976; I thank M. Elizabeth Magill for this information. *National Association of Pharmaceutical Manufacturers v. FDA* ; [487 F.Supp. 412 (SDNY 1980), aff'd, 637 F.2d 877 (2d Cir. *1981*)].

eral Counsel C. Joseph Stetler disparaged the rules and the methods by which they were adopted. Lecturing to food and drug lawyers in January 1963, Stetler vowed that the AMA would "fight hard" for revisions in the law and called openly for changes that would blunt many of the new FDA rules, particularly the IND regulations. The AMA continued to cast doubt upon the legitimacy of the law, and the Association fought the FDA symbolically and procedurally on many particular issues, ranging from the Drug Efficacy Study to proposed regulations for prescription drug advertising. Behind most of these laments lay a continuing fear that the Administration would engage in judgments about the comparative efficacy of drugs and, in so doing, usurp the space for professional autonomy and individual discretion in American medical practice. Anything that touched on drug comparisons—whether it was labeling regulation, the governance of advertising, or the withdrawal of a commonly used drug by dint of its clear inferiority to other marketed compounds—was attacked. "Inherent in the authority to evaluate 'relative efficacy,'" wrote AMA Vice President Ernest Howard, "is a power to designate drugs of choice for a medical indication."[85]

The 1960s and 1970s were a time of wound-licking and massive reform in the global pharmaceutical industry. The industry as a collective entity was poorly regarded in public, scientific, professional, and political audiences, castigated for the high prices of its products, blamed for drug safety problems, and despised for its worldwide political influence. In every industrialized nation with a sizable pharmaceutical sector, politicians and scientists had imposed extensive new regulations upon companies large and small. Many of these regulations were spurred by collective horror of the thalidomide tragedy and wrought from mimicry of the FDA's rules and practices. At the level of research and development practices, a broad ranging deference to the Administration and its pharmacological regime set in, as drug companies universally engaged in product development through sequences of randomized, blinded, and controlled clinical trials, as they adopted FDA-initiated and preferred standards and concepts in their manufacturing and marketing, and as they displayed increasingly obsequious behavior toward Administration officials.[86]

Matters were quite different in American national politics. Led by rebellious firms upset about their treatment by the FDA, American pharmaceutical companies and their conservative allies began a concerted attempt to invert the Administration's image, to display the uglier side of the agency and its new powers. Even as the American consumer protection movement crested in its authority and as the thalidomide memory persisted, libertarians and

---

[85] "AMA Likely to Press for Changes in Law: Stetler," *DTN*, February 4, 1963, 13. Howard to Hearing Clerk, FDA, October 21, 1972, F 0273-04, "FDA Correspondence, 1959—1972," AAMA. The offending regulations for prescription drug advertising appeared at *FR* 37 (163) (August 22, 1972) 16877–8.

[86] Many of these changes in practices are discussed in the following chapter and in chapters 7 , 9 and 11.

neoconservative activists in the United States, combining forces with angered company officials and traditional defenders of the autonomy of medical practice, began to attack the agency and, explicitly, its reputation. The concept of the "drug lag"—the purported slower availability of new medicines in the United States, vis-à-vis European countries—was just one part of a broader and more enduring pattern of anti-regulatory discourse.

The offensive from business conservatives was part of a larger social reckoning with the regulatory state that marked American national politics in the 1970s. The decade witnessed profound disillusionment among American citizens with national government and policies, especially those solutions that entailed a grant of material discretion to federal agencies. At one level, these were political reactions against government in any form, as when anti-tax conservatives helped to pass California's Proposition 13 in 1978. Proposition 13 limited the capacity of local governments and school districts to raise property taxes, and its passage set in motion a wave of similar anti-tax ballot initiatives nationwide. At another level, reactions such as Richard Nixon's New Federalism initiative and growing anti-welfare political sentiment were focused on the growing size and involvement of the national government. This was particularly true among conservatives interested in devolving authority to the states, whether out of concern for decentralized policy solutions or out of disdain for redistributive and racially progressive programs.[87]

While regulatory policies could partially escape the perils of American racial animus and growing societal distaste for redistribution, they could not elude broader currents of libertarianism, business organization, and individualism. The 1970s witnessed growing attacks on national social and economic regulation from both parties, most notably when Democratic President Jimmy Carter commenced a reform initiative that resulted in a wholesale overhaul of federal aviation regulation and the elimination of the Civil Aeronautics Board. Policy analysts began to revisit the entire apparatus of laws and rules erected in the previous decade and cast doubt upon their effectiveness. Simple quantitative analyses—often produced by economists and other policy analysts—demonstrated no abrupt or identifiable change in policy outcomes in the wake of these laws. The null hypothesis of no effect had won out. Libertarian voices, growing in number and pitch, decried the intrusion of federal regulations in the domains of privacy, property, and personal and professional relationships. These anti-regulatory trends would foreshadow the election of former California governor Ronald Reagan as the nation's thirty-ninth president.[88]

[87]Lisa McGirr, *Suburban Warriors: The Origins of the New American Right* (Princeton: Princeton University Press, 2001). For a contemporary view, see Alvin Schorr, "Loose Welds in the Social Compact," *NYT*, July 23, 1979, A17. A *New York Times* poll suggested that 70 percent of voters in 1980 agreed with the statement that "the Government has gone too far in regulating business and interfering with the free enterprise system"; 58 percent of poll respondents agreed with the statement in January 1978. Adam Clymer, "Poll Shows Iran and Economy Hurt Carter Among Late-Shifting Voters," *NYT*, November 16, 1980, 32.

[88]Think tanks also entered the fray over federal regulation. The two most notable were the

Criticism of the FDA was part of a broader anti-regulatory impulse, and the Administration found greater trouble in areas outside traditional pharmaceutical regulation. In some respects, aggressive attempts to ban or stringently regulate chemical additives to foods—mainly saccharin and nitrates—raised doubts and outright defiance from scientific, industry, consumer, and journalistic audiences. Other agencies such as the Environmental Protection Agency (EPA) and the Labor Department's Occupational Health and Safety Administration (OSHA) also witnessed impairment of their scientific credibility in the late 1970s and early 1980s. There was visible damage to the federal government's reputation in matters of science in the post-Watergate period—a contrast to the glory years of previous decades when the national government's scientific regard was sterling.[89]

In other ways, the new torrent of FDA criticism in the 1960s and 1970s simply extended and reproduced earlier laments. In 1963, industry groups and AMA spokesmen combined forces in a way that they had failed to do before the 1962 Amendments. The AMA continued to press for changes in the law and openly advocated the repeal of the efficacy provision. In July 1963, FDA investigators uncovered a rumor campaign by pharmaceutical manufacturers that was designed to discredit the FDA among practicing physicians. The Public Relations Director for the Pharmaceutical Manufacturers' Association began trashing the Administration in speeches to medical audiences. Manufacturers also planned to line up prominent medical authorities behind their drugs and submit them for new indications, waiting for FDA criticism in the hopes of "slaughtering" the agency with "adverse publicity" by contrasting the judgment of world medical authorities and the agency's new medical officers. The FDA responded by carefully scrutinizing supplemental applications and by alerting its field personnel to "the possibility of organized rumor spreading." These early battles underline the centrality of the Administration's reputation as a battleground for industry, medicine, and regulators alike.[90]

---

reliably conservative American Enterprise Institute and the otherwise liberal Brookings Institution. Brookings analysts published numerous critiques of federal regulation, including Roger Noll's *Reforming Regulation* (Washington, DC: Brookings Institute Press, 1979) and Robert Crandall's *Controlling Industrial Pollution: The Economics and Politics of Clean Air* (Washington, DC: Brookings Institution, 1983). For a more popular contribution, see Crandall's "Is Government Regulation Crippling Business?" *Saturday Review*, January 20, 1979. As evidence of the convergence of these two organizations on matters of regulatory policy, AEI and Brookings created a Joint Center for Regulatory Policy in 1998. In the 1980s and 1990s, other think tanks and advocacy organizations would become more prominent, including the Cato Institute, the Heritage Institute, and the Center for a Competitive Economy. Andrew Rich, *Think Tanks, Public Policy and the Politics of Public Expertise* (New York: Cambridge University Press, 2004). There were few if any major think tanks openly advocating more or stronger federal regulation in the 1970s and 1980s.

[89] For a general overview of these troubles, see Jasanoff, *The Fifth Branch*, v, 3, 21-2, 42–43 and the accompanying notes.

[90] Winton B. Rankin confidential memo to BFA and BOM, re "Investigational Drug Regulations," July 17, 1963; BFA-BOM Liaison Group to Rankin, July 31, 1963; FDA General Correspondence, 1963—051.155, B 3422-23, RG 88, NA.

At the same time as business conservatives won allies and seized political and cultural momentum in their attack upon federal regulation, older voices of autonomy of medicine—particularly from general practitioners—were reawakened in response to the Drug Efficacy Study Implementation (DESI). Under DESI, the Administration conducted a review of the thousands of drugs approved between 1938 and 1962, deciding for each drug whether the evidence for its safety and efficacy (as based on the NAS review) justified its continued existence on the American market. At its core, the DESI project was a massive political and economic experiment: the forced withdrawal of hundreds of medicines that were widely utilized and prescribed. It was also a raw projection of the Administration's new powers. With profitable commodities being removed from the marketplace, the FDA's efficacy standard now had tangible bite. While top pharmacologists, medical researchers, and academicians gave little protest to the DESI initiative, general practitioners and family physicians complained loudly of interference in the modes of their profession.

Yet the current of protest that emerged in the late 1960s and early 1970s differed in at least two ways from that of the early 1960s. First, particular drug companies took the lead as others laid back. Second, the object of criticism was less Congress or the efficacy standard per se, and more the Administration.

No single pharmaceutical company was more displeased with the new state of affairs than the Upjohn Company, headquartered in Kalamazoo, Michigan. Company scion Harold Upjohn had been aggressively but privately critical of the 1963 IND rules as they were being formulated. Yet the FDA's regulation of two Upjohn drugs—the antibiotics Lincocin and Panalba—set the company starkly against the agency. The Administration certified Lincocin as an antibiotic in 1965 and within one year it became one of the 200 most prescribed medicines in the United States. Yet Upjohn's advertising for Lincocin failed to disclose what the FDA saw as a crucial side effect—acute, drug-induced diarrhea. In a world with a surfeit of antibiotics, side effects were central to the determination of comparative safety and efficacy. The ad for Lincocin, Administration officials stated publicly, "obscures... the most important information that the physician needs in using this drug—that hematologic toxicity can occur, and that the frequency of severe diarrhea is a unique feature of Lincocin therapy." A week before the FDA's Lincocin statement, General Counsel William Goodrich had scored the advertising campaigns of the major American pharmaceutical companies, who were commonly grouped together and called "The Big Eight." "If the advertising copy for the 'Big Eight' is typical of what is going on, Madison Avenue's new disease of 'Behavioral Drift' is out of hand," Goodrich warned in an address before the Pharmaceutical Advertising Club in New York.[91]

[91]Mintz, *By Prescription Only* (92k).

Upjohn leadership shot back at the Administration and against Goodrich in particular. Speaking from Kalamazoo, Upjohn president R.T. Parfet, Jr., defended the Lincocin advertisement, criticized Administration officials for trying to publicly embarrass his company, and flatly declared that Upjohn "has never intended either to mislead or misinform." Parfet's next steps were less direct but no less visible. Upjohn announced that it would cancel its December 1966 advertising in over thirty medical publications, including *JAMA*. In a swipe at Goodrich, Parfet said that the "constant threat of court action" made his decision necessary. Upjohn's ad cancellation deprived advertising agencies and medical journals of significant revenue, and FDA officials interpreted the move as a broad attempt to provoke Wall Street, Madison Avenue, and medical journal interests to take sides against the Administration. The financial press jumped into the fray first. *Barron's National Business and Financial Weekly*, in its November 14, 1966 issue, blasted the Administration on its front page. *Barron's* readers were greeted by the headline, "Angels of Death," with the subheading "FDA Has Become a Threat to U.S. Health and Welfare." In the accompanying story, *Barron's* unveiled a portrait of tyranny. The Administration, now in "the doctrinaire hands of its new Commissioner, Dr. James L. Goddard," was an emerging "pharmaceutical dictatorship" that the Pharmaceutical Manufacturers Association was brave to resist. Echoing the landmark Supreme Court decision in the speech case *Schenk v. U.S.* (1919), Barron's editors declared the FDA "a clear and present danger to the nation's health and welfare." When understood in the light of proper commercialism, "the medicine men of FDA, all unwittingly perhaps, are angels of death. . . . The 90th Congress should clip their wings."[92]

In several ways, the *Barron's* offensive of November 1966 marked a new moment in conservative rhetoric against the Administration. Like Walter Modell's complaints but much more publicly and brazenly, the *Barron's* story inverted the FDA's imagery of public protection. The Administration was now actively harming the American public, its officials heralding mortality to investors and to patients. Moreover, the story targeted not merely the FDA's leadership but also its careerist structure. It was not just Goddard and Goodrich who came in for censure, but the Administration's "medicine men"—the Bureau of Drugs and its regulation of advertising. The *Barron's* attack was also notable because it signified one of the earliest cases in which the nation's financial press would devote prime news space to the fallout from a single regulatory decision (a pronouncement, actually) and would take sides with a particular company. Since the late 1970s, such prominent news stories have become commonplace.

[92]Morton Mintz interpreted the November 1966 advertising cancellation as "an effort to incite powerful pressures to be brought by diverse sources against the agency" (*By Prescription Only*, 92m). "Angels of Death," *Barron's National Business and Financial Weekly*, November 14, 1966, 1.

Barron's was published by Dow Jones & Company, which also produced the *Wall Street Journal*. The *Journal* had questioned whether the 1962 Kefauver-Harris Amendments were an overreach, but as the regime of Goddard and Goodrich progressed, its criticism began to take on more strident tones. In early 1981, its editorial page argued that the FDA's delay in approving the beta-blocker propanolol had killed 100,000 Americans. The history of the drug raised the question of "whether we should even have an FDA." Floating the idea that "the responsibility for safety" could be "merely returned to the drug makers and doctors," the *Journal* editorial concluded with a portrait of administrative decision making: "It is by now clear that the FDA bureaucrats will never take any risks they can avoid. They have nothing to gain from approving an effective drug and everything to lose from making a mistake. This kind of approach guarantees a huge loss of life. How much longer should it be allowed to prevail?" [93]

The stridency of Dow Jones publications was consequential. It seemed quickly to spill over into the journalism of industry-focused trade reporters, and before long it would influence the internal structure of the Administration itself. First, other publications joined the Wall Street chorus, lamenting (and thereby publicizing) even the most minute of Administration decisions. An earlier generation of trade reporters (exemplified by the *Oil, Paint and Drug Reporter* and the *Food, Drug and Cosmetic Reports* or "Pink Sheet") generally refrained from covering the FDA decisions other than new molecular approvals. Yet in March 1967, after Kelsey's Investigational New Drug branch terminated tests of a cancer vaccine, *Drug Trade News* published an editorial entitled "FDA's Timidity Strikes (Industry) Again." FDA officials responded that the clinical hold was more complicated than the reporter had portrayed it, but the reputational damage was indicative of broader discontent with the slow pace and procedural conservatism of Kelsey's bureau. Faced with growing criticism over a backlog of hindered IND's in Kelsey's division, Commissioner Goddard reassigned his star employee Kelsey in 1967. Goddard placed Kelsey in charge of a new Division of Scientific Investigations, an outfit where Kelsey would investigate possible instances of research fraud and misconduct, including with respect to patient consent requirements of federal law. Goddard effected the Kelsey transfer in the middle of one of his most aggressive and controversial years as Commissioner; in most other respects he had acted to bolster FDA stringency. His move was a demonstration of how the Administration's organizational structure embodied a subtle but transformative politics of legitimacy; the Kelsey transfer appeased two audiences (firms and clinical researchers) while doing so in a way that protected his agency's "sacred cow." [94]

---

[93] "100,000 Killed," *WSJ*, November 2, 1981, 26. See also "Death and Delay," *WSJ*, July 3, 1980; 16 "Dealing with the Drug Lag," *WSJ*, December 22, 1981, 20.

[94] "FDA Timidity Strikes Again," *DTN*, March 27, 1967; Herbert L. Ley, Jr. (Director, Bureau of Medicine), to Paul C. Olson (Editor, *Drug Trade News*), April 10, 1967; FOK. Ley soon would succeed Goddard as Commissioner. On the Kelsey reassignment, see NLM oral history, James Goddard; cited in Daemmrich, "A Tale of Two Experts."

The assault from the business and financial press soon emboldened the political organizations of the U.S. pharmaceutical industry—particularly the Pharmaceutical Manufacturers Association. These entities set out to rehabilitate the image of their industry, in part by contrast with the Administration, now cast as a thoroughly bureaucratic entity regulating American drug companies. The PMA began to describe the ethical drug industry more and more in terms of research and development and less and less in terms of manufacturing. This transformation would become complete when in 1994 the PMA was renamed the Pharmaceutical Research and Manufacturers of America (PhRMA). Already in the late 1960s, PMA communications placed growing emphasis on difficulty of the experimental endeavor. The headings of PMA pamphlets alluded to the "The Unfinished Business of Drug Research," the "Dilemma of Science," "The Painstaking Road," and "The Mysteries within Cells." Ultimately, the Association concluded, the higher calling of drug development is so perilous and so complicated that "Only Industry Can Do the Job." It was the pharmaceutical industry that was shouldering the burden of new medicines development, and in this world, the Administration was a hindrance and not a help. "This is risky business," warned one pamphlet. It is "as varied as it is complex. It is very expensive. It must conform to complicated government regulations, some of which may well be of dubious value in advancing drug therapy."[95]

The voices of dissent from physicians and drug manufacturers would grow louder soon after James Goddard became FDA Commissioner in 1966. Goddard launched his tenure at the agency by publicly berating drug manufacturers, charging that the industry was afflicted with a disease, and "that disease is irresponsibility." Industry observers suspected that Goddard was tarnishing their image in order to enhance his own, and their suspicions became more public as the Commissioner's keep progressed. And Goddard's penchant for speaking incautiously—once on criminal penalties for marijuana possession, later an exuberant remark on how ongoing developments in therapeutics would put the corner drugstore out of business within two decades—secured the opposition of other officials. Nine Republican congressmen called jointly for his resignation in November 1967, and the National Association of Retail Druggists issued another call for his resignation in January 1968. Yet even as Goddard's support within the Johnson administration began to fade, and even as rumors flew in 1968 about the Commissioner's impending resignation, pharmaceutical firms treaded nimbly and continued to approach Goddard with deference and care. One reason, as veteran industry observers noted, was that a robust FDA could help the industry fend off repeated attacks from Congress. Another was that Goddard had many supporters in Congress and was widely seen as having re-energized the FDA, bringing in a generation of career scientists and administrators (including Bureau of Medicine Director Herbert Ley) who shared his regulatory views if not his quick tongue. Under Goddard, Morton Mintz would

[95] "The Unfinished Business of Drug Research," *Commentaries* (Washington, DC: Pharmaceutical Manufacturers Association, October 1968).

write in 1968, "A police agency atmosphere that repelled scientists began changing into one that attracted them."[96]

The AMA's laments were echoed by some in Congress, most notably Senator Edward Long of Missouri. Long took fear and umbrage from an initiative that Larrick's and Goddard's offices had undertaken to publish and distribute information on the agency's prosecutions of American physicians and pharmaceutical manufacturers. The Missouri Democrat decried the Administration's use of "trial by press" as a regulatory tool and held hearings in 1966 and 1967 on these practices. In 1967, he wrote the membership of the American Medical Association, stating a conspiratorial case against the Administration and pleading openly for an organized counteroffensive among American physicians.

> The medical profession as a whole and the [AMA] in particular have expended a great deal of... time and energy in an unsuccessful fight against Medicare....
>
> While this battle progressed noisily to its conclusion, the government (primarily the Food and Drug Administration) quietly stole the march on the medical profession in a much more important battle that may be won without a shot being fired. I refer not to government participation in the financing of medical treatment but rather government dictatorship over all aspects of medical treatment itself.
>
> While few were watching, and fewer were caring, the [FDA] has vastly expanded its powers and duties.
>
> More and more it tells the physician how he is to practice his art.
>
> More and more it tells the pharmaceutical manufacturers how to run their highly complex industry in each and every detail....
>
> Once the harm is undone, it will be impossible to undo.
>
> The process whereby medical judgment is slipping from the hands of the profession into the hands of the bureaucrats is both fast and silent.
>
> Is this process inexorable?
>
> Only the doctors of the nation can supply the answer. As a profession, they should see that Congress tames the FDA before it absorbs what remains of medical freedom.[97]

---

[96] Goddard's opponents in industry and medical society circles reacted with caution to early rumors that the Commissioner was "about to be dropped," telling allies in their network to ignore the reports. "The rumors overlook Goddard's *many powerful friends*. He has revitalized FDA, gotten more funds for basic research. And he has *strong support* among trade unions, consumer groups. Nor is the drug industry in any position to tackle Goddard now. It would look like a hatchet-job, probably *backfire*" (emphasis in original); "Research Institute Recommendations," January 19, 1968; Historical Health Fraud Collection, "FDA, Special Data, 1959–1969," AAMA. On the rumors, see Morton Mintz, "A Guy in a White Hat at FDA," *WP*, January 21, 1968. For industry views that a strong and aggressive FDA could benefit the industry politically as well as economically, see "FDA BuMed Director Dr. Ley Named to Succeed FDA Com. Goddard," *FDCR*, June 10, 1968, 27; Jonathan Spivak, "Ley, Named to Head Federal Drug Agency, Is as Quiet as Goddard was Flamboyant," *WSJ*, June 7, 1968.

[97] Long to Goddard, May 10, 1966; F 0273-04 (FDA Correspondence, 1959–72), AAMA. Long, "The Power of the FDA," in "Letters... As Readers See It," *AMA News*, August 7, 1967, p. 4; corrected for orthography. Long was Chairman of the Subcommittee on Adminis-

Senator Long's brief letter to AMA members was long on exaggeration, but its underlying hypothesis—that through its deep and costly engagement with the politics of the Medicare program, the Association had facilitated the FDA's assertion of regulatory power in the 1960s—was a prescient one. Even as its status and reach had waned appreciably since the 1940s and 1950s, the AMA remained arguably the most powerful organization in American health politics. Yet in legislative, public, scientific, and judicial battles over the power of the FDA, the Association rarely weighed in with vigor or effect. Its energies had been sapped, its credibility diluted, by the Medicare fight.[98]

Longtime AMA staffers and observers saw another transfer of power, not the one that Edward Long was invoking, but one from the AMA itself to the Food and Drug Administration. In the 1950s, the FDA had already begun to eclipse the Association in the practice of new drug evaluation. In the aftermath of the early 1960s, the Administration's public relations wing began an aggressive program of publicity to highlight the Administration's capacities, producing pamphlets like *Your Money and Your Life: An FDA Catalog of Fakes and Swindles in the Health Field* (1963). Even as AMA officials helped with the preparation of these publications, they were later annoyed to see that the pamphlets did not mention the AMA as a source of information on quack treatments. State medical associations and high schools nonetheless eagerly sought out copies of the pamphlets for distribution to physicians and students. Elsewhere, state medical society leaders lamented the increasing prominence of the FDA in consumer protection activities, and the decline in the visibility of their professional organizations.[99]

When the firebrand Commissioner Goddard resigned and was succeeded— first by Herbert Ley and then by Nixon appointee Charles C. Edwards—

---

trative Practice and Procedure of the Senate Judiciary Committee. On the publicity initiatives, see "FDA to Report Unethical MDs," *AMA News*, March 1, 1965, 10.

[98]Such power is difficult to measure, but AMA membership was at its peak in the 1960s in terms of the fraction of American physicians who were members. In a revealing statistical analysis of Washington policy networks, sociologists Edward Laumann and David Knoke produced evidence that in the late 1970s the AMA was the structurally most central and powerful organization in the American health policy domain; *The Organizational State* (Madison: University of Wisconsin Press, 1987). Paul Starr, *The Social Transformation of American Medicine* (New York: Basic Books, 1982); Jacob Hacker, *The Divided Welfare State* (New York: Cambridge University Press, 2002); Jonathan Oberlander, *The Political Life of Medicare* (Chicago: University of Chicago Press, 2003), 21–33, 98; Theodore R. Marmor, *The Politics of Medicare*, 2nd ed. (Chicago: Aldine, 2000).

[99]FDA, *Your Money and Your Life* (Washington, DC: HEW, 1963). Nelson B. Neff (Executive Secretary, Nevada State Medical Association) to Oliver Field (Director, Investigation Division, AMA), February 20, 1964 (requesting information on, and copies of, the FDA pamphlet); Field to Neff, March 2, 1964 (telling Neff that the AMA's pamphlet Beware of 'Health' Quacks was superior); Field to Kenneth L. Milstead (Special Assistant to the Commissioner, FDA), March 10, 1964 (complaining about the FDA's omission of AMA as a source of information); Gordon M. Todd (President, Academy of Medicine of Toledo and Lucas County, Toledo, Ohio) to Field, April 17, 1964; F 0273-04 (FDA Correspondence, 1959–72), AAMA.

industry officials quietly expressed relief but guarded their optimism. Ley was considered to be more moderate, and as a Republican appointee, Edwards was greeted as a leader who would depart from the adversarial approach of Goddard and who would bring more appreciation of industry's troubles to the position. And in his early addresses to the agency's various audiences, Edwards seemed to strike this posture. His speeches to industry and regulatory audiences carried titles of reassurance and empathy—"Toward a New Understanding," "We Must Move On," "The Need for a New Paradigm,"—and he disavowed regulation of the minutiae of drug advertising.[100]

Yet it was under Edwards' Commissionership that Peter Barton Hutt began to engage in his innovative and aggressive construal of the agency's Act. It was in Edwards' Administration that the well-controlled studies rule was not only issued but aggressively applied to efficacy regulation for pre-1962 drugs and new molecular entities. It was under Edwards that the Bureau of Drugs asserted control over institutional review boards. When Edwards stepped out of the Commissioner's Office in 1973, he received numerous letters of commendation and gratitude from food and cosmetic manufacturers, but virtually none from drug interests. Among those drug company officials who did write in, their expressions of gratitude sometimes conveyed profound divisions within the American pharmaceutical industry and the business community. As Francis J. Hailey, Vice President for Medical Affairs of Norwich Pharmacal, wrote to Edwards in February 1973, "To those of us in the pharmaceutical industry who didn't have our vision obscured by an anti-FDA bias it was like a breath of fresh air to have the Commissioner's office occupied by someone who combined the viewpoint of a physician with the skills of a manager and a diplomat."[101]

[100]Edwards, "Toward a New Understanding," presented at the joint New York Pharmaceutical Advertising Club/Midwest Pharmaceutical Advertising Club Annual Luncheon, June 23, 1970, Chicago, IL (during the week of the AMA annual convention); F20, B1, CCE. "The Need for a New Paradigm," presented to the Academy of Pharmaceutical Sciences, April 15, 1970, Speech 10; "FDA: A Positive Approach to Self-Medication," presented at the Proprietary Association Annual Meeting, White Sulphur Springs, WV, May 10, 1971; Speech 16, V2, B2, CCE.

[101]Some sense of many pharmaceutical companies' disappointment in their experience with Edwards can be gauged by comparing the letters Edwards received from food and drug interests upon his departure from the Commissioner's Office in 1973. The letters from food interests are much more laudatory. Tex Cook (Chairman, General Foods Corp.), telegram to Edwards, March 14, 1973; F 7, CCE. Thomas S. Carroll (President, Lever Brothers Co.) to Edwards, March 15, 1973; Clarence C. Adamy (President, National Association of Food Chains) to Edwards, March 21, 1973; Charles H. Adler (Chairman of the Board, Estee Candy Co.) to Edwards, March 16, 1973; Harold S. Mohler (President, Hershey Foods Corp.) to Edwards, March 20, 1973; F 8, CCE. Paul Austin (Coca-Cola Co., Atlanta) telegram to Edwards, April 19; Robert D. Stuart, Jr. (President, the Quaker Oats Co.) to Edwards, March 22, 1973; John C. Suerth (Chairman of the Board—Chief Executive Officer, Gerber Products Co.) to Edwards, March 21, 1973, F 9, CCE. For the quick and praiseless notes from drug company officials, see for example W. H. Consen (President, Schering-Plough Corporation) to Edwards, March 14, 1973; J. Mark Hiebert, M.D. (Chairman of the Board, Sterling Drug, Inc., New York) to Edwards, March 15, 1973; J. N. Cooke (Senior VP, Sterling Drug Co.) to Edwards, March 15, 1973; Hailey to Edwards, February 21, 1973; F 8, CCE.

Hailey's praise of Edwards, and his criticism of the "less progressive" elements of his trade, marks an important but little realized political fact about pharmaceutical manufacturers in the 1960s and 1970s. American and European drug companies were far from united in vigorous opposition to the FDA. This fracture of common interests eased the course of the Administration's initiatives. Indeed, a persistent irony of this period matched contestation with acquiescence in drug companies' responses to the Administration. Along with battles over alternative therapies (Laetrile and nutritional supplements) and the growing discourse of the drug lag, the quarter-century following thalidomide witnessed broad and active company-sponsored litigation against FDA. Yet these cases were largely victories for the Administration's power and reputation, and the period from 1960 to the early 1980s is notable for the facility with which most major pharmaceutical manufacturers adapted to the rule of the Administration over their marketplace and their affairs. This is not to deny that drug companies complained loudly about the 1963 regulations. Nor is it to forget the industry's strong support of deregulatory legislative initiatives such as the ill-fated Drug Regulation Reform Act of 1978. Yet FDA critics perceptively saw the battle being lost in the particulars: the steady and massive obeisance to clinical experimentation guidelines, the widespread adoption (despite considerable protests) of package inserts, the quiet removal of hundreds of formerly quick-selling therapies from the prescription and over-the-counter markets, often at the slightest hint of FDA investigation into their labeling or general effectiveness. When AMA President James Z. Appel spoke to the annual meeting of the American College of Allergists in 1966, he castigated the agency for regulation by "fiat," but reserved his deepest expression of concern for what he perceived as "the tame submission of the pharmaceutical industry to any and every regulatory suggestion or directive... regardless of the medical and scientific facts involved."[102]

Even as these complaints established new patterns of confrontation, they quietly affirmed how much had changed in the world of pharmaceuticals. No one rose to challenge Appel's claim that drug companies had displayed meek compliance with the FDA's advice and edicts. Moreover, Appel's open call for industry and medicine to "cooperate" for meaningful change—and his call for societies like the allergists' College to work together with the AMA—betrayed the underlying weakness of his organization's position. In the 1960s and 1970s, neither "medicine" nor "pharmaceuticals" composed

---

As possible evidence of his regulatory philosophy, consider that Edwards would claim in his 2005 autobiography that he had abandoned his lifelong identification as a Republican, in part because he saw greater energy for consumer protection in the Democratic Party. Edwards (with Mike Ono Benedyk), *Tough Choices: My Extraordinary Journey at the Heart of American Politics and Medicine* (San Diego, CA: Bennett Peiji Design, 2005).

[102] I have characterized language on "progressive" versus other (presumably nonprogressive) elements of the 1960s pharmaceutical industry from reading the trade reporters of the period, particularly the "Pink Sheet" (see for example *FD&CR*, June 10, 1968, 27). Appel, "New Drugs: The AMA and FDA Roles," delivered April 29, 1966; AAMA.

an organic political whole. To be sure, the FDA itself suffered from divisions and inconstancy during the same period, but in relative terms the contrast could not be mistaken. Organized medicine and organized drug manufacture were not speaking or acting with the order, the unity, and the political and regulatory foresight displayed by the FDA. The Administration had not effected the separation, but to the extent that American medicine and global pharmaceuticals were conquered, it was in large part because they were divided.

The Politics of Numerical Imagery and the "Drug Lag." In the aftermath of James Goddard's contentious term of office—and incited by the DESI study and the acrimony coming from the nation's investment and advertising circles—a new critique of the Administration began to take shape. Academic and industry skeptics of federal efficacy standards pointed to the reduced availability of new medicines in the United States and wondered whether the 1962 Amendments were worth their cost. The form of these claims varied, but by the time Gerald Ford ascended to the presidency in 1974, a new term had entered the nation's pharmacological and political vocabulary: the "drug lag."[103]

The drug lag was less a brute fact than a political construction. This is not to deny the underlying institutional patterns—slower development and marketing of novel molecules in the United States, relative to the past and relative to European nations—to which "drug lag" critics pointed. Compared to the United Kingdom, new chemical entities took six months to a year longer to appear on the American market from 1960 to 1982. Yet the rhetoric of the "drug lag" represented these patterns in a certain way, one that synthesized new metrics of evaluation and created a new political reality. The data had existed and had been around since the thalidomide scare. Industry observer Paul deHaen noticed a substantial drop in "new single chemical" approvals—single molecules that have never been marketed alone or in combination in the United States—as early as 1964. From an historic peak of sixty-three such drugs approved in 1959, he calculated, the rate of product introduction had fallen to sixteen new chemicals newly marketed in 1963. While some critics saw confirmation of fears they had voiced during the passage of the Kefauver-Harris Amendments, deHaen saw more favorable trends in the decline. The pace of new drug approvals in the previous fifteen years had been frenetic, he observed, and the result of FDA oversight of clinical development would be "a more measured scientific pace, permitting greater maturity in judgment of product development and marketing." The industry newsletter *Drug Research Reports*, also known as "The Blue

---

[103]In the following section I present a different interpretation of the "drug lag" debates of the past several decades. Yet in my research and understanding of this dialogue I am indebted to Arthur Daemmrich and Philip Hilts. Daemmrich, "Invisible Monuments and the Costs of Pharmaceutical Regulation: Twenty-Five Years of Drug Lag Debate," *Pharmacy in History* 45 (1) (2003): 3–17; Hilts, *Protecting America's Health*, chapters 12 and 18.

Sheet," observed that firms were "concentrating on fewer—and probably better—investigational drugs to make full use of research time, money, and scarce talent."[104]

Financial analysts also began to revise their portraits of the industry's future. One January 1967 projection forecast that, after 1976, the entire U.S. population would have access to federally financed health care and warned that "the FDA will continue to be a limiting factor in new product development, though some improvement over the present situation may develop over the next few years. Clearance of sustained release products, combination products and marginally superior products will be difficult and time-consuming." Pfizer research director Barry Bloom then published a report in 1971 in which he aggregated the number of new drugs produced by the American pharmaceutical industry since 1945. Echoing deHaen's analysis, Bloom concluded that a significant falloff in "development" had occurred since 1960, a drop partially attributable to failures of research productivity but also plausibly accredited to the 1962 Amendments and the FDA's 1963 rules.[105]

In 1970, the collective lament about reduced "innovation" began to relocate, coming less from industry and financial circles and more commonly from academic venues, particularly among two disciplines: clinical pharmacologists who surveyed the development of new medicines, and economists who specialized in industrial organization. The argument from economics was launched by Sam Peltzman, a doctoral student of George Stigler at the University of Chicago who had taken his first academic position at UCLA. In a 1972 article in the *Journal of Political Economy*, Peltzman represented the decline in new chemical entities as a fundamental shift in the industry's "production function," the relationship between "inputs" (such as capital and R&D expenditures) and the "output" of new drugs. Whereas the "input" of pharmaceutical industry investment exhibited a strong correlation with

[104] "Only 800 Pharmaceuticals in Various Stages of Investigation, According to Count by DeHaen from Current Literature; Only Handful Likely to be Marketed," *DRR*, January 22, 1964, 12; "Editorial," *NEJM* 268 (1963): 846; Rising, "The Practicing Physician's Approach to the Evaluation of New Drugs," 1046. It appears to be deHaen who popularized the concept of "new single chemical," a term that later morphed into "new chemical entity" during debates over the "drug lag." Both terms are near substitutes for the Administration's term "new molecular entity," differing to the extent that salts, esters, and diagnostic products were included in the FDA's count but excluded from deHaen's.

The study of this period that best compares "apples" to "apples" —similar molecules across similar regulatory regimes and nations—is Hans Berlin and Bengt Jonsson, "International Dissemination of New Drugs: A Comparative Study of Six Countries," *Managerial and Decision Economics* 7 (4) (Dec. 1986): 235–42. Compared to other countries, Berlin and Jonsson find appreciable American differences only with Great Britain, and not with Sweden, France, West Germany, or Italy; this suggests that perceptions and measurements of the "drug lag" depended greatly upon the reference country against which the FDA was compared.

[105] L. Roden to F. M. Rivinus, "Drug Industry Environmental Expectations," January 8, 1967; LSG. Bloom, "The Rate of Contemporary Drug Discovery," *Lex et Scienta* 8 (1971), 1–11.

new chemical introductions ("output") from 1950 to 1961, the predictive power of investment fell off appreciably for the ten years following the Amendments. From Peltzman's simple analysis of over-time data, one could infer that the fundamental cost structure of the industry had changed, and that the return on capital and other factors of production was far smaller than before the 1962 Amendments.[106]

Whereas Peltzman's article focused on the effects and "costs" of the 1962 law, a series of monographs financed and published by the conservative American Enterprise Institute (AEI) sought to weigh the costs against the benefits. The first of these—*Regulation of Pharmaceutical Innovation: The 1962 Amendments* (1974)—was authored by Peltzman himself. Following standard welfare economics of the time, Peltzman divided the total "welfare loss" from the 1962 Amendments into reduced consumer surplus ($300 to $400 million in 1974 dollars) and higher prices ($50 million). These costs outweighed the gain from "reduced waste on purchases of ineffective new drugs," to produce a total consumer surplus reduction of $250 to $300 million. In later AEI publications, Duke University economist Henry Grabowski would arrive at similar numbers and echo Peltzman's call for ridding the United States of the efficacy standards introduced in 1962. The economic critique soon waned from mainstream academic journals and began to appear more commonly in select, smaller outlets.[107]

The term "drug lag" was coined by University of Rochester pharmacologist William Wardell in an address in a paper presented to the Fifth International Congress of Pharmacology in 1972. Wardell identified a set of new molecules, mainly drugs for cardiovascular, respiratory, and gastrointestinal conditions, that he claimed were introduced into clinical practice in European nations years before their availability in the United States. Focusing on the United Kingdom in particular, he found four times as many new drugs introduced across the Atlantic as in the United States. He then joined with his Rochester colleague Louis Lasagna to produce a series of new reports in the mid- to late-1970s that extended the drug lag critique to a wide series of therapeutic categories. The cardinal sin of the drug lag, Wardell and Lasagna would contend, was the Administration's delay in approving beta-blockers for essential hypertension. By hindering receptors to which adrenaline binds in heart cells, beta-blockers can reduce effective cardiovascular "work-

---

[106]Peltzman, "An Evaluation of Consumer Protection Legislation: The 1962 Drug Amendments," *Journal of Political Economy* 81 (5) (Sept.-Oct. 1973), 1049–91.

[107]Peltzman, *Regulation of Pharmaceutical Innovation: The 1962 Amendments* (Washington, DC: American Enterprise Institute, 1974); Grabowski, *Drug Regulation and Innovation: Empirical Evidence and Policy Options* (Washington, DC: American Enterprise Institute, 1976). Most studies of pharmaceutical regulation were published in a small network of journals; see for instance Grabowski, Vernon, and Lacy Glenn Thomas, "Estimating the Effects of Regulation on Innovation: An International Comparative Analysis of the Pharmaceutical Industry," *Journal of Law and Economics* 21 (1978): 133–63. Like the *Journal of Political Economy*, the *Journal of Law and Economics* was edited by faculty at the University of Chicago.

load." Wardell and Lasagna ascribed many thousands of "excess deaths" per year in the United States to the late introduction of propanolol and practolol as treatments for essential hypertension and angina.[108]

The drug lag was a political construction in one other important sense. It was organizationally sponsored. The American Enterprise Institute linked the two disciplinary critiques—from free-market economists and from renegade clinical pharmacologists—both structurally and rhetorically. Structurally, Robert Helms launched the AEI Center for Health Policy Research in 1974. The Center convened symposia of industry officials, economists from business schools and universities, and pharmacologists. Many of the attendees at the AEI conferences would go on to write important papers contributing to evidence for the drug lag hypothesis. On the advisory committee of Helms' Center were Louis Lasagna, Hoover Institution economist Rita Ricardo Campbell, Duke law professor Clark Havighurst, Michigan business school professor Paul McCracken, and the Cleveland Clinic's Irvine Page, a cardiologist who in 1959 had helped to promote the ill-fated cholesterol drug MER/29. The "drug lag" concept pre-dated Helms' Center, but the networks in which the term was propagated, elaborated, and popularized were girded by the American Enterprise Institute.[109]

The debate over the drug lag and innovation created two numerical metrics—"number of new chemical entities" and "nation of first approval"—that would remain attached to national debates over pharmaceutical regulation. Peltzman's study focused the attention of economists on the number of new molecules being approved by the FDA as the standard measure of aggregate innovation. As critics noted, there were problems with this measure. A single breakthrough drug could provide more therapeutic benefit than twenty other "new molecules." So too, there was a timing issue with the measure; the number of drugs coming to market in a given year is usually a function of decisions made five to ten years beforehand by pharmaceutical companies. Despite this and other problems, and indeed because of the way that the annual "new chemical entities" measure simplified away more nuanced

[108]Wardell, "Introduction of New Therapeutic Drugs in the United States and Great Britain: An International Comparison," *CP&T* 14 (1973): 773–90. In testimony before a congressional committee in 1979, Wardell stated that the three-year delay in a single beta-blocker, alprenolol, had caused more than 10,000 deaths per year in the United States; "Statement of William Wardell, M.D., Ph.D., at Hearings on the Food and Drug Administration's New Drug Approval Process, Submitted to the Science, Research and Technology Subcommittee of the Committee on Science and Technology, U.S. House of Representatives, June 19, 1979"; Gerald D. Laubach, "Federal Regulation and Pharmaceutical Innovation, *Proceedings of the Academy for Political Science* 33 (4) (1980): 71.

[109]The AEI Center for Health Policy Research held its first conference in July 1974. The volume produced from this conference would bring together dozens of academics, industry officials, and industry economists who would later contribute to academic criticism of the FDA; Robert B. Helms, ed., *Drug Development and Marketing* (Washington, DC: AEI, 1975). For the membership of the AEI Center's advisory board, see the front matter of Grabowski, *Drug Regulation and Innovation*. On Page's promotion of MER/29, see Greene, *Prescribing by Numbers*, 159.

measurement, it became perhaps the dominant metric by which the FDA and the American pharmaceutical industry were judged.[110]

The second metric embedded an international contrast. The idea of an "international lag" carried within it a comparison of the FDA's performance relative to similar agencies in other nations. And it created an implicit competition between national regulators to see which nation had first approved a therapeutically novel drug. In this sense, the "drug lag" rhetoric re-expressed decades-old complaints in a new way, quantifying them and establishing European countries as a baseline. Here, too, the accuracy and validity of the measure was in question. A drug could make it to market rather slowly as long as it was available "here" first, which could have been a function of when it was submitted, or perhaps the allure of the United States as a market whose profitability was growing more quickly than that of other countries (most of which have indirect or direct price controls on prescription drugs). So too, in cases where the firm had decided to try to enter a European market first, for reasons unrelated to regulation, the "nation of first approval" statistic could easily mislead.

Perhaps the best evidence that the "drug lag" metrics took hold is that Administration officials began to openly incorporate such considerations into their decisions and communications. In reports issued quarterly and annually, the FDA's drug reviewing division began to announce all new molecular entity (NME) approvals and to make note of whether the annual total of new molecular entities had risen or declined from previous years. The Administration began to issue approval letters in the last weeks of the calendar year—so that the drug could be included in the annual NME tally of that year rather than the next one—giving rise to the phenomenon of "December approvals." Other kinds of approvals such as generic approvals and supplemental approvals were not announced, and their frequency did not spike in December. The Administration began keeping systematic data on whether its approvals occurred before or after those in other countries, particularly Great Britain. And the FDA's response to this criticism created what was known inside the Administration as a "drug lag drug," meaning a drug that had been approved for one year or more in a comparator market and whose delay might be reflecting poorly upon the Administration.[111]

[110]The "victory" of this measure had other causes. For one, the data were available in this form partly because the FDA had separated out "new molecular entities" in its data from 1950 at latest. For another, Paul DeHaen and other pharmaceutical industry analysts had already been using the measure for years. For these reasons, the data for the measure were readily available. Among economists, the idea of measuring innovation by a count of new products introduced also meshed well with the Poisson model of innovation. Jennifer Reinganum, "A Dynamic Game of R and D: Patent Protection and Competitive Behavior," *Econometrica* 50 (1982) (3): 671–88; Rebecca Henderson, and Iain Cockburn, "Scale, Scope, and Spillovers: Determinants of Research Productivity in the Pharmaceutical Industry," *RAND Journal of Economics* 27 (1) (Spring 1996): 32–59.

[111]Arthur E. Hass, et al., "A Historical Look at Drug Introductions on a Five Country Market: A Comparison of the United States and Four European Countries (1960–81)," FDA *Re-*

At more official and visible levels, the Administration's highest officials rejected the premises and implications of the drug lag charge. Commissioner Donald Kennedy wrote a perspective for the *Journal of the American Medical Association* in 1978 entitled "A Calm Look at 'Drug Lag'." Kennedy's essay argued that numerous other variables—patent laws, medical liability, a depleting base of applied knowledge, corporate decision making, and the relative importance of drugs to each nation's health systems—could better explain the "lag" to which Wardell had pointed. Wardell penned a strong and angry reply—"A Close Inspection of the 'Calm Look': Rhetorical Amblyopia and Selective Amnesia and the Food and Drug Administration"—in which he doubted that *JAMA* readers would "regard the 'calm look' as a cogent argument coming from anyone; coming from a respected government agency with a staff of more than 7,600 and a budget of $245 million in 1977, it seriously underestimates the intelligence of [*JAMA*] readers and other taxpayers."[112]

Wardell's praise of the FDA—even as he castigated its leader—points to another, less recognizable feature of the drug lag debate. In many respects, the notion of a drug lag reaffirmed the agency's performance on two dimensions—as a protector of citizens against drug hazards and as a methodical and judicious organization. When Wardell pronounced that articles like Donald Kennedy's would, "if permitted to continue, . . . ultimately destroy the FDA's scientific and medical credibility," he was making a statement that the Administration possessed the sort of credibility that could be lost. In the late 1970s, attributions of "credibility," "respected," and "expertise" to government agencies were few and far between. A similar pattern of praise embedded within blame would occur in libertarian criticism of the drug lag, such as when pundit Sam Kazman of the Competitive Enterprise Institute would decry "Deadly Overcaution" at the FDA. To the extent that delay was occurring in U.S. pharmaceutical regulation in the 1970s, there were numerous causes, sometimes as simple as a cumbersome mail system (see chapter 7). Yet, in the rhetoric of the drug lag, these administrative delays were interpreted as behavioral, as regulatory "caution," "timidity," "risk-aversion" and the like. To be sure, "drug lag" critics saw too much vigilance for drug safety at the Administration and wished to highlight its costs. Yet critics were, in making their arguments, reminding their readers and viewers that the Administration had regulated with prudence and deliberation. An attack on the agency for being overcautious was an affirmation that the agency had in fact behaved cautiously, in accordance with cultural and statutory expectations.[113]

port FDAIACPE-82/55 (Washington: NTIS, 1982). See chapter 7 for a focused discussion of approval timing and its relationship to organizational reputation.

[112]Kennedy, "A Calm Look at 'Drug Lag'," *JAMA* 239 (1978): 423–6; Wardell, "A Close Inspection of the 'Calm Look': Rhetorical Amblyopia and Selective Amnesia and the Food and Drug Administration," *JAMA* 239 (1978): 2004–11.

[113]Wardell, "A Close Examination of the 'Calm Look'," 2011; Kazman, "Deadly Overcau-

One reason that drug lag critics focused upon the agency's behavioral features rather than administrative processes is that the ultimate target of much of "drug lag" rhetoric was the efficacy standards of the 1962 Amendments. To libertarians of the 1960s and 1970s, the idea that a government agency would or could assess the quality of a product was anathema. Quality determinations, they felt, should be left to consumers and the price system of an unregulated market. University of Chicago economists Milton Friedman and George Stigler could tolerate the FDA's judgment of drug safety, but they could not bear its efficacy standard. They both pointed to Peltzman's statistics, questioning not the FDA's enforcement of the 1962 statute, but the statute itself. Hence, the drug lag offensive was one in a long line of arguments made against federal efficacy standards, and many academic studies and policy reports concluded with a call for a relaxation of the 1962 efficacy standard or its disappearance altogether.[114]

The drug lag concept thus grew from industry complaints about innovation, took form as a disciplinary academic concept, and began reverberating in mainstream medical journals. It would soon enter into national politics. In the anti-regulatory moment of the late 1970s and 1980s, national politicians began to single out the FDA as overly intrusive in the doctor-patient relationship and in the entrepreneurial process of drug development. The presidential administration of Ronald Reagan, spurred by the Heritage Foundation and other conservative think tanks, also began to rein in the FDA and to propose far-reaching revisions to the 1962 Amendments. Yet in the main, the political reputation of the Administration was reproduced not so much in election campaigns or in the White House as in the committees of America's national legislature.[115]

An Audience for Vigilance: Sidney Wolfe and the Post-Watergate Congress

The late 1970s and early 1980s saw the rehearsal of an earlier set of laments about the agency's limp governance of the pharmaceutical industry, and

---

tion," *Journal of Regulation and Social Costs* 1 (1990): 35–54. See also the characterizations and ascriptions reported in Daemmrich's summary review, "Invisible Monuments and the Costs of Pharmaceutical Regulation," 6–14.

[114] Wardell and Lasagna, *Regulation and Drug Development*, chap. 13; Yale Brozen, "Foreword" to Grabowski, *Drug Regulation and Innovation*, 8.

[115] John Kelly, "Bridging America's Drug Gap," *NYT*, September 13, 1981; Ray W. Gifford, "Statement of the American Medical Association before the Subcommittee on Science, Research and Technology, Committee on Science and Technology, U. S. House of Representatives," June 21, 1979. File "Research, General, Food and Drug Administration, 1978–1979," 10.1A; RG 1, SG 2 (President's Office Records, 1964–1979), MDAA. From the vantage of political science, the emergence of awareness about the drug lag is familiar as agenda-setting (Kingdon, *Agendas, Alternatives and Public Policies*). From another perspective, it tells us that what political scientists call "agenda-setting" and what sociologists call "problem definition" (Hilgartner and Bosk) is in fact the re-definition or re-framing of an earlier problem. The materials for the conceptual framing of "drug lag" were in place for a decade before the term was popularized. What Wardell and other AEI-affiliated scholars did was to skillfully recombine these materials to create a pressing new crisis that demanded attention and public action.

about organizational malfeasance with regard to drug safety. No voice more cogently or passionately articulated the case for rigorous drug safety standards than that of physician-activist Sidney Wolfe, and no arrangement better amplified the concerns of Wolfe and his allies than the committee systems of the U.S. House and Senate. Wolfe helped to found the Health Research Group, a subsidiary of Ralph Nader's Public Citizen, in 1971. Wolfe surfaced in a 1974 controversy over the transfers of two medical officers in the Bureau of Drugs, when he produced an eighteen-page memo attacking FDA leaders for the decision.[116]

Wolfe's principal weapon was his threat to the Administration's consumer protection image. The credibility of this threat depended on a set of strategies by which Wolfe and his organization could embarrass the agency, extract data from it, influence the FDA's decision agenda, or (less commonly) induce courts to force the agency to take a given action. First, he was adept at using administrative procedures refined in the 1970s, including Freedom of Information Act (FOIA) requests and citizens' petitions, to pry important drug safety and procedural information out of the agency, or to place contentious and uncomfortable items on the Administration's agenda. Second, Wolfe exploited the public comment period of the FDA's advisory committee meetings on drugs, an opportunity that offered a public venue albeit with brief appearances. Third, Wolfe appeared regularly at congressional committee hearings as an invited guest, and his ties to committee chairs and their staff gave him indirect access to committee powers (replete with tools for discovery). In the 1970s and 1980s, Wolfe worked partially in tandem with subcommittee chairmen ranging from Lawrence Fountain, Henry Waxman, and Ted Weiss in the House to Senators Edward Kennedy and Abraham Ribicoff.[117]

Fourth, Wolfe maintained ties to journalists over a period of several decades (Morton Mintz, Christine Russell, Philip Hilts, and others). He used these journalists to publicize actions (such as the taking of surveys of FDA medical officers) that would otherwise not have received much public attention. Finally, Wolfe and his organization shrewdly used lawsuits and the threat of legal action to induce rulemaking and jar the agency into action. The strategies of administrative maneuvering, advisory committee testimony, appearances at congressional hearings, and media access became much more pivotal to Wolfe's leverage over the FDA after 1979, when a federal judge limited the right of Nader's group to sue agencies on behalf of the general public.[118]

[116]Sidney Wolfe and Anita Johnson, "Conflict Against the Public Interest at the Bureau of Drugs," F 7 ("Bureau of Drugs, 1971–1973, n.d."), B12, FOK. The Nestor-Winkler controversy is discussed at greater length in chapter 7. Mintz, "FDA Is Criticized on Consultant Use," WP April 3, 1972, A5.

[117]Morton Mintz, "FDA Plans to Require Drug Test Follow-Ups," WP, September 28, 1974, A2. It was crucial that, during this period, "the proponents of regulatory stringency. . . tended to hold the upper hand within the key authorization committees"; Christopher Foreman, Signals from the Hill: Congressional Oversight and the Challenge of Social Regulation (New Haven: Yale University Press, 1988), 20.

[118]In some cases, media access allowed Wolfe to draw public attention to his group's formal

Wolfe's profile rose further during the Reagan administration, as he accused the Republican president's appointees of favoring business interests over those of the public health. (He would play a similar role, with much more strident rhetoric, during the presidency of George W. Bush.) And Wolfe shrewdly played off the tension, prominent during the Nixon-Ford administrations and the Reagan administration, between the White House and a Congress eager to investigate the executive branch. There were other voices active in drug safety debates, but beside his commanding presence and his diligence, it was Wolfe's facility in congressional, journalistic, and other Washington networks that uniquely positioned him for pivotal influence in American pharmaceutical regulation. From the 1980s onward, there were few if any voices more powerful in public debates over drug safety.

. . .

While Commissioners had always represented the Administration before Congress, the agency began to rely for testimony upon one individual more than any other in matters of pharmaceutical regulation: Robert Temple. For several reasons Temple, who is commonly described as the agency's brightest scientific star in the late twentieth century, would continually testify before Congress on behalf of the Administration. First, as head of the agency's drug review functions, he had passing administrative knowledge of many of the advanced new drug applications—approved, unapproved, accelerated, or delayed—that caught the attention of House and Senate committees. Second, Temple's voice was (and remains) as authoritative as any in American medicine on drug development and clinical experimentation. When, in 1986, Manhattan Democrat Ted Weiss held House hearings on the FDA's approval of nomifensine maleate (Merital)—a novel antidepressant that had been withdrawn from the worldwide market in January 1986 due to its association with severe and fatal immune reactions—it was not an antidepressant specialist or psychiatrist at the FDA who handled most of Weiss's queries, but the "generalist" Temple. Temple spoke as authoritatively on the drug and related therapies as did the more specialized Paul Leber, head of the Administration's Neuropharmacological Products division. He calmly rebutted the arguments of Johns Hopkins immunologist N. Franklin Adkinson that signals from Europe should have cautioned the agency against approval of the drug and that Merital's label failed to disclose its safety risks.

---

letters to federal officials (including in other agencies, for instance the Securities and Exchange Commission); Martha M. Hamilton, "SmithKline Reporting Criticized," WP, September 16, 1981, D8. Christine Russell, "Inside: the FDA," WP, December 17, 1982, A19. Wolfe and his colleagues also petitioned for safety-based drug withdrawals or to reverse over-the-counter conversions; "FDA Urged to Reverse Drug Status," WP, April 18, 1989, A3. Jerry Knight, "Sirica Limits Nader Groups' Right to Sue," WP, March 15, 1979, D10. Wolfe's success in getting federal courts to compel rulemaking action was perhaps clearest in the OTC drug review; "FDA Seeks Stiffer Curb for Nonprescription Drugs," WP, May 13, 1980, A5.

Temple undercut Adkinson's legitimacy by explaining that the efficacy and safety judgments were specific to psychiatry and the needs of the depressed patient. An immunologist could not, Temple implied, make judgments on the marketability of an antidepressant drug. Weiss vigorously disagreed and showed his displeasure with Temple's continual "non-responses" and attempts to complicate what the congressman thought were simpler matters. The tense back-and-forth between Weiss and Temple pitted one of the national legislature's most aggressive interlocutors against one of the federal government's brightest minds.[119]

Celebrity officials like Temple could rebut the criticism, but they could not stop it from starting and coming. The persistent and caustic scrutiny that marked the hearings on MER/29, oral contraceptives, and Merital would remain an ever-present backdrop to the Administration's existence. In 1977, just as the FDA was winning crucial legal battles, as its budget was growing by multiples, and as it was beating back legislative attempts to restrict its discretion, *New York Times* reporter Richard Lyons would write in a front-page story that the Administration stood as "the Federal Government's most criticized, demoralized and fractionalized agency."[120]

Lyons's characterization was impressionary; neither he nor any other journalist had any way of comparing censure, morale, and fractionalization across agencies of American government. Yet Lyons spoke a truth that begets a puzzle. How could the Administration's constant disparagement at the hands of Congress co-exist with the consistently kind portrayal it received in public opinion polls, in journalistic treatments (other than Lyons'), and in general public discussion? Just eight years after Lyons's sentence was published, and in the middle of another episode in which the Administration was being criticized for having "blood on its hands"—the AIDS crisis of the

---

[119] *Oversight of the New Drug Approval Process and FDA's Regulation of Merital*, Hearing before a Subcommittee of the Committee on Government Operations, House of Representatives, 99th Congress, Second Session (May 22, 1986), Washington, DC: GPO, 1986). Weiss is perhaps best known for his attempt to commence impeachment proceedings against President Ronald Reagan after the U.S. invasion of Grenada in 1983. In 1986, Temple served as Director of the FDA's Office of Drug Research and Review. For a revealing biographical portrait of Temple, see Hilts, *Protecting America's Health*, chapter 15. With the development and approval of fluoxetine (Prozac) and subsequent selective serotonin reuptake inhibitors (SSRIs), tricyclic and nontricyclic antidepressants (Merital was a nontricyclic treatment) fell quickly from use in the 1980s. In immune hemolytic anemia, the combination of an antigen and an antibody damages the body's red cells and induces lysis, or removal from circulation. Drugs can cause this condition if they produce drug-induced antibodies in sufficient numbers to remove enough red blood cells. For an influential analysis of this side effect, see Abdulgabar Salama and Christian Mueller-Eckhart, "The Role of Metabolite-Specific Antibodies in Nomifensine-Dependent Immune Hemolytic Anemia," *NEJM* 313 (8) (Aug. 22, 1985): 469–74. The publication of the Salama and Mueller-Eckhart article induced the Administration to revise Merital's labeling in December 1985.

[120] Lyons, "Demoralized F.D.A. Struggles to Cope," *NYT*, March 14, 1977, 1, 49; quoted in Watkins, *On the Pill*, 159, n.99.

1980s—the *Washington Post* would echo Victor Wynn's reminder that Americans, like the citizens of other nations, carried abiding trust in the agency. "Americans are justifiably proud of the regulatory system set up by the government to test new drugs," the *Post* concluded. "Most consumers in this country are satisfied to rely on the FDA's time-consuming evaluations, because when that agency finally approves a drug, it is almost certainly both safe and effective."[121]

The puzzle of blame and confidence is partially explained by the continuing symbolic heft of thalidomide and, less explicitly, of Frances Kelsey and the reformist cohort. Thalidomide was interwoven with a language of consumer protection that established the Administration as one of the most admired yet criticized agencies in all of government—state, national, and international. By the late 1990s, a poll would show that over two-thirds of women over the age of thirty-five had heard of "thalidomide," while a third under that age had heard of the drug. Consistent with this public memory, stories in major newspapers mentioning thalidomide dropped off sharply after 1962–63, but then picked up again through the 1970s and 1980s (figure 5.1). In few of these stories would Frances Kelsey's name be mentioned; in many of them, as in the *Washington Post* editorial, the FDA would be cited, and often approvingly.

Yet there is more to the puzzle of blame and confidence than the figurative persistence of thalidomide. The association between the agency and the concept of "protection" in major American newspapers arose a full decade after the thalidomide tragedy and the Kefauver-Harris Amendments (table 5.7). Doubts about the Administration's organizational capacity were continually expressed but were also displaced by a larger narrative in which success reverberated and fault was reflected to Congress, to the pharmaceutical industry, and occasionally the FDA's leadership, but not its core structure. An implicit equation between the "gold standard" of the double-blind randomized controlled trial and the "gold standard" of the FDA as guarantor of drug safety steadily emerged in American public discourse. Public opinion polls continued to show consistent support for the agency and its mission.

At the center of the FDA's organizational reputation lay the fact that the agency's support was broad and expressed in vague terms, while most of its censure was targeted and specific to particular decisions. Indeed, the specificity of the agency's blame often supported the generality of the confidence Americans and others placed in it. When Victor Wynn reminded Administration officials of the breadth of their trust even as he worried it was misplaced, or when Ted Weiss chastised Robert Temple by stating that "You *exist* to make sure that the medicines you approve are safe and effective," the abiding mission of the agency showed through the temporary rebuke. Even as they produced questions about the Administration's ability and

---

[121] "Drugs for the Dying," *WP*.

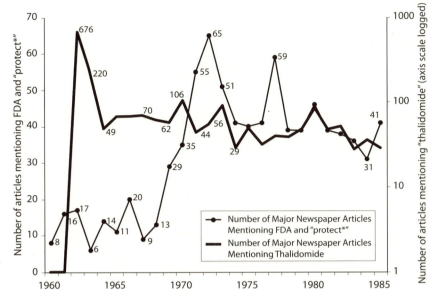

Figure 5.1. Number of Major Newspaper Articles Mentioning "Thalidomide" and Number Mentioning FDA and "Protect," 1960–1985

commitment to uphold its mission in particular circumstances, congressional hearings reproduced a general sense that the FDA served as scientific agency and as protector of the American people. In repeatedly directing public and journalistic attention to the FDA's charge, congressional hearings underscored the formal and cultural basis of the Administration's legitimacy.

The continuous crystallization of an organizational reputation, then, relied upon constant criticism of particular decisions and actions. In retrospect, John Nestor's jarring testimony at the Humphrey hearings in 1963 presaged a growing and persistent pattern of case-specific scrutiny. Like those hearings, congressional inquiries into the Administration's practices tended to focus less upon generalities as such and more upon the agency's performance in regulating a single molecule. In their drug-specific focus, these hearings carried undercurrents of satisfaction and dissatisfaction with the "normal" state of affairs at the agency. For each problem case revealed and publicized by a congressional subcommittee, the Administration's audiences could ask several questions. Is this case indicative of deeper problems at the agency? Or is it the unfortunate exception that proves the institutional rule of regulatory success? When they conveyed the idea that a particular case marked a departure from what the Administration usually did or what it could do, congressional hearings communicated a symbolic message of organizational competence and promise.

TABLE 5.7.
Frequency of Agency Mentions in Major Newspaper Articles, 1960–2007 (with or without the word "protect")*

U.S. Federal Agency	Major Newspaper Articles in which Agency Mentioned, 1960–2007	Major Newspaper Articles in which Agency Mentioned and in which Word "protect*" Appears, 1960–2007	Percentage	Log(mentions) + log(percentage)
Environmental Protection Agency	31,252	536	1.72	2.96
Federal Aviation Administration	28,354	2,840	10.02	4.45
Federal Bureau of Investigation	105,114	9,785	9.31	4.96
Federal Communications Commission	37,256	4,022	10.80	4.64
Federal Deposit Insurance Corporation	8,603	1,531	17.80	4.44
Federal Reserve	117,134	1,660	1.42	3.37
Federal Trade Commission	33,207	6,400	19.27	5.09
Food and Drug Administration	33,927	6,482	19.11	5.09
National Labor Relations Board	10,967	1,483	13.52	4.30
Occupational Safety and Health Administration	5,063	2,237	44.18	4.99
Securities and Exchange Commission	84,014	7,839	9.33	4.86
U.S. Army	36,447	3,763	10.32	4.59

The Political Limits of Gatekeeping:
Battles over Dietary Supplements

Despite its successes in prescription drugs, over-the-counter medications, new molecular entities, and medical devices, the Administration's power over the therapeutic marketplace was anything but absolute and total. Even as the broad vision of the Food, Drug and Cosmetic Act, the IND rules, and the FDA's pharmacological vision were accepted by federal courts, Congress, pharmaceutical companies, academic medical centers, scientific and physician associations and other organizations, the Administration's authority and regulatory power were limited by the concept of a "new drug." The federal courts had spoken quite clearly in the late 1960s and in the *Weinberger* cases of 1973 that the category of "new drugs" encompassed a vast array of compounds, implements, and synthesized substances. Yet an important and popular set of commodities existed and profited in the legal and conceptual space between drugs and foods. These were dietary supplements (for instance, herbal supplements) that purported to be natural while they also offered promises of "health," carefully avoiding claims about activity against a particular disease.[122]

The Administration had possessed pre-market approval authority over food additives since 1958, but that legislation created the exception by proving the rule. In federal statute, only chemicals added to food, not the food itself, were subject to pre-market regulation. Dietary supplements were usually not considered food additives because they fell under the category of "generally recognized as safe" (GRAS). In reality, the distinction is often not so clear cut. Is the synthetic process of including primrose oil in a gelatin capsule with vitamin E equivalent to adding a chemical to food? Courts have denied the FDA's claim that black currant oil is a food additive when encapsulated yet affirmed the oil's status as a food additive when combined with fish oil, vitamins, and minerals. Here the federal courts took a slimmer view of the FDA's powers than they did in drug regulation.[123]

---

[122]In two cases decided in 1968 and 1969, the federal courts interpreted items that appeared to be devices as "new drugs" under the FDCA. In *AMP, Inc. v. Gardner* (389 F. 2d 825, 1968), the Second Circuit held a suture used to join blood vessels surgically as a "drug" under the Act. One year later, in *U.S v. An Article of Drug.... Bacto-Unidisk* (394 U.S. 784), the Supreme Court not only upheld the FDA's declaration of an implanted disc for diagnosis of antibiotic sensitivity as a drug, but also announced the principle that in deciding whether an entity was a drug or device, courts should read the term "drug" broadly and inclusively. Industry officials reacted warily to the decisions; "FDA's Difco Case Victory Foretells Pre-Clearance Demands for Many Devices," *FDCR*, May 5, 1969, 5–8. These interpretations were supplanted by the Medical Device Amendments of 1976, which created a clear statutory basis for pre-market regulation of medical devices. On the distinction between food additives and food, see Lars Noah and Richard A. Merrill, "Starting from Scratch? Reinventing the Food Additive Approval Process," *Boston University Law Review* 78 (2) (April 1998): 329–443.

[123]On primrose oil, see *United States v. 45/194 Kg. Drums of Pure Vegetable Oil* (961 F. 2d. 808, 812, n. 3, (9th Circuit, 1992)). For the contrasting decisions on black currant oil, see

In the years before and immediately following the 1962 Amendments, FDA officials and nutritional supplement makers battled both in open warfare and in quiet legal and compliance struggles. Administration officials announced their intention to regulate supplements as part of a larger program against quackery. Yet they understood that their legal authority in governing these products was tenuous, certainly not as historically or clearly established as their programs of new drug regulation. For their part, nutritional supplement makers presented their therapeutic claims warily. Even during the Krebiozen and Laetrile dramas, few if any supplement makers were going to mount a new claim of effectiveness against cancer, and those that did would not get away with it. Yet the health claims of nutritional supplements varied widely. And much like over-the-counter drugs and pre-1962 drugs, vitamins and nutritional supplements carried the imprimatur of everyday use and familiarity to citizens.[124]

In the spring of 1968, the Administration proposed labeling for dietary supplements. The proposed labeling reflected FDA officials' belief that Americans were wasting hundreds of millions of dollars annually on the preparations. "Vitamins and minerals are supplied in abundant amounts by commonly available foods. Except for persons with special medical needs, there is no scientific basis for recommending routine use of dietary supplements." The labeling initiative had the feel of the FDA's initiative on efficacy regulation of pre-1962 drugs, as the primary targets of the FDA's efforts were the perceived necessity and quality of the products. Along with the rules, the Administration called for hearings on the proposed labels.[125]

Nutritional supplement makers received support from sources both unlikely and famous. The Pharmaceutical Manufacturers' Association (along with a number of individual drug companies) weighed in against the proposed regulations, claiming that the supplements "do much good and no harm." The support of the PMA was odd, considering that the Association had long assisted the anti-quackery initiatives of the Administration, and given that some of the Association's products might well benefit from restricted use of supplements if consumers switched their spending to over-the-counter medications. The most vivid attack on the proposed supplement

---

United States v. 21 Appx. 180 Kg. Bulk Metal Drums (761 F. Supp. 180 (D. Me. 1991)), and *United States v. 29 Cartons of . . . . An Article of Food*, 987 F. 2d 33, 37–39 (1ˢᵗ Circuit, 1993). Cases cited in Noah and Merrill, "Starting from Scratch?" 346–8.

[124]The assertion of intention to regulate supplements as part of an anti-quackery program appears to have been pushed by George Larrick and his appointees. K. L. Milstead (Deputy Director, Bureau of Enforcement), "The Food and Drug Administration's Program Against Quackery," prepared for delivery to the Yonkers Academy of Medicine, Yonkers, New York, May 16, 1962; AAMA. Later Commissioners continued this move, though often with deference to practices of "self-medication" with supplements and over-the-counter drugs; Charles C. Edwards, "FDA: A Positive Approach to Self-Medication," presented at the Proprietary Association Annual Meeting, White Sulphur Springs, WV, May 10, 1971, Speeches Collection, B1, V2, Speech 16; CCE.

[125]"FDA Probes Diet Food Labeling, Drug Claims," *JAMA* 204 (13) (June 24, 1968): 41.

labels occurred when Ronald Reagan, then governor of California and a rising star in the Republican Party, gave a speech to the Pharmaceutical Advertising Club in San Francisco in June 1968. Reagan interpreted the FDA's "march against vitamin pills" as further evidence of the "regulatory nightmare" unfolding in Washington. As he read the proposal labels, the FDA was saying that "You don't need vitamins if you get enough food," to which the governor retorted, "As a customer who prefers to pull the cotton out of his vitamin bottle, I feel better taking a little vitamin C to ward off a cold, and government can take its sticky labels off my pill bottle." Reagan's attack on the FDA's vitamin labeling initiative invoked the consumer-based language of late 1960s and 1970s politics. He could speak rather intuitively about being a customer with respect to vitamin C, but would not as easily have claimed that the government should keep its hands off of an antibiotic label or an antihypertensive drug. It was easier to refer to the FDA as "government" when the target of regulation was considered nutrition than when it was considered therapy. In drawing upon culturally established patterns, Reagan's criticism foreshadowed the constraints facing the Administration in its proposed labeling attempt. The supplement labeling was quietly dropped.[126]

The initiative to regulate nutritional supplements, however, did not disappear. In August 1973, the Administration published fourteen final regulations and five proposed rules that governed the labeling of foods and food supplements. The proposed labels were neither as broad nor as philosophical as those jettisoned in 1968. Yet the August 1973 regulations imposed minimum and maximum standards for the contents of vitamin and mineral products, where the upper and lower bounds were tied to the National Academy of Sciences' recommended daily allowance (RDA) criteria. Products containing 50 percent to 150 percent of the allowance for a substance would be marketed as food supplements and would be required to meet federal standards for purity, identity, and quality. Those products containing more than 150 percent of the RDA would be allowed to remain on the market while the agency studied their safety and effectiveness in a DESI-like analysis. The new regulations also proscribed makers of supplement products from claiming prevention or cure of any disease.[127]

The August 1973 rules brought challenges that were both immediate and long-lasting. The National Health Federation brought a court case, as did the National Association of Pharmaceutical Manufacturers, which represented smaller drug and vitamin makers. Federal courts blocked the rules

[126] "Reagan Hits FDA on Vitamin Pills," *AMA News*, July 1, 1968. Like much of the libertarian and new conservative rhetoric of the late 1960s and 1970s, Reagan referred to "government" and not "the government," dropping the definite article. See also "FDA Probes Diet Food Labeling, Drug Claims," *JAMA* 204 (13) (June 24, 1968): 41.

[127] "Vitamin, Mineral Products Curbed by FDA Over Protests of Health Food Enthusiasts," *WSJ*, August 2, 1973, 10. Safety concerns motivated FDA officials to issue a final order in August placing upper limits on Vitamin A and D preparations, whose excessive use had been linked to adverse mental and physical effects.

from enforcement and remanded the case to the Administration. Separately, supplement manufacturers and enthusiasts began to organize allies in Congress, in state legislatures, and in the general public. The Federation advanced a bill, sponsored by 165 members of the House, to prohibit FDA restrictions on vitamins and minerals except in cases where a clear safety threat had been established. Even as Administration officials released new regulations in 1976, their efforts were being undone in the legislative process. Led by Wisconsin Senator William Proxmire, Congress in 1976 passed an amendment to the 1938 Act which extended the "generally recognized as safe" (GRAS) exemption for vitamins and minerals to dietary supplements. The "Proxmire Amendment" prevents the Administration from restricting the potency of a vitamin or mineral supplement based on either of two criteria: (1) food misbranding charges or (2) on the premise that the supplement would qualify as a drug if it surpassed the agency's desired level of potency. For almost two decades, FDA officials largely backed off from rulemaking on supplements.[128]

Over the ensuing decades, the battle over regulation of dietary supplements continued, and the forces supporting less regulation attracted new allies. Emboldened by the conservative and anti-government forces impelling American politics, and in response to Commissioner David Kessler's new rulemaking initiative in 1993, supplement makers saw their wishes realized in the Dietary Supplement Health and Education Act of 1994. The 1994 law differentiated supplements from food additives and drugs, and placed a safety-based burden of proof upon the FDA in any adulteration proceeding against a supplement manufacturer. These legislative developments created, partially, an interesting cross-national contrast, as the size and diversity of the nutritional supplement industry has been much larger in the United States than overseas, while the safety regulation of these products has been less vigorous in the United States than in Europe.

. . .

Like many government organizations, the twentieth-century Food and Drug Administration was blessed and cursed with multiple publics. The shrewdest of FDA leaders recognized this fact and built strategies that embedded it. Upon taking office in 1970, Commissioner Charles Edwards could speak of the Administration's efforts as constituency building among diverse communities. "We have begun to develop a constituency in the Congress and in

---

[128]The Proxmire amendment established an amended Section 411 of the FDCA. W. Stephen Pray, *A History of Nonprescription Product Regulation* (Binghamton, NY: Haworth Press, 2003), 205–38. In 1991, FDA food regulator Douglas Archer would remark of the Proxmire amendment that "it seemed to signal Congressional intent that supplement-type products not be regulated without indication of real danger to health." Statement by Douglas L. Archer, Ph.D. (Deputy Director, Center for Food Safety and Applied Nutrition, FDA) before the Subcommittee on Human Resources and Intergovernmental Relations, Committee on Government Operations, House of Representatives, July 18, 1991.

the Executive Branch of the Government," he told a meeting of AMA and National Research Council officials, "and I need not remind you that this is essential for any successful agency of government. We are also slowly developing a constituency in the medical and scientific communities." A year later he rendered the point even more consciously, telling a luncheon of drug company officials of his "profound conviction that good communication between FDA and each of its publics are vital to the proper functioning of a regulatory agency in these new times."[129]

The multiplicity of audiences brought both advantages and pitfalls for the Administration and its officials. At its most obvious, multiplicity implied that universal approbation for the agency would never materialize, and that few actors (if any) would express full satisfaction with the Administration's decisions and policies. The sense of operating under rhetorical attack from numerous sides has been a near constant in FDA politics for five decades. Yet it would be wrong to conclude that the persistence of criticism and scrutiny has undermined the agency's reputation and power. It is certainly plausible that criticism has depleted morale, and on occasion publicity and hearings have weakened its leadership. Yet in the American political system, an agency subject to multidimensional criticism is rarely an agency whose fundamental powers get curtailed.

More powerfully, multiplicity meant that different visions of the agency prevailed among different constituencies. The criticism was never cut from a single cloth, and the various depictions of the agency rarely communicated a unifying theme. General practitioners and their representatives in the American Medical Association saw a government agency that ensured and underwrote the minimal safety and efficacy of medicines, but they also saw an entity poised to interfere in the physician-patient relationship and the autonomy of practice. Pharmaceutical firms and economic conservatives saw an entity that they feared and blamed for declining rates of new chemical introduction. Consumer safety advocates saw a promising structure that needed prodding and continual scrutiny in order to behave faithfully with the example of Frances Kelsey and John Nestor. In Ralph Smith, Frances Kelsey, Richard Crout, Robert Temple, and others in the Administration's non-appointed leadership, top pharmacologists and medical specialists perceived diligence, thoroughness of procedure, and the basis of scientific medicine. The U.S. Congress became a structure in which these diverse claims reverberated and filtered to the mass public, as print and television journalists took much of their information from congressional inquiries.

---

[129]Edwards, "Remarks presented on October 18, 1971 at the National Research Council, Joint Meeting with the AMA COD," 4; B3, CCE. Notice that Edwards excluded patients, "consumers," and pharmaceutical companies from this description, as perhaps he was speaking in front of a body of government and scientific officials. Edwards, "Toward a New Understanding," presented at the joint New York Pharmaceutical Advertising Club/Midwest Pharmaceutical Advertising Club Annual Luncheon, June 23, 1970, Chicago, IL, during the week of the AMA annual convention; B 1, F 20, CCE.

The multiplicity of audience created, finally, the opportunity for meaning-ful and advantageous dependencies across the Administration's constituen-cies. As drug firms and clinical researchers complained of an intrusive and intransigent bureaucracy, consumer safety advocates saw in these same la-ments evidence of a "tough cop" regulator. The very image of diligence and thoroughness that firms and researchers propagated would, moreover, assist the FDA in its enforcement and rulemaking efforts, as those same firms and clinical experimenters were reluctant to question the resolve of an Adminis-tration that had continually been depicted as vigorous and rigid. So too, every time that a Ted Weiss excoriated FDA officials for their regulation of a drug like Merital, Robert Temple and Paul Leber were given yet another opportunity to explain the difficulty of their calling and to express their sympathy with practicing psychiatrists. And every time that legislators con-trasted the FDA's behavior in a specific case with the agency's larger commit-ments in law and myth, American viewers and readers perceived once again—all the more powerfully if vaguely—the agency's compelling mission, its promise, and the reason for its existence and endurance.

CHAPTER SIX

Reputation and Power Contested: Emboldened Audiences in Cancer and AIDS, 1977–1992

In implementing the statutory scheme, the FDA has never made exception for drugs used by the terminally ill. As this Court has often recognized, the construction of a statute by those charged with its administration is entitled to substantial deference. *Such deference is particularly appropriate where, as here, an agency's interpretation involves issues of considerable public controversy, and Congress has not acted to correct any misperception of its statutory objectives.* Unless and until Congress does so, we are reluctant to disturb a long-standing administrative policy that comports with the plain language, history, and prophylactic purpose of the Act.

—Justice Thurgood Marshall, *U.S. v. Rutherford*, 1978

Many of us who live in daily terror of the AIDS epidemic cannot understand why the Food and Drug Administration has been intransigent in the face of this monstrous tidal wave of death. Its response to what is plainly a national emergency has been inadequate, its testing facilities are inefficient and gaining access to its staff and activities is virtually impossible. . . . . Indeed, these are understatements. There is no question on the part of anyone fighting AIDS that the F.D.A. constitutes the single most incomprehensible bottleneck in American bureaucratic history—one that is actually prolonging this roll-call of death.

—AIDS activist Larry Kramer, in the *New York Times*, 1987

> The increased flexibility demonstrated by the FDA in the
> case of terminally ill AIDS patients is welcome and will surely
> benefit patients with other serious diseases as well.
>
> —*Washington Post* editorial, 1989[1]

OBSERVERS in journalism and academics have often claimed that American pharmaceutical regulation was irrevocably altered by the AIDS crisis. The clash of dying protesters and white-coated bureaucrats, and the resulting tale of institutional change, have been woven into something of a common parable. In this narrative, a new social movement representing people with nothing to lose aggressively confronted a tradition- and procedure-bound bureaucracy and compelled institutional change. As this telling goes, when the Administration was confronted with tangible sufferers of an illness that promised certain death for them, sufferers who organized into new forms of activism, who made effective moral and political claims upon the Administration through the national media and through professional organizations— once this happened, the agency's modus operandi could no longer persist as it had. In this story, the deliberate, procedurally conservative culture of the FDA's drug reviewing divisions changed, not simply for AIDS drugs but for many others. Rulemaking and administrative procedure followed the lead of administrative practice, bringing new concepts ("Subpart E" regulations, accelerated or "fast-track" approval procedures, "surrogate endpoints") into law, medicine, science, and government.[2]

There is considerable truth in this narrative. The changes struck during the apex of American AIDS politics in the 1980s and early 1990s were lasting. They transformed the agency's image and they sculpted anew its directive, gatekeeping, and conceptual powers. These changes would not have happened or come as they did had AIDS never surfaced. Yet there is much that the story misses.

To begin with, before AIDS there was cancer. Before the Administration was making public and formal exceptions for AIDS patients who sought drugs known as ddI, ddC, Crixivan, and others, the agency was making less visible exceptions to its testing rules for chemotherapy drugs. Before dying

---

[1]Kramer, "The F.D.A.'s Callous Response to AIDS," *NYT*, March 23, 1987, A19; "Drugs for the Dying," *WP*, July 11, 1989, A24.

[2]Philip Hilts (*Protecting America's Health: The FDA, Business, and One Hundred Years of Regulation* (New York: Knopf, 2003), chapters 16 and 17; Hawthorne, *Inside the FDA* (New York: Wiley, 2005), chap. 10; Arthur Daemmrich, *Pharmacopolitics: Drug Regulation in the United States and Germany* (Chapel Hill: University of North Carolina Press, 2004), chapters 2 and 4; Ceccoli, *Pill Politics: Drugs and the FDA* (Boulder, CO: Lynne Rienner, 2004), chap. 5, "The Grand Compromise and the Shift to a New Era." For the AIDS crisis in particular, Hilts and Daemmrich offer excellent, informative, and complementary treatments.

AIDS patients were amassing outside the agency's door, thousands of dying cancer sufferers were defying the Administration's ban on Laetrile. Before communities of immunologists and NIH scientists were pressing the Administration to devise new and more flexible rules under which AIDS treatments could be developed, the NIH-based National Cancer Institute had positioned itself as perhaps the single most effective disease-based lobby in American pharmaceutical regulation. Together, and in strikingly different ways, the intertwined sagas of cancer and AIDS transformed the sufferers of disease into political communities. Differentiation among different diseases (and their variable claims for suffering) became one of the most central facts in the political economy of drug regulation. As with the changes wrought by thalidomide, moreover, the transformations at the Administration in the 1980s and 1990s were more continuous than common narratives suggest.

So too, the AIDS crisis itself embeds a more complicated history, one where FDA officials did not so often carve out legal exceptions to their power as instead exercise administrative flexibility through drug review decisions and rulemaking, thus preserving their legal authority even while projecting ambiguity. Whether this ambiguous adaptation was fully or largely intentional is hard to ascertain, yet the resulting uncertainty was no less real for the fact.

In the contestation brought by cancer and AIDS—among other categories of illness—reputation and power in American pharmaceutical regulation were dually reshaped. Reputation acquired new audiences—federal health agencies, organized activists whose severe illness became their carrying card, new communities of health providers, Hollywood celebrities. Whereas previously the agency's performative and technical reputation had been assailed, it was more the agency's moral reputation under attack in the crises of cancer and AIDS. And these threats to moral reputation were far more powerful than drug lag criticism in changing the behavior of the agency. Management of reputation meant acquiescence with different audiences and with critics, and it meant a management of power. These managerial episodes came variably, in the FDA/NCI clinical testing agreement of 1978, the "Subpart E" regulations of 1988, and the Prescription Drug User Fee Act (PDUFA) of 1992.

The 1980s and 1990s offered another important context of challenge for reputation and regulatory power: a politically conservative era, a time of deregulation, and a time of growing business power in American politics. In many respects, FDA successfully evaded and resisted these threats, and a comparison with other agencies that were disempowered (the Federal Communications Commission, the National Labor Relations Board, and the Occupational Safety and Health Administration) or altogether gutted (the Interstate Commerce Commission) is illuminating. In other ways, FDA was profoundly affected by the deregulatory politics of the time. Its operations suffered from some of the same budget reductions that afflicted other agencies, and the Administration exhibited the common reticence observed among many agencies of this time, behaving fearfully in the face of emboldened business challenges and conservative political ascendancy.

ILLNESS AS A CATEGORY FOR REGULATORY AUDIENCE

Neither the definition nor the politics of a pharmaceutical treatment can be separated from the disease it targets. A chemical entity becomes a "drug" when it is accompanied by a recognized claim that it effectively cures or relieves a particular disease (or symptom of that disease). As medical anthropologists and historians have long recognized, disease is a human concept that lumps together different forms of pathology, experience, and suffering. To draw attention to the subjectivity of disease is not to deny the very material reality and emotional and spiritual disturbance of the underlying human experience. Diseases kill, torment, dismember, maim, dumbfound, bankrupt, weaken, disfigure, isolate, unemploy, dehumanize, emasculate, and haunt people. The combination of objective suffering and subjective definition renders illness a powerful force in modern society. Diseases become political when they morph into public enemies and generate organizational categories. At once they become vilified targets for public policy (as in President Richard Nixon's "War on Cancer") and structures for mobilization (witness the AIDS Coalition to Unleash Power [ACT-UP], or the National Alliance for the Mentally Ill).[3]

Due in part to the FDA's decisions and interpretations, disease has become the most salient category of global pharmaceutical regulation. A drug's disease target—particularly its principal target or "primary indication"—shapes its review, its peer group of competitor therapies (in regulation and in various markets), its politics (those who lobby for it as well as those who oppose it), its chances for approval, and its degree of consensus. Disease arguably shapes these variables more powerfully than any other feature of a drug, including its sponsor or its scientific and clinical history. Much of this force derives from the scientific and medical considerations that accompany any particular designation of a disease. Disease concepts define the targets of drug development—sometimes as broadly as a general state of illness, sometimes quite technologically as a virus or its replication, a pathogen, a metabolic pathway, or a particular protein or enzyme. In part for this reason, disease concepts define the appropriate metrics (the Hamilton Depression Rating Scale, sys-

---

[3] Arthur Kleinman, *The Illness Narratives: Suffering, Healing and the Human Condition* (New York: Basic Books, 1988). For an exemplary study of the concept of disease definition and its relationship to pharmaceutical therapy, see Jeremy A. Greene, *Prescribing by Numbers: Drugs and the Definition of Disease* (Baltimore: Johns Hopkins University Press, 2006). More generally, see Charles Rosenberg, "Framing Disease: Illness, Society and History (Introduction)," in Rosenberg and Janet Golden, eds., *Framing Disease: Studies in Cultural History* (New Brunswick, NJ: Rutgers University Press, 1992); Rosenberg, "Disease and Social Order in America: Perceptions and Expectations," in Elizabeth Fee and Daniel M. Fox, eds., *AIDS: The Burdens of History* (Berkeley: University of California Press, 1988), 12–32; Allan M. Brandt, *No Magic Bullet: A History of Venereal Diseases in the United States since 1880* (New York: Oxford University Press, 1985). As Steven Epstein argues, Susan Sontag has also advanced a more implicit notion of diseases as "frames" in her *Illness as Metaphor* (New York: Farrar, Straus and Giroux, 1978); Epstein, *Impure Science: AIDS, Activism and the Politics of Knowledge* (Berkeley: University of California Press, 1996), 372.

tolic versus diastolic blood pressure, tumor remission) by which the efficacy of treatments is judged. Disease states will also define the essential scientific and medical audiences that must be persuaded if the drug is to gain legitimacy, whether through FDA approval or through other means. Drugs that offer a new mechanism of action for a defined medical condition—serotonin reuptake inhibitors for clinical depression, beta-blockers for angina, cisplatin for advanced ovarian cancer—will be assessed primarily by those with specialization in the disease target (psychiatrists, cardiologists, and oncologists, respectively), even if the mechanism of action is relatively new to them.[5]

Disease states invoke science and medicine, yet the politics of disease is no less real for this reason. Indeed, the force of disease is political precisely because the concept is scientifically constrained. Science and medicine give a factual status to medical conditions (erectile dysfunction, essential hypertension, chronic depression), they create enemies and other culprits in the evolution of disease (carcinogens, high-risk behaviors, the human immunodeficiency virus (HIV), smoking), and they appoint representatives (cardiologists, neuroscientists, oncologists) who officially labor in the service of the afflicted. The politics of disease may be methodological, pitting virology against immunology. The politics of disease may be juridical, pertaining to power and its limits; scientists may disagree about whether a regulation or code of practice can be interpreted flexibly. The politics of disease may be pluralistic, pitting advocates of one disease against another.[4]

The primary dimension of disease politics, however, is organizational. Whenever a drug is developed for a certain disease, the various communities organized about this category quickly become the therapy's most important constituencies. These audiences will include those who suffer from the condition, their advocates, those who claim to treat the disease, and even those who claim that the condition is not a malady, such as when anti-abortion or anti-contraception activists claim that "pregnancy" and "fertility" are not conditions to be treated. The constituencies will not always favor the approval and marketing of the drug in question, though many will.[5]

---

[4]By "political" I mean that a combination of core disagreement and public values structure the way in which the drug is assessed, and that these values derive from worldviews that are associated with other beliefs (though not necessarily partisan ones). A preference for evaluation of drugs via randomized clinical trial evaluation may, for example, be associated with broader doubts about the efficiency and fairness of an unregulated corporate marketplace in minimizing and allocating benefits and risks from pharmaceutical therapy. This notion is broadly consistent with Aristotelian notions of politics (see, e.g., John Cooper, *Reason and Human Good in Aristotle* (Cambridge: Harvard University Press, 1975)), as well a more conflict-based notions (for example, the "friend-enemy" distinction central to the definition of politics in Carl Schmitt, *Der Begriff Des Politichen* (Berlin: Duncker & Humblot, 2002); John McCormick, *Carl Schmitt's Critique of Liberalism: Against Politics as Technology* (New York: Cambridge University Press, 1996)).

For an example of methodological conflict (a school of virology pitted against another school of immunology) in the advancement of the hypothesis that HIV caused AIDS, see Steven Epstein, *Impure Science*, 66–92.

[5]Drugs are often developed long after the essential chemical entity exists, as when a preexist-

For the Administration, the politics of reputation management with these audiences is difficult, complicated, and absolutely necessary. Disease-related organizations and audiences present numerous challenges—potential and actual—to the Administration's organizational image. They can challenge the Administration's expertise. They can jeopardize the Administration's claim to protect the nation and promote the public health. They can subvert the Administration's relations with politicians. Yet these organizations can also provide crucial and enduring support to the FDA. It is for this reason that the Administration has at numerous levels attempted to construct institutions of liaison with these groups, to incorporate them into decision making, and to avoid being surprised by their actions.

In the aggregate, as American medicine has become more specialized, as advocacy organizations have multiplied in American politics, and as American society has witnessed the definition and discovery of numerous new human pathologies, the size and force of disease politics has grown immensely. One implication of seeing disease as a category that structures political constituencies is that patient advocate groups and medical specialties are observed to substitute for and complement one another's activities. The roles and functions performed by a group of organized disease advocates—representation, lobbying, agitation—may have been assumed earlier (and quite differently) by medical practitioners of a certain specialty. What is today carried out by the Breast Cancer Action Network may have been undertaken, albeit partially and imperfectly, by the American Society of Clinical Oncology a decade or generation before.

THE REGULATORY POLITICS OF CANCER IN THE LATE TWENTIETH CENTURY

"Cancer" is an umbrella concept that envelops hundreds of conditions. In modern medicine it is applied to diseases in which abnormal cells divide without control, yielding malignant cells that invade and destroy otherwise healthy ones. Masses of these malignant tissues are called tumors or neoplasms, and most cancers are diagnosed by casual or methodical detection of a tumor. Not all tumors are malignant or cancerous, but most concentrations of malignant tissues fall under the umbrella of "tumor." Tumors and their associated cancer diagnoses are often divided into "liquid" versus "solid" designations. The primary distinction between these categories lies

---

ing chemical entity is examined for activity against the disease target. Prominent examples include azidothymidine (AZT, or Retrovir) for AIDS-related complex and sildenafil (Viagra) for erectile dysfunction; John Lauritsen, *Poison by Prescription: The AZT Story* (New York: Asklepios Press, 1990). And in fact much of drug development consists of bio-assay— the systematic screening of compounds in laboratory settings (in vivo) for activity against a given pathogen, virus, cancer, or other target. Hence, for disease-related audiences I consider the essential moments to be the entry of a compound into clinical trials and the submission of a new drug application. In both cases, a defined health condition (disease) must be specified as a primary indication of the new drug.

in the mobility of the malignant cells. At the more mobile end, liquid tumors encompass lymphomas and leukemias. Most human cancers fall under the heading of solid tumors, which include malignant brain tumors; cancers of connective and structurally supportive tissue such as bone, ligament, and muscle (sarcomas); melanomas and other skin cancers; and neoplasms of the breast and lung, testes, and ovaries. In their research on solid tumors in the late twentieth century, researchers focused ever greater attention upon two sites of general interest: the tumor epithelium (or the outer lining of cells most rapidly dividing) and the tumor vasculature (the nexus of blood vessels supplying the tumor with oxygen and nutrients).[6]

The primary characteristic of a malignant tumor is its spread from a primary site to vital organs and distant locations in the human body. Many cancers will kill a patient not by damaging the organs at the initial tumor site but by traveling to the lungs or the brain, or to the lymph nodes and through the lymphatic system. It is now well established in oncology that sites of secondary growth are nonrandomly determined. This "seed and soil hypothesis" implies that certain types of tumor cells ("seeds") will usually travel to specific organs ("soil"). Deep-tissue sarcomas often travel to the lungs, for instance, while many breast neoplasms often induce metastases in the brain. Since anticancer drugs are usually evaluated with survival as a clinical "endpoint"—an observable signal of the drug's efficacy such as tumor diminution or enhanced viral load—a primary dimension of a drug's clinical value is its potential to reduce metastases or retard the metastatic process.[7]

Scientists have identified over two hundred separable forms of malignancy and there are doubtless many more categories that have yet to be refined. Such vast molecular differentiation at times persists and refracts regulatory politics, and at other times is elided. When a degree of political differentiation exists, as witnessed in the continuing social stigma attached to lung cancer in the United States and its juxtaposition with the social and political sympathy received by breast cancer activism campaigns—the Administration's audiences become more specialized. This specialization yields greater predictability but also stronger political organization, and in the late twentieth century and early twenty-first, more specialized cancer societies have been increasingly armed with more compelling stories and rationales. At other times, the culture and the regulation and the politics lump these different maladies together, as when the Administration's "performance" in

[6]Bert Vogelstein and Kenneth W. Kinsler, "Cancer Genes and the Pathways They Control," *Nature Medicine* 10 (8) (2004): 789–99; *Nature Milestones—Cancer* (April 2006), S36–S37. I have relied primarily upon two background texts as references in narrating modern cancer chemotherapy, one the widely used medical textbook by Vincent De Vita, Jr., Samuel Hellman, and Steven A. Rosenberg, *Cancer: Principles and Practice of Oncology*, 7th ed. (New York: Lippincott, Williams and Wilkins, 2005); the other, William Pratt, Raymond W. Ruddon, William D. Ensminger, and Jonathan Maybaum, *The Anticancer Drugs*, 2nd ed. (New York: Oxford University Press, 1994).

[7]I. R. Hart and I. J. Fidler, "Role of Organ Selectivity in the Determination of Metastatic Patterns of B16 Melanoma," *Cancer Research* 40 (1980): 2281–87.

reviewing and approving "cancer drugs" is assessed and criticized. The NCI's existence as a mouthpiece and lobby for cancer drug development is one part of this reputational lumping of "cancers" into "cancer."[8]

This umbrella understanding of cancer was reflected in social and political organizations, in federal policy, and in the structure of national administration. In the twentieth century, no two organizations figured more prominently in the United States' therapeutic approach to cancer than the American Cancer Society (ACS) and the National Cancer Institute (NCI). The Society—originally the American Society for the Control of Cancer—spearheaded efforts to increase federal funding for basic and applied cancer research. It also functioned as something of an attractor for private philanthropists such as Mary Lasker, and it launched a series of highly memorable public campaigns to increase awareness of cancer and to de-stigmatize the disease concept. Its primary point of interaction with the Food and Drug Administration was in a series of joint efforts to combat quack remedies for cancer treatment.

The National Cancer Institute was established in 1937 and has become the dominant research wing of the National Institutes of Health. No other NIH bureau—neither the National Institute on Aging (NIA), nor the National Institute of Allergy and Infectious Diseases (NIAID), nor the National Heart, Lung and Blood Institute (NHLBI)—has occupied greater public prominence, and no other bureau has consistently received as much money and attention from Congress.[9]

The Society and the Institute weave their way through late-twentieth century health politics as major players in the development and regulation of cancer chemotherapy. Yet in cancer chemotherapy, these muscular organizations witnessed limits to their influence. In part, their dominance in representing cancer constituencies—patients, caregivers, oncologists, and other cancer specialists—has been contested in different ways by more specialized groups. Research centers such as Memorial Sloan-Kettering in New York, M. D. Anderson in Houston, and Roswell Park Memorial in Buffalo have challenged the primacy of the Institute as a beacon of technology. For its part,

---

[8]The cultural and linguistic elision of different forms of neoplasms, and their unification under the umbrella "cancer," is a common starting point for many historical studies. As Thomas Patterson argues, the unification of malignancies under the singular term "cancer" is how "most laymen, as well as many doctors, have tended to describe the various cancerous diseases that afflict the human body" (*The Dread Disease: Cancer and Modern American Society* (Cambridge: Harvard University Press, 1987), x. Legislative and administrative categories in the United States have tended to perpetuate the simplification.

[9]The NCI was the first of the NIH's institutes, of which there are now twenty-seven. Among institutes currently enveloped within the NIH, the next wave was founded in 1948: the NIAID, the NHLBI, the National Institute of Diabetes and Digestive and Kidney Diseases (NIDDK), and the National Institute of Dental and Craniofacial Research (NIDCR). At no point from 1937 to 2005 did any other NIH Institute receive as much in congressional appropriations as the NCI. NIH, "NIH Almanac —Appropriations," *NIH Almanac*, 2006–2007 (Bethesda, MD: Office of NIH History, 2006).

the American Cancer Society has been challenged by disease and patients' associations representing smaller categories of cancer sufferers, most notably breast cancer activists. Yet the biggest challenge to their power came in the Administration's regulation of cancer therapeutics. Before a scheduled détente with the Administration, no amount of money, prominence, or good will at the NCI's disposal could break the impasse over clinical trial design and approval criteria for cancer drugs. Very strongly until the late 1970s, and less forcefully in a manner that continues to this day, the Administration has fundamentally structured and channeled the work of the Institute. The very design of research, the very definition of efficacy and toxicity and their concepts upon which modern chemotherapeutics is based, the very distinction between promising drugs and less-promising ones—all these were shaped primarily by the Administration.

As the politics of cancer unfolded in the 1970s and 1980s, the National Cancer Institute and the American Cancer Society enacted a fascinating inversion of roles. The Institute, a federal government agency, became the most effective and strident voice lobbying for quicker development and approval of cancer therapies and for relaxation and alteration of the FDA's clinical trial requirements. The Society, a civic membership organization, became deeply involved with administrative matters, and its relationship with the FDA was more of administrative cooperation than of lobbying and political pressure. The American Cancer Society saw ever less involvement with cancer drug promotion, and less conflict with the Administration. Moreover, the ACS and NCI rarely allied to combat the Administration, and this pax administrativa represents something of a puzzle. This inversion of roles, while partial, is consequential. It happens because of the way that these groups relate to the FDA, and because of historical patterns of cooperation and conflict.

The NCI-FDA Wars. The promise of some of the new chemotherapeutic agents emerging in the 1970s—such as cisplatin—came in their portent of a new class of chemotherapeutic treatments. Before 1950, most physician-provided treatment for cancer was surgical. With the refinement of radiotherapy and the advent of the linear accelerator, nuclear treatment of cancer became a more common option in the 1960s United States and Western Europe. Chemotherapy advances were slow and highly tumor-specific. Louis Goodman and Alfred Gilman had successfully treated non-Hodgkin's lymphoma patients with nitrogen mustard as early as 1942, and Sidney Farber had administered antifolates to induce remissions in children with acute lymphoblastic leukemia (ALL) in 1948. With these and later compounds, the dominant approach ("modality") in pharmaceutical cancer treatment in the twentieth century was cytotoxic, that is, a strategy aimed at killing malignant cells while inflicting minimal harm on healthy cells. Chemotherapy brought one advantage that neither surgical nor radiological treatments possessed; it offered promise for metastatic cancer. Metastatic human tumors posed several problems for cancer treatment and researchers. For one, they pointed up the limited reliability of animal models of diagnosis and treatment. Human metastases simply behaved in ways that were quite different. Second, because malignant tumors were adaptive, metastatic cancer could recur even after being successfully eliminated by previous forms of therapy, including chemotherapy.[10]

By the early 1970s, chemotherapy had begun to show some promise, albeit with limits, in attacking metastatic tumors. Yet the progress was limited mainly to variants of leukemia and lymphoma, and did not generally apply to the most common types of cancers (lung, breast, prostate, testicular, ovarian) which were usually characterized by solid tumors. It was for this reason, in part, that many observers of the nation's cancer wars considered them to have been lost in some aggregate sense; the most dramatic treatment improvements had not occurred for the most common malignancies. This dearth of options for the broadest illnesses helps to explain the popularity of Laetrile in the 1970s, the excitement that researchers expressed with the BCG vaccine and interferon, and the combination of frustration and desperation witnessed at the National Cancer Institute in the 1970s and 1980s.[11]

As with other forms of cancer drug therapy, combination chemotherapy got its start in the attack upon liquid tumors. In 1965, James Holland and colleagues at M. D. Anderson demonstrated that a combination of methotrexate (an antifolate), vincristine (an alkaloid), the antimetabolite mercaptopurine (also named "6-MP"), and the steroid prednisone—which together earned the acronym "POMP"—could induce long-term remissions in children with ALL. Five years later, Vincent DeVita and a team of researchers showed that a "MOPP" regimen—composed of nitrogen mustard, vincristine, procarbazine, and prednisone—could cure patients with Hodgkin's and non-Hodgkin's lymphomas. The primary advances in solid tumor treatment with combination drugs would not occur until 1975 and afterward.[12]

[10]Alfred Gilman, "The Initial Clinical Trial of Nitrogen Mustard," *American Journal of Surgery* 105 (1963): 574–8; Bruce A. Chabner and Thomas G. Roberts, Jr., "Chemotherapy and the War on Cancer," *Nature Reviews Cancer* 5 (2005): 65–72; *Nature Milestones—Cancer* (April 2006): S43–S50. The limits of the cytotoxicity paradigm became apparent in the development of late twentieth-century research into angiogenesis. Cytotoxic strategies diverted strategic focus from tumors and the way they started and grew, or the way that they metastasized. Chabner and Roberts draw two broad lessons from the history of cancer chemotherapy development: (1) the limited reliability of animal models for human metastatic tumors, (2) adaptability of metastatic tumors that embed "subclones," which generates drug resistance.

[11]As two former NCI officials admit of the 1970s and 1980s, "Cancer drug discovery had gained a reputation for having high risk and little chance of efficacy.... By 1985, the NCI drug development effort had begun to produce a monotonous group of antimetabolites, alkylators, antimitotics and topoisomerase inhibitors" (Chabner and Roberts, "Chemotherapy and the War on Cancer," S-46). Chabner and Roberts regard cisplatin as an exception to this generalization and a "success." R. J. Papac, "Origins of Cancer Therapy," *Yale Journal of Biology and Medicine* 74 (2001): 391–8; Emil Frei III, "The National Cancer Chemotherapy Program," *Science* 217 (1982): 600–606.

[12]Emil Frei III, et al., "The Effectiveness of Combinations of Antileukemic agents in Induc-

The notion of combination chemotherapy was in its infancy at this time. The considerations recommending the inclusion of one drug with a particular bundle of other chemicals were highly empirical. In part this was a result of established procedures at the National Cancer Institute. The NCI's screening program relied upon animal models, particularly liquid tumors in mice, for vetting new compounds. Human tumor screening (and the vetting of drugs against solid tumors more generally) would not begin in earnest until 1976, when the Institute started a xenograft program—essentially transplanting human tumor cells into cell cultures or into mice whose immune system had been compromised. Thereafter, the approach to choosing a particular combination was arguably slipshod and guided as much by side effect considerations as by clinical observations of efficacy. In a strange version of optimization which persists to this day, the combination chemotherapist chooses a recipe of poisons, each of whose most deleterious effects lies with a different organ or system of the human body. In many regimens—the testicular cancer protocol ifosfamide, paclitaxel, and cisplatin (TIP), for instance— one drug induces neutropenia (low neutrophil counts in the blood, inducing greater susceptibility to bacterial infection), another is a myelosuppressant (depressing bone marrow and white blood cell production), while another hurts the kidneys. The other twist confronted by students of combination chemotherapy at this juncture was the sequence and timing of drug administration. With the dawn of "adjuvant" chemotherapy in the 1970s, the cancer patient received drug treatment immediately after surgical resection of the tumor, possibly accompanied by radiation. More recently, the strategy of "neo-adjuvant" chemotherapy has come into favor, whereby the cancer patient receives a combination of drugs *before* surgery and radiation, which amounts to attacking the metastases first. As long as the metastasis is hindered, under this theory, the continued presence of the solid tumor in the human body is of less concern.[13]

---

ing and Maintaining Remission in Children with Acute Leukemia," *Blood* 26 (1965): 642–56. Other pivotal studies in the emergence of combination chemotherapy include J. H. Moxley III, Vincent DeVita, K. Brace, and Emil Frei III, "Intensive Combination Chemotherapy and X-irradiation in Hodgkin's Disease," *Cancer Research* 27 (1967): 1258–63; DeVita, A. A. Serpick, and P. P. Carbone, "Combination Chemotherapy in the Treatment of Advanced Hodgkin's Disease," *AnnIM* 73 (1970): 881–5; M. Levitt, et al., "Combination Sequential Chemotherapy in Advanced Reticulum Cell Sarcoma," *Cancer* 29 (1972): 630–36; D. Berd, J. Cornog, R. C. Conti, M. Levitt, and Joseph Bertino, "Long-term Remission in Diffuse Histiocytic Lymphoma Treated with Combination Sequential Chemotherapy," *Cancer* 35 (1975): 1050–54; Gianni Bonadonna, et al., "Combination Chemotherapy as an Adjuvant Treatment in Operable Breast Cancer," *NEJM* 294 (1976): 405–10. For an insightful study combining cultural and technical narratives of the development of modern cancer chemotherapy, consult Alberto Cambrosio, Peter Keating, and Andrei Mogoutov, "Protocols, Regimens and Substances: The Socio-Technical Space of Anti-Cancer Drugs," in Jean Paul Gaudillière and Volker Hess, eds., *Ways of Regulating: Therapeutic Agents between Plants, Shops, and Consulting Rooms* (Preprint 363) (Berlin: Max-Planck-Institut für Wissenschaftsgeschichte, 2009).

[13] As Chabner and Roberts ("Chemotherapy and the War on Cancer," S-49) summarize, it is precisely the adaptability of most malignancies that calls for combination therapy: "A vast

It was in this context of frustration, new optimism, and conjecture that a new molecule for cancer chemotherapy appeared, one that promised an entirely new mechanism of action and a new way of fighting malignant solid tumors. Platinum-based chemotherapy was a serendipitous discovery of physicist Barnett Rosenberg and his laboratory at Michigan State University in the early 1960s. While experimenting with a procedure to inhibit cell division with electricity, Rosenberg and his colleagues noted that electrical current delivered between platinum electrodes inhibited the replication of *E. coli* bacteria that were suspended in a nutrient broth. Instead of replicating by cellular division, the bacteria had been stretched into long, largely inactive filaments. Upon further examination, Rosenberg found that the bacterial growth inhibition had nothing to do with the electrical current. Instead, the current had released platinum from the electrodes into a solution of ammonium and chloride ions; this solution was necessary and sufficient (in the absence of electrical current) to inhibit cell division. Having established that a platinum-based compound was an effective antibiotic, Rosenberg began to assess its potential anticancer potential. In subsequent tests, Rosenberg's team assessed several platinum compounds against experimental animal tumors (essentially tumors induced in a laboratory setting). They found that a particular platinum-based molecule—*cis*-diamminedichloroplatinum (II), or cisplatin—showed the greatest anti-tumor activity.[14]

Under the direction of the NCI, phase I trials of cisplatin began in 1972.

---

array of resistance mechanisms, involving mutations or amplification of the target enzyme, overexpression of drug transporters, or mutations in cell-death pathways, can defeat single agents, no matter how well designed and targeted." On the NCI's screening programs, see Zubrod, "The National Program for Cancer Chemotherapy," *JAMA* 222 (1972): 1161–2; C. H. Takimoto, "Anticancer Drug Development at the U.S. National Cancer Institute," *Cancer Chemotherapy and Pharmacology* 52 (2003) (Supplement 1): 29–33; Lloyd R. Kelland, "Of Mice and Men: Values and Liabilities of the Athymic Nude Mouse Model in Anticancer Drug Development," *European Journal of Cancer* 40 (2004): 827–36.

On neo-adjuvant chemotherapy, see Bonadonna, et al., "Combination Chemotherapy as an Adjuvant Treatment in Operable Breast Cancer," and Emil Frei III, "What's in a Name—Neo-adjuvant," *Journal of the National Cancer Institute* 80 (1988): 1088.

Theoretical development in combination chemotherapy has come much more recently. See Emil J. Frei III and Joseph Paul Eder, "Principles of Dose, Schedule and Combination Therapy," Section 11, chap. 44 in Donald W. Kufe, et al., *Cancer Medicine* (Hamilton, Ontario: B. C. Decker, 2003), 669–77. Another example of "one poison per organ" regimens is the CVPP protocol (cyclophosphamide, vinblastine, procarbazine, and prednisone) used in advanced Hodgkin's (Pratt, et al., *The Anticancer Drugs*, 143).

[14]Rosenberg, L. Van Camp, and T. Krigas, "Inhibition of Cell Division in *Escherichia coli* by Electrolysis Products from a Platinum Electrode" (letter), *Nature* 205 (1965): 698–9. Rosenberg, Van Camp, E. B. Grimley, et al., "The Inhibition of Growth or Cell Division in *Escherichia coli* by Different Ionic Species of Platinum (IV) Complexes," *Journal of Biological Chemistry* 242 (1967): 1347–52; Rosenberg, Van Camp, et al., "Platinum Compounds: A New Class of Potent Antitumour Agents" (letter), *Nature* 222 (1969): 385–6. Rosenberg, "Cisplatin: Its History and Possible Mechanisms of Action," chap. 2 in Archie W. Prestayko, Stanley T. Crooke, and Stephen K. Carter, *Cisplatin: Current Status and New Developments* (New York: Academic Press, 1980); Jeff Lyon, "Tempo: Winning the War against the Disease Men Fear Most," *Chicago Tribune*, September 19, 1982, I-1.

Rosenberg took particular interest in the drug and followed its clinical trials quite closely. One crucial issue was the purity of the drug. One particular platinum salt or "Magnus salt"—Disodium platinum tetrachloride [K_2PtCl_4]—has highly allergenic properties. Traces of the salt could appear purely as by-products from industrial synthesis of the drug, and so quite particular methods of synthesis had to be followed.[15]

The Phase 2 and 3 trials were overseen by the NCI and the FDA's Division of Oncology and Radiopharmaceutical Drug Products, headed by William Gyarfas. Gyarfas was one of Frances Kelsey's first hires when she took over the Investigational Drug Branch of the Bureau of Medicine in 1963.[16] The Institute's leadership was strongly behind cisplatin, in part because of the favorable results, in part because they were in need of some good news from their Cancer Treatment Evaluation Program. Yet once Institute and Bristol Laboratories officials began making preparations for a new drug application for cisplatin, Barnett Rosenberg's drug got caught up in a larger war between the Institute and the Administration. Robert Young was at this time laying heavy scrutiny upon the NCI's Investigational New Drug applications, often calling to a halt clinical trials that had been under way for weeks or even months. Young's skepticism was not restricted to cisplatin alone. In his first two years on the job, he had identified three antineoplastic drugs—thalicarpine, anguidine, and maytansine, all of them NCI-supported and all in trials at the M. D. Anderson Cancer Center in Houston—whose experimental protocols were, in his judgment, defective.[17]

Young's arrival to the Administration in 1975 had sparked a testy and vitriolic antagonism with NCI officials and M. D. Anderson researchers in particular. Young maintained that antineoplastic INDs in experimental protocols satisfy the same requirements as any other INDs under the purview of the Bureau of Drugs. "In my view," he would later tell the *Blue Sheet* trade reporter, "the risks entailed by having cancer are already taken into account in the risk-benefit equation we make. There is a recognition on the part of the FDA that cancer is devastating—and the level of risk that we deem acceptable is therefore already greater for cancer drugs than it is for other kinds of drugs." On one occasion, NCI Director Frank Zauscher and

[15] As chemist Nicholas Farrell recounted, disodium platinum tetrachloride was sufficiently threatening to patients that one "had to be absolutely sure that none was present." On the salt and methods for its elimination in preparation of aqueous solutions of cisplatin, see Susan J. Berners-Price and Trevor G. Appleton, "The Chemistry of Cisplatin in Aqueous Solution," chap. 1 in Lloyd R. Kelland and Nicholas P. Farrell, *Platinum-Based Drugs in Cancer Therapy* (Totowa, NJ: Humana Press, 2000), 14–15.

[16] Advisory Committee on Investigational Drugs, Summary of Proceedings, 13th Meeting, December 3, 1964, Washington; FOK. Gyarfas is discussed as "a thoracic surgeon in the Investigational Drug Branch." He later became an important medical reviewer and division director.

[17] Gyarfas' Division was within the Bureau of Drugs, and he answered at this time to Bureau Director J. Richard Crout. See the following chapter for Robert Young's review of cisplatin. Radiopharmaceutical products later split into a separate division, as it remains today. The review of cisplatin and the conflict between Young and Gyarfas is presented in chapter 7.

Cancer Treatment Division head Vincent DeVita personally visited FDA headquarters in Rockville to lodge a protest against Young's interference with the IND applications they had sponsored.[18]

On October 1, 1976, at a public meeting of President Gerald R. Ford's Cancer Panel, M. D. Anderson star oncologist Emil Freireich read into the minutes a "bill of particulars" that elaborated a list of complaints about FDA interference in NCI-sponsored trials at his hospital and stopped just short of naming Young as the person responsible. In Freireich's description, the FDA's claims about clinical trial problems at M. D. Anderson lacked plausibility as well as punctuality.

> [They] call the investigator on the telephone and say, "stop what you're doing," without anything in writing, without any document. In several agencies, it takes two or three weeks before we get the letters... and when you get the letters, you find that the comments are of no substance. I don't think we've ever had a comment from the FDA of any substance—that is, in the minds of the investigators—that were significant observations. Then, you respond with those nine-page letters, and there is nothing that motivates them after that. You see, once they have raised a question, there is no way to turn it on again, except to go to a congressman and push [the drugs] through.[19]

Gyarfas' response to Freireich and his fellow lamenters was that the criticism masked problems in the organization of their research. Carping at the FDA and lobbying the Ford administration was, in Gyarfas' view, "a good way to cover up your discrepancies." Benno Schmidt, Chairman of the Ford Cancer Panel, called the rift "the FDA problem."

Robert Young would become a model for understanding and misunderstanding at the National Cancer Institute and the M. D. Anderson Hospital. For Ford administration and Carter administration luminaries such as Benno Schmidt, "the FDA problem" would appear to be the Robert Young problem, much more than the William Gyarfas problem. A rogue individual had come to signify an entire organization. As Freireich explained the FDA's delays:

> Because the success of individuals in these minor positions with regulatory agencies is judged on the basis of how effectively the public regulations are enforced, it is clear that any complaints or errors or unexpected toxicities, which will certainly occur, will be to the detriment of these regulatory individuals... In contrast, a therapeutic triumph will do nothing for the regulator. In the absence of research, a regulator's job will be done perfectly.

---

[18] Young's statement appears in "NCI, FDA Set Early Fall Target Date for Settling New Drug Dispute; Monitoring Pact Approved, but Wide Gaps Remain in Views and on IND Procedure," *DRR* 20 (35) (Aug. 31, 1977): 7. "FDA Nearly Out-Flanked NCI," *DRR* 20 (3) (Jan. 19, 1977): RN-3.

[19] "FDA Blocks Cancer Drug Trials, M. D. Anderson's Freireich Reports; Reasons Unclear, He Tells President's Cancer Panel; Action Pledged," *DRR*, 19 (47) (Nov. 24, 1976): 15. "FDA Nearly Out-Flanked NCI," *DRR* 20 (3) (Jan. 19, 1977): RN-3. It is important, however, that Schmidt did not mention the FDA dispute in his January 1977 *Report to the President on the National Cancer Program; DRR* 20 (7) (Feb. 16, 1977): S-2-11. *DRR* 19 (47) (Nov. 24, 1976): 16.

Lest anyone at the Administration had the impression that Freireich was without sympathy among federal officials, Schmidt immediately labeled Freireich's statement "an eloquent description of the problem." [20]

For his part, Young continued to press forward with an aggressive attempt to rewrite the regulations governing clinical trials of combination chemotherapy. When on January 13, 1977, Young appeared at a meeting of the FDA's Oncologic Drugs Advisory Committee, he introduced a proposal for written guidelines for cancer combination-drug trials. Among the requirements he sought to introduce was stipulating that "all combinations which include agents which may interfere with the catabolism of cytotoxic agents in the combination must be the subject of preclinical studies which define relevant drug interactions." As one advisory committee member noted in questioning, however, the testing of combination regimens relied heavily upon empirically derived variation in drug dosages. Young's rule would have the effect of eliminating this source of variance. The committee voted unanimously to avoid written guidance for the regulation of combination chemotherapy studies.[21]

Young's machinations caught the attention and the concern of Bureau of Drugs head Richard Crout. Crout reined in his subordinate and talked directly with the NCI's DeVita, admitting that Young had exceeded reasonable caution. Crout and DeVita then met fortnightly to hammer out an interagency protocol that would relax FDA regulations for terminally ill patients in NCI-sponsored trials. Crout's moves projected a face of moderation and self-criticism, while also countering the jeopardy of a flank action by NCI that would deprive the FDA of its control over cancer drug development. Yet as Crout knew, the NCI's attempted end-run of his agency was already under way. House Health Subcommittee chairman Paul Grant Rogers (D-FL) released a December 3, 1976 letter from the American Cancer Society calling for full "NCI control over the testing of new anticancer drugs, instead of FDA control" for nonprofit research sponsors. This transfer of power would be accomplished, as ACS representative Nathaniel Polster hoped, by amendments to the National Cancer Act. While NCI officials were largely silent about the ACS proposal, M. D. Anderson's Freireich was not. He openly called for deep "structural changes" so that the "FDA can never again shut down a legitimate cancer research project." This brief union of the Society and the Institute against the FDA posed a new and particular threat. And to Administration officials concerned about the maintenance of their authority over clinical trials, the ACS-NCI proposal raised the specter of debilitation by precedent. Once an exception for one category of illness was carved out of the FDA's power over clinical research, it was feared, demands from representatives of other diseases would soon follow. As if to confirm the FDA's premonitions, Solomon Garb of the Citizens' Committee for the Conquest of Cancer seized upon the NCI-FDA dispute and called for ending FDA power over any clinical trial in which patients have "poor prognoses." Garb's re-

[20]Freireich quotation in *DRR* 19 (47) (Nov. 24, 1976): 16.
[21]"FDA Nearly Out-Flanked NCI," *DRR* 20 (3) (Jan. 19, 1977): RN-3.

marks introduced a different and more formidable voice to the growing chorus of criticism, in part because the Citizens' Committee was an amalgam of union, scientific, corporate, scientific, and civic leaders. Voicing some of the same arguments that were heard in the national debate over Laetrile, Garb argued if such patients "wish to try an experimental treatment, and their physician agrees . . . FDA should not interfere."[22]

With Laetrile politics and antigovernmental energy on the rise, Administration leaders like Crout and Gyarfas knew that an institution with the public clout of the Cancer Institute had to be taken seriously, and with a measure of deference. Even though consumer safety groups such as Ralph Nader's Health Research Group (led by Sidney Wolfe) rebutted the NCI-ACS proposal, the mere existence of that proposal was a serious strike at the agency's image as legitimate governor of pharmaceutical experiment in the United States.[23]

The "NCI-FDA War" ended temporarily in October 1977 with an administrative peace. After four months of regular meetings, DeVita and Crout settled on a new procedure whereby "stop orders" for NCI-sponsored trials for terminally ill patients could be issued only by the Bureau of Drugs chief (Crout himself at the time) or the deputy chief (Marion Finkel, at the time). The two groups later agreed to use the nation's forty comprehensive cancer centers to mediate the surveillance of research protocols. The new arrangement embedded meaningful victories for both sides. For the Institute, the new procedures effectively bypassed Robert Young and, more notably, William Gyarfas, Director of the Oncology Drugs Division. NCI officials and their grantees would now deal more directly with Crout and Finkel, who were more trusted within oncology networks. And the Institute's détente with the FDA helped it to buttress claims that it was being "dominated" by the American Cancer Society, which had called for full relaxation of FDA control over cancer drug studies. Yet the Institute's informal victories were accompanied by a formal triumph for the Administration. A chief goal of the new arrangement, as *The Blue Sheet* trade reporter interpreted it, was "to give the FDA better protection from its critics, who are quick to charge FDA with not fulfilling its statutory obligations in the area of cancer drug development." The Administration would retain full control over cancer trials. The NCI would now officially acknowledge and defer to the IND regulations, and in so doing it would develop a "Master Plan" of drug development that represented a bow to Administration rules and guidance

[22]On Crout's admission, see *DRR* 20 (3) (Jan. 19, 1977): RN-3; "NCI Lists Its Demands on FDA," *DRR* 20 (4) (Jan. 26, 1977): 1. On Crout-DeVita meetings, see "NCI-FDA War," *DRR* 20 (15) (April 13, 1977): 2. "Blue Sheet" reporters rehearsed the logic of the FDA's worries about precedent succinctly: "It's highly doubtful that Rogers' subcmte. or its Senate counterpart will strip FDA of its control over cancer INDs. Members might sympathize with the plight of the cancer drug investigators, but to single them out for special treatment would inevitably trigger similar demands from groups interested in other diseases." "Nader Health Group Leaps into FDA-NCI Dispute over Drug Trials; 'Resist Claims Experimenters Can Regulate Themselves,' Rogers Urged," *DRR* 20 (5) (Feb. 2, 1977): 12. Freireich and Garb statements in *DRR* 20 (7) (Feb. 16, 1977): RN-1.

[23]"Nader Health Group Leaps into FDA-NCI Dispute over Drug Trials," 12.

MEMORANDUM OF UNDERSTANDING RELATIVE TO
ANTICANCER DRUG DEVELOPMENT

The Division of Cancer Treatment, National Cancer Institute, as a result
of its mission, has a substantial and continuing effort of anticancer
drug development, the regulation of which comes under the purview of the
Food and Drug Administration, primarily but not exclusively within the
Bureau of Drugs. A substantial amount of the information available to
the Division of Cancer Treatment and to the Bureau of Drugs, acquired by
each in the pursuit of their missions, is of common interest to these
organizations. In the past, both have been keenly aware of this community
of interest and have had extensive informal and effective interchanges
of views and of information on a wide variety of problems. Such informal
interchanges should and will continue and both organizations encourage
the members of their staff to provide the utmost assistance and cooperation in all appropriate areas. In addition, in order to aid in the
maintenance of a harmonious, direct working relationship between these
two sister organizations, both charged with responsibilities relating to
public health, it is believed that a formal Memorandum of Understanding
is desirable. The following specific agreements between the National
Cancer Institute and the Food and Drug Administration are made to achieve
these objectives:

Figure 6.1. NCI-FDA Memorandum of Understanding (January 1979)

documents. As DeVita's associate Saul Schepartz summarized his agency's concessions, "we've had to take on a whole new set of requirements for IND monitoring and record keeping . . . . we used to be very loose."[24]

By January 1979, the dispute had issued in a document with odd legal status but firm organizational commitments (figure 6.1). An informal procedure for resolving FDA-NCI disputes appears to have been worked out in April 1979. The procedure entailed four steps: (1) first devolving disputes to the lowest managerial level deemed suitable for negotiation—the Associate Director of the Bureau of Drugs (at that time, Finkel) and the Director of the NCI's Cancer Treatment Division (DeVita), then (2) to negotiations between the Bureau of Drugs head (Crout) and the NCI Director, then (3) to negotiations between the FDA Commissioner and NIH head, and (4) finally, determination by FDA Commissioner himself if none of these previous options produced a resolution. The memorandum bound neither agency legally. It was rather an informal institution founded in a political equilibrium, a mutual wish to avoid the spectacle of open, public conflict among two agencies whose reputations generally benefited from being out of the public eye.[25]

The Cultural and Juridical Affirmation of Power: Laetrile

There are many ways of seeing that the layman isn't victimized without according the government the power to control medical research. Such power can't serve science or medicine but can only be abused by medico-politicians playing status and money games.

—*Washington Post* columnist Nicholas von Hoffman, 1971[26]

The stiffest legal and philosophical challenge to the Administration's gatekeeping power in the two decades after 1962 came neither from organized

---

[24]The meetings took place between January 18, 1977 and May of that year. Accompanying DeVita at these meetings was Saul Schepartz, associate director of the NCI's treatment division. Crout was accompanied by his deputy, Marion Finkel. "NCI-FDA Pact Limits Cancer Drug Stop Orders to BuDrugsChief, Top Aide; Final Agreement Coming in Two Months or Two Years? Officials Differ," *DRR* 20 (17) (April 27, 1977): 13–14. "NCI, FDA Set Early Fall Target Date for Settling New Drug Dispute; Monitoring Pact Approved, but Wide Gaps Remain in Views on IND Procedure," *DRR* 20 (35) (Aug. 31, 1977): 7. For his part, Robert Young remained defiant, declaring he would not "give up what by statute we have to do" (*DRR* 20 (17) (April 27, 1977): 13–14) and maintained that "some pretty fundamental significant questions" had yet to be discussed [*DRR* 20 (35) (Aug. 31, 1977): 8]. On alleged ACS domination of the Institute, an accusation vehemently denied as a "red herring" by Benno Schmidt, see *DRR* 20 (29) (July 20, 1977): 1. On the "Master Plan," see "Evolution of the National Cancer Institute Master Plan for Drug Development and Interactions with the Food and Drug Administration," May 15, 1981; Records of the National Cancer Institute 1937-90, RG 433, NA.

[25]"Memorandum of Understanding Concerning Anticancer Drug Development," February 6, 1979; Vincent DeVita to Donald S. Frederickson (Director, NIH), March 15, 1979; Records of the National Cancer Institute 1937-90, RG 433, NA. "NIH, FDA Agree on Four-Step Approach to Resolve Disputes," *DRR* 22 (18) (May 2, 1979): 8. Noncontractual agreements of this nature have received increasing attention in institutional political science; Gretchen Helmke and Steven Levitsky, "Informal Institutions and Comparative Politics: A Research Agenda," *Perspectives on Politics* 2 (4) (Dec. 2004): 725–40.

[26]Von Hoffman, "And If It Works . . . ," *WP* June 6, 1971, B1.

medicine, nor from government cancer researchers, nor from drug manufacturers. It came, arguably, from a naturopathic drug called Laetrile and its odd assemblage of enthusiasts and supporters. Whereas the cures promoted by Harry Hoxsey, Andrew Ivy, and other twentieth-century naturopaths were gaining traction among smaller audiences, Laetrile had the backing of a wide variety of alternative therapy groups, state legislatures (seventeen of whom legalized it between 1976 and 1978), some officials of the National Cancer Institute and the Sloan-Kettering Institute, and national politicians. Compared to the earlier quack cancer therapies, moreover, Laetrile brought not just more people to the contest but also a new set of issues. Laetrile energized critics of the Administration's gatekeeping power and, even more, its power to define and assess the validity and scientific rigor of therapeutic research. The focus of contest was not simply upon therapeutic freedom but also upon the liberty of experiment.[27] Quack remedies had faded in their publicity since Krebiozen's demise, but the ascendance of Laetrile suddenly thrust them into prominence again. Unlike the Hoxsey cure and Krebiozen, however, Laetrile and its votaries faced a vastly altered regulatory environment. Whereas the powers of the FDA against Hoxsey and other quacks were exercised by means of enforcement, the addition of gatekeeping power meant that therapeutic promoters could introduce a new cancer therapy only through experimentation first and marketing later. In the main, the Administration's police power had been redirected from the commercial marketplace to the arena of clinical trials. And just as the target of FDA force changed, so did the political claims involved. The politics of Laetrile were not only a contest over the extent of government intrusion, but also a debate over whether the juridical securities afforded to American citizens would also be available for a new drug. It was in great measure a politics of competing claims as to whether Laetrile would get a "fair trial."[28] Laetrile was also known as "amygdalin" and "Vitamin B-17." Whereas amygdalin is a naturally occurring substance, Laetrile is a compound that was first separated from apricot kernels by self-claimed biochemist Ernst Krebs, Sr. The two names were employed interchangeably by Laetrile supporters, and as FDA Commissioner Donald Kennedy would later remark, the confusion was quite possibly intentional. Laetrile enthusiasts followed Krebs in conjecturing that, upon reaching the tumor site, the compound would release cyanide molecules that had previously been molecularly bound. This cyto-

[27] James C. Petersen and Gerald C. Markle would argue in 1979 that "At no time in American history has there been a more effective challenge to medical expertise and authority than that mounted by the contemporary Laetrile movement"; "Politics and Science in the Laetrile Controversy," *Social Studies of Science* 9 (1979): 139. The states legalizing amygdalin for intrastate commerce were Alaska, Arizona, Delaware, Florida, Idaho, Illinois, Indiana, Kansas, Louisiana, Maryland, Nevada, New Hampshire, New Jersey, Oklahoma, Oregon, Texas, and Washington. "Laetrile: Statutory and Constitutional Limitations on the Regulation of Ineffective Drugs," *University of Pennsylvania Law Review* 127 (1978): 233.

[28] In the wake of Krebiozen's demise, a *JAMA* article in 1967 asked whether non-legitimate cancer treatment had expired from the American medical scene; J. F. Holland, "The Krebiozen Story: Is Cancer Quackery Dead?" *JAMA* 200 (April 17, 1967): 213–18.

toxicity claim had the impressive corollary that only an enzyme present in tumors could "unlock" the cyanide, hence the toxicity of Laetrile was felt only by tumor cells and not elsewhere in the body. Later, supporters of Laetrile would offer other hypotheses, including that cancer resulted from a metabolic deficiency at the cellular level which was corrected by its status as a vitamin. Unlike many of its older cousins, Laetrile had been the subject of experiments at established medical centers at UCLA and the University of Pennsylvania. The compound also had backers of greater national esteem than the Hoxsey Cure and Krebiozen ever did. Laetrile's votaries included AAAS president Chauncey Leake and former National Cancer Institute scientist Dean Burk.

Burk's contribution was more than nominal. In 1971, he had announced his discovery of a molecular model demonstrating Laetrile's anti-tumor activity. Burk had combined an older hypothesis that the cyanide component of the amygdalin molecule was active against tumor cells with a newer claim about the combination activity of cyanide and benzaldehyde. He had also overseen animal studies with Laetrile at NCI, some of which purported to find evidence of anti-tumor activity in cell cultures. Burk continued through the 1970s as a recognizable voice with credentials from government service and in professional medicine, a voice of continued lament about the Administration's approach to cancer and clinical experiment. His remarks to a *Los Angeles Times* staff writer in 1973 were typical of early criticism: "Laetrile is used by a fair number of doctors, FDA or no FDA, and it is being used in Germany and Mexico." Its purported success "doesn't mean [cancer patients] will live forever, but some cancer patients are willing to settle for one more month." Laetrile supporters' furtive attempts at legitimation relied heavily upon these two claims, one that its massive use by cancer sufferers and their doctors was an indication of its test-worthiness, the other that therapy for terminal cancer patients ought to be regulated with greater flexibility.[29]

Laetrile's primary institutional patron was the San Francisco-based McNaughton Foundation, which under the leadership of founder Andrew Mc-

[29]On the nutritional hypothesis, see "Clinica Cydel and the Holistic Approach to the Metabolic Therapy of Cancer with Vitamin B-17," *Cancer Control Journal* 3 (5) (1975). The cytotoxic hypothesis was originally Krebs' claim and later appeared in G. Edward Griffin's *World Without Cancer* (Thousand Oaks, CA: American Media, 1974). For a critique of this hypothesis from within the pro-Laetrile movement, see Michael Culbert, *Vitamin B-17: Forbidden Weapon Against Cancer* (New Rochelle, NY: Arlington House, 1974). Culbert had previously served as editor-in-chief of the *Berkeley Daily Gazette*.

On the confusion between amygdalin and Laetrile, see Kennedy, "Laetrile: Commissioner's Decision on Status," *FR* 42 (Aug. 5, 1977): 39768–806; Petersen and Markle, "Science and Politics in the Laetrile Controversy," 141.

On the studies overseen by Burk, see Nathaniel I. Berlin [Acting Scientific Director, GLAC, NCI] to "Head, Cytochemistry Section, NCI" [Burk], April 9, 1969; Memo from Head, Cytochemistry Section, NCI [Burk] to Berlin, April 16, 1969, Subject : "Response to Memo of April 9, 1969 on 'Amygdalin'" (summarizing results of in vivo and in vitro studies); MSS 78-7, McNaughton Foundation Papers, Archives and Special Collections, UCSF. See also "Doctor Hurls FDA Challenge on Cancer Drug," *LAT*, July 16, 1973, C1.

Naughton began to sponsor research on the compound in 1958. On April 4, 1970, the Foundation submitted Investigational New Drug application 6734 to the FDA's Bureau of Drugs. McNaughton officials and their allies expected an easy approval. The FDA's judgment, in the works of Laetrile promoter Ronald Rakow, would be confined to "simply their allowing us to find out if, how, and to what extent, the material works." As was customary, the Administration issued a summary approval for the McNaughton application while specialists in the IND Branch studied it. Laetrile's summary approval for clinical testing arrived on April 20, but the Foundation's good news was quickly followed by a letter dated April 28 that noted "deficiencies" in the original IND application and mandated their correction within ten days of the letter's receipt. As the Foundation was preparing its response, Administration cancer specialist Earl Meyers telegrammed McNaughton on May 12 to announce the agency's termination of amygdalin's IND. Meyers' declaration meant that McNaughton would not have an "investigational exemption" from the Food, Drug and Cosmetic Act to distribute the drug in interstate commerce for the purpose of research. The Foundation appealed the decision and submitted additional data, but its requests were met with curt refusals. The Administration's stated reasons for ending the McNaughton IND had little to do with amygdalin and everything to do with its promoters and students:

> The Notice fails to provide adequate preclinical studies which may be considered adequate to justify clinical testing or which give proper attention to conditions of the proposed clinical testing. ...
>
> It lacks a bona fide well controlled scientific Phase I protocol. ...
>
> It does not identify a monitor qualified by training and experience to evaluate evidence of safety and efficacy of drug as it is received from investigators. ...
>
> It does not identify a clinical investigator qualified by training and experience to conduct Phase I cancer chemotherapeutic studies. ...
>
> It does not properly identify all facilities and investigators concerned with proposed study.[30]

At no point in the termination letter did Meyers ever voice concern about the animal studies that had been used to support the Laetrile IND. Satisfying Meyers' laments would have required McNaughton to undertake endeavors that no Laetrile supporter was willing (and few supporters were able) to do: find a legitimate sponsor (such as the NCI or a university cancer center) with

[30] "The McNaughton Foundation," *Cancer Control Journal* 3 (5): 3. Andrew R. L. McNaughton (President, McNaughton Foundation), to Earl L. Meyers (Director, Division of Oncology and Radiopharmaceutical Drug Products), February 26, 1971; Meyers to McNaughton, December 18, 1970; Binder "McNaughton Foundation I.N.D., 6734, Response to FDA Letter of 12/18/70," MSS 78-7, McNaughton Foundation Papers, Archives and Special Collections, UCSF. Rakow to Chauncey D. Leake, April 14, 1969; Leake to Rakow, March 30, 1969; MSS 78-7, McNaughton Foundation Papers. "FDA Backed in Barring Cancer Drug," *WP*, August 31, 1971, A12; Leroy F. Aarons and Stuart Auerbach, "Cancer Relief or Cancer Quackery?" *WP*, May 26, 1974, C4.

established pharmacologists and oncologists, name a legitimate monitor for regulation of the trial, and disclose the method and places of manufacture of Laetrile. McNaughton and other "Laetrilists" wanted their own people testing amygdalin, and they did not want to reveal their sources of supply.

Laetrile was neither central to alternative medicine nor entirely on the fringes of the movement. Many homeopathic doctors supported it, but so did many clinical oncologists, including some with impressive organizational affiliations. And many saw the vitality of Laetrile's challenge as an indicator that critics could induce FDA flexibility even in its governance of medicines and cures that had yet to be legitimated pharmacologically.

In the years following Earl Meyers' termination of the Laetrile IND, the compound spread physically through a set of underground networks and ideationally through self-help books, homeopathic and naturopathic societies, and neoconservative foundations and lobbies. Literature that envisioned a cancer-free humanity flowed forth from small, regional presses—including G. Edward Griffin's *World without Cancer* (1974), Michael Culbert's *Vitamin B-17: Forbidden Weapon Against Cancer* (1974) and *Freedom from Cancer: The Amazing Story of Laetrile* (1977). Syndicated editorialists like Nicholas von Hoffman of the *Washington Post* began to ask whether the Administration's prohibitions were converting "citizens" into "wards of the state." Describing FDA officials as "medico-politicians," he surmised that "if Laetrile does turn out to be an important drug... think how many miserable people will have died because some guy in Washington wouldn't issue a permit."[31] Like broader currents of protest in which it coursed, von Hoffman's broadside made the case for Laetrile by mounting a challenge to the reputation and power of the Administration. In most of these arguments, Laetrile supporters framed the central issue not as economic liberty, but as therapeutic freedom. What most bothered many Laetrile supporters and their distant sympathizers was not the absence of Laetrile from the drug marketplace, but the absence of a permit for testing. Appropriating the juridical metaphor of a "fair trial," they linked a populist ethic of self-medication to issues of justice and to more progressive norms of academic and intellectual freedom, the liberty of research and exploration of ideas. The Bureau of Drugs, for its part, responded by declaring that if Laetrile supporters could find a legitimate institution to sponsor a clinical study, a trial would be approved for the claim of pain reduction. "Qualified" here meant technically an FDA-approved organization, but more broadly an entity whose

[31] Griffin, *World Without Cancer*; Culbert, *Vitamin B-17: Forbidden Weapon Against Cancer*; Culbert, *Freedom from Cancer: The Amazing Story of Laetrile* (New York: Pocket Books, 1977). Von Hoffman, "And If It Works... ," *WP* June 4, 1971, B1; "Debating Government Drug Control," *WP* May 21, 1976, B8. In otherwise insightful research, Petersen and Markle overstate this transition as a form of venue shopping: "Defeated, or at least stalemated, at the scientific level, pro-Laetrile forces have expanded the conflict into the ideological, legislative and political arenas" ("Politics and Science in the Laetrile Controversy," 150). Yet popular books and articles voicing the argument for therapeutic freedom were appearing in the early 1970s, and scientific debate over Laetrile continued into the 1980s.

sponsorship of an IND would court less impressionary trouble for the Administration. Lewis Thomas, president of Memorial Sloan-Kettering Cancer Center in New York, had approached Bureau of Drugs director Richard Crout in 1974 about just such a trial, and Crout told the *Washington Post* that "we would be receptive to an IND from them. In return, I don't think they would submit an IND that wasn't first rate."[32]

None of this would satisfy the Laetrile lobby, which regarded large cancer centers like Sloan-Kettering as co-conspirators with the Administration and a host of other offending parties. These included not only the FDA, whose legal power prevented Laetrile from receiving a proper test, but also the American Cancer Society, the American Medical Association, the National Cancer Institute, and the Pharmaceutical Manufacturers Association. Fusing the Administration with these other organizations into a "cancer establishment," Laetrile supporters doubted the very wisdom and capacity of the FDA. As journalist David Rorvik of the Alicia Patterson Foundation hypothesized, "Why does the cancer 'establishment' (generally defined as an alliance of the ACS, FDA, National Cancer Institute, the American Medical Association and various drug companies) oppose even the clinical testing of Laetrile with such ferocity? The easy answer is to surmise that it fears that the substance just might be the magic bullet that will do in not only cancer but (as night follows day) the cancer establishment itself. . . . . [In fact] it is likely that the lockstep resistance of the establishment accrues more from intellectual strabismus and academic catabolism than from any rational, open-eyed concern about money."[33]

Rorvik's rehearsal of the "magic bullet" metaphor—a characteristically American imagery for the therapeutic cure of human disease—demonstrated how the politics of cancer had posed unique challenges to medical research, government policy, and the FDA. As opposed to polio, tuberculosis, and other diseases that had been conquered in Americans' popular imagination, cancer defied the magic bullet model. In the face of metastatic cancer, the dominant strategies of surgical resection and radiotherapy had fallen flat, a point that Laetrile supporters eagerly repeated (NCI antagonist Dean Burk would conjecture in the late 1960s that surgery and radiotherapy "reached their limit" in the broader struggle against cancer). Oncologists now widely understood that most cancer patients were being killed not by their primary tumor but by secondary sites of malignancy. Even as oncologists turned to chemotherapy, moreover, other complications emerged to frustrate the reigning models of medical and pharmacological therapy. For one, the set of

[32]The "FDA has been on record for years as being prepared to approve human tests of Laetrile if experts in cancer found evidence to justify them," "Laetrile: The Making of a Myth," *FDA Consumer* (Dec. 1976–Jan. 1977), 5, 8. FR 42 (1977): 39767, 39781. Leroy F. Aarons and Stuart Auerbach, "Cancer Relief or Cancer Quackery?" *WP*, May 26, 1974, C4.

[33]David M. Rorvik, "Laetrile: The Goddamned-Contraband-Apricot Connection," *Newsletter of the Alicia Patterson Foundation* (New York: Alicia Patterson Foundation, 1976): MSS 78-7, McNaughton Foundation Papers, UCSF.

legitimate chemical treatments was composed of highly toxic compounds. As Laetrile votaries like the NCI's Dean Burk recapped this argument, legitimated chemotherapy's toxic and counterproductive traits were nearly blamable upon the Administration: "all of the anti-cancer agents approved by the FDA are highly toxic, immunosuppressant, meaning that they decrease the body's resistance to cancer and other illnesses, and they all readily produce cancer in mice." For another, new chemotherapy treatments were less likely to rely upon a single drug as upon an array of compounds that were applied before, during or after surgery and radiation. Celebrated combinations included the nitrogen mustard, vincristine, procarbazine, and prednisone (MOPP) regimen with Hodgkin's and non-Hodgkin's lymphoma and other regimens in which chemotherapy was "adjuvant" or administered before surgical resection so as to attack any metastases first. The realization that cancer was "different"—in its resistance to treatments, in the diverse modalities of its therapy, in its challenges to long-held medical and scientific models—was as stark in the 1970s as at any other time.[34]

In this context of a stalemate against cancer, the battle over Laetrile soon took on mass proportions. Even as the Administration was stepping up its legal, scientific, and rhetorical campaign against the drug, thousands of U.S. citizens were rendering a mockery of that stance by seeking supplies of Laetrile from Mexico. In February 1977, federal prosecutors reported that customs officials in San Diego were seizing 40,000 three-gram vials of Laetrile every month. Only narcotics posed a larger detection problem at the Tijuana border crossing. An estimated fifteen thousand Americans were seeking Laetrile-based treatment at the Centro Medico del Mar, a hospital and clinic established by Dr. Ernesto Contreras Rodriguez. These visitors and many others hoped to smuggle the compound into the United States for personal use or distribution. As if to add the imprimatur of state authority to counter the opprobrium of the FDA, Contreras's clinic—which offered radiotherapy as well as more established chemotherapy—was officially backed and regulated by the Mexican government.[35]

The Administration's response to these patterns was as ambiguous as it was manifold. At the level of enforcement, FDA strategy shifted somewhat to seizures and criminal prosecutions. The agency cooperated with state and local governments and U.S. Customs officials to crack down upon Laetrile smugglers and physicians who were actively treating their patients with the compound. The Administration's public justifications for doing so included

[34]Brandt, *No Magic Bullet*; Patterson, *The Dread Disease*. For recognition of the disappointment with the "conquer cancer" drive of the early 1970s, see Aarons and Auerbach, "Cancer Treatment or Quack Drug?" *WP*, May 26, 1974, C4; "The Cancer Drug Dilemma" [editorial], *NYT*, February 11, 1977, A26. Burk statement in Lynn Lilliston, "Doctor Hurls FDA Challenge on Cancer Drug," *LAT*, July 16, 1973, C1.

[35]Aarons and Auerbach, "Cancer Relief or Quackery?" *WP*, May 26, 1974, C1, C4; Bill Richards, "Dying Drug Smugglers: Heavy Traffic in Supposed Anticancer Agent," *WP*, February 14, 1977, A1.

not only Laetrile's inefficacy, but also its status as a black-market entity whose smugglers were making illicit profits. Decrying Laetrile's "slick promoters," Administration spokesman Wayne Pines remarked that "this stuff has a higher markup than heroin." FDA officials also enlisted the help of the American Cancer Society, which launched a renewed campaign in 1975 to expose "unproven" remedies for cancer. In other ways, the Administration engaged Contreras and Laetrile enthusiasts by asking for case records of patients who had been successfully treated with the compound. In each case of purported successful treatment, argued Bureau of Drugs director Richard Crout, there were compelling alternative explanations such as concomitant chemotherapy and radiation. Nor had Contreras or any other Laetrile defender kept systematic records of patients treated with Laetrile that would provide a denominator so that the rate of response could be estimated, or that would permit study of "failures."[36]

Yet the FDA's steadfast opposition on Laetrile had not come without costs. By pressing the case for a total ban, by publicizing its seizures, and by assisting with state and federal prosecutions of Laetrile distributors, the Administration had resurrected a face that had been nearly invisible since the 1950s: the FDA as police. When Californians Donald E. Hanson and Donna Schuster were indicted by a federal grand jury in San Diego in June 1976 for violation of the Food, Drug and Cosmetic Act, the government's united front toward Laetrile received broad media coverage. *Time* magazine gave its Medicine section the title "Laetrile Crackdown," and *U. S. News & World Report* published a summary of the proceedings under the title "Heating Up: Latest Battle over a Cancer 'Cure'." A year later, in an editorial entitled, "When Gods Fail," the *Wall Street Journal* also called into question the Administration's aggressive enforcement strategy, asking "Does the FDA really need to pursue such interests to the point of waging war against the transportation of apricot pits across state lines for immoral purposes?"[37]

By the middle of the 1970s, with growing public animosity toward government, academic, religious, and social institutions, the Laetrile campaign began to attract unprecedented popular support and organized momentum. In 1976, Alaska became the first state to legalize possession of amygdalin within its borders. In April 1977, state legislators in Indiana went further and approved a bill that legalized not only possession of Laetrile, but also production and distribution of the drug within state borders. These libertarian supporters openly avoided the issue of Laetrile's efficacy (or lack thereof).

[36] ACS, *Unproven Methods of Cancer Management* (New York: The Society, 1971). Richards, "Dying Drug Smugglers," *WP*, February 14, 1977, A1. "ACS Acts to Expose Unproven Remedies for Cancer," *WP*, April 20, 1975; Aarons and Auerbach, "Cancer Treatment or Quack Drug?" *WP*, May 26, 1974, C1, C4; "FDA Backed in Barring Cancer Drug," *WP*, August 31, 1971, A12.

[37] For FDA publicity, see "Seized Laetrile Valued at $300,000," *FDA Consumer*, September 1977, 28. For general media coverage, see "Laetrile Crackdown," *Time*, June 7, 1976; "Heating Up: Latest Battle over a Cancer 'Cure'," *U.S. News & World Report*, June 21, 1976; "When Gods Fail," *WSJ*, July 5, 1977, 10.

Frank Solomon, vice president of the San Francisco–based Committee for Freedom of Choice in Cancer Therapy, argued that for any terminally ill patient, the freedom of therapeutic choice was paramount, and that FDA regulation was interfering with the sanctity of the doctor-patient relationship. By early 1977, Solomon's Committee could count four hundred chapters and thousands of members. Other organizations carrying the banner for Laetrile included the Cancer Control Society, the Test Laetrile Now Committee, and the Foundation for Alternative Cancer Therapy in New York. Among the organizations funding and energizing the Laetrile cause was the John Birch Society, a conservative group founded in Indianapolis in 1958 whose members had actively opposed the Equal Rights Amendment and U.S. membership in the United Nations. A nucleus of Birch Society members had started the Committee for the Freedom of Choice in Cancer Therapy in 1972. Following Indiana, Florida legalized Laetrile, and by April 1977, bills on Laetrile legalization were pending in Oregon, Massachusetts, and Minnesota. California—now the nation's most populous state and an increasingly welcoming home to antigovernment politicians and scattered libertarian organizations—became the symbolic center of the Laetrile movement and the principal site of the networks composing the "underground railway" that freighted the drug into the United States.[38] In Congress, Representative Steve Symms of Idaho held hearings on Laetrile and the Administration's attempts to crack down upon its distribution. Symms then sponsored the Medical Freedom of Choice Bill which, among other provisions, would repeal the efficacy provisions of the 1962 Kefauver-Harris Amendments. Symms' bill had 105 congressional co-sponsors by May 1977, and while it never advanced out of committee, its surprising popularity in the House was noted with concern by senior Administration officials.[39]

In the end, the most direct threat to the Administration's legitimacy and power in the 1970s came neither from the states nor from Congress, but from federal courts and the national media. In 1975, cancer patient Glen Rutherford filed suit against the Department of Health, Education and Welfare in the Federal District Court for the Western District of Oklahoma. Rutherford's request—that the federal judge issue an order directing the FDA to desist from Laetrile prohibition—was granted under the principle of "equitable injunctive relief." In *Rutherford v. United States* (1975), Judge

[38]Richard D. Lyons, "Refusal of Many to Heed Government Health Advice Is Linked to Growing Distrust of Authority," *NYT*, June 12, 1977, 55. Richards, "Dying Drug Smugglers," *WP*, February 14, 1977, A1, A7. "Banned Cancer Drug Gains in Some States," *NYT*, April 17, 1977, 28; Lyons, "Laetrile's Legalization in Indiana a Coup for Small Rightist Group," *NYT*, May 15, 1977, 1; Lyons, "Laetrile Networks Become More Open," *NYT*, June 5, 1977, 19; Lyons, "Rightists are Linked to Laetrile's Lobby," *NYT*, July 5, 1977, 30; Aarons and Auerbach, "Cancer Treatment or Quack Drug?" *WP*, May 26, 1974, C1, C4. Lisa McGirr, *Suburban Warriors: The Origins of the New American Right* (Princeton: Princeton University Press, 2001).

[39]Symms, "Don't Ease the Symptom —Attack the Problem," *WP*, June 3, 1977, A27; Von Hoffman, "Debating Government Drug Control," *WP*, May 21, 1976, B8.

Luther Bohannon ruled simply that the Administration had not exercised due process in its Laetrile ban, a finding that was upheld by the Tenth Circuit Court in Denver. For a two-year period from 1977 to 1979, the FDA was enjoined from enforcement of its Laetrile ban. The district court also entered an injunction prohibiting the agency from preventing the use of Laetrile by any patient whose doctor certified a need. At the same time, the number of Americans using Laetrile was publicly estimated at between 50,000 and 75,000.[40]

As the *Rutherford* cases wound their way through the federal court system, Administration officials could properly wonder whether their system of clinical trial regulations (and perhaps with them, efficacy requirements) was being slowly but entirely undone. Bohannon specifically found that Laetrile was nontoxic and was an effective cancer treatment. In *Rizzo v. United States* (1977), the federal court in the Eastern District of New York argued that the burden of proof in the Laetrile controversy lay not with its supporters but with the FDA; the drug was *assumed* safe and the Administration was charged with the dispositive responsibility of showing otherwise. These district courts and the Tenth Circuit Court not only weakened the FDA's formal power, they also implicitly compromised FDA's jurisdiction over safety and efficacy judgments. Federal judges had now done much more than established the libertarian principle that only patients and their doctors can decide whether drugs are safe and effective for life-threatening diseases. They had substituted their own judgment for that of the Administration. While other federal judges would diverge in their findings, prominent newspapers and magazines supported the Bohannon argument. Even as the *New York Times* reported on the "rightist" connections of pro-Laetrile lobbies in the states, its editorial page openly called for relaxation of investigational new drug regulations for cancer patients.[41]

[40]The first case appears at *Rutherford v. U.S.*, 399 F. Supp. 1208 (Western District, Oklahoma, 1975); in 1977, injunctive relief was granted to a broader class of cancer patients in *Rutherford v. U.S.*, 438 F. Supp. 1287 (Western District, Oklahoma, 1977). The Tenth Circuit's second decision, eventually appealed to the Supreme Court, is at 582 F.2d 1234. For a concise review of the early cases, see "Laetrile: Statutory and Constitutional Limitations on the Regulation of Ineffective Drugs," *University of Pennsylvania Law Review* 127 (1978): 233; also Gerald Rosen and Ronald I. Shorr, "Laetrile: End Play Around the FDA," *NEJM* 90 (1979): 418–23. The injunction on the FDA's prevention of individual use lasted ten years, and the Supreme Court's 1978 decision did not dissolve it.

[41]The Tenth Circuit's decision was more complicated than this summary suggests. Chief Judge Oliver Seth of Santa Fe, New Mexico, had overturned Bohannon's more radical finding that Laetrile access was based upon constitutional privacy rights, and instead of permitting universal Laetrile distribution as Bohannon had sought, Seth allowed *intravenous* Laetrile administration only when the patient was "certified" to be terminally ill with cancer. The Tenth Circuit's distinction as to route of administration followed reports that patients taking Laetrile orally were succumbing to cyanide poisoning. *Rizzo v. U.S.*, 432 F. Supp. 356, 359 note 4 (Eastern District, New York, 1977); "Laetrile: Statutory and Constitutional Limitations on the Regulation of Ineffective Drugs," 247–8.

The weakness of the F.D.A. case is the fact that terminal cancer patients are indeed special cases. We doubt that Congress had them clearly in mind in passing drug legislation. To put the matter bluntly, they have little or nothing to lose. A new drug or combination of drugs whose anti-cancer efficacy has been suggested by animal experimentation at least offers them hope—and perhaps even benefit. Some state courts have recently recognized the special status of terminal cancer patients by permitting them to import laetrile... If judges are willing to go that far, it seems only sensible—and humane—to ask the F.D.A. to do so also.

The *Wall Street Journal*, in its "When Gods Fail" editorial, also saw cancer patients as uniquely deserving of exception from the Administration's regulations. "In the case of fatal and incurable disease, the problem of personal choice becomes even more acute, and bureaucratic nuances even more obscene. If a cancer patient should decide simply to die with as much dignity as possible, who is the FDA to second-guess?" In January 1978, the *Times* editorial page went further still. Pointing to "some 75,000 Americans" who were using the drug, the *Times* editors proclaimed that "Laetrile can no longer be dismissed as a quack medicine whose popularity will wane." After legitimizing the drug by dint of its popularity, the *Times* editors concluded that "the risk of circumventing F.D.A. procedures seems worth taking."[42]

In the face of mounting public challenges to its legitimacy, the Administration's ambiguous public stance became with one face more rigid and with another, more flexible. Commissioner Donald Kennedy, his hand forced by the *Rutherford* decision, weighed into the debate with greater heft than ever before, calling Laetrile "worthless," "ineffective," and a "public health problem." Less vocally, he also gestured to the lack of chemical identity between Laetrile and amygdalin (the former is in some sense a purified form of the latter). This point was material not only because it undermined the consistency of the drug's supporters—some of them had tested and distributed one compound, others something quite different—but also because the Administration had for some time demanded "bioequivalence" of any compounds tested and marketed under the same name, as well as methods and facilities for producing equivalent molecules.

On the gentler side, Kennedy and his colleagues did two things. First, they quietly granted greater leeway to the National Cancer Institute for clinical tests of Laetrile. After considerable disagreement within its leadership and its Decision Network Committee, the Institute agreed to study Laetrile in two stages, first by examining records of purported "cures" as part of an initial investigation into claims of the drug's efficacy, then by conducting a Phase 2 clinical trial to assess the drug's efficacy. Despite a fuming battle over cancer therapeutics between the NCI and FDA, no Administration

---

[42] "The Cancer Drug Dilemma" [editorial], *NYT*, February 11, 1977, A26; "When Gods Fail," *WSJ*, July 5, 1977, 10; "No Cure for Laetrile" [editorial], *NYT*, January 29, 1978, E16. For an opposing view, see "The Laetrile Cult," *WP*, July 14, 1977, A26.

official spoke out publicly against the Institute's planned experiments. What is more, the Bureau of Drugs continued to negotiate with the Institute over new protocols that might, one day, win approval. This was a far cry from Commissioner Donald Kennedy's rumored preference, which was to reject the Institute's IND altogether. Second, FDA officials also began to debate their case directly in public media. Following Bohannon's orders in the second *Rutherford* ruling, Kennedy announced public hearings in Kansas City in the summer of 1977. He also testified before the Senate. In ways that Administration officials acknowledged but had hoped to avoid, these public fora—particularly the hearings before Ted Kennedy's Health and Scientific Research Subcommittee—provided Laetrile enthusiasts with a platform of visible equality, a place on the stage next to the Administration. As a *New York Times* reporter would summarize the hearings, "the Laetrile people had won an extraordinary victory," having "come to Washington on virtually equal footing with the leading medical specialists of the day."[43]

So cross-pressured was the Administration that observers in some quarters began to feel sympathetic toward it. "The Commissioner of the FDA is now in an awkward position," concluded Duke University pharmacologists Gerald Rosen and Ronald Shorr. "It is difficult to imagine that the FDA will grant an investigational exemption for laetrile, but political pressures may lead to a different result."[44]

All of these machinations were overshadowed by the Supreme Court's January 1979 announcement that it would hear the government's appeal of the Tenth Circuit ruling in *Rutherford*. In their review of the Tenth Circuit's decision, the Justices were deluged by letter writers asking them to release the drug. The Justices appeared to separate themselves quickly and decisively from what Justice Harry Blackmun termed "Laetrile and all its emotionalism." Oral arguments were heard on April 25, at which Justices Thurgood Marshall, Warren Burger, and William Rehnquist greeted Rutherford counsel Kenneth R. Coe with deep skepticism. Marshall asked Coe, had Bohannon not merely thrown out the findings of the Administration "and substituted his own?" Turning to the exemption for terminal cancer patients from the 1938 Act, Marshall asked Coe, "Where do you get that from? The statute doesn't say it. The regulations do not say it." Before Coe could

---

[43]The Institute had been considering a Laetrile trial since May 1977 at latest; "NCI Mulls Laetrile Trial," *DRR* 20 (22) (June 1, 1977); "NCI Decision on Laetrile Trials Near," *DRR* 20 (28) (July 13, 1977); "HEW Launching Study of Cancer Victims Treated Only with Laetrile; Legal Hurdles Seen in Getting Data; Project Less than Popular at NCI," *DRR* 20 (37) (Sept. 1, 1977): 7. William J. Broad, "New Laetrile Study Leaves Cancer Institute in the Pits," *Science* 202 (Oct. 6, 1978): 33–36; "Laetrile Evaluation Underway at NCI," *JAMA* 239 (1978): 19. B. D. Cohen, "U.S. to Study Laetrile Records," *WP*, January 27, 1978, A1; "U.S. Panel's Review of Laetrile Produces Inconclusive Results," *WSJ*, September 7, 1978, 18; "U.S. Cancer Institute Seeks Laetrile Tests on Cancer Patients," *WSJ*, September 28, 1978, 24. "FDA Official Strongly Contends Laetrile Is Ineffective, Subject to U.S. Regulation," *WSJ*, July 13, 1977, 13; Lee Edson, "Why Laetrile Won't Go Away," *NYT*, November 27, 1977.

[44]Rosen and Shorr, "Laetrile: End Run Around the FDA," *NEJM*.

answer that question, Marshall did it for him. The exemption was judge-made law, Marshall declared, a fiction of the Tenth Circuit and of Chief Judge Oliver Seth of Santa Fe. Coe could do nothing but assent quietly.[45]

By the time of the oral arguments in April 1978, the FDA had one important new card in its hand. No longer was the case for Laetrile's nontoxicity so airtight. Two cases of death after Laetrile treatment were reported to the agency the previous winter, and while the clinical observations in both cases were sparse, they were consistent with acute hydrogen cyanide poisoning. Then in March 1978, the *Journal of the American Medical Association* published the results from a study by University of California-Davis physicians, showing that when taken in conjunction with common health foods such as almonds, Laetrile induced cyanide poisoning and death in dogs. The Administration not only had evidence that Laetrile could induce cyanide poisoning and was nonselective in its toxicity, it also had a credible hypothesis as to why this toxicity might be greater for cancer patients. Cancer patients then and now commonly receive anti-emetic drugs, or medications to prevent vomiting (emesis). The hindrance of vomiting by anti-emetics meant that the body could not react to high cumulative cyanide toxicity by throwing up, hence the poison would accumulate to potentially lethal levels. U.S. Solicitor General Wade McCree, in arguing the FDA's appeal before the Court, willingly recited these new facts and the anti-emetic hypothesis.[46]

The Court handed down its decision in *United States v. Rutherford* on June 18, 1979, and the verdict was literally front-page news. Marshall wrote for a unanimous Court in overturning Bohannon and the Tenth Circuit and finding with the Administration on every issue confronting the high tribunal. Endorsing the Administration's argument about precedent, Marshall concluded that to limit FDA authority over Laetrile for terminal patients would be to restrict its authority "over all drugs, however toxic and ineffectual, for such individuals." Such a "new market would not be long overlooked" by the very unscrupulous quack promoters of whom the Administration had been warning, he reasoned. Marshall also explicitly echoed the equation of safety and efficacy that had been a hallmark of the Ralph Smith

[45]Morton Mintz, "Supreme Court Enters Quarrel Over Laetrile," *WP*, January 23, 1979, A1; "Justices to Rule Whether the FDA May Bar Use of Laetrile as an Anticancer Drug," *WSJ*, January 23, 1979, 10; Morton Mintz, "Justices Voice Skepticism on Laetrile Rulings," *WP*, April 26, 1979, A14. Blackmun handwritten case notes, Case 78-605; Florence Ignoffo, R.N. to Blackmun, May 2, 1977; B295, F4, File 78-605, Harry A. Blackmun Papers, Library of Congress.

[46]Smith, Butler, Cohan, and Schein, "Laetrile Toxicity: A Report of Two Patients," *Cancer Treatment Reports* 62 (1978): 169; Sadoff, Fuchs, and Hollander, "Rapid Death Associated with Laetrile Ingestion," *JAMA* 239 (1978): 1532; Schmidt, "Laetrile Toxicity Studies in Dogs," *JAMA* 239 (1978): 943. Gail Bronson, "Study Finds Laetrile Can Poison if Taken with Certain Foods," *WSJ*, March 7, 1978, 35. Earlier reports had surfaced in 1975 and perhaps as early as 1971. See Townsend and Boni, "Cyanide Poisoning from Ingestion of Apricot Kernels," *Morbidity and Mortality Weekly Reports* 24 (1975): 427; "The Case of the Crushed Kernels," *Consumer Reports* 39 (1974): 514; *Cancer News*, Fall 1973–Winter 1974, 16.

era in the 1950s Bureau of Medicine at the FDA. "A drug is unsafe," he reasoned, "if its potential for inflicting death or physical injury is not offset by the possibility of therapeutic benefit." In granting the agency further legal flexibility, in rejecting with unanimity the libertarian critique of the FDA, in adopting the Administration's logic and rhetoric to the point of duplication—in all these ways and more, the Supreme Court's *Rutherford* decision was in every respect a stunning and total victory for Donald Kennedy and the Bureau of Drugs.[47]

In another political or regulatory universe, the *Rutherford* decision would have ended the cultural and political battle over Laetrile and cancer drug regulation more generally. But this was a politics of belief, a politics of legitimacy, and a politics of reputation. Laetrile lived on, not simply by virtue of its enthusiasts in California and among libertarians, but in part because the FDA kept it alive. Six months after the *Rutherford* decision was handed down, the Administration defied predictions by announcing its conditional *approval* of the NCI's clinical trial application. Even though Rutherford provided legitimation for shutting down the NCI trial—as Kennedy was rumored to want to do—the Administration let it continue. On its face, this decision courted serious risk. If the NCI trial had shown positive results from Laetrile, a decade's worth of stonewalling would have been revealed as erroneous and the experience would have confirmed the most severe criticisms of Steven Symms, John Birch Society devotees, and other radical libertarians. Why, then, did the Administration allow the trial to go forward? One reason for the decision is that Kennedy had departed the Commissioner's office for Stanford University. He had been replaced by UCSF pharmacist Jere Goyan, who was more cordial to the Administration's procedural critics. In part, too, Administration officials saw comfort in the fact that the NCI's chosen trial sites—the University of Arizona, UCLA, the Mayo Clinic, and the Sloan-Kettering Institute of New York—housed strong Laetrile skeptics. Even as his institution prepared to launch the trials, Mayo's Charles Moertel stated that "Laetrile has assumed proportions that no other quack medicine has assumed before." And in June 1977, Sloan-Kettering officials had announced, from a review of case records and from their own pharmacological studies, that they could find no evidence for "preventive, tumor-regressing or curative anticancer powers" in Laetrile.[48]

---

[47] *U.S. v. Rutherford*, No. 78-695, 442 U.S. 544; 99 S. Ct. 2470; 61 L. Ed. 2d 68; 1979 U.S. LEXIS 114. Mintz, "U. S. Laetrile Ban Backed," *WP*, June 19, 1979, A1; Linda Greenhouse, "Ruling in Cancer Dispute," *NYT*, June 19, 1979, A1. J. Brant and J. Graceffa, "Laetrile's Setbacks in the Courts: *Rutherford*, *Privitera*, and *Chad Green*," *American Journal of Law and Medicine* 6 (1980): 151–71. Justice Marshall's echo of the Ralph Smith "safety implies efficacy" doctrine was even more unequivocal, drawing on the Senate report for the 1962 Amendments which noted and affirmed the FDA's pre-1962 practice of applying the doctrine specifically to cancer therapies; *U.S. v. Rutherford*, 442 U. S. 553, fn. 9.

[48] On Kennedy's skepticism toward the NCI's IND, see Broad, "New Laetrile Study Leaves Cancer Institute in the Pits," 36. "U.S. Test of Laetrile on Humans Backed," *NYT*, January 4, 1980, A11; "Cancer Institute Gets Tentative Approval for Laetrile Tests," *WSJ*, January 4,

Yet the reputational politics of the Laetrile IND approval in January 1980 are also evident. The Laetrile affair had projected the police powers of the agency in a way that had not occurred since the 1950s. In seizing shipments and assisting the prosecution of Laetrile distributors and doctors, the Administration was, wittingly or not, resurrecting its Cold War era public image as marketplace cop. Some of Laetrile's votaries thought as much, with one Leroy McNulty of Wichita, Kansas, writing President Carter that the "FDA operates like a special police force for AMA." Taking note of the nation's more conservative mood, and acting in the midst of a general election year, Administration officials wished to enhance their image as a flexible organization, one where enforcement was tangential to science, one whose coercive powers were used sparingly, and one that picked its battles. Consistent with this stance, the FDA's approval was conditional and couched in ambiguity. As one of the animal tests conducted by the NCI showed a possible link with induced fevers, the FDA required another trial in rabbits before any human tests could proceed. And before any comparative clinical trial of the Phase 2 sort could begin, the Institute would have to complete and report from a successful Phase 1 toxicity trial in humans. Accordingly, as Goyan announced his approval of the Institute's IND trial, he deftly negated Laetrile's promise with his next breath. "All the data to date," he declared, "suggests that Laetrile has no effect on cancer, but we will objectively and promptly evaluate any data that is produced by N.C.I.'s study. In the meantime, I caution cancer patients not to delay or abandon conventional cancer therapies by turning to Laetrile as an alternative."[49]

The other event that kept Laetrile politics alive, albeit with grand twists of irony, was the death of Hollywood actor Steven McQueen on November 7, 1980. Diagnosed with mesothelioma in December 1979, McQueen began alternative treatment under the direction of Donald William Kenney, a Dallas-based dentist and orthodontist, in July 1980. At the time of McQueen's treatment, Kenney had been blacklisted by the ACS and his license was suspended in Texas. Laetrile was a small but visible component of Kenney's regimen, which also included pancreatic enzymes, coffee enemas, fifty daily vitamins, psychotherapy, and injections of a cell preparation derived from sheep and cattle fetuses. When that summer McQueen publicly admitted he was receiving treatment for cancer (he had denied it for months be-

---

1980, 6; Victor Cohn, "Cancer Unit Is Starting Laetrile Tests," *WP*, January 4, 1980, A10. The Sloan-Kettering announcement summarized two studies at the center, and the announcement was accompanied by comments by Institute vice president for academic affairs C. Chester Stock and Institute president Robert A. Good. Their participation in the announcement only added to the perception of Sloan-Kettering's organizational unity against Laetrile. "Laetrile Won't Cure Cancer, According to Sloan-Kettering," *WSJ*, June 16, 1977, 26. The papers were eventually published in the *Journal of Surgical Oncology*.

[49] "Cancer Institute Gets Tentative Approval for Laetrile Tests," *WSJ*, January 4, 1980, 6; Victor Cohn, "Cancer Unit Is Starting Laetrile Tests," *WP*, January 4, 1980, A10. Leroy McNulty (Wichita, Kansas) to President Jimmy Carter, December 28, 1977; B 295 (*Rutherford* case files), F 5, Harry A. Blackmun Papers, Library of Congress.

fore), he criticized the American medical establishment and, more implicitly, the Administration: "Mexico is showing the world a new way of fighting cancer through nonspecific metabolic therapies." Yet McQueen, for all of the publicity and rhetoric he brought to alternative cancer treatment, would die less than a year after his initial diagnosis. He died in Mexico, moreover, while he was receiving alternative treatment. Laetrile defenders tried to blunt the impact of McQueen's death, pointing to his post-surgery heart attack as the cause, but media accounts had reported that McQueen's Mexican surgeon had resected a massive, five-pound tumor before he passed.[50]

Slowly but inexorably, the very same networks and media coverage that supported the incredible popularity of Laetrile now contributed to its slow deflation as a viable remedy. Six months after McQueen's death, the National Cancer Institute reported results from its Phase 2 trial. The Mayo Clinic's Charles Moertel issued a blunt summary: "Laetrile has been tested. It is not effective." The response rate of 156 cancer patients to the drug was negligible. Moertel announced the results at the outset of the annual American Society for Clinical Oncology meetings, a propitious venue given that it was a specialty society and unaffiliated with the AMA.[51]

At the very historical moment when the legal powers in its arsenal were strongest, however, the Administration continued to offer an olive branch to votaries of alternative medicine. FDA officials largely backed off Laetrile enforcement, content to let the compound wither on its own. Laetrile use plummeted in the early 1980s, but enough of it persisted that Charles Moertel himself worried that the Administration was not doing its duty to snuff out the drug and its promoters. "In spite of [my] evidence and the Supreme Court decision" in *Rutherford*, Moertel complained to Thurgood Marshall, "regulatory agencies have essentially ceased all efforts to control cancer quackery." So too, as Administration officials saw in Laetrile and related alternative therapies for cancer a problem that would melt away, they projected a face of cooperation to alternative medicine groups. Administration officials called a meeting with top representatives from national homeopathic organizations in Rockville on June 9, 1982. FDA representatives included Deputy Commissioner Mark Novitch, Chief Counsel Thomas Scarlett, and Jerome Halperin, Director of the Office of Drugs. Homeopathy supporters included physicians Wyrth Post Baker, President of the American Foundation for Homeopathy, and Sandra Chase, President of the National Center for Homeopathy. Robert Pinco, legal counsel to the American Cen-

[50]Gary Arnold, "Movie Hero Steve McQueen Dies of Heart Attack at Age of 50," *WP*, November 8, 1980, B4; "McQueen Death Renews Cancer Treatment Debate," *NYT*, November 9, 1980, 21. For a retrospective, see Barron Lerner, "McQueen's Legacy of Laetrile," *NYT*, November 15, 2005, and Lerner's thoughtful chapter 7 in *When Illness Goes Public: Celebrity Patients and How We Look at Medicine* (Baltimore: Johns Hopkins University Press, 2006).

[51]"Laetrile Tests Show Drug Is Ineffective as Cancer Weapon," *WSJ*, May 1, 1981, 5; Victor Cohn, "Laetrile Flunks Test, Is Found As Effective as 'No Treatment'," *WP*, May 1, 1981, A3. Lerner (*When Illness Goes Public*, 156) shows that McQueen's death heightened interest in Mexican treatment clinics, at least for a while.

ter for Homeopathy, would later tell an audience of homeopathy enthusiasts that the June 9 meeting was one of the high points of his entire career. The government, Pinco declared, "is willing to work with us." He stressed the importance of direct contact with legislators in the House and Senate, but underscored the central lesson of recent times as the importance of organization. "If you deal with the FDA, deal through associations, not alone. It hurts. We must show unity." While warning readers that "there is no guarantee that this situation will continue indefinitely," a writer for the American Homeopathic Headquarters summarized the new stance as a "relative regulatory 'hands off' attitude towards homeopathy." The correspondent went even further and portrayed a long-running administrative peace: "FDA in its role of protector of public health, has never felt compelled to either move against individual homeopathic drug products or against the whole industry."[52]

Rethinking the Laetrile Drama. American society seems periodically revisited by quack medicines, and in many respects the Laetrile affair appears as the recital of a much longer and older historical pattern. Yet Laetrile was different in its history, and set apart in its historical legacy. Laetrile presented a rallying cry for previously disparate and scattered organizations and voices. It set nearly two dozen state legislatures against the Administration, and commanded headlines and mass public sympathy in ways that its predecessors failed to do. It is fair to say that no other compound presented as great a symbolic challenge to the FDA's power, and its reputation, in the twentieth century.[53]

In retrospect, an appreciable portion of the hype surrounding Laetrile was due to the reigning modality of cytotoxicity in 1970s cancer treatment. The known therapies of the time were premised fundamentally not upon nutrition, nor metabolism, but upon inducement of cell death. The dual allure that Laetrile brought—one that inspired patients and physicians in Germany, Mexico, the United States, and elsewhere—was its status as a "natural" compound, and the alleged selectivity of its toxicity. By claiming that Laetrile targeted only malignant cells, naturopaths could partake of the cytotoxicity paradigm while avoiding its embedded human costs. The conceptual combination of "apricots" (Laetrile as natural health food) and "cya-

---

[52] Moertel to Justice Harry A. Blackmun, March 9, 1982; B 295 (*Rutherford* case files), F 5, Blackmun Papers, Library of Congress. "Rhetoric Abounds at Preservation Gathering," *American Homeopathy* 2 (9) (Sept. 1982), 1; "Federal Report: The FDA and Homeopathy," *American Homeopathy*, 2 (7) (July 1982): 3. Copies in Records of the McNaughton Foundation, UCSF. The agency's stance toward alternative medicines at this time belies Temin's erroneous and empirically unsupported conclusion that the agency "generalizes the case of Laetrile to other drugs, resulting in a regulatory policy that denies the option of taking "innocuous" drugs to the maximum extent possible" (*Taking Your Medicine*, 205). For additional evidence against this claim, consider the regulation of platinum-based chemotherapy, discussed in chapter 7.

[53] For an account placing Laetrile in a longer line of "cancer quackery," see Wallace Janssen, "Cancer Quackery: Past and Present," *FDA Consumer* (July–August 1977): 27.

nide" (Laetrile as deadly poison) seemed like a patient's dream come true. At some level, it appears, American oncologists and officials at the NCI and the FDA doubted Laetrile because it was not toxic enough.

Historians and observers of American medicine and science have interpreted the Laetrile controversy in various and imaginative ways. From one vantage, Laetrile and its votaries offered a competing paradigm of science and of therapy, one whose claims rested upon its unprecedented popularity, its furtive legalization within and across the borders of the United States, and the simplicity of the hypotheses underlying its alleged curative powers. Laetrile had its own doctors, its own regional culture, its own literature, its own clinics, its own laboratories, its own territory, its own courts. Yet at the intersection of state power and organizational reputation there exists another way to view the struggle. Once it is seen as a larger debate not simply about science but also the power of a particular government agent, a debate that brought the John Birch Society and conservative legislators like Steven Symms into vocal participation, the Laetrile wars can be viewed as a competing paradigm of legitimacy, power, and regulation. Laetrile and its supportive networks promised, in this reading, not merely an alternative form of science. They held out the allure of an alternative mode of governance which, to be established successfully, needed to refute the basis of the Administration's power, namely its legitimacy.[54]

It is in this context of challenges to power and legitimacy that we can divine answers to some difficult questions: Why did Administration officials fight Laetrile so ferociously, if at times ambiguously? And why, once the Supreme Court had granted it legitimation and broad authority, did many of those same officials stay their policing activity and turn a welcoming, moderate face to alternative medicine enthusiasts? One enduring answer lies in the cultural and legal power of precedent. As FDA supporter Philip Schein of Georgetown University's Lombardi Cancer Center summarized the Administration's worries, "We don't live by exceptions, we live by precedents. And [if Laetrile use is legalized] there's absolutely no reason why you or I couldn't come up with a new potion, give it to patients, get testimonials from their families and have it distributed." Once the issue of precedent had been established—through the *Rutherford* decision and through the gradual delegitimation of Laetrile after Steve McQueen's death and the NCI trial results—the Administration backed off in ways that are sensible only from the standpoint of organizational reputation.[55]

By virtue of Laetrile's demise and the *Rutherford* decision, the Adminis-

---

[54]Petersen and Markle, "Politics and Science in the Laetrile Controversy," 156–60, citing arguments by Thomas Kuhn and Everett Mendelsohn. Mendelsohn, "The Social Construction of Scientific Knowledge," in Mendelsohn, Peter Weingart, and Richard Whitley, eds., *The Social Production of Scientific Knowledge* (Dordrecht: D. Reidel, 1977).

[55]Schein quotation in B. D. Coles, "Dispute Over Laetrile Focuses Attention on Rights of Patients," *WP*, May 29, 1977, 18. The Lombardi Center composed a supportive network ally for the Bureau.

tration's power over the modern pharmaceutical world had grown in several dimensions. The lack of a cancer exception to the Food, Drug and Cosmetic Act meant that the agency's formal authorities would extend universally to all areas of therapeutics. No disease, no area of medical practice, no specially appointed or deserving community of sufferers would have immunity from the Administration's purview, its rules and procedures, its concepts and definitions. Even as small tests with Laetrile continued, the federal courts had affirmed the basic legitimacy of the Administration's rationales for halting experiments on a drug. In cases where a medicine's claimed therapeutic mechanism lacked pharmacological plausibility, or where its sponsors were deficient in scientific and medical legitimacy, the Bureau of Drugs could terminate investigational rights with impunity. The agency could quash any such invalid compound that claimed therapeutic benefit against a specific disease. It could do so not merely by denying its entry to the market, but less visibly by preventing experimentation and pointing to the drug's lack of theory or esteem as a rationale for this decision. In this way, the Laetrile case was a powerful message to practitioners of alternative therapeutics that, so far as drug development was concerned, their energies lay profitably in other endeavors. The precedent established one powerful reason for nutritional supplement makers to avoid disease-specific therapy claims, a practice that (in part for other reasons) continues to this day.

A third dimension of the Administration's conquest in the Laetrile affair concerned its status in divining legitimate from illegitimate medicine, valid from invalid experiment, genuine pharmacological theory from unjustifiable speculation. In this sense, the agency's victory over Laetrile was less a scientific triumph than a legal, political, and cultural one. This is not to doubt the ultimate veracity of the Administration's position. There is still no experimental evidence that Laetrile is safe or effective, and enhanced molecular and oncogenetic models of cancer do not support any of the hypotheses offered for its effectiveness. Yet the Administration's main victories were in court—the Supreme Court of the United States and, more slowly, the venues of national media coverage, public opinion, and aggregated medical judgment. Steve McQueen's death and the demise of Laetrile deflated the arguments and visions of Steven Symms, Andrew McNaughton, and others who had sketched out an alternative pharmaceutical world. In resisting the most popular alternative remedy in a generation, the Administration had witnessed its power confirmed in tandem with its reputation.

LIAISON AND THREAT: AIDS AS A METAPHOR
FOR ORGANIZATION AND FOR POLITICS

The emergence of AIDS as a global health crisis—and with it a set of government, business, social, and religious responses to the epidemic—has been extensively documented. Yet there is much that is misleading about the received legend of the FDA's response to AIDS, and much that it misses. The agency was changing and furiously adapting its regulatory processes several years before activists made their most public and memorable protests. The relationship between AIDS organizations and Administration officials was, moreover, one more of liaison and invited participation than of confrontation. Besides overemphasizing the conflict between activists and government, the common parables of AIDS and the FDA miss the deeply ideational struggle fought out by AIDS activists, conservative reformers and journalists, National Cancer Institute scientists, and warring factions within the Administration itself. The primary threat that AIDS activists made—and in the late 1980s and early 1990s they rendered it continually and with great effect— was to jeopardize the FDA's public identity as a public health agency and a protector of the American consumer. The politics of AIDS was, in a different reading, much more than a confrontation of organized consumers versus an intransigent regulator. The AIDS struggle was a multidimensional battle over the reputation and power of the Food and Drug Administration.[56]

An important undercurrent in the early history of the AIDS epidemic is that policymakers and researchers knew neither the exact cause of the epidemic nor how large it might be, and in this vacuum of knowledge swam vast fears that any number of human activities could be contributing factors. In 1981, reports came from Los Angeles, New York, and San Francisco of a previously rare and deadly opportunistic infection (*Pneumocystis carinii*) as well as increased incidence of a form of cancer (Kaposi's sarcoma) among active homosexual males. Together these maladies were killing dozens, and soon hundreds, of otherwise healthy young men. The early reports took infectious disease experts and other physicians by surprise, because both *Pneumocystis carinii* and Kaposi's sarcoma were thought to be easily controlled by the normal functioning of a human immune system. As the number of cases exploded, it became increasingly clear that deep and unanswered questions about the human immune system were in play, that the epidemic would persist and would devastate gay communities, and might well inflict harm on millions more people than was first believed.[57]

AIDS has killed and will kill tens of millions more heterosexual men and women than those who are gay, lesbian, or bisexual. Yet AIDS began its political and social life as a "gay disease," and in particular a gay male disease. Part of the reason is that the early cases and deaths were highly concentrated among sexually active gay men in large metropolitan centers in

[56]For treatments that both reproduce and undermine the common narrative, see Philip J. Hilts, *Protecting America's Health: The FDA, Business, and One Hundred Years of Regulation* (New York: Knopf, 2003), chapter 16 ("The Modern Plague"); Arthur Daemmrich, *Pharmacopolitics: Drug Regulation in the United States and Germany* (Chapel Hill: University of North Carolina Press), 96–115.

[57]Perhaps the most insightful of these narratives for my purposes has been Steven Epstein's *Impure Science*. The medical literature on HIV/AIDS is immense, and I will cite selectively from only those articles or volumes that were of direct consequence to the Administration's regulation of AIDS therapies.

the United States. This fact was perhaps less important than the political and social context in which it was interpreted and broadcast. Homosexuality has consistently been met by pervasive and enduring patterns of stigmatization and subjugation in American society, and in the 1970s and 1980s, these patterns mixed with the resurgence of socially conservative political and religious movements. Hence, the sufferers of AIDS were stigmatized by their sexual identities and relationships long before the disease afflicted them, and their illness exploded in a society in which contempt for their lives and behavior was both publicly and privately sanctioned. This combination of novelty, preexisting stigmatization, and resurgent conservatism meant that AIDS bore a unique and multidimensional politics. In the early 1980s, gay news outlets and mainstream media were similarly awash in casual hypotheses that the primary cause of the illness was sexual promiscuity or something related to it. Even after replication of the HIV virus was identified as the pathological mechanism for the spread of the disease—and hence the proximate "cause" of AIDS—male homosexuality (and what was called the gay "lifestyle") was still identified along with intravenous drug abuse as the most high-risk state behavior, one that implicitly courted the illness.[58]

The reinforced politics of disease and sexual identity combined to render the sufferers of AIDS, together with their advocates, a highly cohesive and well-organized group.[59] The urban centers and networks in which the epidemic had been identified and stoked such vast fear were also populations of younger, whiter, otherwise healthier, better educated, and often wealthier citizens. The personal, political, and collective struggles of these gay men against discrimination and stigma had given them rough but durable skills and templates for politics. These earlier ideational struggles had synthesized

[58] As Epstein remarks, "All speculation about causes [of AIDS] proceeded from the premise of the centrality of male homosexuality," in part because "the epidemic *was* being observed mainly among gay men" (*Impure Science*, 47, 51). This pattern provided plausibility for an early causal story known as the "immune overload hypothesis," wherein the alleged promiscuity of gay men so severely compromised their immune systems that otherwise harmless infections could overwhelm them. For the immune overload hypothesis, and the idea of promiscuity as having plausibility among gay newspapers as well as mainstream media outlets and conservative commentators, see Epstein, 45–66.

[59] In the public narratives that journalists and scholars have produced since the 1980s, it is common to speak of the disease constituency of AIDS as composed of "AIDS groups" or "AIDS activists." The early journalistic accounts of political organization among AIDS sufferers and representatives produced and replicated this portrait; Hilts, *Protecting America's Health*, chap. 16, esp. 237–42, 246–51; Daemmrich, *Pharmacopolitics*, 81–3, 113–14. Some of my own research has relied upon and perhaps perpetuated this simplification; see "Groups, the Media, Agency Waiting Costs and FDA Drug Approval." While accurate in particulars, these terms partially distort the structural diversity of the movement. Long before more militant and attention-getting groups like Project Inform and ACT-UP occupied center stage, there existed a network of infectious disease specialists and researchers, gay men's health groups, gay community press outlets, public health officials at numerous levels of government, concerned journalists from larger media organizations, and others who maintained a vital level of surveillance over the disease and its sufferers. These networks and organizations compose an audience that cannot be reduced to the notion of "AIDS groups" or "AIDS activists" alone.

networks and institutions that were remapped and redirected in the mobilization against AIDS. Hence, it was quickly after the public identification of the epidemic that organizations such as Gay Men's Health Crisis in New York City and the San Francisco AIDS Foundation formed, largely because the essential building blocks of culture, networks, and institutions were, in a sense, already there. After these groups but no less capable or powerful were Project Inform and ACT-UP, among others. For related reasons, lesbian women and their organizations capably assisted gay men's groups in their recruitment and advocacy. The affinity of earlier social networks to later institutions of mobilization gave skills, credibility, and power to AIDS sufferers and their advocates.[60]

The multiplicity and diversity of the organizations representing AIDS patients is partially responsible for the fact that AIDS was etched deeply on the consciousness of FDA officials years before more militant AIDS groups trained their sights upon the Administration. Even though President Ronald Reagan and upper echelons of his administration largely ignored the epidemic, AIDS dominated national news headlines during the early and middle 1980s. Several public events transformed the national and scientific politics associated with the disease. One of the most pivotal moments in the early history of AIDS policy came in 1984, when Secretary of Health and Human Services Margaret Heckler announced that "human immunodeficiency virus" (HIV) had been established as the "cause" of AIDS. For purposes of the public and many AIDS sufferers, Heckler's announcement publicly established AIDS as a viral disease, and the medical and human search for antiviral treatments was under way.[61]

A second event was the revelation that Hollywood actor Rock Hudson

[60]The San Francisco AIDS Foundation was earlier named the Kaposi's Sarcoma Research and Education Foundation. As Epstein summarizes, urban gay communities of the early 1980s "included (and in fact were dominated by) white, middle-class men with a degree of political clout and fund-raising capacity unusual for an oppressed group" (*Impure Science*, 12; see also 49–50). He also remarks that in organizing to meet an earlier pattern of challenges, "lesbians and gay men had developed political and social institutions that were poised to respond to the new threat when it erupted" (65). Later, and with somewhat less precision, he suggests that the primordial networks were partially sexual in nature: "the *same* social networks and institutional linkages that had permitted rapid amplification of a virus also gave rise to the organization of a concerted grassroots response" (78, emphasis mine). Cathy Cohen's imaginative comparison of responses to AIDS in white and black populations suggests that the common parable of AIDS and U.S. pharmaceutical regulation rests upon a vision of AIDS mobilization that was observed much more among white gay communities than among African-American and Latino populations; *The Boundaries of Blackness: AIDS and the Breakdown of Black Politics* (Chicago: University of Chicago Press, 1999).

[61]David C. Colby and Timothy E. Cook, "Epidemics and Agendas: The Politics of Nightly News Coverage of AIDS," *Journal of Health Politics, Policy, and Law* 16 (1991): 215–49. Shalini Vallabhan, *Creating a Crisis: AIDS and Cancer Policymaking in the United States* (Ph.D. diss., Texas A&M University, 1997); Elizabeth Armstrong, Daniel Carpenter, and Marie Hojnacki, "Whose Deaths Matter? Mortality, Advocacy, and Attention to Disease in the Mass Media," *Journal of Health Politics, Policy and Law* 31 (4) (Aug. 2006): 729–72. On the Heckler announcement, see Epstein, *Impure Science*, chapters 2 and 3.

had traveled to France to obtain one of these antiviral treatments, then called "HPA-23." Hudson's saga was heralded along with others in an August 1985 *Newsweek* story on "AIDS Exiles in Paris," which told of wealthy AIDS sufferers who had traveled to France to seek purported therapies available outside of U.S. treatment protocols. This story and others like it appear to have "embarrassed" Administration officials, who quickly announced that HPA-23 and other treatments would be permitted in the United States on a "compassionate use" basis. Yet even as the Administration abruptly changed policy, its public relations officers took pains to disabuse journalists of any notion that the FDA was withholding "a proven treatment." The FDA spokesman complained about the hype that HPA-23 and other unproven treatments were receiving: "Everyone is assuming that this is a panacea, and there is none." The revelation of Rock Hudson's suffering became, for a larger public audience, a social fact of AIDS' familiarity. Millions of American readers could neither identify with nor name any of the suffering and dying AIDS patients they had read and heard about, but now a household name, a celebrity, was infected, was dying, and was desperate. For gay communities and interested observers of the AIDS epidemic, and most powerfully for the Administration, the Rock Hudson story was about something else. It was a story about the deep potential conflict between individuals seeking therapies for an incurable condition, on the one hand, and the contours of the FDA's structure for testing drugs on the other.[62]

It was clear early on that the main pathology of AIDS was the destruction of human immunity to common infections. AIDS patients presented with symptoms whose incidence and aggressiveness could only be explained by a severely compromised immune system. Patients also displayed low "T-cell counts," or quantities of the helper cells that assist the body in fighting common infections. The development and acceptance of a viral hypothesis of AIDS transmission meant in some respects that two diseases were created out of one. There was "HIV infection," and then there was AIDS or "AIDS-related complex" (ARC), an umbrella term to describe the variety of illnesses attending the epidemic including *Pneumocystis carinii* pneumonia. As many popular discussions put it, the clinical and policy problem was not only limiting the spread of HIV—perhaps through public health measures, and perhaps through an "AIDS vaccine"—but also preventing HIV from developing into "full-blown AIDS" among infected patients. Further complicating the matter was the fact that the mechanism of AIDS was not a

---

[62] Mark Clark, et al., "AIDS Exiles in Paris," *Newsweek*, August 5, 1985; Jonathan Kwitny, *Acceptable Risks* (New York: Poseidon Press, 1992). The notion of the Administration having been "embarrassed" by these stories is taken explicitly from Epstein, *Impure Science*, 188. For discussions of the FDA response, see Irvin Molotsky, "French AIDS Drug Due for U.S. Tests," *NYT*, July 31, 1985, A10; Lawrence K. Altman, "The Doctor's World: Search for an AIDS Drug Is Case History in Frustration," *NYT*, July 30, 1985, C1. For these and other references, see Epstein, *Impure Science*, 409. The connection of AIDS suffering and activism to Hollywood and the American entertainment industry is thoughtfully surveyed in Lerner, *When Illness Goes Public*, chap. 11.

standard virus but in fact a "retrovirus." Retroviruses were so named in the
1970s after researchers discovered that some viruses were made of RNA (ri-
bonucleic acid) as opposed to DNA (deoxyribonucleic acid), and that they
replicated not through DNA duplication, like most viruses did, but through
a process called "reverse transcription" in which the viruses copied their
RNA into DNA form for replication, and then copied back again to RNA
form. The extra process of RNA writing its own DNA enabled the duplication of the virus in infected cells, and it also provided a target for drug development. Development of early anti-retroviral therapies focused upon the
enzyme, called "reverse transcriptase," that allowed this nonstandard replication to occur. If reverse transcriptase could be inhibited, the theory of
"anti-retroviral" treatment held, HIV's spread within the body could be
checked and infection would not progress inevitably to AIDS. While anti-
retroviral therapies would not help patients with already weakened immune
systems, they could prevent HIV-infected patients from developing AIDS-
related complex.[63]

The first molecule to receive NDA approval with a primary indication
related to AIDS was azidothymidine, or AZT. AZT was an anti-retroviral
therapy, and in the early 1980s the study of these therapies was in its infancy. The drug had been synthesized years earlier by Burroughs-Wellcome,
a subsidiary of the British giant Wellcome PLC based in North Carolina.
The company first notified the Administration of its possible anti-retroviral
activity in April 1985. The occasion was a "pre-IND" meeting in which a
company presents its plans for clinical research to the Administration and
often vets its research protocol for Phase 1 and Phase 2 trials. Wellcome was
one of the most trusted names in drug development internationally, and its
officers were adept at smoothing the path to clinical testing and regulatory
submission well before the official paperwork arrived in Rockville. The regulatory path to development thus paved, Burroughs-Wellcome submitted an
IND on June 14, 1985, and the Administration approved it in a week. Phase
1 trials—the first legal administration of AZT to AIDS patients, and the first
clinical trial involving AIDS—began July 3, 1985.[64]

In the context of fear and despair among public audiences and particularly in gay communities, the early results from AZT trials were sufficiently
promising as to threaten whatever normality governed drug development in
the 1980s. Phase 1 trials are officially undertaken to determine raw safety
and toxicity. Yet in conveying the Phase 1 results to their readers, journalists

[63] While viral replication through DNA had been well understood, no mechanism was known
for RNA replication until research published in 1970 by David Baltimore and Howard Temin.
For a thorough review of these developments, accompanied by an imaginative and well-
evidenced reading, see Epstein, *Impure Science*, 66–78 and more generally chapters 2 and 3.

[64] Azidothymidine—more properly, 3'-Azido-3'-Deoxythymidine—is a nucleoside analog. It
is structurally similar to the naturally occurring nucleoside thymidine, but has a "zido group"
(N3) in the so-called three-prime position that is normally occupied by a hydroxyl. Irvin Molotsky, "U.S. Approves Drug to Prolong Lives of AIDS Patients," *NYT*, March 21, 1987, A1,
A32. Epstein, *Impure Science*, 192–3; Hilts, *Protecting America's Health*, 243.

at *Science* and the *New York Times*, among other venues, actually focused on the drug's potential *efficacy*. "New Drug Shows Gain in Fight Against AIDS," stated the *Times* headline. The *Science* headline was only a bit more tempered: "AIDS Drug Shows Promise in Preliminary Clinical Trial." By a crude accounting, AZT had stopped HIV from replicating in fifteen of the nineteen patients, T-cell counts had jumped appreciably in these responders, and many of them reported and displayed relief of AIDS-related symptoms. The first randomized clinical study (a Phase 2 trial) started in February 1986, but it was halted in September after stark evidence had surfaced of AZT's short-term efficacy: 19 of 137 patients taking the placebo had died, but only one subject among 145 taking AZT had perished. The termination was a joint decision of Burroughs-Wellcome and FDA officials, and it followed standard protocol of the time. The termination was premised upon the ethical impossibility of keeping patients in a placebo arm when the treatment has demonstrated therapeutic value for a life-threatening illness. With the termination of that trial, the regulatory "data" for azidothymidine's submission to the FDA were essentially truncated. Just as important, AZT's efficacy—more often termed its "promise"—was now regularly trumpeted in numerous articles in the lay press, scientific and medical journals and gay community newspapers.[65]

The NDA for azidothymidine, for the treatment of "serious manifestations of HIV infection," was officially submitted to the Administration's Division of Anti-Infective Drug Products on December 2, 1986. Division Director Edward Tabor assigned the review to Ellen Cooper, a thirty-five-year-old medical officer who then had responsibility for review of most of the drugs for the treatment of AIDS and other forms of HIV infection. Cooper was something of a young star at the FDA. She was an honors political science graduate from Swarthmore College in 1972, and had studied at the medical schools of Yale and Case Western Reserve. A year after getting her M.D. in 1976 from Case Western, she received a master's in public health from Johns Hopkins, and then joined the Children's Hospital National Medical Center in Washington for a five-year stint working on pediatrics and infectious diseases. She had come to the Administration on a vi-

---

[65] "New Drug Shows Gain in Fight Against AIDS," *NYT*, January 26, 1986, A17; R. Yarchoan, et al., "Administration of 3'-Azido-3'-Deoxythymidine, an Inhibitor of HTLV-III/LAV Replication, to Patients with AIDS or AIDS-Related Complex," *Lancet* 8481 (March 15, 1986): 575–80; Jean L. Marx, "AIDS Drug Shows Promise in Preliminary Clinical Trial," *Science* 231 (March 28, 1986): 1504–5. On FDA participation in the decision to terminate the Phase 2 trial on September 19, see the remarks of David Barry, then Vice President for Research at Burroughs-Wellcome, in FDA, *Meeting of the Advisory Committee on Anti-Infective Drug Products*, January 16, 1987 (Bethesda, MD: Baker, Hames and Burke Reporting), 138. Erik Eckholm, "AIDS Drug Prolongs Lives in Some Cases," *NYT*, September 20, 1986, A1; Erik Eckholm, "Test Group for AIDS Drug Is Broadened to Include 7,000," *NYT*, October 1, 1986, B6; Deborah M. Barnes, "Promising Results Halt Trial of Anti-AIDS Drug," *Science* 234 (Oct. 3, 1986): 15–16. For helpful summary discussions, consult Epstein, *Impure Science*, 192–3; Hilts, *Protecting America's Health*, 243.

rology research fellowship in 1982, and Administration officials began to bestow significant discretion and authority upon her as early as 1984. Ellen Cooper would become a central and controversial figure in the regulation of AIDS therapies, but before 1987 she was largely unknown outside the agency.[66]

Cooper's review of AZT effectively started months before the December 1986 submission by Burroughs-Wellcome. Throughout her observation of the clinical trials and her review, Cooper was thoroughly aware of her several audiences. Even though more militant groups such as the AIDS Coalition to Unleash Power (ACT-UP) had yet to form, AIDS patients and their advocates already comprised a visible constituency whose agony was publicly tangible. Administration officials did not, in 1986, feel any direct pressure from organized AIDS patients and advocates for AZT's approval. Yet the imprint of AIDS politics upon Cooper and her Division was no less intense for that fact. Her calculus included not only the "direct effects" of AZT on the health of patients but also the "total cost of caring for patients with AIDS." Among the constituents were not only AIDS sufferers, but also other government scientists as well as researchers and companies developing anti-HIV therapies. She understood that the AZT application bore "major financial implications" for Burroughs-Wellcome. And she knew that she was making history, not just of the fantastic and legendary variety (reviewing the first drug submitted for a global health epidemic), but of the juridical sort. Cooper foresaw that her procedures and recommendations would have "major implications for the testing and evaluation of other drugs in AIDS" as well as "precedents that may be set for the development, evaluation and approval of other drugs for the treatment of HIV infection."[67]

In ironic but meaningful respects, the agony and dire state of AIDS sufferers fostered conditions ideal for a well-controlled study. Human research subjects were ready, available, and plentiful. As Cooper noted, "there certainly has not been a lack of patients interested in participating in clinical trials." Cooper also noticed that the confounding of AZT's effects by virtue of subjects taking other therapies known to be effective was also absent:

[66]Philip M. Boffey, "At Fulcrum of Conflict, Regulator of AIDS Drugs," *NYT*, August 19, 1988, A13.

[67]My impression of the absence of explicit political pressure for the AZT approval was formed in part from interviews I conducted with Administration personnel who worked at the time. According to one public relations officer, pressure from AIDS activists and gay rights groups was not perceived until early in 1988, almost a year after AZT's marketing approval; Interview with Brad Stone, Office of the Commissioner, FDA, February 9, 1990; Rockville, MD. Interview with Ralph Lillie, Chief Consumer Safety Officer, Division of Anti-Viral Drugs, February 9, 1990; Rockville, MD. This interview evidence is consistent with internal Administration documents I have surveyed, which repeatedly mention the "urgency" of the AZT submission but do not discuss or otherwise refer to explicit pressure or lobbying from AIDS-related organizations. See also contemporary reporting in *DRR* and *FDCR*. Cooper's remarks in FDA, *Proceedings of the Anti-Infective Drugs Advisory Committee*, January 16, 1987 (Baker, Hames and Burkes Reporting, 1987), 9–10.

"there have been no limitations imposed by the availability of other drugs or therapies. The latter fact, of course, adds to the urgency of the situation."[68]

In other ways, these conditions frustrated any possibility for a standard operating procedure. The official flaw of the AZT application is that its claims rested upon one and only one clinical trial, and that study had been stopped in midstream after clear differences in survival outcomes emerged between the treatment and placebo arms. Cooper's primary concern, one shared by other Administration officials, was that the requirement for "adequate and well-controlled investigations"—the conceptual legacy of Frances Kelsey and her coterie a generation earlier, explicitly elaborated in statute and in the Code of Federal Regulations—had not been met. There could be subjectivity injected into the terms "adequate" and "well-controlled." The difficulty here was the plurality of the statute's language. Interpreting "investigations" as requiring only one trial necessitated far more than a subjective and creative reading of law and regulation. It required setting aside a long-held requirement for at least two clinical studies in the demonstration of efficacy. The fact that the only trial had been cut short also limited its value as information, in part because longer-term effects from AZT treatment would not be known. Cooper had carefully considered the likelihood that AZT would be prescribed "off-label," as she anticipated "longer administration and use in less-ill patients" after regulatory approval when compared with the study population.[69]

Cooper followed the Phase 2 trial closely through the fall of 1986 and participated closely in the decision to terminate it. While she did not receive the official NDA until December, she had effectively begun the medical review of AZT months earlier. As she completed the review, she also launched two processes in motion, both of them crucial for the Administration's reputation. First, with the enthusiasm of Tabor, Commissioner Frank Young, and Burroughs-Wellcome officials, Cooper led regulatory efforts to make AZT available to over 4,000 AIDS patients before final marketing approval. This uncommon move was announced on September 19, and it saved hundreds if not thousands of lives. Moreover, given the trial stoppage and the publicity it received, Cooper's choice to expand access before final approval, whether wittingly or not, effectively nullified claims that the Administration was moving slowly on the most promising therapy for AIDS patients. Second, well before Cooper had completed her medical review of the azidothymidine NDA, she and Tabor moved to thrust the case of Retrovir in front of the FDA's Advisory Committee on Infective Drug Products. The crucial meeting occurred in January 1987, and Cooper served as something of a

---

[68]Philip M. Boffey, "Thousands in U.S. Receive Treatments in Experiments," *NYT*, January 7, 1986, C1; *Proceedings of the Anti-Infective Drugs Advisory Committee*, January 16, 1987, 12.

[69]"Another issue in the review of AZT, which is fundamentally scientific but has important regulatory implications for labeling, is the expected widespread prescribing of the drug to persons outside of the approved indications, should a general marketing approval be granted." FDA, *Proceedings of the Anti-Infective Drugs Advisory Committee*, January 16, 1987 (Baker, Hames and Burkes Reporting, 1987), 13.

lead prosecutor for the Administration despite the fact that she had not yet formally signed off on the NDA review. In presenting her case for approval to the Committee, Cooper painstakingly outlined the uniqueness of the situation and underscored the novelty and radical nature of the steps that she, Tabor, and her other colleagues had taken. It was for this reason that she and other Administration representatives wanted a clear and unambiguous statement from the Committee that would back up the solidity of her review and the accuracy of her judgments. A statement of intent to the Committee became something of a plea: "We seek a consensus, if at all possible, on whether or not AZT should be approved at this time."[70]

At the Committee and in discussions with media outlets, Cooper and other Administration officials created an informal distinction between "releasing" the drug to desperate patients and "approving" it. Cooper repeatedly remarked that the drug had been released and distributed in September 1986, when the Phase 2 trial was stopped, when massive compassionate use was commenced, and when the Administration all but promised that NDA licensing would occur within months. However, given that access to AZT had been sanctioned through the compassionate-use regulations, satisfying one set of audiences, Cooper and other Administration officials kept their eye on another set of audiences in medicine, consumer protection, Congress, and public health. As they sped AZT to approval, they also insisted on procedural minima, including a measure of public debate among medical, scientific, and regulatory communities. "Because of the complex issues involved in evaluation of the NDA for AZT, we do not want to come to a final decision until the advice and recommendations of the Committee, our distinguished consultants and our colleagues in other sectors of the PHS and, indeed, the scientific community at large, which we trust are well represented here today, are heard in this public forum." While in many respects Cooper and her Administration colleagues had already legitimated AZT, they sought to preserve meaning for the "final decision" that would give scientific and legal imprimatur to the drug. With their official policy and their presentation to the advisory committee, Administration officials in the Anti-Infective Diseases Division and the Commissioner's Office were sending at least two messages. The first was that the agency had acted quickly, differently, flexibly, and radically in response to a public crisis. It was as if the Administration were trying to symbolically disown the label "bureaucracy" in one massive action. The second message was that the case of AZT was so unique as to potentially defy precedent, and that its resolution did not bind the agency's thinking, speech, or behavior in regulating other drugs.[71]

[70]Boffey, "At Fulcrum of Conflict, Regulator of AIDS Drugs"; FDA, *Proceedings of the Anti-Infective Drugs Advisory Committee*, January 16, 1987, 10. At the advisory committee meeting of January 1987, Cooper in fact drew upon the expanded access mechanism in rebutting an argument by National Cancer Institute Director Samuel Broder (a committee member) that the Administration should have done more with the results of the stopped trial (*Proceedings of the Anti-Infective Drugs Advisory Committee*, January 16, 1987, 166–7).

[71]*Proceedings of the Anti-Infective Drugs Advisory Committee*, January 16, 1987, 10. Erik

On the whole, the Advisory Committee gave Cooper and Tabor (and, of course, Burroughs-Wellcome) what they wanted. The vote was twelve to one in favor of approval, with only Committee chairman Itzhak Brook dissenting. Brook placed greater emphasis on a concern that worried Cooper and Tabor, and that many panel members had voiced. The very vitality of AZT could become its primary weakness. Everyone would want the drug, and once "the genie was out of the bottle" upon marketing approval of AZT, as Brook rehearsed an old metaphor, the population demanding and using the drug would explode. Doctors and their desperate patients would not be constrained by even tightly specified labeling and prescription guidelines promulgated by the Administration and Burroughs-Wellcome. Yet on the whole, Committee members spoke of the drug in terms of the disease it sought to remediate, a disease that justified any regulatory or clinical jeopardy induced by AZT's approval. Stanley Lemon of the University of North Carolina talked of "extraordinary measures" for "an extraordinary situation," and consultant Paul Volberding of the University of California at San Francisco concluded that "This is a different situation than most situations. It is a different disease and a different kind of drug."[72]

Even as they highlighted the distinctiveness of the AZT review, Administration officials began to elaborate broader contours of a new regime of development and NDA review, one that would rest upon the exemplar of Cooper and Tabor's sprint with azidothymidine. Some of these moves were symbolic and organizational; Ellen Cooper was quickly promoted up the ladder of the Anti-Infective Drugs Division, and by 1989 she had succeeded Tabor as its director. Yet the most enduring shift was the formal embrace of a "treatment IND" development concept that had run within Administration circles since the 1950s. Agency officials had talked about formalizing the concept since 1983 at latest. On the afternoon of March 10, 1987, a week before the Administration announced formal approval of AZT, Commissioner Frank Young and other officials convened what one reporter called a "hastily called news conference." Young announced that the FDA would soon issue proposed regulations that would ease restrictions on experimental drugs for AIDS, cancer, and other life-threatening illnesses. As Young proposed, and as agency personnel at numerous levels understood, the new rules were intended to formalize the informal, to standardize procedures followed in the regulation of AZT. Crucially, the rules would be limited to those cases where the conditions were "immediately life-threatening" or otherwise "serious" and, in keeping with long-standing administrative practice, where "no alternative therapies exist." Under these parameters, the rules proposed, the Administration would more commonly allow for gen-

---

Eckholm, "License Move Nears for AIDS Drug," *NYT*, January 16, 1987, A12; "Panel Backs Licensing of AIDS Drug," *NYT*, January 17, 1987, I32.

[72]The very informative discussion occurs at *Proceedings of the Anti-Infective Drugs Advisory Committee*, January 16, 1987, 140–217. Volberding remarks at 151, lines 20–21. Lemon remarks quoted in Eckholm, "Panel Backs Licensing of AIDS Drug."

eral distribution of a therapy as early as the Phase 2 stage, and the Administration would bear the burden of proof for denying pre-approval distribution. The rules were finalized and published in the *Federal Register* on May 22, 1987.[73]

The deeper irony of AZT's approval and the 1987 regulations lay in their coincidence with a surge of more confrontational, militant patient-based activism. In other words, just as the FDA had demonstrated measures of flexibility, rapidity, and intended generosity in 1986 and 1987, AIDS-based audiences were expressing their greatest frustration with the agency. Some of the change was witnessed in the synthesis of new organizations. The group AIDS Coalition to Unleash Power (ACT-UP) was formed in 1987, and numerous local organizations dedicated to treatment and testing also emerged. Yet in other ways the transformation came in different behaviors observed among preexisting organizations. Previously "mainstream" organizers now began to foment and participate in a loudening debate about how AIDS drugs should be developed, tested, reviewed, and regulated. Crucially, these voices combined with conservative political entrepreneurs and think tank elites in promoting rapid drug development as a form of "deregulation."

Part of the conflict emerged in the way that the Administration and its audiences interpreted the AZT approval. The Administration had long regarded a life-threatening disease without any approved treatments as a status quo fundamentally different from a disease with even just one legitimated therapy. FDA regulations for the classification of priority NDAs—those receiving a score of 1A as opposed to those receiving 1B or 1C—explicitly referred to "unmet medical need." Although medical need could be flexibly interpreted, the Administration and many American physicians and pharmacologists regarded "need" as appreciably reduced if at least one safe and effective medicine existed. AIDS activists and their organizations did not see it this way. As Larry Kramer wrote in a widely publicized *New York Times* op-ed, one doctor he knew saw AZT's release as only a "sop to the gay community—so they'll shut up. They can't say they haven't been given *something*." To be sure, no one at the Administration or anywhere was under the impression that AZT was a "cure" for AIDS. The question was rather one of whether, in the wake of AZT's approval, further radical measures for changing regulation were justified. For Administration officials, further change modeled upon the development and review of AZT was sufficient.

[73]FR (May 22, 1987): 19466; *HHS News*, May 21, 1987, p. 2. Philip M. Boffey, "U.S. to Relax Rules on Experimental Drugs," *NYT*, March 11, 1987, A24; Interview with Brad Stone, Office of the Commissioner, FDA, February 9, 1990, Rockville, MD. Part of the rationale for formalizing the Treatment IND concept was reputational; writing the term into federal regulations permitted the agency to take public credit for the conceptual innovation during the height of the AIDS crisis; Peter Barton Hutt, personal communication, September 17, 2008. The idea of the AZT review as precedent setting has been developed independently in a study by Donna A. Messner; "AZT as Conceptually Pivotal to U.S. Drug Approval: FDA Therapeutic Drug Rule-Making and Practice, 1987–2000 and Beyond," in Gaudilliere and Hess, eds., *Ways of Regulating*, 247–70.

For increasingly militant audiences of AIDS sufferers and their representatives, much more remained to be done.[74]

Kramer's March 1987 essay—entitled "The F.D.A.'s Callous Response to AIDS"—is exemplary for the way that it voices different features of the AIDS community's critique, as well as for the way it presents a threat to the Administration's organizational reputation of the time.

> Many of us who live in daily terror of the AIDS epidemic cannot understand why the Food and Drug Administration has been intransigent in the face of this monstrous tidal wave of death. Its response to what is plainly a national emergency has been inadequate, its testing facilities are inefficient and gaining access to its staff and activities is virtually impossible.....
>
> Indeed, these are understatements. There is no question on the part of anyone fighting AIDS that the F.D.A. constitutes the single most incomprehensible bottleneck in American bureaucratic history—one that is actually prolonging this roll-call of death....
>
> In addition to ribavirin, why is the F.D.A. withholding Ampligen, Glucan; DTC; DDC; AS 101; MTP-PE and AL 721? AL 721 is not even a drug but a food—a form of lethicin—from Israel that has proved promising at the Weitzmann Institute. Ribavirin, at least, is available at black-market prices in Mexico for those who have the strength and money. None of the other drugs are available anywhere. Doctors wishing to test them have shown me the thick protocols they have submitted to the F.D.A., only to have them returned again and again with petty requests for the rewriting of one sentence, or the reversal of the order of several sentences or the elimination of two words.

Kramer's essay is shot through with inaccuracy and hyperbole. Of the therapies he mentions, only ddC (zalcitabine) emerged as a recognizably and broadly effective treatment for HIV/AIDS in the ensuing two decades—and its development had been accelerated by the Administration at the very time that AIDS activists were expressing strong doubts about it. Furthermore, many who perceived organizational problems at the agency—including journalists at the *New York Times* but also the George H. W. Bush administration—saw less a malady of bureaucracy and more a deficiency of resources. Like other AIDS activists, moreover, Kramer was equating the FDA with the Reagan administration when in fact much of Reagan's and his administration's ignorance of or indifference to AIDS was unrelated to FDA policy or regulations. In other ways, Kramer's tie between the FDA and Reagan was less problematic. They were part of the same executive branch, after all, and Frank Young and other FDA officials had been appointed by Reagan and other executive officials. Yet the FDA caught most of the redirected and highly focused anger of AIDS organizations in the late 1980s, often when they aimed or intended it for the Reagan and Bush administrations.[75]

[74]Larry Kramer, "The F.D.A.'s Callous Response to AIDS," *NYT*, March 23, 1987, A19.
[75]In 1998, a combination of ribavirin was considered by the FDA for approval with two

Yet for all of its shortcomings and simplifications, and indeed because of them, Kramer's essay was politically effective because it projected a simple, accessible, and forceful threat to the FDA's reputation. Like much of the portraiture emerging from AIDS activists, it recast the Administration in terms and symbols diametrically opposed to those fashioned by Young, Cooper, and Tabor in the review and approval of AZT. In some ways, the FDA was being cast as a generalized but faceless bureaucracy, as an inefficient, an "intransigent," "callous," and inaccessible organization. In other ways, it was the Administration's very gatekeeping power—over drugs themselves (the NDA process) and over clinical trials (IND approvals)—that was under attack. By serving as a "bottleneck," a public health agency dedicated to consumer protection was lengthening the "roll-call of death." Instead of raising genuine and substantive issues regarding clinical trial design with AIDS drugs, the Administration was in Kramer's depiction imposing classic "red-tape" constraints upon medical research, nit-picking research protocols, shuffling words and sentences. It was for this reason that, as Kramer portrayed it, the FDA's angry constituencies included not only AIDS patients but also their physicians, whom the Administration had managed to "privately infuriate."[76]

The collective lament of AIDS sufferers and their representatives was manifold, but two claims in particular surfaced. The first targeted the pipeline of drugs in testing for AIDS, while the second targeted the very fundamentals of Administration procedure and power—withholding distribution during clinical experimentation and the placebo-controlled trial. Activists focused upon the pipeline of AIDS drugs—the most notable of which were ribavirin, dideoxycytidine (DDC), dideoxynosine (DDI), and later ganciclovir—because strains of AIDS had arisen that were resistant to AZT. Even when effective, moreover, AZT was also severely toxic, inducing life-threatening anemia and apparently causing numerous heart attacks. Many in the AIDS movement questioned whether AZT was more harmful than therapeutic. Administration spokesmen noted that DDI and DDC were on "the

---

forms of interferon–"Intron A" and Rebetol or Interferon alfa-b–for the treatment of chronic hepatitis C in relapse. At that time, Ribavirin's approved formulation was as a short-term aerosolized therapy for pediatric patients with respiratory syncytial virus infection. DTC stood for diethyldithiocarbamate, DDC for dideoxycytidine. AIDS activists would, moreover, come to express doubts about ddC's approval in January 1994. Mark Harrington of the Treatment Action Group lamented that insufficient attention to efficacy via acceleration of drug approval had been a mistake. As an *Economist* writer summarized matters, "For years, people with AIDS have fought for wider and quicker access to drugs that they thought might help them. They have had the best of intentions; and as one of them told an FDA committee last year, "we have arrived in hell'"; "Beyond Access," *The Economist*, January 8, 1994, p. 79. FDA, CDER, *Meeting of the Antiviral Drugs Advisory Committee*, Open Session, May 4, 1998; Gaithersburg, MD (Washington, DC, SAG Corp, 1998), 9. At the same meeting, Schering-Plough officials noted the existence of acknowledged in vitro data suggesting that the activity of AZT is inhibited by addition of ribavirin. See also Hilts, *Protecting America's Health*, 249.

[76] In Kramer's reading, without any evidence to back up the assertion, many of the physicians were reluctant to speak for fear of retribution by either the Administration or the NIH.

fast track" of the March 1987 regulations, and that AIDS groups had both misunderstood and misrepresented the agency's intent.[77]

The second thrust of criticism was as much circumvention as protest. The AIDS epidemic exposed and rendered personal a set of deep ethical issues implicated in double-blind placebo-controlled clinical trials. Besides claiming that placebo administration was unethical, AIDS activists at the local level—including both patients and doctors as well as alternative treatment organizations—began to consciously undermine clinical trial protocols to the point of hijacking them for therapeutic purposes. Doctors would lie about their patients' previous disease status to secure patient enrollment in a trial. Activist physicians and health-care workers would examine a pill to expose its placebo content. Once a placebo was identified, activists and patients would substitute the genuine treatment for the research subject, using supplies procured underground. In this way, AIDS activists and their organizations were not simply rendering a political critique of the Administration. They were also advancing a scientific critique, complemented by several visions of alternative regimes. When University of California scientists announced in April 1988 that a substance called "Compound Q" inhibited HIV in vitro while leaving uninfected cells healthy, a San Francisco–based group called Project Inform began to import large quantities of the substance and to design a clinical trial of its own. Compound Q followed a pattern of circumvention similar to dextran sulfate, ribavirin, and AL-721, but unlike those drugs Project Inform Director Martin Delaney was explicitly directing a clinical study, albeit one without the controls and prospective designs customary at the Phase 2 and 3 stages of U.S. drug development. Delaney joined Kramer and ACT-UP's Jim Eigo as the most prominent critics of the Administration among AIDS activists. His aim in launching the secret Compound Q trial was not merely to determine the drug's safety and efficacy, but to compel the Administration to rethink its entire approach to therapeutic development. As much as he was treating people in the Compound Q trial, Delaney once said, "We're making a statement here."[78]

As the critics of the Administration became more visible, their targets became more focused and personalized. Ellen Cooper, the medical reviewer for AZT who was now running the new Anti-Viral Drug Products Division, became the face of the FDA not only to the audience of drug companies sponsoring antiviral treatments, but also to AIDS activists. Cooper played a

---

[77]Philip M. Boffey, "New Initiative to Speed AIDS Drugs Is Assailed," NYT, July 5, 1988, C1. Marilyn Chase, "AIDS Patients Press FDA for New Drugs Due to Rise of Viruses that Resist AZT," WSJ, March 16, 1989, B4; Robert Reinhold, "Infected but Not Ill, Many Try Unproved Drug to Block AIDS," NYT, May 20, 1987, B12. On emerging doubts about AZT within the AIDS patient movement, see Epstein, Impure Science, 148–9, 199–200. Boffey, "Campaign to Find Drugs for Fighting AIDS Is Intensified," NYT, February 15, 1988, A1.

[78]Compound Q, or GLQ223, is a purified form of the protein tricosanthin extracted from cucumber-like plants in China. Dennis Wyss, "The Underground Test of Compound Q," Time, October 9, 1989, 18; Gina Kolata, "AIDS Drug Tested Secretly by Group Critical of F.D.A.," NYT, June 28, 1989, A21 (Delaney quotation).

pivotal role in the Administration's decision to deny wider treatment access to ribavirin in 1988 and 1989. ACT-UP manuals targeted her explicitly for pressure. As a caption in the *New York Times* asked, "Is Dr. Cooper a heartless bureaucrat or an 'ideal regulator'?" Martin Delaney found the "heartless" adjective more appropriate and portrayed her as the inflexible bureaucrat: "She's really rigid and adamant in her beliefs," Delaney said, adding that Cooper "clearly places the needs of the research process above the needs of compassion for patients." Beyond criticizing her apparent values, Delaney also openly questioned Cooper's legitimacy, pointing in particular to her age (she was thirty-seven at the time): "It's difficult to see how someone so young can really be responsible for making decisions that affect lives in such a profound way. She shouldn't be given that kind of power." At the Administration, Cooper's colleagues noticed that she was being represented as "some sort of dragon lady" to the general public and to AIDS-based audiences in particular. For her own part, Cooper accurately perceived that agency-wide decisions and behavioral patterns were being reduced and attributed to one person: "I understand the human need to have a scapegoat in frustrating circumstances," she said. An attack on the moral reputation of an organization had become an attack on the insufficient compassion of an individual.[79]

New Protests, New Rules, New Concepts: The Rockville Demonstration, and Subpart E Regulations. The signal event of the new militancy came in an October 1988 demonstration at Administration headquarters in Rockville, Maryland. ACT-UP and other groups considered a protest at the White House as well as at the NIH, but the FDA appeared to be a facile and more identifiable target, and perhaps a more responsive one. Approximately one thousand activists gathered in front of the agency on the morning of October 11 and displayed any number of symbols that seemed to challenge the FDA's public identity as a health agency dedicated to consumer protection and, in the case of AIDS, flexibility and compassion. Various placards exclaimed that "The government has blood on its hands" and "AZT is not

---

[79] In carefully prepared documents on the FDA, ACT-UP members (particularly Eigo) listed different individuals to whom pressure could be applied, including Robert Temple, Carl Peck, James Bilstad, and Cooper. "FDA Action Handbook," 4; "FDA Action Handbook," by Jim Eigo, Mark Harrington, Iris Long, Margaret McCarthy, Stephen Spinella, Rick Sugden, September 21, 1988, 4. Reel 1, Folder "FDA Action"; ACT-UP Papers, New York Public Library. Boffey, "At Fulcrum of Conflict, Regulator of AIDS Drugs," *NYT*, August 19, 1988, A13; Interview with Brad Stone, Office of the Commissioner, FDA, February 9, 1990; Rockville, MD.

On these and other points, Delaney's credibility and appeal were not universal. AIDS drug developer Dannie King, who had played important roles at Burroughs-Wellcome with AZT, expressed his anger about these characterizations of Cooper in a *New York Times* interview. Michael Callen, a founder of the Community Research Initiative, an organization of private physicians who tested AIDS drugs in clinical trials, was "deeply disturbed" by Delaney's secret trial and thought it irresponsible; Kolata, "AIDS Drug Tested Secretly by Group Critical of F.D.A."

enough." Some demonstrators wore white coats with "FDA" on the back with bloody handprints below. As organizers might have hoped, the October 11 demonstration received extensive national news coverage in print and on television.[80]

The irony of the new militancy's timing was noticed by many seasoned observers, including Philip J. Hilts, then a reporter at the *New York Times*. Most of the new oppositional activity occurred not only after AZT had already been reviewed more quickly and radically than other drugs for life-threatening illnesses—cancer and Alzheimer's, for instance—but also after federal procedures had already changed appreciably. At some level, this coincidence of policy success with greater militancy is not so ironic. AIDS activists perceived FDA personnel to be more responsive to public criticism than the Reagan administration, and observers have noted this sort of "success-breeds-more-activism" dynamic in other narratives ranging from civil rights to disability policy. The increased militancy that followed spring 1987's successes (AZT's approval and the treatment IND regulations) sent particular signals to Administration officials, both that earlier efforts had failed in some sense—and this underscores the depth of the ACT-UP threat to FDA reputation—but also that the Administration's earlier changes would need to be trumpeted. Several weeks after the October 11 demonstration, re-trumpeting is exactly what the Administration did. Two weeks before the general presidential election pitting Vice President George Bush against Massachusetts governor Michael Dukakis, Young called a press conference that heralded sweeping new changes in drug regulation in which Bush had participated. In fact, the details of Young's new plan were a restatement of the treatment IND regulations in combination with procedures that had been followed in drug development and review since the AZT submission. Though AIDS groups derided the hearing as a publicity stunt, Young's announcement made the front pages of the *New York Times* and the *Washington Post* on October 20, 1988.[81]

[80]Warren E. Leary, "F.D.A. Pressed to Approve More AIDS Drugs," *NYT*, October 11, 1988, C5 (noting plans for the demonstration). As Hilts aptly summarizes the protest, "Everywhere observers turned, there was something eye-catching. This was not a demonstration like those of the 1960s, in which violence routinely broke out. This was crafted to meet the needs of the media" (*Protecting America's Health*, 248–9). See also Hilts, "How the AIDS Crisis Made Drug Regulators Speed Up," *NYT*, September 24, 1989, E5.

[81]Robert Katzmann, *Institutional Disability* (Washington, DC: Brookings Institution Press, 1986). Katzmann finds that organized advocacy for increased transportation access for the disabled "began after the passage of legislation, particularly section 504" of the Rehabilitation Act of 1973. As Katzmann explains, "The rights orientation of section 504 provided the impetus for the creation of new groups and the building of a coalition among diverse interests" (76).

On the Young announcement, see Warren E. Leary, "F.D.A. Announces Changes to Speed Testing of Drugs," *NYT*, October 20, 1988, A1. HHS News, October 19, 1988, 5; U.S. Congress, HR, Committee on Government Operations, *Therapeutic Drugs for AIDS*, 384–9. The changes that Young announced had been published six months earlier in the *Journal of the American Medical Association*; *JAMA* 15 (259) (April 15, 1988): 2269. On changes over the summer preceding the October 11, 1988 demonstration, see also Philip M. Boffey, "New Ini-

AIDS activists were aware that their demands for access and acceleration dovetailed with a long-running conservative political agenda for pharmaceutical deregulation, including the repeal of the Kefauver-Harris Amendments of 1962. In their internal discussions they consciously expressed fears about becoming a tool of the pharmaceutical industry, the Reagan administration, or any number of conservative voices including the *Wall Street Journal* editorial page. As Jim Eigo wrote to other ACT-UP members in the fall of 1988:

> Aids advocates must be careful to keep their agenda, supporting earlier access to promising life-saving drugs for life-threatening disorders, from being confused with the Bush/Wall St. Journal/Heritage Foundation agenda of sweeping drug industry deregulation. It would be a disaster for all American consumers, including people with HIV infection, if the Kefauver amendments were repealed and drug companies were no longer required to prove safety and efficacy for most drugs. Aids activists want safe and effective drugs, but we want them faster.

As the AIDS battles wore on, this stance would stabilize the group's identity. A crucial element of ACT-UP's credibility resided in its organizational and rhetorical distance from business and pharmaceutical interests, Reagan administration officials, and other conservative voices.[82]

When the Administration responded to these overtures and challenges, it did so less through drug approval than through rulemaking. In May 1987, the FDA had revised IND regulations to formalize the agency's thinking on the concept of a "Treatment IND" or "expanded access protocol" so as to allow for wider access than usual at the clinical trial stage, as long as the treatment followed the experimental protocol. In October 1988, just weeks after the Rockville demonstration, Commissioner Frank Young announced new clinical development rules known as the "Subpart E" regulations. The regulations envisioned a drug development process for "life-threatening and severely debilitating illnesses" that compressed Phase 2 and 3 trials into a single Phase 2 process for the assessment of effectiveness. Conferences with a drug sponsor would occur not as usual after Phase 2 but in a new "end-of-phase 1" meeting. As trade reporters observed when the draft rules were vetted in August, "the plan would basically be a codification of the foreshortened procedure followed for Burroughs-Wellcome's AZT." The rule shift was a major change in the Administration's conceptual architecture of phased experiment, but even as Young announced it, he and others gestured ambiguously at its limits. A compressed Phase 2 trial might be larger than the norm, they hinted. Whereas FDA officials held out the important symbolic possibility that one spectacular clinical trial might suffice for approval

tiative to Speed AIDS Drugs Is Assailed," *NYT*, July 5, 1988, C1; Gina Kolata, "An Angry Response To Actions on AIDS Spurs F.D.A. Shift," *NYT*, June 26, 1988, A1.

[82]Eigo, in "FDA Action Handbook," September 21, 1988; Reel 1, Folder "FDA Action." ACT-UP Papers, New York Public Library. It was common for activists of the time to capitalize only the first letter of the acronym.

of some of these agents, they cautioned that "persuasively dramatic results are rare and that two entirely independent studies will generally be required." The agency also announced that while drugs for symptomatic relief (but not curing) of serious illnesses could possibly qualify for a Treatment IND, such drugs would not be covered by the rules. As with the agency's pronouncements on surrogate endpoints, the Administration was more willing at this time to express its intentions clearly with respect to traditional "cures" than on therapies that offered symptomatic relief.[83]

Commissioner Young and other top FDA officials claimed that they were acting at the urging of a task force headed by Vice President George H. W. Bush (then running for president on the Republican ticket). Yet observers recognized that the regulatory shifts of 1987 and 1988 merely extended and accentuated an earlier and more gradual shift that had been impelled as much by cancer therapeutics as by the AIDs crisis. FDA officials had proposed to formalize the Treatment IND concept in 1983, and various other forms of "compassionate-use" exceptions to the IND regulations had been tried since 1962. Other ideas in the Subpart E regulations had been verbalized by top officials in May 1987, often in discussions of cancer drug development. Other contemporaneous changes, including the formation of the President's Cancer Panel and the splitting of the Center for Drug and Biologics into one center for drug review and another for biologics review, involved therapeutic fields other than AIDS.[84]

The October 1988 demonstration provided a template for future action by AIDS organizations. AIDS organizations would continually and openly intimidate FDA officials with the prospect of another Rockville protest over the coming years, timing their threats to coincide with pivotal FDA deci-

[83]The Subpart E regulations were codified at 21 CFR Part 312, Subpart E, hence their moniker. On the rules as a codification of the AZT review, see *DRR*, August 31, 1988, 2. On other features of the rules, see *DRR*, September 14, 1988, 5–6; *DRR*, October 26, 1988, 2–3. More generally, consult Peter Barton Hutt, Richard A. Merrill, and Lewis A. Grossman, *Food and Drug Law: Cases and Materials*, 3rd ed, (New York: Foundation Press, 2007), chapter 4.F. Some drugs had previously been approved on the basis of one controlled trial; see the example of cisplatin in chapter 7. On surrogate endpoints, see chapter 8.

[84]On the earlier development of treatment IND concepts and the Phase 2–3 compression, see *DRR*, March 25, 1987, 3–5, *DRR*, August 10, 1988, 3. On earlier verbal discussions of these concepts, see *DRR*, May 6, 1987, 2–3. An important discussion concerned more expansive testing of cancer drugs such as interleukin-2 in phase 2 (using the modified "Group C" distribution mechanism for cancer drugs); *DRR*, April 29, 1987, 3–5. See also Hutt, Merrill, and Grossman, *Food and Drug Law*, 653, 656. The August 1988 regulations also provided that Group C drugs would no longer require an advisory committee panel as they had in the past (*DRR*, August 31, 1988, 4). Hutt, Merrill, and Grossman wrongly attribute the Subpart E regulations to AIDS politics alone; *Food and Drug Law: Cases and Materials*, 648. The regulations mentioned both AIDS and cancer (see *FR* 53 (October 21, 1988): 41516. On criticisms over non-AIDS drugs as a crucial context for the drug review reorganization, see Marilyn Chase, "FDA Will Split Up Its New-Drug Unit in an Attempt to Streamline Procedures," *WSJ*, October 2, 1987, 24 (NCI official Bruce Chabner, a severe FDA critic, was quoted in Chase's article); *DRR*, August 19, 1987, 5–6; *DRR*, October 12, 1988, 3. On the President's Cancer Panel, see *DRR*, December 7, 1988, 3.

sions on AIDS drugs. When Bristol-Myers Squibb filed an NDA for DDI, ACT-UP sent a letter demanding that the agency approve the application within thirty days of its filing date. If the drug would not be approved, the letter warned, ACT-UP would plan a demonstration in Rockville. The threat brought ACT-UP a direct letter from CDER Director Carl Peck several weeks later. DDI would be the first drug brought to submission through the reformed approval process, and the first one to be based upon surrogate endpoints (in this case CD4 levels) and historical controls that embedded the patients' previous history. A similar demand was made for approval of the NDA for foscarnet (for treatment of retinal cytomegalovirus (CMV) in AIDS patients, a condition which often caused blindness) by June 2. In this case the drug would not be approved until November. In advancing and strategically timing these warnings, the AIDS groups were revealing the fundamental nature of their threat to the Administration. Their activism imperiled not the FDA's budget, not really the FDA's authority, and no one's job or livelihood, but the FDA's identity.[85]

The difficulty with these threats is that, in order to be credible, they eventually had to be carried out. When the Administration did not respond to the demand for a thirty-day review of DDI, ACT-UP held a one-hour protest in Rockville (this one in front of the building housing the Anti-Viral Division that reviewed AIDS drugs), but only twenty-one demonstrators showed up. And the Administration was ready with a "Talk Paper" noting that Peck had met with ACT-UP on this very issue and that its review of DDI and other AIDS drugs would be completed "as quickly as possible." Relative to the October 1988 demonstration, this was anticlimax, and it underscored the weakening basis of the AIDS constituency's position.[86]

The other limiting factor is that the Administration was not, of course, a hapless or passive bystander in this saga. FDA officials responded to the identity threat from AIDS activism in ways that were moderate, sober, and highly strategic. Beyond rulemaking and its associated rhetoric, they tried to dampen expectations about AIDS therapies, injecting a dose of realism into the debate about treatments and their supposed "promise." Beyond this, the Administration made a series of new decisions from the fall of 1988 to the winter of 1990, most of them rapid NDA approvals. Most of these drugs were not inhibitors of HIV but instead treatments for AIDS and related illnesses such as *Pneumocystis carinii* pneumonia (aerosol pentamidine and trimexetrate), Kaposi's sarcoma (interferon alfa), and AIDS-related blindness (ganciclovir). Many of the chemicals had already been approved for other indications. The most radical move came in September 1989 when the Administration gave treatment IND status to DDI, whose safety and efficacy profile were far less compelling than that of AZT. As the decisions

[85] "ACT-UP requests approval of Bristol-Myers Squibb's new drug application for ddI," *DRR* 34 (15) (April 10, 1991): 11. "DDI Is Scheduled for July FDA Advisory Committee Review, FDA Official Carl Peck Tells ACT-UP," *DRR* 34 (17) (April 24, 1991): 9–10.

[86] *DRR* 34 (19) (May 8, 1991): 8.

poured out of the agency, national news outlets were beginning to describe a changed FDA, one that was potentially crippling under the rush of AIDS, but one that was nonetheless "speeding up" and being "transformed." An alternative narrative of institutional failure emerged, one centered not upon bureaucratic intransigence and inefficiency, but upon organizational neglect and underfunding. In this narrative, whatever blame existed for the slow arrival of AIDS therapies was taken from the Administration and placed on the shoulders of politicians.[87]

FDA officials maintained a complex set of relationships with AIDS organizations. For one, Administration officials realized, as did other observers of the AIDS movement, that there was more than one representative of the disease and its sufferers. Hence, officials kept up correspondence and contact not only with militant organizations, but also with treatment-based organizations such as Mathilde Krim's Foundation for AIDS Research. And the very publicity of ACT-UP meant that the Adminstration could defuse much of the political pressure surrounding it simply by incorporating the group into its functions, including formal and informal meetings and an invited seat to Advisory Committee meetings. By 1991 and 1992, militants began to see a new face to the Administration, even as they knew they were being co-opted. As Larry Kramer later put it, "When we were on the outside, fighting to get in, it was easier to call everyone names. But they were smart. They invited us inside. And we saw they looked human. And that makes hate harder."[88]

---

[87]For FDA pessimism and restraint, see Gina Kolata, "Despite Promise in AIDS Cases, Drug Faces Testing Hurdle," *NYT*, December 13, 1988, C3; Philip M. Boffey, "F.D.A. Is Pessimistic on Drugs to Fight AIDS," *NYT*, July 14, 1988, B9. On alpha interferon and other moves during the winter of 1988–1989, see Lawrence K. Altman, "F.D.A. Approves First Drug for an AIDS-Related Cancer," *NYT*, November 22, 1988, C2; "Five-Minute AIDS Test Is Approved by F.D.A.," *NYT*, December 14, 1988, A21; "F.D.A. Acts to Speed Approval of AIDS Drugs," *NYT*, February 21, 1989, C3. On aerosol pentamidine, see Warren E. Leary, "F.D.A. Approves Drug That Fights Leading Killer of AIDS Patients," *NYT*, June 16, 1989, D16. On ganciclovir and erythropoietin, see Bruce Ingersoll, "FDA to Reconsider Drug for Blindness Connected to AIDS," *WSJ*, March 3, 1989, B2; Gina Kolata, "F.D.A. Gives Quick Approval to Two Drugs to Treat AIDS," *NYT*, June 27, 1989, A1; Larry Thompson, "Growth Drug Gets FDA Nod," *WP*, July 4, 1989, H6. On DDI, see Philip J. Hilts, "Side Effects Noted in High Doses of New AIDS Drug," *NYT*, September 27, 1989, A 20; Marylyn Chase, "AIDS Drug DDI to be Distributed Widely," *WSJ*, September 29, 1989, B2; Hilts, "F.D.A., in Big Shift, Will Permit Use of Experimental AIDS Drug," *NYT*, September 29, 1989, A1; Michael Specter, "FDA Authorizes Unproven Drug For AIDS Cases," *WP*, September 29, 1989, A1. On supplemental approvals for AZT, see Marilyn Chase, "AZT Expected to Be Cleared for Children," *WSJ*, October 26, 1989, B2; "AIDS Drug May Get Wider Use," *Chicago Tribune*, January 31, 1990, 1–5.

On general changes at the FDA, see Michael Specter, "Pressure from AIDS Activists Has Transformed Drug Testing," *WP*, July 2, 1989, A1; Malcolm Gladwell, "Burdened with New Duties, FDA Is Seen Handicapped by Reagan-Era Cuts," *WP*, September 6, 1989, A21; Hilts, "How the AIDS Crisis Made Drug Regulators Speed Up," *NYT*, September 24, 1989, E5; "A Guardian of U.S. Health Is Failing Under Pressures," *NYT*, December 4, 1989, A1; Dick Thompson, "What's the Cure for Burnout?" *Time*, December 25, 1989, 68.

[88]"Foscarnet Approval for Treating CMV Retinitis in AIDS Patients Recommended by FDA

A Contest over Expertise and Image: The FDA and Healing Alternatives Foundation. At the same time that AIDS groups were experiencing a sort of democratic incorporation into U.S. pharmaceutical regulation, other episodes reminded them that the Administration would remain defensive of basic powers and images. At the core of these non-negotiables lay the FDA's claim to pharmacological expertise and drug safety. The FDA's inspection of San Francisco–based Healing Alternatives Foundation in 1992 provides a telling example. As part of the expanded access program for dideoxycytidine (DDC), originally started by Hoffmann-La Roche (DDC's manufacturer) and the FDA, the Administration had decided to look the other way when local AIDS centers acted as buyers' clubs. Many of these buyers' clubs were connected through Project Inform. In San Francisco, the Healing Alternatives Foundation would purchase DDC wholesale from suppliers other than Hoffmann-La Roche and would then distribute the drug to patients, thus bypassing the usual physician and pharmacy conduits for drug access, and of course bypassing Hoffmann-La Roche. But in January 1992, FDA inspectors reported to Rockville that they had obtained DDC from buyers' clubs that had potency variations of up to 300 percent. Healing Alternatives Foundation employee Richard Copeland then received a call from Randy Wykoff, Director of the Administration's Office of AIDS Coordination. Copeland took detailed notes on the conversation and the ensuing affair, notes which reveal the mixture of distrust and credibility between the Administration and the Foundation.

> At about 12:15 p.m. on Friday, January 24, I received a call from Randy Wykoff. He opened by asking if I had talked to Derek Hodel [a representative from a buyers' club in New York] yet that day. I responded that I had not. He said that there had been unconfirmed reports from a lab that some ddC obtained from buyers' clubs had potency variations of up to 300%. He said their interest was for the safety of those taking ddC, not hassling the buyers' clubs. I said that safety was also our concern.[89]

Having traded claims to represent the safety of AIDS patients—a contest that would be repeated in San Francisco, New York, and other urban centers over the coming months, as well as in the national media—Copeland and Wykoff then turned to particulars. Wykoff wanted to send in an inspector "ASAP" to collect samples from the Foundation's supplies of DDC and test for potency variations. He then promised Copeland that he would report back to HAF within a week. While Wykoff did not need Copeland's assent for an inspection, Copeland told him that he would check with the Foundation's Board before giving approval for the inspection. Wykoff

---

Advisory Group," *DRR* 34 (25) (June 19, 1991): 8. Kramer, *The Destiny of Me* (New York: Penguin, 1993), 17; Daemmrich, *Pharmacopolitics*, 100.

[89]Copeland, "Report to the HAF Board of Directors re: the FDA visit for sampling, 1/24/92," Collection of the Healing Alternatives Foundation, UCSF. Dideoxycytidine also had the acronym "ddC" at this time.

agreed to this makeshift procedure. And importantly, he never asked the Foundation to cease or otherwise regulate its distribution of DDC.

Upon hanging up, Copeland's "first reaction was to note the coincidence that [Wykoff] called on a day when many of the main players at buyers' clubs would be in transit to the buyers' clubs meeting that weekend in Florida." At the core of Copeland's conspiratorial fears—fears shared by others, but never directly uttered to FDA leadership—was a notion that the Administration was taking steps to shut down the buyers' clubs. It would be all the easier to launch such a move, he worried, when each club's leadership was out of town.

Copeland quickly called Foundation leadership, other buyers' clubs in New York and San Diego, and people at Project Inform, including Martin Delaney, "who was, as usual, impossible to get a hold of." After discussing the matter with HAF board members, one of whom said "he had met Randy Wykoff twice and that he didn't seem like a guy who would cook up a scheme," Copeland allowed the Administration to send an inspector. In addition, and without the FDA requesting it, HAF Board members decided informally to discontinue all sales of DDC until the FDA inspection report had been returned.[90]

The inspection took place later that afternoon, when Brian Hasselbalch from the FDA's San Francisco office arrived at the Foundation's Market Street offices and greeted Copeland. After showing Copeland his badge, Hasselbalch presented Copeland with two FDA forms: a "Notification of Inspection" and a "Receipt for Samples." The first would establish the legal legitimacy of the inspection, while the second would serve as a receipt for purchase, as the Administration intended to compensate the Foundation in full for the samples that Hasselbalch inspected. After some questioning, Hasselbalch asked Copeland how much DDC the Foundation had in stock, and how recently each shipment had been received, whereupon the two men went to the stock room where the Foundation maintained its pharmaceutical supplies. At this point, Copeland realized that several of the boxes of DDC displayed the address of origin plainly on the mailing label and covered them with his hands. When Hasselbalch disclosed that he knew the origin of the boxes anyway, Copeland removed his hands and started a delicate conversation about how the information could be kept secret. Sources of supply for underground drugs were a source of special anxiety to buyers' clubs. For one, the clubs did not fully trust the Administration with knowledge of these sources as the government might use the information to strike at wholesale suppliers instead of the clubs themselves. For another, buyers' clubs' very therapeutic and social success was predicated upon being able to procure supplies. If the Foundation's supply chain had been broken, its very competitive edge over other buyers' clubs and drug conduits would

---

[90]Ibid. Wykoff was Director of the FDA's Office of AIDS Coordination at the time.

be compromised; AIDS patients might turn elsewhere and begin to patronize other organizations.[91]

Hasselbalch seemed to gain Copeland's trust, but Copeland was not willing to trust those faceless officials who might later be examining the Foundation's supplies. Copeland used a black ink marker to obscure the addresses on the mailing labels and the lot numbers and carried on an open discussion with Hasselbalch about how to allow information in a way that would assist Hasselbalch but that would not disclose the identities of suppliers and other sources.

> He sorted the bottles in the refrigerator by lot and stacked them very neatly, selecting a bottle from each lot, with labels, from the refrigerator, saying he would take those because they had been received earlier and he didn't want to mess up our system. We talked about how the lot numbers might be coded. He suggested it was probably the date, followed by some other information relating to processing only decodable to the manufacturer. He noted that the most recent shipment had an earlier date than the previous shipment and suggested we talk with our distributor about his storage methods. I asked him if his visit constituted the long awaited FDA visit. He said no, that they were still planning to do an inventory, to which he said "Maybe I'm telling you more than you know." He also said they would not do an undercover visit.

By the end of Copeland's notes, Hasselbalch was being called "Brian," with the same sort of familiarity and intimacy with which other board members and buyers' club representatives were being named. The order of official interaction had begun with Hasselbalch's presentation of two forms to Copeland, each of which underlay a different basis to the FDA's legitimacy—law ("Notification of Inspection") and open concern for the Foundation's revenues ("Receipt of Purchase for Samples"). By the end of the inspection, any decorum with which it started had vanished by mutual assent. The two men talked openly about protecting the Foundation's sources.

[91]FDA, "Receipt for Samples," Form FDA-484, signed by Richard Copeland and Brian J. Hasselbalch, January 24, 1992; Copeland, "Report to the HAF Board of Directors re: the FDA visit for sampling, 1/24/92," Collection of the Healing Alternatives Foundation, UCSF. Copeland describes the labels interaction as follows: "I covered the labels discreetly with my hands and asked him if he knew where we got them. He said, 'Down south.' I asked him if he knew more than that. He said 'Corti in L.A.' I said something like 'Well then I don't need to do anything about that.'" "Corti" was Jim Corti, an activist and organizer, who had traveled to China and other countries to procure Compound Q and, originally, dextran sulfate, earning him the moniker "Dextran Man" in AIDS patients' communities in the late 1980s.
Project Inform would later warn that private for-profit suppliers might have been behind the original allegations: "The press should also be aware that one possible origin for this alarming and so far unsubstantiated information might be competitive interests which are currently seeking to gain a toehold in Buyer's Club business as an alternative to the current supplier of ddC." Project Inform, Press Statement regarding "FDA action regarding Buyer's Club ddC," January 29, 1992; Collection of the Healing Alternatives Foundation, UCSF.

They discussed the next steps the regulatory agency would take. The inspector gave the activist a friendly suggestion to inquire about the storage methods of his Foundation's supplier. He took his samples with a concern to minimize any disruption to the Foundation's operations. He admitted to the activist that he had probably told him more than he was supposed to know.

The interaction between Copeland and Hasselbalch is one instance of a dynamic that has been re-nacted hundreds of thousands, even millions, of times in the history of U.S. pharmaceutical regulation. Yet the Administration's January 24, 1992, inspection of Healing Alternatives Foundation is exemplary for what it reveals about the politics of reputation and how they play out in local situations. The inspection was only partially about procuring samples. It was also about trust, about credibility, and about representation. In ways that the FDA inspector Hasselbalch seemed to understand, the Administration was representing itself to the Foundation, face-to-face. Could Wykoff—officially a liaison between the Administration and AIDS organizations—be trusted to present a more compassionate face to the AIDS groups? Was Hasselbalch going to use the information in the inspection for a broader shutdown of the clubs? Was another inspection coming, and how openly and predictably would it arrive? In providing unofficial and personal answers to these questions, Randy Wykoff and Brian Hasselbalch were representatives of the Administration and faces of its reputation to a local audience.

Wykoff and Hasselbalch had approached Healing Alternatives Foundation with sufficient respect that HAF leaders soon deferred to the Administration and defended it in public statements. The *San Francisco Chronicle* and *Herald* reported on January 29 that the FDA had conducted a "seizure" of DDC from the clubs, but Project Inform quickly rebutted the story with a press release that derided the newspapers.

> Contrary to press reports issued in San Francisco today, no "seizure" of ddC has occurred from Buyer's Clubs. Last Friday, FDA representatives asked for voluntary samples of a small quantity (a couple of bottles) from a few Buyer's Club sites to check out what the FDA described as "unconfirmed" stories that the product might have dosage problems. No evidence of a problem was either noted or presented. The Clubs in turn volunteered any samples the agency requested. This absolutely does not constitute as "seizure" as the inflammatory press language implied....
>
> [I]t is clear that no firm information has been presented by any source on this matter. Since apparently anonymous accusations have been made, however, it is appropriate the FDA examine samples of the product. Buyer's Club personnel and community activists welcome this inspection.

Matters became somewhat more serious on February 5, when the Administration informed buyers' clubs that its inspections revealed "potentially serious variations in product potency and quality," resulting from "poor manufacturing conditions." Product samples obtained from New York and

San Francisco demonstrated DDC content ranging from zero percent to 230 percent of the expected content. In simpler terms, some DDC tablets contained no DDC at all, while others contained the equivalent of nearly two and a half doses. At this point, the Administration could have chosen to seize the samples, but FDA officials instead decided to "urge" buyers' clubs to cease sale and distribution of DDC and to notify their clientele of FDA's findings. The enforcement action taken was as cooperative as possible, and the Administration did not issue a talk paper to the press until the following day. Hence FDA officials had respected the autonomy and integrity of the buyers' clubs by warning them privately of their findings before taking them to the public.[92]

In regulating Healing Alternatives Foundation and other "underground" clubs, Administration officials such as Wykoff and Ronald Chesemore (Director of Regulatory Affairs) struck a delicate balance between discipline and flexibility. As they presented their case to HAF and others, they had acted with restraint and "discretion." The message was that "we could have come down hard on you, but did not." To the broader public, the Administration referred to the clubs as "underground" organizations who were procuring "unauthorized" supplies of the drug. Hence, even as Wykoff and Hasselbalch had deferred to the integrity of the groups, FDA officials at Rockville headquarters presented their case in a way that potentially undermined the legitimacy of buyers' clubs.[93]

HAF and its allies realized, too, that a solution to the FDA challenge was not as simple as outright rejection of the Administration's claim. If the Administration's assay results were correct or nearly so, AIDS patients would suffer needless adverse effects (including irreversible nerve damage in the extremities) that could be avoided with proper potency. Just as powerful a consideration was that, if the FDA's claims were correct and the activists chose to deny them categorically, Project Inform's credibility (already weak among some corners of the AIDS activist community) would be further impaired.

Yet the findings of variable potency had opened a new chapter—what Copeland referred to as "Round Two"—in the détente between AIDS groups and the Administration. Healing Alternatives Foundation issued a press release announcing its unconditional discontinuation of DDC sales until the matter had been resolved. Other buyers' clubs and Project Inform issued similar statements to the press and to their clienteles. Yet as quickly as they deferred to the FDA, AIDS organizations questioned the Administration's credibility and began a private campaign to protect themselves from a possible frontal attack. HAF's press release noted that "There are significant

---

[92]FDA Talk Paper, "FDA Urges Buyers Clubs to End Sales of Underground DDC," February 6, 1992; contact, Brad Stone. Ronald G. Chesemore (Associate Commissioner for Regulatory Affairs, FDA) to Richard Copeland (HAF), February 7, 1992; Healing Alternatives Foundation Press Release, February 6, 1992. Collection of the Healing Alternatives Foundation, UCSF.

[93]Collection of the Healing Alternatives Foundation, UCSF.

differences between the independent lab results provided by our distributor and the FDA's test results," and the second press release of February 6 concluded that "The current situation highlights the need for a more effective drug approval process." Project Inform proclaimed itself "surprised and baffled by news of these quality-control problems" and reminded its members and audiences that this was a rapidly changing situation and that the fight for full access to DDC was still under way and entirely unaffected by the FDA's actions. By February 11, Martin Delaney would twice fax messages to buyers' clubs (including HAF) that were inescapably ambiguous, conceding that "it seems likely that quality control mistakes were made in recent months" and that "the current batch developed a problem, although the problem is not nearly as significant as the FDA says."[94]

Privately, AIDS groups took steps to combat a possible enforcement crackdown by the FDA. It was not clear that any Administration official had such aims, but Project Inform and HAF were not taking chances. On February 8, Richard Copeland wrote his Board and warned them that the situation demanded "integrity" more than anything else. Worrying openly about "our credibility," he suggested that the Foundation agree to the FDA's request to make the results of government tests available to Foundation clients. Yet while he did not expect broader action by the Administration, his approach to the FDA was cautious, and he explicitly set aside a section devoted to political strategy vis-à-vis the regulator.

ANTICIPATING FDA MOVES

We should talk to our lawyer. He is, however, on the Project Inform Board of Directors, so we cannot consider him impartial.

Given the chance that the FDA may use this as an opportunity to make moves on the buyers' clubs, I suggest that we rally support from various sectors now, so that we can be ready in case FDA takes drastic actions. Act Up/Golden Gate has been contacted, through Tomas. We should also consider contacting ACT UP/SF, Carole Migden, Roberta Achtenberg, Harry Britt, Nancy Pelosi, Milton Marks, the gay Democratic clubs, as well as coordinating strategies with other AIDS organizations, such as AIDS Treatment News, etc.

Stop selling Clarithrimycin, because it increases our vulnerability.

Copeland's strategy was twofold—to increase the club's credibility and to prepare for the worst—and it was premised upon the privacy of the Foundation's fears. The FDA had never suggested or threatened a crackdown, and HAF and Project Inform officials never elaborated their most explicit fears to Administration officials, in particular that the FDA's enforcement arm might shut down the buyers' clubs. This nuclear option was never mentioned by either party, yet Copeland felt that HAF must be prepared for it.

[94]HAF, "Press Release, 2/6/92"; "Press Release, 2/6/92" (Second Copy, with text about need for "more effective drug approval process"); Project Inform "DDC Bulletin" Fax to HAF, February 7, 1992; Martin Delaney, Fax to Buyers' Clubs, February 11, 1992; Collection of the Healing Alternatives Foundation, UCSF.

If attacked administratively, the Foundation would rally its political support, including militant organizations, wealthy contributors, and members of Congress (Representative Nancy Pelosi was then quickly advancing up the ranks of the Democratic House hierarchy). Copeland's strategy was formulated from a position of mixed trust and distrust—even Project Inform allies were not to be entirely banked upon. Yet in part, Copeland knew that the Foundation was bargaining from a position of weakness. On February 18, HAF discontinued procurement from the supplier of the faulty batches and announced to its clients that it was searching for another source. In this announcement, as opposed to earlier releases, no swipe (implicit or open) was taken at the Administration or its findings.[95]

The FDA never cracked down on the buyers' clubs, and its relations with the Healing Alternatives Foundation and Project Inform would continue in a delicate equilibrium of image over the coming years. The tilt over DDC potency came at the same time that the Administration's relations with AIDS activists were warming considerably. It was for this reason, perhaps, that FDA officials took a very flexible and deferential approach, though one that projected ambiguity. While Chesemore and Wykoff continued to "strongly urge" the Foundation to cease distribution of DDC, they did not further step into the Foundation's operations and never conducted a seizure. Still, in March 1992, Wykoff notified Copeland that the Administration had decided to undertake a series of further inspections of buyers' clubs. Wykoff reminded Copeland that his office had met with a number of the clubs starting in the fall of 1991, hence these inspections would only continue a pattern of gathering "additional information." Moreover, Wykoff took pains to communicate what the inspections were *not* about: "The purpose of these inspections is not to force the cessation of the legal and beneficial activities of buyers' clubs, nor is it to drive their activities underground. Rather, the goal is to maximize the potential positive contributions while eliminating patently illegal and potentially dangerous activities that may exist." Ultimately, Wykoff's message was one of keeping hands off but options open. If the clubs ceased their distribution of DDC in particular, he seemed to say, the Administration would not pursue an aggressive strategy and would continue to look the other way as the clubs distributed other therapies. The ambiguity of Administration's message, while not completely intentional or designed, served dual purposes, both keeping the Foundation sufficiently wary about its distribution activity, and avoiding the presentation of a terrorizing face to the clubs.[96]

The notion that the FDA was turning a blind eye to the buyers' clubs appears to have been something of a longer term strategy. Buyers' clubs for AZT and other medications had existed since the late 1980s, and they had

[95]HAF, "Important Notice to All Clients of Healing Alternatives Foundation (HAF) Regarding ddC," February 18, 1992; Collection of the Healing Alternatives Foundation, UCSF.

[96]Wykoff to Copeland, March 18, 1992; Collection of the Healing Alternatives Foundation, UCSF.

procured massive quantities of AZT, DDI, DDC, Compound Q, AL-721, and just about every AIDS medication that clinical researchers were testing. In generally allowing this underground distribution to occur, and in regulating it only at opportune moments, Administration officials were explicitly conducting a calculus of reputation. The Administration wanted to steer between the Scylla of denying access and roughhousing AIDS organizations and the Charybdis of conferring legitimacy upon a treatment that had yet to be proven.[97]

More broadly, the politics of reputation in the tilt over underground DDC involved competing claims about accuracy and about representation. Both the Administration (Wykoff and Chesemore) and AIDS activists (Copeland, Delaney) advanced claims that they represented the safety interests of patients. Furthermore, HAF members' continued worries about losing clients in early 1992 points to a lack of certainty in the Foundation that their organization could credibly promise safe and potent drugs; the Administration was, in this sense, a serious competitor to representation of patients' health and safety interests. Both parties to the conflict also made claims about what was accurate science. Hence, the Healing Alternatives Foundation and Project Inform were taking aim at more than just the Administration's moral reputation, its negative image of "callousness." These groups were explicitly and openly contesting the Administration's technical reputation, the very fundamentals of its scientific expertise.

The Administration would eventually approve DDC and DDI later in the spring of 1992, but only as part of a combination therapy with AZT. Commissioner David Kessler is reported to have shown great interest in getting the combination therapies approved on the basis of "surrogate endpoints," or data suggesting that the combinations had boosted T-cell counts even where evidence of increased survival was not available. When in the mid-1990s French and American studies revealed that the combination therapy was generally no more effective than AZT alone, and when further research revealed limitations and more toxicity with AZT, AIDS organizations suffered a double crisis. Their members' hope in the pipeline of treatments took a hit, but so did the credibility of the groups themselves. Observers of U.S. pharmaceutical regulation now began to wonder quite openly about why the Administration had approved the combination therapies so quickly. And yet in questioning the 1992 combination approvals, criticism rested more easily and quickly on the shoulders of the AIDS groups than on the Administration itself. The apparent blame lay less with the FDA for turning around these applications so quickly, but rather with the AIDS groups for forcing the Administration's hand. Within the AIDS community, anti-AZT groups such as the Treatment Action Group (TAG) of New York City arose, challenging both the therapeutic claims of earlier groups like ACT-UP, as well as their hostility to placebo-controlled trials and the FDA.[98]

[97]John S. James, "ddC: AZT Combination Approval Recommended," *AIDS Treatment News*, May 1, 1992; Epstein, *Impure Science*, 223–4, 267–9.

[98]Lawrence K. Altman, "AIDS Study Casts Doubt on Value of Hastened Drug Approval in

There was another way in which the politics of AIDS got the Administration off of the hook, and that came in debates about the pricing of AIDS drugs. While "access" to drugs was interpreted as an FDA issue—that is, something for which the Administration and its officials such as Ellen Cooper could be blameworthy—the pricing of drugs was considered an "industry" issue. The price of AZT was undoubtedly influenced by FDA regulations. Yet organized audiences blamed not the FDA but pharmaceutical companies for AZT's steep price. FDA officials repeatedly claimed, as they had for decades, that the pricing of drugs lay beyond their purview. On occasion, however, AIDS groups asked the Administration to explicitly consider pricing in its decisions, as when a large coalition of AIDS groups argued in 1991 that the approval of Fisons' nebulizer *Pneumopent* would reduce the price of competitor therapies for which AIDS sufferers were currently spending thousands of dollars. On the whole, though, when pricing became an issue, the AIDS groups targeted not the Administration, but the companies, as when ACT-UP demonstrators chained themselves to barriers on the floor of the New York Stock Exchange and compelled an appreciable reduction in the wholesale price of AZT.[99]

Today the AIDS crisis seems powerful in U.S. pharmaceutical regulation not just as cause but also as example. The striking demonstration of the power of patient politics was, at the same time, an historical precedent to which other organizations paid heed. Not just in the case of AIDS and HIV, but more broadly for the politics of disease, the politics of AIDS reframed some of the fundamental issues and controversies buffeting the FDA. For cancer activists as well as others, the exceptional disease created a new norm.[100]

U.S.," *NYT*, April 6, 1993, C3. Larry Kramer, "AZT Is Shit," *Advocate*, May 18, 1993, 80; from Epstein, *Impure Science*, 304, 430–31. Tim Kingston, "The Coming Storm Over Expedited Drug Approval," *San Francisco Bay Times*, June 1991, 10–12. The damning evidence on AZT was published in a letter to the *Lancet* in 1991 reporting early results from what was called "the Concorde trial." Jean-Pierre Aboulker and Ann Marie Swart, "Preliminary Analysis of the Concorde Trial," *Lancet* 341 (April 3, 1993): 889–90. On TAG and other AZT doubters, see Epstein, *Impure Science*, 297–9.

[99]In the late twentieth century, the FDA's claims were in large measure rather plausible. Much of the runup in drug costs in the late 1990s and the early twenty-first century, whether justifiable or not, occurred during a period when neither the median length nor the average size of clinical trials was increasing appreciably, and when the approval time for new drugs was declining. Salomeh Keyhani, Marie Diener-West, and Neil Powe, "Are Development Times For Pharmaceuticals Increasing or Decreasing?" *Health Affairs* 25 (2) (2006): 461–8. While these considerations do not rule out FDA regulation as a contributing factor in higher drug prices, they do shed doubt upon it. On Pneumopent, see "Fison's Pneumopent Warrants Approval Based on Advantages Over Lyphomed Orphan Drug—AIDS Groups," *DRR* 34 (15) (April 10, 1991): 9–10. The coalition of groups making this case was quite broad. It included ACT-UP, the AIDS Action Council, the ACLU AIDS Project, the Gay Men's Health Crisis, the Human Rights Campaign Fund, the National Gay and Lesbian Task Force, and the People with AIDS Health Group.

[100]Many commentators have seized upon the AIDS crisis, and the Administration's response to it, as evidence of a new equilibrium or regulatory era in U.S. governance of pharmaceuticals. As Daemmrich suggests, "Pharmaceutical drug regulation took on a more 'postmodern' appearance when government officials recognized that definitions of safety and efficacy would

COMMITTEES, USER FEES, AND THE INSTITUTIONALIZATION OF AUDIENCES

As the protests of the late 1980s and early 1990s died down, the influence of voices contesting the agency's power became less visible but, in a way, more entrenched. An informative example comes in the Lasagna Committee announced in December 1988. The Panel brought many of the agency's critics from the drug lag era and the cancer wars into an institutional fold. Outsiders became insiders of a sort. On the council were Louis Lasagna, Emil Frei III (now at Dana Farber), Samuel Hellman of the University of Chicago, Gertrude Elion of Burroughs-Wellcome, Charles Leighton of Merck, Theodore Cooper of Upjohn, and former general counsel Peter Barton Hutt. Lasagna had been attacking the agency's caution in writing and from his organizational creation, the center for the Study of Drug Development, since the 1970s. Frei was perhaps the most vocal in a network of NCI-connected oncologists who were especially strident in their attack on the agency's effectiveness requirement. Upjohn in the years during and after the Panalba struggle was arguably the single most antagonistic major drug company in dealing with the agency. The Administration's drug review programs also came under scrutiny from Vice President Dan Quayle's Council on Competitiveness. In 1991, echoing a proposal made by the Lasagna Committee, the Quayle Council called for the FDA to begin using external reviewers (including private contractors) in an effort to speed up drug review.[101]

Proposals for "external review" or "third-party review" mounted an attack on the Administration's core functions. If non-FDA review cleared a pathway to market, the Administration's gatekeeping power, conceptual power, and directive power would be radically diminished. Agency officials would not be able to impose its understanding of technical concepts and measures, and companies would not have the necessity of returning with new molecules through a single gatekeeper. Agency officials fought back against this thrust with a parry of rhetoric, internal reform, and acquiescence. Rhetorically, Administration personnel claimed from the late 1980s onward (with great plausibility) that drug review delays were primarily a matter of staffing. Internally, FDA leaders looked at the oncology drug division as an

---

necessarily vary depending on patients' backgrounds and the diseases they were fighting" (*Pharmacopolitics*, 82). While much changed in the regulation of HIV/AIDS therapies, however, much did not, and much that changed had been changing already.

[101]*DRR*, December 7, 1988, 3. On the Lasagna committee recommendations, see Robert Pear, "Faster Approval of AIDS Drugs Is Urged," *NYT*, August 16, 1990; *DRR*, August 22, 1990, 4. Hilts, *Protecting America's Health*, "The Drug Lag Revisited," esp. 277–80, provides an insightful description of this period. See generally "Dan Quayle, Regulation Terminator," *Business Week*, November 4, 1991; two of the Council's most important officials in pushing FDA deregulation were C. Boyden Gray and executive director Allan B. Hubbard. The official title of the Lasagna Committee was the "National Committee to Review Current Procedures for the Approval of Drugs for Cancer and AIDS"; Warren Leary, "Panel Seeks to Streamline F.D.A. for Cancer and AIDS Drugs," *NYT*, January 5, 1989. I gathered crucial information about this period from conversations with former associate commissioner William Hubbard.

exemplar of what quick NDA review could look like, as many of its reviews were completed in less than a year. Oncology drug reviewers were quietly transferred to the anti-viral division, and new medical reviewers were hired. In the late 1980s and early 1990s, drug review times for new molecular entities—perhaps the most important quantitative measure on which the Administration was judged in pharmaceutical politics—began to decline appreciably.[102]

The Administration's primary move of acquiescence came in opening new discussions with pharmaceutical industry representatives, Bush administration officials, and members of Congress about the creation of a "user fee" program for new drug review. The essential idea in a user fee program was to impose a per-application tax on pharmaceutical sponsors, who were the "users" of the NDA review process and would thus pay the fees. The more drugs a company sponsored, the greater in theory would its burden upon the agency be, and the higher would be its immediate fee contribution to the FDA's budget. The fees would cover more full-time employees who were detailed to new drug review. The crucial hitch of the contract was a set of letters in which FDA officials committed to approval time goals for new drug review. Many proposals for user fee arrangements were made before 1992, perhaps most notably in the Reagan administration's budget proposal of January 1987. One reason that the Reagan administration was hesitant to hike direct FDA funding is that it wanted increased staffing tied in a political contract to the agency's adoption of user fees. Largely because an agreement between Congress, the FDA, and the political arm of the pharmaceutical industry (PMA) could not be brokered—and in part because political conservatives thought that rank deregulation was preferable to throwing money in the form of user fees at the FDA problem—user fees were continually discussed but did not take institutional hold.

In 1992, Commissioner David Kessler and his associate commissioners would serve to broker a multidimensional agreement among representatives of industry, patient advocates, committee chairs in congress, Bush administration officials, and his own staff. These negotiations established the basis for the Prescription Drug User Fee Act (PDUFA) of 1992. A key feature of this agreement was that Kessler wrote letters of commitment to Congress in 1992 in which review time goals were elaborated. These review time goals were spelled out not in statute, then, but less formally in written communication. Another crucial feature of the agreement was also an implicit contract

---

[102]*DRR*, January 7, 1987, 4–5. *Business Week* reported that "Administration officials say [Quayle] has been most successful in reining in the Environmental Protection Agency, less so in tempering the gung-ho Food & Drug Administration"; "Dan Quayle, Regulation Terminator." It was well known that the FDA's oncology drug review division had "virtually zero backlog" in the late 1980s and early 1990s; *DRR*, February 8, 1989, 5. On the decline in NME approval times, due significantly to increased staff available from appropriations, see Daniel Carpenter, A. Mark Fendrick, Michael Chernew, and Dean Smith, "Approval Times for New Drugs: Does the Source of Funding for FDA Staff Matter?" *Health Affairs* (Web Exclusive), December 17, 2003, W3-618-624.

by Congress not to exploit the availability of the user fee monies and then reduce FDA appropriations for drug review–related purposes. For most categories of drugs, the Administration committed that by 1997, 90 percent of standard NDAs would be reviewed in twelve months, while 90 percent of priority NDAs would be reviewed in six months. The 90 percent figure reflected what FDA officials would call a "safety valve" so that more problematic drug applications accompanied by greater uncertainty would be allowed to pass beyond the review goal date. A key feature of the new law was its embedded sunset provision—the program would be renewed every five years and hence some measure of past performance would shape whether user fees would be available in the future.[103]

At the level of regulatory practice, the user fee legislation was associated with an appreciable decline in drug review times. To attribute the decline to the user fees or a particular feature of the user fee Act is problematic, however, and academic researchers have debated the causes. Critics of the regime focused increasingly upon the deadline provisions of the law and upon its erosive influence on the agency's culture and independence. "We were on a clock," pharmacologist Elizabeth Barbehenn said in an interview. "We had just so much time to get a review done. I found it extraordinarily frustrating." Observers worried for the agency's culture saw a regulator that was less likely to contest or challenge the actions of large pharmaceutical companies and more likely to do everything possible to achieve the publicly observable goal of quick NDA review. If indeed such a behavioral and cultural shift occurred, it would be difficult to disentangle the effects of the user fee law from the conservative political environment and pro-business culture of the 1990s when the law took shape. In the 1994 midterm elections, a fiercely antigovernment brand of Republicans led by Representative Newt Gingrich of Georgia had won new majorities in the House and Senate. Gingrich and his colleagues called for the elimination of numerous federal agencies and a wholesale commitment to deregulation. Many agencies of the time, not just the FDA, were running scared.[104]

---

[103]The PDUFA law has been capably summarized elsewhere and I emphasize only its general institutional shape and its role in embedding different audiences within the FDA and within pharmaceutical politics here. See Hilts, *Protecting America's Health*, chapters 18–21. On review time shifts and possible safety problems associated with the deadlines, see Daniel Carpenter, Evan James Zucker, and Jerry Avorn, "Drug Review Deadlines and Safety Problems," *NEJM* 358 (13) (March 27, 2008): 1354–61; errata and corrected estimates io *NEJM* 359 (1) (July 3, 2008): 95–98.

[104]Barbahenn's remark comes in Susan Okie, "What Ails the FDA"? *NEJM* 352 (11) (March 17, 2005):1063–6. For a study ascribing the decline in review times to staff (from both appropriations and user fees), see Carpenter, Fendrick, Chernew, and Smith, "Approval Times for New Drugs: Does the Source of Funding for FDA Staff Matter?" For a study attributing the review time decline to the user fee law, see Ernst Berndt, Adrian Gottschalk, Tomas Philipson, and Matthew Strobeck, "Industry Funding of the FDA: The Effects of PDUFA on Approval Times and Withdrawal Rates," *Nature Reviews: Drug Discovery* 4 (7) (2005): 545–54. For a critique, see Daniel Carpenter, Danyank Karl Lok, and Aaron R. Tjoa, "Fundamental Problems in Linear Statistical Analyses of Regulatory Approval Times upon Policy Indicators,"

Perhaps the deeper institutional legacy of the user fee law came in its two-fold influence on the agency's reputation. In image, what was meant to be a tax on drug companies ended up being a mode by which these companies' resources constituted the FDA budget, and (by hiring) the FDA itself. Some would later see this as the definition of capture, not in the sense that the political scientist Samuel Huntington and the economist Stigler had written of the term, but in the sense of a consumer protection agency having lost its way. The second reputational influence came in the way that the law institutionalized different audiences within and surrounding the Administration. The user fee law would be re-enacted in a bargain among the FDA, Congress, and the political arm of the pharmaceutical industry. The user fee law tied the agency to these audiences by tying a critical source of resources to them. And within the agency, as Elizabeth Barbehenn summarized it, the pressure of a ticking clock served as the institutional face of the various voices clamoring for acceleration and drug access. Even as the drug lag criticism of the 1970s and 1980s and the cancer and AIDS protestations of the 1980s and 1990s faded from public light, these voices were echoed within the agency's very procedures and habits.[105]

. . .

The evolution of regulatory power and reputation from the late 1970s to the early 1990s was one of contestation and the shaping of new audiences. Power was contested in its conceptual facet as well as its gatekeeping facet. Both facets were contested in the new regulatory politics of cancer (with variable audiences in NCI officials and votaries of Laetrile), and both facets were contested in the AIDS crisis. Yet both facets of power were partially cemented even as they were challenged. The contested system of phased experiment was reshaped, but even as the notion of surrogate endpoints came into broader use, the act of shaping these measures placed the Administration in the pivotal seat of defining the endpoints and the conceptual architecture used to enforce them. The user fee act restricted the agency's temporal discretion in drug review, but FDA officials responded in part by explicitly and implicitly moving the burden of time and rigor onto the clinical trial stage. And in perhaps the most fundamental legal challenge to the agency's gatekeeping power, the Laetrile decision, the Supreme Court ruled that any therapeutic exceptions to the FDA's rule over the pharmaceutical world be carved by Congress or the Administration itself, not by judicial interpretation of rights or disease severity.

Robert Wood Johnson Foundation Scholars in Health Policy Working Paper, No. 32 (Princeton, NJ: Robert Wood Johnson Foundation, May 2006).

[105] I discuss the reputational fallout of the user fee act and other developments in the past fifteen years in the concluding chapter.

PART TWO

Pharmaceutical Regulation

and Its Audiences

Reputation and the Organizational Politics of New Drug Review

It is a fact of life that, once a drug is approved, it is almost impossible, as a practical matter, to withdraw that approval, unless there is a very serious safety consideration that was not recognized before.

—Edward J. Tabor, Director, Division of Anti-Infective Drug Products, 1987[1]

Citizens may complain when local police fail to curtail unlawful or violent activity, but few believe that even the best-functioning police force can solve, much less prevent, all crimes. FDA is believed to have a different role, a responsibility to prevent harm before it occurs. The law makes it unlawful, without proof of intent or demonstration of actual injury or deception, to market drugs that the agency has not approved. In some sense, the agency becomes a warrantor of manufacturer compliance with the rules that govern drug development and marketing. This responsibility is implicitly acknowledged in the agency's own publications, is frequently referred to in press accounts of its performance, and historically has permeated the dialogue between the agency and congressional oversight committees. FDA is

---

[1] Tabor's remark came in discussions on the approval of azidothymidine (AZT), sponsored as Retrovir by Burroughs-Wellcome; FDA, *Meeting of the Anti-Infective Drugs Advisory Committee*, January 16, 1987; Rockville, MD; transcript produced by Baker, Haynes, and Burkes Reporting, Inc.

repeatedly reminded, and often reminds us, that it shares
responsibility for any drug that causes harm.

—Richard A. Merrill, former FDA General Counsel, 1996[2]

When teams come into each other's immediate presence,
a host of minor events may occur that are accidentally suitable for conveying a general impression that is inconsistent
with the fostered one. This expressive treacherousness is a
basic characteristic of face-to-face interaction. One way of
dealing with this problem is... to prepare in advance for all
possible expressive contingencies. One application of this
strategy is to settle on a complete agenda before the event,
designating who is to do what and who is to do what after
that. In this way confusions and lulls can be avoided and
hence the impression that such hitches in the proceedings
might convey to the audience can be avoided too.

—Erving Goffman, *The Presentation
of Self in Everyday Life*[3]

THE REVIEW of a new drug application marks the pivotal moment in the
transformation of a scientific concept into a therapeutic commodity. The
process seems at first glance to compose a simple, even predictable task.
New drug review denotes the organizational process of deciding whether a
sponsor's New Drug Application shall be deemed "effective" in regulation
and at law. In the United States, a sponsor with an effective NDA can legally
market a molecule in conjunction with a specific claim of healing. If and
when these rights have been conferred upon a sponsor, the Administration's
power—over those sponsors and over their drugs—wanes considerably. When
a new drug application is declared effective, a sponsor becomes a marketer.
Patients, once experimental subjects, become consumers. Physicians and

---

[2] Merrill, "The Architecture of Government Regulation of Medical Products," *Virginia Law
Review* 82 (1996): 1768.

[3] The quotation is from the first edition (New York: Anchor Books, Doubleday, 1959), 227–8.

other medical authorities, once assessors of the probable, become prescribers of actual therapy. The assets of investors and companies move from the expected to the liquid, as sales of a new drug generate millions or even billions of dollars in long-awaited revenue. And whether or not the Administration's officials intend it, the drug and its claims receive the "approval" of an organization, the imprimatur of its legal capacity, its history, and its image.

Because drug review consummates the conversion of idea into product, the process of drug review is accompanied by widespread anxiety and massive scrutiny. It is shot through with subtle politics, with battles over nuance and detail. Experts, advocates, and skeptics engage in debates that consume weeks, months, and even years over whether an experiment has been properly designed, whether the proper technique of data analysis has been used, whether the results justify the particular language in the label or likely advertisements. A drug that has abundant evidence of safety and effectiveness for a given disease will often linger in the regulatory process by virtue of battles over its labeling or its approved dose. What might seem to be good news—a letter from the Administration deeming a sponsor's drug "approvable"—can actually reflect and engender sour prospects for a company and its product. Over the past half-century and more, these battles over nuance, language, numbers, bioavailability, comparability of treatment and control groups, statistical significance, and other issues have received the weekly attention of pharmaceutical newsletters and trade reporters, the earnest scrutiny of congressional committees, searching review by medical journals, and the wary eye of dozens of national media outlets.

The publicity and emotion attached to the review of new drug applications also bestows a politics of reputation upon the process. Regulators often wish to act with fortitude, to inject a note of greater certainty into an inevitably uncertain world. All things considered, they would rather their regulatory decisions appear consensual and, therefore, more "scientific." Yet Administration officials also hedge their claims, so that neither the unpredictable events of the future nor the agency's many gadflies can highlight a prediction gone wrong. Officials wish to fend off and even anticipate political attack from companies, consumer groups, and medical and scientific societies, all of them making various claims about the drug under review. Each claim— that the drug is life-saving and necessary, or that it is overrated—has one or more constituencies. Beneath these politics lies the tension between the breadth of the Administration's authority over new drugs and the political and therapeutic responsibility that comes with it. The Administration's agents eschew the notion that they "approve" drugs—legally they merely permit a combination of compounds and claim to be marketed in interstate commerce—but what does not exist at law nonetheless prevails in fact. Once the Administration has cleared a new drug application, drug companies trumpet the FDA's approval of their products in advertisements to patients and physicians. Doctors, nurses, other health providers, and citizens come to rely upon the agency's decision for greater surety about a therapy. This social and political reality of approval imparts a felt responsibility to the officers of the Administration. It also renders the act of approval irreversible in image even as the declaration is revocable in procedure and law.

Considerations of reputation and science have shaped the administrative organization of drug review, as well as the various ways in which drugs have been evaluated, negated, and affirmed. These considerations can lead FDA offices to treat otherwise similar drugs very differently. Such considerations can affect the timing of decision making as well as the language in which a decision is rendered. Science and reputation are not substitute forces in regulation but interact, complement, and complicate one another. The modern sciences of drug development and evaluation often generate more uncertainty than they resolve, and the forces of organizational image become crucial in giving meaning to complex data, to decisions, and to the implications of otherwise small choices.[4]

The Administration's various and overlapping audiences place impinging pressures upon its officials involved in new drug review. These pressures engender an implicit calculus, one that merges technical and social variables. Different audiences are more or less visible. Drug reviewers see the audience of their superiors, the audience of science (particularly its specialties and subdisciplines), and in part the audience of industry faces with whom they meet. Drug review heads and the agency's Commissioner see the audiences of Congress, the audiences of higher industry officials and organizations, the audiences of patient groups and medical and health specialists who claim to represent those who might be treated with the new drug in question, the audiences of financial and medical publications that follow (and often excoriate) the agency's approval decisions. In advisory committee meetings, a select subset of these audiences meets publicly, and Administration officials must present a case to them, as well as to a wider public.

ADMINISTRATION AND THE MAKING OF MODERN DRUG REVIEW, 1963–1985

The emergence of regulatory power in the American pharmaceutical world was expressed through human organization. Without a bureaucratic structure of human activity to embody and administer the instruments and concepts of power, the Administration's regulatory weapons—the new drug veto and its new armature in the 1962 law, the three-phase system of experiment and the 1963 rules, and the specific regulation of clinical research—would exist only in ideation. In the structure that assigned roles to specific individuals and facilities, and in the patterns and precedents of be-

---

[4]This chapter covers new drug review from the 1960s through the mid-1990s. In the main, it largely sidesteps a central transformation in the agency—the Prescription Drug User Fee Act of 1992—which was discussed in the previous chapter and is examined separately in chapter 12.

havior established in early application of the capacities gained in 1962 and 1963, the Administration's regulatory power became human, visible, and tangible. Most important, it became memorable and self-reproducing.

Administration officials did not redesign the process of new drug review in the aftermath of the 1962 Amendments. Instead, they relied heavily on practices that had emerged in the previous decade, many of them under the leadership of Ralph Smith. When the Bureau of Medicine was "reorganized" in 1965—a move that merely formalized patterns of authority and communication that already prevailed behaviorally—Smith was named leader of the New Drug Division. Within this Division were three branches, the most notorious of which was Frances Kelsey's Investigational Drug Branch that implemented the 1963 IND rules. H. D. Cohn directed the Medical Evaluation branch that evaluated new drug applications, while Earl L. Meyers directed the Manufacturing Controls Branch that examined the control methods that were outlined in sponsors' applications.[5]

While the official topology of the 1960s Bureau of Medicine separated the evaluation of investigational drugs from new drug applications, in practice the two functions ran together. Many of the young scientists who would become the agency's best-known NDA reviewers were hired under Kelsey in her leadership of the Investigational Drug Branch. Kelsey's medical officers, whose primary responsibility lay in evaluating study designs for investigational drugs, also frequently evaluated clinical data for new drug review. These procedural overlaps expressed a notion of continuity of evaluation that stemmed from the Administration's notions of regulatory pharmacology. FDA officials like Smith, Kelsey, and Arthur Ruskin shared a general concern that most pharmaceutical companies lacked genuine experience in clinical pharmacology, so they sought to apply principles of clinical pharmacology to every stage of a drug's development. The IND rules of 1963 required sponsors to delegate their Phase 1, 2, and 3 trials to experts in clinical pharmacology, but Walter Modell conceded in 1963 that among the trained scientists in most companies, "very few can be called Clinical Pharmacologists now." He remarked that the FDA "would have to lower standards to bring more in under [the regulations'] definition."[6] Internally, the Bureau of

---

[5]On Smith and the organizational and philosophical changes to new drug review in the 1950s, see chapter 3. The 1965 reorganization is described in detail and imaged in *FD&CR*, January 11, 1965, Special Section. The role of the Manufacturing Controls Branch was not (and is not now) a trivial one. Then and now, new drug review is not simply an analysis of clinical trial data by in-house scientists but also depends critically upon the perceived consistency of the *manufactured* drug with the one tested in clinical trials. For this reason, the Manufacturing Controls Branch coordinated the review of manufacturing control methods that were outlined in IND and NDA proposals. Its officials analyzed bioassays as well as arranging for FDA laboratories to test new drugs and for FDA inspectors to examine establishments. In the late 1960s and early 1970s, this Branch and its personnel occupied important roles in the evolution of bioequivalence and bioavailability concepts.

[6]Summary of Proceedings, Advisory Committee on Investigational Drugs, October 24, 1963. FOK.

Medicine placed officers with pharmacologic expertise in positions of greater authority. This practice was not formalized, but it reflected the enormous status of Kelsey within the agency's walls, as well as her newfound clout in running the Investigational Drug Branch. "Because of the nature of the work done" in her branch, Kelsey held, "it is highly desirable that the individual medical officers have some experience in the field of pharmacology over and above that ordinarily obtained during the course of medical school, internship, residency and practice." At some level, Frances Kelsey (supported by Ralph Smith) wanted not merely a Bureau of Medicine but a Bureau of Clinical Pharmacology.[7]

The new cohort of medical officers in the Investigational Drug Branch, hired with oversight by Kelsey, matched these criteria almost perfectly (see table 7.1). Without exception they had training in clinical research as well as practice; all were able to evaluate clinical trial data, and all of them cleaved to the standard of double-blind randomized clinical trials. All but one had training in pharmacology, toxicology, or both. Yale-educated Harold Anderson had published research on sulfonamides and penicillin and had directed a streptococcal disease control laboratory. Janos Bacsanyi had conducted studies in animal toxicology and pharmacology at Duke and at the Cleveland Clinic. John Epperson hailed from Johns Hopkins and had analyzed the toxicology of estrogen-based and progestin-based drugs. He had also participated in clinical trials evaluating some of the newest investigational drugs for the treatment of cancer. William Gyarfas had studied toxicology during two years with the U.S. Navy, had developed original medical devices for use in heart surgery, and was among the first U.S. physicians to conduct clinical trials with new radio-isotopes. Robert Hodges came from a clinical pharmacology group at the University of Washington that was among the best in the nation, and studied fetal effects of drugs that crossed the placental barrier. Phyllis Huene, trained at Cornell, pioneered research in the pharmacology of dermatology drugs, and had earned the Bernard Baruch National Essay Award for her article on anti-clotting (anticoagulant) therapy. Irish national Arthur O'Grady was one of the original discoverers of the substance medulin, later synthesized into a drug for hypertension. Michigan-trained Theresa Woo was a Columbia pediatrics resident who was associated with the early trials of penicillin for the U.S. Army. She was also an expert in tetanus.

These officers were not trivial or temporary hires. Some of them—Bacsanyi, Freeman, Gyarfas, Huene, Ochota, Woo—remained with the FDA for two to four decades afterward. Bacsanyi became a pivotal voice in the agency's regulation of AIDS drugs, and was well known for his outreach to the constituencies engaged with AIDS drug regulation. Gyarfas would become director of the agency's anticancer drug division in the late 1970s and early 1980s. Freeman presented a key and different voice in debates about parenteral nu-

---

[7]Memorandum from Joseph M. Pisani, M.D., to Rankin, "Hearings on Drug Safety before the Fountain Subcommittee on May 4, 1965," June 2, 1965; B13, F8, FOK.

TABLE 7.1
Medical Officers in the Investigational Drug Branch, Bureau of Medicine, U.S. Food and Drug Administration, 1964

Medical Officer	Institutions of Medical Training	Training in Pharmacology or Toxicology	Clinical Research Experience	FDA Review Specialty
Harold Anderson	University of Minnesota, Yale University	Sulfonamide drugs, Salicylates	Treatment of rheumatic fever, infectious disease	Infectious disease drugs
Janos Bacsanyi	University of Budapest, Duke University, Cleveland Clinic	Pharmacology of animal preparations	Renal clearance of urea, insulin; kidney function	Animal pharmacologic data, arthritis and rheumatism drugs
John Epperson	University of Maryland, Johns Hopkins University	Toxicity of estrogen- and progestin-based drugs	Obstetrics and gynecology	Obstetrics and gynecology drugs; cancer drugs
Martha Freeman	University of Rochester	none	Nutrition and child development	Pediatric drugs, developmental drugs
William Gyarfas	George Washington University, U.S. Navy	Toxicity of solvents, metals	Medical devices for heart surgery, pulmonary treatment	Anti-cancer drugs, electrolytes used in surgery
Robert Hodges	Wales, University of Ottawa	Effect of drugs that cross placental barrier	Clinical endocrinology, teratogenicity of drugs	Endocrine drugs, cancer drugs
Phyllis Huene	New York Medical College, Cornell University	Pharmacology of skin, drugs for skin conditions	Anti-clotting therapy, skin conditions	Dermatology drugs

TABLE 7.1
cont.

Medical Officer	Institutions of Medical Training	Training in Pharmacology or Toxicology	Clinical Research Experience	FDA Review Specialty
Arthur O'Grady	National University of Ireland, Georgetown University	Distribution of radio-isotopes in kidney	Development of medulin for hypertension	Kidney drugs, endocrine drugs
Laszek Ochota	University of Zurich, Duke University	Toxicity of mercury-based compounds	Allergy and arthritis drugs	Allergy drugs, psycho-tropic drugs
Raymond Uphoff	University of Iowa, University of Indiana	Anti-leukemia medications	Effects of chemotherapy, cancer drugs	Cancer drugs
Morris Weinberger	Tufts University	Drug-induced liver and kidney diseases	Electron microscopy, cortisone in liver disease	Cancer drugs (chemo-therapy), kidney drugs
Theresa Woo	University of Michigan	Metabolism of vitamins in mothers, infants	Penicillin, neonatal tetany	Tropical, pediatric diseases

Source: Memorandum from Joseph Pisani to Assistant FDA Commissioner Winton Rankin, June 2, 1965; B13, F8, FOK.

trition products and artificial sweeteners. Woo stirred controversy when in 1980 and 1981 she recommended against NDA approval of the sedative triazolam (Halcion). Another hire of the Kelsey-Smith era, Marion J. Finkel, became the agency's most authoritative woman officer of the 1970s and 1980s, ascending to deputy director of the FDA's Bureau of Drugs.[8]

The Bureau of Medicine also spelled out the specific roles of pharmacologists in the review of INDs and NDAs. As Bureau regulations stated, there were three types of information on which pharmacologists would be particularly helpful: (1) "pharmacodynamics," (2) toxicology, and (3) metabolism. Pharmacodynamics was then understood as the action of drugs on tissues and organs, usually in nontoxic concentrations. Toxicology was defined broadly as "the study, usually in the intact animal, of a wide range of dosages, extending from the therapeutic level to the one which will produce injury or death." Finally, metabolism was understood to refer to the drug's "fate in the body": how it was absorbed and metabolized and how the body processed the drug and its metabolites. Beyond these traditional specialties, pharmacologists were also relied upon for their expertise in study design and analysis. In an informal manner, clinical pharmacologists served as the Bureau's statisticians before the widespread hiring of biostatisticians and mathematical statisticians.[9]

As in the 1950s, Administration officers in the 1960s and beyond shared particular and enduring doubts about the information and competence available to two agents in the American health-care system: unregulated doctors and unguided patients. FDA medical officers did not have confidence in general practitioners, not out of a concern for their original training, but because of the effects of the pharmacologic revolution of the 1950s. For this reason, early new drug review focused heavily upon labeling. Kelsey remarked that "My duty is to see that all the necessary information is there for

[8] Ibid. For evidence of Smith's involvement in these hires, see Smith and Kelsey to Anthony Celebrezze, October 9, 1964; B1, F3, p. 3, FOK. Freeman ascended to the Commissioner's Office and left in 1987. Gyarfas would later direct the Division of Oncology and Radiopharmaceutical Drug Products and left in the early 1980s. Bacsanyi and Huene remained through the 1990s. Woo appears to have remained in the FDA's drug reviewing center until 1985. Data on later careers from Daniel Carpenter and Susan Moffitt, CDER Personnel Database, Department of Government, Harvard University.

[9] "The Role of Pharmacologists in the Review of IND's and NDA's," Appendix to Memorandum from Joseph M. Pisani to Winton Rankin, June 2, 1965; B13, F8, FOK. In the 1960s when these procedures were elaborated, the typical IND Notice contained "slightly under 400 pages, with a range of 2–16,000 pages" (Ralph G. Smith and FOK to Celebrezze, October 9, 1964, p. 3; B1, F3, FOK). The average number of Notices allocated to each medical officer in 1963–64 was 158 (ibid., p. 4). The role of pharmacologists in IND review was particularly strong because there was "simultaneous review of each Notice by the Division of Toxicologic Evaluation and the Controls Evaluation Branch." The Division had 14 pharmacologists at the time, who devoted "all of their time to a review of investigational New Drug Notices and New Drug Applications." There were at least ten pharmacologists in other divisions that also served as informal consultants (Ralph G. Smith and FOK to Celebrezze, October 9, 1964, p. 3; B1, F3, FOK).

the physician to judge." Few practitioners, the FDA remarked, "have the time or training to evaluate potent new agents, which may not only break new therapeutic ground but also may yield unusual side effects and hazards." Yet the informational basis of the Bureau's distrust of general physicians also provided grounds for the distrust of patients and self-medication. This duality sometimes led FDA officials to engage in the Aristotelian act of "finding the mean" between too little information and too much. As Joseph Sadusk, then Medical Director of the Bureau of Medicine, wrote to a Los Angeles correspondent in 1964:

> Many patients want detailed information regarding their illnesses, even incurable illnesses, and the effects that any drug they are taking may have, whether good or bad. However, there is some question regarding the advisability of complete information for the use of a drug being available to laymen as it may encourage dangerous self-diagnosis and treatment of conditions for which the laymen should be under the care of a physician....You will appreciate that in most situations a layman does not have the training to evaluate the significance of, and in many instances, even the ability to recognize such effects.[10]

Although the statute and the legislative history of the 1962 Amendments did not direct the agency to engage in conscious trade-offs in new drug review, the FDA's drug reviewers nonetheless weighed different properties of drugs against one another, and often compared new drugs against previously approved medicines. In the reviews of the 1960s, these trade-offs incorporated at least two comparisons that spanned drugs. First, a drug's safety profile was more likely to be an issue when a safe treatment alternative was already available for the primary indication of the NDA. Second, drugs administered in hospitals or intravenously tended to receive less scrutiny than self-administered treatments or oral dosage forms. Beyond this, the assessment of efficacy began as early as the IND review and was highly systematized. In order to judge efficacy, the Bureau offered a list of possible outcomes from medicinal treatment (see table 7.2). Bureau officials primarily used this list to judge efficacy, but they also used it more implicitly to assign "grades" to drugs along a linear conceptual scale.[11]

---

[10]Sadusk to Mrs. L. Kerans Moore, Los Angeles, California, October 2, 1964; B1, F3, FOK. "Safety and Skepticism: Thalidomide," *Modern Medicine*, October 15, 1962, 34.

[11]As the randomized and placebo-controlled trial became the standard of evidence for "substantial evidence of effectiveness," the standard became interpreted as statistically differentiable superiority to a placebo control. However, implicit comparisons were often made to other therapies already approved and under development, rendering problematic (and too broadbrush) Marcia Angell's argument that demonstrated superiority to placebo is necessary and (implicitly) sufficient for FDA drug approval (*The Truth About the Drug Companies* (New York: Random House, 2004), 75–6). On this point, see the statistical evidence below and the narrative studies of drug review in this chapter. On the evolution of standards in the 1960s, see "Safety and Skepticism: Thalidomide," 36. Review of NDA 12-831, Ambodryl Hydrochloride Compound (CI-477); B11, F9, FOK. (Ambodryl is an antihistamine closely related to Benadryl.) "Ten Possible Outcomes in Treatment," memorandum of November 6, 1964; B 11, F 14, FOK.

POLITICS OF NEW DRUG REVIEW 475

TABLE 7.2
Ten Possible Outcomes in Treatment

"Cure," future prevention, no residue (polio vaccine)
"Cure," future prevention, residue (cowpox vaccine)
"Cure," no future prevention, no residue (penicillin in pneumonia)
"Cure," no future prevention, residue (penicillin in acute rheumatic fever)
Symptomatic relief followed by spontaneous healing (decongestants in common cold)
Total control with continuing therapy (insulin in diabetes)
Partial arrest with slowing of progress (cortisone in arthritis)
No arrest, with symptom relief (morphine in malignancy)
No benefit
Harm

Source: Frances O. Kelsey Papers, Library of Congress.

The Bureau of Medicine's outcomes ranking reveals the basic premises of the mid-century regime of pharmacological regulation—a "rationalist" therapeutics that greeted new drugs with skepticism and that assessed them by means of conscious trade-offs of their incremental therapeutic "benefits" versus their human costs. The outcomes ranking both expressed this therapeutics and formed the basis for its extensive application in new drug review. In the Administration's drug reviewing divisions, no word was regarded with greater skepticism in the 1960s and 1970s than the word "cure." The idea that a drug could "cure" a disease was a claim permitted only for select antibiotics and vaccines, and even then, a "Cure without residue" left in the human body was appreciably superior to a "cure with residue." Implicitly, this logic made it difficult to apply the concept of "cure" to therapeutic classes other than antibiotics and vaccines. The outcome of preventing death nonetheless appeared more valuable than that of improving the quality of life. Administration officials attached little weight to the relief of symptoms, ranking this outcome lower than the "partial arrest" of an advancing disease with slowing of its progress.

The rank-ordering of therapeutic outcomes was part of a larger process in which the "risks" of drugs were weighed against their "benefits." In the development of this regulatory calculus, the idioms of the past became the basis for the standards of the future. When they revealed their standards of

Kelsey's systematization of IND review was all the more remarkable because it was undertaken in the absence of external pressure and bypassed the rulemaking process. Her Division's "Proposed Outline for IND Review" offered an eleven-point "Description of the Compound," as well as a summary of "Previous Clinical Investigations," published and unpublished. See also "Proposed Outline for IND Review," November 6, 1964; B 11, F 14, FOK.

decision making, Administration medical officers spoke consistently in terms of two metaphors: cancer and birth defects. The first metaphor marked that set of drugs where some acceptance of safety risks to patients and even fetuses was clearly acceptable. The second metaphor expressed and personified the exemplar of a "risk." Kelsey and her coterie repeatedly stressed that the standards of evaluation were flexible and ethically appropriate. "In the treatment of a disease such as cancer," Kelsey told an audience in 1971, "it has generally been accepted that possible ill effects to the child must be weighed against possible benefits to the mother. It would appear difficult, however, to justify the use of known teratogens for the treatment during pregnancy of more benign conditions such as psoriasis or rheumatoid arthritis."[12]

The calculus of reviewing INDs and NDAs was explicit if not entirely quantitative. This formalized calculus expressed both the values at stake and the division of labor involved in drug review. The various "pure" sciences involved in drug review—chemistry and biochemistry—provided information, while the applied sciences of pharmacology and medicine provided judgment. As one internal memorandum put it:

> The medical officer with the recommendation of the pharmacologists before them and information from chemists and others must then conclude: With respect to the IND, whether the clinical testing of a drug is justified in view of the possible risks and benefits.
>
> With respect to an NDA, whether the potential benefit from using the drug as proposed outweighs the potential risk as revealed by the animal and clinical studies.[13]

Even within established fields of medicine represented in the Bureau, pharmacology dominated. Pharmacology reviews seemed to take more time than others, leading to complaints about the extra discretion given to pharmacologists. The status of pharmacologists created an ongoing dispute within the agency about whose information was superior and who was entitled to use it. Pharmacology had formerly occupied its own "Bureau," and after the creation of the Bureau of Science in 1969, it had the status of a "Division" while pathology was a lesser "Branch" in the same Division. FDA pathologists lamented their lack of "proper status" at the Administration, in particular a position that would allow for greater outside voice and an ability to communicate directly with the public, with the American medical profession, and with policymakers.[14] As patterns of decision and scrutiny on new

[12]Kelsey, "Drugs in Pregnancy and their Effects on Pre- and Postnatal Development," address presented at the 1971 Annual Meeting of the Association for Research in Nervous and Mental Disease, December 4, 1971, New York, New York; p. 3 of address, B12, F3, FOK.

[13]"The Role of Pharmacologists in the Review of IND's and NDA's," Appendix to Memorandum from Joseph M. Pisani to Winton Rankin, June 2, 1965; B13, F8, FOK.

[14]Of 2,502 investigational new drugs received in the three years after the 1962 Amendments, chemistry reviews had been completed on 2,018, medical reviews on 1,565, and pharmaco-

drugs developed in the 1960s and 1970s, these seemingly minute issues of professional esteem took on more and more practical importance. In 1967, federal regulations began to express the emerging administrative reality of American drug review, namely that essential decision rights were being vested in government agents (Medical Officers) far down the hierarchical chain from the Commissioner. This devolvement of internal power happened for several reasons. First, at the level of legal authority, the patterns of decentralization that emerged in the 1950s were being formalized through "re-delegation" of approval authority in the Code of Federal Regulations. Over the past three decades, the basic authorities of drug approval and refusal have migrated steadily downward—from the secretary of the cabinet department in which the Administration is located, to the Office of the FDA Commissioner, to the director of the agency's drug reviewing bureau, and more recently to the directors of "offices" of new drug review, and below those offices, to the heads of review divisions. Second, medical officers were using the very detailed requirements governing new drug applications to impose detailed and stringent requirements upon drug sponsors. Lack of compliance with these requirements led to "refusal-to-file" (RTF) judgments where the application was returned without review, or to "non-approvable" letters wherein the application was reviewed but refused. Third, and more symbolically, the agency's drug reviewing division had been hiring more distinguished and authoritative scientists. The commissioner's office and the director of the agency's drug review bureau could less easily overturn lower decisions when they were being made by acknowledged specialists with professional recognition and clout.[15]

In more ways than one, FDA medical officers owed their centrality in new drug review to Frances Kelsey. Her public triumph with thalidomide became the visible exemplar of the agency's capacity, leading Kefauver himself to intone on the Senate floor that "the physicians of the FDA who are trying to protect the American people from drugs with dangerous side effects, such as

---

logical reviews on 1,402. "Status of Review of IND's," Appendix to Memorandum from Joseph M. Pisani, M.D., to Rankin, June 2, 1965; FOK, B13, F8. Pathologist Kent Davis would complain of the "continued fostering of the alterations of pathology through misuse by non-pathologists"; Kent J. Davis, D.V.M. (Division of Pathology) to CCE, May 14, 1970; *CPRPFDA*, 103. On official status disparities between pharmacology and pathology, see Memorandum from Keith H. Lewis, Ph.D. (Director, Bureau of Science), to Commissioner Herbert Ley, November 17, 1969; Howard L. Richardson (Chief, Pathology Branch) to Dale R. Lindsay (Associate Commissioner for Science), December 8, 1969; *CPRPFDA*, 108.

[15]The legal contrast with the pre-1962 regime is noteworthy here. As Hilts discusses (*Protecting America's Health*, 145), "medical officers could approve a drug essentially on their own authority" in 1960. "To turn one down, however, required the unanimous support of the medical officer, the lawyers, the chief of the drug branch, the chief medical director, and the commissioner. This was because the 1938 law said a drug was automatically approved unless the FDA, for good reasons, stopped it. Thus, the legal burden was on the FDA." On the NDA rewrite of 1967, see *FR* 32 (108) (June 6, 1967): 8080. For the elaboration of requirements in regulations, see 21 CFR 314, Subpart B ("Applications"); many of these requirements were cemented in the "NDA Rewrite" of 1985; *FR* 50 36 (Feb. 22, 1985): 7494–7503.

thalidomide... should have an adequate time to assure themselves that the drug is safe." Yet quite apart from her symbolism, Kelsey took an active role in shaping the division of labor in the 1960s Bureau of Medicine. In the heroine's judgment, the medical officer should be apprised of all data—pre-clinical studies, clinical studies (controlled and uncontrolled), data on the investigator, adverse reaction reports, and anything else relevant to the con-tinuing evaluation of safety and efficacy. When in 1966, Commissioner James Goddard proposed rules that would direct incoming adverse event reports to a new unit of the Bureau of Medicine, Kelsey protested.

> I think it is a mistake to place the initial evaluation of adverse reactions in a spe-cial branch or division apart from those who are actually handling the new drugs or supplemental applications or the IND evaluations. The most important consid-eration is that value judgments, even if they be merely the screening out of seem-ingly unimportant adverse reactions, should be the prerogative and the responsi-bility of those ultimately responsible for the day-to-day handling and the initial recommendation concerning the ultimate disposition of these compounds. I be-lieve it should be the aim of the Bureau of Medicine to build up an elite corps of scientists, each of whom is knowledgeable in one or two of the various areas of drug therapy. It is utopian to believe that we could in the foreseeable future build up four such corps in the following areas. 1. Investigational Drugs 2. Medical Evaluation 3. Surveillance 4. Adverse Reaction Reporting.[16]

The historical irony of Kelsey's argument would come decades later, when external skeptics of the agency ranging from the General Accounting Office to the Institute of Medicine would disparage this fusion of pre-market drug review and post-market drug surveillance. The argument was premised upon a simple understanding of the politics of reputation and blame avoid-ance. Putting review of adverse events in the hands (or under the partial or full control) of the same officials who had approved the drug in the first place, argued these critics, created a "conflict of interest."[17]

The Administration's penchant for elaborating requirements for new drug applications both solved core regulatory problems and created new ones. The extensive requirements for NDA submission served to deter lower qual-ity submissions from less thorough sponsors. This act of deterrence was backed up by a very real and tangible veto power. Skeptical medical officers could front-load the information and reporting burden upon sponsors, then issue a "refusal-to-file" judgment or a "non-approvable" letter if the firm failed to comply. Aggregate statistics suggest, in the first decade of drug re-

---

[16]Kefauver remark in CR, July 18, 1962, 12973. Kelsey to Julius Hauser (Executive Officer, BOM), January 6, 1966; B11, F6, FOK.

[17]GAO, *Drug Safety: Improvement Needed in FDA's Postmarket Decision-Making and Oversight Process* (Washington, DC: GAO, 2006); IOM, Committee on the Assessment of the U.S. Drug Safety System, Alina Baciu, Kathleen Stratton and Sheila P. Burke, eds. *The Future of Drug Safety: Promoting and Protecting the Health of the Public* (Washington, DC: National Academies Press, 2007), 83–97.

view under the post-1962 regime, the "bad news" conveyed in non-approvable letters often far outnumbered the "good news" from NDA approvals. In fiscal year 1970, the Administration approved 38 NDAs but issued "not-approvable" letters for 201 different applications. For "supplemental" new drug applications where a previously approved molecule was being reviewed for a new indication or for production by a new manufacturer, the agency's activity was even more robust. The Administration issued about 500 "incomplete" letters per year for supplemental applications in the early 1970s. So too, the NDA requirements disaggregated the evidence on a new drug and allowed the agency's trained specialists to focus on particular data, even to reconstruct the analyses themselves. FDA reviewers and statisticians would occasionally use the original data to produce strikingly different estimates of safety and effectiveness. Representatives of the Pharmaceutical Manufacturers Association (PMA) objected to these elaborate requirements, and to the power they gave to medical officers.[18]

The other dynamic created by voluminous record keeping was that it permitted scrutiny of drugs via scrutiny of their investigators. At Kelsey's initiative, the Bureau of Medicine had embarked upon an enormous effort to track and aggregate the research history of clinical investigators. By 1964, just one year after the IND regulations were issued, the Bureau had already amassed records of "over 20,000 investigators who have worked on either IND's or NDA's." Supplementing this attempt were arrangements to formalize the flow of scientific information across national boundaries; Kelsey consulted with Canadian authorities and regularly received updated lists of investigational drugs from Ottawa. The volume of this information was not accompanied by an efficient system for retrieving it. Yet this information on the research history of the investigator was often sufficient to differentiate quacks from legitimate investigators. When in 1966 Kelsey crossed swords with Stanley Jacob over his experiments with dimethyl sulfoxide (DMSO), she made frequent reference to Jacob's checkered history with other investigational drugs.[19]

[18]Figures on disposition of FY 1969 NDAs taken from HEW, *FDA Quarterly Activities Report, Fiscal Year 1970— 4th Quarter* (Washington, DC: Public Health Service, 1970). Figures on supplements taken from FY 1970 quarterly reports, which average slightly over 125 "incomplete" letters per quarter. For the precedent-setting example of sulfinpyrazone (Andurane), see Hilts, *Protecting America's Health*, 225–7. For a checklist of the different steps of a medical officer's review, along with requirements that an approvable NDA would need to meet, see "Summary and Evaluation of an NDA," 1965, attachment to Bert J. Vos to Donald G. Levitt, "Certified Summary for New Drug Applications," November 26, 1965; DF 505.5, RG 88, NA. The 1965 summary was sent to PMA representatives in order to allow them to comment upon the procedures, but there is no evidence that the Administration changed any feature of this protocol either before or after these comments were received. For another attempt to assuage concerns over the minutiae of NDA forms, see B. Harvey Minchew, "Drug Application Problems," presented at the 1965 Annual Research and Scientific Development Conference of the Proprietary Association, New York, December 9, 1965; DF 505.5, RG 88, NA.

[19]"FDA Letter to Humphrey Subcmte. On International Drug Data," *DRR*, November 28, 1962. On the limitations of the Bureau's database, officials would admit that "At the present

The Bureau of Medicine's voluminous record keeping permitted select and in-depth scrutiny of new drug applications, yet it also satisfied important and nosy audiences in Congress. When asked by an advisory committee why their organization kept such a trove of information, Kelsey and Smith responded that they felt obligated to "maintain voluminous records and write careful summaries" because the Administration had been "criticized in the past by Congressional committees for not doing so." The collection and storage of administrative records on a grand scale thus satisfied logics of function and reputation. Yet the NDA requirements and the Bureau's habit of archiving also created a situation where Administration officials were inundated with paper, slowing down the review process and cluttering office space.[20]

Goddard, Edwards, Crout: The Emergence of Modern Drug Review Organization

While industry insiders and trade newspapers greeted the 1969 resignation of James Goddard with glee and relief, few could anticipate that many of the plans hatched by the outspoken Commissioner would continue under his successors, Herbert Ley and Charles C. Edwards. The most important of these were changes in the organization and procedure of the FDA's drug reviewing bureau, which was reshaped and newly entitled the Bureau of Drugs in 1970. The change in title signified a shift from a professionally based identity ("Medicine") to a product-based identity ("Drugs"). The authority of the Administration's pharmacologist and medical officers did not wane, however. By several mechanisms, the 1970 reorganization of drug review—a remolding whose imprint remains upon the agency today—both centralized and decentralized power at the Administration.

What Charles Edwards and his appointees Henry Simmons and J. Richard Crout would later crystallize, James Goddard started. Goddard's drive to reorganize the Bureau of Medicine began in a struggle with the agency's most visible figure, Frances Kelsey. Kelsey was widely criticized for taking too much time with the review of IND applications. In her administrative

---

moment, all we can do is retrieve manually the name of the investigator and the various drugs that he has worked on"; Smith and Kelsey to Hon. Anthony Celebrezze, Secretary of Health Education and Welfare, October 9, 1964; Kelsey to Sadusk and Ralph G. Smith, January 27, 1966; B1, F3, FOK.

[20] "FDA Letter to Humphrey Subcmte. On International Drug Data," *DRR*, November 28, 1962. "*AFP* 25 Years Ago: FDA's Investigational Drug Branch," *American Family Physician* 38 (4) (1988): 424. Advisory Committee on Investigational Drugs, Summary of Proceedings, 14th Meeting, January 14, 1965; FOK. Crout later recalled that the Bureau was so inundated with paper that "Nobody could find anything. If you made a request, it was days before you got things, so that people—that is the reviewing medical officers and other officers—literally fought over their applications." Ronald T. Ottes and John P. Swann, "Interview with J. Richard Crout, M.D., Director of FDA's Bureau of Drugs, 1973–1982" (Nov. 12, 1997), FDA Oral History Series, NLM.

role, the heroine of thalidomide and the co-architect of the FDA's pharmacological regime experienced a measure of failure. These setbacks were as much symbolic as factual. Kelsey was seen as indecisive and demanding of too much data, much of it irrelevant to decisions about whether an IND should proceed. Sidney Merlis called for a "compromise" between thoroughness and efficiency. Kelsey's unit, he advised, would "have to trust most sponsors and merely scan much of the data." Some of Kelsey's colleagues took the matter further. Medical Director Joseph Sadusk openly ridiculed her in a committee meeting, suggesting that her branch "would be more efficiently carrying out its mission by reviewing 100% of the IND's in '95% depth' rather than reviewing only 20% of the IND's in '100% depth.'!"[21]

When Goddard arrived in 1966, he was generally supportive of Kelsey but quickly grew tired of complaints from numerous quarters that the Investigational Drug Branch was in a state of dysfunction. In 1966, she was removed from the Branch directorship and returned to her "old stand" as a medical officer. By 1967, she returned to drug evaluation for INDs and was appointed assistant to the Director for the Bureau of Medicine. She had lost formal control over investigational drugs and suffered what one reporter would later describe as a "humiliating 'bare-desk' treatment; she was generally ignored and given little to do of consequence." Later that year, in what was formally a promotion but less visibly an attempt to find a place for her, Goddard appointed Kelsey as Director of the Scientific Investigations Staff in the Bureau's Office of Scientific Evaluation. Goddard would later recollect that Kelsey was a "sacred cow" at the time and felt that "Frances could not move people and get things done."[22]

Edwards' new Bureau of Drugs bundled activities of planning, new drug review, post-market surveillance, statistical analysis and efforts to secure industry compliance (see figure 7.1). In a partial realization of Kelsey's wishes, the Division of Epidemiology and Drug Experience remained within the Bureau, but separate from the review divisions. Adverse event reporting, surveillance, new drug evaluation, and evaluation of investigational drugs were now unified in print and in human organization. The six review divisions were broken down by therapeutic specialty and reflected the coarse

[21]Advisory Committee on Investigational Drugs, Summary of Proceedings, 14th Meeting, January 14, 1965; FOK. The exclamation point is in the original minutes, suggesting perhaps that Sadusk had added emphasis or ridicule to his point.

[22]Jerry Kluttz, "The Federal Diary: President Moves to Widen Women's Role in Government," WP, March 9, 1967, A2. Goddard Oral History, NLM; cited in Arthur Daemmrich, "A Tale of Two Experts," *Social History of Medicine* 15 (1) (2002): 156. Kelsey's demotion and transfer were part of a larger self-examination occurring in and around the Bureau of Medicine in the late 1960s. The Modell Committee and other informal consultants perceived an unproductive separation between the review of investigational drugs, on the one hand, and new drug applications, on the other. Bureau leaders, including Kelsey herself, articulated a vision of a more comprehensive process of evaluation in which IND and NDA evaluation overlapped in more synergistic ways. Kelsey would later write that she agreed with this effort, even as she lost some authority in the transition.

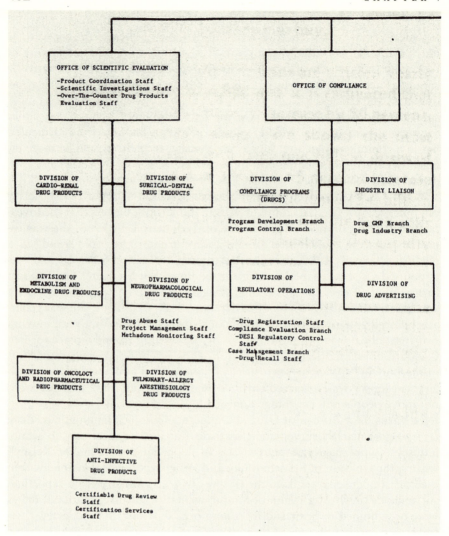

Figure 7.1. Bureau of Drugs Organizational Chart

categories of the time, with cardiology and renal drugs thrown together, oncology and radiopharmaceuticals joined, and surgical and dental products regulated under the same auspices.[23]

The therapeutic division of administrative labor formalized in 1970 set the basis for two more gradual but pivotal developments over the course of the ensuing decades. First, the partitions between review offices became more refined. By 1983, the agency's Center for Drugs and Biologics had established nine offices that reviewed different products, and a decade later the number had jumped to sixteen. This subdivision was not altogether surprising, as it reflected the growing specialization of medicine and of drug development in late twentieth-century American science. Where the subdivision of expertise really mattered was in its coincidence with the diffusion of legal authority. As the number of offices and specialists multiplied, a growing number of federal officials (more and more of them with highly specialized expertise that was less penetrable from above) were empowered with the formal or informal power to govern drug development and approval.[24]

The process of sub-delegation and re-delegation was occurring in numerous agencies from the Kennedy administration through the Reagan administration. The significance of these patterns varied by the power of the organization. Where the authority being re-delegated was that of issuing reports, planning, representing the organization in inter-agency discussions or to Congress, sub-delegation was a re-allocation of labor but not necessarily of power. Within the FDA's Bureau of Drugs and its successor offices, sub-delegation diffused power in its three faces. Entry-level medical officers could affirm and negate new drugs almost entirely on their own, in part because IND and NDA review overlapped to an unprecedented degree. In 1975, review divisions became formally empowered to terminate investigational drugs. The formal authority rested with the division director, but medical reviewers and officers could often induce a firm to abandon its drug before the FDA would need to act. Medical officers and other officials could and did formulate standards and concepts informally that would later become

[23]The new Bureau of Drugs was announced in *FR* 35 (38) (Feb. 25, 1970): 3689–92. It followed a reorganization order of HEW Secretary Robert H. Finch in January 1970 that delegated reorganization authority to the Commissioner, among other officials; *FR* 35 (11) (Jan. 16, 1970): 606–7. Edwards brought management expertise from Booz Allen and tightly controlled the bureaus through a project management system and weekly meetings with each of them; personal communication from Peter Barton Hutt, September 17, 2008.

[24]"[FDA]: Statement of Organization, Functions, and Delegations of Authority," *FR* 38 (99) (May 23, 1973): 13574–7. "National Center for Drugs and Biologics," issued September 2, 1983; copy in FOK. The CDB fused the previously separate organizations of drug review and biologics review, which had long been distinct by virtue of the legal foundations of their authorities (federal authority over biologics stemming from the Biologics Act of 1902). The Office of Drug Research and Review (previously the Bureau of Drugs) housed the review of (1) cardiorenal drugs, (2) neuropharmacological drugs, (3) oncology and radiopharmaceutical drugs, and (4) surgical-dental drugs. The Office of Biologics Research and Review housed the review of (1) blood and blood products, (2) bacterial products, (3) metabolism and endocrine products, (4) anti-infective drugs, and (5) certification (which housed antibiotics review).

formalized, natural, and accepted by the "scientific community." Peter Barton Hutt could later remark, with hyperbole but little inaccuracy, that "the lowest medical reviewer in the FDA has as much power over the future of a pharmaceutical company as does that company's CEO."[25]

The extent of sub-delegation within the Bureau of Drugs—and later in its successors, the Center for Drugs and Biologics and the Center for Drug Evaluation and Research—would emerge more clearly in FDA rules published in 1982, 1984, and 1985. The last of these, often called the "1985 NDA Rewrite," signified the practices of the past and the constraints of the future. As with other federal regulations, these rules were meant to establish policies governing the future behavior of the Administration and the industries it regulates. And, as with other regulations, particularly interpretive regulations, they codified a mass of long prevailing sub-delegation patterns. The FDA rules of the early 1980s appear today less as a vision for the future than as a summary of practices and understandings that had already crystallized. The 1982 proposed rules sought to limit the production of excess data by limiting agency requirements for NDA sponsors to produce "case report tabulations" and "case report forms." These report documents essentially created individual-level data so that Administration officials could replicate statistical analyses or investigate individual outcomes in greater detail. Yet the final rule in 1985 did little to inhibit medical officers' access to disaggregated data. Information from a sponsor's pivotal clinical trials was still required, as were data from any case where an adverse drug experience or death was observed. More than this, the official constraints on case report tabulations and case report forms actually formalized and legitimated their use in new drug review. Two years later, the 1984 rules spelled out patterns of sub-delegation of NDA review; the power of negation and approval for supplemental NDAs was located in directors and deputy division directors of the various drug review divisions. Among many other achievements, the 1985 rules added requirements for comparability of treatment and control groups above and beyond that achieved by randomization. The "rewrite" rules also allowed limited use of foreign data, but left FDA officials with ultimate say in whether such data would be appropriate.[26]

[25]Sub-delegation of IND termination authority appears at *FR* 40 (12) (Jan. 17, 1975): 2979–80. General principles of sub-delegation appear at *FR* 38 (99) (May 23, 1973): 13574–7. The line came from an interview with Hutt at the offices of Covington & Burling in August 2000. Since June 8, 2001 (*FR* 66 (2001): 30992–31025), these provisions of sub-delegation have been embedded within CDER's Manual of Policies and Procedures (MAPP), Guides 1410.102 (IND termination), 1410.104 (NDA Approval), and 1410.106 (refusal and withdrawal of NDA approval), among others.

[26]The proposed rules appear at *FR* 47 (202) (Oct. 19, 1982): 46622–66. See particularly 46642–44 (foreign data) and 46648–9 (CRTs and CRFs). The sub-delegation rules appear at *FR* 49 (74) (April 16, 1984): 14931–5; the proposed rules appeared on March 19. The final rule for the 1985 NDA rewrite appears in *FR* 50 (36) (Feb. 22, 1985): 7452–7519. See particularly 7494–8 (required content and format, CRTs and CRFs, and sub-delegation to review division directors to request additional disaggregated data), 7500–7503 (adverse event report-

As the history of ongoing new drug review reveals, moreover, the rule-making of the early 1980s probably overstated the degree of centralization of power. In crucial cases—the review of beta-blockers, platinum-based chemotherapy, triazolam, and other benzodiazepine tranquilizers—medical reviewers exercised significant "property rights" over new drug applications. Their judgments were not easily, and never quickly, reversed. In this respect, the 1985 NDA rewrite conveyed an impression of NDA drug review that was more hierarchical, more disciplined, more structured, than its factual course in regulatory behavior. Regulatory behavior did not neatly obey the mappings of formal authority and, therefore, neither did regulatory power. The formal trees of hierarchy and the elaboration of standard operating procedures, while not inconsequential, served to elaborate and project an organizational image of rationality and order. In these rules, as Erving Goffman might have read them, the Administration was managing face, showing its legal, congressional, and scientific audiences a portrait of drug evaluation where stability ruled, where formal authority conformed to the boundaries of expertise, but where neither action nor power were so diffuse as to promote chaos.[27]

Patterns of sub-delegation placed greater and greater importance upon the hiring and recruiting practices that were used to fill the positions of Administration officers who exercised ever more authority and power. It was in employment and personnel that Frances Kelsey's influence would persist even as her Division of Scientific Investigations was often ignored. By the late 1970s, two of her hires—Marion J. Finkel and William Gyarfas—held director status and were recipients of the capacities accorded them by the sub-delegation provisions of regulatory practice and federal rule. While Kelsey was no longer involved as centrally in drug review, her many recruits were. Below Finkel and Gyarfas, dozens of physicians and pharmacologists she had hired remained with the agency. This persistence of hires from the early 1960s helped to cement the generational shift from the 1950s and the dominance of clinical pharmacology as a structure of thought and perception in the late twentieth-century FDA.

Whether or not it was Kelsey's influence, women physicians composed a higher fraction of FDA scientists than they did in the nation at large. In 1970, 6–8 percent of American physicians were women, depending on the

---

ing requirements), 7505–7 (foreign data, "approvable letters," and redefinition of "adequate and well-controlled studies" in terms of comparability of treatment and control groups).

[27]The merger of review organization for biologics and drugs was announced on June 22, 1982; *FR* 47 26913. On the difference between interpretive and substantive rules, see Thomas W. Merrill and Kathryn Tongue Watts, "Agency Rules with the Force of Law: The Original Convention," *Harvard Law Review* 116 (2) (Dec. 2002): 467–592. Goffman, *Interaction Ritual: Essays in Face-to-Face Behavior*, particularly the first chapter, "On Face Work" (New Brunswick, NJ: Transaction, 2005 [1967]). The classic interpretation of organizational structure as a legitimating fabric appears in John Meyer and Brian Rowan, "Institutionalized Organizations: Formal Structure as Myth and Ceremony," *American Journal of Sociology* 83 (1977): 340–63.

estimate. At the Bureau of Medicine, over 16 percent of medical officers were women. The Bureau continued to outpace American society and many universities in the fraction of its medical and scientific officers who were women. This may have been because the Bureau was hiring younger physicians, among whom women composed a greater proportion, but it also appears to have been assisted by the hiring of specialist physicians, as it was in general practice where women were most outnumbered at the time.[28]

The persistence of these early cohorts and the common identity they shared did not necessarily engender an amicable setting. Just as internecine conflicts between skeptical drug reviewers and pressure-impinged office directors had characterized the late 1950s, such battles suffused the 1960s and 1970s as well. Perhaps the most infamous of these struggles became public when consumer advocates, journalists, and Senator Edward Kennedy publicized the demotion of medical officers John Nestor and John Winkler from the Bureau of Drugs in 1974. Nestor had arrived to the agency in 1961 and was clearly aligned with the reform cohort of the late 1950s, including Frances Kelsey. He was outspoken and showed neither deference nor respect to the pharmaceutical companies who brought their new drug application to his bureau. Nestor had once famously asserted that "I have never found an honest drug company—although I haven't dealt with all of them. Even those who would like to be honest find out that they are all at a competitive disadvantage and can't afford to be." His reputation for extreme skepticism was earned, and it was widespread through the pharmaceutical world. "The Pink Sheet" trade reporter would continually refer to him as "John 'I've Never Met an Honest Drug Company' Nestor."[29]

[28]Calculated by author from Medical Officer list in FDA, *Bureau of Drugs Weekly*, Special Edition, May 1, 1972; copy in FOK. For gender composition of American physicians in 1970, see AMA Women Physicians' Congress, *Women in Medicine: Celebrating our Past, Present and Future*, 25th Anniversary Presentation (Chicago: AMA, 2002). This estimate is repeated in John Dorschner, "Growing Number of Female Doctors Changing Medical Profession," *Miami Herald*, March 23, 2003; for a slightly larger estimate, see Perri Klass, "Are Women Better Doctors?" *NYT*, April 12, 1988. Figures on gender composition in 1981 refer to a slightly different sample, namely Bureau of Drugs personnel with advanced degrees (M.D., Ph.D., or a doctoral equivalent), of whom 21.7% were women. Daniel Carpenter and Susan Moffitt, CDER Personnel database, 1981–99 (Harvard University).

[29]When reports of birth deformities began to flow in from Europe, Nestor had arranged the pivotal meeting between Kelsey and Johns Hopkins pediatrician Helen Taussig. Nestor also testified before the Fountain committee in the early 1960s. For a detailed (if somewhat one-sided) account of the controversy over Nestor and Winkler, see Sidney Wolfe and Anita Johnson, "Conflict Against the Public Interest at the Bureau of Drugs," F 7 ("Bureau of Drugs, 1971–1973, n.d."), B12, FOK. Hilts' account (*Protecting America's Health*, 187–90) of the Nestor-Winkler demotions is nuanced and compelling, but like Wolfe's it misses the Bureau's uneasy position at the nexus of different audiences — consumer safety advocates, clinical researchers (particularly cardiologists and oncologists), demands from different legislators for stringent regulation of safety risks and for reduced regulatory burdens (not only upon drug companies but also upon clinical researchers). The call for relaxed standards was coming not only from "business," the "industry," and "conservatives." It was also coming from important audiences in medicine (e.g., oncology and the National Cancer Institute; see chapter 6) and,

Nestor's aggressive and shrill demeanor brought renewed conflicts with his superiors when the Bureau of Drugs was organized in 1970. The reorganization and its attendant patterns of sub-delegation gave medical reviewers even more formal authority than they had enjoyed in the mid-1960s, and Nestor was not shy about using this authority. At the same time, the more business-friendly Nixon administration was beginning to have an imprint in upper-level appointments, and two Charles Edwards appointees, Henry Simmons and J. Richard Crout, were running the Bureau of Drugs. Beginning in 1971, Simmons and Crout, joined by a Nixon political appointee named George Leong and a rapidly rising personality from the early 1960s cohort, Marion J. Finkel, began to challenge Nestor's decisions and his deportment. In 1972 and 1973, Nestor and Winkler were abruptly shuttled from the Cardio-Renal Division to other work. The official reason, widely doubted among investigators of the controversy, was that Nestor was "needed elsewhere," namely in the Office of Compliance. Around the same time, as many as eleven other medical officers were also transferred.[30]

When Massachusetts Senator Edward Kennedy held hearings in August 1974, the Nestor-Winkler controversy was soon broadcast upon a Washington-wide canvas, albeit one overshadowed by President Nixon's resignation that same month. At Kennedy's hearings, nine medical officers testified to a pattern of asymmetric oversight from Bureau of Drugs superiors: when they recommended approval of an NDA, they saw no challenge from Crout, Finkel, and Simmons, but where they counseled rejection or delay of an application, their recommendations were sometimes overruled. When they questioned the overruling decisions, these medical officers alleged, they were on occasion removed from review of the drug in question. They also claimed that they were subjected to patterns of "harassment." Kennedy's hearings combined with other allegations to create a public relations crisis for Administration leaders, and Commissioner Alexander Schmidt quickly announced an investigation into the matter, overseen by a congressionally appointed panel. Schmidt's report offered a sanguine portrait of his Bureau—there were conflicts but no improper drug approvals, no systematic bias in favor of industry or new drugs. The congressionally appointed panel overseeing Schmidt's investigation reached a somewhat different conclusion. From 1970 onward, the Panel concluded, the Bureau had taken a stance "less adversarial towards and more cooperative with drug manufacturers," and tried "to neutralize

---

indeed, from Democrats in Congress (e.g., Sen. Edward Long and, by 1978, Edward Kennedy himself).

[30]Abraham, "Scientific Standards and Institutional Interests," 441–2; Hilts, *Protecting America's Health*, 188–9. Simmons was appointed personally by Edwards in 1971 with Crout's appointment as Deputy Director of the Bureau coming the same year; *DRR* (July 9, 1980): 18; Crout Oral History, NLM. See also records in B6, F 14, CCE. Finkel had been Deputy Director before Crout and remained in various leadership positions in the Bureau in the 1970s before heading up the Office of New Drug Evaluation in the early 1980s; *DTN*, February 22, 1971, 51.

reviewing medical officers who followed a different philosophy." These patterns of behavior were described as part of an explicit and conscious policy, a "program."

> The program to neutralize the more adversarial reviewers was carried out by various devices, including a systematic pattern of involuntary transfers to positions which the incumbents did not want, and, in a few cases, removal from the review of particular drugs. FDA management generally concealed the truth about the reasons for the transfers from the persons affected.[31]

The Nestor-Winkler controversy has been interpreted in various ways by its chroniclers—as a part of "Partisan Politics," as evidence for "partial industry capture"—but the episode speaks more to complications than to a world bifurcated by alliance to party or to industry. To be sure, Nestor's demotion occurred in a world of sharp antagonism between Nixon administration Republicans and congressional Democrats, and the medical officer's prickly carriage was not irrelevant. Yet in important ways the controversy of the early 1970s was also suffused by the politics of disease and therapeutic specialty. Nestor worked in the Cardio-Pulmonary Division (later called the Cardio-Renal Division), and his outfit was handling investigational new drugs for hypertension and arrhythmia, not least the class of new compounds known as beta-blockers. Nestor was particularly concerned that cardiovascular drugs had not demonstrated sufficient safety in animals; Finkel and Crout disagreed on scientific grounds and saw larger problems in Nestor's regulatory approach. Crout had been a Clinical Associate at the NIH Heart Institute in the late 1950s, so had credible expertise in cardiology drugs. In terms of the risk-benefit trade-offs that Crout and Finkel had witnessed from the 1950s and 1960s, moreover, the beta-blockers promised in their view a clear advance over previous medicines. All this while beta-blockers had become the exemplar molecules to which FDA critics—not only conservatives but also cardiologists—gestured. Most of the beta-blockers had been available in Great Britain five to ten years before their approval in the United States.[32]

---

[31]For contemporaneous coverage of the hearings, see "Kennedy's Investigation of FDA Continuing with 3-Man Team that Hit Headline 'Paydirt' at Aug. 15 Hearing," *FD&CR*, September 2, 1974, 3–5, 7–8. For later publications and reports, see Alexander M. Schmidt, *The Commissioner's Report of Investigation of Charges from Joint Hearings (Summary)* (Washington, DC: GPO, 1975), 901. Review Panel on New Drug Regulation, *Summary of Special Counsel's Conclusions* (Washington, DC: GPO, 1977); this is also known as the "Dorsen Report." Special Counsel to Review Panel on New Drug Regulation, *Investigation of Allegations Relating to the Bureau of Drugs, Food and Drug Administration* (Washington, DC: Department of Health and Welfare, April 1977). The Review Panel, appointed by HEW Secretary F. David Mathews, also alleged improper action by Senator Kennedy in conducting the hearings, namely that those testifying were misled about the eventual questions and subject of their testimony.

[32]Hilts describes the controversy in a chapter entitled "Partisan Politics," while Abraham ("Scientific Standards and Institutional Interests," 427) argues that "key regulatory personnel at the FDA have assimilated some of the perspectives of the pharmaceutical industry," so much so that "the agency may be *partially* 'captured' by the industry" (emphasis in original). For

POLITICS OF NEW DRUG REVIEW

The Nestor-Winkler transfers demonstrate as well that the power of medical reviewers in the age of sub-delegation was not merely technical and procedural, but reputational and political. Senator Kennedy's 1974 hearings occurred not exogenously, but after consumer safety activists Sidney Wolfe and Anita Johnson had publicized the transfers, and after Nestor and other reviewers had taken their case to Wolfe, to journalists, and to Congress. In the American regulatory world of the 1970s, where consumer safety interests were better organized than before and where congressional committees were highly decentralized, medical reviewers constrained from above could "go public." The complex of networks and audiences in which the Administration's organizational image was suspended also provided retreats and shelter for the more aggressive and spirited regulators within the agency.[33]

So too, Nestor's demotion gestured as much to the formal power of the FDA medical officer as to the weakness of that position. One solution to Nestor's behavior, after all, was to continually overrule him and remove drugs from his purview. Nothing in the regulations prevented Simmons, Crout, and Finkel from doing this, and indeed they sometimes engaged in these practices. Yet the transfer of Nestor, Winkler, and other reviewers—and their replacement by anonymous officers—was a tacit acknowledgment that supervision from above could not entirely control recalcitrant officers below. Once in place, medical reviewers had significant authority and discretion in individual decisions. In order to stabilize the division under their purview, Crout and Finkel needed something well beyond the powers that their formal authorities had bequeathed to them. They needed new people in positions that embedded broad discretion.

The congressional review panel later charged that Nestor was transferred in order to break up the Cardio-Renal Division, because the Division displayed "pronounced anti-industry bias" and brought "constant complaints

---

summary numbers on the delayed introduction of beta-blockers in the United States as compared to Europe (particularly the United Kingdom), see William M. Wardell and Louis Lasagna, *Regulation and Drug Development*, (Washington, DC: American Enterprise Institute, 1975), 60 (chap. 7, table 2). On the review of beta-blockers such as Inderal in the Division at the time, see Wolfe and Johnson, "Conflict Against the Public Interest at the Bureau of Drugs," 12; also Daemmrich, *Pharmacopolitics*, chap. 4. The interpretation here is not that Nestor's criticisms of the beta-blockers and other molecules were clearly wrong or unfounded. The claim instead is that credible audiences other than Wardell and Lasagna, in clinical circles, and the PMA, in industrial circles, were critical of the Cardio-Renal division and its actions. The politics of reputation was multidimensional, and the actions of Simmons, Crout, and Finkel were undertaken to address numerous public and private audiences. In the end, none of these audiences came away well satisfied, a fact which implies in some measure that none of them dominated the agency.

[33] Wolfe and Johnson, "Conflict Against the Public Interest at the Bureau of Drugs," F 7 ("Bureau of Drugs, 1971–1973, n.d."), B12, FOK. Hilts beautifully renders the intricate political construction of the Nestor-Winkler controversy and the Kennedy hearings (*Protecting America's Health*, 189). The notion of "going public" comes from studies in the U.S. presidency in political science; see the classic work of Sam Kernell, *Going Public: New Strategies of Presidential Leadership* (Washington, DC: CQ Press, 1986).

from industry." This is part of the explanation, but not all of it. The affair
was never so simple as an array of Nixon appointees and "industry-friendly"
FDA superiors versus the scientists and the Kelsey regime. For one, Crout
and Finkel were not industry loyalists. Their careers matched well with
other members of the pharmacological regime of the 1950s and early 1960s.
Finkel was hired in 1963 by Ralph Smith, and arrived just months before
Kelsey hired William Gyarfas, Phyllis Huene, and Theresa Woo. Crout came
to the agency not from industry but from the NIH—where he worked with
luminaries Albert Sjoerdsma and Sidney Udenfriend—and as director of
clinical pharmacology at the University of Texas Southwestern Medical
School. For another, the transfer itself was multidimensional, as was its public justification. Crout would later admit that he and Finkel did have organizational and philosophical reasons for transferring Nestor, but given the
scrutiny received by the Bureau, the least important reason for the transfers
became their public validation. As a matter of procedure, just one "valid"
rationale was sufficient for the transfer. As a matter of reputation, Crout
and Finkel did not wish to expose the messy scientific politics internal to the
Administration.[34]

Issues of reputation had also figured in Sidney Wolfe's investigation into
the Nestor-Winkler affair. Wolfe was at the time establishing himself as the
premier consumer activist critic of the Administration's drug programs; in
effect he represented one of the agency's more opaque audiences. Moreover,
Wolfe's vision of consumer protection rested in part upon an understanding
that the FDA's reputation itself would enhance the agency's consumer protection work. To the extent that the Administration was believed to behave
with neutrality, scientific commitment, and pursuit of public interest, Wolfe
thought, its essential tasks would be more successfully attained. Appearances of "conflict of interest," on the other hand, would cast "a shadow" on
"the integrity of the entire agency." Wolfe's vision of consumer protection
was one including substantial redelegation of the tasks of the agency to its
medical officers, who would stand institutionally apart from the regulated
industries and who would form the nation's bulwark against hazardous
drugs. "FDA staff functions must be rigidly protected from the influences of
special interest groups," he warned. "Medical officers must be left in peace
to evaluate the data, without the influences of insinuating friendships and
unspoken threats of appeal to superior officers."[35]

The final, perhaps determinative complication was that of inter-branch
tension. The Nestor-Winkler controversy and the Dorsen report were played
out in a setting of stark institutional hostility. The year 1974 was the height

[34]Finkel arrived to the Bureau of Medicine in May 1963; "Bureau of Medicine: Probationary and Temporary Medical Officers," April 12, 1964, FOK. On Crout's career, see Crout Oral
History, NLM. Crout essentially admits in this interview that issues of philosophical disagreement and personal behavior were involved in the transfer, but maintains that he was compelled
to provide only one "valid reason" for the transfer, not all of the reasons.

[35]Wolfe and Johnson, "Conflict Against the Public Interest at the Bureau of Drugs," 15, 17.

of the Watergate scandal, a struggle far more than partisan and indeed a battle of great and precedent-setting proportions between the executive and legislative branches of American government. Edwards and Schmidt were Nixon appointees, and by most accounts Schmidt was more industry-friendly than his predecessor. Most visible Nixon appointees of the early 1970s were subject to searching congressional and public scrutiny, but Schmidt's relationship with Congress was even more confrontational than Edwards' had been. In this respect, the controversies at the early 1970s FDA should be read and remembered in light of the larger pattern of conflict between a particularly assertive executive branch and a particularly distrustful legislature. So too, testimony from current and former government officials, speaking openly against their superiors, was a common refrain in congressional hearings of the time. And Nestor's willingness to speak directly with journalists, with activist groups, and with Congress was an evolving pattern of subterfuge among federal bureaucrats in the early 1970s, a pattern best exemplified in the Watergate scandal.[36]

For their part, Crout and Finkel would go on to take some of the more risky postures and launch some of the more aggressive initiatives in the history of American pharmaceutical regulation. Crout became Director of the Bureau of Drugs in 1973, and Finkel became Director of the New Drug Evaluation Division. It was Crout who hired Robert Temple—who would become the agency's (and the nation's, if not the world's) clinical trials guru—from the NIH in 1972. It was Crout and Finkel who collaborated with William Beaver in their assertive effort to define "adequate and well-controlled investigations" in terms of randomized clinical trials with a placebo arm. Crout and Finkel oversaw the promulgation of new regulations governing institutional review boards, regulations that met with strong criticism from medical researchers around the world. Crout directed much of the Administration's response to Laetrile, and he defended his Bureau against the charges of testy oncologists at the NCI. In 1977, Crout and Finkel introduced a priority ranking system for drugs: an "A"-"B"-"C" ranking system that scored drugs by their degree of innovation over existing medicines. This system received many criticisms from industry representatives, who argued that the therapeutic marketplace and not the Administration ought to rank drug effectiveness. Yet the A-B-C scoring system prevailed for more than a decade, and created a logic of differentiating more important "priority" drugs that persists to this day.[37]

[36] On the larger conflicts, see James Sundquist, *The Decline and Resurgence of Congress* (Washington, DC: Brookings Institution Press, 1981). Keith Whittington and Daniel Carpenter, "Executive Power in American Institutional Development," *Perspectives on Politics* 1 (3) (Sept. 2003): 495–513. In a statement that would be widely quoted, Schmidt had chided Congress for criticizing only questionable approvals, not questionable non-approvals and delays.

[37] On the IND regulations and the criticism they received, see "FDA's Preference for Placebo Controls in Concept Papers Could Evolve into 'Rigid' Regulatory 'Hierarchy,' Squibb Exec Asserts at Public Forum on Regs," *DRR* 22 (46) (Nov. 14, 1979): 8; "NRC-FDA Radiopharmaceutical Regulatory Officials to Meld," *DRR* 22 (46) RN-3. On the ranking system, see

The Administration under Charles Edwards and his appointees, moreover, hardly behaved as an industry stand-in. Edwards and Simmons completed the initiative to promulgate stringent rules governing fixed-combination drugs in 1971. Crout took the lead in removing older drugs from the market under the Drug Efficacy Study; while most of the NAS/NRC studies had been completed before Crout's arrival, many of the messy drug removals had not. Another Edwards appointee, General Counsel Peter Barton Hutt, led the legal charge for more aggressive agency enforcement and interpretive powers. For his part, Crout hired not only Robert Temple from NIH, but also James Bilstead, who would later run the agency's biologics evaluation programs. Neither Bilstead nor Temple would emerge as soft regulators. The tensions of the early 1970s are well understood not merely in the context of industry-government antagonism, but also in terms of a battle over the decentralization of authority in the agency. Increasingly, formal and informal authority diffused downward, coming to rest partially among the medical officers and principally in the middle layer represented by the Bureau of Drugs Director and the directors and deputy directors of the review offices. Nestor and Winkler were governed from above, no doubt, but Alexander Schmidt, Donald Kennedy, Jere Goyan, and future FDA Commissioners in the 1980s and 1990s became increasingly bound by decisions "below."[38]

Patterns: Administration, Organization, Interpretation

American pharmaceutical regulation settled into something of a procedural equilibrium in the 1970s and early 1980s. No one at the time would have confused this equilibrium with a happy stasis, for the Administration was continually buffeted by criticism from numerous sources, and legal and political challenges to the agency's authority continued apace. Yet for a number of reasons—some related to overt politics surrounding the Administration, others having more to do with varying degrees of consensus among some scientific communities about efficacy standards and clinical trial procedures—the weekly and monthly rhythms of new drug review were as steady

---

Crout Oral History, NLM. Robert Temple would also play a role in the definition of adequate and well-controlled trials through the issuance of guidance documents in the 1970s through the 1990s.

[38]On fixed-combination rules, see "Stringent Rules for Combinations Issued by FDA," *DTN*, February 22, 1971, 25. In the continuing implementation of the Drug Efficacy Study in the late 1970s and early 1980s, authority for revocation or withdrawal shifted from the Commissioner to the Director of the Bureau of Drugs (this was later codified in 21 CFR 5.82; *FR* 49 (74) (April 16, 1984):14935). See for example the withdrawal of approval for NDA 4-681, Ciba-Geigy's Trasentine-Phenobarbital Tablets, *FR* 45 (13) (Jan. 18, 1980): 3670–71. For a theoretical understanding of the importance of middle-level officials in a differentiated bureaucracy, see Daniel Carpenter, *The Forging of Bureaucratic Autonomy: Reputations, Networks and Policy Innovation in Executive Agencies, 1862–1928* (Princeton: Princeton University Press, 2001), chap. 1.

at this time as any other in the past half-century. The procedural stability of this era—expressed in and continued by the NDA rewrites of 1982 and 1985—had the additional effect of shaping patterns of review that would endure for decades afterward.[39]

The Administration's veto power over new drug applications rested at the core of the procedural equilibrium. In order for the various faces of regulatory power to work, the agency would have to negate an appreciable fraction of new drug applications. If approval became so happily predictable as to become perceivably deserved, the incentives for drug companies to conduct exhaustive, careful, and clinical trials would vanish. Every NDA that was withdrawn or rejected as "not approvable" converted sponsors' hope and energies—millions of dollars in experiment, thousands of hours of time, millions or billions in financial asset prices that reflected judgments about the regulatory as well as commercial viability of the drug—into expenditure that was vastly depreciated or altogether wasted. Vetoes could happen for numerous reasons, but functionally they occurred whenever (1) the Administration declared an application "incomplete" or refused to file it for consideration, (2) the Administration issued a "not approvable" letter to the sponsor, or (3) the sponsor withdrew the application. The last of these outcomes—abandonment of the NDA—was not the official doing of the FDA but was often induced by doubts raised among FDA officials as to the submission or one or more parts therein. In 1962, an estimated 30 percent of all new drug applications were withdrawn or were terminated as incomplete. Many of these would ultimately be resubmitted and perhaps approved, but the lost time meant lost money and added uncertainty. And by 1995, the General Accounting Office estimated that nearly half of all NDAs submitted in the previous decade had not been approved.[40]

Matters were somewhat more generous for what the Administration called "new molecular entities" (NMEs), or those drugs that had never before been marketed in the United States in whole or in part. NMEs were then and remain now the lifeblood of the industry, as they carry the greatest patent protection against competition. For these drugs, which had been the focus of much of the debate about the drug lag, approval rates were higher, in part because their applications reflected much more research, in part because they often targeted diseases characterizing "unmet medical need," and not least because criticism of the agency focused on the number of new NMEs entering the market per year as a measure of the health of the

[39]The final rules for the NDA rewrite came in 1985; the 1982 rules were proposed rules but had the effect of announcing in print what was already stable in practice.

[40]For a highly simplified mathematical model of regulatory vetoes as creating incentives for research on new products, see Daniel Carpenter and Michael M. Ting, "Regulatory Errors with Endogenous Agendas," *American Journal of Political Science* 51 (4) (Oct. 2007): 835–52. "Safety and Skepticism: Thalidomide," *Modern Medicine*, October 15, 1962, p. 26. GAO, *FDA Drug Review Time Has Decreased in Recent Years* (Washington, DC: GAO, 1995).

pharmaceutical industry and an index of the Administration's "performance." The issuance of "refusal-to-file" judgments for new molecular entities became increasingly rare as firms adapted to FDA requirements. Nonetheless, an appreciable fraction of NME applications failed in their "first try" at the review process (figure 7.2). For NME applications submitted from 1976 to 1998, the annual percentage that were withdrawn or deemed "not approvable" ranged from 6 percent to 31 percent, with an average of 16.8 percent. For any given year, then, about one in six submitted NMEs failed in the review process, and most of these failures were withdrawals (10.1 percent of NME submissions, or 60 percent of those not receiving approval).[41]

The other primary dimension of variation was the time taken to review the drug. Here comparison is more difficult because the Administration has not consistently published review times for NDAs not receiving approval. Reasonably complete data are available, however, for approved drugs. The Administration's responsibilities in evaluating drugs grew significantly in the wake of the 1962 law. Its resources also grew, but more slowly and unpredictably. In 1965, the Bureau of Medicine was reviewing over one thousand new investigational drug plans per year and was applying stringent new standards of evaluation to new drug applications. The FDA's budget had tripled in the six years preceding the 1962 Amendments. Yet from 1967 to 1972, the agency lost authorization for over four hundred employees; and hiring in the Bureau of Drugs stagnated. There were also inefficiencies as the agency adapted to the new rules and as drug sponsors acclimated to new standards of development.

The upshot of this mismatch between responsibilities and resources and learning was an extended administrative delay in the review of new drugs. For new molecular entities—the sort of medicine that observers regarded as the definition of innovation—median approval times rose from just under sixteen months for drugs submitted in 1962 to more than thirty-three months for drugs submitted in 1966. Review times then stabilized in the late 1960s, and the annual average approval time generally stayed between eighteen to twenty-four months from 1967 to 1981.

Resource constraints and the adaptation of regulators and sponsors to new standards, then, render over-time comparisons problematic. Among the population of ever-lengthening drug reviews conducted by the Administration, however, there were significant and telling differences in the time to

---

[41]The comparison is limited by the data available. The Administration does not regularly publish data on non-approved NDAs, but did so for a twenty-year period from 1976 to 1998 when its drug reviewing division issued annual reports with summaries of non-approved drugs; see for example *New Drug Evaluation Statistical Report*, 1987 (Rockville, MD: FDA, April 1987; reproduced by National Technical Information Service, Department of Commerce).

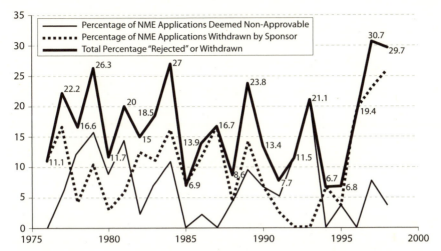

Figure 7.2. Percentage of NME Applications "Rejected" or Withdrawn,
1976–1998

approval. These data suggest important differences prevailed among drugs,
most prominently by therapeutic category.[42]

The most notable change in the wake of the 1962 Amendments was a
dramatic lengthening of review time for new molecular entities. Examination of NMEs approved from 1950 through 1986 suggests that the set of
transitions surrounding the 1962 law and the 1963 rules was associated
with the addition of twelve to fifteen months to the average review time,
which climbed from approximately six months to an average of two years
by the end of the period. It is, however, difficult to assign a causal role in
this deceleration to the 1962 Amendments or the 1963 rules, much less to
any specific feature of them. For one thing, the lengthening of approval
times for NMEs was a continuous process that had begun in the mid-1950s
with the assertion of standards by the pharmacological regime in the FDA's
Bureau of Medicine. This had occurred even as the agency's resources tripled in the years following the 1955 Citizens' Advisory Committee report.
Depending upon the measurement, median approval times had risen from
about three months for each NME in the early 1950s to nearly one year for
each NME by 1961 and 1962. For another, a larger set of pharmacological
standards was being elaborated in the 1960s, including the rise of randomized clinical trials, placebo controls, and more sophisticated statistical measurements. Some of these were advanced by the Bureau of Medicine, but
more generally they were developments that occurred at the intersection of

[42]Some of the more striking and persistent differences among firms and noncommercial
sponsors, as well as some variables which seem to account statistically for some of these differences, are examined in chapter 10.

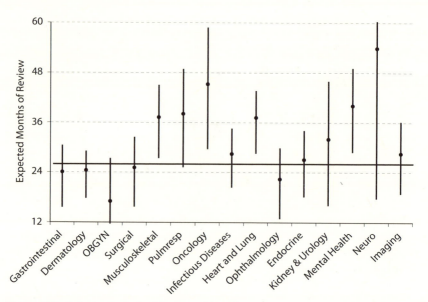

Figure 7.3. Relative Speed of Approval by Therapeutic Category, Approved NMEs Submitted 1962–1985. [Note: Bold dot indicates estimated average review time for category, and vertical lines encompass 95%confidence intervals.]

science, regulation, and more progressive elements of the pharmaceutical industry.[43]

From the 1962 Amendments to the completion of the NDA rewrite in 1985, the average NME approval time was about two years (25.2 months). As figure 7.3 shows, however, it was appreciably higher for drugs in several therapeutic categories, most notably medicines for pulmonary and respiratory conditions (37 months of NME review), musculoskeletal conditions (38 months), and cardiovascular conditions (37 months), and much higher for anticancer drugs (an average of 45 months of NME review) and mental health therapies (40 months). It merits comment, however, that it is impossible in statistical examination to control for the relative safety and efficacy of these

[43]The statistical "effect" estimates of 12 to 15 months for the set of events in 1962 and 1963 is retrieved from parametric duration regressions of NME approval times upon a set of covariates, including random effects for each primary indication of the NME. The estimates are larger for Weibull duration models (which embed an assumption of monotonic duration dependence) than for lognormal duration models (which embed an assumption of non-monotonic duration dependence). The 1962 effects are statistically significant in more flexible semi-parametric Cox hazard models as well, but these models are not well equipped for the expression of marginal effects in terms of additional months of approval time. The Cox models suggest that the changes beginning in 1962 were associated with a 67 percent decline in the month-to-month approval rate of drugs ($p < 0.0001$), with a 95 percent (model-dependent) probability of the estimate lying between 75 percent decline to 55 percent decline.

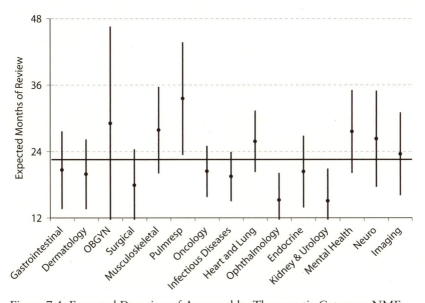

Figure 7.4. Expected Duration of Approval by Therapeutic Category, NMEs Submitted 1986–2004 [Note: Bold dot indicates estimated average review time for category, and vertical lines encompass 95% confidence intervals.]

drugs. It is therefore impossible to rule out the hypothesis that the variations in review time were being driven by the particular quality of evidence adduced for each drug.[44]

In the two decades following the NDA rewrite, these differences by therapeutic category waned (figure 7.4). One reason was that the mean review time had declined by six to nine months, mainly as a result of increased staffing at the agency. As the average review got smaller, so too did the variance of review time across drugs, and differences among therapeutic categories waned accordingly. Yet meaningful reductions occurred in the review of cancer drugs, with a drop of almost two years in average review time from the pre-1985 period to the last two decades. Among other therapeutic categories, musculoskeletal, pulmonary/respiratory, cardiovascular, and mental health drugs still had review times significantly longer than the average.

One feature of therapeutic categories is that they are subject to varying degrees of public attention, not least coverage in the national media or in

[44]These averages are retrieved as statistical estimates from parametric duration models (the Weibull, with similar effects from a log-normal model). The models control for important covariates of review time, including a linear time trend, the number of staff in the FDA's drug-reviewing bureau, and the order of entry of the drug into its therapeutic class. The models also control for the submitting firm as a random effect.

congressional hearings. A reputation-based perspective suggests that this coverage enacts an audience pressure on regulatory organizations. Much as the Administration reacted quickly and decisively to the pressure of AIDS activists and the National Cancer Institute, the agency has generally accelerated its drug review processes where the drug in question is intended to treat a disease with greater public attention. One rough measure of public attention comes in the stories run by major newspapers—the *Washington Post*, the *Wall Street Journal*, and the *New York Times*. Statistical estimates displayed in figure 7.5 suggest that for every one standard-deviation increase in the four-year moving average of *Washington Post* stories on a drug's primary indication over the period 1976 to 1998, the associated FDA review time for that drug was nine to eleven months shorter. This relationship prevails in the presence of controls for severity of the disease, FDA staffing resources, political and partisan oversight of the agency, orphan drug status, and other covariates of approval time.[45]

Another dimension of observed response to public attention comes in the Administration's decision of whether or not to formally consult one of its many advisory committees. The decision to do so often eases many later approval or rejection decisions, insofar as the agency's committees have already pronounced their judgment on the matter and so the agency's choice has not been made. Observers of FDA advisory committees often detect that the Administration chooses to invite an advisory panel's judgment when the case before the agency is scientifically or politically more difficult. The statistical estimates presented in figure 7.6 add support to this characterization. For every one standard-deviation increase in the four-year moving average of *Washington Post* stories on a drug's primary indication over the period 1992 to 2004, the associated probability of pre-market advisory committee consultation increased by six percentage points. It is important to realize that, when an advisory committee is called into action on a new drug review before the drug is approved, the drug review necessarily gets slower; the association between increased media coverage of disease and FDA advisory panel consultation (figure 7.6) becomes all the more salient when viewed in light of the association between media coverage and reduced NME approval times.[46]

[45] For an examination of varying amounts of media coverage to disease conditions, see Elizabeth Armstrong, Daniel Carpenter, and Marie Hojnacki, "Whose Deaths Matter? Mortality, Advocacy, and Attention to Disease in the Mass Media," *Journal of Health Policy, Politics and Law* 31(4) (2006): 729–72. For the Administration's response to publicly salient disease communities, see chapter 6 and Carpenter, "Groups, the Media, Agency Waiting Costs and FDA Drug Approval," *American Journal of Political Science* 46 (3) (July 2002): 490–505, from which these results are taken.

[46] The argument that patterns of FDA advisory committee consultation reflect legitimacy and reputational considerations is well established, primarily by Sheila Jasanoff, *The Fifth Branch: Science Advisors as Policymakers* (Cambridge: Harvard University Press, 1994), chap. 8, esp. 154–65. See also Susan I. Moffitt, *Inviting Outsiders In: The Political Economy of Federal*

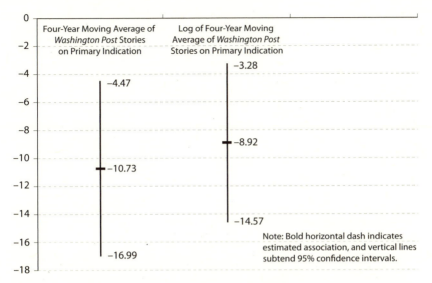

Figure 7.5. Change in NME Review Time (months) for Every Standardized Increase in Media Coverage of NME's Primary Indication Disease, 1976–1998

Beyond differentiating molecules from one another, therapeutic categories also provided for comparisons of each new drug to those that had already been approved. Over the past half-century, the order of entry into a therapeutic class has been consistently and positively associated with longer review times, such that the first few drugs to treat a given medical condition receive quicker review times than "later" therapies. The behavioral and organizational mechanisms that contribute to this relationship are numerous—later entrants to a therapeutic class are less likely to receive "priority" ratings that designate a drug as deserving of scarce resources and quick action, more likely to receive intense scrutiny because other treatments for the condition exist, and less likely to be accompanied by intense patient advocate pressure. In terms of expected approval time (figure 7.7), the first four entrants to a therapeutic class averaged 13.2 months of approval time, while the eleventh through the fourteenth entrants to a therapeutic class averaged 17.9 months. Additional statistical examination suggests that the pattern depicted in figure 7.7 follows not a strictly linear trend but rather a log-linear relationship. In other words, the review time advantage of an approved drug over the next few entrants grows smaller

Agency Advice (Ph.D. diss., University of Michigan, 2003); I acknowledge Susan Moffitt for providing me with the data used for this analysis; I assume all responsibility for any errors and interpretations with the data.

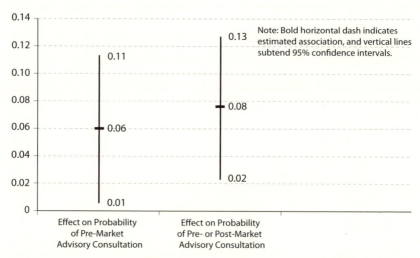

Figure 7.6. Change in Probability of Pre-Market Advisory Committee Consultation for Every Standardized Increase in Media Coverage of NME's Primary Indication Disease, 1992–2004

over time, such that the earliest drugs in a therapeutic class not only have quicker approval rates, they also have larger relative advantages relative to their followers.[47]

Over the past half-century, the pattern by which one approved drug displaced the medical need and reputational pressure for others in its therapeutic category was robust. Yet early-entrant advantage also varied markedly by therapeutic category in ways that aggregate statistics can conceal. Put differently, the displacement of later drugs by earlier ones was more severe for some therapies than for others. Table 7.3 displays these variable relationships as "elasticities," such that an estimate of 0.5 implies that a 10 percent increase in order of entry is associated with a 5 percent increase in NME approval time. The higher the elasticity for the therapeutic category, the greater the extent to which one approved drug displaced the need or

[47]The parameters in figure 7.5 are jointly estimated and drawn from a Cox proportional hazards model in which statistical controls are included for the year of submission (as a linear time trend) and the number of staff in the FDA's drug-reviewing bureau. For details on the data and estimation, see Daniel Carpenter, et al., "Early Entrant Protection in Approval Regulation: Theory and Evidence from FDA Drug Review," *Journal of Law, Economics and Organization* 26 (2) (Fall 2010) [doi:10.1093/jleo/ewp002]. In addition, the equation adds a random effect (or "frailty") for each of 194 primary indications. The joint estimation of these parameters means that, under reasonable assumptions about their joint posterior distribution, the parameters can be compared statistically. The differences in expected approval time are retrieved from a Weibull duration model. The difference between the expected approval time of the first four entrants and the expected approval time of the eleventh through fourteenth entrants is statistically significant ($\chi^2(1) = 5.46$; $p = 0.0195$). In separate Cox proportional hazards models, the first three drugs to enter a therapeutic class generally had a month-to-month approval rate three times as high as an NDA representing the fourteenth or twentieth entrant into a class.

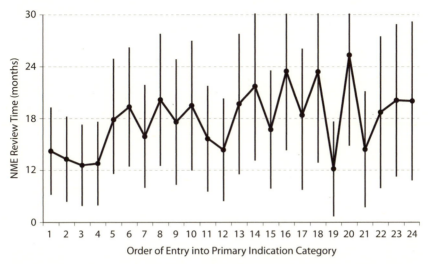

Figure 7.7. Average Approval Times by Order of Entry, 1962–2000 [Note: Bold dot indicates estimated average review time for entry order, and vertical lines encompass 95% confidence intervals.]

pressure for a later one targeting the same disease. There was nothing perfectly systematic about those therapeutic categories bearing the highest elasticities—antibiotics and other anti-infective drugs, drugs for depression, thrombosis, or anti-stroke medications, cardiovascular medications for congestive heart failure and arrhythmia, and anti-inflammatories. Yet the estimates are broadly consistent with narrative evidence of particular drug reviews where the set of previously approved drugs served to constrain the perceived necessity or political demand for new therapies.[48]

The comparison set defined by available drugs in a therapeutic category figured in different ways, but almost always pivotally. A pattern of regulatory advantage for early entrants to a category defined by the drug's primary indication arose and persisted across the four decades following the 1962 Amendments. The pattern of early-entrant advantage suggests that, despite the absence of an affirmative mandate to compare efficacy across drugs, the Administration found it impossible to avoid implicit efficacy comparisons of new drugs with their previously approved rivals. Yet the pattern also points to

[48]It important here to acknowledge a basic limitation of the measurements used in the statistical estimation generating figure 7.5. The measurement differentiates by primary indication disease, but not by the basic mechanism of the drug. So, for example, tricyclic antidepressants (imipramine or amitriptyline) are lumped together with selective serotonin reuptake inhibitors (SSRIs, such as fluoxetine) under the therapeutic category "depression" or "anti-depression drugs." To some degree these drugs are differentiated by their submission at different times so that controlling for linear trends and other historical variables helps to differentiate them partially. The estimates also control for cross-drug measures of safety and efficacy constructed from medical literature; see Carpenter, et al., "Early Entrant Protection in Approval Regulation."

TABLE 7.3.
Disease-Specific Entry-Order Gradients, Expressed as Elasticities
(Robust standard errors in parentheses)

Disease [# of molecules]	Elasticity	Disease [# of molecules]	Elasticity
Arthritis [8]	**−3.5449** (0.5379)	Bacterial infections [43]	**3.9300** (0.4674)
Arthritis, rheumatic [9]	1.2553[+] (0.5689)	Respiratory infections, acute [6]	**2.2228** (0.3360)
Inflammation [20]	**2.7380** (0.3494)	Urinary condition/UTI [6]	3.4429 (5.5621)
Migraine [8]	3.1460[+] (1.2409)	Overactive bladder, incontinence (5)	1.0454 (0.5863)
Pain (chronic, non-analgesic) [10]	**2.3303** (0.5777)	Alzheimer's (5)	5.2355 (1.2663)
Spasticity, muscle spasms [10]	0.3451 (0.8569)	Anxiety [13]	**1.0313** (0.4452)
Allergic rhinitis, hay fever [14]	**1.3739** (0.3766)	Depression [19]	1.1134[+] (0.6261)
Asthma, incl. pediatric [14]	1.5586[+] (0.7253)	Insomnia [12]	−0.0228 (0.2184)
Respiratory distress syndrome (baby breathing problems) [5]	1.4860[+] (0.1611)	Psychotic disorders [12]	**1.6464** (0.6668)
Cancer (general) [10]	1.7025[+] (0.7086)	Schizophrenia [8]	0.1984 (1.0976)
Breast cancer [12]	−1.5379 (1.1331)	Dermatosis [12]	**0.8240** (0.2914)
Chemotherapy/nausea [10]	**1.7781** (0.6161)	Psoriasis [6]	−0.6093[+] (0.0624)
Leukemia [13]	−0.0809 (0.5616)	Tinea pedis [6]	0.6602[+] (0.2084)
Ovarian cancer [7]	4.1381 (2.2320)	Ulcer [16]	−0.7159 (0.9082)
Prostate cancer [8]	**1.2932** (0.4112)	Constipation [7]	1.0906 (0.7150)

TABLE 7.3.
cont.

Disease [# of molecules]	Elasticity	Disease [# of molecules]	Elasticity
Allergic conjunctivitis [5]	0.8005 (0.2400)	Analgesic [8]	−1.2575 (0.2264)
Glaucoma [14]	**0.8632** (0.2376)	Anesthesia [21]	0.5629+ (0.2819)
Angina (incl. chronic stable) [7]	0.9408 (0.5019)	Anesthesia(surgery-specific) [10]	**1.5429** (0.0846)
Arrhythmias [17]	**1.2479** (0.5270)	Parkinson's [15]	**0.6730** (0.2635)
Congestive heart failure [8]	**1.4793** (0.1124)	Diabetes [23]	**0.8861** (0.2682)
High cholesterol [13]	**2.5758** (0.9842)	Obesity [9]	0.7301+ (0.2890)
Hypertension [77]	**0.6876** (0.2264)	Epilepsy [9]	−0.7285 (1.1816)
Thrombosis [7]	**1.5961** (0.0434)	Seizures, partial [8]	−1.0843 (1.2281)
HIV/AIDS [20]	−0.6830 (0.5520)	Diagnostic [97]	**1.6369** (0.4734)
Inter-ocular pressure [3]	0.0882 (0.2290)	Contraceptive [9]	**3.6235** (0.7323)

Note: Elasticities in boldface connote statistical significance at the $p < 0.05$ level. + indicates significance at the $p < 0.1$ level. (All tests are two-tailed.)

a logic of politics and of reputation. It evinces the agency's continued awareness of disease-based constituencies—not simply the vocal patient advocacy groups that are so familiar today, but also medical specialty organizations such as cardiology societies, pediatricians' colleges, and oncologist groups. For these audiences, the visible demand and perceived necessity for new therapies waned where previously approved medicines were more abundant or more effective.[49]

---

[49] On legal and regulatory bases for efficacy comparisons, whether explicit or implicit, see Thomas E. Knauer, "The Regulation of Drugs on the Basis of Relative Effectiveness," *FDCLJ* 42 (1987): 323–45.

Drug reviewers voiced abiding concerns about how newer therapies matched up with older ones, and the case was clearest in antibiotics. Given the lack of patient-based organization in infectious diseases, support for further antibiotics would have come, if anywhere, from physicians with expertise on the drugs and the illnesses for which they were prescribed. Yet far from leading the cry for new antibiotics, infectious disease specialists in the 1960s and 1970s voiced frequent and public doubts about the newer anti-infectives. These specialists were newly organized in 1963 under the Infectious Disease Society of America. Neither in corporate nor in informal voices, however, did they press the Administration for rapid approval or gentle treatment of the new generation of antibiotics in the 1960s and 1970s. Concerns about the quality of second-generation anti-infective medications were voiced by numerous infectious disease specialists, most notably Harry Dowling and Maxwell Finland. The state of satisfaction with existing drugs, and the lack of enthusiasm for new varieties, translated into slower consideration for antibiotic submissions. At Frances Kelsey's Investigational Drug Branch in the 1960s, antibiotics constituted 10 percent of all submissions but 20 percent of the set of drugs that received a delayed medical review. In NME review, antibiotics also lagged in the 1970s and 1980s, with an average review time of two years despite immense standardization in antibiotics review during the preceding decades. With so many broad-spectrum antibiotics having been introduced in the World War II and post-War years, it was perhaps to be expected that reduced perceptions of unmet medical need generated reduced emphasis on later antibiotics.[50]

In different ways and at a different time, anti-inflammatory drugs also began to experience delays in review. From 1963 through 1985, new anti-inflammatory molecules required about thirty-four months for approval, on average. The average review time for those with a newer mechanism (so-called non-steroidal anti-inflammatory drugs or NSAIDs) was lower, at twenty-seven months, but still lay above the median review time of twenty-four months for the period. With the advent of Richard Crout and Marion Finkel's A-B-C priority ranking system in the late 1970s, however, anti-inflammatory drugs of all varieties began to receive less official and unofficial emphasis. From 1984 to 1991, NSAID drugs took an average of fifty-three months for NME review, and those in the lowest "C" category (accounting for seven of the twelve NSAIDs reviewed in this period) aver-

[50]FOK to Joseph Sadusk (Medical Director, Bureau of Medicine), "Current Status of IND Review," undated [probably June 25, 1965]; B13, F8, FOK. For some of Maxwell Finland's doubts about the state of antibiotic therapy, as expressed to NIH officials, see Finland to William Jordan, January 5, 1979; B4, F 1 ("National Institute of Health"), MF. Finland to Owen (NRC), March 9, 1957; B4, F3 NRC, 1938–1978), MF. Finland had cooperated with the Bureau of Medicine in the early 1960s in their attempt to remove Eaton Labs' Altafur (furaltadone) from the market. Conversations with Jeremy Greene were very helpful in developing this point.

aged fully seventy-three months. The slowest of these—Wyeth-Ayerst's et-
odolac (Lodine)—spent over eight years (97 months) in the review process,
from its submission in December 1982 to its final approval in January 1991.
In the 103rd Congress, Wyeth-Ayerst sought to introduce private legislation
to extend the term of its patent on Lodine, arguing that the slow FDA approval process deprived the firm of its rightful patent protection. Among the
reasons for Lodine's delay, concluded the General Accounting Office, were
safety concerns raised about the NSAID class from 1982 to 1985 and Canadian regulatory alerts about possible carcinogenicity in the drug. Yet the
GAO rightly noted that with comparable drugs already on the market, Lodine received a low official priority rating and even lower informal emphasis, and that its fate was not dramatically different from that of other anti-
inflammatory drugs reviewed at the time.[51]

Comparisons and Subjectivity: Drugs for Epilepsy and Parkinson's Disease.
Whereas a surfeit of approved and perceptibly effective medications can
delay new drugs, a vacuum in a particular therapeutic area often creates
regulatory advantages for the company that promises to fill it. In the 1980s,
the Administration did not approve a single new molecule for the treatment
of epilepsy. When Burroughs-Wellcome submitted an NDA for its anti-
epileptic drug Lamictal (lamotrigine) on December 31, 1991, FDA officials
found the application "disorganized" and sloppy in its statistical analyses.
Division of Neuropharmacology Drug Products director Paul Leber considered a refuse-to-file action, but decided against it. Since "no new anti-
epileptic product had been marketed over the previous 12 years," Leber
reasoned, "a refuse to file action, although justified, could have untoward
political consequences for the agency." [52]

Paul Leber's administrative writings show an open logic of organizational
reputation at work. In memoranda to other officers, most frequently to Robert Temple, Leber often wrote of his wish to avoid controversy and his preference for projecting an image of stability. Such reputation-based calculus
was on display in Leber's review of SmithKline Beecham's Requip (ropinerole)
for symptom management in Parkinson's disease. Parkinson's disease is a
complex set of conditions that generally entail loss of basic motor control
and increasing rigidity and slowness of muscle activity. Since the 1970s,
Parkinson's patients have been treated with a combination of dopamine

[51]GAO, *FDA Premarket Approval: Process of Approving Lodine as a Drug* (Report to Congressional Requesters), (Washington, DC: GAO, April 1993). Wyeth-Ayerst's attempt to pass
remedial patent term legislation (appearing first in H.R. 4896, 102d Cong. (1992)) never succeeded; Jane Fritsch, "When the Secrecy Was Lost, So Was the Favor," *NYT*, August 6, 1996;
Richard M. Cooper, "Legislative Patent Extensions," *FDLJ* 48 (1993): 59.
[52]"Lamictal Efficacy Comparable to Carbamazepine in First-Line Epilepsy, Glasgow Study;
Lamotrigine in Phase III for Monotherapy, Pediatrics," *Pharmaceutical Approvals Monthly*
(Jan. 1996): 29.

agonists—these moderate the neurotransmitter dopamine in the brain—and, most commonly, with synthetic dopamine drugs known as levidopa and carbidopa (marketed at present under the trade name Sinemet). At this writing, there are only symptomatic treatments, and no approved medicine reverses the course of Parkinson's disease progression. The agency had approved two new molecules in the late 1980s for Parkinson's, but neither took hold in clinical settings.

The context of therapeutic comparison for ropinerole was especially stark because a pharmacologically similar drug—Pharmacia & Upjohn's Mirapex (pramipexole)—was being reviewed at the same time. Indeed, the Mirapex NDA was filed with the Administration on December 28, 1995, one day before the arrival of the Requip NDA. The Requip NDA embedded a lot of data pointing to potential safety problems, and the clinical data and its analysis by SmithKline Beecham were greeted with doubt by the Administration's statistical reviewer. Researchers had employed the "UPDRS motor score"—one of eight portions of the Unified Parkinson's Disease Rating Scale—a commonly used index of basic motor performance by Parkinson's patients, in their studies. SmithKline Beecham argued that, on the basis of the clinical data, ropinerole not only was effective as monotherapy, but also carried an added boost when combined with selegiline. The sponsor's analysis of the clinical trials pointed to a 24 percent reduction in UPDRS motor score for ropinerole-treated patients compared to those treated with a placebo. Yet SmithKline Beecham admitted that the data were affected by "non-normality," a violation of the bell-shaped-curve pattern that is often assumed or approximated in conducting statistical tests upon clinical trial data. The company suggested some alternative statistical methods for correcting this problem, but the FDA statistical reviewer perceived that the violation of normality was not the sort of issue that could be corrected by statistical technique. It was being caused by the presence of six "outliers." In statistics, an "outlier" is an observation that lies so far from the mean of its sampling distribution that it is considered suspect to include it in the analysis. The intuition is that an outlier's departure from the sample mean renders the observation so different that it is useful to think that it was produced by a different experiment, one whose results are not comparable to the true sample. Because of their extremity, outliers can also influence the computation of simple averages, correlations, and statistical comparisons. In a sample where the estimated effect of the drug was a 24 percent change in the motor score, six patients experienced changes in motor score ranging from 94 percent to 250 percent of the baseline. When the FDA statistician removed these six observations from the analysis, the apparent interactive boost that selegiline received from ropinerole disappeared. Although generally supportive of the application, the reviewer added a troubling note about why simpler techniques of addressing the non-normality issue were not used. "The real reason" that

SmithKline Beecham used a more sophisticated method in accounting for the non-normality, "this reviewer thinks, was that the alternative [simpler] method made the interaction 'disappear' by their model." SmithKline officials were, by this reading, selectively presenting the most favorable evidence to the agency.[53]

Further scrutiny by medical officers and statisticians produced pleasant surprises and identified further problems. The statistical reviewer noted strong evidence that patients receiving ropinerole needed less l-dopa for Parkinson's symptom management. Since long-term l-dopa therapy is associated with uncomfortable and potentially dangerous side effects—low blood pressure, nausea, confusion, dry mouth, dizziness, and dyskinesia—this regulatory affirmation came as good news for Requip. The medical reviewer saw evidence from the clinical trial data that higher doses might be called for, as the most commonly tested doses in the studies did not reduce the cyclic nature of symptom expression in Parkinson's. Neurologists often refer to phases of symptom expression in Parkinson's as "on periods," as contrasted with "off periods" where the patient's motor skills are at or near normal. At the doses tested, ropinerole reduced the severity of symptoms when expressed, but did not effect a statistically significant reduction in the fraction of "awake time spent 'off.'" This would have spelled a stronger problem for the Requip application, but its simultaneous competitor Mirapex lacked any measurement whatsoever of patient "on-off" time, an omission that troubled the FDA medical reviewer.[54]

When Paul Leber wrote his summary memorandum on Requip to Robert Temple on December 13, 1996, he perceived a new drug application that was less than the sum of its parts. The data were not impressive—SmithKline Beecham's statistical analyses were suspect and flatly inaccurate on several occasions, and there were worrisome safety events. He began his conclusion with a note of the uncertainty and circumspection that buffeted any such judgment as the one he was about to offer.

[53]Russell Katz (Deputy Director, Division of Neuropharmacological Drug Products), "Supervisory Review of NDA 20-658, for the Use of Ropinerole as Mono- and Adjunctive Therapy for Patients with Parkinson's Disease," November 25, 1996; Janeth Rouzer-Kammeyer, "Review and Evaluation of Clinical Data," NDA 20-658 (Ropinerole (SK&F 101468-A) Requip Tablets), July 15, 1996; 11–21, 56–7. Within the Division of Neuropharmacological Drug Products, Rouzer-Kammeyer was the principal medical reviewer, while Gregory Burkhart reviewed the effectiveness trials and Kun Jin of the Division of Biometrics acted as statistical reviewer for a subset of the effectiveness studies; all in NDA File 20-658, FDA.

[54]Katz, "Supervisory Review of NDA 20-658, for the Use of Ropinerole as Mono- and Adjunctive Therapy for Patients with Parkinson's Disease," November 25, 1996; NDA File 20-658, FDA. The principal medical officer in the Mirapex review was John Feeney. Burkhart was also involved in the review safety data, just as he had been involved in the safety review of Requip; "Pharmacia & Upjohn Mirapex Advanced Parkinson's Trials Should Have Measured Duration of Patient 'On-Off' Time, FDA Reviewer Says," *Pharmaceutical Approvals Monthly* (August 1998): 28–33.

Because no pharmacologically active drug substance is entirely free of risk, the conclusion that a drug has been shown to be "safe for use," is actually no more than an opinion, albeit one offered by an individual reasonably knowledgeable in the management of the condition that is the intended target of treatment, that the benefits associated with the use of the drug are sufficient to outweigh its known risks of use.

Accordingly, risk to benefit assessments are inherently arguable, all the more so because each turns not only on personal sentiments about the nature of risks and the benefits of a drug, but upon incomplete and imperfect information concerning the drug's risks.[55]

In the inescapably subjective calculus of ropinerole's risk and benefit, Leber found several facts about the regulatory context crucial for making his decision. First, all of the "treatments" for Parkinson's disease were "effective" only in remediation of symptoms. In the absence of a "cure," symptom management became all the more important. Second, there were adverse events associated with ropinerole use, but he perceived the drug as "reasonably free of a potential/capacity to cause death and/or serious injury at an unacceptably high incidence." The risk of mortality was the central "red flag" measure, and other adverse events paled in comparison during the safety evaluation. Third and perhaps pivotally, Leber perceived that his agency's past decisions constrained its future choices, less on matters of law than on matters of image. In its review of other anti-Parkinsonian therapies—not least Mirapex itself, for which his Division was about to issue an approvable letter—the Administration had established precedents in reputation even though no such standards held at law. It was crucial, he felt, for the agency to retain and project a modicum of consistency.

> On the other hand, past agency actions document that this risk is readily acceptable in a treatment for PD. Specifically, dopamine agonists already marketed for the management of PD (i.e., bromocriptine, pergolide) cause the very same set of presumably autonomic nervous system mediated adverse events. Like these marketed drugs, ropinerole also causes hallucinations, nausea, vomiting and a host of other not so troubling AEs....
>
> I am mindful that, in light of this view, a case could be made for declaring the NDA not approvable. I am persuaded, however, that although such an approach is defensible, it is less desirable than an approvable action conveyed in the company of the caveats and requests enumerated in the draft labeling and action letter.[56]

---

[55]The clinical trials and Phase 1 studies suggested syncope, caused by orthostatic hypotension and bradycardia. No sooner had Leber written that ropinerole was "reasonably free" of death and risks at "an unacceptably high incidence" than he inserted a caveat in a footnote: "I am fully mindful that I have begged the definition of what does or does not represent 'an unacceptably high incidence.'" Neither Leber nor any other officer could point to an established standard or cutpoint for making such decisions. Leber to Temple, December 13, 1996; 6–7 (incl. footnote 11), 9; NDA File 20-658, FDA.

[56]Ibid.

Robert Temple brought greater skepticism to Requip and he learned different lessons from comparing the drug with others in its therapeutic category. He saw clear evidence of ropinerole's effectiveness, but comparing it with Mirapex raised concerns. Orthostatic hypotension and syncope were "more prominent than usual" and "far more prominent than a contemporaneously evaluated drug of similar pharmacology." The data were, moreover, much more variable in the Requip NDA than in the Mirapex NDA, and Temple felt that SmithKline Beecham had rushed its application. "Part of the problem" with the safety data, he remarked, "seems likely to be SKB's avoidance of well-designed dose-finding efforts." There were few red flags from the safety data, but "syncope and falls in the elderly and infirm are not trivial and the combination of hypotension and bradycardia is capable of killing." Temple concluded that an approvable letter should issue, but it should be injected with "a note of somewhat greater uncertainty" and with the possibility of "a conspicuous warning" (namely a black-box warning) attached to the eventual approved labeling.[57]

Mirapex received final approval in July 1997, and Requip would be approved in September of the same year, with significant concessions in its approved labeling. The simultaneous review engendered cross-pressures upon the respective applications—the Requip NDA offered data that the Mirapex application had not, but Mirapex presented a gentler safety profile. These comparisons allowed the Administration's officers some leeway in their treatment of the two drugs. Yet the simultaneity of the Mirapex and Requip drug reviews also created pressures for procedural and behavioral consistency at the Division of Neuropharmacological Drug Products. Communities of neurologists were watching, so were Parkinson's disease organizations, and so were two deeply interested companies and the audiences of global financial markets. The drug applications were not so different as to permit full-scale rejection of one while embracing the other, so the differences emerged in the details of labeling and the timing of approval.

Safety, Red Flags, and Irreversibility. The structure of new drug review in the last four decades is one where questions of safety continue to be paramount. In part this reflects the continuity of law and regulatory culture from the pre-1962 period. Discussions about what is "safe" and what is "toxic" lie at the heart of organizational conversations, and these discussions form the basic concepts of regulatory science. In part the primacy of safety comes from the widespread concern that the most severe safety problems are most difficult to detect in pre-market clinical studies. Questions of potentially adverse effects upon the developing fetus (or teratogenicity) were largely skirted

---

[57]Temple to Leber, January 7, 1997; NDA File 20-658, FDA. An approvable letter had been sent to Pharmacia & Upjohn for Mirapex on December 23, 1996. It was common in this period for CDER officials to ask the company to produce a "dosing algorithm" to reduce the risk of adverse events; "Pfizer Pursuing Tikosyn Ventricular Arrhythmia Indications," *Pharmaceutical Approvals Monthly* (May 1999): 8–9.

by the decades-long exclusion of women, particularly women of child-bearing age, from U.S. clinical trials. And as drug development has become more complicated, and as the tools for detecting safety and toxicity issues in pre-market studies have become more refined, the dilemmas facing the Administration have become not lighter but in fact more pressing. It was with a sense of painful irony that Bureau of Drugs Director Richard Crout could say, in 1977, that the agency's successes had in fact helped to generate a context in which decisions were now harder. The easy decisions on new drugs were generations gone, Crout reminisced, and new technologies of development and review meant that the choices of the present were increasingly more difficult ones.[58]

Among the rare events that can derail a new drug application, liver toxicity (or hepatotoxicity) is paramount. Drugs act intentionally and unintentionally through their metabolites, and the process of metabolism can generate metabolites and enzymes that damage liver cells. Examination of liver enzymes to see whether they are elevated (and how much) beyond normal levels is often undertaken. Even a few instances of such elevation among patients in a clinical trial can become "sentinel cases" or "flagging events" that induce the agency to ask for more data, different labeling, restricted primary indications, or some combination of restricted measures. In the agency's 1995 review of Duract (bromfenac sodium), submitted by Wyeth-Ayerst for rheumatoid arthritis and osteoarthritis, agency reviewers openly discussed the significance of rare but troublesome cases of liver toxicity. They initially decided against approving the drug, wondered whether it should eventually carry a boxed warning for liver toxicity, and sent an "approvable" letter to Wyeth-Ayerst that underscored their worries. Slightly over two years later, the agency would approve the drug without a boxed warning. In reviewing the liver data on Duract, FDA officer Rudolph Widmark offered a candid admission of uncertainty in the endeavor of divining safety problems from rare events in clinical trial data. "In our safety review of NDA studies," he wrote, "we usually do not get definitive answers based on unequivocal data but are forced to interpret 'flagging' events. We think that in the case of bromfenac, we have seen a 'liver flag' that can only be fully explored through responsible marketing of the drug." The agency approved Duract in July 1997, only to see it withdrawn from the market for liver toxicity in June 1998.[59]

[58]Crout, "The Nature of Regulatory Choices," *FDCLJ* 38 (1978): 413.
[59]Medical Reviewer John Hyde expressed the uncertainty about the "sentinel cases" in the Duract NDA as follows: "While these may have been unlucky events that might be diluted with greater exposure experience, it is hard to tell with the data currently available. Just as there is room for downside correction with greater exposure experience, there is ample opening for upside correction as well"; Hyde (Medical Officer, Anti-Inflammatory, Analgesic and Ophthalmic Drug Products Division), "Review of DURACT Labeling Revision," July 31, 1996 (p. 3 of Review); also Hyde, "Overview of Chronic (OA and RA) Studies," December 19, 1995; Widmark's remarks come in his "Memo regarding hepatotoxicity of bromfenac," November 14, 1996; all in NDA File 20-535, FDA. "Wyeth-Ayerst Duract Hepatotoxicity Boxed Warning

Another characteristic red flag comes in the potential carcinogenicity of drugs, especially those that are destined for long-term, continual use as primary therapy for chronic conditions. In the Administration's review of benoxaprofen (Oraflex) in 1979 and 1980, FDA medical officers William Gyarfas and Manfred Hein imposed exacting standards for carcinogenicity tests upon the drug's sponsor, Eli Lilly. A long and wide-ranging debate continued within the Bureau of Drugs about how to interpret Lilly's carcinogenicity tests on animals. Based on Gyarfas and Hein's evaluations and other data, Oraflex was declared not approvable in the United States in February 1981, even though it had been previously approved by British authorities. By April 1982, these concerns had been allayed among leaders in the Bureau of Drugs, and the Oraflex NDA was cleared by Marion Finkel, but not without considerable anxiety.[60]

Administration officers' deepest tremblings about safety stem from the possibility that a drug will come to dash the agency's and sponsor's hopes, and that safety concerns written and unwritten during the review process will later be revealed to be much worse. Medical officers have long felt and behaved as if they bear some responsibility for any approved drug that goes awry, particularly when there were warning signs in the clinical and preclinical data that are observable during NDA review. The legal, political, and economic contexts of new drug approval also generate a perceived permanence to the approval decision. And during many NDA reviews and advisory committee hearings, there are spoken and unspoken cues of what Edward Tabor reminded his colleagues in the azidothymidine (AZT) review in 1987: "It is a fact of life that, once a drug is approved, it is almost impossible, as a practical matter, to withdraw that approval, unless there is a very serious safety consideration that was not recognized before."[61]

Yet the irreversibility of new drug approval is less a procedural, legal, or economic fact than an ideational one. As former General Counsel Richard Merrill would write two decades after his time in office, a sense of perceived and collective responsibility for a new drug pervaded the culture of the late twentieth-century Administration. This culture was the constructed amalgam of beliefs that impinge upon the agency from American society, international expectations, professional standards, and congressional scrutiny and internally held ideals that were symbolized in the thalidomide case. Unlike those "cop-like" agencies of state that police the marketplace, Merrill

---

Was Suggested During NDA Review; Dysmenorrhea Claim Dropped for Study Irregularities," *Pharmaceutical Approvals Monthly* (April 1998): 34. "Wyeth Positioning Duract as Opioid Alternative in Outpatient Post-Op; Dosage, Treatment Length Were Issues in 18-Month 'Approvable' Phase," *Pharmaceutical Approvals Monthly* (Sept. 1997): 3–5.

[60] John Abraham, "Scientific Standards and Institutional Interests: Carcinogenic Risk Assessment of Benoxaprofen in the UK and US," *Social Studies of Science* 23 (1993): 402–3, 405.

[61] Tabor's remark came in discussions on the approval of azidothymidine (AZT), sponsored as Retrovir by Burroughs-Wellcome; FDA, *Meeting of the Anti-Infective Drugs Advisory Committee*, January 16, 1987; Rockville, MD; transcript produced by Baker, Haynes and Burkes Reporting, Inc.

writes, the "FDA is believed to have a different role, a responsibility to prevent harm before it occurs." Through law, its own projection of image, and its relations with Congress, "the agency becomes a warrantor of manufacturer compliance with the rules that govern drug development and marketing." Drug companies will be sued in court for safety problems, but the agency is reminded by its many audiences, and its own cultural conscience, that it too is at fault. "FDA is repeatedly reminded, and often reminds us, that it shares responsibility for any drug that causes harm."[62]

There is some evidence that this irreversibility of drug approval in reputation generates a similar irreversibility in dialogue. A number of medical officers and division directors have argued that the agency—particularly the drug-reviewing divisions—exhibits great reluctance to revisit previous approval decisions. Perhaps the earliest of these complaints was directed at none other than the pharmacological regime of the 1950s, and it came during the hearings chaired by Senator Hubert Humphrey in 1963, voiced by none other than John Nestor. Nestor pointed to a culture in which the decisions of the past were not easily re-examined.

> Unfortunately, although my frankness was acceptable before I was hired, after joining the organization I found that any medical opinion that raised issues that involved reappraisal of past decisions, past policies, or past commitments to the pharmaceutical industry would be challenged—not in a healthy scientific atmosphere, but, rather, with indifference, disapproval, or even hostility. This, unfortunately, was frequently the case with drugs for pediatric use.

When asked by Humphrey to clarify this statement, Nestor elaborated that "in making present decisions, it was sort of a sacrosanct situation that we were not to question decisions made in the past."[63]

The Construction of Efficacy: Standards, Measures, and the Case of Platinum Chemotherapy

The continued primacy of safety issues in new drug review did not imply that the effectiveness requirements of the 1962 legislation were trivial. Preceding that law were patterns of regulatory behavior in which "efficacy" became a criterion of review along with safety in the middle 1950s. The law, for its part, imposed a set of requirements upon the Administration that required fresh action and interpretation. Not least of these were the definition of clinical trial standards and the efficacy-based review and eventual market removal of hundreds of drugs approved before 1962 under the Drug

---

[62] Merrill, "The Architecture of Government Regulation of Medical Products," *Virginia Law Review* 82 (1996): 1768.

[63] Nestor remarks at *ICDRR*, 783, 790. Humphrey himself emphasized these points in a review of the MER/29 case; "Memorandum from Senator Hubert H. Humphrey on Background to Exhibits on MER/29," Exhibit 127 in *ICDRR*, 822.

Efficacy Study Initiative. Shot through all of these endeavors was the thorny question of how to translate a philosophy of "efficacy" founded in clinical pharmacology and regulatory precedent into the legal and more familiar terms of "effectiveness." Nothing in the statutory law defined what therapeutic properties a drug would have to have in order to qualify as "effective" for a given medical condition. There were allusions to "general recognition" and "qualified experts," but these concepts invited subjectivity and discretion. They did little to bind the Bureau of Medicine and its successor, the Bureau of Drugs. So too, nothing in the law (which spoke of "effectiveness" requirements) directly mandated the use of randomized and placebo-controlled trials (the residue of "efficacy" discussions in medicine, pharmacology, and statistics). The construction of efficacy—in part the transformation of regulatory and scientific practices into legal realities—was an ongoing and contingent affair in the decades after the Kefauver-Harris Amendments.[64]

The Evolution of Experimental Control Standards. One relatively stable pattern of interpretation came in the insistence of Administration medical officers upon randomized clinical trials with a placebo arm as the principal form of evidence on which drugs could be deemed effective for their intended uses. Randomization had long been accepted as the basis for comparability of treatment and control groups, but placebo controls—the assignment of some research subjects to an "arm" or group of the experiment where they received an inert treatment that resembled the actual treatment as much as possible—had not. As early as the 1950s and quite clearly in the 1960s, Administration officials voiced their strong preference for (but did not require) randomized, placebo-controlled trials for demonstration of efficacy in Phase 3 studies. Then, in a gradual transformation accelerated by the Drug Efficacy Study and its regulatory conflicts, the randomized, controlled trial (RCT) became a near-absolute standard of regulatory evidence, and increasingly randomization and placebo control were expected in Phase 2 as well as Phase 3 studies.

FDA officials' preference for randomized, placebo-controlled trials predated the 1962 Amendments. The idea of accounting for placebo effects was tied up with the idea of assigning subjects to treatment or control by chance—randomization and the placebo ran together in regulatory conversation. With newfound authority from those Amendments and the 1963 rules, however, and with the legitimation of the federal court rulings of the early 1970s upholding the 1969 "adequate and well-controlled investigations" rule, FDA officials' stance became more assertive and insistent.[65]

---

[64]I am grateful to legal scholars Richard Merrill and M. Elizabeth Magill for their suggestion that the DESI study was not simply an exercise in the regulation of "old" drugs but also a standard-setting exercise in the regulation of "new" drugs developed and submitted in the 1960s and later.

[65]The 1969 rule placed emphasis on randomization but did not state a strong preference for a placebo control. Much of the elaboration of the placebo-control standard would come in the

In the redrafting of regulations and guidance documents for INDs and NDAs in the mid- to late 1970s, William Beaver, Crout, Finkel, and Temple began outlining a plan for placing emphasis on placebo controls. Temple, who was then head of the Cardio-Renal Division that had once housed John Nestor, ran an internal task force charged with redefining the phrase "adequate and well-controlled studies." This effort was undertaken as part of the late 1970s and early 1980s "IND/NDA rewrite." Temple wrote concept papers pointing to placebo-controlled trials as a "scientific standard," mainly because in such studies there "are no assumptions that really need to be made." Other forms of clinical experiment—positive controls, no treatment, and historical controls—ranked "scientifically below" placebo-controlled studies, Temple argued, and any IND protocol or new drug application relying on something other than a placebo-controlled trial would need to offer a separate justification stating why the standard could not be met. Temple's initiative expressed pharmacological thinking that was regnant in academic networks and had been popular in the 1950s Bureau of Medicine. In the 1970s, it met with public resistance but private deference. Publicly, Squibb vice president Norman Lavy expressed his fear that Temple's "preference" was for all intents and purposes a rule, and that it would enact a "rigid regulatory hierarchy" of experiments, leading evaluators away from the actual data. To these and other criticisms, Temple responded that "high-quality data" were paramount, and that it was the task and prerogative of the Administration to see that clinical experiments produced it. Privately, firms and noncommercial drug sponsors began to regard the placebo control arm as an absolute requirement, and to design their IND studies (especially the trials they hoped would become "pivotal" at the NDA stage) accordingly.[66]

The dominance of the placebo-controlled trial became nearly complete. The Administration's expectations for placebo controls were applied to drugs treating fatal diseases, so much so that diverse audiences comprising

---

evaluation and removal of drugs under DESI. See *FR* 34 (152 (Aug. 9, 1969): 12966 [Panalba and novobiocin combinations]; *FR* 34 (180) (Sept. 19, 1969): 14596–9 [antibiotics, especially in fixed combination]; *FR* 35 (33) (Feb. 17, 1970): 3073–4 [general regulations and antibiotics]; *FR* 38 (45) (March 8, 1973): 6296–6300 [oral steroids]; *FR* 38 (185) (Sept. 25, 1973): 26748–9 [anorectic combinations].

[66]See chapter 3, and particularly William Weiss, "Long-Range Planning in the Scientific Areas," attachment to memorandum from Grey to "Directors of Bureaus, Divisions and Districts," subject "PPA Presentation at 1961 Bureau, Division and District Directors' Conference," October 16, 1961; in *ICDRR*, 374. On Temple's working group and the criticism that its guidance publications received, see "FDA Preference for Placebo Controls in Concept Papers Could Evolve into 'Rigid' Regulatory 'Hierarchy,' Squibb Exec Asserts at Public Forum on Regs," *DRR* 22 (46): 8. Jean Seligmann, Mary Haver, and Dan Shapiro, "Drug Test Creates Doctor's Dilemma," *Newsweek*, July 14, 1980, 52D. Temple appears to have been influenced by the work of Louis Lasagna, whose papers he cited often and pivotally in making his case for placebo-controlled trials. Lasagna, "Placebos and Controlled Trials Under Attack" (Editorial), *European Journal of Clinical Pharmacology* 15 (1979): 373–4. See also Marks, *The Progress of Experiment*, part 2, esp. chapters 5 and 6.

scholars in bioethics, patient advocates, and journalists began to worry that the application of placebo controls was inhumane. When in 1980 the Bureau of Drugs reviewed isoprinosine for the treatment of a rare but deadly form of encephalitis, an advisory committee recommended that the drug proceed to NDA review. Temple initially refused, saying that no application for isoprinosine could be submitted unless and until the sponsor had conducted a placebo-controlled trial. His decision met with protest from infectious disease specialists and was covered in national media outlets. The controversy compelled Temple and his FDA colleagues to publicly elaborate an ethical and scientific logic of when it was appropriate to demand placebo controls. Temple acknowledged that when existing treatments had a recognized ability to "prevent death or irreversible deterioration, or to control pain, we would never ask for a placebo test." Instead, the "positive control" (or "active control") technique of assigning patients to the new drug or to the effective standby would be permitted. The question then became one of "demonstrated efficacy" or common scientific beliefs about a drug's effectiveness. In many cases, such beliefs had not congealed from randomized, placebo-controlled trials but from widespread utilization and clinical observation. In the case of isoprinosine, there were international audiences that weighed in silently but compellingly. The drug had been marketed in thirty-five nations, including the three nations most commonly cited by drug lag critics: England, France, and West Germany. Within weeks of Temple's initial refusal, *Newsweek* reporters would announce that "the FDA has quietly modified its position: it will still insist on controlled studies, but they need not involve a placebo." And fully seven years before the Administration announced new rules permitting compassionate use in trials during the AIDS crisis, the Bureau in July 1980 permitted physicians to use isoprinosine for critically ill patients.[67]

The isoprinosine case presaged a more general attack on placebo-controlled trials from different audiences in science, medicine, and bioethics in the 1980s and 1990s. Ethicists began to argue that in a wide variety of cases extending well beyond life-threatening or critical medical conditions, the use of placebos was unethical. They seized upon language in a 1975 amendment to the Helsinki Declaration calling for patients in clinical studies, including those in experimental control groups, to be "assured of the best proven and diagnostic therapeutic method." By the end of the century, the World Medical Association and the International Conference on Harmonization had articulated principles that cast doubt on the propriety of placebo-controlled trials whenever there was an existing treatment of proven efficacy and the disease in question was associated with serious harm. For less serious medical conditions, these bodies called for informed consent for placebo assignment, a procedure which often created genuine sample selection issues

---

[67]Temple's initial refusal was reported in *Newsweek*, July 7, 1980. "Drug Test Creates Doctor's Dilemma," *Newsweek*, July 14, 1980, 52D. In fact, different forms of compassionate use had evolved since the 1950s; see Hutt, Merrill and Grossman, *Food and Drug Law*.

in trials as wary patients opted out of the study. As enthusiasm waxed for "active control" studies where patients were assigned by chance to the new drug or to an existing medicine, Temple and his FDA colleagues began to propose modified procedures for placebo-controlled studies and to remind the medical and statistical audiences of when active control trials were complicated with insuperable barriers to inference. Temple and others in the Administration, including neuropharmacology specialist Paul Leber, continued as the most vocal proponents of the enduring use of placebo arms in clinical experiment. As skillfully and rigorously as any participant in the larger debate—and in an apparent attempt to convey the scientific and logical prowess housed in his organization—Temple weighed the ethical and statistical properties of placebo-controlled trials together and suggested novel solutions to the emerging dilemma.[68]

From the standpoint of procedure, the debate over placebo controls in clinical studies pointed to something deeper, and often unrecognized, about new drug review: its continuity from clinical experiment to regulatory evaluation. The Administration's officers usually had abundant knowledge of a drug and the design of its clinical studies, knowledge possessed years before the submission of a formal NDA. Indeed, the very decision to submit a drug to the agency was often undertaken in consultation with the directors of FDA review divisions and subordinate medical officers. From the 1970s onward, these overlaps between NDA review and IND progression became more regular and, later, formalized in "End of Phase 2 conferences."

Along with other provisions, the effectiveness clause of the 1962 legislation assigned the burden of proof clearly to the drug's sponsor. The inevitably subjective question was how exactly to conclude when the adduced evidence somehow aggregated to meet the burden of proof imposed by law. These decisions inevitably involve trade-offs and considerations that take medical officers and other FDA officials well beyond the clinical evidence into discussions of who will be affected (and how) by a given assignment of

[68]The debate over placebo controls and their ethicality is much larger and more complicated than can be adequately covered here. For an excellent summary and review, see Harry A. Guess, Arthur Kleinman, John W. Kusek, and Linda W. Engel, eds., *The Science of the Placebo: Toward an Interdisciplinary Research Agenda* (London: BMJ Books, 2002). A seminal paper is Kenneth J. Rothman and Karin B. Michels, "The Continued Unethical Use of Placebo Controls," *NEJM* 331 (1994): 394–8. World Medical Association, "Declaration of Helsinki. Ethical Principles for Medical Research Involving Human Subjects," *JAMA* 284 (2000): 3043–5. For the ICH statement, see "International Conference on Harmonization: Choice of Control Group in Clinical Trials," *FR* 66 (2001): 24390–91. For FDA contributions, see Leber, "Hazards of Inference: The Active Control Investigation," *Epilepsia* 30 (Supplement 1): S57–62; Robert Temple and S. S. Ellenberg, "Placebo -Controlled Trials and Active-Control trials in the Evaluation of New Yreatments. Part 1: Ethical and Scientific Issues," *AnnIM* 133 (2000): 455–63; Ellenberg and Temple, "Placebo Controlled Trials and Active-Control Trials in the Evaluation of New Treatments. Part 2: Practical Issues and Specific Cases," *AnnIM* 133 (2000): 464–70. My sense of Temple's apparent concern for his agency's reputation comes from a recollection of Arthur Kleinman, who helped to organize the 2001 NIH conference at which Temple spoke. I assume all responsibility for its use here.

the burden of proof. An early example comes from the FDA's application of efficacy standards to medicines for the treatment of influenza. In the late 1960s, epidemiologists documented a substantial flu epidemic attributable to the so-called Hong Kong strain of Type A influenza. The Dupont Company proposed use of amantadine for prevention and treatment of the strain. At first, Administration officials took the position that amantadine must be proven to be effective in man against each specific influenza strain prior to marketing. This stance brought immediate and fierce criticism from virologists, most notably Ernst Herrmann of the Mayo Clinic. Herrmann argued that if this policy were followed, drug development would always fall behind changes in the antigenic constitution of bacteria or viruses. Infectious diseases were moving targets, Herrmann implied, and FDA policy needed proper recognition of that fact. Herrmann counseled reliance on bird (*in ovo*) studies that had shown amantadine's action against the Hong Kong strain. The issue reached the FDA's Medical Advisory Board, which discussed whether in vitro data would be sufficient to permit labeling of amantadine for efficacy against a particular strain, or "should every strain variation be tested for clinical effectiveness prior to recommendation for use in humans."[69]

In the regulatory debates that followed, the question came down not to whether Dupont's data were valid, but what standard of evidence should be applied. There were human trials with amantadine, but they were undertaken by Russian investigators, and the Bureau of Medicine had long regarded foreign trials of anti-infective drugs with suspicion. FDA official Harvey Minchew noted a difference of opinion on this question among virologists. Along with Herrmann, many investigators felt that "the burden of proof is on those who say that the changes in this strain are not correlated with changes in the effectiveness of the chemical agent." Harry Dowling suggested "a cautious approach." Amantadine, after all, was "the first drug of its type," and there was substantial "uncertainty about the significance of antigenic drift in viral populations; one cannot necessarily reason by analogy from the situation with bacteria." William Kirby of the University of Washington School of Medicine disagreed with Dowling and worried about the "disservice" to drug development and to flu sufferers that such an approach would entail. The following day, the committee examined data from the Russian clinical trials. These were "relatively small clinical trials in volunteers inoculated intra-nasally with mixed influenza viruses and then treated with amantadine." Kirby and Dowling now concurred that Dupont should receive the go-ahead for revised labeling stating the efficacy of amantadine against Hong-Kong strain Type A influenza.[70]

[69]FDA-BOM, Medical Advisory Board, Seventeenth Meeting, December 16th and 17th, 1968, p. 2; Harry F. Dowling Papers, NLM.

[70]FDA-BOM, Medical Advisory Board, Seventeenth Meeting, December 16th and 17th, 1968, pp. 2–3; Harry F. Dowling Papers, NLM. Amantadine was approved for general use against influenza in 1976, and sold later under the trade name Symmetrel.

Efficacy also carries normative connotations that have constrained more technocratic judgments about research design and statistical significance. In her review of Flolan (epoprostenol), a drug developed for primary pulmonary hypertension by Glaxo Wellcome, FDA medical reviewer Eugenie Triantas saw major problems in the construction of the efficacy studies. The treatment and control groups were not balanced, and she argued that the randomization of patients to arms of the experiment should have been conditioned upon their prior health (in summary, how well they had walked at the time they entered the study). Yet Triantas' reservations about the drug were outweighed by her superiors and by a unanimous advisory committee vote. The pressure for approval had much to do with the severity of the disease targeted. "The medical officer has a strong belief that the drug should not be approved, and this perspective must be considered," wrote division director Stephen Fredd. Yet while Flolan was not "benign therapy," he continued, "I think the consequences of the disease are worse, and since I believe the drug improves hemodynamics, exercise capacity and the chance for survival in severely affected individuals, I think the drug should be approved." Similar trade-offs were made several months later when the Administration approved Rhone-Poulenc Rorer's Rilutek (riluzole) for amytrophic lateral sclerosis (ALS)—a progressive and ultimately fatal condition often known as "Lou Gehrig's disease," after the New York Yankees baseball player who succumbed to it in 1941—despite wide acknowledgment that Rorer's efficacy data were "substandard." In this case, the drug's effectiveness in clinical trials was not statistically significant at customary levels—the p-value was 0.076, meaning that seven or eight out of one hundred times the result observed would have been generated by chance alone. This value was above but "reasonably close to the usual standard" limit of 0.05—the "one in twenty" criterion that has become a global standard for statistical significance in medical and social science applications. Yet the severity of ALS and the apparent consensus on Rilutek's safety profile generated a narrow but real victory for the sponsor and its drug—the FDA's advisory committee voted five to four in favor of the drug's efficacy, and Rilutek was approved in December 1995. [71]

Chemotherapy Goes Platinum: The Political Career of Cisplatin. At the same time that organizational and ideological battles over Laetrile were being fought out, federal officials and university scientists were testing a promis-

---

[71] The division director was Stephen Fredd, Division of Gastrointestinal and Coagulation Drugs. The trade journal *Pharmaceutical Approvals Monthly* concluded that "approved labeling for Flolan presents the most favorable analysis of mortality results." Fredd to Temple, March 25, 1995; in "Glaxo Wellcome Flolan Mortality Benefit in Primary Pulmonary Hypertension Was Questioned by FDA Reviewer: Imbalance in Study Groups Cited," *Pharmaceutical Approvals Monthly* (June 1996): 29–32. "Rhone-Poulenc Rorer Rilutek's Survival Benefit in ALS Demonstrated Despite Failure of Studies to Meet FDA's Usual Efficacy Standards, Agency Says," *Pharmaceutical Approvals Monthly* (Aug. 1996): 26–34. On the "$p < 0.05$" standard, see Marks, *The Progress of Experiment*.

ing new class of platinum-based compounds for their action against malignant tumors. Unlike Laetrile, platinum-based chemotherapy received little national or global media attention before the 1979 approval of cisplatin as first-line treatment for testicular cancer. Perhaps more than any other drug, however, cisplatin and its relatives (platinum coordination complexes such as carboplatin and oxaliplatin) posed lasting dilemmas and challenges to the drug development paradigm in the United States, and to the thinking of the Food and Drug Administration. Perhaps the most notable challenge was the difficulty of thinking about the efficacy of a drug as part of a combination to be employed with other forms of non-pharmaceutical therapy. The other challenge was in thinking flexibly about what it means for a trial to be "controlled." The Administration's adaptation to these challenges is notable for the way it undermines common perceptions—images prevailing at the time, and that remain with us today—of the agency's rigidity and inflexibility. When contrasted with the "hard line" FDA regulation of illegitimate cancer treatments, including Laetrile, the regulatory experience of platinum-based chemotherapy demonstrates the Administration's capacity for taking a "soft line" regulatory stance when treatments with high legitimacy were in development.

Cisplatin and Laetrile are two drugs that were never considered together procedurally, but collided in ideation and reputation. Pharmacological conservatives approached cancer drugs with Laetrile in mind. Given the abundance of drugs that lacked an established molecular mechanism against malignant tumors but that could induce tumor remission in animals, therapies with merely empirical support were not viewed favorably by many Administration officials. Procedural liberals in the FDA, at M. D. Anderson, the NCI, and other venues approached cancer drugs as a field with inherent promise, easily differentiable from quack remedies.

The main safety challenge facing cisplatin—one that nearly ended its career as cancer therapy—was its toxicity to the kidneys. The drug's "nephrotoxicity" was not only immediately hazardous to cancer patients, it was also "dose-limiting," meaning that the higher doses at which cisplatin showed greater efficacy were rendered off-limits by massive and irreversible kidney damage. Nephrotoxicity was addressed by pre-hydrating patients before cisplatin administration and then by giving cisplatin in a slow saline-based infusion (mannitol and saline being the most common). There was also considerable damage to the ears (ototoxicity) from cisplatin administration, and this damage, like that to the kidneys, was cumulative. Compared to other cytotoxic drugs, cisplatin had appreciable side effects as well, including a high degree of nausea and vomiting as well as neuropathy, though none of these issues seems to have played a significant role in the drug's eventual FDA review.[72]

---

[72]On the preclinical development of cisplatin, see the previous chapter. John R. Durant, "Cisplatin: A Clinical Overview," in Prestayko, Crooke, and Carter, *Cisplatin*, 317–22. When the concept is rendered literally, every drug will have a side effect that is "dose-limiting"; the relevant question becomes whether dose-limitation interferes with the dosage administered for

With the conclusion of Phase 1 trials for cisplatin, sponsorship rights were assigned (at first to the Johnson Matthey Company and the Institute of Cancer Research in Sutton, England, later to Bristol Laboratories). The National Cancer Institute continued to provide cisplatin to investigators under its effective IND application, and as positive clinical reports and quasi-experimental data flowed in, the Institute began to back cisplatin with increasing energy and fervor. Bristol-Myers officials also saw considerable promise in the chemotherapy market, and placed high hopes on Platinol as part of its "stable" of chemotherapy drugs (which also included cyclophosphamide, bleomycin, and mitomycin C). At this point, the principal question facing cisplatin was one of therapeutic efficacy, and it was with Phase 2 and 3 trials that platinum chemotherapy experienced its first regulatory politics.[73]

Bristol Laboratories submitted its first New Drug Application for Platinol on July 21, 1977, for treatment of ovarian and testicular cancers. The director of the Oncology Drugs division, William Gyarfas, assigned the application to a review team headed by medical officer Robert Young, and Young swiftly informed Bristol and the NCI that the application was inadequate. Bristol withdrew its Platinol NDA and re-submitted in the spring of 1978. The company and the NCI pointed to seven studies that provided evidence of cisplatin's effectiveness, but chief among these was a study conducted at Indiana University under the direction of Lawrence Einhorn. Using protocols developed by the Southeastern Cancer Study Group—one of the regional cooperative cancer chemotherapy groups that had been set up by the NCI—Einhorn administered cisplatin in combination with vinblastine and bleomycin to fifty patients with "disseminated" (or advanced metastatic) testicular cancer. The control for Einhorn's study was both historical and counterfactual. The "cure rates" observed—74 percent complete remissions and 26 percent partial remissions for a 100 percent response rate—were contrasted with the fact that in the early 1960s, testicular cancer was generally 100 percent fatal, and that a previous combination of vinblastine and bleomycin was associated with complete remissions in 19 percent of pa-

---

effective therapy. D. J. Higby, H. J. Wallace, Jr., James F. Holland, "*Cis*-diamminedichlororplatinum (NSC-119875): A Phase I Study," *Cancer Chemotherapy Reports* 57 (1973): 459–73; A. H. Rossof, R. E. Slayton, C. P. Perlia, "Preliminary Clinical Experience with *cis*-diamminedichloroplatinum (II) (NSC 119875, CACP)," *Cancer* 30 (1972): 1451–6; R. W. Talley, R. M. O'Bryan, Jordan U. Gutterman, et al., "Clinical Evaluation of Toxic Effects of *cis*-diamminedichloroplatinum (NSC-119875) —Phase I Clinical Study," *Cancer Chemotherapy Reports* 57 (1973): 465–71. It was only in the latter part of the Phase 3 studies that feasible solutions to nephrotoxicity were discovered; Stephen D. Williams and Lawrence H. Einhorn, "Cisplatin Chemotherapy of Testicular Cancer," in Prestayko, Crooke and Carter, *Cisplatin*, 324.

[73] Among the Bristol-Myers officials centrally involved with the Platinol submission were Stanley Crooke (Bristol Labs Associate R&D Director) and Archie Prestayko (at Bristol Labs and the Baylor College of Medicine in Houston); "B-M Developing Unique Business in Cancer Chemotherapy Based on Formula of Small Volume Products Which Work Together to Form Full Line and Reduced Sales & R&D Costs," *FDCR*, November 20, 1978, 12.

tients. By May 1977, nearly three years after the Einhorn trial had started, forty-three of the fifty patients (86 percent) were "disease-free." The results were sufficiently breathtaking that the study was published in the *Annals of Internal Medicine*, a mainstream medical journal that stood quite apart from the oncology journals where most chemotherapy studies appeared in print.[74]

By the time the Division of Oncology Drugs was asked to deliver judgment on cisplatin, the Administration faced two quandaries that would become all too familiar in succeeding years. There were not, literally speaking, two randomized, controlled, and double-blinded studies, independently conducted, that had demonstrated cisplatin's efficacy. Cisplatin had been evaluated as single-agent therapy in more than one study, but none of these studies had been randomized or double-blinded. Second, the highest response rates and "cure rate" (complete response rates) were being observed in combination therapy, and the effective combination for testicular cancer was different from that for ovarian cancer.[75]

In his initial August 1978 review of the drug, Robert Young seized upon these weaknesses and recommended flat rejection of the Platinol NDA. Young was something of a loose cannon in the Division, and his caustic interactions with NCI officials and researchers at M. D. Anderson hospital in Houston had already led to high-level talks between Richard Crout and NCI officials about how to smooth relations between the organizations. Young took a literal approach to the statute, declaring that "the Act requires that I recommend that this NDA be made non-approvable because the sponsor has failed to submit the data required for approval." The comparisons between treatment and control groups were undertaken not within the same study, but across studies. The studies had not been run concurrently, and the essential principle of "comparability" of treatment and control groups had not been met. Initially, biostatistical reviewers agreed with him. Following guidances developed by Robert Temple and consistent with developments in statistics at the time, Young's notion of a proper controlled experiment was one that produced groups comparable in "all pertinent variables" but of course for the treatment.[76]

[74]Lawrence H. Einhorn and John Donahue, "*Cis*-Diamminedichloroplatinum, Vinblastine and Bleomycin Combination Chemotherapy in Disseminated Testicular Cancer," *AnnIM* 87 (1977): 293–8. A previous article in *Annals* that served to introduce the drug to general practitioners was Marcel Rozencweig, Daniel D. von Hoff, Milan Slavik, and Franco M. Muggia, "*Cis*-Diamminedichloroplatinum (II): A New Anticancer Drug," *AnnIM* 86 (1977): 803–12. The 19 percent response rate was observed in an M. D. Anderson study; M. L. Samuels, E. E. Johnson, and P. Y. Holoye, "Continuous Intravenous Bleomycin Therapy with Vinblastine in Stage III Testicular Neoplasia," *Cancer Chemotherapy Reports* 59 (1975): 563–70. For an update to the study that began in 1974, see Stephen D. Williams and Einhorn, "Cisplatin Chemotherapy of Testicular Cancer," in Prestayko, Crooke, and Carter, eds., *Cisplatin*, 324–5.

[75]R. Osieka, U Bruntsch, W. M. Gallmeier, Siegfried Seeber, and Carl G. Schmidt, "cis-Diamino-dichloro-platinum (II) in the Treatment of Otherwise Treatment-Resistant Malignant Testicular Teratoma" [author's translation from German], *Deutsche medizinische Wochenschrift* 101(6) (Feb. 1976):191–5, 199.

[76]Notice that there were no placebo controls in the cisplatin studies, reflecting the already

Separately, Bristol Laboratories then submitted their proposed labeling and advertising materials in a supplement on August 28. Just after returning from a two-week hiatus, Robert Young wrote another memorandum recommending rejection of the NDA. Young first seized upon the advertising materials that Bristol had included with their latest submission. Young directed his attention to the following components of the proposed brochure and medical journal advertisement for Platinol, elaborating five transgressions in the proposed marketing materials.

A. Brochure
   1. "Initial investigators have documented its usefulness in combination with other agents as a major, first-line chemotherapeutic for disseminated testicular and ovarian carcinoma." (page 1)
   2. "Perhaps, in fact, Platinol has cured some patients of their disease as data below would indicate." (page 9).
   3. "Therefore, many of the disease-free survivors who were treated with Platinol, Blenoxane (sterile bleomycin sulfate) and Velban (vinblastine sulfate) may be cures." (page 10).
B. Ad
   1. "Introducing a major new antineoplastic agent."
   2. "Cisplatin... one of the most promising anti-cancer chemotherapies under investigation, is now commercially available from Bristol Laboratories."[77]

The one component of Bristol's rhetoric that seemed to bother Young most was the word "cure," used variably as noun and verb in the proposed advertising materials. Young's skepticism of the term was founded in a longer vein of deeply embedded organizational skepticism in the Bureau of Drugs and its predecessors. "Cure" had been the favored noun and verb of cancer quackery for decades, and furnished the product name for the popular remedies of the 1950s ("Harry Hoxsey's Cancer Cure"). Beyond this, the Bureau's procedures had long reserved the word "cure" only for those therapies, like antibiotics, that completely rid the patient of the disease without residue or strong side effects (table 7.2). This notion was not merely theoretical but bore implications for clinical trials and the duration of patient follow-up. Unless a clinical trial (even one without rigid controls) could track patients for a period of several years after treatment at least, the idea that any patient had been cured was a statistical misnomer.

Having identified sins in the proposed advertising, Young went further

---

well-established practice at the time of dropping the placebo arm in cancer clinical studies. On Young's battles with the NCI and M. D. Anderson, see chapter 7 of this book. Robert S. K. Young, "Group Leader's Review of NDA 18-057," August 23, 1978; Approval Letters, NDA 18-057, FDA. Young's notion of experimental control was an exacting one, albeit one around for some time, and echoed ongoing research in "matching" and other techniques to render arms identical in all respects but the treatment.

[77] Robert S. K. Young, "Group Leader's Review of NDA 18-057, Submission of August 28, 1978," August 31, 1978, page 1; Approval Letters, NDA 18-057, FDA.

and condemned the entire drug application. He continued to press his claim that the clinical studies were lacking proper controls.

> There is no substantial evidence in the form of adequate and well-controlled studies that show that this drug is able to cure or mitigate any human disease. As I review this jacket it seems to me that other reviewers have missed the fact that the ovarian data was reviewed by biostatistics and found wanting. I reviewed the ovarian data and it is grossly deficient....
>
> I review and discuss this material because on face value it makes a strong and convincing case for approval of the drug. Unfortunately, the approval of drugs is conditioned on the scientific data submitted, not on the undocumented and unvalidated claims that people make. If the latter were the standard for approval, Laetrile would have been approved a long time ago.[78]

Young's stance was quite overblown, and his question may seem arcane and packaged in 1970s red tape. Yet at the time, his point did not entirely lack resonance or scientific plausibility. Given what oncologists knew in 1979, what exactly differentiated cisplatin from Laetrile? Three decades later the difference is obvious and clear, but at the time neither drug had the imprimatur of an established molecular model demonstrating its probable activity. Put more bluntly, while none of the hypotheses for amygdalin's anticancer activity were theoretically plausible, nobody knew with precision how cisplatin worked either. (The best hypotheses for cisplatin's effectiveness would come from literature in the late 1980s and 1990s, well after the Platinol battle had ended.) In the case of cisplatin, Bristol Laboratories was offering one informally controlled clinical study, other noncontrolled studies undertaken in the adjuvant chemotherapy paradigm, and the vigorous support of the NCI. Beyond this, the most salient brute fact of the discussion was that unlike Laetrile, cisplatin killed cancer cells (as well as noncancerous cells), but no one could demonstrate how. In this vacuum of mechanical knowledge, Platinol's demonstrated cytotoxicity and the power of its side effects became, ironically, favorable evidence in regulatory consideration.[79]

[78]Robert S. K. Young, ibid.; Approval Letters, NDA 18-057, FDA.

[79]About a year after Platinol's approval as an NME, Barnett Rosenberg would write an essay for a state-of-the-art cisplatin therapy volume in which he admitted that cisplatin's mechanisms of action were obscure; Rosenberg, "Cisplatin: Its History and Possible Mechanisms of Action," chap. 2 in Prestayko, Crooke, and Carter, eds., *Cisplatin: Current Status and New Developments*, esp. 14–18. Rosenberg would offer a similar admission in a 1982 interview; Jeff Lyon, "Tempo: Winning the War against the Disease Men Fear Most," *Chicago Tribune*, September 19, 1982, I-1. A commonly cited paper that offered a hypothesis for cisplatin's molecular mechanisms was H. C. Harder, R. G. Smith, and A. LeRoy, "Template Inactivation: The Mechanism of Action of *cis*-dichlorodiammineplatinum," *Proceedings of the American Association of Cancer Research* 17 (1976): 80. As recently as 2000, cancer researchers Daniel Fink and Stephen B. Howell could conclude of cisplatin that "the molecular details of how it causes cells to die are largely unknown" and that "its effectiveness varies quite markedly in different tumor types." Fink and Howell, "How Does Cisplatin Kill Cells?" chap. 7 in Lloyd R. Kelland and Nicholas P. Farrell, *Platinum-Based Drugs in Cancer Therapy*, (Totowa, NJ: Humana

In October 1978, Robert Young's division director, William Gyarfas, made a recommendation to approve cisplatin for use in adjuvant therapy in ovarian and testicular cancer. Gyarfas was hardly an apologist for the NCI or for Bristol Laboratories or any other pharmaceutical company. He had come into the agency as one of Frances Kelsey's hires in the Investigational Drug Branch in 1963. Like John Nestor and others, he had gone to Congress with his complaints about FDA's top management in the 1970s. Yet in a manner that points to the complications of the time, it was Gyarfas who overruled Robert Young by emphasizing the fundamental subjectivity of the applicable law and regulation, and the essential vacuum of treatment options for testicular cancer. After reviewing the various studies and constructing a table from several studies comparing the efficacy of cisplatin versus other chemotherapies as monotherapy against testicular cancer, Gyarfas turned to the ultimate question of whether the drug met the requirements of the law. He first transferred the burden of proof from cisplatin's sponsor to its critics.

> It is believed that NDA 18-057 is adequately complete and contains sufficient data and information to permit experts qualified by scientific training and experience to reach a conclusion that Cisplatin is safe and effective as claimed under part 130 of CFR. Specifically, under CFR 314.111 (Refusal to approve the application), all criteria and requirements of the Act are adequately met so that NDA 18-057 is approvable.

By invoking Section 314.111 of the Code of Federal Regulations, Gyarfas was interpreting the application (as "adequately complete") and its evidence in such a way that it would receive an "approvable" designation as opposed to a "non-approvable" judgment. He then turned to the two core concepts of the law—whether the investigations were "adequate" and whether the evidence was "substantial." In a creative and ethically based reading of the applicable law and regulations, and with a bow to organizational practices of the NCI and the FDA, Gyarfas presented a nuanced case for cisplatin's approval (figure 7.8).[80]

From the standpoint of a strict reading of the law and the regulations, William Gyarfas was conducting emergency surgery on the Platinol new drug application. The cisplatin NDA was stitched together from numerous clinical trials, few of which were controlled, none of which were explicitly set up to be commensurable with one another. Young and others in the Bureau

---

Press, 2000), 149. The dominant hypothesis in the literature for cisplatin's mechanism is that it effects a cross-strand linkage of DNA adducts, basically straight-jacketing or gluing strands of tumor DNA together so that malignant cells cannot divide and ligands are displaced. But this mechanism does not explain cell death, nor does it provide explanatory space for how some tumors acquire resistance to cisplatin.

[80]Gyarfas, "Addendum to Division Director's Evaluation of NDA 18-057," October 24, 1978; NDA File 18-057, FDA. Along with Nestor, Gyarfas had testified at Edward Kennedy's Senate hearings in 1976 to draw attention to what he saw as worrisome "bedfellow" relations with the pharmaceutical industry; *FDAPP*, 126.

The investigations of Cisplatin are reported and do show that the drug is safe and effective under conditions recommended. The reports of clinical investigations may not be as complete or optimal as desired, often just abstracts not "raw" data, but are adequate to permit evaluation and reaching conclusions. Since the word "adequate" is not defined in the Act other than that permitting experts qualified by scientific training and experience to reach conclusions, there is information and data in NDA 18-057 sufficient for the conclusion that Cisplatin is safe and efficacious as claimed. The key or pivitol studies have been identified. (Also, see Addendum to Medical Officer's Review of October 18, 1978).

Since 1965, Cisplatin has been under investigation under NCI control and following NCI's essentials of adequate and well-controlled clinical studies, they do provide substantial evidence to support claims of safety and effectiveness. Again, the Act does not define "substantial" so referring to Webster's Dictionary, substantial is defined as real, true, important, essential, ample to satisfy, and being that specified to a large degree or in the main. The information and data available in the NDA is substantial to permit reaching supportable conclusions regarding the safety and efficacy of Cisplatin.

In clinical investigations of Cisplatin, principles that have been developed over a period of years and are recognized by the scientific community for the evaluation of oncologic agents were utilized as set forth in NCI's and other recognized oncological investigators. In certain circumstances such as cancer that have high and predictable morbidity and mortality, historical as well as some preceding study data was used in control. This is scientifically, morally, ethically proper in oncological drug studies.

Figure 7.8. Paragraphs from William Gyarfas' October 24, 1978 Recommendation for Approval of Cisplatin (Platinol) for Testicular and Ovarian Cancer

of Drugs wanted more studies, and Rosenberg would later recall that the agency was "antagonistic to the whole idea" of cisplatin. In the end, however, Robert Young was overruled, and Barnett Rosenberg himself would later credit intervention with Congress for breaking the stalemate. For Rosenberg, "the FDA" was Robert Young, not Gyarfas, and not Marion Finkel, who would issue the final letter of approval for Rosenberg's promising laboratory child.[81]

Cisplatin's December 1978 approval was nearly silent and highly conditional. The Administration authorized Platinol as "palliative therapy" for metastatic testicular cancer and metastatic ovarian cancer. In ways that represented stark departures for the Administration, cisplatin was approved for use *only* in combination chemotherapy regimens, but still as "first-line," palliative therapy. Previous approvals of this sort were limited to therapies for liquid tumors such as lymphoma and leukemia. For solid tumors, combination therapy had been approved as "second-line" treatment when other modalities—surgery, radiation, and chemotherapy—had failed. Prescribing cisplatin as stand-alone therapy would have been, at least literally, a violation of its labeling requirements. Beyond this, the FDA included a recommended combination therapy in its approval literature and on the labeling of the document. For testicular cancer, cisplatin would be combined with bleomycin sulfate (Blenoxane) and vinblastine sulfate (Velban). For ovarian cancer it would be combined with doxorubicin hydrochloride (Adriamycin). In light of all the flexibility that Gyarfas and Finkel displayed in moving Platinol through the Oncology Drugs Division and the Bureau of Drugs, it is interesting the approved indications for cisplatin in January 1979 were those for which at least one randomized study had been completed.[82]

[81] On the lack of raw data in the application, see H. L. Walker, "Medical Officer Review NDA 18-057," March 14, 1978, 5; in Medical Officer Review (MOR) File, NDA 18-057, FDA. Unlike Young, Walker recommended approval contingent on Bristol's completion of more refined statistical analyses.

In a November 2006 interview, Rosenberg recalled that the FDA was "very much antagonistic to the whole idea" of platinum-based chemotherapy. "FDA said no, we want another trial to verify. We want repeat testing. My thought was that if you do this, a number of people are going to die. And I had to go to a number of Congressmen and Senators and ask them to put pressure on the FDA. We succeeded. We made enemies at the FDA." Rosenberg did not wish to revisit the situation or to make his records available for perusal. Author Phone Interview with Barnett Rosenberg (Barros Research Foundation, Holt, Michigan), November 13, 2006. I have not at this writing been able to verify (1) Rosenberg's claim that he (and possibly others) contacted members of Congress and (2) whether these contacts were at all influential in the eventual decision to approve cisplatin, or in the over-ruling of Robert Young.

[82] On the limited fanfare, see "New Cancer Drug Is Approved," *WP*, December 21, A32. The final approved labeling for Platinol appears in Final Printed Labeling (FPL) file, August 1978; NDA 18-057, FDA. The Administration's own records contain a second-guessing of this restriction, as a summary of the pharmacology review described cisplatin as "intended for intravenous administration in the palliative therapy of metastatic testicular and ovarian tumors *mostly* in conjunction with other modalities" (italics added); "Summary Basis of Approval," NDA 18-057, Cisplatin (copy completion date: May 22, 1991). For a summary of the approval, see "Bristol's Platinol (Cisplatin) Anti-Cancer NDA Approved," *FDCR*, January 1, 1979, T&G 8.

Cisplatin is today widely recognized as one of the most effective anti-tumor agents in the entire arsenal of chemotherapy. It is now complemented by other platinum-based agents, most notably carboplatin and oxaliplatin. The controversy over its development and approval seems antiquated now, and can be appreciated perhaps only in the historical context in which it was evaluated, and chief in that context was the presence of Laetrile politics. Laetrile and cisplatin were something like pharmaceutical strangers, passing each other in the hallways of the Administration at the same time but never being properly introduced. Both drugs were governed by the FDA primarily in the regulation of their testing. Both drugs pitted the National Cancer Institute partially or wholly against the Administration. And as Robert Young's review of cisplatin shows, Laetrile was on the minds of FDA reviewers and officials in their evaluation of cisplatin. In both cases, moreover, regulators rejected the theoretical basis of the drug's anti-tumor action as weak, at least at the time of development.[83]

The simultaneous regulatory careers of Laetrile and cisplatin also point to another question. What explains the FDA's deference to cancer therapies at the same time that its stance on Laetrile was so fierce, at the same time that its regulation of other drugs continued apace? The reasons lie not in any inherent severity of cancer as a disease, but more contingently in the status of the Institute as a bureaucracy-cum-lobbyist backed by the imprimatur of

---

As far as I can establish, cisplatin was the first NME approved by the Administration for first-line solid tumor therapy, but only in combination with other approved agents. Carmustine—also from Bristol Laboratories and approved in 1977—was approved as stand-alone therapy in addition to palliative combination therapy for brain tumors. In the 1960s and 1970s, several other agents had been approved as part of combination therapy regimens, but always for use against liquid tumors. These combination approvals included *methotrexate* (1953), *vincristine* (sanctioned for use in combination regimens against non-Hodgkin's lymphomas), and *procarbazine* (1969), which was authorized for use with the MOPP regimen. Before cisplatin, drugs for solid tumor therapy had largely been approved on stand-alone basis, as with *fluouracil* in 1962. For solid tumors, *mitomycin* had been approved in 1974 for pancreatic and stomach cancer (both solid tumors), but as "second-line" therapy when previous modalities had failed. Similarly, *lomustine* had received approval in 1977 for use after surgery and radiotherapy in brain tumors. Drugs for second-line therapy were subject to different approval criteria because only a select subset of patients would receive them.

Earlier combination drugs—in particular fixed combination antibiotics— functioned only as a distant metaphor for the development of clinical trial standards for combination therapy, but they were not irrelevant. As discussed in chapter 3, fixed-combination antibiotics posed difficulties to Bureau of Medicine evaluation standards in the 1950s because the partial or marginal contribution to treatment "efficacy" was difficult to establish. In antibiotics and other cases, a single agent could have appreciable efficacy. Although the genetic bases of the hypotheses had not yet been established, oncologists knew in the early 1970s that, in confronting the adaptive properties of tumor cells, particularly metastatic tumors, single agents often prove futile.

Vincristine was submitted by Eli Lilly with the trade name Oncovin. Procarbazine had been sponsored by Sigma-Tau Pharmaceuticals under the trade name Matulane.

[83]David H. Johnson, "Evolution of Cisplatin-Based Chemotherapy in Non-Small Cell Lung Cancer," *Chest* 117 (4) (April 2000) (supplement): 133S–137S. B. D. Evans, K. S. Raju, A. H. Calvert, S. J. Harland, E. Wiltshaw, "Phase II Study of JM8, a New Platinum Analog, in Advanced Ovarian Carcinoma," *Cancer Treatment Reports* 67 (1983): 997–1000.

the National Cancer Act. As Crout saw matters, the IND/NDA system had been established to regulate free enterprise, but "the cancer business is different. The cancer institute . . . has a public trust to get new drugs into the medical system as soon as possible." The fact that much cancer drug development was not commercially sponsored, combined with the Institute's stated mission, created the basis for an informal exception to the Administration's power over clinical research.[84]

Pressure to Approve: The Calculus of the Drug Lag and the December Effect

The construction of safety and efficacy often served to delay new drug approvals, to dash sponsors' hopes with new requests for studies, with non-approvable letters, and with skepticism. Yet as William Gyarfas' embrace of cisplatin shows, there were energies impelling many drugs toward approval, energies that operated within and upon the Administration long before the carnage and the politics of Acquired Immune Deficiency Syndrome (AIDS) transformed FDA politics in the 1980s. In some cases, these pressures came from the government itself, not least the National Cancer Institute and other NIH organs. In some cases, particularly well-heeled and legitimated companies could bring pressure from Congress and medical communities for drug approval. Yet the pressure for approval—and the calculus of reputation so central to the FDA's drug review behavior—was never so apparent as in the Administration's response to criticisms that it was responsible for the "drug lag" by which valuable new therapies were available in Europe years before being marketed to Americans. Even as top FDA officials publicly denied the existence of a drug lag, even as they minimized its significance or justified American skepticism by pointing to Laetrile, their organization was systematically reviewing drugs so as to present its audiences with a mechanical portrait of continuous innovation.

The precise nature of the drug lag has never been defined. In some measure, international differences were attributable to differing clinical trial standards, in some measure they were due to home-country favor for European pharmaceutical manufacturers, and in some cases the FDA was taking longer to review new drug applications than their counterpart agencies in Europe were taking. The British Medicines Control Agency, for instance, was accustomed to reviewing manufacturers' summaries of clinical trials, not the painstakingly disaggregated data that were passed on to the medical officers of the FDA. To the extent that the "drug lag" stemmed from delay in new drug review, it was mainly a product of the mismatch between the new legislative demands thrust upon the FDA in the 1960s and the meager congressional appropriations given to the agency in the ensuing decades. Over the long run, there has been a generally negative relationship between

---

[84]Crout remark in *DRR* 20 (17) (April 27, 1977): 14.

the duration of new drug review and the level of staff resources available to the FDA. As the level of resources at the Bureau of Drugs rose in the late 1970s, and as the staffing of the Center for Drug Evaluation and Research rose in the late 1980s and early 1990s, review times for NMEs came down accordingly.[85]

Whatever its reality or its causes, the drug lag became a political fact by the mid-1970s. Congressional critics ranging from Steven Symms to Edward Kennedy pointed to it, the AMA and renegade clinical pharmacologists decried it, and by mid-decade the term had entered the parlance of mainstream journalism. So too, specialty medical societies bemoaned the particular drugs that were already available by a physician's prescription in Europe—cardiologists and beta-blockers for essential hypertension, allergists and Albuterol for asthma control. The story behind the drug lag ran together with currents of strong anti-government criticism, the language of "red tape," and the increasing aversion of American citizens and politicians to anything bureaucratic.[86]

Whereas clinical pharmacologists and social scientists pointed to the 1962 regulations and their burdens as the cause of the drug lag, politicians increasingly began to gesture to broader patterns of bureaucratic regulation and the emotional distance of FDA officers from the patients who needed the drugs they were reviewing. A stock narrative—one that has since been repeated thousands of times in press accounts, everyday conversation, trade publications—was expressed by Steven Symms, Republican representative from Idaho. In this account—at times psychoanalytic, at others philosophical—the drug lag was a creature not of bureaucracy, but a lack of organizational compassion and the overwhelming audience of consumer activists.

The FDA is not faced with the urgencies of patient care and, therefore, finds it easier to say no than yes. It is unquestionably open to attack if it approves an ineffective or unsafe drug, but the greater damage done by delaying approval of an effective drug will not be laid at its door. The value of a new drug is often clear to an expert in the clinical field before it is formally recognized by a reviewer at the

[85]There were also administrative problems associated with the mail room; see the remarks of Sidney Merlis at the January 1965 meeting of the Modell Committee; Advisory Committee on Investigational Drugs, Summary of Proceedings, 14th Meeting, January 14, 1965; FOK. For statistical evidence on the long-run relationship between increased FDA staffing levels and reduced drug approval times, see Daniel Carpenter, A. Mark Fendrick, Michael Chernew, and Dean Smith, "Approval Times for New Drugs: Does the Source of Funding for FDA Staff Matter?" *Health Affairs* (Web Exclusive), December 17, 2003, W3-618-624. Hilts argues that elements of industry were responsible for the new backlog of NDAs in the early 1970s. "It was the drug companies themselves that had created the new backlog by successfully lobbying Congress to halt the recruitment of additional Public Health Service doctors. The new FDA officials had assumed incorrectly that a backlog had been caused by the sluggishness of overcautious reviewers" (Hilts, *Protecting America's Health*, 186).

[86]On the drug lag as an inversion of the agency's reputation for caution and precision, see chapter 5 of this book. Statement of the American Medical Association before the Subcommittee on Science, Research, and Technology, Committee on Science and Technology, by Ray W.

530 CHAPTER 7

FDA. The [Washington] *Post* fails to realize and appreciate that stringent drug regulation for society as a whole limits therapeutic choice by the individual physician, who is better able to judge the risks and benefits for his patients.[87]

Leaders in Congress and in the top ranks of the Administration began to talk ever more assertively about the importance of drug "approval" as well as drug "review." Representative Garry Brown of Michigan argued in congressional hearings that the FDA's functions were of "affirmative as well as regulatory obligation," which included the requirement that "the law should not be interpreted in a technical, irrational way so as to preclude the use of [a] drug if it can be shown to be effective." FDA General Counsel Peter Barton Hutt reminded audiences that "we have two duties: to regulate bad drugs off the market, certainly, but also to regulate good drugs, useful drugs, lifesaving drugs on to the market." Other top officials, girded by enthusiasm from HEW Secretary Joseph Califano, began to make a practice of publicizing new drug approvals in 1978.[88]

Less visibly, reviewers and managers within the Bureau of Drugs and, later, the Center for Drug Evaluation and Research (CDER) kept tabs on which of the NDAs in front of them had been approved in Europe, Canada, Mexico, or Japan. Certain applications became known as "drug lag items" and were unofficially designated for special treatment. The enforcer (and perhaps the author) of these standard operating procedures appears to have been J. Marion Finkel. Finkel was in the habit of making "administrative rounds" to different medical reviewers in the Bureau of Drugs, and no later than 1975 she and other officials were in the habit of reminding medical officers about foreign drug approvals. If a drug had been cleared in England, in particular, it quickly acquired fresh emphasis and energy in the Bureau, and fresh attention from Finkel. When Americans began to travel to Mexico

Gifford, Jr., M.D., "Re: the FDA New Drug Approval Process," June 21, 1979; microfiche copy in RG1, SG2— President's Office Records, 1964–1979, 10.1A— Research, General, Food and Drug Adm., 1978–1979"; Research Medical Library, University of Texas— M. D. Anderson Cancer Center, Houston.

[87]Steven D. Symms, "Don't Ease the Symptom—Attack the Problem," *WP*, June 3, 1977, A27. In a deeply perceptive address in 1978, Bureau of Drugs Director J. Richard Crout noted that accounts like Representative Symms' served as one of two stock "stories" about the FDA, the other being that the agency was bought off by the pharmaceutical industry and organized medicine; the address is reprinted in Crout, "The Nature of Regulatory Choice," *FDCLJ* 33 (1978): 413–15.

[88]*Consumer Protection: FDA Regulation of the New Drug Serc*, Hearings before the Intergovernmental Relations Subcommittee of the House Committee on Government Operations, 62. Wayne Pines directed the FDA's public relations efforts in 1978, and it was Pines who (according to Richard Merrill) initiated the practice of publicizing new approvals. "A generation later, FDA misses no opportunity to remind the public, and a critical Congress, that it is busy approving, not just reviewing, new treatments"; Merrill, "The Architecture of Government Regulation of Medical Products," 1768, n. 46. Until 1996, the FDA published a "summary basis of approval" (SBA) identifying the pivotal trials that were used to adduce evidence for the drug's safety and efficacy; Abraham and Sheppard, "Clinical Risk Assessment of Triazolam," *Social Studies of Science* 29 (6) 808.

and Canada to obtain albuterol (Proventil), sponsored by Schering Corporation for asthma management, and already approved in England, Finkel renewed organizational pressure for the drug's approval, despite clear weaknesses in the application.[89]

Giving quicker clearance to drugs already approved in other nations, particularly in Canada and the United Kingdom, was one organizational response to the drug lag discourse. The other metric used by industry, financial, and congressional audiences to evaluate the Administration was the number of new molecular entities approved in any given year. Over the long run, the Administration on its own could do little to influence these dynamics, as they were influenced mainly by aggregate patterns of science, research, and development, and by the contours of the Food, Drug and Cosmetic Act. Yet beginning in the late 1970s, the FDA began to take short-term measures to pack as many plausible molecular candidates for approval into the calendar year as possible, producing a "December effect" that was noticed by financial analysts and congressional observers. Cisplatin was one instance of this pattern, and there were many others. The dynamics of the December effect are best portrayed statistically, however (figure 7.9). As criticism related to the concept of a "drug lag" began to crest, so too did the fraction of approvals packed into the final month of the calendar year. And critically, this pattern prevailed for new molecular entities—whose annual numbers were being tallied by the Administration and its critics—but not for supplemental NDAs or for generic drugs, whose numbers were less salient to Administration audiences. The December effect stands as enduring evidence of the Administration's attention to its external image, and how this attention shaped some of its most important decisions. It also demonstrates that the rhetorical logic of the "drug lag" was less about average approval times and more about the general availability of new molecular forms.

The December effect was noticed by congressional overseers in the 1980s, particularly those legislators more friendly to consumer safety such as California Democrat Henry Waxman and Manhattan representative Ted Weiss. In a 1986 hearing on the agency's approval of the antidepressant Merital (nomifensine maleate), Weiss asked Robert Temple why so many new molecules

[89]At the 1976 hearings, Kennedy quoted an October 23, 1975 note from Finkel to a medical reviewer that stated: "Use our SOP for drug lag drug, viz approval if that firm submits a protocol for a phase 4 study"; *FDAPP*, 141. Minutes before Kennedy's quotation, John Winkler had refered to the term "drug lag item" (140). Finkel later asked about the relative therapeutic profile of albuterol (Proventil) and whether it had been approved in Canada and any other European countries besides England; Margaret A. Clark to John Winkler, September 19, 1975. According to the medical officer, Finkel wanted to know "what is the basis for the apparent opinion among some of the medical community that this drug is an important addition to the physician's armamentarium" (ibid., *FDAPP*, 189). Even as she acknowledged weaknesses in Schering's studies and its NDA, Finkel later identified albuterol as a "drug lag drug." Winkler resisted this characterization, but only on the basis that albuterol was not a valid example of what truly constituted a "drug lag item"; Winkler, "Memorandum of Meeting," November 3, 1975; *FDAPP*, 211.

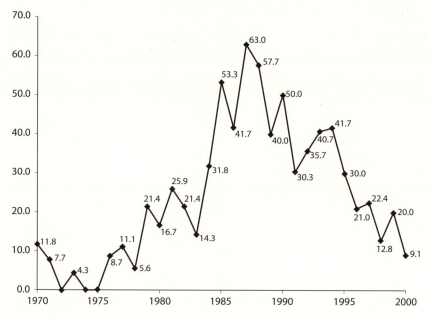

Figure 7.9. Percentage of NME Approvals in December, 1970–2000

(like Merital) had received their approval in December, and why so few drugs were receiving approval in January. Weiss stated his hypothesis rather frankly to Temple: "You have established increased numbers of approvals as a means of demonstrating success. And when you get down to December and are not satisfied with your numbers, and you go pell-mell about approving drugs in December." Temple shot back that Weiss's notion was "just fantasy." The key decision was not the date of approval but the date at which an application received an "approvable" letter. And even if he wanted to time approvals according to the logic of reputation, "I don't have that sort of control" over the approval process, Temple declared, "and I wouldn't want it if I did." Weiss was not persuaded. He offered a brusque critique of Temple's management.

> You do not exist to churn out approvals. You exist to make sure that the medicines that you approve are safe and effective. And I think, regardless of your attempt to explain away the huge statistical difference concerning the timing of approvals, that it is the date that FDA finally approves a drug, not that it declares a drug approvable, that counts. I don't know how you can possibly explain to anyone's satisfaction the vast discrepancy between what happens in January and what happens in December.[90]

[90] *Oversight of the New Drug Approval Process and FDA's Regulation of Merital*, Hearing before a Subcommittee of the Committee on Government Operations, House of Representatives, 99th Congress, Second Session (May 22, 1986), (Washington, DC: GPO, 1986), 69–74,

While the December effect was real, there is no primary source evidence to support a hypothesis advanced by some "drug lag" critics, namely, that FDA medical officers were purposefully allowing drugs to be approved earlier in England and other countries, then following post-market experience in those nations to gather further evidence on the drug's safety. In the crucial drug lag cases, FDA officials discussed the drugs extensively, yet without reference to post-market experiences in other nations. Instead, their conversations focused entirely upon the official application and the evidence produced from clinical trials. Where Canadian, English, or other European markets were discussed, the conversation was uniformly about the fact of the drug having already been approved. The continued attention to "drug lag items" in the 1970s and 1980s suggests that the opposite was occurring; considerations of international reputation were inducing the FDA to move faster where possible, and not to slow down the process in hopes of observing safety data from abroad.[91]

The Power of Gatekeeping: NDA Supplements, Approvable Letters, and Pre-Market Bargaining over Labels

The pre-market review process is undertaken in the shadow of regulatory power. Despite pressures for approval of new drugs, the Administration has the final say on whether and when a drug will be marketed. Given that pharmaceutical companies often plan marketing campaigns months or years in advance of a drug's approval, delays mean not only lost sales but organizational disruption, both of which firms are eager to avoid. It is in the power of negation—and in continued interaction between sponsors and regulators—that the faces of the Administration's pre-market power come into fuller and clearer view. These interactions occur in minute bargaining over the details of approval, concerning issues such as what the content of the labeling will be, whether a drug is approved for stand-alone use (monotherapy) or in conjunction with other drugs, and whether the drug is approved as "primary" therapy or as "secondary" therapy when the first

---

esp. 71. The FDA throughout this period would keep tabs on which country had first approved an NME.

[91] The notion that FDA officers were waiting for post-market evidence from other countries before approving in the United States comes from Henry Grabowski and John Vernon, *The Regulation of Pharmaceuticals: Balancing the Benefits and Risks*, (Washington, DC: American Enterprise Institute, 1983). The FDA's reluctant post-market regulation of oral contraceptive medications suggests the opposite pattern. After the 1950s, the FDA was in many cases less attentive to post-market patterns than its foreign counterparts, and failed to follow up on foreign data until they were brought to the agency's attention; see chapter 9. I cannot rule out that FDA medical officers may have done this in one case, but after reviewing dozens of "drug lag" candidates from the 1970s and 1980s I am unable to find an example where medical officers were keeping track of foreign post-market drug experience during the NDA review in the United States.

course of attack upon a disease has failed. These interactions also occur over the long run, as the Administration does not entirely relinquish its power over a new drug once it is approved, especially when the manufacturer seeks to market the drug for new therapeutic uses.

While most of the academic ink spilled on FDA drug review is devoted to new molecular entities, some of the most important decisions rendered by the agency concern new uses for previously approved molecules. These new drug applications are a particular kind of supplemental NDA—the "efficacy supplement"—in which a sponsor requests the right to amend the drug's labeling and regulatory status so it is deemed "effective" for a new indication. In effect, the sponsor officially adds a new therapeutic market to the drug. Given the previous approval of the molecule, this market could have been accessed through "off-label prescribing." Off-label prescribing occurs when physicians prescribe a medicine to a patient to treat a disease different from those diseases for which the FDA has deemed the drug effective. There is nothing in federal law preventing physicians from prescribing drugs for uses other than those approved. The Food, Drug and Cosmetic Act does prohibit the marketing of drugs for off-label indications, and pharmaceutical companies have paid fines in the hundreds of millions of dollars for violating these provisions of law. With the ever growing reliance of drug companies on advertising and marketing—both to physicians and directly to the consumers—the supplemental NDA takes on added importance, and demonstrates that the Administration does not relinquish all gatekeeping power when it approves a new molecular entity.[92]

Administration officials have long recognized the significance of their regulation of supplemental applications. Well before the 1962 Amendments, FDA official Julius Hauser had been writing new regulations for the review of supplemental applications since at least 1959. As soon as the 1962 Amendments passed, FDA medical officers sought to apply increased scrutiny to drugs and supplements that had been approved in years before the amendments, and to apply the efficacy standard much more rigorously to supplements than before. Upon the passage of the 1962 legislation, Commissioner George Larrick fired off a memorandum to Ralph Smith and directed him to apply renewed scrutiny to supplemental applications. "If... you do not have adequate evidence of efficacy," Larrick wrote, "the applicant will be informed that he does not have an effective new drug application and that it will be necessary for him to submit the needed information on efficacy. We would suggest a review of all pending 'conditionally effective' new drug applications in this category so that a letter may issue promptly to each applicant where this paragraph applies." Smith followed suit by announcing new guidelines in November 1962 and again in January 1963. By

---

[92] There are numerous kinds of supplemental NDAs, including applications to permit a previously approved molecule to be manufactured by a new company. The "efficacy supplement" is a particular kind of amendment to the approved NDA. On off-label prescribing more generally, and the regulatory problems it creates, see chapter 9.

managing supplemental NDAs internally by directive, Larrick and Smith avoided the trouble of a *Federal Register* statement, preferring instead to deal "on a product-by-product basis with individual applicants." Larrick and other top officials preferred to regulate supplements by means of case-based decision making and the accumulation of reputation-based precedents. The resulting form of governance was neither adjudication nor rule-making. It was instead the informal establishment of behavioral patterns.[93]

The Power of Supplemental Regulation: The Case of Enovid for Acne. In the years following the Kefauver-Harris Amendments and the new IND rules, the Administration found itself revisiting some familiar molecules, sponsored and represented by some familiar faces. In 1965, G. D. Searle approached the FDA with a proposal to market Enovid as an acne therapy. It was a time of massive wealth accumulation and strategic market protection for Searle. Being first to the oral contraceptive market had brought immense profits and a dominant market share. Of the 1.75 million women taking the pill in 1963, 90 percent of them were using one or another dosage form of Enovid. Searle's bid to redefine its star molecule was part of a broader pattern in the 1960s, popular in pharmaceutical firms and university medical centers, to try out synthetic-hormone contraceptives for new disorders, including menopause and related symptoms, coronary disease, and breast cancer. One reason for this push, at least on Searle's part, was that the market for oral contraceptives was quickly becoming saturated with competitors. Within four years of Enovid's regulatory approval, three major pharmaceutical firms—Johnson & Johnson with Ortho-Novum (1962), Parke-Davis with Norlestrin (1964), and Syntex with Norlutin (norethindrone) (1964)—had entered the oral contraceptive market with their own alternatives. Others from Eli Lilly, Upjohn, and Mead Johnson were on the way. Hence, with Searle's "Enovid for Acne" application, a molecule that began its regulatory and medical life as a treatment for dysmenorrhea, a drug that had effected a social transformation as great as any other in the twentieth century, came to the Administration once again, this time under auspices that were even more commercialized.[94]

[93]Memorandum from Jean L. Harvey, Deputy Commissioner of Foods and Drugs, to Directors, Bureau of Biological and Physical Sciences and Bureau of Medicine, subject "Revised Regulations Affecting Supplemental Applications," August 10, 1959; FDA Decimal Files, RG 88, NA. Larrick memorandum to Ralph G. Smith, October 19, 1962, Subject "New Drug Application Procedures"; FDA Decimal Files, RG 88, NA. Smith, "New Drug Policies—Supplements," Memorandum of January 16, 1963; DF 505.5, RG 88, NA. Updates to the Kirk-Larrick-Smith policy on supplements were issued in 1965 and 1966, but the essential policy of re-evaluation changed. J. Kenneth Kirk, Memo to Director, BOM, "Policy on Supplemental NDAs," October 12, 1966; DF 505.5, RG 88, NA.

[94]Herbert G. Lawson, "Birth Control Push: Drug Companies Press Development of New Oral Contraceptives," *WSJ*, November 1, 1963, 1. The Johnson & Johnson compound was produced by its subsidiary, Ortho Pharmaceutical Corporation. "Drug Manufacturers Step Up Drives to Get Share of Market for Oral Contraceptives," *WSJ*, March 2, 1964, 7.

The FDA's regulation of Enovid as a potential acne medication offers a stark historical juxtaposition of two different ways of regulating the same molecule in different therapeutic niches. Put simply, the FDA exhibited both laxity and caution with the same chemical at the same time. As oral contraceptive, Enovid was treated with deference. As acne therapy, it met with disdain. The Administration had in 1963 spoken publicly to deflate concerns about thromboembolism. By the time Searle proposed to market Enovid as an acne medication, the ballgame had changed. If Searle's application had been granted, Enovid would be given to men as well as women. An acne indication for Enovid would hence open up a vast new population of users, a population whose gender was doubtless more familiar and relevant to most FDA officials, and a population on whom little if any data were available. Despite all sorts of denials from 1963 to 1965 about the thromboembolic risk of Enovid and other estrogen-progestogen combinations taken as oral contraceptives, risks that the Administration would later explicitly acknowledge and publicize, the approach to Searle's acne application for Enovid was much more cautionary.[95]

Searle submitted a supplemental NDA for Enovid on June 10, 1965. The application was not a rigorous one. Searle medical director J. William Crosson had asked a number of allied physicians to try Enovid as an acne treatment, but no protocol was developed beforehand and the study lacked uniform measurement and any sense of control. The reports from physicians throughout the country were short on statistics and on particulars, and long on casual observation. Dr. Murray Zimmerman of Whittier, California, wrote Searle with "a rough summary of my results" in March 1965. Zimmerman had primed his patients by giving them a working theory of acne— "telling them that the basic cause of acne is an imbalance of sex hormones which results in an excessively oily skin"—and then explaining how Enovid "turns off the faucet" by restoring hormonal balance. As a summary of his efficacy results, Zimmerman said only that "my results in acne were much better than those previously reported by other investigators." In summarizing safety, he offered no numbers but said that "In giving female acne patients Enovid, Murphy's Law has followed through, i.e., 'Everything that can go wrong, will go wrong.'" Dr. Samuel Bluefarb of Chicago reported that "the results are not encouraging," noting "improvement" in "two girls" and exacerbation of acne in six others. When Boston University dermatologist John Strauss offered a detailed breakdown of his subjects in his report to Crosson, it stood out as a rarity in Searle's application.[96]

[95] On the initial approval of Enovid, see chapter 3. For discussion of the thromboembolic risks of oral contraceptives, see chapter 9.

[96] Murray Zimmerman, M.D. (Whittier, CA), to G. D. Searle & Company, March 11, 1965; Samuel H. Bluefarb, M.D. (Chicago, IL), to J. William Crosson (Assistant Medical Director, Searle), April 27, 1962; John S. Strauss, M.D. (Associate Professor, Department of Dermatology, Boston University School of Medicine) to Crosson, June 6, 1962; NDA 10-976, V121, RG 88, NA. Zimmerman's theory was a common one at the time, and appears to have its origins

At first Helling and Searle heard promising news. Officials in the Drug Surveillance Branch first warned Helling that the issues raised by Searle's submission were of sufficient regulatory weight that the "supplement" had been given its own NDA number, and that the application would be evaluated not by the Drug Surveillance Branch (DSB), but by the Medical Evaluation Branch. Yet one day later, the agency reversed this jurisdictional decision, sending the drug to the DSB. This decision appears to have provided relief and satisfaction to Helling, who expected a more positive outcome in the postmarket arm of the Administration and who had tried to place the review there in a casual act of venue shopping.[97]

Herbert Helling's optimism proved to be unfounded. One month after the FDA's venue decision, Helling called the Drug Surveillance Branch to inquire about the status of the "Enovid for Acne" submission. The FDA's Pierce was now considerably less committal and hinted that the application had raised concerns. In a move that likely troubled Helling and his associates at Searle, Pierce proposed a "personal conference" in Washington a week later. At this time, face-to-face meetings between company representatives and Administration officials were rarely if ever convened for the purpose of exchanging good news or pleasantries. The calling of such a meeting usually meant that there were difficult, complex issues to be worked out, and it was often a signal of expected delay in the approval (if any) of the application. When FDA dermatologist Donald Mitchell communicated his concerns to Helling—a lack of controlled studies, no defined dosage level, and a lack of attention to subgroup differences in the clinical results—it was clear to Searle that approval for Enovid as an acne drug was many months if not years away. The Administration declared the application "incomplete."[98]

Searle submitted another supplemental application in March 1967, and it would take another fifteen months for the FDA to deliver another "incomplete" ruling on the application. This time the bad news was delivered not by an epidemiologist, nor by anyone in drug surveillance, but by John Jennings of the Bureau of Medicine. In essence, the favorable venue decision of August 1965 had been reversed. The Administration felt it "important to reevaluate Enovid on its own merits," and hence "Enovid for Acne" was being treated as a completely new drug. Searle's new application was reviewed by a medical officer in the Metabolic and Endocrine Division and a pharmacist. The FDA endocrinologist noted that fundamental terms were

---

in the hypotheses of New York dermatologist Laurance Palitz. "Hormones & Health: New Medical Uses Seen for Sex Hormones and Synthetic Derivatives," *WSJ*, October 26, 1964, 1.

[97] A. Grace Pierce, M.D. (DSB/DMR), "Memo of Telephone Interview" (with Herb Helling, Searle), August 3, 1965; "Memo of Telephone Interview" (with Herb Helling, Searle), August 4, 1965; Donald E. Mitchell, M.D., "Memorandum of Conference" (with Helling and Pierce), September 28, 1965; NDA 10-976, V 121, RG 88, NA.

[98] Donald E. Mitchell, M.D., "Memorandum of Conference" (with Mr. Herb Helling, G. D. Searle & Co.), Subject: "Enovid" (NDA 10-976), September 28, 1965; NDA 10-976, V 121, RG 88, NA.

never defined, and that Searle's new efficacy scale—a five-point grading system ranging from "E" for "Excellent = complete clearing of the skin" to "W" for "Worse = exacerbation of acne despite treatment"—was uninformative and had been essentially ignored by "the majority of investigators." In concluding his "incomplete" letter, Jennings chided Helling for including duplicate reports from the 1965 application.[99]

Searle never resubmitted an "Enovid for Acne" application, and the company's star drug was never approved or marketed for acne vulgaris in the United States. The company's failure to open a vast new market for its oral contraceptive is telling not merely because the Administration was keeping an industry giant at bay, and not merely because a profitable market for a known drug did not translate into regulatory leniency, but because it heralded a different facet of the new era in U.S. pharmaceutical regulation. The Administration's approach to new drugs was not merely a stringency applied to new molecules. It was also an austerity applied to new claims for old molecules. And this austerity had a pervasive effect upon the strategies of drug development and marketing. Developers of synthetic estrogen-progestogen compounds limited their proposed labeling for new drug applications solely to the primary indication of "contraception," mainly because the regulatory route to market was much easier and more legitimized for oral contraception than for other indications.[100]

Oral contraceptives illuminated the organizational politics of supplemental review in two other ways. One common pattern in the late twentieth century is that several sponsors have sought entry to a new therapeutic market at the same time. In some cases, this simultaneous pressure for added entry comes through so-called me-too drugs—technically original molecules whose mechanism of action is similar to that of the "pioneer" molecule. Oral contraceptives presented the FDA with just such a dynamic. Most of the second-generation oral contraceptives, such as Johnson and Johnson's Ortho-Novum and Syntex's norethindrone, differed little if at all from Enovid. With this influx of oral contraceptives, FDA officials faced a thorny and inevitably political decision about how to prioritize them. Syntex was so similar to Enovid that it was cleared quickly. "Yet there are other applica-

[99]John J. Jennings, M.D. (Acting Associate Director for Marketed Drugs, BOM) to G. D. Searle & Company (attention: Helling), June 24, 1968; F. Connelly, "Pharmacist's Review," NDA 10-976, April 29, 1968; L. J. Trilling (Division of Endocrine and Metabolic Products), "Summary of Supplement," February 14, 1968; NDA 10-976, V130, RG 88, NA. Jennings copied the Office of New Drugs, the Medical Evaluation Division, and the Office of Marketed Drugs on the correspondence, and FDA officials from four separate offices signed off on the "incomplete" notification letter.

[100]Ortho's Ortho Tri-Cyclen, a combination of ethinyl estradiol and norgestimate, is today one of the very few oral contraceptives with FDA approval for the treatment of acne vulgaris in females. For evidence of its efficacy, see G. Redmond, et al., "Norgestimate and Ethinyl Estradiol in the Treatment of Acne Vulgaris: A Randomized, Placebo-controlled Trial," *Obstetrics & Gynecology* 89(4) (1997): 615–22. "Drug Manufacturers Step Up Drives to Get Share of Market for Oral Contraceptives," *WSJ*, March 2, 1964, 7.

tions for new types of pills," wrote one officer, "that have been before the FDA for several months but which because of their newness require more extensive review by the agency than the Syntex pill." Under the crunch of competing regulatory pressures, and constrained by limited resources, the Bureau of Drugs was faced with an explicit policy decision: "whether to clear the pills on a first-come, first-served basis or whether to clear the pills as rapidly as possible." Given the size of the market at stake, these problems subjected the Administration to considerable lobbying, and the decisions about prioritization often came down to seemingly minute matters such as the ambiguity of the labeling.[101]

Perhaps the most forceful pressure for approving efficacy supplements comes when large-scale clinical trials convincingly demonstrate new therapeutic uses. These trials—sometimes sponsored by the manufacturer, sometimes paid for by the government, sometimes bankrolled by philanthropists and social organizations— receive extensive publicity and often appear in high-profile medical journals. The chief example of this dynamic in recent years comes in the drug tamoxifen (trade name Nolvadex), which had been approved for adjuvant treatment of metastatic breast cancer in 1977. Tamoxifen is thought to have its effect by depriving breast tumors of the estrogen they rely upon to grow. In the early 1990s, scientists and the drug's manufacturer, AstraZeneca, saw evidence from earlier studies that tamoxifen might be helpful in reducing the risk of breast cancer among women who were already "at risk" but for whom no tumor had appeared. The implied metaphor coursing through breast cancer debates was transformed from chemotherapy to "chemoprevention." In 1992, scientists led by Bernard Fisher began enrolling thousands of women in the Breast Cancer Prevention Trial (BCPT). The BCPT was a study of 13,388 otherwise healthy women aged thirty-five and over who were considered to be "at risk" for breast cancer. The study was closely watched and returned encouraging results for those who believed that a strategy of early screening and preventative pharmaceutical medicine would reduce many women's risk of developing metastatic breast tumors. The NCI stopped the trial early when examination of ongoing data showed that the rate of expected breast cancer development in the tamoxifen group was 1 in 236, compared to 1 in 130 for the placebo arm.[102]

---

[101] "Drug Manufacturers Step Up Drives to Get Share of Market for Oral Contraceptives," *WSJ*, March 2, 1964, 7. A Grace Pierce, "Memo of Telephone Interview" (with Herbert Helling), August 3, 1965; NDA 10-976, V 121, RG 88, NA.

[102] The powerful and sometimes controversial role of tamoxifen in the nation's struggle with breast cancer is far more complex and intricate than can be adequately covered here. Barron Lerner offers a perceptive account in his *The Breast Cancer Wars: Fear, Hope and the Pursuit of a Cure in Twentieth-Century America* (New York: Oxford University Press, 2001), 263–6. Bernard Fisher, "Highlights of the NSABP Breast Cancer Prevention Trial," *Cancer Control* 4 (1) (1997): 78–86; James S. Olson, *Bathsheba's Breast: Women, Cancer and History* (Baltimore: Johns Hopkins University Press, 2002), 258–9. On the political organization of breast cancer activism, see Maureen Hogan Casamayou, *The Politics of Breast Cancer* (Washington, DC: Georgetown University Press, 2001), particularly chap. 5.

In the wake of Fisher's announcements, often criticized by doubters of chemoprevention and by scientists wary of the corporate backing of tamoxifen, the National Cancer Institute began distributing computer software to patients that was designed to assess breast cancer risk. The software was premised upon the BCPT study results and offered quantitative estimates to patients of when and where tamoxifen preventive therapy was likely to be helpful. The NCI's massive distribution (accompanied by a publicity campaign) came while the Administration was still considering the supplemental NDA for tamoxifen, and it underscored how the NCI could be as forceful a lobby as any for new drug approval. The BCPT did not, however, clear an entirely easy path for tamoxifen's approval as a risk-reduction therapy. The Oncology Drugs Advisory Committee, following cues from the Oncology Drugs Division headed by Richard Pazdur, took issue with AstraZeneca's attachment of the term "preventative" to tamoxifen. Given that the trials had a short follow-up period, it was entirely possible that instead of "preventing" cancer, tamoxifen was treating preclinical tumors, thereby selecting for more aggressive cancer. This issue also emerged in AstraZeneca's advertising for tamoxifen in 2000.[103]

Approval decisions have also been affected by publicized clinical trials because these studies influence future clinical practice. Long before it was withdrawn in Europe and temporarily in the United States, Warner-Lambert's Rezulin (troglitazone) was the subject of debate at the FDA about whether it should be approved as monotherapy or strictly as used in combination with sulfonylurea. At the core of this debate was the medical reviewer's perception, backed by superiors, that the clinical results for the combination were much stronger than the data supporting monotherapy. Rezulin had also received a priority rating, based on results from the ten-year Diabetes Control and Complications Trial. Division leader Alexander Fleming argued for approval of Rezulin, stating that "We urgently need new therapies for this condition in order to achieve the potential that the Diabetes Control and Complications Trial has suggested." Yet part of the decision was a bow to what FDA medical officers saw as expected clinical practice. It was likely that Rezulin would "soon be used widely," and that "physicians will probably begin to prescribe troglitazone as monotherapy." Because physicians were likely to prescribe Rezulin as monotherapy anyway, FDA medical officers reasoned, the FDA should approve it for the condition and include specific instructions on the label so it would be used properly as monother-

---

[103]"Tamoxifen Breast Cancer Risk Analysis Software is Being Distributed by NCI; FDA's User Fee Goal for Nolvadex Supplemental NDA is Oct. 30," *Pharmaceutical Approvals Monthly* (Oct. 1998): 13–15. The risk assessment campaign also came in for scrutiny because it was associated with wider efforts by AstraZeneca to popularize the drug and condition that it treated; AstraZeneca has long been the main corporate sponsor of Breast Cancer Awareness Month; Samantha King, *Pink Ribbons, Inc.: Breast Cancer and the Politics of Philanthropy* (Minneapolis: University of Minnesota Press, 2006), 81–2; Lerner, *The Breast Cancer Wars*, 249.

apy, namely with a higher dose and with proper expectation of a lower treatment effect.[104]

Bargaining, Arm-Twisting, and the Approvable Letter. The other domain of continued gatekeeping power appears in the capacity of the Administration to extract concessions from firms in the last stages of drug approval, as it becomes clear that the molecule will be approved but when some of the crucial details have yet to be determined. These interactions provide an opportunity for Administration officials to exercise some of their starkest power, for the drug sponsor wants approval in favorable terms, but usually wants approval earlier than later. Pre-approval bargaining over labels, marketing materials, and other features of the drug places drug companies in a position of relative powerlessness, and this position has given rise to numerous complaints over the past decades. In communications with the Modell Committee in 1964, officials from Burroughs-Wellcome acknowledged that their relations with the FDA were generally productive, but he lamented that "FDA often *dictates* to industry regarding the phrasing of warning letters, labels, brochures, etc." He hoped that "with greater representation of industry on FDA committees, these problems would wane." Besides pointing to "the problem of 'conflict of interests' in such a set up," FDA officials did little to address these concerns. Associate Commissioner Winton Rankin instead repeated the decades-old refrain that the "FDA is always willing to sit down with industry and discuss mutual problems."[105]

These industry complaints have persisted since the 1960s, in part because the underlying dynamics of regulatory power have not changed appreciably. Medical officers and Division Directors often reserve their greatest battles for labeling. And control over labeling gives these officers, by virtue of subdelegation and informal practices of deference to lower-level expertise, significant regulatory power. Paul Leber, long-time director of the Neuropharmacological Drug Products Division at the FDA, began to attach caveats to labels of pain and migraine medications in the 1990s. For the approved labeling of the anti-migraine drugs Imitrex, Migranal, and Amerge, Paul Leber's division added the following strong warning.

> Comparisons of drug performance based upon results obtained in different clinical trials are never reliable. Because different studies are conducted at different times, with different samples of patients, by different investigators, employing different criteria and/or different interpretations of the same criteria, under different conditions (dose, dosing regimen, etc.), quantitative estimates of treatment re-

[104]Robert Misbin, Medical Review of NDA 20-720, June 3, 1997; NDA File 20-720, FDA. "Warner-Lambert Rezulin Study Shows 54%–65% Response to Monotherapy; sNDA for Monotherapy and Sulfonylurea Combo Use Submitted," *Pharmaceutical Approvals Monthly* (March 1997): 3–6.

[105]Advisory Committee on Investigational Drugs, Summary of Proceedings, 7th Meeting, February 27, 1964; FOK.

sponse and the timing of response may be expected to vary considerably from study to study.

Leber apparently took some pride in this caveat, noting in correspondence that it grew out of innovations that he had made to neuropharmacological drug products labeling. Leber held that "an anti-migraine drug product will be misbranded if its labeling fails to advise that the data adduced in controlled clinical investigations of the drug product cannot be validly compared with that adduced in trials of other anti-migraine drug products." Firms resisted the generic warning, arguing not only that the statement was not always applicable, but also that the Division lacked authority to request the introduction of such a statement.[106]

It would be wrong to assume, however, that companies always want as permissive a label as can be achieved. On Duract, Widmark's memo on hepatotoxicity contributed to an internal dispute about how to handle the drug. "The company proposes a label that states that bromfenac is for short-term management of pain; when given longer than 30 days, the patient should be monitored for liver abnormalities. The company would like a label that actually puts the onus on the prescribing physician because, if severe and maybe fatal liver toxicity of bromfenac will occur in treatments longer than 30 days, the physician will be sued and will be found liable if he/she did not 'monitor' for liver damage. Wyeth-Ayerst will be in the clear, because 'it is in the label.'" Like Wyeth-Ayerst, drug companies sometimes want more aggressive warnings in the FDA-approved labeling, as a way to head off or constrain tort lawsuits in case of adverse events.[107]

Use of approvable letters became more common after the passage of the Prescription Drug User Fee Act of 1992, in which review decisions were mandated under timelines. Instead of issuing a final decision at the deadline, FDA officials often issued an "approvable" letter. By this shift, what once heralded the imminent marketing of a commodity had now become a marker of delay and the absence of regulatory commitment. Such cautious logic showed in the writing of FDA official Russell Katz in the approvable letter for Lamictal: "I believe the data support the conclusion that Lamictal is effective against secondarily generalized seizures. The lack of more robust findings is likely the result of the relatively small sample sizes." Katz's colleague Paul Leber disagreed, writing that small samples indeed composed "the most probable explanation for the failure," but that "it is imprudent to base a regulatory decision on an assumption in any situation in which the question can be resolved definitively through the conduct of a randomized controlled clinical trial." The agency's advisory committee recommended

---

[106] "Migraine Nasal Sprays Approved without ICH-Specified Long-Term Data, Higher Rate of Attacks Offsets Lower Patient Enrollment, FDA Says," *Pharmaceutical Approvals Monthly* (July 1998): 27–9. "Indeed, the sponsor [Novartis, for Migranal] goes so far as to specify steps that the Division should follow before requiring the introduction of such a statement."

[107] Rudolph Widmark, "Memo Regarding Hepatotoxicity of Bromfenac," November 14, 1996; NDA File 20-535, FDA.

approval of the Lamictal for adjunctive therapy, but denied an indication for monotherapy in epilepsy and for use in children. The agency followed these recommendations, approving the drug in December 1994 as adjunctive therapy in treatment of partial seizures in adults with epilepsy.[108]

. . .

The power over medicinal details retained by Administration medical officers and division directors is significant and enduring. Its continuance has led scholars in administrative law to ask whether the gatekeeping authority wielded by the FDA and other agencies translates into other powers that Congress has not expressly authorized for regulatory bodies and their subordinate officers. The existence of such a multifaceted issue, and its continual appearance in legal and academic circles, demonstrates that in the past half-century of new drug review, regulatory power was more complicated and intricate, but no less forceful, than it would otherwise appear.

[108] "Lamictal Efficacy Comparable to Carbamazepine in First-Line Epilepsy, Glasgow Study; Lamotrigine in Phase III for Monotherapy, Pediatrics," *Pharmaceutical Approvals Monthly* (January 1996): 27–8.

The Governance of Research and Development: Gatekeeping Power, Conceptual Guidance, and Regulation by Satellite

> There is a feeling that the regulations that emanate from and are promulgated by the Food and Drug Administration are intended to regulate the therapeutic human research as it is currently executed in academic and private research centers. This feeling is rapidly becoming a reality, solely because it is widely believed. Institutions go into defensive postures to accommodate Food and Drug Administration regulations.
>
> —Oncologist Jan van Eys, M.D., to President Charles LeMaistre, M. D. Anderson Hospital and Tumor Institute, Houston, Texas, 1978

> I don't think it is FDA's role to define standards for therapy [for diseases] for which we have no therapy.
>
> —NCI Division of Cancer Treatment Director Bruce Chabner, 1989 [1]

A REGULATOR'S authority over admittance to the pharmaceutical marketplace has become—contingently, gradually, and forcefully—a set of powers over the research and development that precedes market entry: its conduct,

---

[1] J. van Eys, "Food and Drug Administration Regulations and Research in Cancer Centers (Conceptual construct for Dr. LeMaistre)," May 29, 1979; Felix L. Haas to LeMaistre, "Material from Dr. van Eys for Your Consideration in Response to F.D.A. Proposed Regulations Regarding IRBs," May 29, 1979; RG1, President's Office Records, 1964–1979, 10.1A—"Research, General, Food and Drug Adm., 1978–1979"; MDAA. Chabner remark in *DRR*, February 8, 1989, 4.

its practitioners, its essential concepts and ruling structures. The Administration now governs the qualification of clinical investigators and can essentially debar researchers from the practice of drug research. It has cleaved the process of drug experimentation into four "phases" and has all but defined the notions of "effectiveness," "safety," "efficacy," "adequate," "bioequivalence," and "bioavailability" by which drugs are compared and judged. In a series of rules elaborated over one half-century, the Administration has forcefully reshaped the meaning of human subjects protection, and has formally defined the elements of "good clinical practice." And the visible implements of the FDA's authority are everywhere, as two generations of researchers have become intimately and agonizingly familiar with such institutions as the quality assurance monitor, the project control team, the data safety and monitoring board, and the institutional review board (IRB).[2]

The Administration's regulation of medical research is expressed mainly in rulemaking and stems from two sources of authority. The first is a vacuum of legislative content that former FDA general counsel Richard Merrill has called "statutory indirection." Before 1997, the Federal Food, Drug and Cosmetic Act did not expressly authorize the FDA to regulate experimental drug trials. Instead, it prohibited interstate distribution or transportation of a new drug not yet approved by the FDA. Yet in order for any drug to be tested, interstate distribution is a near certain prerequisite; a drug tested at the Mayo Clinic of Rochester, Minnesota or at the M. D. Anderson Center in Houston, Texas, would require such an exemption because the drug may be manufactured in other states, or because the drug may be administered by physicians in provider networks in other states. The result is that any experimental drug must receive an exemption from federal law as an "investigational new drug." The lack of congressional specificity on this term gave interpretative authority to the Administration to define what these drugs were. A second and related source of authority is the gatekeeping power of the FDA. Since most clinical trials with drugs are designed to produce results that can justify regulatory approval, the Administration can and does powerfully shape clinical trials simply by amending its approval criteria. Any set of clinical experiments that does not satisfy the Administration's regulations can and usually will result in a New Drug Application that is rejected or delayed at a later stage.[3]

The Administration's directive and gatekeeping power over research and development support a broader conceptual power. Conceptual power in American pharmaceutical regulation appears as the ability to define the terms and concepts in which human agents think, experiment, and infer. It

[2]More recently the title of "data safety and monitoring board" has become the "data monitoring committee." With the advent of a "Phase 0," there are now technically five IND phases.

[3]Merrill, "FDA Regulation of Clinical Drug Trials," in Marc Hertzman and Douglas E. Feltner, eds., *The Handbook of Psychopharmacology Trials: An Overview of Scientific, Political, and Ethical Concerns* 61 (New York: New York University Press, 1997), 62.

is the power to shape the categories by which scientists, physicians, and others organize their learning, and to define these concepts, categories, and institutions in ways that make them seem natural or, in this case, "scientific." Indeed, so much research is done on drugs that the portion of research directly regulated by the FDA spills over heavily on to research that is not directly regulated: research on psychiatric therapy and interventions, surgical techniques, public health policies and interventions, and much quantitative and ethnographic inquiry in the contemporary social sciences.

The story of clinical study regulation told here is a story of transformations in the practices of the FDA and its audiences from the 1960s to the early 1980s. It is largely a story of clinical research, that is, research on human subjects in a context (the "clinic") where the ultimate aim is superior therapy. These constraints—the periodization adopted in this chapter and its clinical focus—partially obscure a wider ambit of FDA influence. The Administration has asserted rather broad authority over animal drug trials, the stuff of more classical pharmacology. And the narrative of change does not stop in the 1980s, as crucial concepts have developed since. It is arguable, however, that the principal and most enduring changes to the regulation of clinical drug trials in the last half-century were adopted from 1963 to 1981. These include good clinical practices ("GCPs"), good laboratory practices (or "GLPs"), the technologies and procedures of human subjects protection (including the patient consent form and the institutional review board, IRB), the quality assurance monitor, the quality control unit, and others.[4]

PROJECTIONS OF POWER: THE PROTECTION OF HUMAN SUBJECTS, THE REGULATION OF THE LABORATORY

Clinicians and clinical researchers are well aware of the importance of human subjects regulations in medical research. Just about any study conducted at a university medical center, a hospital, a contract research organization, or elsewhere must now pass the muster of an institutional review board. IRB approval is necessary before the project is begun, in some cases before investigators can even apply for funding. This is as true of social science projects in anthropology, economics, epidemiology, political science, and sociology as it is of clinical or experimental research in medicine and psychology. The aggregate activity conducted under human subjects protections is staggering: every year thousands of IRBs in the United States examine over 20,000 research proposals, and hundreds of thousands of experimental subjects and patients are presented with their legal human subjects' rights and sign con-

[4]The 1963 IND regulations and their pre-history are discussed in chapters 3 and 4. On animal drug trials and their regulation, see Merrill, "FDA Regulation of Clinical Drug Trials," 68. What observers call "clinical research" is what others call "drug development" or "pharmaceutical R&D."

sent forms stating that they understand these rights as they participate in the experiment.[5]

Exactly how modern science and government arrived to this point—the evolution and maintenance of human subjects protections in clinical research—is not well understood. A casual understanding, available from some published histories and a brief tour of the World Wide Web, is that current human subjects protections in medical research followed from the Nuremburg Code of 1947 and the World Medical Association's Helsinki Declaration of 1964 and have been supported by the evolution of ethical standards in the medical profession. These impressions are half-true and miss the more important feature of human subjects protections: their partial (and political) authorship and their historical enforcement by the U.S. government, especially the FDA. The breadth and rigor of human subjects regulations that govern clinical research in the United States and much of the world are as attributable to the Administration as to the AMA or the National Institutes of Health.[6]

Because the Administration is the primary enforcer of human subjects protection in the United States, its officers also shape the authorship of those protections. The agency's role as gatekeeper to the American prescription pharmaceutical and device markets, combined with the implied powers that come with that role, make the Administration an incredibly consequential force for human subjects protection. The FDA's veto power over product development gives pharmaceutical firms and researchers compelling incentives to cleave tightly to federal regulations and rigorous ethical standards. Just as important, the FDA has interpreted its authority over clinical research quite broadly, issuing detailed and comprehensive rules and aggregating inspection forces to monitor clinical investigators, laboratories, and IRBs and even to interview human subjects enrolled in clinical trials. The Administration has a life-or-death say, not just about products but also about IRBs, clinical investigators, individual studies, and the firms and universities that sponsor them.[7]

[5]For some rough estimates of the number of IRBs, the number of federally sponsored or regulated clinical trials, and the number of human subjects participating, see GAO, *Protecting Human Research Subjects*, (Washington, DC, March 8, 1996; GAO/HEHS-96-72), 2, 6. In the past half-century, the total number of human subjects in medical and pharmacological research easily exceeds 10 million and is perhaps much larger.

[6]Casual and academic treatments of human subjects protections, including informed consent and the evolution of IRBs, generally ignore or accord trivial treatment to the role of the FDA. For example, the National Cancer Institute's "A Guide to Understanding Informed Consent" (available at www.cancer.gov) discusses the Nuremburg Code, the Declaration of Helsinki, the 1979 Belmont Report, and the unified 1991 Federal Code for the Protection of Human Subjects, but not the FDA. For more prominent academic treatments, see Ruth Faden and Tom Beauchamp, *A History and Theory of Informed Consent* (Oxford: Oxford University Press, 1986); David J. Rothman, *Strangers at the Bedside* (New York: Basic Books, 1991).

[7]Given that it is impossible to receive an NIH grant without IRB approval at the sponsoring institution, it is important not to overstate the Administration's power over academic research; the point here is to detail the Administration's effect on shaping the behavior and structure of modern IRB.

As with the efficacy provisions of the 1962 law, the human subjects protections in federal regulation were proposed in FDA rulemaking before they were codified into statute in the Kefauver-Harris Amendments. The pivotal proposed rules were signed by Commissioner George Larrick on August 7, 1962 and were published three days later in the *Federal Register*. In the August 1962 rules, the Administration's power over clinical research was expressed in much the same way that its power over new drugs was codified in 1956: by publication of a form. The 1962 proposed rules received their expression in the shape of two federal forms. The first, Form "FD-1571," the "Notice of a Claimed Investigational Exemption for a New Drug," provided the sponsor with an opportunity to apply for interstate distribution of the drug for research purposes. The second, Form "FD-1572," was a "Statement of Investigator" that permitted the Administration to assess the qualifications of the person proposing the study. Along with the NDA form authored in 1956, form FD-1571 would quickly become the primary structure upon which clinical research in the United States (and many other countries) is based. In ensuing years it would embed regulation of preclinical studies, human subjects protections, standards for clinical pharmacology and statistics, guidelines for research design, and procedures for establishing an institutional review board. While the Kefauver-Harris Amendments would thoroughly structure the Administration's early regulation of medical research, the primary referent for regulation of clinical investigations in the 1960s was not the new statute, but the proposed rules of August 1962.[8]

In part because New York Senator Jacob Javits had made it a priority, even more because Frances Kelsey assumed control of the Investigational New Drug Branch in the FDA's 1963 reorganization, the Administration became directly involved in human subjects protection immediately after the 1962 Kefauver-Harris Amendments. The 1962 Amendments added a Section 505(i) to the Food, Drug and Cosmetic Act which required investigators to "obtain the consent" of patients or their representatives in drug trials, except where consent was infeasible or where, in the "professional judgment" of the investigator, obtaining consent would be "contrary to the best interest" of the patient. Administration officials drafted rules published

[8]HEW/FDA, "New Drugs for Investigational Use: Proposed Exemptions," *FR* 27 (155) (Aug. 10, 1962): 7990–92; "New Drugs; Procedural and Interpretative Regulations; Investigational Use," *FR* 28 (Jan. 8, 1963): 179–82. President John F. Kennedy signed the Drug Amendments into law on October 10, 1962. Comparing these two sets of rules suggests that the Kefauver-Harris legislation added very little to the August 10 proposed rules.

As far as I can establish, it was political scientist David Weimer who first documented the fact that IND requirements in rulemaking preceded the enactment of the Kefauver-Harris Amendments ("The Regulation of Therapeutic Drugs by the FDA: History, Criticisms, and Alternatives," Discussion Paper No. 8007, Public Policy Analysis Program, University of Rochester). Weimer's observation was picked up by a NAS-NRC report on the competitiveness of the U.S. pharmaceutical industry, *The Competitive Status of the U.S. Pharmaceutical Industry: The Influences of Technology in Determining International Industrial Competitive Advantage* (Washington, DC: National Academies Press, 1983), 59–61.

in 1966 that accounted for the first appearance of the term "informed consent" in U.S. regulations. The 1966 rules required investigators to inform patients of the administration and dosage of the drug and "all inconveniences and hazards reasonably to be expected," including the possibility that the person would receive a placebo or control. And in perhaps the most important and consequential statement of the 1966 rules, the FDA required for the first time that "informed consent" must be obtained in writing. As historian David Rothman observed of the 1966 rules, the Administration had advanced the most forceful, definitive and consequential statement yet for human subjects protection. "The FDA regulations unquestionably represent a new stage in the balance of authority between researcher and subject," Rothman concluded. "The FDA's definitions of consent went well beyond the vague NIH stipulations, imparting real significance to the process."[9]

Regulation by Satellite: The Institutional Review Board as a Political Creation. Internal review bodies had been emerging indigenously at many research institutions in the middle twentieth century. While the development of the IRB was not uniform, the prototype of the IRB concept was in place at some top research hospitals and academic medical centers several years before the FDA mandated its attachment to clinical studies. And federal legislation in 1966 required any institution receiving Public Health Service funding to create a "local" board for oversight of human subjects research. Yet perhaps the key institutional change supporting the standardization of IRBs came in 1969, when the Administration published proposed rules in the *Federal Register* requiring every investigational new drug application to have passed an institutional review committee before being submitted to the agency. Proponents of human subjects' rights lambasted the proposed rules as "grossly inadequate, hopelessly fragmentary and vague." The Pharmaceutical Manufacturers Association worried about costs for clinical sponsors and suggested that IRB approval be left to the discretion of the sponsoring organization. Despite these protests, physician-researchers at clinical research centers like the Mayo Clinic resigned themselves to the inevitability of FDA control over IRBs and began preparing to adapt. FDA commissioner Charles Edwards and general counsel Peter Barton Hutt gave little ground in responding to consumer and industry comments. In reaction to medical rights organizations, the new rules mandated IRB approval for all three

[9]See FFDCA, Section 505 (i). On Javits, see Rothman, *Strangers at the Bedside*, 64–7. The Administration's 1966 rules appear at "Consent for Use of Investigational New Drugs on Humans; Statement of Policy," *FR* 31 (168) (Aug. 30, 1966): 11415. Rothman also argues that "The blanket insistence on consent for all nontherapeutic research would have not only prohibited many of the World War II experiments but also eliminated most of the cases on [Henry] Beecher's roll"; Rothman, *Strangers at the Bedside*, 92; William J. Curran, "Governmental Regulation of the Use of Human Subjects in Medical Research," *Daedalus* 98 (1969): 542–94. Beecher's concerns were elaborated in "Experimentation in Man," *JAMA* 169 (1959): 461–78.

phases of clinical testing (the 1969 proposed rules had required IRBs for Phases 1 and 2 only). Yet in most other respects the Administration refused deference to its critics. The Drug Review Board of the National Academy of Sciences had implored the Administration to rely upon the Declaration of Helsinki—a code adopted in 1964 by the World Medical Association that embraced the concept of informed consent—but in the 1971 rules the Administration offered no endorsement of previous thinking on human subjects. "The Declaration," the new rules announced, "is a general statement regarding protection of the humans used as research subjects. More specific guidance is necessary and in some instances more rigid requirements are needed." The 1971 rules required the listing of the relevant IRB in the investigational new drug application, in other words, form FD-1571. With the new rules, the Administration had seized international ascendancy in making human subjects protection a concrete organizational and institutional reality. And at least symbolically, by its relegation of the Helsinki Declaration to mere literary status, Administration officials had declared human subjects protection to be their turf. Fully three years before Congress passed the National Research Act of 1974 (Public Law 93-348) requiring institutional assurances of human rights protection and IRB review, then, the Administration had accomplished most of what Congress set out to do through rulemaking and revision of the IND form.[10]

Some of the most pivotal changes in the application of human subjects protections occurred as the Administration began to assert its authority under the 1971 rules. In 1976, the General Accounting Office (GAO) issued a report of its inspections of clinical study sites throughout the United States. As is typical with GAO reports, the principal message was conveyed in the title: *Federal Control of New Drug Testing Is Not Adequately Protecting*

[10]I thank Jeremy Greene for discussions on the indigenous growth of many IRBs. *World Medical Association Declaration of Helsinki*, adopted by the 18th WMA General Assembly, Helsinki, Finland, June 1964; "Human Experimentation: Code of Ethics of the World Medical Association," *BMJ* 2 (177) (1964); Faden and Beauchamp, *A History and Theory of Informed Consent*, 156. HEW/FDA, "Peer Group Committee Review of Clinical Investigations of New Drugs in Human Brings," *FR* 34 (161) (Aug. 22, 1969): 13552–3. At least part of the IRB proposal issued from the Bureau of Medicine's Medical Advisory Board; FDA-BOM, Medical Advisory Board Minutes, Twenty-First Meeting, December 18 and 19, 1969, pp. 3–4; Harry F. Dowling Papers, NLM. The 1969 proposed rules, authored by J. Kenneth Kirk (then Associate Commissioner for Compliance), applied only to Phase 1 and 2 studies, which were deemed to be "the most hazardous phases" of experimentation. This restriction raised the ire of Council of Health Organizations, a coalition of coalitions that included the Medical Committee for Human Rights, the Physicians Forum and Physicians for Social Responsibility. On preparations at the Mayo Clinic in response to the 1969 proposed rules, see Minutes, Committee on the Safety of Therapeutic Agents (CSTA), Mayo Clinic, Friday, October 3, 1969 (noon); Minutes, CSTA, Friday, October 24, 1969; Minutes, CSTA, Monday, November 10, 1969 (noon); MAYO. The "final" rules appear at HEW/FDA, "Institutional Committee Review of Clinical Investigations of New Drugs in Human Beings," *FR* 36 (52) (March 17, 1971): 5037–40. Hutt served as General Counsel at the FDA from 1971 to 1975. Current FDA regulations are summarized in 21 CFR Part 50 (Informed Consent), part 56 (IRB Standards), part 312 (rules on Investigational New Drugs), and parts 812 and 813 (investigational devices).

Human Test Subjects and the Public. Some of the Office's most stunning and visceral findings were aided by the FDA's own investigations. FDA inspectors uncovered one study in which an experimental drug was given to mentally retarded children without the consent of their parents. In another trial, a radioactive drug was administered without consent to thirty-seven elderly patients. The biggest problems, however, lay not in ethical breaches in starkly visible cases, but in the debility of the procedures and institutions governing research. Violations of the Administration's IND regulations occurred frequently, including unreported protocol changes, drug administration prior to submission of an IND application, and continued drug treatment after the completion of a study. Even when they were used properly, the GAO reported, patient consent forms were inadequate to protect patient rights. Many consent forms failed to describe the relevant details of the pharmaceutical treatment, how long the drug's effects would last, or what the possible or expected effects of the drug might be. Consent forms also routinely excluded the results of previous tests with the drug, risks associated with the drug, nonmedical details of the proposed study, and even the possibility that a placebo might be used. When these deficiencies were taken into account, fully 85 percent of clinical investigators in the FDA's sample had failed to obtain adequate consent for their studies.[11]

The GAO report was part of a larger investigation directed by the Senate's Subcommittee on Health, chaired by Edward Kennedy of Massachusetts. At hearings in April 1976, Kennedy and other Senators focused on deficiencies in drug testing, including not only human subjects violations but also difficulties in identifying rare but lethal events. The GAO report identified various culprits, including the Administration's rules for their ambiguity and confusion. Yet the principal moral targets of the report were IRBs and the sponsors of the research. Even though the GAO had asked the Administration to conduct most of the investigations, the agency was nonetheless criticized severely for presiding over a system in which lapses of the sort that its own investigators had uncovered could occur.[12]

It was a public relations war on multiple fronts for the Administration. Bureau of Drugs gadfly John Nestor elaborated his perceptions of pro-industry bias at Senate hearings that year. The Administration uncovered evidence that G. D. Searle may have falsified animal data in one of its new

---

[11]GAO, *Federal Control of New Drug Testing Is Not Adequately Protecting Human Test Subjects and the Public* (Washington, DC, July 15, 1976), HRG-76-96. "GAO Finds Informed Consent Violations Widespread, Most Consent Forms Inadequate," *DRR* 19 (29), July 21, 1976, 19; Morton Mintz, "Drug Test Monitoring Called Lax," *WP*, January 23, 1976, A1.

[12]The Kennedy hearings of April 1976 are published in *Food and Drug Administration Practice and Procedure:* Joint Hearing Before the Subcommittee on Health, United States Senate Committee on Labor and Public Welfare, and Subcommittee on Administrative Practice and Procedure, Senate Committee on the Judiciary, U.S. Congress (Washington, DC: GPO, 1976). GAO, *Federal Control of New Drug Testing Is Not Adequately Protecting Human Test Subjects and the Public*, 36–41.

drug applications, prompting criticism of the FDA as well as of Searle. Senators Gaylord Nelson and Kennedy, meanwhile, were still clamoring for relabeling of the oral contraceptives. Combined with ongoing controversies over the sweetener cyclamate, the safety of veterinary drugs, and the agency's review of the safety of common food dyes, it was little surprise that even the *Wall Street Journal*'s front page seemed to call into question the consumer protection capacities of the FDA.[13]

> **Lax Protector?** The FDA draws growing attacks as laggard, slipshod. Staffers' complaints aired at Senate hearings rock the agency. GAO reports alleging laxity in supervising drug tests sap public confidence. Important projects bog down. A review of food dyes' safety drags on for over a year. New warning labels for oral contraceptives are long overdue.

Partially as a response to the GAO report and other criticisms, and partially as an extension of organizational power over vast networks of clinical research that had begun in 1974, Administration officials in August 1976 announced plans for a "Bio-Research Monitoring Program." The new program would include $16 million in funding for research monitoring. FDA plans were hammered out in five task groups composed of top officials, each group headed by a bureau chief. The groups proposed systematic monitoring of animal tests, clinical tests, bioavailability tests, research sponsors, and institutional review boards. The monitoring strategy required the agency to compile an inventory of all firms submitting INDs and every institutional review board reviewing research proposals. Such a store of information would commit the Administration to a greater surveillance of firms (and a greater capacity in sheer information storage) than would ever have been thought feasible just years earlier.[14]

The situational politics governing the Bio-Research Monitoring Program suggested an organization deeply aware of its public and congressional constituencies. In fact, FDA drug regulators had launched an informal new program of "on-site visits" with clinical investigators in 1969, but it was small and remained so through the early 1970s. By 1976, there were thousands of pharmacological studies under way, and in the face of congressional criti-

---

[13] "FDA Proposes to Ban 4 Veterinary Drugs in Bid to Upstage Congressional Hearing," *WSJ*, March 15, 1976, 10; "Washington Wire," *WSJ*, August 13, 1976, 1; Mintz, "Drug Test Monitoring Called Lax," *WP*, January 23, 1976, A1; Mintz, "Broad Conflict of Interest," *WP*, July 1, 1976, A1, A18. For a more thorough discussion of the FDA's relationship with Searle during the 1960s and 1970s, see chapters 7 and 9 in this book; "FDA Calls for Grand Jury Investigation of G. D. Searle's Drug-Testing Practices," *WSJ*, April 9, 1976, 30.

[14] "FDA 'Bio-Research Monitoring Program' Plans Nearing Completion; Studies Backing Pending New Drug Applications Get Top Priority," *DRR* 19 (33) (Aug. 18, 1976): 17–19. "Blue Sheet" reports suggest that Bureau of Drugs officials had been planning greater investigator oversight "since at least 1974, when a comprehensive plan was adopted to study and develop regs for institutional review cmtes., patient follow-up, and clinical and pre-clinical labs" (18). The GAO report and the Kennedy hearings provided both the timing and a broadening of the regulations that Bureau of Drugs officials had already planned.

cism, Administration staff knew that tens of thousands more had been completed since 1938. Even with two hundred new personnel and $16 million in funding for the program, the Bureau of Drugs would be faced with genuine trade-offs. Crout and other bureau leaders voiced two rules of thumb in discussions with media. For ongoing studies, the FDA would examine studies that were used to support new drug applications. As one source remarked, "You figure that before we make a risk-benefit decision to suddenly release the drug to a much larger population our first priority is to substantiate those studies if we can." For drugs that were already approved, Administration inspectors would revisit those that received the most attention from Congress in the 1976 Kennedy subcommittee hearings.[15]

At the core of their efforts, the Administration's 1976 task forces intended to elaborate a set of "good laboratory practice" (GLP) rules for animal studies and "good clinical practice" (GCP) regulations for human studies. Both would be modeled on the agency's "good manufacturing practice" rules from the 1940s. The "good practice" regulation of clinical testing sites would serve at least two purposes. First, it would create a template for routinizing compliance among future investigators. Whereas targeted monitoring would examine studies for pending new drug applications and would revisit approved drugs from the past, the "GCP regs," as they are still called, would lay the basis for regulation of future studies. Second, in the context of various radical ideas being proposed within the agency and being suggested from without (by Ralph Nader's Public Citizen group), the GCP regulations would enact a moderate form of governance. Alternative forms of laboratory regulation considered by the Administration included shifting part or all of preclinical testing to the Administration, licensing of all test facilities, full-time, on-site monitoring by FDA personnel, or voluntary, industry-wide guidelines. Compared to these alternatives, the GLP and GCP rules had appreciable cost advantages—they would require far fewer staff to enforce, would not insert the visible presence of the federal government at a time of rising anti-government sentiment, and would leverage the FDA's gatekeeping authority. FDA bureau leaders stated that the new clinical research regulations would merely "put into regulatory form" the agency's existing practice "so it's not as loose as it is now." Still, Administration officials and industry observers noted that "existing FDA policy" was neither a static nor a known entity. The agency's practices were in part inherited from experience under the IND regulations of 1963. Yet the ongoing experiments

[15] On the 1969 program, which would have occurred under Frances Kelsey's reign as head of the IND division, see "Bureau of Medicine Weekly Items of Interest," October 2, 1969; B5, F "Bureau of Medicine Activities," Harry F. Dowling Papers, NLM. The Bureau planned for initial visits to be carried out by medical officers and division directors, in combination with field personnel. Only later would medical officers visit on their own. *DRR* 19 (33) (Aug. 18, 1976): 17–19. Senator Kennedy would soon criticize the lab inspection program for "covering the waterfront" instead of focusing on the cases where inspection would have the greatest impact, namely "for-cause" inspections that Crout had de-emphasized. "Kennedy Hits FDA Clinical Lab Inspection Program, Asks 'Wiser Targeting'," *DRR* 20 (11) (March 16, 1977): 11.

under the Bio-Research Monitoring Program would provide additional data and administrative experience from which to build the new regulations.[16]

Perhaps strategically, the Administration floated its proposed Good Laboratory Practice regulations for animal studies two weeks after the November 2, 1976 election in which Democrat Jimmy Carter defeated incumbent President Gerald Ford. The Carter administration had eagerly courted the support of consumer activists, to the point of hinting that his health, safety, and environmental appointees might be vetted with Nader himself. Trade reporters saw the GLP regulations as "impressively detailed and sweeping"— animal facilities were for instance required to avoid "excessive noise levels" that might contribute to errors—but two features of the code received the most attention. First, the regulations mandated the creation of two positions—a "study director" and a "quality control unit"—for each laboratory conducting preclinical studies. FDA officials drew explicitly from the Good Manufacturing Practice regulations in requiring the control unit, which would establish "a focal point for FDA inspection of studies." Violation of GLPs was essentially equivalent to production of invalid research for purposes of the new drug application. Second, the new codes provided for unconditional disqualification of preclinical investigators. The possibility of disqualification was mentioned in the preamble to the regulations as "the ultimate administrative action for serious noncompliance," but the very statement of its possibility was a warning to readers that the text of the new regulations was backed up by legal authority and the Administration's gatekeeping power. Failure to follow the Good Laboratory Practice rules (including the failure to appoint a study director and a control unit) became stated and sufficient grounds for disqualification. With publicized penalties and the creation of laboratory control units as an organizational venue for regulatory strategy, the GLP rules had codified the target and consequences of FDA power. And as the GLP rules were quickly adopted in other nations, once again the Administration's conceptual architecture diffused well beyond its official boundaries.[17]

[16]On the GMP rules, see John P. Swann, "The 1941 Sulfathiazole Disaster and the Birth of Good Manufacturing Practices," *PDA Journal of Pharmaceutical Science and Technology* 53 (3) (May–June 1999): 148–53; Dale E. Cooper, "Adequate Controls for New Drugs: Good Manufacturing Practice and the 1938 Federal Food, Drug, and Cosmetic Act," *Pharmacy in History* 44 (1) (2002): 12–23. Robert Temple was pivotal in the development of the GCP regulations. Important actors in the GLP initiative were Richard Lehmann of the Bureau of Veterinary Drugs and John Petricciani, deputy director of pathology at the Bureau of Biologics. "FDA Sets Nov. 1 for Start of Big New Scientific Monitoring Program; 42 Animal Labs Are First Targets; Data Sought for Good Lab Practices," *DRR* 19 (41) (Oct. 13, 1976): 9–10; *DRR* 19 (33) (Aug. 18, 1976): 17–19.

[17]The proposed GLP rules appear at FDA, "Nonclinical Laboratory Studies: Proposed Regulations for Good Laboratory Practice," 21 CFR Parts 3e, 8, 121, 312, 314, 430, 431, 414; Docket No. 76N-0400; *FR* 41 (225) (Nov. 19, 1976): 51206ff. For trade reaction, see "Regulation of All 'Nonclinical Laboratory Studies' Proposed by FDA; Basic Research, Human Testing Not Covered in Good Lab Practice Regs," *DRR* 19 (47) (Nov. 24, 1976): 1, 4–5; "FDA Unveils Preclinical Testing Regs," *DRR* 19 (46) (Nov. 17, 1976): 2. Extension of the GLP principles

Yet just as laboratories could be disqualified from submission of materials in support of an NDA, so could scientific investigators and sponsors. The Administration had carried the right of disqualification since the 1962 Amendments but had used it sparingly. Disqualification meant that an investigator could not receive an "investigational exemption" under the Food, Drug and Cosmetic Act, and hence could not legally conduct research on drugs or devices. From 1963 to 1976, a total of twenty-three investigators were disqualified, creating what Louis Goodman would call an implicit "blacklist" of rogue medical researchers. In the summer of 1976, however, Administration officials moved to bestow greater legitimacy, discretion, and authority upon their regulators (including Frances Kelsey) who governed medical researchers. On August 20, the agency promulgated eleven standards whose violation was sufficient for disqualification. Grounds for disqualification would include beginning a study without prior approval from the Administration and an IRB, deviating from the protocol so as to "adversely affect the rights or safety of the subjects or the validity of the study," any violation of human subjects provisions, deficiencies in recordkeeping (including tardiness in submitting reports), and refusal to permit an inspection. The August 1976 rules applied to devices and in vitro diagnostics, but four months later new draft regulations had extended the principles to drugs and biologics. What most startled industry observers about the new rules was a sub-delegation provision allowing lower-level FDA monitors to initiate disqualification proceedings without waiting for the permission of the deputy bureau director. The stated rationale for this provision was one of procedural justice. Since the Bureau's leadership would preside over the required disqualification hearing, the new rule would separate "prosecutory" and "judicial" functions of research monitoring. When combined with the eleven new "trigger" standards, however, the predominant reading of the sub-delegation rule was as an extension of organizational force. Emil Freireich of M. D. Anderson warned that the disqualification provisions of the August 1976 rules "puts in the hands of hierarchically low-level individuals... the power... to completely stop drug development as it is now practiced and has been experienced."[18]

---

from preclinical to clinical studies appears in "Obligations of Sponsors and Monitors of Clinical Investigations: Proposed Rules," *FR* 42 (187) (Sept. 27, 1977): 49612–30; "Proposed FDA Regs Require Clinical Studies Sponsors to Maintain Close Watch Over Investigators; Violators Could Be Disqualified," *DRR* 20 (39) (Sept. 28, 1977): 15. On Carter's courtship of Nader and the consumer protection lobby, see "BuDrugs' Nestor Gets Head-Table Seat at Lunch," *DRR* 19 (33) (Aug. 18, 1976): 18. "Carter's Miami Speech Holds Major Clues to Research, Delivery Policies His Administration Will Pursue if He Wins Nov. 2 Election," *DRR* 19 (43) (Oct. 27, 1976): 4. On foreign adoption of GLP rules, see Jasanoff, *The Fifth Branch*, 260–61.

[18] Frances Kelsey ran the Division of Scientific Investigations from 1966 onward, and she was responsible for most of the investigations and disqualifications, including ten disqualifications by July 1968; FDA-BOM, Medical Advisory Board, Minutes of Sixteenth Meeting, July 18 and 19, 1968; Minutes of Eighteenth Meeting, March 27 and 28, 1969; Harry F. Dowling Papers, NLM. "L.G.'s Testimony & Council of Drugs Dismissal," undated, LSG. The 1976

The specter of disqualification induced tremors among many in the pharmaceutical research community. While researchers like Freireich saw the August 1976 rules as making disqualification easier, the September 1977 extension of disqualification procedures to sponsors and monitors aroused new fears among company-employed scientists and contract research organizations who worried that their errors could doom entire organizations. In the feedback received during the notice and comment period of the rulemaking process, critics conjectured that trivial, "insignificant deficiencies in investigator conduct" would trigger disqualification proceedings. Famed pharmacologist Louis Lasagna declared the threat of IRB disqualification a "draconian measure" and stated that "scientific reputations deserve better than kangaroo courts and *pro forma* hearings." And despite the Administration's written assurances that disqualification would be used sparingly—repeated in the preamble to the 1976 and 1977 regulations as well as in public and media statements accompanying the release of the draft rules—commentators insisted that, under the proposed rules, disqualification would happen far more often than FDA officials were sanguinely predicting.[19]

Other audiences were scoring the Administration for failing to govern early clinical trials with rigor. Senator Edward Kennedy of Massachusetts interpreted the shortcomings of early clinical trials as criminal in nature—Commissioner Donald Kennedy admitted them to be "horrible" but did not mention possible criminal penalties—and introduced a "consensus bill" in March 1978 that would have limited the FDA's powers over Phase 1 and 2 trials to human subjects protection only. The American Society for Clinical Pharmacology, represented by FDA critic William Wardell, proposed instead that Administration authority over Phase 1 and 2 studies be "decentralized" to local peer review committees themselves. In response, the Administration announced it would step up its inspection of IRBs and clinical research facilities, boosting visits to three hundred annually from two hundred the year before.[20]

---

rules appear at *FR* 41 (163) (Aug. 20, 1976): 35282–313 (esp. 35305–9 [IRBs], 35311–12 [disqualification]). "Tough New Research Rules Pushed by FDA," *DRR* 19 (34) (Aug. 25, 1976): 2–3. "FDA Blocks Cancer Drug Trials, M. D. Anderson's Freireich Reports; Reasons Unclear, He Tells President's Cancer Panel; Action Pledged," *DRR* 19 (47) (Nov. 24, 1976): 16. On extension of August 1976 rules to all products regulated by the agency, see "Draft FDA Clinical Investigator Regs are Agency-Wide," *DRR* 20 (15) (April 13, 1977): RN-3. "Proposed Drug Sponsor Regs to Include Disqualification," *DRR* 20 (21) (May 21, 1977): RN-3.

[19]*DRR* 20 (39) (Sept. 28, 1977): 16. Lasagna statement in *DRR* 21 (13) (April 19, 1978): RN-4.

[20]"FDA Blasts 'Horrible' Violations of Subjects' Rights in Drug Firm Research; Sen. Kennedy Sees Abuses as Cause for Criminal Penalties in New Law," *DRR* 21 (10) (March 8, 1978): 10–11. "Drug Bill Removes FDA Scientific Oversight for Phase 1 and 2 Testing," *DRR* 21 (12) (March 22, 1978): 11. "FDA Will Beef Up Inspections of Institutional Review Boards Soon," *DRR* 21 (18) (May 21, 1978): 10. "Groups Seek Local Peer Review of Phase I and II Drug Studies," *DRR* 21 (26) June 28, 1978): 11. The proposal to relieve the FDA of Phase 1 authority resurfaced in the following Congress, the fall of 1979; *DRR* 22 (40) (Oct. 3, 1979): 7.

Separately, Administration officials began writing rules to use the institutional review boards as satellite regulators of early phase clinical trials. The FDA's designs upon the IRB set up something of a national contest in the late 1970s over how these committees would operate and over who would control them. Two months before the congressionally established Belmont Commission issued its recommendations for use of institutional review boards in October 1978, Administration officials published rules governing IRBs in the *Federal Register*. The proposed rules mandated a quorum for procedures, declared that the boards were expected to assure "the validity or reliability of the scientific data" produced by the proposed study, empowered the boards to suspend or terminate the study, and compelled the boards to copy "records that identify the human subjects" in the trial at the FDA's request. Since identifiable records for Phase 3 trials would often include patient histories, the privacy implications of this last provision were far-reaching.[21]

Perhaps more than any set of FDA rules proposed during the turbulent 1970s—and perhaps as much as any rules floated since—the FDA's August 1978 IRB regulations met with stinging criticism and rebuke. Human subjects protection expert Robert Levine of Yale University found the Administration's rules "contrary to the letter and the intent" of the Belmont Commission's report.

> The FDA proposal expects the IRB to perform some functions for which it is incompetent—e.g., assure the validity or reliability of scientific data. It instructs the IRB to collaborate in such dubious activities as facilitating access to patients' medical records. It burdens the IRB with the requirement to perform various tasks of dubious value. And it prescribes heavy penalties for noncompliance with its requirements.

Officials at the M. D. Anderson Hospital and Tumor Institute in Houston wrote to Commissioner Kennedy and expressed their mixed enthusiasm. "Our procedures and safeguards which are presently in place," President Charles LeMaistre declared, "have been shown to effectively prevent abuses. Accordingly, we do not welcome the imposition of very detailed standards for IRB's which do not allow for the necessary flexibility based on local conditions and which do not allow continuance of procedures proven effective over time." LeMaistre's star researchers Jan van Eys and Emil Freireich

---

[21]National Commission for the Protection of Human Subjects of Biomedical and Behavioral Research, *Report and Recommendations: Institutional Review Boards*, DHEW Publication No. (OS) 78-0008 (Washington, DC: GPO, 1978); reprinted at *FR* 43 (231) (Nov. 30, 1978): 56174–98. FDA, "Standards for Institutional Review Boards for Clinical Investigations: Proposed Establishment of Regulations," *FR* 43 (153) (Aug. 8, 1978): 35186–208. For the various requirements, see Section 56.82 (quorum provisions), Section 56.2 (assessment of validity and reliability of data), Section 56.92 (suspension/termination of an investigation), and Section 56.15 (access to patients' medical records). "FDA Asserts Its Right to Inspect IRBs, Including Patient Records; Proposed Rules Require IND [IRB] Review Before Application Goes to Agency," *DRR* 21 (32) (Aug. 9, 1978): 20–21.

saw in the rules a constitutional violation and an affront to academic freedom. Another manager found the prospect of disqualification for noncompliance "offensive and highly threatening." Two organizations representing pharmaceutical research facilities—the American Association of Medical Colleges (AAMC) and the American Federation for Clinical Research (AFCR)—sent official letters of protest and called for one-on-one meetings with top FDA and NIH officials. At public hearings on September 14, 1979, John Adams of the Pharmaceutical Manufacturers' Association voiced his doubt that the Administration possessed even the statutory authority to disqualify IRBs.[22]

Faced with a growing torrent of criticism, Kennedy took the rare and embarrassing step of announcing—by leak to interested organizations in May 1979 and then publicly in the *Federal Register* of August 14—that his agency was withdrawing its proposal to establish IRB standards. "I am inclined to be optimistic," wrote Yale's Robert Levine in November, expressing his hope that the Administration was at last responding in genuine good faith to the Belmont Report's recommendations, and that FDA officials were truly cooperating with Health, Education and Welfare officials. Officials at the American Association of Medical Colleges, the American Federation of Clinical Research, and M. D. Anderson and other research sites expressed their public and private relief.[23]

Yet even as they were celebrating, clinical research facilities and their representatives began preparing for a regime shift in the way they went about

[22]Robert J. Levine, "Changing Federal Regulation of IRBs: The Commission's Recommendations and the FDA's Proposals," *IRB: A Review of Human Subjects Research* 1 (1) (Jan. 1979). On AAMC and AFCR strategy, see the "Update on FDA Regulations for Institutional Review Boards," AAMC *Weekly Report* #79-22, 1–2. Charles LeMaistre (President, M. D. Anderson Hospital and Tumor Institute) to Kennedy, June 4, 1979; Felix L. Haas (Office of Research) to LeMaistre, May 29, 1979; van Eys to LeMaistre [undated]; Haas to LeMaistre and Charles Brown (Executive Assistant), May 30, 1979, "Comparison of National Commission Recommendations and FDA Proposed Rules Regarding Institutional Review Boards"; Felix L. Haas (Assistant to the Director for Research) to LeMaistre, May 8, 1979, "Response to F.D.A. Proposed Regulations"; 10.1A; RG 1, SG 2 (President's Office Records, 1964–1979), MDAA. The federal docket for the August 1978 IRB rules was No. 77N-0350.

[23]FDA, "Standards for Institutional Review Boards for Clinical Investigations: Withdrawal of Proposal," *FR* 44 (158) (Aug. 14, 1979): 47688-98. The AAMC reported the impending withdrawal in its *Weekly Report* for June 5, 1979. The AAMC report described a letter sent by Commissioner Kennedy and Don Frederickson (NIH Director) to the American Federation for Clinical Research and received May 23, 1979; "Update on FDA Regulations for Institutional Review Boards," AAMC *Weekly Report* #79-22, 1–2. Upon seeing the AAMC report, M. D. Anderson administrator Beverly Ross contacted the FDA's John Petricciani to verify the report, and Petricciani confirmed it; Beverly Ross memo to Jan van Eys and Felix Haas, June 14, 1979; 10.1A; RG 1, SG 2 (President's Office Records, 1964–1979), MDAA. For reaction to the withdrawal, see Levine, "Changing Federal Regulation of IRBs, Part II: DHEW's and FDA's Proposed Regulations," *IRB: A Review of Human Subjects Research* 1 (7) (Nov. 1979); Felix L. Haas to Charles A. LeMaistre, "Proposed FDA Regulations for IRB's," June 18, 1979; File "Research, General, Food and Drug Administration, 1978–1979," 10.1A; RG 1, SG 2 (President's Office Records, 1964–1979), MDAA.

their business. Administration officials had quietly informed M. D. Anderson officials that, along with the withdrawal of the August 1978 IRB rules, a new set of rules would be forthcoming. M. D. Anderson researcher Jan van Eys messaged top hospital leadership that "I believe we need to go forward with a 'model' plan for IND's although regs rescinded!—it is our best interest to work out a model with FDA before new regs issued." As it turned out, the Administration would release its new rules more quickly than even the prescient van Eys had anticipated. Donald Kennedy published his agency's "second try" at IRB regulation in the same August, 14, 1978 issue of the *Federal Register* in which the first set of standards had been retracted. Whereas the aborted 1978 standards had been published under the title "Standards for Institutional Review Boards," the 1979 rules referred first to human subjects protection, and only then to IRBs: "Protection of Human Subjects: Standards for Institutional Review Boards for Clinical Research."[24]

The imbroglio over new FDA rules in 1978 and 1979 suggests, if nothing else, that Administration officials wanted IRBs to do far more than monitor clinical trial protocol for human subjects issues. In reviewing the first set of rules from August 1978, M. D. Anderson officials voiced a widely shared suspicion that the Administration wanted fundamental control over the IRB for purposes of extending its regulatory reach. "It is apparent that the F. D.A. wishes to take over supervision and monitoring of Institutional Review Boards from HEW," Jan van Eys wrote. Yale's Robert Levine similarly perceived a turf battle between HEW and FDA and accused the Administration of converting the institutional review board to purposes and designs that it could not possibly satisfy. In revising the regulations, the Administration acknowledged that "actual evaluation of the scientific merits of a proposal is not intended as a major function of an IRB." Yet as Levine noticed with dismay, the revised 1979 rules continued to mandate IRB review "for assuring the validity or reliability of the scientific data." And the new rules had barely altered the record-copying requirements from the 1978 rules; the IRB was obligated to permit copying of medical records, even as Administration inspectors would carry out the actual reproduction. In many salient respects—the breadth of IRB responsibilities and the threat of disqualification in particular—the revised August 1979 proposal formed the basis for the rules finalized two years later, in January 1981.[25]

[24]FDA, "Protection of Human Subjects: Standards for Institutional Review Boards for Clinical Research," *FR* 44 (158) (Aug. 14, 1979): 47699–712; "Protection of Human Subjects: Informed Consent," pp. 47713–29. *DRR* 22 (34) (Aug. 22, 1979), 1–12. John Petricciani had warned M. D. Anderson's Beverly Ross that the withdrawn IRB standards would be quickly replaced by new proposed rules; Beverly Ross memo to Jan van Eys and Felix Haas, June 14, 1979; van Eys written note to "CRB" (Charles R. Brown, Executive Assistant to LeMaistre), on van Eys memo to M. D. Anderson Task Force Committee for Research Management, June 18, 1979; 10.1A; RG 1, SG 2 (President's Office Records, 1964–1979), MDAA.
[25]Felix Haas urgent memo to LeMaistre, May 4, 1979; 10.1A; RG 1, SG 2 (President's Office Records, 1964–1979), MDAA. Levine, Changing Federal Regulation of IRBs" (Jan. 1979); Levine, "Changing Federal Regulation of IRBs, Part II" (Nov. 1979). FDA, "Protection of

In ways that have yet to appreciated or narrated, the Administration effected a far-reaching transformation of research practices in the two decades
before its clinical research rules were temporarily cemented in 1981 and
1985. At Burroughs-Wellcome in the 1970s, President Fred Coe instituted a
system of internal monitors whose job it was to anticipate FDA criticism. As
he later summarized his experience with early clinical trials, when "you finally get to the point where you have a possible product, and you go the
F&DA and say, 'This is what we've got, evidence to show that this product
is safe.' That's the primary thing they care about." After contracting with
experienced universities or research organizations, the most important task
of his organization became monitoring trials for potential regulatory issues.
Coe so perfected his system that anticipation of the FDA's scrutiny became
thoroughly routinized within Burroughs-Wellcome.

> In my time it was relatively easy. You'd get some hospital probably where they had
> a number of these patients, and you'd get somebody who was in charge of taking
> care of them, to accept the idea of running these trials, and he's run 'em. And he'd
> do them the way you told him to do them, or he agreed to do them. And then,
> you'd start with monitoring, you'd send people out from the office to check on the
> results, and try to make sure that everything had been done the way you wanted it
> done, so that there's no question with the F&DA that something screwed up.[26]

Among research institutions, the Mayo Clinic and M. D. Anderson Cancer Center provide signal and influential examples of organizations that
transformed their procedures and structures in anticipation of impending
FDA rules and regulatory initiatives. In the wake of the 1969 rules on IRBs,
Mayo officials overhauled their Committee on the Safety of Therapeutic
Agents (CSTA) to perform an institutional review function. Even as early as
1965, Mayo administrators began centralizing their record-keeping and
monitoring of clinical trials in an attempt to establish and maintain a positive
reputation with the Administration. The CSTA created a subcommittee to
generate proposals for the internal regulation of clinical trials, and ongoing
discussions turned toward the centralization of research oversight at Mayo.

> Dr. Maher ... again stressed the need for a central registry for all new drugs, with
> facilities for record keeping and storage facilities for drugs as a staff service. He
> believed that the volume of new drugs would be greatly increased in the immedi-
> ate years ahead and felt that the Clinic's image with the F.D.A. and other agencies
> would be enhanced with a uniform procedure which provided for protection for
> the patient, the Clinic and the investigator.[27]

Human Subjects: Standards for Institutional Review Boards for Clinical Research," *FR* 44 (158)
(Aug. 14, 1979): 47699–712. For the 1981 rules, see *FR* 46 (17) (Jan. 27, 1981): 8975–9.
    [26]Coe was president of Burroughs-Wellcome in the United States in the 1970s and oversaw
American operations from Wellcome's offices in Research Triangle Park, North Carolina. Fred
Coe Oral History Interview, April 2001, p. 38; Burroughs-Wellcome Oral Histories, WLUK.
    [27]Minutes, CSTA, July 1, 1965; MAYO.

At M. D. Anderson, the reaction seems to have been more varied. The Administration's reach into governance of clinical research induced a divide between those who wished to fight the agency at every step and those who saw time, power, and organizational image on the FDA's side. The latter group included LeMaistre, Glenn Knotts, Felix Haas, and eventually, Jan van Eys.

M. D. Anderson had raised the suspicion and concern of Administration officials for several reasons. In the middle 1970s, cancer vaccine researcher Jordan Gutterman began to report positive clinical trial results for the "Bacillus Calmette-Guérin" (BCG) vaccine, a tuberculosis relative, in breast cancer and melanoma. BCG was an immune system stimulant that, in the hopes of some researchers, promised to create a "fourth modality" of cancer immunotherapy to complement the existing troika of surgery, radiation, and chemotherapy. Yet other studies of BCG had produced results starkly different from those Gutterman had detailed. In reporting positive results with BCG in melanoma, Gutterman's clinic was alone among centers testing the drug in the United States.[28]

The standoff between the federal government and M. D. Anderson grew from a simple institutional fact: most human subjects inspections were then, and are now, carried out by officers of the Administration. Inspector Richard Aleman of the FDA's Houston Office first visited Gutterman's labs in February 1978, then again in August and September. When Aleman asked Gutterman to turn over copies of patient records and signed consent forms, Gutterman announced he would do so only if the inspector would first sign a waiver of liability that had been created by Freireich, the fiery oncologist who had publicly criticized the Administration in 1976. Aleman refused to sign the form, hence Gutterman refused to turn over his records. From the

---

[28]Gutterman's studies, which operated under Bureau of Biologics INDs 588 and 794, used a "fresh frozen" form of BCG obtained from the Trudeau Institute of Saranac Lake, New York; Gutterman memo to R. Lee Clark, August 1, 1978; Boland Shepherd (Supervisory Manager, Houston District, FDA) to R. Lee Clark, June 22, 1978; RG1, SG2—"President's Office Records, 1964–1979, 10.1A," MDAA. In Toine Pieters' thoroughly documented narrative, the failure of BCG created a structural opening for interferon; *Interferon: The Science and Selling of a Miracle Drug* (London: Routledge, 2005), 135–6. Robert Teitelman, *Gene Dreams: Wall Street, Academia and the Rise of Biotechnology* (New York: Basic Books, 1989), 29; Ilana Löwy, *Between Bench and Bedside: Science, Healing, and Interleukin-2 in a Cancer Ward* (Cambridge: Harvard University Press, 1996), 112. Gutterman's early research with BCG appears in "Chemoimmunotherapy of Advanced Breast Cancer: Prolongation of Remission and Survival with BCG," *BMJ* 2 (1976): 774–7; and in Gutterman, "Immunotherapy for Recurrent Malignant Melanoma: The Efficacy of BCG in Prolonging the Postoperative Disease-Free Interval and Survival," in M. Sela, ed., *The Role of Non-Specific Immunity in the Prevention and Treatment of Cancer* (Rome: Pontificia Academia Scientarum, 1977), 57–65. Gutterman would eventually build a stellar career from his interferon studies; Gutterman, et al., "Leucocyte-interferon-induced Regression in Human Metastatic Breast Cancer, Multiple Myeloma and Malignant Lymphoma," *AnnIM* 93 (1980): 399–406. See more generally the Jordan Gutterman Papers on Interferon, MDAA. On Gutterman's eventual stature in biological cancer therapeutics, see Pieters, *Interferon*, 2. On the hype shed upon immunotherapy in the mid-1970s, see Teitelman, *Gene Dreams*, 31; Löwy, *Between Bench and Bedside*, 110; Pieters, *Interferon*, 224.

records that he could examine, Aleman documented four pages of alleged code violations. Aleman found that two of Gutterman's protocols had never been approved by M. D. Anderson's IRB, that Gutterman had allowed patients' relatives and friends to administer BCG vaccine to them outside of the clinic, and that twenty-one melanoma patients had been treated with the vaccine before IRB approval of one protocol. Various patient consent forms were incomplete or missing, Aleman observed, and the forms that were signed were inadequate in that they had failed to convey the risks and discomforts expected from the drug, as well as the patient's right to revoke consent and withdraw from the trial at any time. Gutterman wrote an angry response to the Aleman report and insisted that not one of his patients had either protested or been visibly harmed. In response to Aleman's contention that Gutterman had permitted his treatment to be distributed and administered outside his possession—a clear violation of the IND rules, which permitted possession of investigational drugs only by the principal investigator who was testing them—Gutterman shot back that "The literal interpretation of some regulations, [namely] that a lay person could not administer this test article, would lead to a serious obstruction of cancer research." In a summary memorandum written October 13, 1978, Gutterman's superiors admitted to careless record keeping but otherwise defended their researcher.[29]

These protestations were of little consequence. M. D. Anderson officials' claims that no patient was harmed from Gutterman's slapdash procedures, and that none of them had protested, fell on unsympathetic ears in FDA offices in Houston and Rockville. Sensing his organization's dimming status in the eyes of the Administration, Hospital President Charles "Mickey" LeMaistre invited Bureau of Drugs Director Richard Crout to come to Houston for a full-day meeting on November 24, 1978. LeMaistre expected good behavior and "special involvement" from his researchers and promised Crout that M. D. Anderson would use the meeting to create a "model information system" that would remedy the discrepancies uncovered in the Ale-

---

[29]Before Aleman's in-person visit to Gutterman, he had phoned Gutterman to request an inspection of all patient records and raw data covering work with IND 794; Gutterman memo to R. Lee Clark, August 1, 1978; FDA, Form FD-483 (7/75), "Inspectional Observations," signed by Aleman; Memo from "Sue" to Gutterman, September 25, 1978; Albert E. Gunn (Assistant Director, M. D. Anderson Hospitals) to LeMaistre and Joseph T. Painter (VP for Administration), October 13, 1978; 10.1A; RG 1, SG 2 (President's Office Records, 1964–1979), MDAA. Gutterman further defended family-based administration of the vaccine on the basis that its method of administration was better taught to family members than to the patient's doctor: "The principal investigator could not administer BCG to every patient on every occasion. Since the FDA officials refused to see how BCG is administered, they fail to understand that the best person to administer BCG on a weekly basis is the patient or one of the patient's relatives. Administration of BCG by scarification cannot by taught over the phone to a doctor." Gutterman's reference to scarification is historically contingent; it was the predominant mode of BCG administration, consisting of multiple cuts to the melanoma site and direct application of the BCG vaccine to the incisions. See M. R. Desner, J. L. Lichtenfeld, C. L. Dennison, K. O. Kalmbach, and M. R. Mardiney, Jr., "A New Apparatus for BCG Scarification," *Journal of the National Cancer Institute* 54 (1) (Jan. 1975): 57–60.

man investigation. In the coming months, M. D. Anderson officials would admit—to themselves and to the FDA—that their own procedures were to blame for Gutterman's shortcomings and for the whole touchy affair. As Research Director Felix Haas would recount:

This investigation was initiated primarily because results reported for investigations carried out here using a particular drug issued on an IND could not be duplicated by investigators elsewhere using the same drug on other INDs. The only clearly favorable results were being obtained at our institution. This was the reason that the FDA delved so thoroughly into our record-keeping and inspection systems and were so critical of them. I do not know whether the investigator [Gutterman] falsified or shaded the results being reported or not; but I do know that he was never inspected [by M. D. Anderson] during his research, and that the results he reported during periodic reviews were taken at face value. Neither the Office of Research nor the Surveillance Committee has at present any system for checking on the veracity of results reported by investigators.[30]

LeMaistre and M. D. Anderson had blinked, and their deference quickly established an administrative peace. Anderson pharmacologists again invited Crout for a visit in January 1979 with a promise of "local media coverage, so that the FDA (and our medical students) would at least get some good publicity out of the deal." Crout declined for scheduling reasons but he did so graciously, sending his warmest regards to "many friends and colleagues in Houston." The results of the tacit understanding would come not by announcement, but by the strange juxtaposition of two events in March 1979. First, LeMaistre appointed a "Task Force to Recommend Procedures for staff and Institutional Compliance with FDA and NIH Regulations." Jan van Eys chaired the task force, which was known informally as the "FDA Response" committee. Second, on March 16, 1979, FDA Bureau of Biologics official Sam Gibson sent Gutterman a warning letter politely detailing the deficiencies unearthed in the Aleman inspection, and thanking Gutterman for the "cooperation that you gave to our staff members during their visit." The Administration had slapped Gutterman's hand, avoiding much more intensive investigations that LeMaistre and his staff wanted desperately to avoid.[31]

[30]Felix Haas memo to van Eys, May 18, 1979, "Discussion of Points Made By Task Force at April 11, 1979 Meeting"; RG1, SG2— "President's Office Records, 1964–1979, 10.1A," MDAA.

[31]LeMaistre memo to Drs. Bodey, Gunn, Hill, Jackson, Painter, van Eys, Zimmerman, and Hostetter, November 24, 1978; "Itinerary for Dr. J. Richard Crout, Director, Bureau of Drugs, FDA," November 28, 1978. The initial composition of the Task Force appears in "Committee to [be] Proposed," noted as "FDA Response" Committee, undated. For the second Crout invitation, see G. Alan Robinson (Professor and Chair, Pharmacology, University of Texas) to Louise Patterson (Director, Speaker's Bureau, FDA), January 22, 1979; Crout to Robinson, February 15, 1979. The warning letter is Sam T. Gibson (Director, Division of Biologics Evaluation, Bureau of Biologics) to Gutterman, March 16, 1979; RG1, SG2—"President's Office Records, 1964–1979, 10.1A," MDAA.

To be sure, the March 1979 exchange was real. Gutterman escaped further investigation, even as Edward Kennedy and other national politicians were calling for tougher criminal penalties for human subjects and other clinical research violations. For his part, LeMaistre committed M. D. Anderson to a genuine and far-reaching reform of its research procedures. To remedy the hospital's deficiencies, Office of Research Director Felix Haas proposed a substantial overhaul and centralization of the way that M. D. Anderson oversaw its research. He first recommended the creation of a Quality Assurance Board to supervise all clinical studies at M. D. Anderson. This board would exist outside of the IRB and in addition to the quality control unit that each and every study would have as a result of the Good Clinical Practice regulations. The board was essentially a checking device to ensure that suspicion-raising issues were discovered by Anderson officials before the FDA discovered them; it would "check all protocols or INDs reporting unexpected results or reactions, and all controversial protocols or INDs, or those on which inquiries are made by FDA or NIH." Second, Haas called for central record keeping of all research protocols and much more detailed records of any meetings at which these protocols were hammered out. "If this had been done when we were inspected by the FDA," he surmised, "we would have forestalled two of their criticisms." Third, Haas advocated a fundamental change in the way that Anderson departments kept track of their research. The behavior and health of each patient would now be documented by a flow chart, and anything out of the ordinary, from "changes in approved protocols" to "unexpected reactions" to "mistakes in protocols or INDs," would now be reported immediately to the hospital's previously dormant Surveillance Committee.[32]

At the core of LeMaistre's fears was the specter that, if his organization earned the distrust of the Administration, its very livelihood could be in jeopardy. The reorganization plans of April and May 1979 were an admission that two crucial audiences—the FDA and the NIH, the latter getting

<hr/>

[32] "FDA Blasts 'Horrible' Violations of Subjects' Rights in Drug Firm Research; Sen. Kennedy Sees Abuses as Cause for Criminal Penalties in New Law," *DRR* 21 (10) (March 8, 1978):10–11. Haas had called for similar reforms in the fall of 1978 when the Aleman-Gutterman affair was just beginning. Reading the FDA's proposed IRB rules of 1978 and the Belmont Commission Report, he proposed to his M. D. Anderson colleagues that "although these [rules], at this stage, are only recommendations, it has become quite apparent that they will be adopted—almost in toto—by Presidential Executive order in the immediate future." Faced with the impending rules, Haas suggested that "we might as well start now getting our House in order." Haas interoffice memo, November 17, 1978. Felix Haas memo to van Eys, May 18, 1979, "Discussion of Points Made By Task Force at April 11, 1979 Meeting"; RG1, SG2—"President's Office Records, 1964–1979, 10.1A," MDAA. A bullet-pointed summary of Haas's recommended changes appears on pages 5–6 of the document. The patient-specific flow chart replaced a previously informal system of "progress notes." See also Haas to LeMaistre, "Response to F.D.A. Proposed Regulations," May 8, 1979"; RG1, SG2—"President's Office Records, 1964–1979, 10.1A," MDAA. The Surveillance Committee at M. D. Anderson, which functions as its IRB, continues at this writing.

reports from the former—did not look upon M. D. Anderson research procedures with favor.

> When the FDA was here looking at a particular drug that they issued an IND on, they were less than enthused at some of the institutional systems that were in place to assure that the investigators at this institution do indeed comply with the requirements that we ourselves have imposed in our General Assurance Statement to the NIH for human subjects investigation.... One ultimate consequence is that if we continue to be in violation, and *do not show an effort to address those problems in getting compliance*, they can and do have the opportunity to withdraw all grant and federal contract funds to this institution. Therefore, we jeopardize all extramurally supported research programs.[33]

LeMaistre's 1979 overhaul of M. D. Anderson was a departure from the hostile approach of his predecessor, R. Lee Clark, a rebuff to the irritable Emil Freireich, and an elaborate curtsy to the Administration. It was, in addition, an ostentatious and ceremonial display of procedure of the sort that LeMaistre hoped would assuage the concerns of Crout and the FDA's Houston inspectors. The structural overhaul was accompanied by a noticeable shift in rhetoric and decorum. M. D. Anderson doctors began taking a more deferential tone with the FDA, and they were rewarded internally for it. The Administration's Houston office began to sponsor week-long conferences outlining and clarifying compliance requirements, and Anderson officials now faithfully and punctually attended every session.[34]

By 1980, clinical research at M. D. Anderson, Mayo, and many other cancer institutions was far more centralized, planned, monitored, and documented than it had been just five years earlier, and the impetus for structural change was not congressional statute, not a federal rule, but the *anticipation* of future FDA behavior. The Aleman-Gutterman incident at M. D. Anderson was in fact one instantiation of a much larger regulatory pattern. FDA inspectors had encountered similar problems at Boston University, Georgetown, Indiana University, UCLA, and research hospitals in Boston, New York, Philadelphia, Minneapolis, New Orleans, Salt Lake City, Phoenix, and Puerto Rico. Both National Cancer Institute officials and pharmaceutical trade reporters noted the increasing stringency and greater presence of FDA inspectors at clinical research sites and IRBs. The Administration boosted the number of investigator disqualifications from three in 1978 to twenty-six in the first five months of 1979. The overwhelming reaction of research organizations to this initiative was to restructure observably, to centralize, to empower top officials and their committees with oversight

[33]Italics added. Minutes, Task Force Committee Meeting, April 11, 1979; RG1, SG2—"President's Office Records, 1964–1979, 10.1A," MDAA.

[34]On the task force, see Felix Haas memo to van Eys, May 18, 1979, "Discussion of Points Made By Task Force at April 11, 1979 Meeting." FDA, Schedule for "Houston Section Conference," May 7th–May 11th, 1979; RG1, SG2—"President's Office Records, 1964–1979, 10.1A," MDAA.

powers *within* the hospital, the clinic, and the medical school. Observing the "defensive postures" that M. D. Anderson and other organizations took in anticipating FDA regulations, van Eys soberly documented a widespread "feeling that the regulations that emanate from and are promulgated by the Food and Drug Administration are intended to regulate the therapeutic human research as it is currently executed in academic and private research centers." "This feeling is rapidly becoming a reality," he concluded, "solely because it is widely believed." Through inspection, rhetoric, the force of disqualification, and the power of conceptual definition, the Administration had established a self-sustaining equilibrium of belief, and of compliance.[35]

An Organizational Interpretation of IRB Expansion. Institutional review boards are often taken at the words for which they were created, viewed as providing additional safeguards to the vulnerable patient in research with human subjects. This procedural interpretation of the IRB is a sensible one, and review boards undoubtedly do serve these purposes. Yet an organizational lens provides a different and illuminating take on the proliferation of IRBs and, more importantly, their many functions. The review board propagated for the purpose of human subjects protection, to be sure, but in ways that have yet to be narrated or fully appreciated, the diffusion of IRBs became a (partially unintended) mode of more thoroughly and efficiently regulating pharmaceutical development. The Administration might, in 1969, have chosen to review and inspect each and every research protocol itself, both for human subjects issues and for research quality issues. By implicitly

In a May 1979 meeting between M. D. Anderson staff and officials at the FDA's regional office in Houston, Albert Gunn, who served as Medical Director for Anderson's Rehabiliation Center, took a very deferential tone that seemed to defuse the antagonism. As Knotts summarized the meeting, "While it was clear at the outset that the session might become testy, Dr. Gunn disarmed the audience with complimentary remarks about the FDA's efforts and reviewed its salutary effects on society since its inception.... He represented our institution very forcefully, after establishing a very cordial atmosphere with the group. He fended their questions with straightforward answers and assured our willingness to cooperate reasonably with the FDA in our research activities"; Glenn R. Knotts to LeMaistre, May 17, 1979. Anthony Whitehead, Director of the FDA's Houston Section, wrote that Gunn's address "reflected a sincere effort to generate and promote better understanding between this office and a research institution"; Whitehead to Gunn, May 16, 1979. Gunn then received a letter of commendation from LeMaistre on May 24.

[35]van Eys, "Food and Drug Administration Regulations and Research in Cancer Centers (Conceptual construct for Dr. LeMaistre)," May 29, 1979. On NCI officials' attention to the growth of unannounced visits, see memorandum from Vincent DeVita, Jr., to FDA Clinical Monitors, April 4, 1979; Cheri Stadalman (Group Administrator, Southwest Oncology Group) to Principal Investigators of the SWOG, April 20, 1979; RG1, SG2—"President's Office Records, 1964–1979, 10.1A," MDAA. "FDA Urged to Tone Down Its IRB Reviewers," *DRR* 21 (29) (July 19, 1978): 2–3. On the hike in disqualifications and other FDA initiatives, see *DRR* 22 (22) (May 30, 1979), 17; *DRR* 22 (42) (Oct. 17, 1979), 6. For a selected list of institutions at which major violations of the IND regulations and human subjects codes had been unearthed in the 1978 and 1979 inspections, see "Examples of Fraud, Abuse in New Drug Tests on Human Subjects Found by FDA," *DRR* 22 (42) (Oct. 17, 1979): 8.

delegating this task to the IRB, a resource-poor agency was able to effect a vast expansion in its governance of medical research while effecting minimal direct intrusion into clinical settings. Of course, for the system to work, the Administration must itself inspect and monitor IRBs, clinical investigators, and research sponsors, and in the late 1970s, federal budget politics both constrained and liberated the FDA's regulation of its satellite regulators.[36]

Perhaps the best evidence for this reading comes from the ceaseless contestation of the FDA's perceived intentions for IRB function. In the decades since the 1981 IRB rules were finalized, laments have flowed continuously from clinical trials and pharmacology quarters about IRBs taking on tasks they are constitutionally ill-equipped to handle. The Inspector General of the Department of Health and Human Services hinted in 1998 that the capacity of the institutional review system to protect human subjects was in fundamental "jeopardy" because the boards had been overworked. Other analysts of IRBs have warned that they cannot serve effectively as data and safety monitors, and that they cannot take the inevitable and rightful place of the FDA in regulating clinical investigators. At some level, whether these arguments are right is beside the point. Perhaps IRBs can handle these functions, perhaps they cannot. Yet the very rehearsal of these warnings—from human subjects ethicists, from the GAO, from Congress, from IRB heads themselves—would not occur in a regime where the Administration had not placed massive additional pressures upon institutional review boards. The sort of demands borne by IRBs are, moreover, small-scale versions of the larger tasks that Congress has delegated to the Administration: overseeing the quality of clinical research in support of new drugs, monitoring safety information, adverse events, and data quality from clinical trials.[37]

The empowerment of IRBs has projected the Administration's veto power to universities, institutes, contract research organizations, and ultimately to small committees within these organizations. From one vantage the empowerment of review boards seems to decentralize, because the officials carrying out the review of research protocols are at distant remove from federal officials. In other ways, however, IRBs profoundly expand the regulatory reach of the FDA, for two reasons. First, the Administration has created a

---

[36]For more traditional accounts of the IRB, see Faden and Beauchamp, *A History and Theory of Informed Consent*; Rothman, *Strangers at the Bedside*. See also the many writings of former Yale School of Medicine professor Robert J. Levine, who edited the principal journal covering human subjects protection, *IRB: A Review of Human Subjects Research*. Frances Kelsey shrewdly perceived the Administration's powers and limits; "The FDA's Enforcement of IRBs and Patient Informed Consent," *FDCJ* 44 (1989): 13–20.

[37]Former FDA General Counsel Richard Merrill concludes that the "FDA's expectations for IRBs have progressively expanded since the agency first mandated their participation in 1971," to the point that the IRB now functions as "FDA's onsite deputy"; Merrill, "FDA Regulation of Clinical Drug Trials," 76–8. Elizabeth Bankert and Robert Amdur, "The IRB Is Not a Data and Safety Monitoring Board," *IRB: A Review of Human Subjects Research* 23 (6) (Nov.–Dec. 2000): 9–11. David A. Kessler, "The Regulation of Investigational Drugs," *NEJM* 320 (1989): 281–8.

series of veto points—more than five thousand of them, according to one recent estimate—over clinical research while still retaining its own ability to place a clinical hold upon the research, to reject the IND application for a later phase, or to reject the eventual new drug application. The structure of potential vetoes embedded within IRBs is consistent with this interpretation. The Administration's rules allow for an appeal of a positive recommendation by an IRB, but not for appeal of a negative recommendation. A rejected study remains rejected, in other words, but an approved study still risks future negation. Second, because each board is monitored by the Administration and can be potentially disqualified by the agency, strong reputation-based incentives exist to toe the line on FDA rulemaking. Because IRB disqualification is tantamount to disqualification of an entire research institution—firms will avoid universities and contract research units whose IRBs have been disqualified, and these organizations will face difficulty in procuring grants—review boards and the universities they serve have incentives to remain thoroughly and fearfully accountable to the Administration.[38]

From another vantage—that of organizational image—the institutional review board keeps the FDA out of (and symbolically "above") the fray of protocol approval and study monitoring. Some of the most difficult, antagonistic, and "red-tape"-laden features of clinical research regulation are hence carried out not by the Administration itself—a distant federal agency—but by a local institution. In the aggregate, these local institutions impose appreciable direct costs upon the institutions that house them; from $170,000 to $5 million per year for academic medical centers alone, according to one recent analysis. Indirect costs such as paperwork and diverted time are likely much higher and defy measurement, but like monetary figures they gesture to the impact of the FDA's rules. The satellite regulators not only do most of the work, but they also bear much of the brunt of criticism from scientists whose aspirations are constrained by federal regulations. The built-in intellectual and methodological diversity of IRBs—the FDA has long expected and required them to include "lawyers, clergymen, or laymen as well as scientists"—relocates conflict from the sphere of federal regulation to the organization in which the research takes place. Because the Administration helped to foster them and has by rulemaking and inspection placed them securely within its regulatory orbit, the institutional review board has shouldered burdens far surpassing explicit human subjects protection.[39]

[38] On the number of IRBs, see Jastone, *Federal Protection for Human Research Subjects*, 52. On the asymmetry of appellate rights from IRB decisions, see *FR* 36 (52) (March 17, 1971): 5039, revision of paragraphs in Form FD-1571. To my knowledge this asymmetry is not apparent in NIH regulations or in the U.S. government's Common Rule.

[39] Jeremy Sugarman, et al., "The Cost of Institutional Review Boards in Academic Medical Centers," *NEJM* 352 (17) (April 2005): 1825. I summarize the costs of these procedures only as a way of documenting some of the effects of FDA rulemaking upon local institutions. The "benefits" of these regulations are incredibly hard to measure—patient autonomy, the liberty of human subjects, the added quality of medical research from more carefully designed protocols—and I intend no conjecture here on the desirability of the IRB rules vis-à-vis alternative institutions.

It would be inaccurate and careless to conclude that the Administration intended to conspiratorially rig clinical research monitoring and the IRB system to convert these institutions into bald projections of the regulatory state. The original intentions of Frances Kelsey in heading the IND Branch, intentions shared by many of her colleagues and by HEW superiors, were to create institutional guarantors of patients' rights. Yet once the institutional review board had been created, it was difficult to ignore its regulatory possibilities. The thrust and parry of rulemaking in 1978 and 1979 was consistent with other actions and the agency's frank rhetoric that its officials sought greater control over medical research, not just the human subjects issues arising in clinical studies, but issues of data safety, the credentials of clinical investigators, and the rigor of research plans. In 1977, speaking to an audience at the annual Institute of Medicine meeting, Donald Kennedy admitted openly that his agency did in fact regulate both medical research and medical practice, despite long-standing protestations to the contrary. "If you monitor informed consent, the composition of institutional review committees, the qualifications of clinical investigators, and the adequacy of protocols," he concluded, "you equally surely regulate clinical research." Once the foray into human subjects protection had been made, Kennedy and other FDA officials inferred, regulation of clinical research could not be avoided. More forcefully, the Administration's various audiences—the Kennedy, Fountain, and Nelson committees chief among them—had begun to expect as much from the agency. For a resource-strapped regulator answering demands from ever more demanding and disagreeable constituencies, mandating research institutions such as quality control units and IRBs was a supple adaptation that would last.[40]

The Aftermath: Research Monitoring and IRB Regulation Since 1981. After harmonization of the Administration's clinical regulations with the Department of Health and Human Services in 1981 and 1985, the federal government's *Federal Policy for the Protection of Human Subjects* (the "Common Rule") was adopted in 1991. At the time of its adoption, the Common Rule applied to research funded or governed by sixteen federal agencies. It represented the long-held wish of federal officials and clinical trials experts to have a unified federal policy across agencies. Its three pillars were sections on "informed consent" and "minimal risk," requirements for IRB review of research proposals, and institutional assurances of compliance with the Rule. In many ways, the Common Rule codified practices and collected rules that were adopted decades earlier by the FDA.[41]

The Administration mandated nonscientific authorities on the board "to assure complete and adequate review of the research project"; *FR* 36 (52) (March 17, 1971): 5039, revision of subparagraph 12 of Form FD-1572.

[40]On Kennedy's speech to the IOM audience, see *DRR* 20 (43) (Oct. 26, 1977): 7–8.

[41]Lee O. Jastone, ed., *Federal Protection for Human Research Subjects: An Analysis of the Common Rule and Its Interactions with FDA Regulations and the HIPAA Privacy Rule* (New York: Novinka, 2005).

The FDA's formal capacity in regulating clinical research is uniquely complemented by the day-to-day field and enforcement activities that the agency devotes to human subjects protection. No agency at any level of government conducts more inspections of clinical researchers and IRBs than does the FDA. Again, this practice began quite early. After a trial monitoring program was run and observed from 1972 to 1974, the FDA launched its Bioresearch Monitoring Program in 1977, which included inspections of clinical investigators, biopharmaceutic laboratories, toxicology laboratories, and IRBs.[42] Such inspections reports consume the time of more than thirty FDA employees at headquarters and in field offices. When deficiencies are found, the FDA may issue a warning letter to institutions detailing "significant deficiencies" in IRB oversight. If the deficiencies are serious enough, the FDA can disqualify both the IRB and the clinical investigator. At this writing, whereas human subjects protections are officially governed by the Office of Human Research Protection in the Department of Health and Human Services, the FDA still conducts most of the inspections.

Just how intensive or exhaustive has Administration oversight been? Data are insufficient to permit a good answer to this question, but some patterns from the past two decades can be gleaned from FDA and congressional reports. From fiscal year 1986 to fiscal year 1995, for instance, the FDA's Center for Drug Evaluation and Research conducted 1,712 inspections of establishments for compliance with FDA informed consent requirements. From 1991 to 1995, the FDA issued an average of 158 IRB inspection reports per year. In the early 1990s, such inspections uncovered numerous violations of federal rules, most of them minor. Almost half of IRBs (48 percent) inspected from October 1992 to September 1994 failed to keep adequate minutes of their meetings, while more than one-third (36 percent) failed to promulgate adequate written procedures. Almost half (48 percent) were found to have operated without a quorum of members present.

From January 1993 to November 1995, the FDA found violations serious enough to merit a warning letter in thirty-one cases. The agency has never disqualified an IRB, but in response to FDA findings of serious noncompliance with federal regulations, research institutions have disbanded their IRB more than sixty times in the past two decades. The FDA can also disqualify clinical investigators for serious or repeated violations of agency regulations. This too has happened only rarely—just nineteen times from 1978 to 1994, according to one FDA report—but this number understates the reach of FDA regulation. Over the same period, more than 110 clinical investigators were sanctioned or have signed consent agreements with the FDA, a serious and embarrassing admission of negligence in clinical research that can hamper researchers' ability to attract further funding. The threat of harm to reputation is sufficiently harrowing for clinical researchers and

[42] See "FDA Institutional Review Board Inspections," *FDA Information Sheets*, October 1, 1995; Rockville, MD, U.S. Food and Drug Administration.

medical centers that even rare sanctions present sufficient incentives for most researchers to rigorously maintain human subjects protections.[43]

The FDA cannot, of course, disqualify physicians from medical practice, nor can it prohibit universities from engaging in research. What backs up the FDA's human subjects regulations is its authoritative gatekeeping role in the pharmaceutical and medical device marketplaces. Universities, medical centers, and research organizations that violate FDA regulations will simply lose business from sponsors that must conduct clinical studies to receive FDA approval. Since funding is the lifeblood of any research endeavor, FDA sanctions can do enormous implicit and explicit damage to the careers and livelihoods of researchers and research organizations that violate federal law.

Before approving an Investigational New Drug application, the FDA requires researchers to submit and sign a formal statement that they will uphold prevailing ethical standards and that their institution's relevant parties will be notified of their study. FDA officials have the power to reject or terminate INDs (and hence terminate clinical studies) when the proposal presents "unacceptable risk" to human subjects.

The Administration's power over medical research is quite general, and hence issues that might have seemed the parochial property of another agency have come to fall under FDA purview. In human subjects protection, the regulation of research on prisoners provides a compelling example. Under Secretary Joseph Califano, the federal Department of Health, Education and Welfare (HEW) sought to rewrite the regulations on research with prisoner subjects in 1977. Califano was well known in the Carter administration for trying to centralize policymaking at the top of his Cabinet department, in part because he feared (correctly) that his organization would be split and his power would be muted by Carter's ambition to create a Cabinet-level Department of Education. Initial draft rules came out of the HEW Office for Protection from Research Risks in September 1977, but they were quickly routed to the FDA, where they took on a new form. The rulemaking "ballgame" changed because Administration officials proposed, and Califano's deputies agreed, that "since the bulk of the research done on prisoners—testing of new drugs—fell under the control of the FDA, FDA should write up its own regs concerning the ethics of such research." The Administration's power over pharmaceutical research translated, contingently on the assent of Califano, to partial authority over prisoners' rights in the clinical laboratory.[44]

[43]Nightingale S. Bagley GP, "FDA sanctions for practitioners for violations of clinical trial regulations and other misconduct," *Bulletin of the Federation of Scientists* 81(1994): 7–13. Different figures for disqualification—more than 50 disqualified from 1977 to 1990—are presented by CDER medical officer Bette Barton in *DRR*, April 25, 1990, 7. On the role of Frances Kelsey in some of these investigations, consult *DRR*, April 25, 1990, 6–7.

[44]On how the FDA referral changed the "ballgame," see "Prisoner Research Regs Were Routed to FDA," *DRR* 20 (37) (Sept. 14, 1977): RN-3. On Califano's moves toward centralization, see "Califano Opens a Drive for Clear Regulations," *NYT*, September 13, 1977, 61; David Rosenbaum, "To Know Califano Is to Respect Him: The President Is an Admirer," *NYT*,

The emergence and enforcement of human subjects protection in the United States has been the product of efforts by many organizations, institutions, and individuals. Neither the National Institutes of Health nor university research committees nor medical associations (as general as the AMA and as specific as the American College of Cardiology) can be ignored. Yet to think of the Administration as just one more player in the political and scientific arena of human subjects protection would also be inaccurate. With its gatekeeping power over medical products, its considerable inspection force, and its long-held statutory authority, the FDA is one of the pivotal organizations shaping the form, content, and aspirations of modern clinical research.

The Shaping of Statistical Measure: An Interlude on Intermediate and Surrogate Endpoints

The paradigmatic form of the modern clinical trial embeds the documentation of a human research subject from treatment to the time that an index event (a measurement point, death or heart attack, for instance) is observed. Often the endpoint is structured within the trial, for example in mental health studies where depression rating or functioning scores are measured three months, six months, or a year after the initiation of a treatment. The occurrence of measurements at the time points of three, six, and twelve months in such a study is an artifact of the research design. Yet for a wide variety of clinical trials, the endpoint is itself determined by an event that reflects a significant outcome for the patient. A cancer clinical trial may examine survival after treatment, in which case patient death is the endpoint. Trials for a drug treating patients who have suffered a previous heart attack or congestive heart failure may use subsequent heart attack or a subsequent heart failure episode as endpoints. In these and many other kinds of trials, the essential act of statistical inference comes from comparison of survival times in the treatment group versus the control group. An entire branch of modern biostatistics is dedicated to the analysis of such data under various assumptions, constraints, and experimental designs.[45]

In the 1980s and through the 1990s into the twentieth century, the determination of endpoints in clinical trials became a subject of material controversy. Questions of measurement and ethics have prompted many analysts

---

March 19, 1978, E6; "Califano Moves Strip Richmond, PHS of Many Major Responsibilities; FDA, NIH Chiefs Report Directly to Secty.; Can He Keep HEW Intact?" *DRR* 20 (37) (Sept. 22, 1978): 9. On President Carter's wish to avoid any single Cabinet official gaining too much influence, see Clyde H. Farnsworth, "Diffusion of Economic Power," *NYT*, August 4, 1977, 62; Califano, *Inside: A Public and Private Life* (New York: Public Affairs, 2004). Upon the creation of the U.S. Department of Education in 1979, Califano was fired by Carter.

[45] A classic introduction to this literature, as well as to the measure-theoretic and statistical assumptions that undergird these analyses, appears in Thomas R. Fleming and David P. Harrington, *Counting Processes and Survival Analysis* (New York: Wiley, 1991).

to suggest "biomarkers"—measured physiological, pathogenic, or biological processes such as viral load, counts of certain blood cells or other cells, clot formation, or tumor regression—as a substitute for the ultimate endpoints of serious morbidity or mortality. Debates over "surrogate" and "intermediate" endpoints for clinical trials have attracted much scientific and statistical debate and they have invited social-science and historical analysis as well. What merits additional reflection is how the Administration's gatekeeping and conceptual power have allowed FDA officials and bureaus to influence the definition of endpoints. By shaping the construction of an endpoint, Administration officials model the very data that are used to assess a medical treatment, not only in regulation but also in studies that form the basis for physicians' clinical guidelines and insurance determinations. As with the case of tissue plasminogen activator, conceptual power in the definition of endpoints amounts to conceptual power in the definition of what counts (literally) as a cure.[46]

The debate over surrogate endpoints is often associated with the AIDS crisis but, like many of the institutional and policy responses to AIDS, has earlier roots in the struggles over cancer therapeutics. Interest in methodically defining intermediate endpoints in cancer clinical trials arose at the National Cancer Institute in the mid-1980s, where officials in 1987 created an early detection branch dedicated to "intermediate endpoints." Charles Smart, the branch's director, spoke boldly about a new therapeutics of surrogate measures, in terms that could not have been lost on FDA officials: "I think the day of the gold standard of the randomized clinical trial with mortality as an endpoint is through." An important stimulus for the NCI's effort came in its continuing battle with Administration officials over concepts and standards for the approval of oncologic agents. Bruce Chabner, then Director of NCI Division of Cancer Treatment, repeatedly voiced his dissatisfaction with the slow and uncertain pace of approval for NCI-sponsored drugs. If the Administration would not adjust its approval standards for cancer drugs, he threatened in October 1987, NCI officials would "consider the option of doing it ourselves, making a strong public statement about what we think the approval criteria should be for oncologic drugs." In response to these and other statements, Robert Temple shot back, warning that the determination of alternative endpoints would require a "trade-off" that Chabner and his colleagues had ignored or poorly considered. Besides, Temple argued, his agency already considered alternative endpoints, and he expressed openness to the idea of palliation as an endpoint, wondering why NCI-sponsored drugs were not tested using this measure.[47]

[46]On disputes over surrogate endpoints for AIDS trials, see Steven Epstein, "Activism, Drug Regulation, and the Politics of Therapeutic Evaluation in the AIDS Era: A Case Study of ddC and the 'Surrogate Markers' Debate," *Social Studies of Science* 27/5 (1997): 691–726. I emphasize that the discussion here merely connects the surrogate endpoint debate to reputation and regulatory power; a fuller analysis of this would require at least one or two monographs. I thank Harry Marks, Richard Merrill, and Robert Temple for suggesting this discussion.

[47]*DRR*, January 14, 1987, 3–4 (NCI branch and Smart's remark); *DRR*, October 14, 1987,

At the core of the new NCI-FDA dispute was not whether Administration officials would consider surrogate endpoints, but whether they would *commit* to a set of endpoints before a trial was designed or conducted, particularly in a published guidance or regulation. FDA officials like Temple were inclined to express flexibility, but were reluctant to tie down their organization by issuing a published rule. Temple's most important pronouncements on the issue would come in speeches, concept papers, and medical journal articles, all of which were enormously influential in the subsequent course of biostatistics and clinical trial design. In response to what they perceived as ambiguity, NCI officials lamented that the gray areas left by regulation always yielded a preference on the part of researchers to test for survival. "There's absolutely no doubt," remarked one NCI critic in a February 18, 1988 meeting, "that the way the regulations are commonly interpreted and the whole tone of the way the agency tends to deal with the sponsors . . . is couched in terms of survival. So sponsors feel that that is the surest route to FDA approval." Chabner and others called for the wholesale redefinition of endpoints. Procedurally, Chabner was demanding a reversal of the customary informal-to-formal progression of concepts from administrative practice to guidance documents to rulemaking; Chabner and NCI officials wanted the explicit concept first, the applied concept later. By the summer of 1988, Center for Drug Evaluation and Research director Carl Peck offered a compromise solution; "complete response" rates could be used for cancer drug approval, but the particular application of this shift would depend on the type of tumor. Chabner pressed Peck to render the "complete response" standard as universal as possible. "I think complete responses and quality of life are important no matter what tumor you have," said Chabner, "and you ought to accept the general principle that patients who experience improvement in quality of life or good responses are benefitting, no matter [what type of cancer] they have." Possibly sensing an opening in Peck's proposal, Chabner also pushed the agency to consider "historical controls" (in which a patient receiving treatment was compared to her own pre-treatment experience) for cancer drug approvals. Peck resisted this overture and refused to commit his agency to a shift away from prospectively designed trials with separate treatment and control populations.[48]

4–6 (Chabner-Temple debate). For endpoints and practices governing the regulation of oncologic drugs, see John R. Johnson and Robert Temple, "Food and Drug Administration Requirements for Approval of Anticancer Crugs," *Cancer Treatment Reports* 69 (1985):1155–9.

[48]*DRR*, February 24, 1988, 9 (on February 18 meeting). *DRR*, June 1, 1988, 5; *DRR*, June 8, 1988, 3–4 ("complete response" proposal and feedback). It is notable that the controversy between the two agencies persisted despite the fact that personnel flowed freely between the two organizations, with Edward Tabor (formerly director of the FDA's anti-infective drug products division) named associate director of the NCI biological carcinogenesis program in the spring of 1988; *DRR*, March 2, 1988, 10. FDA reviewers also participated in clinical protocol reviews at NCI's Cancer Therapy Evaluation Program; *DRR*, December 13, 1989, 3. The agencies also hosted joint advisory committee appointees; *DRR*, October 17, 1990, 9.

By 1989, with President George H. W. Bush about to be inaugurated, Peck and Chabner openly discussed the possibility of a joint agency task force. Samuel Broder had just been appointed as head of the Institute, and observers of the biomedical research community in Washington surmised that Broder would bring "a more conciliatory approach" to NCI/FDA relations than his predecessors. Broder broadened the subjects of inter-agency discussion from endpoints and approval criteria to "protocols" more generally. Yet even as Broder and other NCI officials opened up the umbrella of discussion, they recognized that endpoint definition would remain the central crux of dispute. "I think this is an area where there are strongly held philosophies and two different worlds," Broder recognized. "I don't believe FDA recognizes and accepts complete response rate as an indication for approving [cancer drugs]... Therefore, we are caught in the track of having to do survival data, which, in effect, is another way of denying access to [a] drug." As Broder struck a more mollifying tone, Chabner continued to challenge the Administration's regulations on issues ranging from supplemental NDA approval (these "should not require extensive review by FDA," he claimed) to animal toxicology requirements for IND applications.[49]

The Administration's first material act of compromise came not in rule-making but in discussions over an impending drug review. Just as the review of cisplatin had established important precedents and exceptions in the 1980s, the review of the second-generation platinum-based chemotherapy treatment for solid tumors (carboplatin (Paraplatin)) would serve to establish benchmarks for cancer therapeutics. Temple offered an olive branch in February 1989, claiming that carboplatin could be approved without survival data for later stages of ovarian cancer, but maintained that approval as first-line therapy would require survival data. Since cisplatin was the standard for ovarian cancer treatment at the time, Temple wanted an implicit benchmark with which to compare carboplatin to its ancestor, which was approved on the basis of survival data just a decade before.

> The reservation I would have is if one approved [carboplatin] for unvarnished, unmodified front-line therapy without knowing that detail, I think there is a potential for serious loss until you have reasonable evidence that survival is comparable [to cisplatin].

As the debate over carboplatin and related drugs raged on—in part impelled by challenges from the Lasagna Committee formed by President Bush—Temple also drew attention to what he regarded as quick NDA approvals for a number of cancer therapies—mitoxantrone, ifosfamide, mesna, and (he hoped) carboplatin itself. Even as industry and biomedical observers were predicting approval of carboplatin by late summer or fall 1989, the Administration announced its approval for recurrent ovarian cancer in March. Rather quickly, the carboplatin decision became a template for other

---

[49]*DRR*, January 11, 1989, 7–8.

endpoint discussions. As the Administration gave with one hand, it took away with another. Three months after carboplatin's approval, the agency's Oncologic Drugs Advisory Committee announced that survival would remain the critical endpoint for approval for breast cancer drugs.[50]

As these debates in the context of cancer therapy unfolded, NIH and FDA researchers began to discuss appropriate endpoints for AIDS clinical trials. The two most common biomarker candidates of the late 1980s were CD4 levels and p24 antigen levels. Argument persisted over whether treatment-induced changes in these markers qualified as a measure of the "effect" of the drugs in question. Yet even as the debate over surrogate endpoints in AIDS developed, AIDS activists and infective disease researchers recognized that in the battle of concept formation, they were significantly behind the network of cancer therapeutics. In an April 1990 meeting, Carl Peck noted what was obvious to many following the saga of AIDS clinical trials. There was much greater research experience in the cancer field and, not least, his agency's advice was "accepted more often." In the examination of AIDS study protocols, Peck remarked, "we're amazed at times at how we have to wrangle with all parties on simple things like getting the dose regimen, using body weight to determine a dosage, and working on the kinetic and dynamic concepts."[51]

Even as the NCI/FDA pattern of collaboration was praised, moreover, the two organizations found themselves at odds over particulars. The Lasagna Committee (and Louis Lasagna himself) intervened in the dispute, though only rhetorically since the Committee carried only the authority of recommendation. In his view of the debate over surrogate endpoints, Lasagna simplified matters considerably, seeing two sides: the FDA and "everybody" else, with the added remark that the Federal Food, Drug and Cosmetic Act clearly favored the FDA's critics. The Lasagna Committee further roiled the waters of conceptual politics in August 1990 by proposing that tumor regression—as opposed to complete response or palliation measures that the FDA had favored—should be an acceptable endpoint for cancer drug approval. Administration officials rejected this overture and relied instead upon the compromises they had hammered out with the NCI in the working group. In October 1990, the FDA/NCI working group announced five accepting endpoints for demonstration of oncologic drug efficacy:

---

[50]Chabner pointed to the development and review of carboplatin as an example of a drug that could be approved without survival data; *DRR*, January 11, 1989, 9. See also *DRR*, February 8, 1989, 4. Carboplatin for injection (NDA 19-880) was approved on March 31, 1989 for advanced ovarian carcinoma. The carboplatin approval was announced March 3; *DRR*, March 15, 1989, 11. The public nature of this debate was accompanied by one of the very first academic articles that connected surrogate endpoints theoretically to cancer therapeutics; Susan S. Ellenberg and J. Michael Hamilton, "Surrogate Endpoints in Clinical Trials: Cancer," *Statistics in Medicine* 8 (4) (April 1989): 405–13. By May 1989, the FDA/NCI working group was using the carboplatin case (as well as pentostatin, mitoxantrone, and flutamide) for more general discussions of "appropriate endpoints"; *DRR*, May 17, 1989, 3–4. On the breast cancer decision, see *DRR*, June 14, 1989, 8.

[51]*DRR*, June 21, 1989, 4.

- Survival benefit
- Time-to-treatment failure and disease-free survival
- Complete response rate
- Response rate
- Beneficial effects on disease-related symptoms and/or quality of life[52]

The "five endpoints" announcement was marked by ambiguity as well as clarification. At no time did the NCI/FDA working group state clearly that any trial or two demonstrating a statistically significant difference in treatment and control groups on these measures would be approved. Yet the announcement was accompanied by indications from Carl Peck and others that AIDS drugs—particularly ddI (Videx)—would also be considered for approval based upon surrogate endpoints, in this case CD4 counts, and historical controls. Peck's announcement followed a threat by AIDS activists for a Rockville protest if the agency did not meet the group's demands. And when in June 1991 the agency approved carboplatin as first-line therapy for ovarian cancer, FDA officials pointed both to survival data and to the endpoint of 'time to progression" as the basis for their decision. Even as clarity emerged in decision making, however, ambiguity was projected from choice. An Administration advisory panel explicitly rejected the use of CD4 counts as an efficacy endpoint for AIDS vaccines in November 1991; biotechnology stock values plunged in response to the decision.[53]

In the years following the Administration's initial decisions on carboplatin, ddI and other cancer and AIDS drugs, something of a cottage industry dedicated to the discovery of biomarkers and surrogate endpoints arose and flourished within American academics. Academic discussions of intermediate and surrogate endpoints did not precede but accompanied and followed the FDA's statements and precedents. The evolution of surrogate endpoints cut in at least two directions. It accelerated and eased the development and marketing of some drugs, while hindering others where poor results were obtained on surrogate measures. And, much as FDA officials had feared in the late 1980s and early 1990s, the partial carving of "exceptions" to the agency's previous insistence on final clinical endpoints has been copied in

[52]DRR, August 22, 1990, 2–5. It was at this time, too, that the Lasagna Committee proposed the use of external reviewers for NDAs. On the five endpoints, see DRR, October 24, 1990, 7. It is telling that whereas the FDA's enabling statute used the term "effective," virtually all of the discussion in Drug Research Reports ("the Blue Sheet"), and other trade reporters (such as FDCR, or "the Pink Sheet") used the term "efficacy." In cancer therapeutics as with many other areas of pharmacology, attention to the strict concept of "effectiveness" was largely a legal fiction. For evolution of endpoint concepts in regulatory oncology after this period, consult John R. Johnson, Grant Williams and Richard Pazdur, "Endpoints and United States Food and Drug Administration Approval of Oncology Drugs," Journal of Clinical Oncology 21 (2003): 1404.

[53]DRR, April 24, 1991, 9–10; DRR, July 10, 1991, 3. The FDA's Antiviral Drugs Committee also decided in July 1991 that CD4 levels would be an appropriate endpoint for judging the efficacy of Bristol-Myers Squibb's ddI (Videx) for AIDs; DRR, July 31, 1991, 8–9. Regulatory affairs officer David Rosen argued that "innovative approaches were employed in analyzing the [ddI] data, and additional efforts were made to facilitate communication with the sponsor."

realms far away from cancer and AIDS. In recent years, even antibiotics researchers have come to regard "time to defervescence" (fever response) as an appropriate endpoint in clinical trials in infectious diseases.[54]

RULES, GUIDANCE, AND CONCEPT FORMATION

Robert Young's ill-fated attempt in January 1977 to rewrite the rules for the conduct and evaluation of combination chemotherapy was emblematic of another development gaining steam in the 1960s and 1970s. Young was attempting to influence not federal rules of the substantive or legislative form, and not merely "descriptive" rules, but a novel form of administrative governance. As the Drug Efficacy Study Initiative shifted into a more administrative realm, the Administration's effective rules for clinical trial planning, design, procedure, and analysis were not statements of the sort that would run through an elaborate process of notice-and-comment rulemaking. They were instead published by the Administration itself, usually (though not always) with tacit or explicit approval from a relevant advisory committee, and only later in the *Federal Register*. The FDA's issuance of successive "guidelines" for clinical experimentation was one of the most notable forays into a regulatory pattern that has become government-wide in the United States—the issuance of "guidance documents."[55]

The Administration's reliance upon documents that conveyed informal advice was a pattern that preceded the 1962 Amendments. Indeed, British government officials had been issuing guidelines for experimentation since the 1930s. Yet it was in the 1970s—in the administrative collaboration of J. Richard Crout and Peter Barton Hutt—that these structural forms began to displace formal rulemaking as a means of communicating structures of clinical experiment and drug development to the global pharmaceutical industry and the American medical profession. The context in which these documents emerged and came to dominance was one of political conflict and regulatory ambiguity. The Administration, along with other federal regulatory agencies, was receiving complaints that new regulations were coming without warning, or that important rules were taking too long to cement. At the same time as these laments acquired greater and greater pitch, the Ad-

---

[54]Not a single article indexed in the electronic search engines PubMed or J-STOR mentioned the concept "intermediate" or "surrogate" endpoints until April 1989; see the collection of articles in *Statistics in Medicine* 8 (4) (April 1989). Jon Cohen, "FDA Committee Raises AIDS Vaccine Hurdles," *Science* 254 (5035) (Nov. 22, 1991): 1105. For a theoretical and historical reflection on the debate over surrogate markers in AIDS, see Thomas Fleming, "Evaluating Therapeutic Interventions: Some Issues and Experiences," *Statistical Science* 7 (4) (Nov. 1992): 428–41. On antimicrobial drug development, see John H. Powers, "Antimicrobial drug development—the past, the present, and the future," *Clinical Microbiology and Infection* 10 (Suppl. 4) (2004): 23–31. Susan S. Ellenberg, "Surrogate Endpoints: The Debate Goes On," *Pharmacoepidemiology and Drug Safety* 10 (2001): 493–6.

[55]On Young and the oncology trial rules, consult chapter 6.

ministration's senior officers were quietly launching an initiative to revise the Investigational New Drug regulations more substantially than at any time since 1963. The Administration was buffeted by a slew of proposals—many from within, many from firms and the clinical pharmacology community—to revise the Phase 1, 2, and 3 concepts. And, in response to the concerns of cancer activists and the Laetrile controversy, FDA officers began to revise the concept of a "Treatment IND," a study approval that would permit commercial sponsors to distribute the drug in question to patients with terminal illness.[56]

The emergence of nonbinding clinical testing guidelines dates from the 1960s, as Division Directors of the FDA's Office of New Drugs began to elaborate informal codes of practice for clinical testing. Once these draft guidelines had been distributed to manufacturers and scientific societies, Administration officials sought input on the guidelines from the National Academy of Sciences. The Academy prepared a proposal for collaborative development of guidelines with the Administration. The Pharmaceutical Manufacturers Association also expressed interesting in cooperating in a joint venture, with the cautious understanding that industry involvement would be limited and many of the drug-specific "guidances" would emerge from the FDA's system of advisory committees. Administration officials predicted in 1969 that even informal elaboration of nonbinding guidelines would produce much greater uniformity in industry and academic research practices.[57]

Yet even when it was developed in consultation with voices from drug companies and medical specialties, the guidance document could still trigger cries of heavy-handed regulation. One example comes in the efforts of FDA leaders in the 1970s, led by Robert Temple, to increase the use of placebo-controlled trials in drug experiments. When in 1979 the Gastrointestinal Drugs Advisory Committee, chaired by Nicholas Hightower of Scott & White Memorial Hospital in Texas, noted the "enormous placebo response" associated with gastrointestinal drugs, Temple and other FDA officials seized upon the declaration and called for a broader requirement for placebo control

---

[56]In Britain, the guidelines were issued by the Committee on Clinical Trials, formed by the Medical Research Council of Great Britain in 1931; see Marks, *The Progress of Experiment.* "FDA Asked to Give Health Professions Prior Notice of Reg-Writing; Agency Promises Small, In-Depth Quarterly Meetings, Maps Other Efforts," *DRR* 22 (26) (June 27, 1979): 6. "Investigational New Drug Reg Changes Readied by FDA for Unveiling at a September Public Meeting; Formal Proposal Planned by Year's End," *DRR* 22 (30) (July 25, 1979): 11–12.

[57]The vision elaborated in the Office of New Drugs and in collaboration with the National Academy of Sciences would shape much of the subsequent development of the guideline documents. The FDA/NAS protocol was divided into two parts, the first entailing the elaboration of "general guidelines for clinical investigation of drugs," and the second "the development of specific protocols by class of drug." FDA-BOM, Minutes of the Medical Advisory Board, Twenty-First Meeting, December 18 and 19, 1969, pp. 7–8; Harry F. Dowling Papers, NLM. The agency's advisory committees also participated in the development of guidelines; see the discussion of trial design and reporting standards for anti-arthritis drugs in Transcript, Arthritis Advisory Committee Meeting, May 15, 1975, vol. I, 10-41; RG 88, NA.

in gastrointestinal drug study protocols. The Temple proposal opened fresh divisions among the diverse audiences in drug development and medical experiment. The agency's own advisory committee and medical specialists were calling for exactly the kind of advice that Temple was offering, as they preferred more clarity and formality in placebo considerations. At the same time, drug company executives worried openly that the character of medical experiment was being dictated by a "regulatory hierarchy." Companies were worried that "guidance" would become law.[58]

In part because the Administration spoke with greater and greater legal authority in the 1970s, and in part because its veto power over drug development was really never in doubt, the various *Guidelines for Clinical Evaluation* and *General Considerations for Clinical Evaluation* bound companies and researchers in fact even where they did not at law. As scholars and observers in food and drug law would continually notice, gentle FDA suggestions for clinical trial design were highly likely to be followed, given that the officials dispensing advice were highly likely to be involved in the eventual NDA review. Backed up by reputation and by gatekeeping authority, guidances enacted a conceptual "third" face of regulatory power over the pharmaceutical world to a degree that is perhaps unequaled in other realms of regulation.

The sequence of documents that became formalized in the 1970s—*General Considerations for Clinical Evaluation of Drugs* (1977), *General Considerations for the Clinical Evaluation of Drugs in Infants and Children (1977)*, *Guidelines for the Clinical Evaluation of Analgesic Drugs (1979)*—represented some of the most forceful assertions of rules without rulemaking in all of federal regulation in the late twentieth century. Like so many other features of American pharmaceutical regulation, the approach of these documents was shaped elaborately by Richard Crout (then Director of the Bureau of Drugs) and Marion Finkel (Associate Director for New Drug Evaluation) with assistance from the various top agency legal counsel of the time, principally general counsels Peter Barton Hutt and Richard Merrill. In introducing these documents, Crout and Finkel couched the agency's recommendations within a language of advice, legitimacy, and a lack of binding legal compulsion.

> The purpose of these guidelines is to present acceptable current approaches to the study of investigational drugs in man. These guidelines contain both generalities and specifics and were developed with experience from available drugs....
>
> These guidelines are not to be interpreted as mandatory requirements by the FDA to allow continuation of clinical trials for investigational drugs or to obtain approval of a new drug for marketing. These guidelines, in part, contain recommendations for clinical studies which are recognized as desirable approaches to be

[58] "Put 'Behavioral Factors' in G-I Guides, FDA Is Urged," *DRR* 22 (43) (Oct. 24, 1978): 22. "FDA's Preference for Placebo Controls in Concept Papers Could Evolve into 'Rigid' Regulatory 'Hierarchy,' Squibb Exec Asserts at Public Forum on Regs," *DRR* 22 (46) (Nov. 14, 1979): 8.

used in arriving at conclusions concerning safety and effectiveness of new drugs; and in the other part they consist of the views of outstanding experts in the field as to what constitutes appropriate methods of study of specific classes of drugs....

Under FDA regulations (21 CFR 10.90(b)) all clinical guidelines constitute advisory opinions on an acceptable approach to meeting regulatory requirements, and research begun in good faith under such guidelines will be accepted by the Agency for review purposes unless this guideline (or the relevant portion of it) has been formally rescinded for valid health reasons. This does not imply that results obtained in studies conducted under these guidelines will necessarily result in the approval of an application or that the studies suggested will produce the total clinical information required for approval of a particular drug.[59]

The Administration's guidance documents were not immune from court review, as the landmark decision in *Washington Legal Foundation v. Kessler* (1998) would demonstrate. And as more and more federal and state government agencies in the United States began to rely upon the guidance document for making policy, politicians began to rein in the ability of agencies to issue them without prior authorization. Yet the consensus among regulatory observers and administrative law scholars that a new mode of policymaking had emerged—one used as aggressively at the Administration as in any other organ of American government—meant that the modern pharmaceutical world was being governed by a new and legitimated instrument of regulatory power.[60]

GATEKEEPING AND PRODUCT ABANDONMENT: A BRIEF STATISTICAL PORTRAIT

The incidence of conceptual power that appears in regulation of clinical trials, investigators, and statistical measures is premised greatly upon the Administration's gatekeeping authority and the power that comes with it. A rarely witnessed consequence of that gatekeeping power comes in the many drugs and therapeutic projects that are never submitted to the Administration as a new drug application or a biological license application. The visibility of these drug abandonment decisions is reduced in part by companies'

---

[59]FDA, *Guidelines for the Clinical Evaluation of Analgesic Drugs* (Nov. 1979); HEW Publication # (FDA) 80-3093 (Washington, DC: GPO, 1979), iii (Crout and Finkel general statement). *General Considerations for the Clinical Evaluation of Drugs in Infants and Children*, HEW (FDA) 77-3041, September 1977 (Washington, DC: GPO). Some sense of Finkel's role in producing these documents comes from her essay, "The Role of the FDA in the Clinical Development Process," in Gary M. Matoren, ed., *The Clinical Research Process in the Pharmaceutical Industry* (Informa, 1984), chap. 23.

[60]*Washington Legal Foundation v. Friedman*, 13 F. Supp. 2d 51 (D.D.C., 1998); Richard Abood, *Pharmacy Practice and the Law* (Sudbury, MA: Jones & Bartlett, 2004), 95. Janet Pelley, "President Bush Expands Influence over Regulatory Agencies," *Environmental Science and Technology*, April 11, 2007. Michael R. Asimow, "Guidance Documents in the States: Toward a Safe Harbor," *Administrative Law Review* 54 (2002): 631.

reluctance to publicize their bad news to investors. The investors will observe the news eventually, but it then makes little sense for the company to devote scarce publicity resources to its dead product lines.

Beyond this, the problem of causal inference is even harder—it is difficult if not impossible to know whether a drug was abandoned because it was considered insufficiently promising on the sponsor's own terms, or whether the drug was abandoned because it was considered profitable enough by the company but unlikely to gain success in the American regulatory process. Only in the second case, at least theoretically, would a drug's abandonment count as induced by the regulator. The problem then comes in separating drugs that would have been abandoned even in the absence of FDA regulation from those that would not have been abandoned but for the necessity of regulatory approval.[61]

One statistical glimpse into this dynamic comes from examining firms' response to FDA rejections or delays at the drug approval stage. When the Administration announces that a drug is not approvable, or asks for more data, the message conveyed by such a decision probably affects many drugs that are "upstream" in the development process and have yet to be submitted. Some drugs that are already on the market or that promise to compete against the drug being rejected or delayed may face enhanced prospects, but for most drugs, a regulatory rejection likely signals a higher barrier. In the face of such rejections and the longer odds communicated by them, many drug sponsors may abandon marginal projects.

One possibility for focusing the glimpse is that many drug rejections come as a surprise to the firms submitting them for approval, and relatedly, to the community of investors who are positioned to buy or sell publicly traded shares in the company. When a drug is rejected and the share price of the sponsoring company drops by 35 or 70 percent, for example, it is likely that for everybody but the FDA officials making the decision, the rejection came as something of a surprise. These surprises and their financial size then encode something of the degree to which a rejection or delay was not anticipated beforehand by drug-developing firms. If the shift in asset prices is due to unanticipated FDA rejection, these perturbations to stock prices measure something of the "shock to the system" that is conveyed by an FDA rejection or delay. A plausible strategy for examining the influence of FDA decisions on drug abandonment lies in correlating these stock price "shocks" with subsequent observed decisions by drug sponsors to discontinue drug projects, either in the clinical trial stage or beforehand.[62]

[61]For a mathematical model of "equilibrium abandonment," see Carpenter and Ting, "Regulatory Errors with Endogenous Agendas," *American Journal of Political Science* (2007).

[62]In previous studies of market reaction to FDA decisions, financial economists have found that "The large price changes associated with approval and rejection decisions suggest that a significant amount of uncertainty about FDA decisions is present almost up to the announcement day"; Jean Claude Bosch and Insup Lee, "Wealth Effects of Food and Drug Administration Approval Decisions," *Managerial and Decision Economics* 15 (6) (1994): 589–99. The

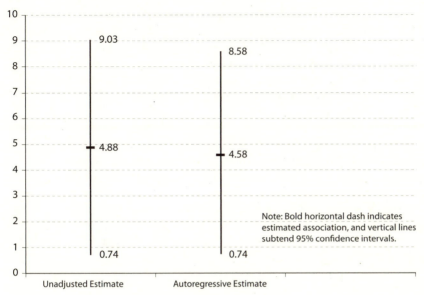

Figure 8.1. Additional Drug Projects Abandoned for Every Standardized Shock in Sponsor Firms' Asset Price Induced by FDA Rejection or Delay

The administration rejects and delays drugs all the time, but the more surprising decisions are usually covered. For the period 1989 to 2003, the *Wall Street Journal* reported on forty-eight different instances in which the FDA or one of its advisory committees rejected or delayed a drug. When these instances are multiplied by the percentage decline in share price on the day of the FDA decision, and the incidents are combined by month, there was an average change of 4.5 percent in stock price per month during the period. The day-of-rejection shocks varied widely, however, with a standard deviation of 14.8, meaning that one month's shocks differed from another's by an average of almost 15 percentage points. The largest drop in combined share prices was 87 percentage points for two companies in a single day.[63]

Figure 8.1 displays the estimated number of drugs abandoned in the month following every standardized (downward) shift in the asset price of the sponsor whose drug was rejected, as recorded in the *WSJ*. The statistical

statistical estimates presented here are a "glimpse" from a much more complicated and technical exercise in estimation; see Daniel Carpenter, et al., "Estimation of Equilibrium Drug Abandonment with Asset Value Perturbations Induced by Regulatory Decisions," manuscript, Department of Government, Harvard University (2008).

[63]The data are taken from the Pharmaprojects database. Measures for FDA decisions are taken from a search of the *Wall Street Journal* for the phrase bundles ("FDA" and "reject"), ("FDA" and "deny"/"denied"), and ("FDA" and "more data"). There are, of course, other ways to measure the asset price disturbance, including the examination of the change in total asset value of the company. In other research, findings are similar using this measure; see Carpenter, et al., "Estimation of Equilibrium Drug Abandonment with Asset Value Perturbations Induced by Regulatory Decisions."

estimates suggest that, for the period from 1989 to 2003, a standard-deviation reduction in stock price following a "surprise" FDA rejection or delay was associated with the abandonment of five additional drugs by other sponsors. Perhaps intuitively, the statistical estimates suggest that this effect is observed in the month of or month following the FDA's decision, not the second to sixth months following the FDA decision.

. . .

The statistical glimpse is exactly that: a glimpse. There are many more drugs abandoned than are accounted for by asset price shocks detailed in major financial newspapers; yet the existence of this phenomenon shows the reach of the Administration's drug approval power. The glimpse nonetheless demonstrates the minute and less visible imprint of the FDA's gatekeeping power, whereby development projects that aim to transform ideas into commodities are affected by sponsors' anticipation of the decisions of the regulator far into the future.

CHAPTER NINE

The Other Side of the Gate: Reputation, Power, and Post-Market Regulation

> It seems incredible that if the Pill is not safe we
> should have to wait till the British tell us so.
>
> —Drew Pearson and Jack Anderson,
> *Washington Post* columnists, 1969

> I could bore you with a long list of prominent and not-
> so-prominent safety issues where CDER and its Office
> of New Drugs proved to be extremely resistant to full and
> open disclosure of safety information, especially when it
> called into question an existing regulatory position. In these
> situations, the new drug reviewing division that approved
> the drug in the first place and that regards it as its own
> child, typically proves to be the single greatest obstacle
> to effectively dealing with serious drug safety issues.
>
> —David R. Graham, M.D., in testimony
> before the U.S. Senate, November 2004[1]

ONCE the Administration declares a New Drug Application "effective," a drug legally enters the U.S. market. At this point, the agency's statutory and public responsibilities continue. An effective NDA is still the object of regulation. Federal law, Congress, and the public still hold the agency responsible for ensuring drug safety, and the agency's work is now called "post-market regulation." But the powers of the Administration have changed. And its

[1]Pearson and Anderson, "FDA Lags on Data for 'Pill' Fatalities," *WP*, March 19, 1969, D15. Testimony of D. Graham, *The FDA, Merck and Vioxx: Putting Patient Safety First?* Hearings before U.S. Senate Finance Committee, November 18, 2004. Available online at: http://finance.senate.gov/hearings/testimony/2004test/111804dgtest.pdf. Accessed July 31, 2009.

incentives have changed. And hence the ballgame has changed. What was once caution about the drug itself is now aversion to bad news about a product that has the imprimatur of federal approval. What was once a formidable veto authority over millions of dollars and thousands of hours of research and development has been reduced to a small set of feeble tools—tools underfunded and little used—for badgering and coaxing a company into compliance with Administration wishes. A drug that is past the gate is a legal entity whose controllability and associated politics differ starkly from those of the New Drug Application.

What is called "post-market" is upon further examination a regulatory artifact. It means, legally and for all intents and purposes, "after NDA approval." Post-market regulation comes, simply enough, when the Administration has relinquished its gatekeeping power over a drug.[2] The agency has granted rights to a sponsor, rights to market a chemical entity, and a set of claims associated with that entity. Post-market regulation may be conceived as the set of governance relationships that occur once a product-claim combination has been approved, has become formally legal. Though this conception may be straightforward, the world it simplifies is not. The world of post-market regulation is a vast one. It encompasses labeling, advertising, drugs sold "over-the-counter" without a prescription, "surveillance" monitoring of drugs for adverse reactions, risk management, the mandating of further clinical studies by the sponsor and monitoring the progress and results of those trials, the inspection of production and storage facilities, and the potential seizure and confiscation of products found in violation of the law.

The FDA has coincident weaknesses and strengths in this world. The weaknesses are glaring and are the subject of extensive study and lament in contemporary medicine and politics. They have motivated hundreds of articles and editorials in the world's health and medical journals, dozens of books and government policy reports, and numerous congressional hearings in the past decade. Once a drug is approved, the FDA assumes a set of new stances—legal, political, and scientific—toward it. The Administration is criticized for placing so much weight on pre-market review and too little on surveillance after approval. FDA officers, particularly the more powerful managers in higher echelons, are disparaged for the slowness and timidity with which they examine and question past decisions. The agency's powers and resources in new drug review, however inadequately they are perceived by some critics, appear cosmic when contrasted with the tools available for post-market regulation.

In the late twentieth century, reputation and power—and their historical interplay—animated and subtended the post-approval regulation of pharmaceuticals. Within the Administration, there emerged a pervasive and enduring cultural conflict between those who approve drugs and those who

---

[2] The possibility of "off-label" prescribing and supplementary approvals renders even this boundary a porous one. See James M. Beck and Elizabeth D. Azari, "FDA, Off-Label Use, and Informed Consent: Debunking Myths and Misconceptions" *FDLJ* 53 (1998): 71–104.

monitor them after approval. The conflict was in part about reputation. The epidemiologists who populated the FDA's Office of Drug Safety (ODS) gained their positions, their prestige, and their reputation from identifying unsafe drugs. The organizational and individual reputations of gatekeepers stood diminished when their previous approvals became the target of scrutiny from medical journals, journalists, and committees of Congress. Yet the conflict was also about power. The Administration's fundamental statutory authority was more of gatekeeping than of surveillance. Within the FDA, the reputational conflict was reproduced in the structures of formal organizational authority. The gatekeepers directed and oversaw the monitors, who were subsumed within the offices of the gatekeepers. The methods of pharmacologists (gatekeepers) were considered superior to those of epidemiologists (monitors), and the pharmacologists dominated the epidemiologists in terms of authority and organizational status. Power mattered, too, not only within the agency but outside it, at the interface of state and market. The legal and reputational object of agency policy is the firm that develops and manufactures drugs, not the physician or other health-care provider who prescribes them or the hospitals, pharmacies, and other facilities where drugs are dispensed.[3]

What strength the Administration does have in the world of post-market regulation is itself embedded within and constrained by reputation and power. Initially, the New Drug Application is an explicit contract that keeps firms in line, and agency officials have, upon detecting obvious violations to the NDA in the post-market phase, purposefully "made an example" of different firms. In some cases the unfortunate recipients of FDA animus have been small, new entrants to the pharmaceutical world, but in many others they have been large, established companies. In making examples of the elites, the reputational aims of the Administration are better served, even if the action is more costly. Second, the dependence of firms' profits and valuation upon the company's "pipeline" of future patent-protected drugs means that firms will with necessity appear before the Administration to present new molecules for regulatory approval. The success of these future appearances will be in part conditioned by past behavior, specifically by behavior with respect to post-market regulation. Hence, the firm's current reputation with Administration officials will come to bear upon its future regulatory success, which is a key determinant of its present value.[4]

[3] I refer generically to the "Office of Drug Safety" (ODS) and the "Office of New Drugs" (OND) at different points in this chapter. These entities have taken different forms and have had various names over the past four decades. Where appropriate I will use the historically specific titles.

[4] The idea of repeated interaction between the Administration and a firm is a blunt simplification. In reality there is repeated interaction between different officials of the Center for Drug Evaluation and Research, on the FDA side, and representatives in a company's regulatory affairs office, on the firm side. Turnover on both sides of the relationship creates new uncertainties and new identities.

Yet the fact that most companies have regulatory affairs offices—offices through which most

Issues of regulation after new drug approval have waxed and waned in publicity and importance over the past five decades, but they have recently acquired much more heft. The withdrawal of Merck's rofecoxib (Vioxx) in September 2004 sparked a series of discussions about the institutions of pharmaceutical regulation in the United States and around the globe. The Senate Finance Committee, under the chairmanship of Iowa Republican Charles Grassley, held several high-profile hearings into the issue. In April 2006, the U.S. General Accounting Office (GAO) published a report that was highly critical of existing policy and offered several reforms, including expanded FDA authority to require that post-market studies be carried out by drug companies.[5] These ongoing policy initiatives were accompanied by proposals from prominent medical academics and medical journal editors for the creation of a drug safety office or commission that is independent of the FDA, or at least of its drug approval divisions. The large-scale debate over these proposals reached a temporary culmination in the Food and Drug Administration Amendments Act of 2007 (FDAAA). Among other changes, the FDAAA accorded greater authority to the Office of Drug Safety and required drug sponsors to prepare Risk Evaluation and Mitigation Strategies—essentially pre-marketing commitments for post-marketing surveillance and possible adjustment of marketing plans—and include them in new drug applications.[6]

The current dilemma—and its embedment in the conflict between pre-market approval and post-market surveillance—has a long history. Since the

---

FDA communications and new drug applications are routed—creates an organizational permanence and identity for the company. The regulatory affairs office becomes the "face" of the company to the Administration. One sees this in the role of Herbert Helling and associated officials at Searle in the narrative of oral contraceptives, presented in chapter 7. A similar story could be told with more recent officers, whether of Bruce Burlington, Ronald Chesemore, Alison Lawton at Genzyme, or Philip Crooker at AstraZeneca. The existence of a professional society for regulatory affairs officers (at this writing entitled the Regulatory Affairs Professional Society), combined with the existence of a network of regulatory affiliations among companies and between firms and the Administration, imparts a greater familiarity to these interactions than an atomistic understanding of firm-regulator interactions would suggest. Of course, these networks are shaped in part by the flow of people from the FDA to the companies or to independent regulatory consulting firms, as in the case of Burlington, Theodore Klumpp, and prominent industry consultants such as Wayne Pines.

[5]U.S. General Accounting Office, *Drug Safety: Improvement Needed in FDA's Postmarket Decision-making and Oversight Process*, GAO-06-402 (2006), p. 36. For a summary theoretical review of recent issues in FDA post-marketing regulation, see D. P. Carpenter and M. M. Ting, "The Political Logic of Regulatory Error," *NRDD* 4(10) (Oct. 2005): 819–23.

[6]Jerome J. Avorn, *Powerful Medicines* (New York: Knopf, 2004); Philip B. Fontanarosa, Drummond Rennie, and Catherine D. De Angelis. "Postmarketing Surveillance—Lack of Vigilance, Lack of Trust," *JAMA* 292 (21) (Dec. 1, 2004): 2647–50; Simon Frantz, "How to Avoid Another Vioxx," *NRDD* 4 (1) (Dec. 12, 2004): 5–7. Alastair J. J. Wood, C. M.Stein, and Raymond Woolsey, "Making Medicines Safer: The Need for an Independent Drug Safety Board," *NEJM* 339 (25) (1998): 1851–4. For a recent and unapologetic rehearsal of the ideas from the Joint Committee Report of 1980, see Brian L. Strom, "How the U.S. Drug Safety System Should Be Changed," *JAMA* 295 (17) (May 3, 2006): 2072–5. The FDAAA (Public Law 110-85) appears at 121 Stat. 823.

1960s at latest, critics and observers of U.S. pharmaceutical regulation have targeted the post-market surveillance system for complaints. And their conclusions, while varied in some respects, have often revisited the perceived conflict between pre-market and post-market processes. Consider for example the late 1970s and early 1980s. In September 1979, Senator Edward Kennedy's "Drug Regulation Reform Act of 1978" passed the Senate. Kennedy's bill would have equipped the FDA with authority to require post-market surveillance studies for up to five years after approval, and would also have loosened the standards for market withdrawal. The bill would never pass the House and hence never became law. One year later, the Joint Commission on Prescription Drug Use proposed a national "Center for Drug Surveillance (CDS)"—an agency independent of the FDA's new drug review divisions—which would "perform and encourage research into drug effects." In the 1980s, 1990s and early twenty-first century the General Accounting Office issued reports critical of post-market drug safety policy in the United States, all of them sounding the familiar refrain that the Administration's post-market surveillance system needed strengthening.[7]

The post-approval regulation of pharmaceuticals can be studied conceptually and narratively, and this chapter combines several methods of analysis in its study. It begins in a narrow historical fashion, describing a set of methods and tools for post-market regulation—the adverse event report and pharmaco-epidemiology—and their evolution. It follows this discussion with a narrative on the regulation of oral contraceptives in the 1960s and 1970s. The saga of oral contraceptives regulation provides lessons and forms a benchmark set of developments that shaped post-approval regulation in the 1980s and beyond. It also forms the basis for a general discussion of the politics of post-market regulation, including some statistical analyses of how the Administration has revisited previously approved drugs in the past several decades. The chapter concludes with an inquiry into the symbolism and choreography of drug withdrawal, the most stark and halting event in post-approval regulation.

EPIDEMIOLOGY AND THE ADVERSE-EVENT REPORTING SYSTEM

Just as the new drug application has historically governed the gatekeeping operations of the FDA, so too the Administration's post-market safety system has been premised largely upon a single document: the "adverse event

---

[7] For a concise and summary historical review of 1970s efforts to reform post-marketing regulation, see U.S. Congress, Office of Technology Assessment, *Postmarketing Surveillance of Prescription Drugs* (Washington, DC: GPO, 1982). After hearings before the Subcommittee on Health of the Senate Committee on Labor and Human Resources in 1974, the Department of Health Education and Welfare created a Review Panel on New Drug Regulation, which issued its report in May 1977. Lawmaking in the Senate followed this report in the subsequent session of Congress. Report of the Joint Commission on Prescription Drug Use, *Final Report* (Rockville, MD: Joint Commission on Prescription Drug Use, 1980). GAO, *Drug Safety: Improvement Needed in FDA's Postmarket Decision-making and Oversight Process*, GAO-06-402, 36.

report." As the General Accounting Office recently concluded, "Adverse event data are the primary basis for postmarket safety reactions ranging from labeling changes to withdrawal." Even when federal officials use data from controlled clinical trials, observational analyses of data from large government or company databases, or "meta-analyses" in which previous clinical studies are lumped together and analyzed as if they were part of a single, broader experiment, they still use adverse event data to form hypotheses for these more sophisticated methods.[8]

Like so much of the modern pharmaceutical regime, the contemporary system of adverse event reporting has its roots in the 1950s FDA, and like so much else with American pharmaceutical regulation, the system has been keenly observed (and in some cases copied) by foreign governments. One impetus was the painful moral of problems with chloramphenicol and aplastic anemia. The drug that turned "blood into water" and killed hundreds (perhaps thousands) of otherwise healthy patients did so with public silence; it was not until Albe Watkins and other chloramphenicol critics began aggregating data from the nation's hospitals that medical and regulatory authorities suspected a wider problem. Yet the adverse event reporting system owes its existence not just to a crisis, but also to a network of sponsors centered by FDA officials Albert "Jerry" Holland and Irvin Kerlan. It was Kerlan—then essentially the FDA's head medical librarian—who gathered a diverse network of interested hospital administrators, pharmacists, and medical record librarians and who elaborated a vision for an adverse event reporting system. A five-hospital pilot program in 1956 had become, by 1960, a nationwide program explicitly under FDA auspices. This was in some respects a failure, insofar as Kerlan wished to use the expanding U.S. hospital network to collect information. In 1963, FDA officials would admit that "relatively few hospitals" were affected. The adverse events flowed not from hospitals, but overwhelmingly from manufacturers who were compelled by statute to report them.[9]

[8]GAO, FDA *Postmarket Drug Safety*, (GAO-06-402), 24, n.42. Robert Temple, "Meta-analysis and Epidemiologic Studies in Drug Development and Postmarketing Surveillance," *JAMA* 281 (9) (March 3, 1999): 841–4.

[9]Holland, "Drugs, Records, and You," *Journal of the American Association of Medical Record Librarians* 26 (April 1955): 109–14. Kerlan was head of the Bureau of Medicine's Research and Reference Branch in the 1950s; Kerlan, "Reporting Adverse Reactions to Drugs," *Bulletin of the American Society of Hospital Pharmacists* 13 (July–August 1956): 311–14. William W. Goodrich (FDA General Counsel), "Follow-Up on New Drug Applications, Reporting of Clinical and Other Experience, and Removal of Drugs from Market," speech delivered at the Federal Bar Association Brief Conference on the New Drug Law, Washington, DC, June 27–28, 1963; DF 505.53, RG 88, NA. On Kerlan's program as launched in January 1960, see Kerlan, "Adverse Drug Reaction Reporting: Approach to Better Patient Care," *Hospitals: The Journal of the American Hospital Association* 34 (Nov. 1, 1960), 65; "FDA... Physician Protection of Foods, Drugs, Devices and Cosmetics," *Medical Times*, December 1960 (HEW Reprint, FOK); "Why FDA Set Up a Program to Assemble Reports on Drug Reactions," *Materia Medica*, December 1961. A portrait of the hospital reporting program appears in Memorandum from A. D. Davis (Acting Chief, Management Surveys Branch) to Leo L. Miller (Assistant

Lacking sticks, the FDA relied on carrots. The Administration's attempts to entice hospitals into more consistent adverse event reporting depended mainly upon a network of research and reporting contracts. Because the AMA had developed a reporting system for hospitals that were unconnected to medical schools, the Administration focused on research and teaching hospitals. Through this network, the Administration was for a brief period able to improve reporting from hospitals. In 1965, the FDA's adverse event reporting arrangement involved over 250 hospitals and amassed over 6,000 reports per year. Yet these aggregates conceal the low informational value of the individual reports, as well as an experience of frustration among reporting hospitals. At Mayo Clinic, where the FDA regulated pre-approval clinical research and contracted for post-approval pharmaceutical reporting, Mayo officials saw a stark contrast between the efficiency and image of pre-market and post-market modes of regulation. The FDA's governance of clinical research was developed, intricate, and capable of inspiring fear. Mayo officials met monthly to review clinical research protocols, all the while keeping a close eye on developments in FDA rules and policy statements. Yet in post-market drug utilization, Mayo officials were characterized not by fear but by frustration and confusion. FDA officials continually tinkered with payments and incentives to induce hospitals to report more events. At Mayo in 1964, the hospital received $50 for participating and $5 per report; two years later, the $5-per-report incentive remained but two Mayo administrators were now paid $250 per year for participation. Meanwhile, hospitals sent reports to the agency but wondered what was becoming of them; they wanted aggregate data from which to learn. Mayo staff physicians worried that the Administration's program was duplicating nearby state-level efforts and even hospital-based programs to tally drug experience. The low reporting rate persisted despite the expansion of the adverse event reporting network.[10]

Commissioner for Administration, FDA), Subject "Factfinding Survey of the FDA Adverse Reaction Reporting Program," November 30, 1962; NYU pediatrician Charles May singled out the Administration's adverse event reporting system for praise in the Senate's Humphrey Committee hearings of 1963; *ICDRR*, 1108–14. In the 1970s, the West German government would commission pharmacologist Helmut Kewitz (Freie Universität Berlin) to travel to the United States and examine FDA institutions for post-market surveillance. Kewitz's travels are documented in an unpublished report recommending that the West German government establish a system for reporting adverse events modeled partially on that of the United States; Bestand B 189, Akten 11561, BK.

[10]On the tension between AMA and FDA systems for post-market surveillance, consult the excellent narrative of Harry M. Marks, "Making Risks Visible: The Science and Politics of Adverse Drug Reactions," in Jean-Paul Gaudillière and Volker Hess, eds., *Ways of Regulating: Therapeutic Agents between Plants, Shops, and Consulting Rooms* (Berlin: Max Planck Institut fur Wissenschaftsgeschichte, Preprint 363, 2008). For an early acknowledgment of the variable reporting from different hospitals and research medical centers, see "Tabulation of August 31, 1962, by Food and Drug Administration of Information Furnished Under Adverse Reaction Program —July 1961 to June 1962"; Exhibit 67 in *ICDRR*, 399.

The structure of the modern adverse event reporting form—Form FDA-1639—was cemented in 1968. Separately, the Administration issued regulations that year to bring uniformity to reports of general clinical experience with pharmaceuticals, reports that concerned not adverse events but new animal and clinical data, as well as promotional literature and medical journal advertising. With these required periodic reports, the FDA could, at least in principle, monitor post-market experience of the drug and the post-market behavior for the company. The AER system was computerized in 1970 and has been continually revisited in the years since. The basis for an individual report is a "serious" or "unexpected" adverse drug reaction. A *serious* reaction is defined as one that involves death, injury, hospitalization, disability, or other significant adverse outcome, one that is not currently listed on the label of the medication. An *unexpected* ADR occurs when the adverse reaction is not in the drug label or the frequency of adverse reactions rises to a rate greater than that anticipated on the basis of the new drug application and the labeling. Since 1963, Administration rules have required firms to submit these to the agency within fifteen days of their receipt.[11]

As the AER system has aged, the dilemma faced by Irvin Kerlan in the 1950s has become clearer and more stubborn. ADR reports come overwhelmingly from manufacturers, and far less from physicians, hospitals, and

---

In the 1960s, these contracting and voluntary efforts were managed by FDA physician Albert F. Esch. Minutes, Committee on the Safety of Therapeutic Agents (CSTA), Mayo Clinic, December 1, 1966; Minutes, CSTA, July 11, 1969; *MAYO*. On close monitoring of FDA statements on investigational new drug research, see Minutes, CSTA, December 10, 1964; February 18, 1965; July 1, 1965; September 22, 1966. On FDA tinkering with payments, compare Minutes, CSTA, March 26, 1964; May 28, 1964; August 27, 1964; December 1, 1966. Rochester Methodist Hospital (one of the constituent hospitals of the Mayo system) started to conduct a "Drug Reaction Study" in the late 1960s, comparing their statistics to those of St. Mary's Hospital (another constituent institution) and conducting a rudimentary statistical analysis; Minutes, CSTA, February 7, 1969, MAYO. Mayo officials would complain in 1967 that their compliance with the Administration was solid but that little was coming of it; "Doctor Peters has had no answer from F.D.A. about their retrieval methods for drug reactions. Systematic and immediate access to reaction reports should be available." Mayo officials also worried about duplicating an effort by the State of Iowa, many of whose citizens were Mayo patients. Minutes, CSTA, October 26, 1967; Minutes, CSTA, November 30, 1967; MAYO.

[11] FDA, "Approved New Drugs and Antibiotic Drugs: Proposed New Forms to Accompany Records and Reports on Experiences," *FR* 33 (April 12, 1968): 5687–8; this rule extended earlier rulemaking at *FR* 32 (108) (June 6, 1967): 8087. (I thank Arthur Daemmrich for this information.) Efforts to establish a compendium of reports were based on the form commenced in 1969; FDA-BOM, Medical Advisory Board Minutes, Twentieth Meeting, October 2 and 3, 1969, pp. 4–5; FDA-BOM, Medical Advisory Board Minutes, Twenty-First Meeting, December 18 and 19, 1969, p. 3; Harry F. Dowling Papers, NLM. For general surveys of the development of the AER form and reporting system, see FDA Division of Drugs and Biologics Experience (Center for Drugs and Biologics), "Draft Guideline for Postmarketing Reporting of Adverse Drug Reactions," August 23, 1985; FDA Docket No. 85D-0249. L. Beulah and W. M. Turner, "The Food and Drug Administration's Adverse Drug Reaction Monitoring Program," *American Journal of Hospital Pharmacy* 216 (June 28, 1971): 2135–6. F. E. Karche and L. Lasagna, "Toward the Operational Definition of Adverse Drug Reactions," *CP&T* 21 (1977):

other agents in the U.S. health-care system. In 1985, of 36,931 ADRs received by the Administration, 70 percent came from manufacturers, whereas only 8 percent came directly from health professionals, and 2 percent came from patients. This is not to say that physicians and health-care providers have not participated in the process. They have, but their communications have generally been limited to the manufacturer, and epidemiologists and other researchers have long known that adverse events with drugs are woefully underreported. One 1988 study estimated that only 5 percent of all adverse drug reactions observed by physicians are reported to the FDA's Surveillance Reporting System (SRS). Due to a combination of "complacency," "fear," "guilt," "ignorance," "diffidence," and "lethargy," physicians themselves often failed to report adverse events.[12]

The heavy institutional reliance upon pharmaceutical manufacturers for adverse event information is a historical legacy of reputation and power. Upon receiving ADRs, firms are required to report them to the FDA under the agency's regulations. Yet no such mandate governs the behavior of physicians or hospitals, and the Administration's efforts are hampered by lack of authority and an inability to rely upon a reputation of fear. As in so many forms of pharmaceutical regulation in the United States, the subjects of government power are the producers of drugs, not the human providers of care. The political lodging of post-market authority in the Administration—as limited as that authority was—also accounts for the slow but certain death of the American Medical Association's role in post-market drug surveillance. The AMA was never able to compel American physicians to report adverse drug events. As the share of American physicians who counted themselves Association members steadily declined, and as the FDA's regulatory grip upon the pharmaceutical industry tightened in the 1960s, the AMA's program became ineffectual and meaningless. The AMA terminated the registry of its Adverse Event Reporting Committee in 1970.[13]

247–54. R. C. Nelson, "Drug Safety, Pharmacoepidemiology, and Regulatory Decision Making," *Drug Intelligence and Clinical Pharmacy* 22 (April 1988): 336–44. Daemmrich (*Pharmacopolitics*, 137) wrongly attributes the fifteen-day requirement to 1985 regulations; by then the rule was over two decades old. Goodrich, "Follow-Up on New Drug Applications, Reporting of Clinical and Other Experience, and Removal of Drugs from Market"; DF 505.53, RG 88, NA.

[12]GAO, *FDA Can Further Improve Its Adverse Drug Reaction Reporting System*, Report to the Secretary of Health and Human Services, GAO-1.13: HRD-82-37, March 8, 1982. G. A. Faich, "Adverse Drug Reaction Monitoring," *NEJM* 314 (24) (1986): 1589–92. M.D.B. Stephens, *The Detection of New Adverse Drug Reactions* (New York: Stockton Press, 1985). For 5 percent estimate, see A. S. Rogers, E. Israel, C. R. Smith, et al., "Physicians' Knowledge, Attitudes, and Behavior Related to Reporting Adverse Drug Events," *ArchIM* 148 (July 1988): 1596–1600.

[13]The disparity between requirements for firms and the "encouragement" aimed at physicians and hospitals was noted explicitly in the Administration's elaboration of new labeling rules in June 1979. Under federal regulations (21 CFR 300.310), holders of NDAs approved under Section 505 of the FDCA "are required to submit information concerning the quantity

The other side of the post-market reporting coin is that pharmaceutical firms are generally quick and rather thorough in reporting adverse reactions, not least because their regulatory affairs officers know that serious regulatory and legal trouble awaits the company if this pattern is not followed. Moreover, while physicians often fear tort liability if they do report aggressively, a firm invites serious liability issues if reporting is negligent.

REGULATING ESTROGEN: ORAL CONTRACEPTIVES ON THE MARKET

In the wake of the FDA's approval of Enovid (norethynodrel) as an oral contraceptive in 1960, "the pill" became one of the most quickly diffusing technologies in human history. In the United States alone, 1.75 million women were taking the pill by November 1963, and by end of the decade, an estimated 8.5 million American women took oral contraceptives on a monthly basis. The use of oral contraceptives among younger women was particularly robust. Statistical estimates suggest that among women born in 1948, fully 85 percent would use the pill at some point during their lifetime. In a 1999 article entitled "Oral Contraceptives: The Liberator," the *Economist* magazine identified the pill as the twentieth century's greatest technological advance.[14]

Oral contraceptives confronted the Administration with a set of issues surrounding post-market regulation that the agency had never before faced. Millions of American women were swallowing a synthetic hormone combination on a daily basis, and FDA officials and epidemiologists hence knew

---

of the drug distributed and reports of clinical experience, studies, investigations, and tests conducted by, or reported to, the NDA holder." By contrast, "the FDA encourages individual physicians to submit reports to the agency of adverse experiences that they observe with marketed drug products" (*FR* 44 (124) (June 26, 1979): 37453). R. H. Moser, "The Obituary of an Idea," *JAMA* 216 (June 28, 1971): 2135–6; R. R. Miller and S. Shapiro, "Detection and Evaluation of Adverse Drug Reactions," *JAMA* 220 (May 15, 1972): 1011.

[14]For estimates on early usage patterns, see "Johnson & Johnson Puts Birth Control Pill on U.S. Market," *WSJ*, February 5, 1963, 9; "Johnson-Johnson Unit Aims to Sell Cheap Oral Birth Control Pill Soon," *WSJ*, October 15, 1963, 18. For the 8.5 million estimate, see Charles C. Edwards, M.D. (Acting Commissioner of Food and Drugs), "Dear Doctor" Letter, January 12, 1970; in *CPRPFDA*, Hearings before the Intergovernmental Relations Subcommittee of the Committee on Government Operations, HR, June 9, 1970, 27. Herbert G. Lawson, "Birth Control Push: Drug Companies Press Development of New Oral Contraceptives," *WSJ*, November 1, 1963, 1. By 1976, fully 73 percent of single women who had *ever* used contraception of any form had used oral contraceptives. Bernard Asbell, *The Pill: A Biography of the Drug That Changed the World* (New York: Random House, 1995); Elizabeth Siegel Watkins, *On the Pill: A Social History of Oral Contraception, 1950–1970* (Baltimore: Johns Hopkins University Press, 1998); Charles F. Westoff and Norman B. Ryder, *The Contraceptive Revolution* (Princeton: Princeton University Press, 1977). For economic and career effects of the legal expansion of oral contraceptive availability to single women in particular, see Claudia Goldin and Lawrence Katz, "The Power of the Pill: Oral Contraceptives and Women's Career and Marriage Decisions," *Journal of Political Economy* 110 (4) (2002): 730–70. "Oral Contraceptives: The Liberator," *Economist* (Dec. 31, 1999): 102.

that even small relative risks and side effects could aggregate to death and suffering for thousands of women. The pill became in some respects the epitome of twentieth-century pharmaco-therapy: a drug used for a chronic condition—essentially the primary indication of "fertility"—and expected to be used for years, even decades. In the early 1960s, with the international thalidomide experience weighing upon the Administration and the medical profession with the symbolic heft of an albatross, oral contraceptives posed the specter of another cultural, medical, and regulatory disaster. Safety and efficacy issues for oral contraceptives received mass media coverage out of all proportion to that received by other objects of FDA regulation. Yet because they had effected a massive social, cultural, economic, and political transformation, oral contraceptives were not going to be removed from the marketplace. The genie was out of the bottle, and the experience underscored the political and social irreversibility of new drug approval for FDA officials.[15]

Amid all the tales of far-flung diffusion and immense profit, there were reports trickling in from Great Britain of thromboembolism—the potentially fatal obstruction of a blood vessel by a clot that has been dislodged from the vein in which it formed—among pill users there. By the summer of 1962, the FDA had received twenty-eight reports of thromboembolic events—at least five of them fatal—associated with Enovid use in the United States. The Administration's first public response was to request in May 1962 that Searle issue a warning statement to physicians, customarily known as a "Dear Doctor Letter." Searle did not act on the request, and when the *British Medical Journal* published further reports on thrombosis among British women taking oral contraceptives in early August, the FDA sent another request to the Chicago-based company. This time, however, the Administration made its request public, infuriating Searle officials, who lamented that a "supercharged atmosphere over thalidomide" was inducing the Administration to press forward with an unnecessary warning.[16]

So began a public drama about drug safety with a familiar choreography, one re-enacted many times over the past half-century. An initiative for risk disclosure or full market withdrawal comes from the FDA. An official warning or withdrawal announcement issues from the company, which reluctantly accepts the FDA's judgment and communicates (more or less severely)

[15]In 1969, the Administration's Advisory Committee on Obstetrics and Gynecology would take note of this peculiar status of oral contraceptives: "The current aggregate pharmacological experience with the oral contraceptives is unique... in that large numbers of healthy young women are using potent drugs for a purpose other than the control of disease"; *Second Report on the Oral Contraceptives* (Washington, DC: GPO, 1969), 1.

[16]Thromboembolic disease included, in the categorization of the time, intravascular (venous or arterial) thrombosis as well as coronary or cerebral thrombosis, as well as pulmonary embolism. See, for instance, P. E. Sartwell, A. T. Masi, F. G. Arthes, G. R. Greene, and H. E. Smith, "Thromboembolism and Oral Contraceptives: An Epidemiologic Case-Control Study," *AmJEpid* 90 (1969): 365–80.

its disagreement. Then the Administration follows the company's move with a more moderate gloss, in some cases an ambiguously optimistic read, on the news. In the case of Enovid, Searle and the Administration would repeat this pattern several times in the 1960s and 1970s. On August 3, 1962, the very day that major news outlets announced that Searle would send warning letters to American doctors, the agency advised reporters that the Bureau of Medicine could not establish a definitive link between Enovid and blood clots, and that the Bureau was actively studying the relationship. So tepid was the FDA's announcement that the *Wall Street Journal* reported "varied rumors" that the Administration "in some manner had 'endorsed' the use of Enovid." Searle's common stock price rose in response to the FDA announcement, which was certainly not the expected result of an FDA requirement to inform physicians about new health risks.[17]

One year later, the Administration made a similarly ambiguous move. In a letter from Commissioner George Larrick to Searle, the agency asked Searle to issue a public warning about an "apparent hazard" with the Enovid among women over the age of thirty-five. Whereas the August 1962 warning was restricted to physicians, the August 1963 warning delivered potentially troubling news directly to Enovid's users and consumers, millions of American women who were both current and potential future users of the drug. Searle officials were privately dismayed about the warning, fearing that otherwise healthy older potential users would shy away from their product. Yet at the same time as his agency forced Searle's hand, Larrick said that the drug should remain available for a prescription. Enovid's "apparent hazard," Larrick reasoned, must be balanced against "the demonstrated hazard of pregnancy." And that very day, less publicly but far more significantly, the FDA extended the maximum period of Enovid use from two years to four. On a day when health risks associated with its star mol-

---

In the United Kingdom, the estrogen-progestogen combination was sold under the trade name "Conovid." Howard Simons, "Drug Link to Clotting Is Studied," *WP*, August 4, 1962, A1; John A. Osmundsen, "British Issue Warning on Oral Contraceptive Pill," *NYT*, August 4, 1962, 20. In some of the newspaper accounts of the report, five women had died as a result of the thrombotic event, while in others, six had perished. "6 Women Die; Birth Control Pills Probed," *Chicago Tribune*, August 4, 1962, 1; "Pill Maker Accused on Warning Doctors," *NYT*, August 5, 1962, 65; "Searle Agrees to Warn Doctors, Pharmacists on Use of Enovid Pill," *WSJ*, August 9, 1962, 7; Nate Haseltine and Morton Mintz, "Safety of Birth Control Pill Questioned: FDA May Ask Study by Outside Experts," *WP*, December 23, 1962, A1.

The scientific literature on oral contraceptives and their safety is immense. Some of the earliest studies include G. Pincus, "Control of Conception by Hormonal Steroids," *Science* 153 (July 29, 1966): 493–500. G. Pincus and C.-R. C Garcia, "Symposium on Long-Term Safety of Progestin-Estrogen Combinations: Studies on Vaginal, Cervical and Uterine Histology," and J. Donayre and G. Pincus, "Symposium on Long-Term Safety of Progestin-Estrogen Combinations: Effects of Enovid on Blood Clotting Factors," *Metabolism* 14 (March 1965, pt. 2): 344–47 and 418–21, respectively. For an accessible review of studies in the last two decades, see Lisa A. Edwards, "An update on Oral Contraceptive Options," *Formulary* 39 (Feb. 2004): 104–21.

[17] "Searle Agrees to Warn Doctors, Pharmacists on Use of Enovid Pill," *WSJ*, August 9, 1962, 7. "AMA Finds No Pill Link to Blood Clot," *WP*, August 11, 1962, A1.

ecule were being publicized worldwide, Searle announced itself "quite pleased" with the Administration's statement, and company officials glee-fully predicted that "the sales curve will accelerate." The *Washington Post* reported that the agency had "cleared" and "approved" Enovid for general prescription use, as if a new drug application had been made effective when in fact the agency was only announcing a conclusion from its advisory com-mittee. With one hand, the FDA had forced Searle to caution millions of American women about the pill. With the other, the agency seemed to wel-come them back to the drug.[18]

No sooner had the Administration imparted a murky hue to the issue of Enovid's safety when, one month later, its own advisory committee muddied the waters further. In September 1963, the Wright Committee—so named because it had been chaired by Dr. Irving S. Wright of Cornell University Medical College—admitted a mathematical error in the computation of relative risks from oral contraceptive use. The short-run consequence of this admission was an effective retraction of the August 1963 warning. The committee's reversal stung the Administration, which, as the *Wall Street Journal* described it, found itself "in the embarrassing position of having promulgated stricter warning labeling for the drug last month." The agen-cy's short-run tactic was to quickly announce the error and shift blame to the advisory committee. The longer-run strategy was to give a default regu-latory imprimatur to oral contraceptives. Despite lingering doubts at nu-merous levels of the Bureau of Medicine, the Administration committed it-self to a policy that Enovid was safe for "longtime continuous use." At several junctures in 1963 and 1964, FDA officials would state that they could neither confirm nor deny a connection between oral contraceptives and thromboembolism. The package insert for the 10-milligram form of Enovid in 1964 acknowledged "the occasional occurrence of thrombophle-bitis and pulmonary embolism in patients taking estrogen-progestogen com-binations" but added that "a cause and effect relationship has not been demonstrated."[19]

---

[18] "FDA Asks Searle to Warn Women Over 35 of 'Apparent Hazard' in Birth Control Pill," *WSJ*, August 5, 1963, 22. On Searle officials' private dismay, see "Researchers Call FDA Warn-ing on Enovid Wrong, Blame Own Mathematical Error," *WSJ*, September 18, 1963, 28. Nate Haseltine, "Enovid Cleared for Use: FDA Gives Approval to Birth Control Pill," *WP*, August 4, 1963, A1. Robert C. Toth, "Birth Pill's Sale Upheld by U.S.," *NYT*, August 4, 1963, 57. The referral to an advisory committee was sparked by a report delivered by Dr. Helmo Trees to the Division of New Drugs on December 18, 1962. Five days later, the *Washington Post* leaked the story of Trees' report, apparently inducing Commissioner George Larrick to appoint an outside advisory committee. Haseltine and Mintz, "Safety of Birth Control Pill Questioned: FDA May Ask Study by Outside Experts," *WP*, December 23, 1962, A1.

[19] *Ad Hoc Committee for the Evaluation of a Possible Etiologic Relation of Enovid with Thromboembolic Conditions: Final Report on Enovid*, September 12, 1963 (Washington, DC: FDA). The Wright committee essentially muffed a hypothesis test, neglecting to equate the com-parison samples for the "treated" population taking Enovid and the "control" population not taking the drug. "Researchers Call FDA Warning on Enovid Wrong, Blame Own Mathematical

The Administration's 1963 rhetoric appears to have quieted some of the storm over Enovid's risks. Among major metropolitan newspapers such as the *Chicago Tribune*, the *Los Angeles Times*, *New York Times*, the *Wall Street Journal*, and the *Washington Post*, there would be no further coverage of clotting issues associated with the pill until 1968. Yet among clinical researchers, epidemiologists, and cardiologists, there was continued uncertainty over oral contraceptives' causal relationship to stroke and related conditions. Searle continually underlined the absence of consistent evidence and highlighted a 1966 World Health Organization technical report that found little general evidence of a causal link between oral contraceptives and stroke.[20]

Still, Searle officials were well aware of the possibility of regulatory action, and they made surplus efforts to show appropriate deference to the Administration. Searle regulatory affairs director Herbert Helling continually submitted reports from the medical literature, and from the company's clinical trials and animal studies, to the Office of Drug Safety (ODS). In an awkward equation of market utilization with clinical research, Searle officials also reminded the ODS that Enovid's widespread use was an experiment in and of itself, and that "the efficacy and safety of the drug in extended use is still under surveillance." In 1966 alone, they reasoned, "the users of Enovid added 1,599,900 woman-years of experience to the drug's record." FDA pharmacologists were not, however, buying the equation of market experience and clinical study. Agency officials aggressively required Searle to conduct animal and clinical studies to check for a variety of conditions associated with estrogen-progestogen use. Many of the animal studies generated further concern in the Bureau of Medicine, not least over the possibility of birth defects and spontaneous abortion among pregnant women taking the steroid-based oral contraceptives. ODS pharmacologists quietly battled with Searle pharmacologists over labeling, first in 1966 over the agency's suggestion that Searle amend its Enovid and Ovulen labels to strengthen the warnings against use by pregnant women, then a year later over how much information from the animal studies should be included on the label. In 1967, upon receiving reports that primates taking an oral estro-

Error," *WSJ*, September 18, 1963, 28; "FDA Says G. D. Searle Can Drop Its Warning About Taking Enovid," *WSJ*, September 23, 1963, 5. "Enovid Held Safe for Regular Use," *WP*, November 21, 1964, A4. See proposed labeling for Enovid in NDA 10-976, V 124; RG 88, NA.

[20] F. Schaffner, "The Effect of Oral Contraceptives on the Liver," *JAMA* 198 (Nov. 28, 1966): 1019–21. In summarizing a WHO report on oral contraceptives, J. William Crosson (Assistant Medical Director of Searle) and William Stewart summarized the WHO consensus as saying that "The consensus of the scientific group was that departures from normal values in the various categories are seldom of proven pathological significance. Discussing such serious consequences as thromboembolic phenomena, the authors point out that no relationship of these to the use of oral contraceptives has been established." "Clinical Aspects of Oral Gestogens," World Health Organization Technical Report Series, no. 326: 1–24 (1966). J. William Crosson, M.D., and William C. Stewart (Division of Clinical Research), G. D. Searle, *Enovid —Annual Post-NDA Report*, April 7, 1967; NDA 10-976, V131, RG 88, NA

gen-progestogen combination developed atypical breast hyperplasia—signaling a possible link to tumor formation in oral contraceptive users—Administration officials required Searle to undertake long-term animal studies for Enovid and all other estrogen-progestogen combinations under development. Goddard's order left Searle with little leeway. The agency enclosed a recommended protocol for the mandated studies which required daily observation of monkeys and dogs for five years. Within two years, these mandatory tests would be applied to all contraceptives—whether approved or under development—and the timelines increased to seven years for dogs and a lifetime for primates.[21]

As Searle's efforts continued, company officials began to see a new facet of the Administration. Agency officials were irritated by Searle's continual trespass on the boundary between information provision and raw market promotion. Fearing declines in profits and market share in the wake of the imminent arrival of other estrogen- and progestin-based compounds from its competitors, G. D. Searle attempted to strengthen its hold on the oral contraceptive market through a combination of advertising and physician education. The education initiative was in reality an advertising campaign, and it highlighted Enovid's historic role as the first oral contraceptive approved for marketing in the United States. Searle published a booklet entitled "A Prescription for Family Planning—The Story of Enovid" and circulated a documentary film entitled, "Enovid—A Documentary of Ten Years' Research in the Service of Medicine."[22]

By 1966, the Bureau of Medicine had seen enough. Bureau officials pressed the Administration's Office of General Counsel to prosecute Searle for misbranding and for failure of full disclosure. FDA attorney B. T. Myers considered the request of his agency's physicians and decided against prosecution.

---

[21]J. K. Lamar, Ph. D. (ODS), to E. M. Ortiz (Metabolic and Endocrine Division, ODS), August 23, 1966. E. M. Ortiz, M.D., Intra-Administrative Referral, to Jennings (ODS), March 30, 1967; NDA 10-976, V126, RG 88, NA. Ortiz declined to recommend a written request to Searle merely because "our pharmacologists have not requested it." In the investigation of spontaneous abortions, ODS pharmacologists wanted larger studies—using a smaller (10-to-1 or 25-to-1) ratio of progestin to estrogen than Searle was using (67-to-1). On the specificity of pharmacologic data to be included in Enovid labeling, see Ortiz, "Memorandum of Telephone Conversation" between Herbert Helling (Director of Regulatory Affairs, G. D. Searle), July 27, 1967, "Subject: Labeling for Enovid"; also Crosson and Stewart, G. D. Searle, *Enovid—Annual Post-NDA Report*, April 7, 1967; NDA 10-976, V131, RG 88, NA. Paul A. Bryan, M. D. (Acting Associate Deputy Director for Drug Surveillance, BOM) to Helling, July 20, 1967; all in NDA 10-976, V126. RG 88, NA. JLG to G. D. Searle (William L. Searle), July 5, 1967; Attachment: "Recommended Protocol for Chronic Oral Contraceptive Studies"; NDA 10-976, V131, RG 88, NA. Searle also conducted studies of breast and other tumors among rats. See Herbert Helling to OSE, BOD, FDA, November 16, 1970; D. Hertig, "Pharmacology Review of NDA 10-976, Amendment (dated 16 Nov 70) to Last Annual Report (dated 14 April 1970)," NDA 10-976, V 139.1, RG 88, NA. *Second Report on the Oral Contraceptives*, 6.

[22]T. E. Myers (Division of Case Guidance, BRC) to Director, BRC, January 4, 1967, Re "Proposed Prosecution of G. D. Searle & Co. for Alleged Misbrandings by Medical Journal Advertising and Promotional Labeling," NDA 10-976, V 124; RG 88, NA.

As Myers wrote, "we believe that forwarding this matter for prosecution would no longer be timely and would be punitive rather than corrective." Yet Myers also saw things that concerned him and left open the possibility that "if objectionable practices are encountered we could then proceed via seizure, to more forcefully bring to the firm's attention our objections." He understood, though, that "since the proposed disposition of this matter may not meet with Bureau of Medicine concurrence," the Office of the Commissioner would need to resolve the issue. Myers thus hewed to a moderate line of regulation, wishing to avoid seeming "punitive" but also wanting to send proper signals to the firm. Although the case against Searle was never pursued, it sent a chilling message to the company, and other criminal cases against Searle were considered in the 1960s and 1970s.[23]

The Administration had not entirely lost its gatekeeping power. Enovid was irretrievably on the market, yet every new indication for the drug still needed the FDA's approval, as did the new molecules in the company's development pipeline. When in 1970 Searle wished to develop and publish a new patient information brochure for Enovid, the company submitted a copy of its patient brochure *Planning Your Family* to the FDA as a supplement to the Enovid New Drug Application. Bernard St. Raymond of the Division of Metabolic and Endocrine Drug Products reviewed the proposed brochure and declared it "unacceptable in its present form." St. Raymond complained that Searle's booklet implied that menstrual spotting was much more common and "natural" without Enovid use than clinical studies had shown, and that the brochure implicitly slighted another publication—*What You Should Know About "the Pill"*—prepared by the AMA and the American College of Obstetricians and Gynecologists.[24]

Nor was regulation of promotional literature limited to the publications of a drug's producer. In 1967, the New York publishing firm Simon & Schuster contacted the FDA's Bureau of Regulatory Compliance (BRC) and expressed concern that its volume by Dr. Robert Wilson, *Feminine Forever*, might violate federal rules. Simon & Schuster had already gotten into trouble with its book, *Calories Don't Count*, and Wilson was under well-publicized investigation by the Administration for his claims that continued usage of Enovid would forestall menopause. D. W. Johnson of the BRC told Simon & Schuster lawyers that "it is our opinion that the book does seem to list indications for use. Therefore, any use of the book in a promotional way for the drugs would cause the drugs to be misbranded." The FDA's Johnson did,

[23]T. E. Myers to Director, BRC, January 4, 1967, Re "Proposed Prosecution of G. D. Searle & Co.," NDA 10-976, V 124; RG 88, NA. Donald Kennedy (FDA Commissioner) to Thomas P. Sullivan, Esq. (U.S. Attorney, Northern District, IL), April 11, 1979; B11, F 7, FOK.

[24]G. D. Searle, *Planning Your Family*, Brochure # OA18 (dated September 1, 1970). See also *FR* 35 (113) (June 11, 1970), 9001-3. By 1970, with the weight of physician opinion behind lower dosages of estrogen-progestogen combinations, most of Searle's amendments were directed to its 5-milligram tablets. Notice of Approval: New Drug Application or Supplement, NDA 10-976/S-024, February 10, 1971; St. Raymond, "Summary of Supplement," September 14, 1970; NDA 10-976, V 138.1, RG 88, NA.

however, allow Simon & Schuster to make the book available on the shelves of a drug store as long as it was not coupled with any prescription item.[25]

Then the thrombosis link resurfaced. Although the FDA and Searle had downplayed the pill's connection with stroke from 1963 to 1965, the evidence began to mount for a connection as the politically turbulent decade wore on. The support now came both from adverse reaction reports and, more forcefully, from studies in the rapidly developing field of "pharmacoepidemiology." In the calendar years 1966 and 1967, the Bureau of Medicine received approximately nine thousand adverse reaction reports on oral contraceptives, over one thousand of these involving serious injury or fatality. The Bureau analyzed data from these reports, which were submitted by oral contraceptive manufacturers. It was the most elaborate data set on post-market safety ever amassed by the Bureau, and its analysis produced tentative but potentially far-reaching conclusions. Bureau officials tallied 1,023 cases of "serious and fatal" disease attributable to oral contraceptive use, and of the 115 known fatalities, 84 involved thrombosis of some variety. They also presented preliminary evidence that the risk of different medical conditions varied systematically across the brand names and dosage forms of the pill. The Bureau of Medicine turned the reports over to the FDA's Advisory Committee on Obstetrics and Gynecology, chaired by Louis Hellman of SUNY–Brooklyn. Commissioner James Goddard then charged the Hellman committee with the preparation of a report on the safety of oral contraceptives.[26]

Additionally, in 1968 and 1969, epidemiological analyses in Great Britain and the United States produced new statistical evidence of a pill-thrombosis association. These studies relied on retrospective case-control methods, which compared hospital records of women on oral contraceptives with interview-based records of "control" subjects who were similar in most respects except that they had not used the pill. The American study had been conducted by Johns Hopkins epidemiologist Philip Sartwell with a grant from the Administration and encouragement from FDA Medical Director Joseph Sadusk. The studies concluded that oral contraceptive use was associated with substantially higher risks of deep vein thrombosis, and that the risk was greater at higher doses. All of these analyses were subject to possible false inferences, due mainly to the fact that they did not (and usually could not)

[25]Robert A. Wilson, M.D., *Feminine Forever* (New York: Simon & Schuster, 1966); D. W. Johnson, "Memorandum of Telephone Conversation" (with Selig J. Levitan, representing Simon & Schuster), June 19, 1967; NDA 10-976, V 131; RG 88, NA. "FDA Investigating Doctor Who Wrote 'Feminine Forever,'" *WP*, August 15, 1966, A12.

[26]Morton Mintz, "FDA Reveals 77 Deaths, 336 Illnesses in Users of the Pill," *WP*, April 14, 1968, A3; Drew Pearons and Jack Anderson, "The Washington Merry-Go-Round: FDA Lags on Data for 'Pill' Fatalities," *WP*, March 19, 1969, D15. Among the figures suggesting cigarette smoking as a confounder was Anruth K. Jain, a biostatistician at the Population Council; Mintz, "FDA Works Up Final Draft on What 'Pill' Users Should Know," *WP*, September 6, 1977, A7. Advisory Committee on Obstetrics and Gynecology, FDA, *Report on the Oral Contraceptives*, (Washington, DC: GPO, August 1, 1966).

control for cigarette smoking among women. Since women who smoked were also more likely to be using oral contraception, a pattern of strokes attributed to oral contraceptive use may in fact have been caused by smoking and related behaviors. As the epidemiological literature developed, researchers would acknowledge and frankly discuss this possibility. By the early 1970s, the reigning hypothesis was that oral contraceptive use may have interacted with smoking to raise stroke risk. Yet quite apart from the hypothesized interactions with smoking, and in part because of the suggestive nature of studies in animal pharmacology, American and British regulatory and medical communities largely concluded that the stroke risk of oral contraceptive use was real.[27]

These epidemiological studies formed something of a pivot in the regulation of oral contraceptives, and their publication became a turning point for postmarket surveillance generally. In the case of each study, the Bureau of Medicine learned of the results about four or five months before its actual publication. Bureau officials learned of the British results in December 1967 (they were officially published in April 1968), and in June 1968, the Administration ordered U.S. manufacturers of the pill to relabel their product. The FDA's labeling requirements compelled uniformity among the labels of different oral contraceptives. The rules were promulgated and finalized without any official input from drug manufacturers, even though the Hellman Committee had explicitly asked for an FDA-industry labeling conference. The new labels made direct reference to case-control studies, warning of a "seven- to ten-fold increase in mortality and morbidity in women taking oral contraceptives." A follow-up on the British study by Philip Sartwell and colleagues at Johns Hopkins—a study funded by the FDA—reported very similar risk ratios.[28]

[27]Among the early studies documenting a link between oral contraceptive use and increased risk of deep vein thrombosis and pulmonary embolism, see Royal College of General Practitioners, "Oral Contraception and Thromboembolic Disease," *Journal of the College of General Practitioners* 13 (1967): 267–79; W. B. Jennett and J. N. Cross, "Influence of Pregnancy and Oral Contraception on the Incidence of Strokes in Women of Childbearing Age," *Lancet* 1 (1967): 1019–23; W.H.W. Inman and M. P. Vessey, "Investigation of Deaths from Pulmonary, Coronary and Cerebral Thrombosis and Embolism in Women of Child-bearing Qge," *BMJ* 2 (1968): 193–9; M. P. Vessey and R. Doll, "Investigation of Relation between Use of Oral Contraceptives and Thromboembolic Disease: A Further Report," *BMJ* 2 (1969): 651–; P. E. Sartwell, et al., "Thromboembolism and Oral Contraceptives: An Epidemiologic Case-control Study." *Second Report on the Oral Contraceptives* 2, 21 (funding of the Sartell study), 3–5 (labeling revisions without industry input). Consult Avorn, *Powerful Medicines*, 111–14 for an accessible discussion of how retrospective case-control studies work. Another study using Kaiser Permanente records from Lawrence County, Pennsylvania was launched but FDA support was discontinued halfway in. Expert testimony in civil liability cases also suggested a link; "Expert Links Blood Clots to Birth Pills," *Chicago Tribune*, May 14, 1969, B10.

[28]Pearson and Anderson, "FDA Lags on Data for 'Pill' Fatalities," *WP*, March 19, 1969, D15. Mintz, "The Pill: What Are the Risks?" *WP*, April 17, 1972, B1. On the Bureau's early notification of the studies, see Mintz, "FDA Watered Down Pill Warning: Ex-Aide Testifies in Oral Contraceptive Suit," *WP*, August 5, 1973, A16. "Oral Contraceptive Labeling," document attachment to Edwards "Dear Doctor" letter; *CPRPFDA*, 27–33. It was later charged

By 1969, Administration officials realized that their apparatus for monitoring and ensuring the safety of oral contraceptives had rusted considerably. To confirm the point, the Hellman committee's *Second Report on Oral Contraceptives* (1969) found that, despite progress on a number of regulatory fronts, the Administration had yet to improve in any way upon its surveillance and record-keeping systems which had been criticized in the 1963 report. Less than one month into his post, FDA Commissioner Charles Edwards took the rare step of publicly intervening in the decentralized prescription practices of American physicians, counseling in a national press release that doctors prescribe oral contraceptives with the lowest possible dose of estrogen. Newer forms of oral contraceptives had lower doses of estrogen, but many doctors were prescribing older preparations. Edwards also published a revised package insert in the *Federal Register*.[29]

Steady and unrelenting criticism followed from journalistic quarters and from committees of Congress. "It seems incredible," wrote *Washington Post* watchdogs Drew Pearson and Jack Anderson, "that if the Pill is not safe we should have to wait till the British tell us so." Widely publicized congressional hearings in the House and Senate, the latter still known as "the Nelson hearings," brought widespread criticism of the agency, less for its resolve (its moral reputation), and more for its institutional capacity (its performative and technical reputation). Congressional investigators termed the FDA's record-keeping "chaotic," so much so as to render conclusive judgments "impossible." This was a criticism that new Commissioner Charles C. Edwards would accept. These and other negative judgments were rehearsed with even greater publicity at Senate hearings held by Gaylord Nelson. In the view of the Nelson committee and many of those testifying before it, the Administration had grossly underestimated the safety problems with oral contraceptives. It was perhaps the most severe reputational price paid by the agency and its

---

that this warning had been diluted under pressure from Searle. In testimony before a Multnomah County, Oregon jury in the summer of 1973, Robert S. McCleery, who had served as special assistant for medical communications to Commissioner Herbert L. Ley, stated that in February 1968, Bureau of Medicine physicians drafted a more emphatic warning, stating a "cause and effect relationship" between contraceptive use and thromboembolic events, and recommending discontinuation of oral contraceptive use after suspected problems. After contraceptive producers complained, Commissioner James Goddard approved labeling that met the companies' demands; "Mintz, "FDA Watered Down Pill Warning."

[29]Advisory Committee on Obstetrics and Gynecology, *Second Report on the Oral Contraceptives* (Washington, DC: GPO, 1969). Edwards' recommendation followed a similar appeal from the British Committee on the Safety of Drugs, released December 11, 1969. The British proposal was more specific than that of Edwards, as the Committee advised physicians to limit their prescriptions to products containing 0.05 milligrams or less of estrogen. Charles C. Edwards, "Dear Doctor" Letter, January 12, 1970; *HEW News*, April 24, 1970; *FDA: Current Drug Information*, April 24, 1970; *CPRPFDA*, 27–33. The earliest contraceptives (including Enovid) contained 9 mg of progestin and 0.15 mg of synthetic estrogen, but the most recent arrivals to the market by 1970 contained 0.5 mg progestin and 0.05 mg or less of estrogen; "Report of the Task Force on Utilization, Effectiveness, and Current Investigations," *Second Report on the Oral Contraceptives*, 15.

officials since the thalidomide episode. One reason that it did not pay a large price before 1970 is that other events and processes were dominating the news.[30]

In some respects, Edwards' gesture was a licking of public wounds. The Administration began to take a tougher tone with oral contraceptive manufacturers, began to draw more policy-relevant inferences from adverse event report data, and began to call for more case-control epidemiologic studies of drug safety. Edwards would testify before the Fountain subcommittee of the House that "FDA shouldn't play the role of doctor," yet in sending his own "Dear Doctor" letter, in mandating a specific package insert, and especially in his broadcast recommendation for physicians to minimize estrogen in their contraceptive prescriptions, Edwards and the Administration had done just that. Doubts also began to mount about the credibility of Searle, and there was visceral and sustained criticism of the general medical profession, particularly the *Journal of the American Medical Association*. The *Journal* had published two articles by Searle's director of medical research Victor A. Drill, one concluding that "the U.S. data did not reveal a clotting or death risk." Drill's articles and the *JAMA* editors were publicly castigated by epidemiologists and pharmacologists in the United States and Britain, and at the FDA the *Journal*'s pages became ever more suspect in the eyes of Bureau of Medicine officials.[31]

Whether this displeasure spilled over into other regulatory practices is difficult to say. New drug approval times offer entirely circumstantial but telling evidence. In 1967, the year before the British reports, Searle submitted supplementary NDAs for two Ovulen dosage forms, and the Administration approved the first in two weeks, the second in three months. In the ten years following the April 1968 report, Searle's experience with new drug

[30]In the House, hearings were held before the Intergovernmental Relations Subcommittee of the Committee on Government Operations, also known as "the Fountain committee." Edwards admits a "poor recordkeeping system, *CPRPFDA*, 119. The Senate Committee, chaired by Wisconsin Democrat Gaylord Nelson, organized the more famous hearings. Pearson and Anderson, "FDA Lags on Data for 'Pill' Fatalities," *WP*, March 19, 1969, D15. Anderson, "The Washington Merry-Go-Round: Hill to Get Warnings on 'the Pill,'" *WP*, January 15, 1970, F1.

[31]Edwards' disavowal of "playing doctor," June 9, 1970; *CPRPFDA*, 100. Contraceptive manufacturers wanted the package insert to be introduced at the discretion of the prescribing physician. William Goodrich, long-time FDA attorney and the agency's General Counsel at the time of the Fountain hearings, argued that a voluntary program ran "contrary to the overall policy of the [FDA] of requiring some patient information in print"; *CPRPFDA*, 100. Anderson, "The Washington Merry-Go-Round: Hill to Get Warnings on 'the Pill,'" *WP*, January 15, 1970, F13. Mintz, "The Pill: What Are the Risks?" *WP*, April 17, 1972, B1. On doubts about Searle and its credibility, see Mintz, "FDA Watered Down Pill Warning: Ex-Aide Testifies in Oral Contraceptive Suit," *WP*, August 5, 1973, A16. V. A. Drill and J. W. Calhoun, "Oral Contraceptives and Thromboembolic Disease," *JAMA* 206 (1968): 77–84. British epidemiologists responded viscerally to the Drill-Calhoun study; R. Doll, W. H. Inman, and M. P. Vessey, *JAMA* 207 (1969): 1150–51.

TABLE 9.1.
Searle's Experience with New Drug Approval before and after the 1968 Report

	Year Submitted	Approval Time (months)
Searle Oral Contraceptives		
OVULEN-28	1967	½
OVULEN-FE-28	1967	3
DEMULEN 1/50-28	1970	7
DEMULEN-FE-28	1970	12
CU-7	1973	14
DEMULEN 1/35-28	1978	43
DEMULEN 1/35-21	1978	42
Searle's Norpace compared with other anti-arrhythmia treatments		
Norpace (NME)	1973	54
Bretylol (American Critical Care) (NME)	1976	20
Pronestyl (Squibb) (supplement)	1972	20
Median FDA Review Time, all NMEs	1971–1976	20
Mean FDA Review Time, all NMEs	1971–1976	28

review was not nearly as positive or punctual. The FDA took four years and six months to review Searle's anti-arrhythmia treatment disopyramide phosphate (Norpace). As table 9.1 shows, Norpace's review time was well over double the expected review time for other new molecules, and also well over double the review times for other anti-arrhythmia treatments submitted in the same period: Squibb's procaine hydrochloride (Pronestyl) and American Critical Care's bretylium tosylate (Bretylol). Nor were Searle's problems limited to new drug review. In response to concerns raised by Frances Kelsey herself that Searle had falsified animal data for new drug applications, Commissioner Charles Edwards appointed a Task Force dedicated explicitly and solely to monitoring of Searle's research. The Task Force recommended criminal prosecution, but the U.S. Attorney for the Chicago district declined to pursue the case. For the second time in a decade, Searle had narrowly dodged a legal bullet.[32]

[32]Norpace (NDA 17-447) was submitted February 28, 1973 and approved September 1, 1977. Bretylol (NDA 17-954) was submitted October 22, 1976, and approved July 18, 1978. Both were given a summary efficacy rating of "1B" by the Administration, and Bretylol had

An innovative study by the Collaborative Group for the Study of Stroke in Young Women, published in the *New England Journal of Medicine* in 1973, raised the specter that reports of cerebral ischemia and thrombosis—what popular outlets had been calling "brain stroke"—were indicative of a causal relationship. Even more chilling than the raw result was the size of their reported "risk ratio." The Collaborative Group concluded that the relative risk of cerebral ischemia or thrombosis was *nine times* higher among women using oral contraceptives than among those avoiding the pill.[33]

In the wake of a more adversarial posture from the Administration, Searle's response to the Collaborative Group study was altogether different from anything witnessed in the early 1960s. Regulatory Affairs director Herbert Helling and other company officials acted quickly, firing off a supplemental NDA to change the labeling for its oral contraceptives Enovid, Ovulen, and Demulen. Helling implicitly criticized the Collaborative Group study but never hesitated in asking for a label amendment. Helling wrote that "such a revision would be consistent with the policy of G. D. Searle & Co. and FDA of bringing reports of significant adverse information to the attention of the medical profession in a timely and responsible manner." At this point, Helling's proposed labeling revision went beyond anything that the FDA had proposed or required. In an underlined sentence, the proposed labeling repeated (and slightly raised) the risk-ratio from the Collaborative Group study: "In an American study of cerebrovascular disorders in women with and without predisposing causes, it was estimated that the relative risk of thrombotic stroke was 9.5 times greater in users than in non-users." In light of its earlier approach to the reports of thrombotic stroke in the 1960s, when Helling himself was already head of regulatory affairs, Searle's aggressive publicity for the Collaborative Group study evinced a new corporate vigilance about product risks, a strategy that showed every sign of deference to a regulator that the company now feared. Helling's new rhetoric proposed a revelation program as a matter of joint and shared policy. He was simultaneously genuflecting to the Administration and partaking of the agency's status.[34]

---

taken six years longer to bring to market. Pronestyl (NDA 17-371) was submitted as a supplementary NDA on July 5, 1972 and approved on February 28, 1974. FDA New Drug Approval Database, Center for American Political Studies, Harvard University. J. Richard Crout to FOK, July 22, 1975; Thomas P. Sullivan (U.S. Attorney, Northern District of Illinois, Chicago) to Donald Kennedy (FDA Commissioner), January 29, 1979; Kennedy to Thompson, April 11, 1979; B11, F7, FOK.

[33] The Collaborative Group for the Study of Stroke in Young Women, "Oral Contraception and Increased Risk of Cerebral Ischemia or Thrombosis," *NEJM* 288 (1973): 871–8.

[34] Searle Laboratories, NDA supplement (FD Form 356H), May 18, 1973; amended labeling appears in Exhibit B of the NDA. Herbert Helling (Director of Regulatory Affairs and Quality Assurance, Searle Laboratories) to Division of Endocrine and Metabolic Drugs, OSE/FDA, May 18, 1973; NDA 10-976, V 145.1, RG 88, NA. In the abstract and parts of the text of the 1973 *NEJM* study, the Collaborative Group reported that the risk was "about nine times greater"; "Oral Contraception and Increased Risk of Cerebral Ischemia or Thrombosis," *NEJM* 288 (1973): 871.

By the late 1970s, there was no longer any question about the link between oral contraception and thromboembolism. The issue was not whether a link existed, but of what nature and causal mechanism it was, and how to fashion a regulatory policy to respond to it. The Administration had withdrawn trust from Searle and other contraceptive manufacturers, and the ability of the organized medical profession to communicate risks to patients was held in even lower regard. Beginning in 1975, the Administration began to recommend alternative forms of contraception, particularly and explicitly to older women. In 1976, the FDA compelled the withdrawal of so-called sequential oral contraceptives on the basis of evidence suggesting a link to uterine cancer. Finally, when in 1977 the Administration revisited its requirements for patient warnings, it bypassed the AMA and substituted its own language and literature for the companies' previous warning. The FDA now required that doctors and pharmacists provide a copy of a brochure— *What You Should Know About Oral Contraceptives*—each time a prescription for the pill was written or refilled. The Administration's document explicitly stated that some women should not use the pill—the strongest proscription to emerge since the approval of Enovid in 1960. Whereas earlier FDA literature had met with criticism for its opacity, Morton Mintz found the new brochure "notably free of technical jargon," and thought it would "faithfully reflect" the new labeling requirements.[35]

The early issues facing oral contraceptives are largely forgotten now, displaced by the politics of abortion and by wider consensus in American society. Yet the very facet that renders oral contraceptives so revealing—their durability in use for a newly defined chronic condition—also obscures. Oral contraceptives introduced a wide array of issues, but a host of others never came to the fore. Simply put, the dominant oral contraceptives of the late twentieth century were never withdrawn, and never came close to being withdrawn.

Reputation and the Political Structure of Postmarket Regulation

In the fifteen years following the Kefauver-Harris Amendments, oral contraceptives confronted the United States with its most durable and critical questions on post-market drug safety. The governance of oral contraceptives

[35]*FR* 41 (236) (Dec. 7, 1976): 53630. Mintz, "FDA Works Up Final Draft on What 'Pill' Users Should Know," *WP*, September 6, 1977, A7. The 1975 warnings came in response to British studies suggesting that the added risk of heart attacks among pill users increased with age. The adjective "sequential" was applied to oral contraceptive formulations in which tablets with an estrogenic compound were taken for 14 to 16 days of the cycle, followed by 5 to 7 days of taking both estrogen and progestin. The new warnings also came from FDA concern about continuing education programs by oral contraceptive manufacturers that Administration officials feared were masking an advertising campaign by Ortho and the University of Southern California; Crout "Regulatory Letter" to Robert R. Wilson (Group Vice President, Ortho), June 14, 1977; *DRR* 20 (33) (Aug. 14, 1977): 8–9.

illumined larger currents of regulation: a reduction in stringency once drugs are approved, the Administration's hold upon its gatekeeper identity (and hence its avoidance of responsibility for hazards that arise through utilization after approval), the public choreography of drug withdrawals and revelation of hazards, and the high reliance on labels as a post-market regulatory device in the United States. Yet the history of oral contraceptives also changed those patterns, in part because some very deeply etched lessons were learned by firms, by medical communities, by the Administration, and by diverse observers of the pharmaceutical world.

Gatekeeping. The form of the Administration's power over pharmaceuticals constrains and enables the agency once drugs are approved. The constraints work through statute and fact, and they work through identity and projection. In statute, the agency's formal authority wanes upon new drug approval. The Administration cannot *directly* regulate prescription practices, physician behavior, and many other determinants of the safety and efficacy of drugs. In identity, officials have actively relinquished control over approved drugs under the view that the Administration's role is drug approval, not post-market regulation. In essence, this view of identity places something of a temporal limit on the agency's powers, and upon its responsibility. Once a drug is approved, the agency's job is heavily reduced. Indeed, by some interpretations, the job is complete.

When American physicians began to prescribe estrogen extract as long-term hormone replacement therapy in the 1970s, Administration officials largely ignored the issue, as the compound in question—synthetic estrogen extracted from the urine of pregnant mares, manufactured as Premarin by Wyeth—was approved for menopausal symptoms. Only in the 1990s would large, randomized clinical trials produce abundant evidence that estrogenic hormone replacement therapy was associated with higher rates of breast cancer and heart disease. In reviewing the tale of Premarin, pharmaco-epidemiologist and long-time FDA observer Jerry Avorn wrote in 2004 that, "Until very recently, the agency didn't see its role as monitoring how drugs are used in practice; rather, it stuck closely to its authority to simply say yes or no to the initial entry of a given product onto the market. What doctors and patients did with it after that decision, FDA believed, was none of its business." Avorn's portrait oversimplifies, yet it testifies roughly to a culture of gatekeeping's dominance in pharmaceutical regulation.[36]

The form of government power in pharmaceutical regulation also limits

[36] Avorn, *Powerful Medicines*, 35. The history of oral contraceptives regulation, among other narratives, suggests that Avorn's characterization is too simple. Officials distributed throughout the FDA hierarchy—from Commissioner Charles Edwards to medical reviewer John Nestor and epidemiologist David Graham—attempted to study and regulate drugs that were previously reviewed but that had been prescribed for a growing list of non-approved indications, and in some cases these interventions were successful. Yet the procedural and cultural resistance that met these efforts lends some support to Avorn's characterizations.

the targets of that power. Because regulation and law establish the firm as the fundamental subject of FDA authority, the Administration can shape the incentives and behavior of drug companies much more easily and durably than that of nurse-practitioners, pharmacists, physicians, hospital administrators, and others whose decisions influence how drugs are utilized. Again, most of the reports on adverse reactions come not from physicians, nor from hospitals, but from manufacturers. Hence, the gatekeeping legacy is one that structures the flow of information about post-market safety. And it underscores the limits of the gatekeeping metaphor as an unconscious solution to pharmaceutical issues in the United States. From the standpoint of control, the Administration generally lacks broad and effectual sway over physician behavior. Physicians can and do prescribe "off-label," and tort liability is a much greater deterrent to abuse of this practice than anything that the FDA can do. Premarin as long-term hormone replacement therapy again provides an illuminating example. Not only was Premarin past the gate, its expanded uses resulted from "off-label" prescribing by physicians. Since off-label prescribing cannot be directly regulated under the Food, Drug and Cosmetic Act, Administration officials sometimes wish to ignore it entirely. The possibility and prevalence of off-label prescribing renders the initial molecular approval the most pivotal one.[37]

Because the New Drug Application is the central document, and in some ways the central procedural institution, of U.S. pharmaceutical regulation, the FDA's power is temporally and spatially limited. Temporally, once an NDA is approved, the Administration's gatekeeping power over the firm weakens. With gatekeeping power lost—at least for the drug in question— so are the incentives of pharmaceutical companies to behave in strict conformity with FDA wishes. Spatially, many of the powers FDA has are powers that exercised through control of the NDA. When the FDA wishes for a company to tweak a Phase 2 or Phase 3 trial, or to gather additional information on a drug *before* an NDA is approved, pharmaceutical sponsors respond quickly and completely. Once the drug is "past the gate," however, firm behavior changes. The best example of this lies in the low initiation and completion rate of "Phase 4" studies. Of the 1,682 Phase 4 post-marketing study commitments that FDA documented firms had agreed to carry out, only 38 percent of the studies had even been commenced by October 2007.[38]

As it was endowed until 2007, the FDA could do little about such pat-

---

[37] Avorn, *Powerful Medicines*, 25, 28, 35. See also the discussion on regulation of off-label prescribing, below.

[38] Data on Phase 4 completion appear in *FR* 73 (80) (April 24, 2008): 22157-9; Similar statistics appear several years earlier, at *FR* 70 (33) (Feb. 18, 2005): 8030. See *Comments of Consumers Union before the FDA Science Board*, April 14, 2005, pp. 8-9; available at http:// www.fda.gov/ohrms/dockets/ac/05/slides/2005-4136OPH_02_01_Consumer's%20Union.pdf [accessed September 8, 2005]. Thirty percent of the Phase 4 studies either were ongoing or were already submitted (completed, in terms of federal regulations). See also GAO, *Postmarket Drug Safety* (GAO 06-0402), 28.

terns. The set of punishments available to the FDA was brute. Faced with a noncompliant firm that refuses to honor its Phase 4 commitments, the FDA could not, until the Amendments Act of 2007, issue fines. It still cannot restrict advertising, and cannot administer any administrative penalty save that of suspending the company's NDA; what powers over advertising the agency now has are largely contained within the Risk Evaluation and Mitigation Strategies (REMS) toolkit. The political incentives weighing against NDA suspension—as well as the punishment this delivers to patients and their physicians—render Phase 4 commitments nearly unenforceable.

It is interesting in light of these conflicts that, in the wake of the Vioxx tragedy of October 2004, higher FDA officials (including many long-term careerists) engaged in an organizationally motivated embrace of the status quo by defending randomized controlled trials and by disparaging pharmacoepidemiology. For different reasons, Deputy Commissioner Scott Gottlieb, CDER officials Sandra Kweder, Robert Temple, and others did not want to cede more control of the pharmaceutical market to David Graham and his colleagues at ODS. Yet it was also an extension of the familiar, an area where the agency had already developed capacity. Clinical trials have advantages when they are randomized and placebo-controlled. They also have drawbacks. Often tests are done on homogenous patient populations, among patients who differ in many ways from the patients who will utilize the drugs in clinical situations. Clinical trials usually have an endpoint, and can often be too brief to allow analysts to detect whether the drug in inducing adverse events, particularly for toxicity, hepatotoxicity (or liver damage), and cardiovascular outcomes.[39]

Reliance upon Labeling. The Administration's weakness in post-market regulation is tempered somewhat by its conditionally aggressive approach to labeling revisions for drug products. The saga of oral contraceptives regulation starkly revealed this pattern, as the struggle with Searle focused heavily upon the content of revised labeling and how prominently thromboembolic risks should be highlighted. It was during the 1970s that the attention of the Bureau of Drugs became more tightly focused upon labeling as a form of policy, not only for governance of companies, but implicitly for the practice of pharmaceutical therapy. In addition to revisions and package inserts required of oral contraceptives, the Bureau required the listing of negative findings (a "possibly effective" or "questionable" rating) from the NAS/NRC Drug Efficacy Study, and the warning of birth defects associated with tranquilizer use in early pregnancy. And in response to the publication of results from the University Group Diabetes Program (UGDP) study that shed negative light on oral antidiabetic drugs such as Upjohn's Orinase and Pfizer's Diabinese, the Administration compelled labeling restrictions that established the drugs as third-line therapy. The FDA's required label explic-

---

[39]GAO, *FDA Postmarket Drug Safety*, (GAO-06-402), 26.

itly stated that dietary regulation and weight loss were the preferred treatments for "adult onset" diabetes, and that oral antidiabetics should be used only after insulin-based therapy had been unsuccessful or rejected by the patient. This move brought sustained protest from many endocrinologists, 250 of whom organized as the "Committee on the Care of the Diabetic," as well as a preemptory lawsuit from Boston's Joslin Clinic. The controversy focused less on the disagreements about the UGDP study and more on questions of whether FDA labeling requirements were unduly interfering in the doctor-patient relationship. These procedural and interpretive moves coincided with an organizational initiative at the Bureau of Drugs, undertaken in cooperation with the American Society for Hospital Pharmacists, to draft labeling for twenty different classes of drugs.[40]

As the concept of the appropriate label came under debate, Administration officials began to rely more and more thoroughly upon the notion of a "layman." The Food, Drug and Cosmetic Act requires that labeling provide "adequate directions for use"; Administration officials interpreted this to mean directions that a layman would need to have in order to use a drug safely and effectively. At one moment the emphasis on a pharmaceutical laity bespoke the emergence of consumerism in American medicine; at another moment it gestured to the transformative effects of oral contraceptives on regulatory notions of therapy and its regulation.[41]

Since these originary moves in the early 1970s, the Administration has depended heavily upon labeling revisions as a form of regulatory policy. The frequency of labeling revisions can be gleaned from supplementary new drug applications (sNDAs). Since a labeling revision would result in a drug that differs from the one approved in the original new drug application, each label change requires a supplemental NDA. Hence, the supplemental NDA process creates a sort of archive of revisions to each drug after its approval. Quite apart from the utility of these data, their very existence is telling. The

---

[40] "FDA Rules Labels, Ads On Prescription Drugs Give Adverse Findings," *WSJ*, June 8, 1971, 10; "Pharmaceutical Group Criticizes FDA Ruling On Drug Labels and Ads," *WSJ*, June 9, 1971, 3; Jonathan Spivak, "FDA to Tell Makers of Oral Diabetes Drugs to Curb Ad, Label Claims, Include Warning," *WSJ*, May 10, 1972, 3; Jerry E. Bishop, "FDA Nears Ruling on Whether to Require Warning Labels for Antidiabetes Pills," *WSJ*, March 19, 1979, 23. The UGDP ran a randomized controlled trial assessing the drugs over an eight-year period. For a thorough discussion of this trial and some of its clinical, scientific, and regulatory implications, see Harry Marks, "Anatomy of a Controversy: the University Group Diabetes Program study," Chapter 7 in *The Progress of Experiment* (New York: Cambridge University Press, 1997). On the prescription drug labeling project and cooperation with the ASHP, see *FR* 44 (124): 37439, 37454. The drug classes included digitalis glycosides, thiazide diuretics (but not all diuretics), cephalosporins, corticosteroids, oral anticoagulants, and tetracyclines.

[41] The labeling requirements of the FCDA appear in Section 502(f)(1). On the concept of "layman" in pharmaceutical therapy, see FDA, "Labeling and Prescription Drug Advertising; Content and Format for Labeling for Human Prescription Drugs," *FR* 44 (124): 37438. The official language of the interpretation (21 CFR 201.5) is that "adequate directions for use" implies "directions under which a layman can use a drug safely and for the purposes for which it is intended."

received structure of official data on labeling revisions points to the centrality of the new drug application process as an apparatus for managing and
documenting therapeutic change after product approval.

In the aggregate, and since 1970, labeling revisions have been at least as
common as a wide variety of other changes to drugs that are politically
easier for the Administration to secure. Table 9.2 displays the frequency of
different drug changes that are documented by a supplemental NDA. In the
aggregate, firms and the Administration have revised labeling for approved
products over twenty-five thousand times since 1970. From 1970 to 1990,
only chemistry changes to an approved NDA were more frequent than labeling changes, and since 1990, no form of regulatory revision to an approved
drug has been more common. Moreover, the frequency of labeling changes
dwarfs the frequency of other revisions to products, not least manufacturing
and packaging revisions and control supplements. The Administration's reliance upon labeling reflects the limited means of compulsion at its disposal,
as well as the lower administrative costs and burden of pursuing changes to
a drug's label as opposed to pursuing withdrawal or a change in advertising
and prescribing practices. Yet from the standpoint of reputation, labeling
provides a form of legitimation, a form of political insurance to the Administration, in the case of post-market safety problems. Time and again when
safety problems have arisen with an approved drug—increased cardiovascular mortality associated with oral antidiabetics in 1972, congenital malfor-
mations attributed to tranquilizer use in 1976, links between Reyes' Syndrome and children's aspirin formulations in the 1980s, Propulsid and
COX-2 inhibitors in the 1980s and 1990s —the FDA's first policy response
has been to change the product's labeling. And when confronted by criticism
that the approval was faulty or that the surveillance of the product after approval was lax, the Administration's first rhetorical response to critics is
often that the relevant safety issues have been identified in the labeling. Once
the label officially states the existence of a threat, an official record of the
problem exists. The Administration can argue—and has at length argued—
that the problem has been revealed, that the public has been notified, and
that responsibility for the problem has been delegated at least partially to
the prescribing physician. And with labeling revision, the possibility of having been surprised by a drug's safety issues wanes. The fact of surprise and,
more important, public and professional audiences' perceptions of the FDA
having been surprised, would present real damage to the Administration's
organizational image. The admission of surprise is tantamount to the admission of a lack of control, a lack of power, and a lack of protective ability. Labeling revision reduces the prospect and appearance of regulatory surprise.[42]

[42]On labeling revision as a "first resort," see Spivak, "FDA to Tell Makers of Oral Diabetes
Drugs to Curb Ad, Label Claims, Include Warning"; Jerry E. Bishop, "FDA Nears Ruling on
Whether to Require Warning Labels for Antidiabetes Pills." For later examples, see "FDA to
Require Label on Some Drugs Warn of Use in Pregnancy," *WSJ*, July 23, 1976, 3; "U. S. Health
Agency Is Delaying on Plan for Aspirin Warning," *WSJ*, November 19, 1982, 16.

TABLE 9.2

Drug Changes Requiring a Supplemental NDA, 1970–2006

	1970–1974	1975–1979	1980–1984	1985–1989	1990–1994	1995–1999	2000–
Chemistry Revisions	2	376	3,710	7,728	5,664	8,520	258
Manufacturing Revisions	0	492	910	1,045	1,063	2,229	1,936
Package Changes	38	465	757	733	573	847	994
New or Modified Indications	3	6	7	76	121	273	294
Control Supplements	242	2,516	3,710	2,138	1,902	2,885	4,357
Labeling Revisions (SLR)	529	1,968	2,005	2,360	1,909	2,341	4,472
Other Label Changes	0	0	168	1,998	3,588	2,923	1,672

Source: FDA, Drugs@FDA database.

It merits attention that this is a conditional pattern, contingent both in history and in behavior. Behaviorally, the FDA's aggressiveness in labeling seems to emerge as a tool only once the agency's initial reluctance to address and publicize a safety problem has been overcome. FDA officials have consistently sought to limit the uses of labeling, inveighing for instance against the inclusion of cost-effectiveness and economic information. The Administration's stated fear is that if drug labels included everything that some consumer safety advocates wanted in them, they would become "small textbooks of medicine."[43]

Historically, the Administration's reliance upon labeling is a partial legacy of the 1938 Food, Drug and Cosmetic Act, which gave the FDA control over labeling but left jurisdiction over advertising in the hands of the Federal Trade Commission. With limited authority to govern firm promotion, Administration lawyers began to press for expanded authority and interpretation of the meaning of labeling. By and large, the courts assented, not least in *United States v. Kordel* (1948), in which federal courts interpreted material

---

The Administration's data on these changes are partial. In particular, information on different forms of drug changes is available beginning in different years (1950 for most labeling revisions, 1954 for modified indications, 1960 for package changes, 1964 for manufacturing changes, and 1970 for control supplements). Hence, a proper comparison requires, at a minimum, that the same years are compared for the different supplemental changes.

[43] On labels as potential "small textbooks," see *FR* 44 (124) (June 26, 1979): 37436.

"accompanying" the label—and therefore subject to regulation under the 1938 Act—to include written information shipped separately from the product. From this basis a large number of materials such as brochures, reprints of scientific papers, and press releases have come under FDA jurisdiction.[44]

The other pivotal contingency was the nation's experience with contraceptives regulation. Two crucial foundations of the governance of modern drug labeling—the uniform labeling regulations of 1979 and the compulsory patient package insert—emerged in the Administration's struggle to regulate the pill. As part of a response to dilemmas encountered with oral contraceptives, uniform standards for drug labeling were proposed in 1975 and finalized four years later. The June 1979 rules were the product of considerable antagonism and debate, but they required a fixed format for each drug label with eleven different "sections" (see table 9.3). Along with the patient package insert, these sections and their contents reflected the degree to which American women as the "ultimate consumers" of prescription drugs had come to define the concepts and assumptions of post-market regulation. Yet under continuing concerns about teratogenicity in the shadow of thalidomide, the rules also reflected a reigning conception of women as mothers, potential or actual. The rules created five different categories of evidence, ranging from "Pregnancy Category A" in which adequate and well-controlled studies had failed to demonstrate fetal risk, to "Pregnancy Category X" in which studies had shown risks to the fetus. The Administration also required firms to list inactive ingredients.[45]

The patient package inserts that were required with Enovid and other oral contraceptives were also standardized as part of regular administrative requirements. Package inserts were used for a select variety of medications in the late 1960s and 1970s, but they were used most commonly for estrogen- and progestin-based products directed to women patients. Then in September 1980 the Administration attempted once again to codify regulatory practice, announcing that inserts would be required for virtually all new drug

---

[44] U.S. v. Kordel, 335 U.S. 345 (1948). In the Administration's 1979 interpretation, "labeling or advertising" included "newspapers or lay periodicals that are supported or influenced by pharmaceutical manufacturers" as well as "printed matter issued or caused to be issued by the manufacturer or distributor of a drug." This authority did not, however, include "articles about specific drugs in newspapers and lay periodicals," saying that "substantial constitutional questions" would be involved. FR 44 (124) (June 26, 1979): 37438. Kleinfeld, Kaplan, and Becker, "Human Drug Regulation: Comprehensiveness Breeds Complexity," in Richard M. Cooper, ed., Food and Drug Law (Washington, DC: Food and Drug Law Institute, 1990), 287.

[45] The proposed rules appear at FR 40 (April 7, 1975): 15392. FR 44 (Dec. 18, 1979): 74817; 21 CFR 202.1(e)(6)(ii),(vii). The GAO remarks that the 1979 uniformity regulations accelerated a "gradual trend toward greater standardization." GAO, FDA Drug Review: Post-approval Risks, 1976–85, Report to the Chairman, Subcommittee on Human Resources and Intergovernmental Relations, Committee on Government Operations, USHR (Washington, DC: GAO/PEMD-90-15, April 1990), 27–8. For a thorough and conceptual review of comments on the 1975 proposed rules and the FDA's response to them, see "Labeling and Prescription Drug Advertising; Content and Format for Labeling for Human Prescription Drugs," FR 44 (124) (June 26, 1979): 37434–67. For pregnancy category elaboration, see ibid., 37464–5.

TABLE 9.3
Required Label Sections from Uniform Labeling Requirements from 1979

Description

Clinical Pharmacology

Indications and Usage

Contraindications

Warnings

Precautions

- General
- Information for patients
- Laboratory tests
- Drug interactions
- Carcinogenesis, mutagenesis, impairment of fertility
- Pregnancy (with evidentiary categories A, B, C, D, and X)
- Labor and delivery
- Nursing mothers

Adverse Reactions

Drug Abuse and Dependence

Overdosage

Dosage and Administration

How Supplied

Source: Federal Register 44 (124) (June 26, 1979) 37462; 21 CFR 201.56(d)(1).

products. The September 1980 regulations—soon whittled to apply to ten drug products only—targeted two legal entities: pharmaceutical firms and legal dispensers (mainly pharmacies). The former were required to publish a legible and accessible package insert, the latter to include this literature with any dispensed drug product. When the Reagan administration took office, these changes were stayed, and the Administration's use of patient package inserts has been uneven ever since.[46]

The emergent irony of prescription drug labeling in the United States is

---

[46] Along with Enovid, the first drugs to which patient package inserts were mandatorily attached were the beta-agonist isoprotenerol inhalation products used for bronchodilation. Isoprotenerol was associated with increased heart rate, onset of arrhythmia and, occasionally, induced heart failure; *FR* 33 (June 18, 1968): 8812. Kleinfeld, Kaplan, and Becker, "Human Drug Regulation." Over-the-counter contraceptives were regulated through somewhat different advisory mechanisms, not least by advisory panels associated with the DESI initiative; "Tentative Findings of the Advisory Review Panel on Contraceptives and Other Vaginal Drug Products," November 1978, vol. 13; 88.85.0057 (NN3-088-99-001), B 3, RG 88, NA.

that it increasingly depends upon pre-market decision making rather than post-market surveillance. Administration officials have acknowledged and facilitated this development since the early 1970s. In 1972, Commissioner Charles Edwards described pre-market approval of labeling as a core responsibility of the FDA, every bit as central to the 1962 Drug Amendments, and just as equivalent in stature and burden, as the evaluation of safety and efficacy in new drug review. As Commissioner Donald Kennedy admitted in elaborating the June 1979 rules, "the final labeling for a drug is often the result of interactions between FDA and the manufacturer when a manufacturer seeks approval for a prescription drug." By 1979, Kennedy's acknowledgment confirmed what many American physicians already knew and lamented. Throughout the 1970s, some physicians had been complaining that the most significant labeling decisions excluded physician participation, instead being negotiated entirely between firms and the government. Food and drug lawyers read the Administration's shift more broadly. Attorneys for the Washington law firm Kleinfeld, Kaplan and Becker wrote in 1990 that "labeling for many drugs is now *controlled* through the new drug approval process. This process has reduced the significance of the general labeling controls that would otherwise apply under the misbranding provisions of the act." The Progressive-Era misbranding and fraud provisions of the 1906 legislation are, in other words, being subsumed under the gatekeeping provisions of the 1938 statute. What was formerly construed as a post-market endeavor has become a pre-market responsibility.[47]

The oral contraceptives saga illustrates some dynamics behind this shift. The Administration's ability to compel labeling changes wanes after NDA approval, reflecting its reduced bargaining power. It is facile at law, but difficult in practice, to compel firms to add a warning. And the parameters of the FDA's legal authority over the product label have never been clearly and consensually understood. As Morton Mintz described negotiations over contraceptives labeling in 1977, "The process was something like collective bargaining between a company and a union, although the purpose was to instruct physicians purely on the basis of scientific facts." And the oral contraceptives regulation convinced Mintz that "The results were sometimes bizarre." The Norinyl brand of norethindrone and mestranol contained a broad warning against use by women with a history of clinical depression. Johnson and Johnson's Ortho-Novum was essentially identical as a chemical entity, but in its label there was only a mild precaution that patients with a history of depression be "carefully observed." The discrepancy stemmed from differences in individual negotiations with the companies. The Administration's labeling revisions—both the 1977 rules compelling uniform risk reporting among the oral contraceptives and the 1975–79 effort to stan-

[47]Edwards stated that "As the law now stands, therefore, the [FDA] is charged with the responsibility for judging the safety and effectiveness of drugs and the truthfulness of their labeling"; *FR* 37 (158): 16504. Kennedy acknowledgement at *FR* 44 (124) (June 26, 1979): 37437. Kleinfeld, Kaplan, and Becker in Cooper, ed., *Food and Drug Law*, 289; emphasis added.

dardize labels in general—reduced these disparities. Yet they did so, ironically enough, by transferring more power and agency to the pre-market stage of drug regulation.[48]

Reliance on labeling has its own pitfalls. Even in the midst of more aggressive governance of off-label utilization, the practice continued apace, in part because the institutional structure of the industry had changed. Survey-based studies have also cast doubt upon the effectiveness of labeling. A 1997 analysis reported that fully 85 percent of American physicians responded that FDA labels have either "little influence" or "practically no influence at all" in their treatment decisions. It is for this reason that a behavioral analysis of FDA reliance upon labeling is so instructive. Labeling has been shown repeatedly to be at best a weak factor in shaping physician and patient behavior.[49]

Regulation of Prescription and "Off-Label" Usage. The practice of off-label prescribing and utilization creates another set of issues for post-market regulation. When approved molecules experience what physicians call "prescription creep"—the expanded use of a drug beyond the medical conditions for which it was originally developed and approved—the power embedded in supplementary new drug approval wanes. One implication of the practice is that the initial approval of a new molecular entity represents a substantial loss in gatekeeping power over the drug, and this fact has given the Administration further incentives to regard NME approvals with a sense of irreversibility. More generally, FDA officials have recognized that much drug utilization takes place independently from, and occasionally in defiance of, the approved labeling. Hence, the approach to off-label usage compels some delicate political balancing, and the resulting equilibrium is one shaped by power and reputation, and their limits.[50]

To the extent that it exists, the FDA's governance of off-label prescribing can be categorized by whether the target of regulation is a physician or a drug company. The Administration has little or no formal authority over physicians and their prescribing behavior. The historical complication here is that the FDA lacks this authority in part because agency officials have not wanted it. As part of a long-running projection of identity in which the agency is publicly differentiated from the AMA and other professional bodies, Administration officials have eschewed anything resembling "the regulation of

[48] Mintz, "FDA Works Up Final Draft on What 'Pill' Users 'Should Know,'" *WP*, September 6, 1977, A7.

[49] Marlene Cimons, "FDA's Approval Process Faces Challenge in New Senate Bill," *LAT*, July 22, 1987, A5.

[50] "Use of Approved Drugs for Unlabeled Indications," *FDA Drug Bulletin* 12 (1982): 4–5. As legal scholars have recognized, the term "off-label" is perhaps not so precise as "extra-label." The absence of an indication for a drug on the approved labeling implies only that the claim has not been approved. It does not imply that the Administration has evaluated the claim negatively or has decided that the drug should not be used for the given medical condition. James M. Beck and Elizabeth D. Azari, "FDA, Off-Label Use, and Informed Consent: Debunking Myths and Misconceptions," *FDLJ* 53 (1998): 71, n.2.

medical practice." In part this reflects a shared understanding of the Food, Drug and Cosmetic Act. In rulemaking, in congressional hearings, and in correspondence with congressional committees, Administration officials have openly stated that the Act does not limit physician use of an approved drug. Indeed, quite apart from relations with Congress, the agency's legal and enforcement offices have followed this rule, citing "a well-established and long-standing FDA policy to refrain from initiating enforcement action against physicians who prescribe medical products for unapproved uses."[51]

Yet this policy of official indifference to off-label prescribing has not bought the agency predictable immunity from censure. Critics in Congress, medical academia, and the media have disparaged the FDA for failing to exert greater control over off-label prescribing practices. Stuck in this bind, the Administration has come to rely upon other means. Chief among these is the occasional and gentle reminder to physicians that they may face greater tort liability when they prescribe a drug for any indication other than those expressly approved in the new drug application process. As Commissioner James Goddard hinted in a letter to hospitals in 1969:

> Any physician is, of course, free to use a marketed drug for his own patient as his best judgment directs. When he departs from the conditions of safe and effective use established through the new drug clearance procedure described in the package insert, he should understand that he may be using the drug investigationally, and if a patient suffers an untoward reaction, the physician may be called upon to justify his use of the drug contrary to the prescribing information. This will be a matter between the physician, the patient, and the court that hears the case.

FDA Commissioners after Goddard, including Charles Edwards and Donald Kennedy, issued similar warnings, and agency officials have repeated these admonitions in *Federal Register* announcements, in guidance documents, and in speeches to industry groups. Implicitly assisting the Administration, financial newspapers and industry trade reporters have echoed these cautions. From the 1970s to the present, several outlets have informed their readers that failure to comply with labeling restrictions invites greater tort

[51]The FDA's proposed rule in August 1972 explicitly acknowledged that no attempt to regulate the practice of medicine was intended or desirable. "Legal Status of Approved Labeling for Prescription Drugs; Prescribing for Uses Unapproved by the Food and Drug Administration," *FR* 37 (158) (Aug. 15, 1972): 16503–4. In public comments on the April 1975 proposed rules for uniform labeling, physicians lamented that the labeling requirements were an incursion upon their turf. The FDA vigorously rejected this argument, stating that "these regulations specifying the content and format of prescription drug labeling do not infringe on a physician's right to practice medicine, nor do they attempt to regulate the practice of medicine" (*FR* 44 (124) (June 26, 1979) : 37436; see also *FR* 48 (June 9, 1983): 26720, 26733; *FR* 52 (March 19, 1987): 8798, 8803). Commissioner Charles Edwards insisted before the Fountain committee that his agency should not be "playing doctor," June 9, 1970; *CPRPFDA*, 100. "Use of Approved Drugs for Unlabeled Indications," *FDA Drug Bulletin* 12 (1982): 4–5. FDA, "Memorandum of Points and Authorities in Opposition to Plaintiff's Motion for Summary Judgment at 13, *Washington Legal Foundation v. Kessler*, C.A. No. 94-1306-RCL (filed Dec. 24, 1997); Beck and Azari, "FDA, Off-Label Use, and Informed Consent," 78, n.64.

liability. As the *Wall Street Journal* summarized matters in 1976, "The drug labeling constitutes recommendations from the FDA to physicians on how to use drugs. While the doctors aren't required to follow the recommendations, they run the risk of malpractice suits if they don't."[52]

Where the Administration does have greater authority—over pharmaceutical companies themselves—it takes a much harder line with off-label promotion and has occasionally tried to set examples with aggressive criminal and civil prosecution. To bring charges against physicians for off-label prescription is legally difficult and politically risky. To prosecute drug companies for off-label *promotion* is much easier because questions of interstate commerce are involved, and because the modern apparatus of U.S. pharmaceutical regulation leashes companies to the FDA in a tight cycle of repeated interaction. When off-label prescribing began to consume a greater share of prescription dollars in the 1980s, FDA Commissioner David Kessler launched an enforcement initiative aimed at reining in promotions. His main target was not the physician, but the firm. Some of the nation's most prominent companies, including Johnson & Johnson, were targeted. Kessler's motives were debated in the trade press, but many felt that he was trying to induce companies to pursue more supplemental NDAs, that is, to expand drug indications through the legitimate channels of the Administration's gatekeeping mechanism. The off-label campaign's most notable success came in 1999, when San Francisco-based Genentech pleaded guilty to off-label promotion of its growth hormone drug Protropin, paying $50 million to the federal government. The Administration's Division of Drug Marketing, Advertising and Communications (DDMAC) had commenced investigations in 1994, and the aggressiveness of the investigation startled industry observers. The threat of criminal prosecution for off-label promotion," food and drug lawyers concluded in 1998, "is a real one."[53]

---

[52] Goddard's announcement was widely circulated both among hospitals and within them. Mayo Clinic administrators sent a verbatim copy of the statement to all of its staff physicians; Minutes, CSTA, Mayo Clinic, March 28, 1968; MAYO. For references to the possibility of tort liability, see *FR* 37 (158) (Aug. 15, 1972): 16504. "FDA to Require Label on Some Drugs Warn of Use in Pregnancy," *WSJ*, July 23, 1976, 3; see also Jerry E. Bishop, "FDA Nears Ruling on Whether to Require Warning Labels for Antidiabetes Pills," *WSJ*, March 19, 1979, 23. In October 1996, Deputy Commissioner Mary K. Pendergast reportedly told attendees at a Food and Drug Law Institute luncheon that if off-label utilization continued without restraint, "the doctors of this country are not going to have to worry about FDA because they are going to have to worry about the tort lawyers who will come in and say that the kind of switch that you allowed was not a really good idea for the patient and you ought to be liable." Pendergast's speech was reported by industry observer James G. Dickinson, "As I See It: FDA Letter, Deputy's Speech, Define a Dilemma," *Medical Marketing & Media* 31 (10) (Oct. 1996): 18. Avorn (*Powerful Medicines*) remarks that the tort system is currently the strongest regime of regulation for off-label prescribing.

[53] As the Administration stated in a 1972 policy statement on off-label uses, "A prescription new drug may not be shipped in interstate commerce when intended for uses not contained in the currently approved labeling"; *FR* 37 (158) (Aug. 15, 1972): 16504. John Carey and Joseph Weber, "The FDA Is Growling at Drugmakers, Too," *Business Week*, July 1, 1991, 34. For a

In recent history, the most notable and costly case of criminal prosecution for off-label promotion is the near half-billion-dollar judgment paid by Warner-Lambert (parent company Pfizer) for off-label promotion of gabapentin, trade name Neurontin. This case was brought not by the FDA, but by the Department of Justice. Its resolution nonetheless eased FDA enforcement of off-label marketing restrictions. Neurontin was approved in 1993 for treatment of epileptic seizures but was found by federal investigators to have been promoted for attention-deficit disorder, migraine, (psychiatric) bipolar disorder, various pain disorders, amyotrophic lateral sclerosis (ALS, or "Lou Gehrig's disease"), drug and alcohol withdrawal seizures, and restless leg syndrome. The statute under which Warner-Lambert was prosecuted was not the Food, Drug and Cosmetic Act but instead the False Claims Act—a nineteenth-century statute covering criminal cases in which the federal government (in this case, Medicaid) has been defrauded—and in 2004, Pfizer paid what was at the time the second-largest punitive fine in U.S. history for a health-related case, approximately $430 million. The FDA was not the instigator of the Neurontin case, but Administration officials backed and assisted the prosecution. As the Neurontin verdict was announced, the FDA and the Department of Justice launched criminal investigations into numerous "big pharma" companies, including Eli Lilly, Schering-Plough, Wyeth, Bristol-Myers Squibb, Johnson & Johnson, and Forest Laboratories. So expansive was the government's criminal canvass of the industry that *Pharmaceutical Executive* magazine wondered, "Is Everyone A Target?"[54]

The Administration's authority to govern off-label promotion was curtailed in an important court decision in 2002. In response to FDA regulations limiting the distribution of clinical studies that shed favorable light upon the manufacturers' therapy, the Washington Legal Foundation brought suit, claiming First Amendment violations. A generation earlier, such a case might have been dismissed. But in the wake of the federal judiciary's growing penchant to interpret the First Amendment as protective of commercial speech, a tendency underscored in the 1996 Liquormart decision, a different result was to follow. Federal judge Royce Lamberth, in a surprising opinion,

---

somewhat conspiratorial take, see Alan R. Bennett and Mark E. Boulding, "The Hidden Agenda Behind FDA Regulation of Enduring Materials," *Medical Marketing and Media* 30 (6) (June 1995): 26. On the Protropin case, see "Putting a Mistake Behind It, Genentech Pays a $50 Million Fine," *Business Week*, April 15, 1999 (published online at http://yahoo.business-week.com/bwdaily/dnflash/apr1999/nf90415c.htm [accessed June 21, 2006]); Tamar Nordenberg, "Investigators' Reports: Growth Hormone Maker Feels Long Arm of the Law," *FDA Consumer* 33 (5) (Sept. –Oct. 1999); Jill Wechsler, "Whither DDMAC?" *Pharmaceutical Executive* 19 (7) (July 1999): 18. Paul E. Kalb and I. Scott Bass, "Government Investigations in the Pharmaceutical Industry: Off-Label Promotion, Fraud and Abuse, and False Claims," *FDLJ* 53 (1998): 63–9.

[54] Megan Barnett, "The New Pill Pushers," *US News & World Report*, April 26, 2004; Michael D. Lam (Associated Editor), "Is Everyone A Target?" *Pharmaceutical Executive* 24 (3) (March 2004): 56.

argued that limitation of off-label information was an unconstitutional violation of companies' free speech rights.[55]

The Persistence of Lament, and the Debility of Post-Market Regulation. If nothing else, the saga of oral contraceptives also reminds us that public and congressional criticism of the post-market "surveillance system" has been something of a constant feature of pharmaceutical politics in the past half-century. The FDA has been criticized repeatedly for its failure to upgrade its surveillance system. Official complaints were made by the Hellman Committee on Oral Contraceptives in 1966 and again in 1969, by the Fountain Committee of the House in 1970, by the General Accounting Office in 1974 and again in 1982.[56]

The durability of this critique signifies a number of things, not least the ease with which congressional and professional bodies can heap blame upon an agency without providing the authority or resources for the problem to be solved. The lack of an effective surveillance system has been easier perhaps for agency critics to identify, especially when contrasted against the massive and more intricate regulatory apparatus of pre-market review. Yet the durability of the critique also testifies to the reputational forces shaping the FDA.

From the vantage of history and the stylized images of Max Weber, the interesting feature of the Administration's post-market surveillance system is that it is less classically "bureaucratic" in its operation. The FDA's post-market surveillance system, particularly information storage and retrieval, has been consistently and thoroughly excoriated as insufficiently organized, rational, and systematic over the last five decades. Charles Edwards was compelled to acknowledge the point before the Fountain subcommittee in 1970.[57]

Pre-Market versus Post-Market. The fundamental politics of post-market regulation is one that maps the temporality of action ("before" versus "after" approval) onto positions, offices, and status. Pre-market approval occupies "reviewers" and "officers" whose training was traditionally in pharmacology and related fields, whose dedication to the randomized clinical trial is particularly strong, and whose perch at the top of the organizational hierarchy of pharmaceutical regulation is secure. Post-market regulation and surveillance employs epidemiologists, "drug safety specialists," "communications officers" and other officials, all of whom occupy a lower rung in the

---

[55] *Washington Legal Foundation v. Kessler,* 880 F. Supp. 26 (D.D.C. 1995). "WLF Case Dies," *Medical Marketing and Media* 36 (1) (Jan. 2001): 8.

[56] Among the central recommendations of the Hellman Committee report in 1969 was "Strengthen the surveillance system of the Food and Drug Administration." The committee noted, however, that "This recommendation from the previous report has not been satisfactorily implemented." *Second Report on the Oral Contraceptives,* 9.

[57] Edwards in 1970: "The scientific recordkeeping system of the Food and Drug Administration is not good"; *CPRPFDA,* 100.

Administration's official and symbolic hierarchies. In identity and in practice, the Administration's drug safety specialists are mere "consultants" to the drug reviewing divisions.[58]

FDA officials whose job it is to monitor drugs after approval are generally housed in one of two offices: the Office of Drug Safety (ODS) or the Division of Drug Marketing, Advertising and Communications (DDMAC). Both of these offices are housed within the Center for Drug Evaluation and Research, and both are superintended by officials from the agency's drug reviewing divisions. When DDMAC began in the 1990s to review off-label promotional materials submitted by industry, the review program was overseen by none other than long-time medical officer Robert Temple, the clinical trials guru who was now running a new "Office of Medical Policy" within CDER. Similarly, when epidemiologists in the Office of Drug Safety have proposed labeling revisions or even product withdrawals, their views are first vetted within CDER before reaching the Commissioner's Office or the public. The symbolic hierarchy is particularly constraining when issues of representation and participation arise. As the General Accounting Office has noted, CDER officials often prevent Office of Drug Safety officials from presenting their views to relevant advisory committees. In these meetings, the Administration is represented by CDER officials to the exclusion of ODS personnel, whose more aggressive views on post-market regulation are frequently omitted from committee discussions. In select professional and public fora, then, the Administration is signified by its gatekeepers, with the monitors kept from view.[59]

The conflict of identities becomes, in some measure, a conflict of incentives. Reviewers may wish for less labeling revision after approval, wishing to rely on the extensive negotiations and textual adjustment effected before the drug's approval. Unless safety problems were severe, moreover, reviewers may wish to avoid a case where market withdrawal was necessary. When drug safety officials discover potential problems with marketed drugs, they ineluctably draw attention to the possible errors in earlier decision processes. Any success of post-market epidemiology threatens to demonstrate a failure of pre-market clinical trial design and review. This is not to say that drug safety officers seek media or congressional attention, or that they are motivated by one-upmanship. Rather, the organizational setting and the professional context of drug safety officials, together with surrounding medical and public attention, generate a role and set of associated scripts that place the epidemiologist in direct and symbolic conflict with the enthusiast of ran-

---

[58] As the GAO summarized in a 2006 report, "ODS staff take a population-based perspective in their work, which ODS staff we spoke with contrasted with the clinical perspective of OND" (*FDA Postmarket Drug Safety*, GAO-06-0402, 15).

[59] Jill Wechsler, "Whither DDMAC?" *Pharmaceutical Executive* 19 (9) (July 1999): 19–20. Clifford Rosen, "The Rosiglitazone Story—Lessons from an FDA Advisory Committee Meeting," *NEJM* 357 (9) (August 30, 2007): 844–46. In recent years, epidemiologists and other Office of Drug Safety specialists have received greater formal and informal testimony rights at advisory committee meetings.

domized controlled clinical studies. An institutionalized mixture of publicity and opacity accompanies this conflict of pre-market and post-market regulators. Most disputes tend to be hidden from public view and, when they are revealed, are often referred initially to an advisory committee. In those memorable cases where stark controversy surfaced, drug safety officers have testified not so much at advisory committee meetings but at congressional hearings, essentially "going public" with their views and complaints.[60]

The influence of pre-market decisions upon post-market regulation also emerges in differential patterns of labeling across drugs. Drugs undergo labeling revisions with variable frequency, and an instructive look at the conflict between pre-market and post-market processes comes from examining how drugs are relabeled depending on which office or division approved them in the first place. Between 1980 and 2000, over four thousand individuals served at some point in the FDA's Center for Drug Evaluation and Research (CDER), and CDER officials approved nearly seven hundred new molecular entities during the same period. Applying the most stable measure of general labeling revisions to these drugs, the average NME received five labeling revisions after approval during this period, about one for every three years of marketing after approval. About one in four drugs had no labeling revisions, but another one in four experienced twenty-eight or more revisions, with the maximally revised drug (indinavir sulfate, or Crixivan) receiving thirty-seven.

Approving offices also differ in the composition of their personnel, particularly with respect to tenure. Employee turnover has long been a worry of Administration officials and advocates, and while turnover affects the agency as a whole, some offices and divisions experience greater levels of turnover among careerist officials than do others. In the 1980s, the average staff tenure increased most appreciably in three divisions: the Divisions of Neuropharmacological Drugs, Anti-Infective Drugs, and Surgical-Dental Drugs. By the year 2000, all three of these CDER divisions still had longer-than-average staff tenure, but the Cardio-Renal Division, headed by Raymond Lipicky, was far and away the most tenured division.

As a hypothesis, it is historically and psychologically plausible that reputational considerations will be enhanced—in ways that are conscious and perhaps unconscious—where length of service is greatest. Historically, some of the career officers who have contributed most to the agency's reputation—Frances Kelsey and Robert Temple, for example—were long-tenured individuals. Statistically, average tenure is a product of the number of new arrivals and the length of stay for those officials who do matriculate. While the relationship is more complicated than any multivariate analysis can incorporate,

---

[60] Associate Commissioner for Science Dale R. Lindsay stated the importance of taking "such steps as were necessary to insure that there was expert agreement as to the interpretation of results." Lindsay to John Jennings (Assistant to the Commissioner for Medical Affairs), May 15, 1970, Re: "Dr. Richardson's charges that pathology data have been altered by FDA officials"; CPRPFDA, 105.

it is reasonable to hypothesize that the greater the number of new arrivals (people whose identification with the organization is probably weaker) to an office, the lower the attachment to an organizational reputation. Similarly, the longer tenure of officials who do matriculate likely implies a greater attachment to organizational image. The mechanism is what social scientists would call a "selection effect": those who remain at the agency have done so at steadily increasing opportunity cost financially—mainly by forgoing more lucrative employment in the private sector—which suggests they are likely more motivated by other considerations and have greater organizational identification.

Tenure may also be an indicator of other mechanisms pertinent to reputational concerns. Two related mechanisms are organizational power and deference. Due to seniority rules in the federal civil service, those officials with longer internal careers probably enjoy greater authority within their bureaus, which may imply that divisions with greater tenure will have greater say over the choice to revisit an approved drug. Less directly but perhaps more plausibly, drug safety officials may be less likely to press for revised labeling on a drug when the product was first approved by a senior CDER official. In ways that are conscious or unconscious, the decisions of longer-tenured officials may be less likely to be questioned.[61]

If tenure is an indicator of attachment and reputational concern, then drugs approved in reviewing divisions with longer-tenured staff may be less likely to undergo labeling revisions than drugs approved in offices with shorter-tenured staff. It is possible to gauge the association between office tenure and the post-market regulation of drugs by analyzing data on labeling revisions and staff tenure aggregates. Figure 9.1 offers a summary representation of the relationship between (1) the tenure of a staff in a reviewing division at the time of the drug's approval, and (2) the frequency of general significant drug warnings in the years after approval. The estimated associations are based upon statistical analyses of labeling revisions to 327 molecular entities submitted to the Administration from 1980 to 2000. The measure for a significant labeling warning is taken from a 2002 study by epidemiologist Karen Lasser and published in the *Journal of the American Medical Association*.

The analyses include the total number of staff in a division in a given year, as well as the annual change in staff totals for the relevant division, as statistical controls. The hope is that in including these variables in the analysis, the estimated association between tenure and labeling is purged of reductions in tenure that occur through the arrival of new members (as, for instance, when an office expands in size). The analyses also control for the tenure (in years) of the relevant division director, a yearly time trend to dif-

---

[61] Still, decisions to revisit or not to revisit an approved drug are fruitfully viewed within the context of reputation-based considerations. Authority alone as a variable cannot explain the variance of labeling revisions, and deference is a mechanism that often invokes and relies upon reputation and related concerns.

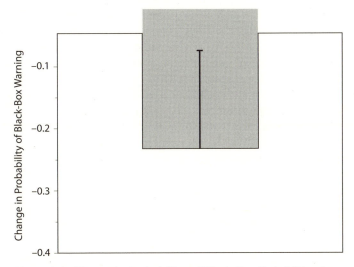

Figure 9.1. Change in Probability of Black-Box Label Warning when Average Tenure of Approving Division Moves from Minimum to Mean [Note: Bold horizontal line indicates estimated association, and vertical line encompasses upper 95% confidence interval.]

ferentiate drugs submitted early in the 1980–2000 period from those submitted later, and for fixed characteristics of the drug's primary indication and the sponsoring firm.[62]

The estimated relationship depicted in figure 9.1 also includes lower "confidence interval," which gives some sense of statistical significance of the association. For every year increase in average staff tenure of the division that originally approved the drug, the drug is 6.9 percent less likely to experience a black-box warning. Given the average probability of a black-box label warning (11.6 percent for drugs in the sample), this means that a one-unit increase in average staff tenure is associated with a reduction in the probability of a black-box warning from 11.6 percent to 4.7 percent. When the tenure variable moves from its minimum to its mean, as in figure 9.1, a larger shift in the likelihood of a black-box warning is observed.[63]

[62] More specifically, the analyses are "probit" analyses where the dependent variable is scored "1" if the drug received a black-box warning as measured in Lasser's article, and zero otherwise. The probit regression assumes that the "link function" that translates a vector of values into a probability estimate is given by the cumulative distribution function of the normal distribution. As in any such analysis, it is important to stress that only static characteristics of the drug's sponsor and primary indication are analyzed. If there is a feature of the target disease or the sponsoring firm that influences labeling, and these features change over time, the estimated model cannot account for these effects.

[63] As with any statistical analysis of observational data, there exist other possible explanations for this result. One possibility is that FDA staff tenure is lower in those divisions that regulate product markets characterized by greater technological change (oncology drugs versus

Once a drug has been cleared for marketing, labeling issues require the Administration to revisit a molecule it previously sanctioned. It would appear that regulatory practices of re-examination are less frequent or severe when the officials who originally approved the drug had greater tenure (and, perhaps, greater stature and greater organizational power). This finding may well be historically contingent, and the available personnel data allow for a test only with data from 1980 to 2000. Yet the pattern is consistent with a broader organizational reluctance to revisit past decisions—not just labeling but also product withdrawal. It also underscores the irreversibility of new drug approval with respect to reputation and politics.

In several respects, this conflict of incentives is healthy and quite possibly benefits the American public. As it is currently structured, the Administration places implicit advocates for approved drugs in the reviewing divisions, and places potential "detractors" in the Office of Drug Safety.

Reputation and the Symbolic Politics of Product Withdrawal

The removal of a drug from the therapeutic marketplace proceeds as a reversal of the process by which the drug first gained entry. As the drug's admission was premised upon an effective New Drug Application, the drug's departure occurs when the Administration suspends or withdraws approval of the NDA. Safety-based drug withdrawals reveal organizational and scientific politics more starkly than any other event. Discord among scientists—between medical authorities in universities and those employed in the pharmaceutical industry, between FDA pharmacologists and FDA epidemiologists—is cast into public view.

The oddity of product withdrawals in the United States is that an agency that has often regarded approval so cautiously also treads carefully in removal. At one end of the political spectrum, libertarian critics of the Administration have relentlessly lampooned what they perceive to be the agency's

---

anti-infective drugs, for instance). Rapid changes in technology and medicine may make FDA service more valuable to pharmaceutical companies who wish to speed these drugs through the regulatory approval process; hence, these reviewers may be drawn into industry at a higher rate. Yet these also may be the very drugs that are more likely to experience labeling revisions because the stock of medical and pharmacological knowledge is less. Put another way, drugs approved in more tenured divisions might be characterized by less technological advance, which would account both for less labeling revision and for the fact that reviewers in these divisions are less sought after by drug firms. This explanation has plausibility and cannot be ruled out entirely, but it is worth noting that two of the reviewing divisions with the most advanced tenure in recent years—Cardio-Renal and Neuropharmacological Products—governed rapidly changing technologies. In the case of the Cardio-Renal Division, numerous orphan drugs for rare disorders such as pulmonary arterial hypertension and Amyloid A Amyloidosis have appeared before the division. In the case of Neuropharmacological Products, a generation of selective serotonin reuptake inhibitors beginning with Prozac and continuing through Effexor has made for some difficult reviews.

extreme risk-aversion and "deadly over-caution." If these criticisms are on the mark, one would be tempted to think that a very cautious and slow-to-approve agency would, given any adverse signal, quickly pull a drug from the market. Indeed, this principle is enunciated in the legislative history of the 1962 Amendments. The first Kefauver bill to clear the Senate in 1962 was a measure to "keep unfit drugs off the market . . . and speed their removal should they reach the market." Yet, if anything, the Administration has generally approached the prospect of drug withdrawal with trepidation. For most of the past half-century, withdrawal has been characterized by much of the organizational conservatism that has accompanied initial drug review.[64]

It is worth remembering that, in the decades following the thalidomide episode, the Administration received severe and sustained criticism from numerous quarters for its lax oversight of drug products. As the controversies surrounding oral contraceptives continued to occupy public space, the FDA's reluctance to revisit its decisions with several other medications raised sporadic but heated congressional ire. Perhaps the most pointed controversy came with Unimed Corporation's drug betahistine hydrochloride, trade name "Serc," which received FDA approval on November 11, 1966, mainly because a pivotal clinical study, published in *JAMA* in 1966 by Reno, Nevada physician Joseph C. Elia, reported that the compound reduced the severity of vertigo episodes in patients suffering from Ménière's syndrome. Yet Elia's results were so positive as to draw suspicion from within and outside the Administration, including a public rebuke from the *Medical Letter on Drugs and Therapeutics*. So central was Elia's analysis to the Administration's approval decision that in April 1967, two weeks before the *Medical Letter*'s expression of doubt, FDA investigators descended upon the doctor's offices to review his records. In an implicit swipe at the beleaguered American Medical Association and its flagship journal, agency officials found the data "inadequate" to support the study's conclusions, and in 1968 the FDA published a notice of intent to withdraw approval of Serc's new drug application.[65]

---

[64]See the first Kefauver bill of the 87th Congress: S. Rep. No. 1744, Part I, 87th Congress, 2nd Session, p. 8. On the slowness of Administration action in the post-market phase, see GAO, *FDA Postmarket Drug Safety* (GAO-06-0402): 36.

[65]Ménière's syndrome is a disease of the inner ear which, besides causing vertigo, can induce a ringing in the ears called "tinnitus," a feeling of fullness or pressure in the inner cochlea, and variable hearing loss. At the time of Serc's approval, its pathogenesis and pathology were considered unknown; H. H. Merritt, *Textbook of Neurology*, 4th ed., (Philadelphia: Lea and Febiger, 1967), 788. Other records have the approval at November 17, 1966. For the original study, see J. C. Elia, Jr., "Double-Blind Evaluation of a New Treatment for Meniere's Syndrome," *JAMA* 196 (2) (April 11, 1966): 187–9. "Betahistine hydrochloride (serc) for Meniere's syndrome," *MLDT* 9 (8) (April 21, 1967): 29–30. B. D. Minchew (Acting Director, Bureau of Medicine) to Commissioner Herbert Ley, Memorandum, May 2, 1969, Subject "NDA 14-241 Serc (betahistine hydrochloride)"; in *Consumer Protection: FDA Regulation of the New Drug Serc* (hereafter *Fountain Serc Hearings*), Hearings before the Intergovernmental Relations Subcommittee of the Committee on Government Oversight, U. S. House of Repre-

Yet the order was stayed by Henry Simmons, Director of the Bureau of Medicine, and Peter Barton Hutt, the agency's general counsel. Administration officials instead compelled Unimed to design and implement a new randomized controlled trial to reassess efficacy. Over a three-year period, Unimed representatives and FDA officials corresponded, with the company engaged in a trial-and-error procedure to determine just what Simmons' bureau would accept as a valid protocol. Finally, in September 1972, Simmons approved the company's new study design, and Serc was allowed to remain on the market while being studied.[66]

The Administration's deferral of market withdrawal for Serc brought hearings and condemnation from North Carolina Democrat Lawrence Fountain, who saw the Serc's regulation as "one of the most blatant cases we have seen" of FDA error. Pointing to Section 505 (e) (3) of the Food, Drug and Cosmetic Act, which provided that the Secretary of Health, Education and Welfare "shall" withdraw a product if the agency determines that there is a "lack of substantial evidence" for its efficacy, Fountain and other critics demanded Serc's immediate market removal. In a pointed exchange in hearings before Fountain's House subcommittee, Simmons vigorously denied that his agency was under a statutory obligation to immediately withdraw the product: "We are not in an inflexible position where fact A inevitably leads to action B." Meanwhile, Fountain and his staff argued that the agency had no administrative discretion over the matter. Fountain's staff physician accused FDA general counsel Hutt of enacting "a government of men, not of laws." He then mocked Simmons by comparing his remarks about Serc and its studies to "the testimonials that FDA makes companies prove for the effectiveness of their products."[67]

---

sentatives, 35, 102–3. Notice of intent to withdraw: *FR*, July 17, 1968. In subsequent investigation, Morton Mintz reported that Serc allies, including several New York investment bankers, had lobbied the Administration and Congress, including Speaker of the House James McCormack, to try to derail the Administration's withdrawal decision; "Lobby Tries FDA Bypass; Promoters of Serc Drug Press Hill," *WP*, August 4, 1968, E1. Martin Sweig, a top aide to McCormack, later pleaded guilty in an unrelated case to perjury and conspiracy counts.

[66]The Elia study and almost all of Unimed's proposed alternatives in the dialogue with the FDA from 1968 to 1972 followed a "double-blind crossover design." Under a crossover design, all patients receive both the treatment and the control, but sequentially. Patients are randomized into one of the following two sequences: (1) administration of the treatment, then the placebo, or (2) administration of placebo, followed by the treatment. The dominant alternative to a crossover protocol is a more conventional "parallel" design in which some patients receive only the treatment, and others only the control. Elia, "Double-Blind Evaluation." Philip R. Jacoby, M.D., Memorandum of Conference (with Unimed, Inc.), Morristown, N.J., April 14, 1971. Simmons, Memorandum to Gerald F. Meyer (Director, Office of Legislative Services), September 22, 1972; *Fountain Serc Hearings*, 44–5. Throughout this period, Unimed was seeking other indications for the marketing of betahistine hydrochloride, including for memory enhancement in the elderly; "Heard on the Street," *WSJ*, March 14, 1968, 31.

[67]*Fountain Serc Hearings*, 58 ("most blatant"), 62 ("inflexible position"), 33 ("government of men, not of laws"), 53 ("testimonials"). Mintz, "FDA Assailed on Anti-Dizziness Medicine," *WP*, October 1, 1972, F6. Hutt had previously served as counsel for some of the nation's

Just beneath the politics of withdrawal lurked a politics of reputation, and a criticism of the original approval. The original medical reviewer, Dr. David Lidd, had testified before the Fountain committee that he opposed the drug's approval. Commissioner Herbert Ley would also admit that the Administration's dependence on the Elia study contradicted a "rigid" reading of the 1962 law's "substantial evidence" for provision for data on efficacy, which was widely interpreted as requiring two controlled clinical trials.[68]

The FDA terminated Serc's new drug application on December 21, 1972, five days after the Consumers' Union sued the agency for failure to remove Serc from the American marketplace. Betahistine hydrochloride has not since been available for prescription in the United States. It is used sparingly among Ménière's sufferers in Europe, Asia, Latin America, and Canada. The FDA's regulation of Serc is remarkable in that, even during a period of pronounced procedural conservatism—the very era that libertarian critics of the FDA identify as "the drug lag"—the Administration demonstrated a stark reluctance to revisit a past approval decision. From 1967 on, Administration officials had severe doubts about Serc's efficacy—doubts that were magnified by Unimed's furtive attempt to bypass the Administration and directly lobby members of Congress against withdrawal—and no top official doubted the agency's authority to remove the drug from the American marketplace. The final withdrawal decision came, symbolically enough, in response to challenges to the agency's reputation and power—the many broadsides of the Fountain hearings and the pointed Consumers' Union lawsuit.[69]

The event of safety-based drug withdrawal almost always occasions a probing inventory of the drug's pre-market review. In cases that have been reviewed most intensively by Congress, whether Serc for Ménière's syndrome in the 1970s, Merital for clinical depression in the 1980s, Propulsid for gastrointestinal reflux disease in the 1990s, or for a host of drugs whose NDAs were cleared after 2000—Arava for rheumatoid arthritis, Baycol for high cholesterol, Bextra for general inflammation and rheumatoid arthritis—discussions of product withdrawal seem universally accompanied by a debate about the propriety and rigor of the original NDA decision.[70]

---

larger pharmaceutical companies, and was roundly criticized during the Serc affair as being too cozy with the industry; Jack Anderson, "FDA Hit on Failure to Ban Drug Serc," *WP*, November 24, 1972, D19.

[68] Mintz, "FDA Assailed on Anti-Dizziness Medicine," *WP*, October 1, 1972, F6. The first approved labeling for Serc was, in Mintz's words, "extremely modest," indicating to FDA critics the weakness of the underlying evidence.

[69] Mintz, "Lobby Tries FDA Bypass," *WP*, August 4, 1968, E1. "Serc, Vertigo Drug, Ordered Off Market," *WP*, January 5, 1973, E16. Mintz, "Consumer's Union Sues U.S. on Drug," *WP*, December 17, 1972.

[70] *Oversight of the New Drug Review Process and FDA's Regulation of Merital*, Hearing before a Subcommittee of the Committee on Government Operations, House of Representatives, 99th Congress, Second Session, May 22, 1986 (Washington, DC: GPO). See also "regulatory chronologies" for Propulsid, Arava, Baycol, and Bextra in GAO, *FDA Postmarket Drug*

In these revisitations, organizational discord is played along the dimensions of official and symbolic hierarchy, too. More elevated officials in CDER, who are drawn from the ranks of reviewers, often resist pressures for relabeling and withdrawal when ODS officials suggest it or when Public Citizen or another advocacy organization demands it by means of a press release or a citizens' petition. In some cases, interestingly enough, these FDA post-market conservatives are the same officials who delayed NDA approval in the initial review. Hence, different concerns will be voiced, and different incentives faced, by the same individuals at different times (pre-approval versus post-approval), and at the same time at different levels of the hierarchy.

The FDA's public reputation as patient and consumer protector in the American health-care system is a powerful one, and the incentives for its protection consciously and unconsciously influence much regulatory behavior. Indeed, while the usual "conflict of interest" debates in drug regulation pertain to advisory committee representatives who have received industry money, the embedment of authority over post-marketing surveillance in the Office of New Drugs creates a different but no less real "conflict of interest" that current policy has just begun to recognize. The very office of the FDA that approves new drugs—and which therefore has the least reputation-based incentives to revisit its past approval decisions—is also the office with legal authority over post-marketing. As the General Accounting Office has recognized, the ODS, which houses the agency's epidemiologists and its major capacities for post-market surveillance, is only a weak "consultant" to the Office of New Drugs (OND).[71]

It is perhaps audacious to claim, and certainly difficult to prove, that reputation-related incentives weaken the Office of New Drugs' willingness to scrutinize drugs that have already been approved. Yet at the level of plausibility, characterizations to this effect have been with us for fifty years, and they have usually been advanced by FDA officers themselves. In 1963, John Nestor testified before Congress that FDA medical reviewers were discouraged from revisiting past approval decisions: "What the problem seemed to be was that in making present decisions, it was sort of sacrosanct situation that we were not to question decisions made in the past." Four decades later, Office of Drug Safety epidemiologist David Graham would testify in front of the Senate Finance Committee. "My experience with Vioxx," Graham stated, "is typical of how CDER responds to serious drug safety issues in general." In a riveting metaphor that endures long after his testimony concluded in 2004, Graham lamented that "the new drug reviewing division that approved the drug in the first place and that regards it as its own child, typically proves to be the single greatest obstacle to effectively dealing with serious drug safety issues."[72]

While the reluctance of FDA officials to revisit the Vioxx approval may

Safety, GAO-06-0402, 39–57. See also the discussion of the Vioxx approval and controversy in chapter 12, "A Reputation in Relief."

[71]GAO, FDA Postmarket Drug Safety, GAO-06-402 (2006), 19.

[72]See Nestor's remark in 1963 that "although my frankness was acceptable before I was hired, after joining the organization I found that any medical opinion that raised issues that

have been exceptional, reflection suggests that the Vioxx episode is not without precedent. In the fifteen years before Vioxx, Graham and his ODS colleagues attempted to remove ten other drugs from the market. It is fair to say that not one of these product withdrawals was uncontroversial within the agency's ranks. Graham and his colleagues have received at least some opposition from within the FDA whenever his office has supported market withdrawal for a specific drug.

An absolutely critical caveat merits discussion here. Discord between the Administration's drug reviewing divisions and the Office of Drug Safety does not imply that a drug was wrongly approved, or that the ODS is right. Yet Graham's remarks are telling because they point out an essential and underlying conflict between the identity and the incentives of those who approve and those who monitor. The conflict of identity is also a conflict of methodology, between clinical pharmacology (and its legacy) and epidemiology, between the methodology of randomized clinical trials and the methodology of observational studies.

FDA observers and FDA officials themselves have consistently pointed to institutional reluctance to revisit past decisions. One need not agree entirely with either Nestor's or Graham's broader arguments to see the plausibility of their depictions of the FDA. Conflicts about reputation thus get built into the very structure of the Administration. The reputation-based identities and incentives governing CDER's drug approval offices (not to draw public attention to regulatory error) conflict directly with the identities and incentives governing the Office of Drug Safety (ODS) to scrutinize the products that CDER has approved.[73]

Because the Office of New Drugs controls the agenda of an advisory committee meeting, it can and does exclude skeptical voices from the ODS. In March 2003, the Arthritis Advisory Committee met to review the safety and efficacy of Arava (leflunomide) in the context of other medications available for the treatment of rheumatoid arthritis. The OND review division that had approved Arava presented its own analysis but did not allow the ODS staff—who had recommended that Arava be removed from the American market—to present their analysis. About one year later, in February 2004, the Psychopharmacologic Drugs Advisory Committee excluded an ODS epidemiologist who had intended to report an association between SSRIs and suicidality in teenage and adolescent patients, particularly for the drug Paxil (paroxetine).[74]

---

involved reappraisal of past decisions, past policies, or past commitments to the pharmaceutical industry would be challenged—not in a healthy scientific atmosphere, but, rather, with indifference, disapproval, or even hostility." See *Interagency Coordination in Drug Research and Regulation*, Hearings before the Subcommittee on Reorganization and International Organizations of the Committee on Government Operations, U.S. Senate, 89th Congress, 1st Session, March 20, 1963, Part 3, "The Bureau of Medicine in the Food and Drug Administration," pp. 783, 790. D. Graham, The FDA, Merck and Vioxx: Putting Patient Safety First? [online], http://finance.senate.gov/hearings/testimony/2004test/111804dgtest.pdf.

[73]GAO, *FDA Postmarket Drug Safety*, (GAO-06-402), 22.

[74]Ibid., 21–2. The term "suicidality" has been much misunderstood. Properly speaking, it

In April 2006, a GAO audit found the Office of Drug Safety's role unclear. ODS staff raised issues about drugs on the American market, but some felt their advice was falling into a "black hole" or "abyss." The system of post-market regulation is characterized by informal procedures, and by consultation, whereas the pre-market approval system is highly routinized, with a stable division of labor and fixed roles, much as the German sociologist Max Weber described the typical bureaucracy in his 1920s writings.[75]

The withdrawal of a product is nonbureaucratic in other ways, insofar as withdrawal bespeaks a symbolic message to the Administration's public audiences. It signifies awareness and action on the part of the Administration. An illustrative case comes in the FDA's 2005 response to reports of progressive multifocal leukoencephalopathy (PML) in multiple sclerosis patients taking Tysabri (natalizumab). Tysabri was withdrawn from the market in February 2005. Following Tysabri's withdrawal, the Administration also stopped Phase 2 clinical trials of another drug in its class—GlaxoSmith-Kline's 683699. As David Feigal, by then former director of the FDA's Center for Devices and Radiological Health, stated to a *Nature Medicine* reporter, "the FDA and the companies had to take some sort of action to show the public that they are committed to safety." Karl Kieburtz, the chairman of the advisory panel for Tysabri and a professor of neurology at the University of Rochester, applied a sort of regulatory Hippocratic oath to the case: "Nobody knew the scope of the problem," he said, and "In the absence of information you have to act on the principle of 'do no harm.'"[76]

Withdrawal and warnings are symbolic in another way, for they are often initiated by the Administration, but the dirtier work is performed by the company sponsor. FDA officials have long presented their policy as one of providing "publicity" and "public warnings" for drug withdrawals. This is not a lie. Yet it conceals a deeper pattern whereby the withdrawal action (and its original announcement) is attributed to the firm.[77]

The choreography of product withdrawals in the United States has an implicit structure, one founded in regulatory practice. The events of drug

refers not just to suicidal "thinking" but to suicidal "ideation," the visualization of an attempt of suicide such as when a depressed person envisions himself entering a tall building, taking an elevator to the top, and jumping off of the roof. In contemporary psychiatric treatment guidelines, doctors, psychologists, and social workers are encouraged to intervene actively—including temporary institutionalization of the patient—when such ideation is reported.

[75]GAO, *FDA Postmarket Drug Safety*, (GAO-06-402), 23. For informal norms and networks in formal organizations, see Peter Blau, *Dynamics of Bureaucracy* (Chicago: University of Chicago Press, 1955).

[76]These issues surrounding the Tysabri withdrawal were reported in Emily Waltz, "US Drug Approval Ignores Science's Subtleties," *Nature Medicine* 12 (4) (April 2006): 373. Waltz errs considerably in stating that "Once a treatment is on the market, the FDA cannot pull it off the shelves unless the information on its label is fraudulent. But the agency can use its power to persuade a company to withdraw it."

[77]Goodrich, "Follow-Up on New Drug Applications, Reporting of Clinical and Other Experience, and Removal of Drugs from Market," June 27–28, 1963, p. 5; DF 505.53, RG 88, NA.

warnings and withdrawals are highly sequenced, even predictable from the vantage that retrospection provides. After some internal agency debate about the matter, perhaps coupled with a demand from Public Citizen and like organizations, the Administration requests the company to withdraw the drug, the company makes an announcement that it is withdrawing, and the Administration then follows the company's announcement with a public health advisory. Another sequence is seen in the Vioxx episode: a company alert to FDA, followed by a company announcement, accompanied by a moderating and reassuring Administration statement. Here the silences and absences speak louder than do the actual pronouncements. What we do not see in the United States is an FDA announcement followed by company moderation. As Israeli political scientist Moshe Maor has carefully documented, regulatory sequences in which the difficult news (and a sense of culpability) is delivered only by the agency are common in Australia, Canada, Great Britain, and New Zealand.[78]

To say that drug safety dramas possess a structure and a choreography is not to say that the Administration has somehow rigged or manipulated the system. There is no conspiracy here. There are numerous purposes and interests served by the present structure, and it has evolved if not organically, then somewhat contingently through regulatory contest and practice. In this arrangement, the company and not the FDA incurs the physical costs of printing hundreds of thousands of letters. Yet the structure is one which places the Administration above the fray, that identifies the company with the bad news, and that permits major media outlets (newspapers, television channels, and websites) to rehearse these images—and their assignments of responsibility—in their coverage.

. . .

In 1963, at a Federal Bar Association conference on the new drug statute passed into law the previous year, FDA General Counsel William W. Goodrich offered a sober review of post-market drug regulation at his agency.

> We in FDA have long recognized the problems of new drug control after the application has become effective. There has been no affirmative requirement that we be kept informed about clinical experience as it emerged, or indeed that we be supplied with the promotional material prepared by the sponsor or his ad agency after the so-called final printed labeling was made a part of our new drug file. Upon receipt of this printed labeling, the problem became an inspectional one to maintain surveillance over promotional material and a job of medical detection to dredge up the most obscure note or minor comment that may furnish the first sign that the drug was performing as expected or that some unexpected side effect or untoward reaction might attend the use of the drug in actual clinical practice.[79]

[78] Maor, "Organizational Reputation and the Public Observability of Drug Warnings in 10 Countries," manuscript, Department of Political Science, Hebrew University, Jerusalem, 2006.
[79] William W. Goodrich, "Follow-Up on New Drug Applications, Reporting of Clinical and Other Experience, and Removal of Drugs from Market," speech delivered at the Federal Bar

Viewing Goodrich's portrait four decades later, it presaged much of the federal government's quandary in post-market regulation. By and large, the Administration's problem in the late twentieth century remained "an inspectional one," sifting through data that were unsystematic, scattered to the far ends of the continent and the globe. Many of the agency's (and the nation's) problems stemmed from the general limitation of FDA power to pharmaceutical firms, and its lack of power over others who might inform the agency about clinical experience, not least American physicians and hospitals. William Goodrich went on to laud the new requirements of the law— the multiform requirements placed upon pharmaceutical companies that they submit adverse event data to the FDA, that they comply with dozens of new FDA rules, that they relabel their products with ever greater frequency and care. Yet in complimenting the new law for its changes, Goodrich unwittingly told a very plausible tale of why, in the ensuing four decades, post-marketing regulation would prove so difficult and ineffectual. In the main, the Administration's power remains embedded in the new drug application, and the vast share of that power is directed toward firms.

Recent changes in the Food and Drug Administration Act of 2007 and other initiatives have, at least officially, shifted the institutional focus of the FDA toward different lenses of post-market surveillance. The agency now has authorities at its disposal for requiring NDA sponsors to plan and complete Phase 4 studies, for mandating the company-led execution of Risk Evaluation and Mitigation Strategies, for continually querying and analyzing large-scale electronic claims and prescription databases (a set of patterns embedded in a new "Sentinel Initiative") and, at least in statute, for imposing genuine penalties upon firms that do not comply with the letter or the spirit of the new federal legislation. Yet the very proposal and enactment of these institutional reforms and others—whatever their ultimate effect— flowed from a far-reaching and broadly shared critique of the twentieth-century regime of American pharmaceutical regulation. In that critique, voiced repeatedly over the past half-century, observers lamented the asymmetry of regulatory power on the two sides of the regulatory gate—the state-governed interface between scientific development and commercial market.

Association Brief Conference on the New Drug Law, Washington, DC, June 27–28, 1963; DF 505.53, RG 88, NA.

The Détente of Firm and Regulator

> The manner in which a thing is done has more influence than
> is commonly imagined. Men are governed by opinion; this
> opinion is as much influenced by appearances as by realities;
> if a Government appears to be confident of its own powers,
> it is the surest way to inspire the same confidence in others;
> if it is diffident, it may be certain, there will be a still greater
> diffidence in others, and that its authority will not only
> be distrusted, controverted, but contemned.
>
> —Alexander Hamilton, letter of 1780[1]

ASTRIDE the Administration itself, there is no more central or powerful agent in the development, evaluation, production, and marketing of medicines than the organization commonly known as a "drug company." Most of the sponsors of investigational drugs and new drug applications are for-profit entities. Among these are both privately held companies and publicly owned (stock) corporations. There are, to be sure, important roles played by nonprofit, academic, and government organizations in drug development and distribution. There are telling cases of national and academic sponsorship—numerous antibiotics of the middle twentieth century serve as examples, and many of the drugs in the arsenal of modern cancer chemotherapy, having been first investigated by the National Cancer Institute, are also reminders of the significant government and academic role in drug development. So too, a meaningful debate has raged for decades, concerned with just how much credit for medical innovation should be assigned to the global pharmaceutical industry. The precise contribution of any one organization to a drug's development is difficult to ascertain. In terms of money invested, pharmaceutical companies have over the past two decades clearly expended the greatest fraction of resources in pre-market development of drugs. Indeed, the fraction of drug development accounted for by for-profit entities arguably has been increased by the Administration's investigational

---

[1] Hamilton (writing at Liberty Pole) to James Duane, September 3, 1780; in Joanne B. Freeman, ed., *Hamilton: Writings* (New York: Library of America, 2001), 86.

new drug regulations. Yet the centrality of the pharmaceutical industry in drug development is perhaps best reflected in the structure and behavior of the FDA itself. Most of the agency's regulatory procedures and administrative patterns have been designed or adapted for interaction with for-profit entities, for engagement with pharmaceutical firms and the researchers with whom they contract.[2]

As property holders in dynastic Europe approached the crown in supplication, so do pharmaceutical firms appear as petitioners of sorts before the Administration. They come asking for rights conferred only by the sovereign: the legal permission to produce, distribute, and make particular claims about a chemical entity in the national commerce of the largest and most profitable drug market in the world. One mapping of the supplication metaphor is ceremonial. The act of developing a drug is a regulatory and legal process, and it establishes something of a ritual, including a detailed list of procedures to be satisfied and followed. These hurdles, and the real probability of a wish denied, are barriers that deter or delay many weak applications from being submitted. Another mapping of the supplication metaphor comes in the partial equality of petitioner and sovereign. Not unlike the crowns of early modern Europe, the regulator is partially dependent upon its sponsors. If the regulator acts so harshly that the pipeline of new drugs dries up, the Administration will invite a good portion of the resulting blame. More ominously, if the petitioners revolt and attack the legal and political authority of the sovereign, the sovereign's power can be undermined. The petitioners desire the good will of the sovereign, but the sovereign needs theirs as well.[3]

The metaphor of supplication is revealing in its failures as well as in its correspondence. Pharmaceutical firms in the United States are no mere petitioners but form some of the wealthiest and most powerful organizations on the planet. Company by company over the past half-century, pharmaceutical firms have established and nurtured entire "regulatory affairs departments"—staffed with hundreds, and with hundreds of others employed by contracts—to present the case for drug approval to the Administration and to its advisory committees, to resolve issues pertaining to manufacturing and inspections, and to fend off or smooth regulation of marketing. The new drug application process has become embedded in organizational rou-

[2]There are important exceptions to the engineering of FDA structure for the regulation of for-profit entities, not least the agreements hammered out between top NCI and FDA officials in the late 1970s (see chapter 6). Yet they form the exception that proves the rule. The agreements were necessary because the NCI was so distinct in its political authority and scientific legitimacy from pharmaceutical firms.

[3]Gwylim Dodd, *Justice and Grace: Private Petitioning and the English Parliament in the Late Middle Ages* (Oxford: Oxford University Press, 2007). User fee legislation may have increased this dependence, insofar as much of the FDA budget now comes from per-application taxes on NDA submissions. If the amount of NDAs submitted were hypothetically to decline, then so would the user fee portion of the Administration's budget and staffing resources.

tine, and the individuals who negotiate and manage this process successfully are some of the most sought-after personalities in global business.

At its core, the new drug application process defines an identity, an existence at law, and a dimension of expertise. Since 1938 and forcefully since the middle 1950s, U.S. regulation has converted the pharmaceutical firm from a "producer" to a "sponsor." This transformation of economic identity amounts to much more than a purely interpretive matter. Over the past half-century, the variable capacity of firms to negotiate the regulatory process and to present credible cases for drug approval has become a crucial determinant of profit and survival. For pharmaceutical firms and biotechnology companies, "success" consists not merely in the discovery of new molecules or in finding new uses for old molecules. Success demands much more than this: a reputation of credibility with the regulator and with allied professional communities, and a durable capacity to petition the sovereign for rights. Firms differentiate themselves from one another in their variable abilities to make a good case, to convey believably the products of their research. These differences, it is plausible to say, account for vast disparities in wealth—easily tens of billions of dollars worth, perhaps much more—among firms and their shareholders. Over the past half-century, large disparities in regulatory success have evolved and persisted among firms, larger than can be plausibly explained by some of the factors that are often invoked to account for such variability.

The structure of the American pharmaceutical market dictates that firms must interact repeatedly and successfully with the gatekeeper if they are to generate profits and remain profitable. In the United States, drugs lose patent protection after a specified period of time—now twenty years from the patent date, occasionally extensible by various legal maneuvers—and when they do, they lose nearly all of their profitability. They lose even more in the United States, where the prices under patent protection are constrained neither by government regulation nor by the government's monopsony power as the sole purchaser in a national health insurance system. In 2006, for instance, generic drugs accounted for 50 percent of all prescriptions—that is, all drug regimens taken by Americans—but only 15 percent of the spending. Pharmaceutical companies generate most of their revenues and nearly all of their profits from the sales and valuation of molecules whose patents have yet to expire. Because all drugs will lose their patent protection, then, the profitability (and capital market valuation) of pharmaceutical companies depends in great part upon their pipeline of therapies: the new drugs that have not yet made it to market and that will need a successful NDA process to get there. Yet this fact just compels the firm to appear before the gatekeeper once more. This necessity of repeated interaction has some properties that convey advantages for the regulator and for the longer-lived firm, as repetition helps to surmount the difficulties that attach to one-shot interaction. The firm can renege on informal agreements and misbehave only if it never expects to come before the regulator again. But every firm that wants to make a long-term profit will have to come before the regulator repeatedly. Except for some recent companies in the biotechnology industry model, very few firms are established to produce and market one drug only. Indeed, as will become clear in the following pages, a political economy of credibility ensures that there are few such firms. Moreover, firms with a successful NDA often intend to market one drug in many therapeutic markets, thus necessitating a supplemental NDA, and another appearance before the regulator.

This continual dependence of firms on the regulator begets a kind of obedience and fear among individual companies, and Administration officials have at times recognized and even exploited this fact. In order to establish meaningful precedents and to secure compliance with objectives, it is necessary for the agency occasionally to "make an example" of individual firms when the evidence is clear that they have transgressed FDA regulations. This occasional but real bullying is at once a form or reputation-making and a form of *divide et impera* strategy, in that firms castigated in harsh fashion are set apart from the larger industry.

The relationship between firms and regulator is more complicated, though, because pharmaceutical firms have a political existence as "industry." Firms are collectively organized in the United States, primarily (but not entirely) under the Pharmaceutical Research and Manufacturers of America (PhRMA). In the past several decades the political resources and organization possessed by the global pharmaceutical industry have grown immensely. Speaking hyperbolically, Vermont Senator Bernie Sanders recently declared that in American politics and policymaking, "As powerful as the oil companies are, as powerful as the banks are, as powerful as corporate America, in general, is, in influencing legislation, the pharmaceutical industry stands as a world unto itself. They never lose."[4]

A regulator animated and constrained by reputation carries on a set of complicated and multidimensional relationships with pharmaceutical firms whose content is also laden with reputation and image. Firms balance their desire to market drugs in profitable ways with their need for regulatory credibility. Administration officials acknowledge the need to project an image that inspires a moderate degree of fear among firms, but not so much antagonism that the firms as a collective (as "industry") mobilize to weaken the regulator's essential authorities. The "bad cop" face of enforcement and induced obedience must be balanced by the "good cop" face of assistance in development and recognition of valid research. In the politics of reputation, pharmaceutical regulation becomes a complex and multidimensional process of equipoise. Regulation establishes and perpetuates forceful ambiguity.[5]

[4] Sanders statement in interview with journalist Bill Moyers, "Bill Moyers Journal," "Congressional Ethics," aired June 1, 2007 on Public Broadcasting System; transcript available at http://www.pbs.org/moyers/journal/06012007/transcript1.html [accessed July 22, 2009].

[5] For mathematical models that simplify much of this logic, see Daniel Carpenter and Michael Ting, "Regulatory Errors with Endogenous Agendas," *American Journal of Political*

FROM PRODUCER TO SPONSOR: THE REGULATORY REMAKING
OF THE MODERN PHARMACEUTICAL FIRM

Understanding the modern pharmaceutical firm requires, among other things, concepts developed in law, economics, the sociology of networks and organizations and, not least, politics and culture. The notion of a firm in law and finance—as a holder of property and as claimant to the aggregated residual (profit or loss) separating marginal revenue from marginal cost—certainly applies. Ideas from classical industrial organization are also essential; drug companies integrate research and development and production, and they fold within one organization what can be more profitably "internalized" than purchased upon the marketplace. This helps to account for why many drugs are developed not within the laboratories of the companies selling them, but by other companies whose products are purchased by the firm that eventually becomes the drug's sponsor. Integration helps explain why in the middle of the twentieth century, many pharmaceutical companies grew out of bulk chemical manufacturers, but why today modern pharmaceutical companies employ many thousands more sales than manufacturing personnel and why they purchase most of their bulk ingredients from other firms.[6]

In pharmaceuticals as in many other areas, the firm serves as a nexus of contracts and a connective network webbing together various nodes of information and expertise. As scholars and students of urban space have observed of cities and their role in political, economic, and social development, pharmaceutical firms have become meeting places for ideas and methods from academia, medicine, in-house labs, and notions aggregated from the global medical literature. This fact of connectivity underscores the dependence of the drug company on other organizations and structures (academics, professions, public sector investment), just as it gestures to the companies' pivotal role in integrating the ideas and factors produced by these nonprofit sectors.[7]

Science 51 (4) (Oct. 2007): 835–52; Steven Callendar and Daniel Carpenter, "Ambiguity in Approval Regulation," manuscript, Northwestern University.

[6] At the core of "institutional" scholarship in economics over the past three decades, scholars have asked "What is a firm?" and "Why is economic production organized within a firm as opposed to a market?" For a classic take on this question from the perspective of "transaction costs," see Oliver Williamson, *Markets and Hierarchies* (New York: Free Press, 1979). There is a vast literature on the nature of the firm in economics, sociology, organization science, and management, not to mention other disciplines.

[7] A series of studies of inter-organizational networks has linked "centrality" and "brokerage" properties of firms to superior market and durability outcomes; Woody W. Powell, Douglas R. White, Kenneth W. Koput, and Jason Owen-Smith, "Network Dynamics and Field Evolution: The Growth of Inter-organizational Collaboration in the Life Sciences," *American Journal of Sociology* 110(4) (Jan. 2005):1132–1205. For insightful historical treatments of the role of external networks in the development of pharmaceutical firms, see John Swann, *Academic Scientists and the Pharmaceutical Industry: Cooperative Research in Twentieth-Century America* (Baltimore: Johns Hopkins University Press, 1988); Geoffrey Tweedale, *At the Sign of the Plough: Allen & Hanburys and the British Pharmaceutical Industry, 1715–1990* (London: John Murray, 1990); Nicolas Rasmussen, "The Drug Industry and Clinical Research in Interwar

Firms are also literal "brand names." They are carriers of variable status and legitimacy, and these symbolic residues of a firm rest inevitably upon its members, contractors, and produced commodities. These extensions of the firm usually enter a marketplace where the firm's reputation precedes them. The effects of image are crucial in the pharmaceutical realm, in part because the primary consumers of drugs include not only patients but also their physicians. Drug companies and biotechnology firms gain and lose, survive and go bankrupt as holders of reputations. They bear reputations not simply with respect to a community of prescribers but a community of evaluators in academic medicine and another community of evaluators in finance. Among these audiences, the firms' various dimensions of performance— manufacturing, R&D, marketing—receive endless and painstaking assessment. In all three of these dimensions, particularly the last two, the firm is often defined by its reputation: by its perceived expertise, rigor, subtlety, caution, or lack of these virtues.[8]

The role of the firm as regulatory sponsor defines perhaps the most central and durable identity for contemporary pharmaceutical companies. Since the middle of the twentieth century, the sponsor function has established a primary basis of difference, status, and wealth among firms. Simply put, those companies that better develop their products and negotiate the regulatory process take up a position of economic superiority vis-à-vis their competitors, actual and potential. Other things equal, effective sponsors profit and endure while firms that poorly manage regulation are more likely to fail. The firm's status as sponsor recasts the regulator as an audience, a constant evaluator of the firm's intentions and capacities. And like other audiences, the regulator picks apart the firm in the continual act of assessment; the Administration's officers may trust a company's research and development but doubt that same company's marketing branch. These judgments will, sooner or later, have an important and asymmetric influence upon those of other audiences. Financial analysts in New York and Hong Kong may value a drug company's R&D pipeline highly, but if the Administration values it less, it is the financial valuation that will drop, not the regulatory judgment that will rise.

So central is regulation to the existence and endurance of pharmaceutical firms that many global drug companies have become regulatory carriers, operating primarily as sponsors of the research and production that other companies have sold to them. Research can be done elsewhere, by entire companies that are later purchased (themselves or their star products) by

America: Three Types of Physician Collaborator," *BullHistMed* 79 (1) (2005): 50–80. Louis Galambos, *Networks of Innovation: Vaccine Development at Merck* (New York: Cambridge University Press, 1997). Alfonso Gambardella, *Science and Innovation: The US Pharmaceutical Industry during the 1980s* (Cambridge: Cambridge University Press, 1995), particularly chap. 4.

[8] Neil Fligstein, *The Transformation of Corporate Control* (Cambridge, MA: Harvard University Press, 1990).

larger entities. Manufacturing can be contracted out and is often done half a world away from the laboratories in which the drug is developed and tested. Increasingly over the late twentieth century, what qualifies firms like Merck and Pfizer as "drug companies" is their marketing organization and their central role in the process of bringing a drug to and through the Administration's review processes, negotiating with the regulator about marketing, labeling, manufacturing, and future development of the drug for other therapeutic markets. This is not a trivial identity, for legal rights to market a drug in interstate commerce are rights vested with the sponsor. The sponsor becomes an owner of property rights that are bequeathed by the regulator.

These different concepts of the firm help in tracing out the ecology of pharmaceutical companies over the past half-century. Historically, the "drug companies" have not been a monolith, and important divisions have endured among companies that compete against one another, as well as between producers and developers of different types (biotechnology companies versus older, chemically based drug makers). All of these firms have been fundamentally reshaped by developments in science, political economy, and regulation over the last half-century, but along with the changes there are some continuities. Pharmaceutical firms emerged from different types and their hybrids. They evolved from large chemical manufacturers that created laboratory divisions in the interwar period (Pfizer; Merck, Sharp and Dohme). They grew from old-line drug houses (Abbott Laboratories, Upjohn, and Parke-Davis). The firms that emerged at mid-century were able to blend chemical innovation with marketing capacity. Marketing, in particular the existence of a vast and geographically dispersed sales force, defines the competitive advantage of many modern pharmaceutical firms, and marketing accounts for the largest fraction of employees among some of the notable giants of the industry.[9]

CREDIBILITY AND FIRM STRUCTURE IN THE TWENTIETH CENTURY

The sponsorial role of the modern pharmaceutical company evolved from regulatory as well as scientific forces. The creation of pre-market approval processes, combined with the architecture of the modern clinical trial, compelled

[9]This narrative is much more complicated than can be attempted here, so the points registered are but précis's of other, more capable summaries. See Alfred Chandler, *Shaping the Industrial Century: The Remarkable Story of the Evolution of the Modern Chemical and Pharmaceutical Industries* (Cambridge, MA: Harvard University Press, 2005); Viviane Quirke, *Collaboration in the Pharmaceutical Industry: Changing Relationships in Britain and France, 1935–1965* (London: Routledge, 2008). These narratives are valuable but many of them (particularly Chandler's) ignore the significance of regulation in shaping the structure of the modern pharmaceutical industry. For a careful and compelling analysis of how drug companies negotiated crucial relationships between academic medicine and marketing forces in the twentieth century, consult Jeremy Greene, *Prescribing by Numbers: Drugs and the Definition of Disease* (Baltimore: Johns Hopkins University Press, 2007).

drug companies worldwide to overhaul their development processes in short order, particularly during the two decades spanning the mid-1950s to the mid-1970s. Many firms of an earlier generation (Dover Laboratories, Eaton Laboratories, the William S. Merrell Company) did not survive this ecological shock, and those that survived did so by abandoning many drugs that would have been considered profitable bets just fifteen years earlier. As firms refocused their efforts on the drugs that would make it to market in a new world order, they also adopted various structural and procedural reforms that redefined the notion of a drug company and its "company man."[10]

The most suggestive changes were those that, both intentionally and unintentionally, conveyed signals of respectability to audiences in academic medicine, science, and the federal government. Companies established new programs in pharmacology, and they increasingly formalized their links to academic pharmacologists and therapeutic reformers, particularly in the infectious diseases field. Top names like Alfred Gilman and Louis Goodman became ever more sought after for their expertise, for their students, and for their casual judgment on firms' multiyear R&D plans.[11]

Companies began to create separate initiatives and organizations for the management and planning of pharmaceutical research and development. In 1968, Abbott established its "Operation Expedite," which focused on more rapid development of promising "target" drugs and the principle that "Best Drug Leads Get Priority." Like other companies of the time, Abbott was narrowing its search for the most promising compounds, discarding less alluring development projects, in large measure because the Administration's standards had compelled a focus on those products most likely to clear the regulatory bar. At Abbott, this sort of planning was soon assigned to specific managers and administered by particular offices. So too, in January 1971, Smith, Kline and French announced "a major realignment of the corporate organization" (table 10.1). The company configured its global organization along product lines and slowly phased out its international division that had managed product lines in foreign markets. At the center of the transformation was the creation of a division (and an associated position) with centralized global responsibility for all human ethical pharmaceutical R&D. The firm created a new "vice president for pharmaceutical research and development." New occupant Bryce Douglas had not only taken over the responsi-

---

[10] In the United States especially, the pharmaceutical world of this time—scientists, engineers, marketing personnel, middle managers, and corporate leaders—was an overwhelmingly male one. In this light, Frances Kelsey's centrality to the regime of pharmaceutical regulation in the United States (and much of the world) in the late twentieth century is all the more noteworthy.

[11] I acknowledge conversations with Jeremy Greene and Scott Podolsky for several of the insights in this paragraph. I bear full responsibility for the statements and any errors. William N. Creasy (President, Burroughs-Wellcome) to Goodman, May 14, 1965; B11, F "Burroughs-Wellcome," LSG. For Goodman's (solicited) advice on Smith, Kline and French's R&D operating plan, see Goodman to Harold A. Clymer (Vice President, R&D, Smith, Kline and French), January 27, 1971; B11, F "SK&F," LSG. For SK&F's solicitation of names for a research management post, see Bryce Douglas to Goodman, August 8, 1979; B11, F "SK&F," LSG.

TABLE 10.1
Smith Kline and French Corporate Leadership after 1971 Reorganization

President and Chairman of the Board (Tom Rauch)

Executive Vice President (Robert F. Dee)

Group Vice President, Pharmaceuticals (Donald van Roden)

Vice President, Pharmaceutical Research and Development (Bryce Douglas)

Group Vice President, International Operations (Stanley Fenwick) [scheduled
to be phased out, responsibilities transferred to other Group VPs, except in
pharmaceuticals, where they are transferred to VP of Pharmaceutical R&D]

Group Vice President, Ultrasonic Products and Corporate Technical Services
(Alfred J. D'Angelo)

President, Branson Instruments (Walter Bleistein)

President, Branson Sonic Power (Stanley Jacke)

Group Vice President, Medical Services and Instruments, and Animal Health
Products (Lewis E. Harris)

Vice President, U.S. Consumer Products Division (Peter Godfrey)

Vice President, Corporate Business Development (Harold A. Clymer)

Note: **Boldface** denotes new position. Charge: "will direct all human pharmaceutical re-
search and coordinate human pharmaceutical development throughout the Corporation."
Source: SK&F announcement, untitled, January 25, 1971; B11, F "Smith Kline and French,"
LSG.

bilities of his predecessor, but nervously confessed that "I must now become
the architect for the worldwide R&D structure within the broad concept of
product line management." One of the most powerful rationales for centralization was the regulatory climate. As drug development in general was
slowing down, the competitive value of speed and selectivity was increasing.
Companies began to establish positions of authority where new products
could be negated internally during the IND process, in response to clinical
results, in anticipation of FDA actions, or in response to agency signals.[12]

---

[12]For a summary discussion of the "Expedite Plan," see Abbott Laboratories, *Annual Report 1969* (Abbott Park, IL: Abbott Laboratories), 20. SK&F announcement, untitled, January
15, 1971; Douglas to Goodman, March 5, 1971; B11, F "SK&F," LSG. The post of vice president of human pharmaceutical R&D was first given to Bryce Douglas. Similar transformations
occurred at Warner Lambert Company, which established a Research Division with a Health
Care Group; Bryce Douglas to Goodman, B 11, F "SK&F," LSG. Burroughs-Wellcome also
sponsored a "scholars program" in clinical pharmacology and had been granting Clinical Pharmacology Awards since 1959; George Hitchings (President, Burroughs-Wellcome Fund) to
Goodman, April 17, 1972; "New Officials for the Burroughs-Wellcome Fund," news release
(copy), June 11, 1971; B1, F16, LSG. SK&F had been at the vanguard of structured firm-FDA
liaisons since the 1950s, under the leadership of CEO Francis Boyer. See the organizational
changes detailed in *FDCR*, March 9, 1959, pp. 22–3.

At the same time that they produced forward-looking plans for research and development, companies also created new offices of liaison with the Administration. In 1965, Abbott Laboratories created two new vice-presidential positions (and associated divisions): a Vice President for Corporate Planning and a Vice President for Regulatory Affairs. Other global firms such as Squibb and Upjohn soon followed this pattern, creating regulatory affairs positions and offices in their U.S. pharmaceutical operations (though not in operations for foreign markets). In 1968, Upjohn copied Abbott's pattern, establishing a regulatory affairs department along with a "research planning" department. Global giants like Merck, Pfizer, and Wellcome also established regulatory affairs offices in the 1970s. The ongoing transformation in the organization of research and innovation was accompanied by a transformation in the structure of approach to government. It is not coincidental that these dual, co-evolving reforms came with the cementing of FDA regulatory structure and with the British Medicines Act of 1968, implemented in 1971.[13]

In companies large and small, the regulatory affairs department became one of the most powerful offices in the entire corporate organization, and regulatory affairs directors became ever more vital to the firm's success. Just after submitting three copies of a 32-volume NDA to the Bureau of Drugs, Robert J. Bever, regulatory affairs manager for Mallinckrodt, explained the nature of his division's work to other Mallinckrodt employees. "Although we are involved in the research period," Bever stated, "the Regulatory Affairs Section is the last step for all of the information acquired before it is compiled and sent to the FDA." Older companies like Mallinckrodt, submitting new drug applications under the new regime, were astonished at the size of the applications and saw in the NDA process a fundamental restructuring of their investment and marketing. "This NDA is the largest we have prepared to date," Bever continued, "but it is small compared with what some companies have had to prepare. The nature of our research has expended in the last several years, and many of our future NDA's will likely be this large or even larger."[14]

Some companies, including global giants like Wellcome, came more slowly to the concept of a separate organization for dealing with regulatory matters. The long-time head of regulatory affairs at Wellcome, former chemist

[13] Abbott Laboratories, *Annual Report 1966* (Abbott Park, IL: Abbott Laboratories), 3–4. Squibb-BeechNut, *Annual Report 1968* (New Brunswick, NJ: Squibb), 37. Upjohn Company, *Upjohn Annual Report 1968* (Kalamazoo, MI: Upjohn), 4. Warner-Lambert, *Annual Report 1973* (Morris Plains, NJ: Warner-Lambert), 35. Sterling Drug (which had taken over the reins of Winthrop Laboratories) added this position in 1976; *Annual Report 1976* (New York: Sterling Drug Company), 20. Merck, *Annual Report 1978* (Whitehouse Station, NJ: Merck & Co.), 20.

[14] "Size of NDA's to Increase," *The Benzene Ring*, Mallinckrodt Company Employee newsletter, March-April 1972; Mallinckrodt Company Scrapbooks, University of Missouri, St. Louis. Significantly, Bever's official title was "Manager, Regulatory Affairs, Pharmaceutical R&D Division"; at Mallinckrodt the work of regulation was folded within, but also inseparable from, a distinct organization given to drug R&D.

Don Knight, had started his career in regulatory affairs at Norwich Eaton. Dissatisfied with Eaton's legalistic approach to regulatory affairs, he decided to apply openly for a job whose identity was being created as he wrote.

> So after eight years at Norwich I decided I had better go look for another job and I wrote letters to companies, looking for a position in what I called regulatory affairs, and that was a word that was being used sparingly in some companies. And I got a letter back from Burroughs-Wellcome, basically said what's that? This was in 1970, late '70 or possibly early '71, and they told me they were building a new facility in Research Triangle Park, North Carolina, and it might be a good idea if I came down and talked to them about my thoughts about this regulatory affairs or whatever that is.[15]

At Wellcome in 1971, Don Knight hired paralegal Mary Lou Shenck from the company's legal affairs office, and together the two formed the company's first regulatory affairs department. Knight and Schenk would remain with the company into the 1990s, providing Burroughs-Wellcome with stability in crucial positions for almost three decades. From the early 1970s onward, moreover, Knight occupied what Burroughs-Wellcome executives perceived as a crucial position in product development; he reported directly to top corporate leaders. In 1972, just one year into his new position, Knight used his expertise on the FDA to help Wellcome officials establish a regulatory affairs office in Britain. As Burroughs-Wellcome turned its gaze to global pharmaceutical markets, the power of Knight—and at other companies, those like him—grew immensely. The management of regulatory affairs was perceived as hand-in-hand with corporate planning and the "globalization" of research and development. In Knight's memory, the perch of regulatory affairs director allowed a unique vantage on the entire corporation.

> One of the interesting things about regulatory affairs is that it is the one place in the company where you can get the opportunity to see everything. People in various areas of research see their own piece, the pharmacology, the chemistry, and that's what they are focusing on. The medical people are focusing on the clinical work and the marketing people are focusing on how we are actually going to market a product. Regulatory affairs is the one area in the company that sees the whole picture, that when we put a new drug application together you have an opportunity to get all the pieces from the various sections of the entire R&D process and

---

[15]Don Knight Oral History, interview February 6, 2002; in *Oral History of the Wellcome Foundation and Burroughs-Wellcome*, WLUK. Knight's dissatisfaction with Eaton was in part based upon his deference to the Administration and scientific standards of drug development: "And so I started to visit the FDA in Washington and meet some of the people, and then over time Norwich Eaton began to look at it as a legal challenge, the FDA was pushing the boundaries of what they were supposed to be doing, and therefore the people interacting with the FDA probably should be lawyers, or if I were to go the FDA, a lawyer should probably go with me, and I got very upset about it, and felt that this was not what we were there for. Science was the issue, not legal issues, and if we were going to bring new products to the market, it should be based on scientific evidence and not challenged legally at every step."

put it together to make a submission to a regulatory agency, whether it's in the US or somewhere else in the world, to be able to market the product. So regulatory becomes for me an opportunity to oversee the entire R&D process globally and as I gained more and more friends in the UK then I began to get more and more support to go the global route.[16]

The credibility-based transformation of the pharmaceutical company also came to marketing. CIBA, Robins, Syntex Laboratories, and Warner-Chilcott Laboratories were among the smaller firms that attempted to bestow "certification" upon their sales personnel. The companies contracted with the Certified Medical Representative's (CMR) Institute, which promised to subject sales personnel to the "approximate equivalent of 600 college classroom hours of intensive study." Upon completion of this program, the Institute promised, "They will be well-versed in advanced pharmacology, pharmaceutical history, bio-chemistry, research methodology, and other vital areas." Larger companies like Hoffmann-La Roche built these programs within their organizational structure. Company officials created the Roche Board-Certified Salesman Program in 1967, holding out the vision of a two-year effort that every certified salesman would need to endure in order to receive certification. At the peak of Roche's program was a National Certification Board established in 1971, chaired by none other than Louis Goodman himself.[17]

Like the Administration's own reformation, the transformation of the pharmaceutical industry composed a set of elaborate gestures meant to appeal to several audiences. At a time of growing technical complexity in drug development, accompanied by widespread distrust of the pharmaceutical industry among better-trained physicians and pharmacists, the education of salesmen and the observable strengthening of links to top pharmacologists were crucial status-boosting moves. As earlier in the century, drug companies turned to academic scientists to get some of their best ideas, and often proposed new products or combinations in "trial balloon" correspondence with academics. So too, changes in corporate investment practices, including the rise of new, prospective financial instruments, contributed to pharmaceutical companies' emphasis on corporate planning as a way of attract-

[16]Knight oral history, *Oral History of the Wellcome Foundation and Burroughs-Wellcome*, WLUK. It is important, in using these texts, to recognize that narrators may be prone to inflate their own significance in the history of the organization. This is a possibility with Knight's interview, and I perceive no way of entirely confirming or disconfirming his impressions. Support (not confirmation) for his portraiture comes from other Burroughs-Wellcome oral histories and from narratives of other regulatory affairs directors and their role in corporate planning and globalization initiatives.

[17]Certified Medical Representative's Institute (Roanoke, VA), undated advertisement entitled "We know of five companies that are putting as much into their men as they put into their products"; Roche Laboratories flyer, *Board Certified Health Services*; Stanley E. Kleiner (Associate Director, Career Development) to Goodman, February 17, 1971; in F 16 ("Hoffmann-La Roche"), LSG.

ing capital. These patterns were not limited to American firms but were actively copied overseas. In particular, British firms such as Imperial Chemical Industries actively incorporated regulatory affairs and testing structures into their corporate forms, in part out of mimicry of American arrangements.[18]

While the salience of the Administration as audience for firm structure should not be inflated, neither should it be gainsaid. Upon Louis Goodman's suggestion, Roche's curriculum for certified salesmen included a heavy dose of regulatory awareness. Among the required topics of Roche's training (on which salesmen were tested) were the history and structure of the FDA, the impact of the 1962 legislation, the NAS/NRC drug review, the movement toward name standardization that had been supported by the FDA, and "fixed-dose drug mixtures." The other mark of the Administration's centrality in these company-by-company reforms appears in the joint assembly of regulatory affairs departments and R&D or planning divisions for pharmaceuticals. Separate R&D posts and organizations were not established as frequently for medical devices and other consumer product lines. And the simultaneous creation of corporate planning and regulatory affairs units—the biggest wave of these arrivals coming from five to fifteen years after the 1962 Amendments—reveals how the regulatory era of the 1960s and 1970s generated a congeries of pressures for organizational reform in the pharmaceutical industry.[19]

The Limitations of Size: A Tale of Two California Start-Ups

The firms that successfully negotiated the transition to a new regulatory world traveled much more stable and predictable paths to drug development. Success in managing the transition was equivalent to the establishment of trust, in part through networks, in part through institutions, in part through reputation. New companies, particularly "biotechnology" firms

[18]Swann, *Academic Scientists and the Pharmaceutical Industry*. For numerous examples of firms suggesting new product possibilities to pharmacologists, see the "Burroughs-Wellcome" folder (B1, F14) and the "Hoffmann-La Roche folder" (B3, F8) in LSG. Roche's primary scientific contact with Goodman (and other academics) was Barney V. Pisha (Assistant Director, Professional Services); Pisha to Goodman, March 7, 1974; B3, F8. On the increasing pace of American investments in French laboratories and academics in the 1970s, see Sophie Chauveau, *L'Invention pharmaceutique: La pharmacie francaise entre l'Etat et la societe au XXe siecle* (Paris: Institut d'edition Sanofi-Synthelabo, 1999), 584–92. Fligstein, *Transformation of Corporate Control*; Chandler, *Shaping the Industrial Century*. Viviane Quirke, "The Impact of Thalidomide on the British Pharmaceutical Industry: The Case of Imperial Chemical Industries," in Jean-Paul Gaudillière and Volker Hess, eds., *Ways of Regulating: Therapeutic Agents between Plants, Shops and Consulting Rooms* (Berlin: Max Planck Institut für Wissenschaftgeschichte, Preprint 363, 2009), 125–41. Quirke, "Anglo-American relations and the co-production of American hegemony in pharmaceuticals," in H. Bonin and F. de Goey, eds, *American Firms in Europe* (Geneva: Droz, 2008).

[19]Goodman to Kleiner (Roche), February 22, 1971; B3, F 8, LSG.

whose pipeline was filled with novel therapeutic mechanisms, lacked the familiarity advantages of older firms that had made the necessary adjustments. The ability to liaison and project credibility—with personal and scientific familiarity, and with a structure of interface through "regulatory affairs" departments and executives—separated durable and profitable companies from those that faltered.

As California-based Genentech, now considered one of the "pioneer" firms of the biotechnology era, developed its human growth hormone therapies (somatostatin) and its heart treatment tPA in the late 1970s and early 1980s, its principal difficulties were regulatory ones. Genentech held numerous patents, dozens of them with promising therapeutic and economic potential, but the problem, as legal counsel admitted, was one of pushing "an elephant-sized body of rights... through the keyhole of the FDA regulatory process." For Genentech analysts, the concepts of "clinical development pipeline" and "FDA regulatory process" were essentially interchangeable. The dilemma of drug development was increasingly the saga of regulatory negotiation.

Genentech's early experience in these processes was one of alternating success and frustration, and one of powerful lessons. Genentech developers had defined surrogate endpoints in clinical trials for tPA; these endpoints were intermediate markers of health (dissolution of blood clots and improvement in patients' measured blood flow) that served as substitutes for the ultimate measure of therapeutic improvement, which was whether heart attack sufferers survived at higher rates. Genentech developers had, however, defined these endpoints without first passing the idea by the Bureau of Drugs. In testing their human growth hormone, Genentech had run out several clinical trials for a year longer than their scheduled duration. These procedural lapses met with robust skepticism among FDA reviewers and advisory committees. For the company's chief financial officer of the time, Fred Middleton, it was clear that Genentech's future success required familiarity and trust between the company and its regulator.

> We were just naive. The big drug companies had close relationships with the reviewers, they go to meetings, talk to them continuously, take them out to lunch. They know how they think. We were showing up in Washington, for the first time, with the guidebook, learning how to fill out the forms. People in Washington, being bureaucratic, being skeptical of this small company from California—took a very tough and somewhat adversarial position with us. Their attitude probably was "We're going to show these kids a thing or two about what you have to know to get a drug approved in this country." [laughter] All that's changed in the succeeding years. The FDA works pretty well with small companies today.[20]

---

[20]Genentech's early products relied upon recombinant DNA technology and monoclonal antibodies. "Thomas D. Kiley, *Genentech Legal Counsel and Vice President, 1976–1988, and Entrepreneur*," oral history conducted by Sally Smith Hughes, Regional Oral History Office, The Bancroft Library, University of California, Berkeley, 2002 (p. 53 of transcript). "Fred A.

Middleton's reflections reveal his ignorance as much as his knowledge. His impressions of the FDA, based on "probable attitudes" of the agency, were more projections than evidence-based judgments. And the fact that a chief financial officer was one of the primary liaisons for the FDA pointed to the company's structural weakness: its lack of an experienced regulatory affairs officer. Genentech CEO Robert Swanson took primary responsibility for these relationships. Middleton's relationship with the Administration also pointed to the raw necessity for any firm's executives and financial managers to keep apprised of regulatory developments affecting their products.[21]

On the whole, the advantages from establishing formal liaison positions accrued to larger companies that could devote significant resources to the creation and maintenance of regulatory affairs offices. Advantages in regulation were hence correlated with the size and age of the company. This fact imposed substantial limitations and disadvantages upon smaller, newer companies like Genentech. The fledgling California outfit saw the economic potential of one of its best products, human growth hormone, damaged from Eli Lilly's successful appeal to receive orphan drug protection on its own growth hormone. There were plausible differences between the Genentech and Lilly products, but the former company was much less capable of a credible regulatory appeal in the early 1980s, when the orphan drug designation application process was just being established. Limitations of size also led Genentech to sell some of its most promising products and ideas to larger companies, companies bearing the wherewithal to approach the sovereign and take a drug through the regulatory process. As longtime company scientist Daniel Yansura recalled of Genentech's development of recombinant insulin, later sold to Lilly, "It was pretty clear that we wanted to give insulin away because we didn't have the ability to market it. There's no way we could have scaled it up and gone to the FDA with it. We only had a very small fermenter. You need a tremendous army of people to take a drug through the FDA."[22]

Yansura's "army of people" was but an aspiration at Genentech in the late 1970s. In larger companies, such a force would have been manned by

Middleton, *First Chief Financial Officer at Genentech, 1978–1984*," oral history conducted by Glenn E. Bugos for the Regional Oral History Office, The Bancroft Library, University of California, Berkeley, 2002 (p. 39 of transcript).

[21]On Swanson's reputed skill in dealing with the Administration, see Thomas J. Perkins, *"Kleiner Perkins, Venture Capital, and the Chairmanship of Genentech, 1976–1995,"* oral history, Regional Oral History Office, The Bancroft Library, University of California, Berkeley, 2001.

[22]Genentech later sued Lilly for patent infringement on its growth hormone product and won, so the company's economic damage was limited. "Thomas D. Kiley, *Genentech Legal Counsel and Vice President, 1976–1988, and Entrepreneur,*" oral history, 64. "Daniel G. Yansura, Senior Scientist at Genentech," oral history conducted by Sally Smith Hughes for the Regional Oral History Office, The Bancroft Library, University of California, Berkeley, 2002 (p. 71 of transcript).

clinical trial managers and regulatory affairs personnel. As Genentech matured through the 1980s, "regulatory people" began to exercise an increasingly greater role in the design of clinical trials. Yansura's superior David Goeddel remarked that the company's drug development process became one in which the discovering "bench" and "lab" scientists nearly stopped participating once the company designed animal studies and Phase 1 trials. This abdication came in part by choice, but also from the bench scientists' having been eclipsed by their lack of development expertise: their inexperience in trial design and analysis, and their inability to deal with the officers of the Administration on the terms of federal regulation. Asked in 2002 about his interactions with company officials in other specialties, Goeddel answered that he had "quite a bit" of interaction with process specialists in the firm who took the essential concepts from molecular biology and "scaled them up" into viable drug candidates, but from the point of manufacture onward,

> no, we didn't have any interaction; it was the process science guys that worked with the manufacturing people. Every scientist feels they have an idea of what clinical trial should be done. So I'm sure the clinicians always got too much advice and probably didn't listen to much of it; they knew what they wanted to do. Then you would get regulatory people to deal with the FDA. By the time something entered the clinic and got in the first patients, I usually completely quit going to the project team meetings. That reached the goal: We had discovered something, made it, the first patient was treated. From then on the project team meetings were largely regulatory, manufacturing, time lines, commercialization, and things like that.[23]

While the dominance of "regulatory people" in drug development begrudged Genentech scientists, they understood well that the firm's skill in navigating regulation was widely considered a central factor in its success. From the very beginning, chairman Tom Perkins and CEO Fred Swanson focused on regulatory approval as the key variable defining triumph or failure in drug development. "We were so sensitive to the potential for delays within the FDA, that Genentech worked that side of the equation aggressively," Perkins later recalled, crediting Swanson for his skill in "handling of the political side of the FDA." The "political side," for Perkins, was not the Commissioner or a partisan appointee but the drug reviewers who demanded stiff adherence to Administration clinical trial standards and reporting requirements. Swanson and Genentech's R&D leaders "learned quickly, and learned very well, how to design the clinical trials with the FDA very fully informed as to what was going to go on. What would be the efficacy benchmarks, and so forth." Swanson also placed regulatory viability at the center of his strategy for selecting products for development. The company's decision to develop insulin and human growth hormone was based not simply

[23] "David V. Goeddel, Ph.D., Scientist at Genentech, CEO at Tularik," oral history conducted by Sally Smith Hughes for the Regional Oral History Office, The Bancroft Library, University of California, Berkeley, 2003 (pp. 45–6 of transcript; see also 72–3).

upon the therapeutic and economic potential of the drugs, but upon a bet
that the path to regulatory approval would be easier.

> Clearly, from the beginning the goal was to try and find a product that could be
> reviewed and approved easily by the FDA. At that time, insulin was actually regu-
> lated under a different set of rules than new chemical entities, and so I thought
> that might be helpful. We didn't have a lot of experience, obviously, but we did a
> little homework to try and figure out what would be the end point for approval.
> In the insulin case, it was easy to say, Okay, is it safe? Is it reducing the level of
> glucose in the blood? As opposed to some of the other FDA criteria which were
> more difficult to satisfy at the time. At the time, they were requiring survival to
> prove a new cancer drug, so you had to do long studies and show survivals. Even
> arthritis: is your hand feeling a little bit better? It's not as easy to measure, and
> probably would be longer and more difficult for approval. So thinking about how
> quickly something could go through the regulatory process was a key part of the
> product selection.[24]

While Genentech experienced delays in product development, and while
its leaders would later acknowledge naïveté in their approach to the Administration, the company in fact fared well in comparison to other start-up and
biotechnology enterprises. At the same time that Genentech was maturing
its human growth hormone and insulin products, pediatrician and immunologist Robert Hamburger, working five hundred miles to the South in the
burgeoning biotechnology hub of San Diego, was experimenting with a potential therapy nicknamed HEPP (Human IgE Pentapeptide). Hamburger
had hypothesized and found animal evidence that HEPP could block hista-
mine production in skin cells, thereby serving as a potent anti-allergy medication. In 1981, the rights to Hamburger's product were bought by Immunetech, a small company incorporated that year.[25]

Hamburger's regulatory trouble started early and reappeared often. Having applied for an IND exemption to examine HEPP in clinical studies in
December 1979, Hamburger was visited by William Lieberthal from the
FDA's Los Angeles field office. Lieberthal inspected Hamburger's laboratories in April and May of 1980 and found several violations of Good Laboratory Practice regulations. These violations and the act of remedying them
appear to have consumed more than fifteen months; clinical trials did not
start until September 1981, by which time the Administration had warned
Hamburger that his go-ahead for studies in human patients was premised
on a strict requirement to exclude women of child-bearing age from his experiments. Studies continued until February 1982, when they were stopped

---

[24]Perkins oral history, 26; Swanson oral history, 41; Bancroft Library, UC-Berkeley.

[25]Chris Kraul, "Immunetech's Future Hinges on FDA Approval," *San Diego Business Journal*, June 13, 1982. Herbert Lockwood, "Immunetech Uses Peptide to Intercede," *San Diego
Daily Transcript*, March 6, 1984. Gary S. Hahn, "Immunoglobulin-derived Drugs," *Nature*
324 (20 Nov. 1986): 283–4.

(and the IND exemption halted) after a female patient complained of side effects. Hamburger asked for a meeting in June 1982 and expressed his wish for the "the continuation of the study of our IND." As of October, FDA division director James Mann was informing Hamburger of numerous problems in his study protocols and in his application for a continuation of the IND. By January 1983, FDA officials had permitted Hamburger to proceed with further Phase 2 trials, using different dosages of HEPP and different methods of administration. The earliest and least costly stages of clinical study had already consumed three years, and Hamburger's outfit was running out of money.[26]

Despite the regulatory issues, in part because of them, Hamburger's product fared well in early clinical trials. In the fall of 1981, a randomized and double-blinded Phase 2 study comparing HEPP to placebo for allergy showed an absence of toxicity for HEPP and a statistically significant difference in outcomes based upon reports. This was a small study that enrolled forty-none patients, and Hamburger asked for the go-ahead to do another trial with different dosage levels and more patients. By the summer of 1983, Immunetech was ready to launch large Phase 3 trials using physicians in private practice. The *San Diego Business Journal* headlined its June 13, 1983 edition with an ominous fact: "Immunetech's future hinges on FDA approval." The prospect of regulatory legitimacy for HEPP was under active discussion at Immunetech, and genuine but cautious optimism had emerged among the company's investors and watchers, even though the largest clinical studies had yet to begin.[27]

Until early 1984, Immunetech's liaison with the FDA was primarily Hamburger himself. It was Hamburger who dispatched the clinical results to James Mann. It was Hamburger who drafted and sent study protocols and numerous revisions of those protocols to Mann and his staff. It was Hamburger who bore the bad news of another delay in the continuation of his Phase 2 trials. It was Hamburger who supplied materials for the FDA's Pulmonary-Allergy Drug Advisory Committee in its 1983 review of the studies and its consideration of the HEPP IND. Hamburger knit together his own

[26]Commissioner Jere Goyan, letter to Hamburger, March 17, 1980 (announcing GLPs and inspection to come); Hamburger to Goyan, telegram, March 21, 1980; B13, F1, RNH. "Inspectional Observations," Form FD 483 (7/75), filled out by inspector William R. Lieberthal; the form is undated but the inspections occurred on April 21–23 and May 1–2, 1980; B13, F3, RNH. Hamburger on occasion lamented the delays in the continuation of his IND. "It seems inappropriate for your staff to have time to inspect my facilities and not to have the time to respond to my letter regarding IND 12,291 since the 5th December 1979." James P. Mann was Director of the Division of Surgical and Dental Drug Products at the time. On the patient with side effects, see Hamburger to Mann, May 3, 1982; B3, F21, RNH. On the problems with the application for IND continuation, see Mann to Hamburger, October 12, 1982; B 14, F 1. Kraul, "Immunetech's Future Hinges on FDA Approval," *San Diego Business Journal*, June 13, 1982.

[27]Hamburger to Mann, February 18, 1982; B13, F21, RNH. Kraul, "Immunetech's Future Hinges on FDA Approval," *San Diego Business Journal*, June 13, 1982.

research team, grabbing biostatisticians and chemists from UCSD to help replicate and assess essential results in their labs. By 1984, correspondence between Immunetech and FDA was handled by Kathryn Rangus, newly appointed as Immunetech's Vice President for Regulatory and Technical Affairs. Hamburger became a "Clinical Monitor" for Immunetech's development of HEPP, and he was one of many Immunetech representatives in meetings with Administration officials.[28]

Although Immunetech's progress was painstaking, it was real. By 1985, the company was preparing to submit a new drug application, and it met with FDA representatives in early 1986 to discuss its impending submission. The company lobbied for a "1A" classification, a priority ranking that would grease the path to approval if granted. And by this juncture, Rangus had fine-tuned Immunetech's presentation and preparation for the meeting, preparing for all possible contingencies. Her agenda revealed a strategy to use multiple personnel to address any possible issue that the FDA raised—to show that behind Hamburger's drug was a viable and legitimate organization.

1. Purpose of Meeting
    a. Answer questions from reviewers
    b. Therapeutic classification of NDA
    c. Inclusion of women of child-bearing potential in future clinical studies....
4. Status of review
    a. Pharmacologists review completed.
    b. Be prepared to answer possible questions on applicable sections of NDA:
        Manufacturing—S. Richieri and M. Verlander
        Toxicology—A. Kung
        Pharmacology and metabolism—G. Hahn
        Clinical—R. O'Connor and K. Rangus
5. Potential questions from FDA—Anything and everything.[29]

By 1990, the regulatory story of Human IgE Pentapeptide had ended favorably for HEPP but not for Immunetech. Drained of resources (and possibly optimism) by years of regulatory review, the company agreed to sell its rights to HEPP to the Japanese outfit Tanabe Seiyaku in 1989. Immunetech had spent $50 million on HEPP, but if the drug was going to receive approval, it would have to occur with another company. The terms of the sale

[28]Hamburger to Peter Pallai, Ph.D., Immunetech (San Diego), February 9, 1983: "Dear Peter: Could I get your help in drafting a response to Dr. Mann concerning item #1 in his letter of 11 January 1983"; B14, F1, RNH. "Annual Report of the Pulmonary-Allergy Drug Advisory Committee for the period July 1, 1982 through June 30, 1983," 3; copy in B14, F1, RNH. Kathryn Rangus (VP for Regulatory and Technical Affairs) to Patricia H. Russell, M.D. (Acting Director, Division of Surgical-Dental Drug Products, Office of Drug Research and Review, National Center for Drugs and Biologics, FDA), April 17, 1984; Rangus to Conrad Ledet (Consumer Safety Officer, Office of Drug Research and Review, National Center for Drugs and Biologics, FDA), June 28, 1984; B14, F1, RNH.

[29]"AGENDA for October 30, 1985. Preparation for FDA Meeting December 3 or 4 regarding HEPP NDA"; Immunetech Memorandum, October 31, 1985; B24, F13, RNH.

were not disclosed, but from the statement that its payment would be nominal, observers guessed that Immunetech received an insignificant sum. Three years later, Tanabe Seiyaku would discontinue development of HEPP, and the drug has not at this writing been resurrected. According to San Diego business reporters, Immunetech's saga underscored the lessons of therapeutic development for small and inexperienced firms: "Stand on the cutting edge of technology and you stand a good chance of bleeding to death."[30]

In the annals of pharmaceutical history, the silent and brief roles played by companies like Immunetech and their products are as compelling and as important as those played by more notable firms who sped to market and survived. The decade-long saga of Robert Hamburger and Immunetech was shaped throughout by a number of factors. Immunetech did not lack for investors, for famous scientists, or for plausible bets that its star project would become a commodity. An investment weekly published in 1988 reported that "FDA approval is now pending for an injectible form of the compound." Immunetech scientist Gary Hahn echoed this optimism and sketched out the company's marketing schedule and possible revenues: "Assuming the product is approved, we expect to be selling it in 1989 and selling other new compounds in the 1990–1991 timeframe, or right beyond that. These are products with market potential that ranges in the hundreds of millions of dollars." What Hamburger, Hahn, and Immunetech lacked was the capacity to deliver a regulatory commodity with the necessary credibility. This capacity marked the essential organizational skill of the late twentieth-century pharmaceutical company, and without it firms and their products were far less likely to appear and endure in the therapeutic marketplace.[31]

GOOD COP VERSUS BAD COP—THE MULTIPLE FACES
OF REGULATORY REPUTATION

Regulatory politics requires a delicate balance between fear and facilitation. The sheer aggregate of activities in which drug companies engage—among them laboratory development, clinical experimentation, regulatory submission, synthesis and mass production, packaging and distribution, marketing and advertising, and post-marketing surveillance—is impossible for the FDA or any other government agency to fully survey. As with other forms of policing, pharmaceutical regulation depends upon deterrence. By occasionally projecting a fearful image, and by symbolically reminding drug companies who is in charge of the modern pharmaceutical world, Adminis-

[30]Steven Findlay, "New Drug Hives Relief of Allergies," USA Today, April 1, 1987. Craig D. Rose (biotechnology columnist), "Hard Cell: Immunetech's Fate Is Example of Life at Science's Cutting Edge," San Diego Union, December 18, 1990. "ProVenture Company Profile, Immunetech Pharmaceuticals," ProVenture Report, First Quarter 1988.
[31]"ProVenture Company Profile, Immunetech Pharmaceuticals," ProVenture Report, First Quarter 1988.

tration officials establish boundaries of appropriate action, secure compliance with low effort, and can induce firms to abandon strategies of contestation and to ditch questionable therapies. Deterrence—and behind it, a measure of fear—becomes a central tool of regulation.

Deterrence is complicated, ambiguous, and not entirely strategic, however. Many of the Administration's most dreaded actions are not undertaken with the express intent to create fear. Sometimes strong FDA enforcement or legal action results from an inspired defense of the agency's legal prerogatives, and a perception that a firm has clearly broken the law's spirit as well as its letter. Sometimes the agency unpredictably issues a "not approvable" letter for a new drug because of a felt sense that the safety profile of the drug merits further study. Sometimes drug company officials shudder with regulatory anxiety when the Administration has not attempted to scare them.

Further impelling this ambiguity is the need for the agency to avoid appearances of "over-regulating." Among the many reasons that agency officials have offered (publicly and privately) for this avoidance, a chief concern is the goodwill relationship that the FDA hopes to carry on with most pharmaceutical companies. Faced with the massive private activity under their purview, the agency's officers understand that effective regulation requires some measure of trust. Beyond the imperatives of regulation, moreover, there are compelling political reasons for the agency to facilitate as well as frighten drug companies. Combined with particular criticisms of the Administration, the anti-government rhetoric of the late twentieth century subjects many FDA actions to open and public criticism. Strong enforcement activity that could under plausible framings appear draconian, can and often will be publicized by numerous trade reporters and national media outlets. The pharmaceutical industry's allies in Congress and in lobbying circles can and will rally to the defense of particular companies, and there is always the prospect of a difficult congressional hearing on aggressive enforcement patterns. The growing organizational and political power of drug companies in the late twentieth century (discussed below) amplifies these factors.[32]

The politics of fear, then, runs from industry to regulator as well as from regulator to firm. Individually, firms (sponsors) fear the FDA. Yet Administration officials also fear the industry as a political collective and its capacity to weaken the agency both with respect to reputation and formal authority.

The deterrence embedded in modern pharmaceutical regulation takes at least two forms, each with tangible effects. First, firms are prevented, in part by fear, from breaking the law or exerting only lax efforts in those areas of safety and quality control where their effort matters. One such area may be pharmacovigilance, namely, the prompt and thorough reporting of drug adverse events to the FDA, upon having received physicians' reports of these

[32]For one such hearing, held soon after Republicans took majority control of the House of Representatives in the 1994 elections, see *Allegations of FDA Abuses of Authority: Hearings before the Subcommittee on Oversight and Investigations of the House Committee on Commerce*, 104th Congress, 2nd Session (Washington, DC: GPO, 1995).

events. Here, especially with clinical trial regulations but also with marketing practices and reporting of adverse events, Administration officials can display a fierce countenance. A second role played by deterrent effects is to prevent firms from developing (and eventually submitting) substandard products.

Deterrence in Legal and Enforcement Action. It is difficult to produce solid, unambiguous evidence that the FDA and its officials have consciously and consistently engaged in scare tactics and in reprisals. It is abundantly clear, however, that many firms and many individuals in the employ of drug companies harbor deep and abiding fears of the Administration and its functionaries. It is also clear that drug company officials hold widespread perceptions of the agency's propensity to manipulate fear and engage in payback.

One of the earliest and memorable cases of FDA aggression came in the agency's attempted prosecution of the William Merrell Company in 1962. Merrell was the American sponsor of thalidomide, but its less publicized troubles came with its product MER/29, an anti-cholesterol drug. MER/29 had been associated with cataract formation in rhesus monkeys in preclinical studies, but Merrell never reported the adverse animal events to the Administration. Having been tipped off by a former Merrell employee, FDA inspectors raided the Merrell Company's laboratories in August 1962. Numerous officials in the Bureau of Medicine and the General Counsel's Office saw the MER/29 falsification as evidence of a more widespread problem, and these officials began to discuss the need to "make an example" of Merrell. As the "Pink Sheet" trade reporter commented in November 1961, "Adverse reactions withheld by manufacturers disturb FDA-ers who mumble about need for criminal prosecution to get full and prompt reporting." The Administration turned the MER/29 case over to the Department of Justice for criminal investigation and possible prosecution. It was the first time the agency had ever exercised its power under law to refer a case involving experimental falsification to the Justice Department. In related speeches and remarks to reporters at the time, Administration officials emphasized that the Merrell prosecution could become part of a larger campaign. In a May 1962 speech to the Yonkers Academy of Medicine, Bureau of Enforcement Deputy Director Kenneth Milstead decried the production of "rigged" and "tailored" scientific research as another form of "quackery." As the *Drug Trade News* put it, "Dr. Milstead said FDA is going after physicians who participate in furnishing false information in support of NDAs." Another FDA source told *Drug Trade News* that "a few 'big' manufacturers may get caught up in the net." [33]

[33] Barbara Yuncker, "United States Presses Probe of Heart Drug Sales," *New York Post,* August 7, 1962, 2. *FDCR* 23 (46), (Nov. 13, 1961): 26. Milstead, "The Food and Drug Administration's Program Against Quackery," delivered at the Yonkers Academy of Medicine, May 16, 1962; DF 505, RG 88, NA. "FDA Reviewing NDA Claims of Called-In Drugs," *Drug Trade News,* June 11, 1962. Memorandum from John D. Archer to "Medical Officers, DND,"

Combined with other "tough cop" facets of FDA enforcement that would continue through Commissioner James Goddard's tenure to 1969, the Merrell prosecution conveyed several new signals to the pharmaceutical industry. It crystallized the harsher facets of the agency's image, sending the message that even marginal cases of record and experiment falsification would be pursued with vigor and criminal means. The agency's occasional pursuit of physicians—later institutionalized in Frances Kelsey's Office of Scientific Investigations—broke apart the cozy links between doctors and pharmaceutical companies, as physicians became much more aware of the legal risks of supporting untrustworthy firms through careless research. Kenneth Milstead's speech skillfully reframed the language of quackery, applying the term anew to shoddy clinical research as opposed to its earlier meaning of unscientific treatment. Along with the Lincocin prosecution, the MER/29 case also signified that the Administration would now target some big and established manufacturers instead of restricting itself to the "easier" cases of small-time mail-order quacks or local and regional drug firms.

In the coming years, most of the Administration's enforcement actions would be directed at firms like William S. Merrell Company—firms whose research operations were smaller and, most important, whose operations lacked scientific legitimacy and credibility. Corporate researchers for Eli Lilly released a report in 1978 documenting that, during the preceding three years, the best known, "research-intensive" companies were least likely to be targeted with Class 1 and 2 product recalls and with court action. A research-intensive company was four times less likely than other companies to experience a recall, and twenty-four times less likely to be named in legal action. When the writers controlled for the volume of sales or prescriptions, these disparities became much larger. Smaller but still appreciable differences were seen in the adverse drug reporting system. Products of less research-intensive companies were three times more likely to experience an adverse event report, controlling for millions of prescriptions or millions of dollars in sales.[34]

September 8, 1961, "Subject: Clinical Investigators Contributing Incredible Data for NDA's"; *ICDRR*, 975–7. Administration officials also considered criminal referral in the matter of Belleville, New Jersey drug maker Wallace & Tiernan's new drug application for Dornwall; *ICDRR*, 528.

[34]Lynn M. Pauls and Baldwin E. Kloer, *FDA Enforcement Activities within the Pharmaceutical Industry: Analysis of Relative Incidence* (Indianapolis: Eli Lilly and Company, 1978). At the time, Class 1 recalls were considered those in which the disputed product might cause "serious health consequences," while Class 2 products threatened "temporary health consequences." The Lilly writers used their numbers to shed doubt upon "equivalence" claims of generic manufacturers (p. 22). The research-intensive companies in the Pauls-Kloer report were: Abbott, American Cyanamid, American Home Products (including Ayerst Labs and Wyeth Labs), Bristol-Myers, Wellcome Foundation (including Burroughs-Wellcome), Ciba-Geigy, American Hoechst, Hoffmann-La Roche, Johnson & Johnson, Eli Lilly, Merck, Pfizer, Richardson-Merrell, A. H. Robins, Sandoz, Schering-Plough, Searle, SmithKline, Squibb, Sterling Drug, Syntex, Upjohn, and Warner-Lambert (including Parke-Davis). It is important to

Still, these numbers and ratios aggregate what is perhaps not countable—the emotive and informational impact of a single prosecution. Over the ensuing decades, the Administration would occasionally pursue criminal charges against large and otherwise reputable pharmaceutical manufacturers, and the usual effect (at least as observed in trade reporters) was to awaken notice and to stoke fears in financial circles as well as corporate and company boardrooms. In the past two decades, the most alarming regulatory action was the Administration's closure of Warner-Lambert operations in 1993. In its consent decree, the agency never pointed to a "critical health risk," yet as one observer remarks, "a variety of complaints against the company had accumulated without effective remedy." The previous year had witnessed fully fourteen recalls of Warner-Lambert products. The firm had failed to report mandated quality control test results to the Administration and had repeatedly employed laboratory workers who were not legitimately trained. Under the decree, entered in U.S. District Court in New Jersey, Warner-Lambert was permitted to sell its existing stock of commodities, and it was allowed to manufacture drugs without bioequivalent substitutes under strict FDA supervision. But the damage was real, not simply to the reputation but to the bottom line: an estimated $150 million in forfeited revenue.[35]

Whether aggregated or not, publicized enforcement activity and documented legal action do not illuminate the broader power of the Administration to induce compliance by implied or actual threat. Observers have described patterns in which product recalls are officially voluntary but are in fact somewhat forced, because the Administration threatens to generate adverse publicity about the company or its products. In other cases, Administration attorneys have used the threat of legal sanctions to induce companies to create new institutions of compliance. Along with its request to Syntex to run "corrective" advertisements for its nonsteroidal anti-inflammatory product Naprosyn (naproxen), Administration attorneys in 1992 threatened to seize the company's entire stock of the drug. Syntex quickly launched the corrective publicity campaign in medical journals and on cable television. Similar threats led Bristol-Myers Squibb to agree to "preclear" its oncology advertisements with the FDA in 1991. In response to another set of purported threats, Kabi Pharmacia signed a consent decree in 1993 with the agency that committed the company to an FDA-approved training program for all of its sales representatives.[36]

---

underscore that this heavier regulation of smaller and newer firms does not in any way bespeak "capture" of the Administration by larger, older firms. For a mathematical argument to this effect, see Daniel Carpenter, "Protection without Capture: Product Approval by a Politically Responsive, Learning Regulator," *APSR* 98 (4) (Nov. 2004): 613–31.

[35] Roger Sherman, *Market Regulation* (New York: Pearson/Addison Wesley, 2008), chapter 23.

[36] Administrative law scholar Ernest Gellhorn observed in 1973 that, with limited statutory power to compel recalls, "the FDA ensures compliance by threatening seizure, injunction, and

Firms do not lack some means of defense in these interactions. They can in theory argue. They can in principle contest the agency's actions legally. They can, in concept, call the agency's bluff in response to its threats. Yet the deterrence power of the Administration—a showing of the second face of regulatory power—operates to stop most such challenges before they begin. Company officials seem continually haunted by the possibility that their argumentative and legal challenges will bring reprisal in the form of aggressive enforcement action, adverse publicity, arbitrary delays in current product submissions, or negative decisions on future submissions. Whether or not these fears are well-founded and rational is a separate question; such tremblings have been widely shared and expressed in the past half-century. J. K. Weston of Burroughs-Wellcome stood before Walter Modell's committee on advisory drugs in 1964 and boldly stated that the FDA often "dictates to industry" regarding the phrasing of warning letters, labels, brochures, and other features. Most of the potential debates went unargued by virtue of companies' "general reluctance" to argue with the Administration because of "fear of reprisals and arbitrary delays." In other matters, Weston confided, "FDA purposely 'leaks' the information it wants to the 'Pink Sheet' (*F-D-C Reports*) and the press," a practice to which he "expressed strong objection." Decades later, discussing what he had learned from former CEO Kirk Raab, Genentech chairman Thomas Perkins would issue a similar warning about the possibility of bringing suit against the Administration. Perkins had argued for legal action against the Administration on two separate occasions, but was twice talked out of the strategy by Raab. "In both cases, I learned, you don't sue the FDA. They'll crucify you for ever after." Perkins never produced evidence to suggest this is true, but his perception was clear and stable. "There were some mistakes that the FDA made, that Genentech could have publicized to embarrass the FDA for short term tactical advantages," Perkins would later recall. But Kirk Raab "perceived that that's not the way you play the game. You just cooperate, and love 'em, and eventually it will work out."[37]

By the 1990s, the possibility of regulatory payback had become something of a mythical specter. In part the myth persisted because of ideological politics. Claims of retaliation echoed libertarian and antigovernment con-

---

the issuance of publicity"; "Adverse Publicity by Administrative Agencies," *Harvard Law Review* 86 (1973): 1408. See generally Lars Noah, "Administrative Arm-Twisting in the Shadow of Congressional Delegations of Authority," *Wisconsin Law Review* 1997 (5): 889–90. Noah argues that the agency "continues to rely on explicit or implicit threats of disseminating adverse publicity as a method of encouraging compliance with its various demands" (890).

On the Syntex case, see *FDCR*, October 14, 1991, 8. On Bristol cancer drug promotions, see *FDCR*, June 3, 1991, 6. On Kabi Pharmacia's consent decree, see *FDCR*, August 9, 1993, 17. All quoted in Noah, "Administrative Arm-Twisting," 892–3.

[37]Advisory Committee on Investigational Drugs, Summary of Proceedings, 7th Meeting, February 27, 1964; FOK. Thomas J. Perkins, *Kleiner Perkins, Venture Capital, and the Chairmanship of Genentech, 1976–1995* (Regional Oral History Office, University of California, Berkeley, in 2001), 45.

servative arguments that no federal government agency should be trusted with such broad power as the Administration possessed. *Forbes* magazine reported the results of a 1993 survey that found that 84 percent of respondents declined to advance "potentially legitimate complaints" against the Administration for fear of reprisal. The myth of retaliation also became encoded in law. In negating the Administration's attempt to regulate discussions of off-label prescribing in continuing medical education programs, the D. C. Circuit Court in 1995 bought wholesale the Washington Legal Foundation's argument that court intervention was necessary because the FDA's de facto power through reputation-based fear outran its delegated authority. The "reality of the situation," the Court concluded, was precisely as the plaintiff had claimed, namely that

> few if any companies are willing to directly challenge the FDA in this manner. In the first instance, the company must expose itself to the FDA's power to seize an entire product line.... In addition, FDA wields enormous power over drug and medical device manufacturers through its power to grant or deny new product applications. It is evident that manufacturers are most reluctant to arouse the ire of such a powerful agency.[38]

Firms' reluctance to challenge FDA decisions reveals a second face of regulatory power. The set of problems confronting the Administration—its political and regulatory "agenda"—has been narrowed considerably by these fears. It warrants a reminder that firms can collectively challenge the agency through their industrial organization (the Pharmaceutical Research and Manufacturers of America, or PhRMA), or collect allies in Congress, among physicians and other health providers, or among patient advocacy groups. Yet the collective and indirect route with which these challenges are occasionally pursued points to the firms' relative legitimacy (or lack of it), as well as to the continual operation of regulatory fear.

Deterrence and Drug Development. The harsher side of the agency's reputation supports another appearance of regulatory power's second face. The agenda of challenges and problems facing the Administration is narrowed not only in law and argumentation, but also in research and development, in the restricted set of new products submitted to the agency. In part from the high barriers imposed by federal regulation of clinical trials and stan-

---

[38]Peter Brimelow and Leslie Spencer, "Food and Drugs and Politics," *Forbes*, November 22, 1993, 115; James Dickinson, "Will Anybody Sue FDA?" *Medical Marketing & Media*, October 3, 1993. The case was *Washington Legal Foundation v. Kessler*, 880 F. Supp. 34 (D.D.C. 1995); cited in Noah, "Administrative Arm-Twisting," 922–3 (n. 185, 186). To be clear, my assignment of mythic status to companies' fear of retaliation is not a denial of the possible truth or plausibility of these claims. The difficulty is that evidence supporting payback arguments is incomplete and, more important, subject to numerous interpretations (see for instance the arguments of Representatives Henry A. Waxman and John D. Dingell in *Allegations of FDA Abuses of Authority*). The more relevant (and durable) point is that the fears are widely stated and that the perception engenders its own reality.

dards for new drug applications, but also from the fear of rejection even where those barriers are formally satisfied, many questionable (possibly promising) therapeutic products are abandoned well before they could possibly be submitted. In some ways, then, the Administration can effectively reject a new drug without ever formally taking action on it (establishing a form of gatekeeping power). There is nothing illegal about this arrangement. The standards of evidence in the 1962 Kefauver-Harris Amendments were partially intended to deter producers of subpar drugs from developing and submitting them in the first place. And, as with policing activity in other forms of regulation, as well as presidential veto power over legislation itself, there is nothing illegitimate about deterred action. The shaping of the pharmaceutical agenda by the regulator's own projections and companies' fears is nonetheless a central mechanism of American pharmaceutical regulation. By a subtle conveyance of doubt—sometimes given at the investigational new drug stage, often expressed after the conclusion of Phase 2 trials, more rarely but gravely communicated during the NDA process itself—the Administration's drug regulators can quickly induce companies to abandon riskier therapies, and in so doing render the reputation-based challenges of regulation much easier. The resulting mix of therapeutic products submitted to the agency may then contain fewer "hard cases."[39]

The second face of power also works to create an ironic but pervasive criterion of success within the global pharmaceutical industry and among its investors. Those firms that are considered successful are not the ones that generate numerous product submissions alone, but those whose submissions meet with smooth and likely approval. As observers of the late twentieth century's most celebrated pharmaceutical company—Merck and Company of Rahway, New Jersey—have noted, it is credibility and not mere productivity that is most handsomely rewarded in financial markets. The strategy of drug development depends in some measure on some sort of wisdom—and, quite possibly, strategies of randomization—that prevail in the play of poker. In particular situations, an early departure ("fold") from one's product development will reduce the likelihood of much more costly and unsuccessful development down the road. So too, Administration officials may wish to induce sponsors to abandon drugs with marginal experimental records, as in a sort of "bluff." Success at Merck and other companies comes not simply in the art of development, but in the craft of wise abandonment. And this craft is one that is occasionally welcomed by the

---

[39] Again, the intentionality of these patterns should be neither overstated nor gainsaid. On one hand, Administration officials often have purely technical reasons for conveying doubts, and legitimate and persistent differences of opinion on a product's worth prevail within the agency's drug reviewing divisions, as well as between the agency and a sponsor. So doubts may be expressed for reasons having nothing to do with deterrence. On the other hand, Administration officials at the upper reaches of the drug reviewing divisions and in the general counsel's office display shrewd (sometimes anxious) awareness of the precedent-setting possibilities of their actions and utterances. See chapters 4 and 6 for more extensive discussion of this second point.

Administration itself, as the agency sets its official criteria high enough, and its informally conveyed projections rigidly enough, so that many marginal drugs that would present difficult cases are deterred from development and submission.[40]

REPUTATION MANAGEMENT, THE ADVANTAGES OF SIZE, AND THE SUCCESS OF MERCK

Organizational image forms the basis of FDA power, but as drug companies are organizations too, reputation figures centrally in the behavior and performance of private entities as well. The imperatives of reputation management are multidimensional for pharmaceutical firms as they are for the agencies and officials who regulate those companies. Reputation management is observed in the continual crafting and revision of a company's brand name, which for drug companies involves audiences such as investors, physicians, hospital administrators, and pharmacies and pharmacy chains, and research clinics and academic medical centers as well as patients. The administration of organizational image also involves the supervision of performance by those who represent the company with suppliers, purchasers, investors, physicians, and others. And companies establish reputations with and among their competitors: those firms whom the company may wish to deter from contesting a particular market, or whom the company might welcome into partnership for long-term product development.

When the institutions of government and the political economy of a marketplace compel the sort of involvement that the Administration has with drug companies, private reputation management establishes the regulator as a crucial audience for the firm. As when Frances Kelsey conducted a moral calculus of the Merrell company during her review of thalidomide; as when the FDA judged Searle's intentions for the surveillance and marketing of oral contraceptives; as when Bureau of Drugs personnel wondered about Bristol-Myers Squibb's promotion of its oncology drugs; as with the Administration's frequent battles with the Upjohn Company—agency officials frequently take conscious and unconscious stock of the intentions and subtle expressions of company representatives. The relevant company officials include not merely those of the top management, but also those of researchers, regulatory affairs officials, and allied professionals. It is for this reason that regulatory affairs personnel in drug companies have become so important—

---

[40]The discussion here gestures to a somewhat strategic equilibrium in which "mixed strategies" (or strategies that embed the play of two or more simple strategies, each with a given probability) are employed both by the sponsor and by the regulator as a veto player. For a formalization of such a model, which is nonetheless limited by its brute simplification of the dynamics of pharmaceutical development and regulation, see Carpenter and Ting, "Regulatory Errors with Endogenous Agendas." On Merck, see Fran Hawthorne, *The Merck Druggernaut: The Inside Story of a Pharmaceutical Giant* (New York: Wiley, 2003), 62.

they help coordinate various members and units of the company into a unified and coherent "face" for presentation to the FDA. Regulatory affairs specialists reconcile conflicting claims, they preserve credibility by making sure that no one speaks too optimistically of the product, they make sure that compliance means the same thing to all internal arms.

Different firms carry different reputations with the FDA. Some firms are trusted more, others less. Yet reputation is not merely a monotonic property that firms have more or less of. Firms are known for different traits, different histories, different capacities. And in crucial ways, reputation decomposes the firm itself. The politics of reputation can induce FDA officials as well as investors to figuratively break apart a firm and analyze which parts of the organization it trusts more. FDA officials might have high expectations for a company's research divisions but harbor strong doubts about the organization and training of its sales personnel. A company might have a weaker regulatory affairs division but may also promise excellent prospects for compliance due to sound manufacturing operations with strong quality controls.

Firms' reputations matter in part because a resource-constrained and uncertain regulator is compelled to rely partially upon trust. No tripling or more of the FDA's budget would obviate this fact. In part because of the Administration's regulations, and in ways that support its organizational legitimacy and power, the modern pharmaceutical world defies simple surveillance. In such a complex and highly publicized world, the Administration and its identified officials are greatly concerned that once they release a drug onto the marketplace, any number of things may go awry. Observable errors and plausible mistakes come in many forms, but those where firms are most implicated are matters of product safety and regulatory compliance. The Administration's own reputation management generates attention to the reputations of the firms it governs. And this dynamic often leads to greater regulatory trust of larger and older firms, the companies whose histories and professionals are better known to FDA officials. This trust does not create a permission slip for big companies. It does not enable the Administration to purposefully ignore the mistakes of an established corporate behemoth. It is rather a form of greater cognitive dependence placed upon well-oiled company structures and persons with whom FDA officials have professional and social understanding.

The logic of regulatory familiarity is widespread and vaunted in the global pharmaceutical arena. Firms covet the solid relationships of those few sponsors that continually win the FDA's confidence. Smaller, newer companies seek out these firms for licensing agreements, hoping that a recognized firm with a predictable "machine" for generating regulatory approvals will allow them to shepherd a new product to market. A trusted company's approval machine need not be a quick-working one, just one that offers credibility and a higher probability of eventual success.

The logic of regulatory familiarity also shapes the very structure and hiring of drug companies. Companies seek out former FDA employees for many reasons, not least the uncommon expertise, experience, and inside knowledge that these individuals possess from their service with the Administration. Yet the logic of reputation gives companies another reason to hire former FDA employees. When Administration officials attend an end-of-Phase 2 meeting and see one of their former colleagues representing the sponsor on the other side of the conference table, they may be, all things equal, more likely to be persuaded of the sponsor's claims. Former FDA employees can speak the same vernacular, and they can appeal to the sort of concerns (including their emotional components) that current FDA officials are likely to harbor and to express. When a company has as its officer or consultant an individual with lengthy and valued employment at the Administration—Theodore Klumpp, J. Richard Crout, Wayne Pines, Peter Honig—its case may well be more credibly conveyed, and the Administration's uncertainty about the company is correspondingly reduced.[41]

This premium upon previous FDA service within the global pharmaceutical industry establishes a collective phenomenon otherwise known as "the revolving door." Students of regulation have long observed that particular individuals work at a regulatory agency, then leave to take employment with the very industry they once regulated. In some cases such as telecommunications, the observed circuits are complete: high-level regulatory officials usually come from the industry to the agency, and then return to the regulated industry after their service with the regulator. Numerous commentators have argued that this pattern of employment is evidence of regulatory capture, yet the evidence for such an interpretation is weak if not altogether absent. In highly specialized industries, what appears to be a revolving door may be due to the fact that the agency and the regulated firms are drawing from the same pool of trained professionals. More likely, companies value the information, expertise, and legitimacy that former regulatory officials bring to their organizations. The revolving door is an artifact, not of capture but of mutually sustaining organizational relationships.[42]

---

[41]It is entirely possible that an official who has "jumped ship" may incur the resentment of remaining FDA staff, yet numerous conversations suggest that this state of affairs is the exception rather than the rule.

[42]From the vantage of the firm, the expertise of a former FDA official becomes a firm-specific form of asset which is industry-specific in its application. (One might also speak of FDA experience as a form of specific "human capital.") The firm specificity of FDA knowledge comes from the fact that one cannot gain precise knowledge of regulatory affairs simply by working in the industry; there are some things that FDA employees know about the Administration and its procedures that long-serving industry officials simply do not. The industry-specificity of this knowledge means that working for the FDA has much less experience value in those industries that are not regulated by the agency.

On the revolving door, see William Gormley, "A Test of the Revolving Door Hypothesis at the F.C.C.," *AJPS* 23 (Nov. 1979): 665–83. Among many other capture theorists, Stigler wrongly interpreted "revolving door" phenomena as per se evidence of capture; *The Citizen and the State*, 163–6.

The purchase of legitimated individuals from the regulator itself is only part of a much larger set of strategies in which pharmaceutical companies have engaged for most of the twentieth century. Reputation management also entails alliances with prominent scholars and academics. This is especially so in the pharmaceutical industry, where persons with scientific and intellectual prominence bring not only new ideas for technology, but also credibility. In the late twentieth century, the continued efforts of drug companies to ally themselves with academic scientists and clinicians have amounted to much more than surface painting. These alliances have fundamentally transformed the business. Firms like Merck and Hoffmann-La Roche have placed academic stars in integral roles in the monitoring of the firm. Academics were hired and appointed not merely for their contributions to scientific innovation, but for their oversight of marketing and sales, employee training, manufacturing, and many areas outside their specific competence. Hoffmann-La Roche, for example, appointed Louis Goodman as chair of its sales personnel training program in 1971. Seven years later, the firm asked Goodman to serve on the board of its Drug Literature Evaluation Program, but Goodman flatly refused, perceiving little value in the effort. Roche officials built the program anyway, and the company assembled an oversight committee of big names: Yale biostatistician Alvan Feinstein, UCSF pharmacologist Kenneth Melmon, San Francisco pharmacologist Carl Peck (who was well known to FDA officials in the 1970s), Tulane pediatrician Harry Shirkey, and pharmacy specialists Ann Amerson and Philip Hansten. In addition, Roche continued to rely upon its Editorial Advisory Board, of which Goodman, Harvard pharmacologist Jan-Koch Weser, and Emory cardiologist Leon Goldberg were prominent members.[43]

The Exemplar: Reputation Management at Merck. In assembling teams of prominent academics for prominent advisory and even leadership positions, American drug companies were often emulating the history of a business and scientific paragon: Merck and Company, headquartered in Rahway, New Jersey. If there is one company that stood out on numerous dimensions

[43]Swann, *Academic Scientists and the American Pharmaceutical Industry*; Quirke, *Collaboration in the Pharmaceutical Industry*. Memo to "Roche Sales Force," May 1973; Glenn Horstdaniel (Associate, Career Development, BCRS Program) to Goodman, March 23, 1972; B3, F8, LSG. On the literature evaluation program, see Susan D. Roeder (Health Professional Education, Professional Services, Roche Laboratories) to Goodman, February 17, 1978; B3, F8, LSG. Goodman wrote Barney V. Pisha in 1978 that he wanted no part of the literature program: "The purpose of this note is to ask you to quietly but firmly convince her [Roeder] that I do not want to take part in the program—in any way whatsoever. I thought I made this clear when the two of you visited here some months ago. Despite the impressive roster of participants, I remain most skeptical. As the late dear friend Walter Loewe used to say, "What's all about it?"; Goodman to Pisha, March 9, 1978; B3, F8, LSG. Carl Peck would become Director of the FDA's National Center for Drugs and Biologics— the successor to the Bureau of Drugs— in the 1980s.

in the late twentieth-century pharmaceutical industry, it was Merck. Journalist Barry Werth noted that the company displayed a dual reputation for vigor and warmth; Merck in the 1980s and early 1990s "was both the Arnold Schwarzenegger and Mother Teresa of American businesses." Perhaps with hyperbole, financial writer Fran Hawthorne could remark in 2002 that "Simply put, whether in terms of product or philanthropy, numbers of niceties, no other pharmaceutical company, and perhaps no other U.S. company of any sort, has ever had a reputation like Merck's."[44]

Merck is an American company with a celebrated past in Europe and the United States alike. Founded by the Merck family of Darmstadt, Germany, the company had its roots in pharmacy and alkaloid preparations. George W. Merck moved much of the business to the United States, purchasing large plots of land for expanded chemical manufacturing in Rahway, New Jersey, in 1900. Like other pharmaceutical giants of the twentieth century, it started as a bulk chemical manufacturer, and pharmaceutical development and production was something of an acquired taste which expanded greatly in the 1930s with investment in vitamins, sulfa drugs, steroids, and antibacterials. The company's wartime contributions to the United States formed the raw material of legend. Along with Pfizer and other companies, Merck had jump-started the mass production of penicillin for the American military effort in the Second World War. Leading more than sixty other companies, Merck in December 1962 donated $2.5 million in medical supplies to the national ransom paid to Fidel Castro's Cuba that freed American prisoners captured during the failed Bay of Pigs invasion. At mid-century, the company consistently tendered top appointments and board directorships to celebrated scientists—Alfred Newton Richards, Max Tishler, Vannevar Bush. The company also provided crucial assistance to Rutgers professor Selman Waksman in his development of streptomycin in the 1940s. When the anti-tuberculosis potential of streptomycin was demonstrated, the company waived its patent rights, thereby giving Rutgers and an allied foundation a windfall of tens of millions of dollars. Waksman and other Merck scientists won Nobel Prizes in Medicine in 1950 and 1952 for the development of streptomycin and cortisone. Merck had won an image projecting both philanthropic concern and scientific purity.[45]

---

[44]Barry Werth, *The Billion-Dollar Molecule: One Company's Quest for the Perfect Drug* (New York: Simon & Schuster, Touchstone Paperback, 1995); quoted in Hawthorne, *The Merck Druggernaut*, 13. Schwarzenegger became governor of California in 2002 but in the 1980s and 1990s was best known as a champion body-builder and a star in Hollywood action films such as *Terminator*, where he projected strength and ferocity in defense of the human race. Mother Teresa of Calcutta won the Nobel Peace Prize in 1979. Hawthorne, *Merck Druggernaut*, 11.

[45]American pharmaceutical and medical supply companies donated over $50 million in therapeutic supplies to Castro in December 1962, with Merck giving $1 million more than any other company. Merck and other companies wrote off the donations as "charitable contributions" against their tax liabilities. "In the Black," *Time*, March 29, 1963. G. Pascal Zachary, *The Endless Frontier: Vannevar Bush, Engineer of the American Century* (Cambridge, MA:

Business historians and journalists have identified the tenure of Roy Vagelos as pivotal in Merck's evolution in the late twentieth century. Vagelos became head of the company's research laboratories in 1976, and served as chief executive officer from 1985 to 1994. Vagelos made his mark by pouring millions more dollars into research and development than his predecessors had. He is reported to have argued that the company's research laboratories should have the feel of a university, and his contemporaries describe him as cautious and fretful over different facets of the company's image: philanthropic, competitive, scientific, profitable, pure. *Fortune* magazine would rank Merck as the most admired company in the nation for seven years straight, from 1987 to 1993. Some part of this celebration surely stems from the fact that at the time of Vagelos' leadership, Merck's public asset value exploded. From 1985 to 1990, its aggregate stock value rose fivefold, twice outpacing the runup of the Dow Jones Industrial Average during one of the headiest surges in American financial history. And propelling these massive profits (and reflecting and contributing to the company's reputation) was its much-envied stream of new molecules: the blockbuster cholesterol drugs Mevacor and Zocor, the popular antihypertensive drug Vasotec, the heartburn treatment Pepcid (now sold over-the-counter), the AIDS drug Crixivan, and others.[46]

Merck's legitimacy translated into a positive regulatory reputation, and that reputation in turn shaped Merck's general public, financial, and scientific esteem. Observers have perceived that Merck enjoys a high success rate in its new drug applications, for which part of the reason is that it knows whether and when to abandon a marginal drug. These abandonment patterns are not merely singular choices. They reflect the composite result of structured internal deliberations in which new product ideas are vetted in a formal and occasionally adversarial system. "One reason Merck hasn't had products killed by the FDA," observes financial writer Fran Hawthorne, "is probably that it kills them early itself." Merck's art of abandonment is

---

MIT Press, 1999); Hawthorne, *Merck Druggernaut*, chap. 2. The company's move to Rahway was both marker of and contributor to a broader trend in the location of pharmaceutical companies in the early 1900s; Maryann Feldman and Yda Schreuder, "Initial Advantage: The Origins of the Geographic Concentration of the Pharmaceutical Industry in the Mid-Atlantic Region," *Industrial and Corporate Change* 5 (3) (1996): 855–8.

[46]The tenure of Vagelos and his predecessors Henry Gadsden and John J. Horan has been capably documented by historian Louis Galambos, who is also known for his innovative contributions to the "organizational synthesis" in American history. Galambos, "The Authority and Responsibility of the Chief Executive Officer: Shifting Patterns in Large US Enterprises in the Twentieth Century," *Industrial and Corporate Change* 4 (1) (1995): 187–203. For accounts based on interviews with contemporaries, see Hawthorne, *Merck Druggernaut*, chap. 2; also John A. Byrne, "The Miracle Company," *Business Week*, October 19, 1987. For a corporate sponsored history, see Jeffrey L. Sturchio, ed., *Values and Visions—A Merck Century* (Rahway, NJ: Merck, 1991). On Merck's economic performance, see Gardiner Harris, "How Merck Survived While Others Merged—Drug Maker Relied on Inspired Research," *NYT*, January 12, 2001; also Werth, *The Billion-Dollar Molecule*, 271.

structural and behavioral; perhaps more than any other company of the late twentieth century, the company had anticipated and internalized many of the constraints and scrutinies imposed by the Administration. In so doing, Merck could more credibly present its case to FDA reviewers, and company officials could conserve a form of political capital by saving their best energies for those battles where effort and lobbying mattered—disputes over labeling, marketing, and late-stage clinical trial design. In its behavior and its structure, Merck had established a face of deference to the regulator. In the 1980s and 1990s, when one asked virtually any company official which firm was the best practitioner of the craft of regulatory affairs, the overwhelming answer was Merck.[47]

Merck's experience with federal regulation was not always a positive one, however. Its deference to the Administration was learned, and its reputation often generated high expectations that its product applications did not meet. One of the company's most bitter disappointments in the post-Kefauver era came in its 1968 tangle with the Bureau of Medicine over its potassium-conserving agent Colectril (amiloride hydrochloride). Colectril was a mild diuretic whose safety and efficacy had, in the opinion of its sponsor, been well established in company-sponsored studies. Yet shortly after submitting its new drug application, Merck received some harsh news. Not only was the Bureau declaring the Colectril NDA "incomplete," Kelsey's Investigational New Drugs branch was prepared to terminate its IND. Bureau of Medicine officials saw "very casual planning" in Merck's Phase 3 studies;

[47]Hawthorne, *Merck Druggernaut*, 62. Two other European companies with a solid scientific reputation and generally favorable regulatory experiences were ICI and Glaxo, particularly the latter's pipeline of products developed in the laboratories of Allen & Hanburys. Consult Geoffrey Tweedale, *At the Sign of the Plough: Allen & Hanburys and the British Pharmaceutical Industry, 1715–1990* (London: Glaxo Pharmaceuticals, 1990), particularly chapters 7 and 8. ICI and Glaxo's pattern of within-firm development supplemented (and later partially displaced) earlier patterns of development through academic collaboration; Quirke, *Collaboration in the Pharmaceutical Industry*, 207–40, esp. 235, 239.

Even Merck's face of deference was partial, however. In dealing with, many firm officials, including at Merck, favored interactions with FDA officials they could trust. A revealing portrait emerges from Edward Skolnick's electronic messages to other personnel at Merck Research Laboratories about a labeling issue in 1999: "If I am right I think the ONLY way to handle is to GO THERE AND INVOLVE LUMPKIN and word by word agree to final circular next mon/tue. I DID THIS WITH TEMPLE ON VASOTEC IN 1985. At the end of session I signed the hand changed circular; he signed it and we were done, all that was left was making it pretty .THIS GROUP IS DYSFUNCTIONAL AND WILL NOT RESPOND TO YOU NOT IN PERSON TELECONS. DELAPP IS TOO WEAK VS GOLDKIND ET AL" [capitalization in original]; Skolnick to David Blois and Bonnie Goldman, May 14, 1999, subject "vioxx us circular"; document oxx10x10, UCSF-DIDA.

Temple is Robert Temple, discussed elsewhere in this book. Robert DeLap was a former Review Division director; Leonard Goldkind directed the agency's anti-inflammatory drugs reviewing division; Murray Lumpkin was Director of the Agency's Anti-Infective Drug Products Division. Skolnick was arguing that Goldkind would be a road block to the company's objectives with Vioxx and that Lumpkin would be a more powerful ally within the agency than would DeLap.

many Colectril patients were being co-treated with other medications, so the tests were not properly controlled. The Phase 3 studies were also poorly documented; although 193 investigators were recruited, Merck reported no data from 75 of them, another 57 reported on ten patients or less, and the rest of the investigators reported on 20–25 patients each. Perhaps most troubling, Merck had failed to report promptly the adverse events and deaths that it had observed in its Colectril trials. University of Minnesota luminary Wesley Spink expressed his concern that "such a large company" displayed "such loose control over its investigational studies and the delays in reporting deaths in patients under study with this drug." The Bureau's Medical Advisory Board saw a disconnect of esteem and fact: "There seemed to be a great gap between the very fine renal physiology group at Merck, the very qualified investigators who performed the study, and the very poor data which were available."[48]

Merck's renal group was indeed "very fine," composing perhaps the world's top group of renal physiologists. Merck's renal group descended from the laboratories of Sharpe and Dohme, where renal specialist John Shannon trained such future luminaries as Julius Axelrod, Karl Beyer, Bernard Brodie, John Baer, Robert Berliner, and Sidney Udenfriend. After the merger with Merck, the renal group housed chemists James Sprague, Frederick Novello, Everett Schultz, Edward Cragoe, and Carl Ziegler. Its pharmacologists included Baer, Horace F. Russo, L. Sherman Watson, and George M. Fanelli. The same group that produced Colectril had also produced innovations such as Diuril and HydroDiuril, two thiazide diuretics that transformed the diagnosis, conceptualization, and treatment of hypertension in the 1950s and 1960s. Karl Beyer, a Lasker Award winner for his work with Diuril, was intimately involved with Colectril.[49]

The problem was one not of capacity, but adherence to regulatory wishes and instructions. Whereas in 1966 the Bureau had recommended to Merck that the company restrict its Colectril trials to "careful phase 1 and phase 2 studies," FDA officials and advisers later observed that the number of Phase 3 studies for Colectril had actually grown during the following two years. So too, Merck had foregone the customary practice of holding a large, formal conference with its participating physicians where the various study results could be openly discussed in the context of academic medical dialogue, with possible participation and input from Administration officials. Most distressing to FDA officials was the perceived "attitude of the Company... that FDA should accept the pronouncements of Merck" concerning pharmacology and toxicology "on faith." Associate Commissioner Harvey

[48]FDA-BOM, Medical Advisory Board, Sixteenth Meeting, October 3, and 4, 1968, p. 12; Harry F. Dowling Papers, NLM.

[49]Karl Beyer, Jr., "A Career or Two," *Annual Review of Pharmacology and Toxicology* 17 (1977): 1–10. On Merck's development of the thiazide diuretics, see Jeremy Greene, *Prescribing by Numbers: Drugs and the Definition of Disease* (Baltimore: Johns Hopkins University Press, 2007), chapters 2 and 3.

Minchew commented that although Merck had used "some of the best investigators" available, the agency did not feel compelled to accept poorly designed and reported studies. Minchew and Harry Dowling concurred that "very broad responsibility for providing the data" rested not with the investigator but with the "sponsor" of a new drug."[50]

The FDA held a conference on Colectril studies on November 27, 1968. The meeting was chaired by Arthur P. Richardson, Dean of the Emory University School of Medicine. Administration officials and medical academics were surprised to discover that over two hundred investigators were collaborating on studies of Colectril. It was daunting to these audiences to learn that no one outside the company knew of the full array of ongoing Colectril trials. This dearth of information raised questions of whether Merck was in a position to selectively report its clinical findings with the drug. At the conclusion to the conference, Richardson gently chided the assembled group of renal physiologists as well as Merck; all of them needed to "take responsibility for setting standards in the field as well as to improve investigational practices." Echoing the Bureau's emerging preference for public conferences at which the results of clinical experiments were discussed and openly debated, Richardson called the November Colectril meeting "an excellent precedent for the future."

When Merck convened its Colectril investigators for a meeting two weeks later, a culture of apologia and deference suffused the proceedings. Cardiothoracic specialist and hypertension luminary John Henry Laragh emphasized the lack of information on dose-time relationships and extra-renal effects of Colectril. Arthur Richardson was in attendance, as were members of the Bureau's Medical Advisory Board. They noticed "many fractions of studies were spread over many investigative groups," and that Merck's studies had failed to illuminate Colectril's mechanism of action. Participants at the Merck meeting also concurred with Administration claims that Merck needed to disclose more scientific information from its trials to the Bureau of Medicine.[51]

At the conclusion of its conference, Merck understood that its new drug application would not survive, and that the entire Colectril development plan needed revisitation. The Bureau of Medicine, and Frances Kelsey in particular, had identified glaring weaknesses in the company's research program. In the ensuing years, Colectril would quietly be dropped. Among the

[50]FDA-BOM, Medical Advisory Board, Sixteenth Meeting, October 3 and 4, 1968, pp. 12–13; Harry F. Dowling Papers, NLM. Prominent voices in the Board's discussion of Colectril were Allan D. Bass, of the Department of Pharmacology at Vanderbilt University School of Medicine and Wesley W. Spink of the University of Minnesota School of Medicine. Bass and Spink were members of the Medical Advisory Board.

[51]Merck held its conference on December 9 and 10, 1968. Minchew later commented that "there was obvious influence of the FDA conference on the proceedings of the Merck meeting." FDA-BOM, Medical Advisory Board, Seventeenth Meeting, December 16 and 17, 1968, p. 5; Harry F. Dowling Papers, NLM. Less than a year after the meeting, Laragh would be awarded the Stauffer Prize in High Blood Pressure Research.

many reasons were the weakness of the results and the fact that the company's sponsorship of the drug had marred its otherwise sterling reputation with the agency. Still, the stars of the company's award-winning renal physiology group were incensed. In an essay published shortly after his commercial retirement, Merck celebrity Karl Beyer mockingly noted that "This compound is marketed in the principal countries of the world except the USA."[52]

The imbroglio over Colectril sent powerful signals to Merck and to other companies in the global pharmaceutical industry. Merck's reputation had in some respects raised the bar for the quality of its new drug application submissions and its clinical trial protocols. Beyond this, the Administration served notice that drug development was now an organizational responsibility, and that the Bureau of Medicine was in some sense "deconstructing" pharmaceutical companies in their evaluation of new drug products. A company could possess a "very fine renal physiology group" but a weak regulatory affairs operation, and it was the weaker of the two links that dashed the hopes of Colectril. From the Administration's vantage, if a large company with reputable renal physiologists would not produce high-quality data in a systematic way, then there was little reason to believe that less established companies would do so.

In conceding the Colectril battle to the Bureau (and in part to Kelsey), Merck may have gained crucial advantages in a larger struggle for regulatory legitimacy. Merck's deferential posture of focused, scientific, and exhaustive preparation of regulatory documents was widely perceived to have won the company esteem in the eyes of FDA officials. By the late 1970s and early 1980s, Merck's name was consistently mentioned as the exemplar of what it took to get a drug through the FDA review process. Looking back at the difficulties of his early tenure, former Genentech CEO Robert Swanson remembered that Administration officials saw apt comparisons and contrasts between his fledgling company and Merck. Like Merck, Genentech was perceived by the FDA to have competent scientists in its laboratories. Unlike Merck, they did not have a mature and respectable operation of drug development and regulatory submission. "I think the FDA in those days felt that we had some of the best science. They compared us to Merck in terms of the quality of the science that we came in with. But they thought we were incredibly naïve in terms of what it took to get a drug approved."[53]

What made a company naïve in regulatory affairs was not simply its lack of a regulatory affairs operation, but also its attitude, its face. To veterans of the early biotechnology struggles, deference to the FDA meant first that companies would supply 100 (and perhaps 110) percent of what Administration officials had asked of them. Reports, statistical analyses and summaries, and communications all had to follow prescribed regulations or unstated

[52]Beyer, "A Career or Two," 9.

[53]Robert A. Swanson, Co-founder, CEO, and Chairman of Genentech, Inc., 1976–1996, Oral History by Sally Smith Hughes (Regional Oral History Office, The Bancroft Library, University of California, Berkeley, 2001), 80.

FDA preferences. "If that's what they want," Genentech's Robert Swanson later remembered, "that's what they're going to get. And delivered exactly as they want us to do it and in fact almost to overdo them." Deference also implied an option for cautionary labeling and understated promotion, as when Merck decided upon the most conservative label warnings for women of child-bearing potential for its anti-cholesterol blockbuster Mevacor. The annals of 1980s and 1990s drug development are indeed filled with long and occasionally acerbic debates within companies over how best to credibly submit a new application.[54]

For many reasons, even this portrait of firms with variable reputations is far too simple. In the 1970s and 1980s, many new drugs were developed not within companies (Merck-style) but at the interface of corporate organizations. One driver of this development was the failure of many larger pharmaceutical companies to engage in the "biotechnology revolution." Large pharmaceutical companies in the 1970s and early 1980s were making their biggest investments in microbial biochemistry and in the mechanism of enzyme inhibition. This failure opened up space for firms like Amgen, Genentech, and other companies that acquired the scientific and financial identity of "biotechs." Yet as the smaller firms experienced troubles in go-it-alone R&D, they often turned for strategic development alliances to the larger, more established firms of the time. And the "big pharma" companies usually welcomed them. Firms like Merck and DuPont in the United States and Glaxo in Great Britain had begun to master "discovery by design" processes aided by computer models. The big companies, moreover, had scientists and instruments that could help demonstrate a drug's plausible pharmacological or biochemical mechanism, thereby conveying scientific rigor to financial and regulatory audiences. The big companies had the resources to take bets on unknown but possibly blockbuster molecules. And, as important as anything else, "big pharma" companies had the resources to "over-experiment" with drugs and hence generate reassurance at the Administration and among academic physicians that a molecule had been thoroughly studied. Patterns of collaboration among firms and between firms and scientists in the global pharmaceutical industry were not merely a by-product of exogenous economic forces. At least partially, they were induced by the constraints and demands of the Administration and other national regulators, and by the heavy burdens of what drug development had become: the organizational sponsorship of new molecules.[55]

[54] *Robert A. Swanson, Co-founder, CEO, and Chairman of Genentech, Inc., 1976–1996,* 80. Swanson shortly admitted that the FDA's requests often proved his company officials had been wrong in their preferences about trial design, statistical reporting, and the like. Hawthorne, *Merck Druggernaut,* 157–8; Werth, *The Billion-Dollar Molecule,* 243–4.

[55] For a detailed and technical discussion of how Glaxo and Merck used computer models and other novel techniques to discover and synthesize drugs such as Losartan (losartan potassium, Merck's antihypertensive developed with DuPont) and Acyclovir (a herpes medication developed by Glaxo with activity against cytomegalovirus, which often affects AIDS patients), see Walter Cabri and Romano Di Fabio, *From Bench to Market: The Evolution of Chemical*

Reputation and Aggregate Patterns
in Development and Regulation

The narratives at Genentech, Immunetech, Merck, Glaxo, Roche, Upjohn, and other companies were variably and often repeated over the course of the late twentieth century. Their repetition was not uniform, to be sure, and considerable differences prevailed in company success and failure, even within a set of products developed by a single company or partnership. At the same time, aggregate patterns of development, submission, and regulatory decision making help to bear out the meaning of the narratives and to shed light upon the dynamics of reputation.

In new drug development, the ultimate outcome in which sponsors are emotionally, financially, and politically invested is the approval of a new drug application. Every new drug starts off unapproved, and the aim of a sponsor during NDA review is to procure an "approvable letter" that carries minimal requirements for full NDA approval (the declaration that a firm's NDA is "effective"). When the sponsor expects quick approval, or approval with high probability, an approvable letter can actually deliver bad news because it upsets more optimistic expectations and may compel significant additional testing before final approval. Whereas approvable letters can deliver good and bad news, then, "non-approvable letters" almost invariably carry adverse judgments and poor prospects for eventual marketing.[56]

If, as many observers claim, there is large-firm advantage in the FDA new drug review process, one would expect larger and older firms to be less likely to receive non-approvable letters. Yet if a sponsor's number of previous INDs can proxy for its size and experience, then over the past three decades, smaller and less experienced firms have been less likely to receive

---

Synthesis (Oxford: Oxford University Press, 2000), chapters 6 and 8. For an accessible and summary narrative of these developments, see Gambardella, *Science and Innovation*, 32–9 (discovery by design and the role of computers and other instrumentation), 61–81 (networks and the division of labor in innovation), 146–58 (quantitative analysis of "external linkages" in drug development). For a skilled analysis of some of the collaborations that emerged in the 1980s and 1990s, see Louis Galambos and Jeffrey L. Sturchio, "Pharmaceutical Firms and the Transition to Biotechnology: A Study in Strategic Innovation," *Business History Review* 72 (Summer 1998): 250–78. For an interpretation and analysis based upon network analysis of patterns of collaboration, consult Walter W. Powell, Douglas R. White, Kenneth W. Koput, and Jason Owen-Smith, "Network Dynamics and Field Evolution: The Growth of Inter-organizational Collaboration in the Life Sciences," *American Journal of Sociology* 110 (4) (Jan. 2005): 1132–1205.

[56]In 2008, the "approvable letter" was replaced by "complete response letters" that either rejected the NDA or accepted it. It is important to understand that a "non-approvable" judgment does not mean "never approvable." Nothing at law or regulation prevents a sponsor from later re-submitting an NDA earlier deemed non-approvable. It is also possible, though less common, for an NDA to receive multiple non-approvable judgments; much more commonly the firm either abandons the application or later corrects the deficiencies of the FDA so that it receives an approvable designation. In the statistical analyses that are reported here, a drug is coded as receiving a non-approvable letter if it receives one or more such letters and has not been approved by the end of the sample.

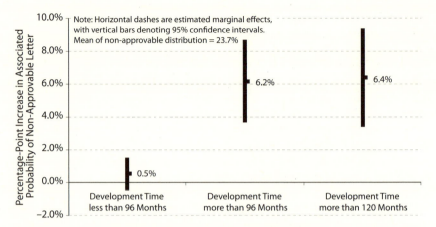

Figure 10.1. Change in Probability of Non-Approvable Letter Associated with One-Standard-Deviation Increase in Sponsor's Previous INDs

non-approvable letters than more experienced ones. Figure 10.1 displays the shift in the probability associated with a standard-deviation increase in a sponsor's number of previous INDs. When the sample is restricted to those drugs whose development phases (usually the IND phase, sometimes more) consumed over eight years (96 months), firms with greater experience developing investigational drugs are appreciably more likely to receive a non-approvable judgment. The relationship is slightly larger for drugs that take over ten years to develop before NDA submission, and the relationship essentially disappears for those drugs that take less than eight years.

The "small-firm" (or "newer firm") advantage, then, is a property of particular conditions of drug development. When a newer and smaller firm submits a new drug application for a molecule that it has taken longer to test, the duration of experiment becomes a marker for the sponsor's investment. This is all the more true for smaller and newer firms because, by their lack of economies of scale and learning by doing, the financial cost of additional experimentation is almost certainly higher for them. By pouring their scarce resources into a drug, smaller firms can transmit something of a "costly signal" of their beliefs about the product. Costly development and experimentation becomes a showing of credibility, a risky demonstration to be sure, but one that many firms are willing to undertake. Once these smaller firms have borne this risk, their products are less likely to be rejected by the Administration, in part because cost has established a form of brute credibility. A similar logic governs many firms' decisions to "over-experiment" with a drug, as Pfizer did when it ran and reported the results of seventy-one Phase 3 studies in its original NDA for the erectile dysfunction treatment sildenafil citrate (Viagra).[57]

[57]The logic of "costly signaling" has been a staple contribution of informational game theory for several decades (see, for example, Michael Spence, *Market Signaling: Informational*

The evidence in figure 10.1 is, to be sure, that of statistical association. There are other possible explanations for the result, including the possibility that smaller and newer firms like biotechnology companies tend to invest in riskier drugs with novel pharmacological mechanisms. Such drugs may both take longer to develop and, at the same time, represent the sort of promising new technologies that are less likely to be rejected by the Administration's reviewing divisions. Yet a credibility-based explanation helps to account for some patterns that other explanations cannot. The Administration's drug reviewing divisions appear to take more chances with the NDA submissions of smaller firms. In the 1970s through the 1990s, drugs with longer development times that were submitted by less experienced firms were, upon approval, significantly more likely to experience a safety-based market withdrawal in the United States or other industrialized countries, and significantly more likely to have longer black-box warning labels.[58]

Some patterns of drug review, then, give very conditional advantages to the smaller and newer firms in the bunch. Even if credibility is not the mechanism underlying the smaller-firm advantage in approvals, the observed statistical association nonetheless complicates the empirical picture of FDA-sponsor relationships. Put simply, not every pattern of FDA drug review is one in which larger companies possess clear advantages.

Another outcome of great interest to pharmaceutical sponsors is the speed of the review, particularly for those applications eventually approved. All other things equal, sponsors usually wish to market their drug as quickly as possible. Earlier marketing means an earlier chance to generate cash flow and to recoup the costly outlays of investment in the development phases. It is also crucial to mechanisms of sales and marketing competition in the pharmaceutical industry, as drug marketing depends heavily upon advertising to physicians and, more recently, to consumers. Earlier approvals and earlier product launches translate into more time in which the company can acquaint doctors, pharmacists, and patients with their product, at the expense

---

Transfer in Hiring and Related Screening Processes, (Cambridge, MA: Harvard University Press, 1974). The metaphor of costly credibility expressed here is more contingent—the demonstration of credibility through expensive and durable experimentation can only work for particular kinds of firms. The logic expressed here has been expressed in a simple model; see Carpenter and Ting, "Regulatory Errors with Endogenous Agendas."

[58]Put technically, there is probably unobserved correlation between which sorts of firms develop novel-mechanism products and which sorts of firms are newer and have less IND experience. The statistical techniques used to generate the estimates in figure 10.1 account for these patterns only partially, by controlling for the primary indication disease of the drug and by controlling for the particular firm that sponsors the application. Hence, the associations are leveraged statistically by over-time increases in experience for the same firm. All in all, however, the evidence summarized in figure 10.1 is not of the sort produced by a randomized controlled experiment where some feature of credibility could be randomly assigned to different firms or drugs.

For evidence based upon safety-based market withdrawals and black-box warnings, see Carpenter and Ting, "Regulatory Errors with Endogenous Agendas."

of competitor treatments. Indeed, the speed of approval was a major reason that pharmaceutical firms and industry organization supported user fee legislation in 1992 that was widely expected to reduce new drug review times.

In drug review times, the expected advantages of larger and more experienced firms reappear. For a sample of NMEs approved from 1977 to 2000, a consistent negative relationship prevails between the sales of the sponsor at the time of the product's submission and the speed of the subsequent NME approval. In short, larger firms with higher sales can expect quicker new drug approvals. At the mean of the sales variable for this period—where the annual *Sales* variable equals $2.1 billion in 1990 U.S. dollars—a one-unit increase in the natural logarithm of sales (to $5.8 billion) is associated with a two-month reduction in expected review time. Going from the minimum to maximum of sales (zero about $43 billion) is sufficient to generate a two-year expected differential in review time for the larger firm. [59]

The general negative correlation between firm sales (at the time of NDA submission) and the duration of the subsequent is a statistical statement that masks a more complicated set of relationships. In table 10.2, the rate of approval by time of review is presented for a sample of drugs reviewed from 1977 to 2000. The sample is stratified by different quantiles of the firm sales distribution, from the "poorest" firms (lowest decile) to the richest (top decile). While the approval rates generally rise with sales, there are some interesting inversions. For most of the review cycle, firms in the very top decile of the sales distribution have appreciably lower approval rates than do firms in the 75th to the 90th percentile of the distribution. This is not a slight inversion, as firms in the top decile averaged more than two-and-a-half times

[59]The quantities here are retrieved from maximum likelihood duration models. Sales are from total sales of the firm and not simply pharmaceutical sales; hence, a company such as Johnson & Johnson that sells many billions of dollars in non-drug medical products such as band-aids and children's shampoo, among many others, is measured as having more "sales" than another company that sells just as many prescription pharmaceuticals but lacks these other products.

The measure of sales used in the survival regression is not linear sales but the natural logarithm of firm sales [ln(*Sales*)]. At the mean, this variable equals 7.66. A linear specification of large-firm advantage (using non-logged sales (in millions of 1990 U.S. dollars) instead of logged sales in the model) yields a negative but statistically negligible coefficient ($\beta = -2.67$; SE(β) = 1.79). A model with non-logged sales produces a log-likelihood of -501.082 and likelihood ratio of 2.23 (Pr = 0.1354), while the model with logged sales yields -493.036 and a likelihood ratio of 18.32 [Pr = 0.000]. In other words, the association between increased sales and reduced FDA approval times is better described as log-linear than as linear. The intuitive inference from this result is that whatever advantages larger firms enjoy in pharmaceutical regulation may be characterized by decreasing marginal returns to size.

The analyses used to generate these estimates also show that estimated large-firm advantage is considerably suppressed when the sample excludes non-approved drugs. The coefficient on sales approximately doubles, from -0.0350 to -0.0678, when non-approved drugs are added to the sample. Because marginal effects of a variable are not a linear function of the estimated coefficient, moreover, the marginal effects more than double. Adding non-approved drugs to the sample increases the estimated marginal effect of firm sales upon duration by over 250 percent.

TABLE 10.2
Approval Probabilities (Expressed in Percentages), by Quantiles of Firm Sales Distribution NMEs Reviewed, 1977–2000

Months of NME Review	Lowest Decile of Firm Sales (Below 10%)	From 10% to 25%	From First Quartile to Median of Firm Sales	From Median to Third Quartile of Firm Sales	From 75% to 90%	Top Decile of Firm Sales (Above 90%)
3	0.0%	0.0%	0.0%	2.1%	1.8%	2.9%
6	5.0%	1.9%	6.3%	9.5%	19.6%	8.8%
9	20.0%	15.4%	10.4%	21.1%	32.1%	14.7%
12	50.0%	23.1%	18.8%	34.7%	42.9%	38.2%
15	50.0%	42.3%	31.3%	42.1%	51.8%	44.1%
18	50.0%	50.0%	42.7%	49.5%	58.9%	52.9%
21	60.0%	53.9%	51.0%	58.0%	71.4%	58.8%
24	60.0%	65.4%	61.5%	65.5%	82.9%	67.7%
30	70.0%	84.6%	67.7%	73.2%	88.6%	88.2%
36	70.0%	86.5%	71.9%	85.5%	90.9%	97.1%

Notes: Estimates are Kaplan-Meier "failure" rates, stratified by quantiles of firm sales distribution. Sales aggregates are scaled by interest rates (to 1990 U.S. dollars) and deflated using implicit price deflators. For each time interval, cell of sales quantile with largest approval rate is shaded.

the sales of firms in the category below ($38.9 billion to $14.3 billion). Yet the six- and nine-month approval rates for these slightly poorer firms are more than double those for the richest firms. So too, the poorest firms in the sample—those in the lowest decile of annual sales—have higher approval rates than many richer companies, particularly from the ninth to the eighteenth months of the review cycle. The association between firm wealth (or profitability) and regulatory speed is therefore a rough one. On average, larger firms do better, but the relationship is full of complications and twists. As one former big pharma employee later working for a biotechnology company remarks, "size brings so many things with it" that it is difficult to specify a single reason or two why larger firms prosper.[60]

When particular therapeutic categories are examined, the heterogeneity of larger-firm advantage appears further to be contingent upon the therapeutic categories in which a particular drug is developed and submitted. For the years 1977 to 2000, the association between larger firms and reduced approval times is most pronounced in pulmonary-respiratory and anti-viral/anti-infective, gastrointestinal, and dermatological drugs. It is much smaller for cancer and cardiovascular drugs.

The apparent advantage of size masks a related advantage of larger and older firms: dual familiarity. Firms that have regulatory experience better know how to negotiate the regulatory process, and they know the proper deference and thoroughness that the FDA review process demands. So too, FDA officials will be more familiar with firms that have continually appeared before them. One marker of regulatory experience comes in the number of previous new drugs that a firm has successfully shepherded through the review process. Generally, firms with more submissions receive shorter review time, an effect that is robust across repeated estimations. For the sample of NMEs approved from 1977 to 2000 reviewed earlier, every additional NME approved in since 1962 is associated with a week's reduction in expected approval time for the next NME submitted. Put differently, a standard-deviation increase across firms in number of previous submissions (6.3 NMEs approved) is associated with a 1.6-month reduction in expected FDA approval time. In figure 10.2, the average NME approval time ("detrended" by accounting for general over-time patterns) is plotted as a function of the number of previous NMEs accepted during the period under study. The trend is downward and the relationship depicted closely approximates the relationship estimated in more complex statistical models. Still, the graph shows the messiness of the statistical relationship; firms with seventeen or eighteen NMEs accepted do considerably worse, on average, than firms with six or nine previous drugs accepted.[61]

Still, the rough relationship between experience and speed of drug approval

---

[60]The estimates presented in table 10.2 are derived from "non-parametric" (Kaplan-Meier) methods of calculating the approval rate that rely upon a minimum of assumptions regarding the statistical distribution governing the data.

[61]The measurement of regulatory experience by previous NMEs accepted from 1963 poten-

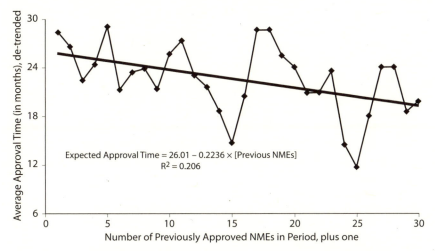

Figure 10.2. Average NMEs Approval Time by Sponsor's Previous NMEs

persists and, perhaps as important, it helps to account for large-firm advan-- tages more generally. Accounting statistically for previous firm submissions is sufficient to reduce the estimated statistical effect of firm sales by 30 percent. Almost one-third of statistically measurable large-firm advantage in the late twentieth century, then, can be explained by reference to the greater regula- tory familiarity that large firms enjoyed. Another pattern observed in the data is that the association between experience and approval times appears to be smaller (to the point of possible reversal) for firms that merged one or more time during the 1977–2000 period. Exactly why merged firms would benefit less from previous experience is not clear, though it is plausible that firms lose some experience when they merge two previously distinct business and devel- opment operations. In these cases, the economic advantages of a merger may recommend themselves to firms for reasons less intimately related to regula- tion, such as production, marketing, and preclinical development.[62]

Even accounting for size, experience, and structural history, there are cru- cial differences among firms that cannot be explained by reference to ordered statistical variables. In the late twentieth century, lasting differences appeared among the better-known pharmaceutical companies. In table 10.3, a list of twenty-eight global drug firms is rank-ordered by the aggregate review time advantage they appear to have enjoyed (or lacked) over the late twentieth- century (1977 to 2000) sample. This advantage can be calculated in very

---

tially understates large-firm advantage, insofar as some larger firms like Merck had also intro- duced important NMEs before 1962.

[62]The difference between the experience effect for merged firms and non-merged firms is retrieved from a Cox proportional hazards of NME approval time; the Cox model makes fewer assumptions about the distribution governing approval times than does a "parametric" model, but more than the Kaplan-Meier model does. The difference between the coefficients for sub- missions and submissions for merged firms is statistically significant at conventional levels of interpretation (χ^2 (1) = 4.31; p = 0.038).

TABLE 10.3
Rank Ordering of Aggregate Advantage for Firms Sponsoring More than 1% of Approved NMEs, 1977–2000

Sponsor	Months of Advantage per NME	Portion of Sample Sponsored	Probability for Statistically Significant Firm Effects ($p < 0.10$)	Aggregate Firm Advantage (in months of review time, 1977–2000)
Merck	-8.76	5.1%	0.003	-183.91
SmithKline/SKB	-6.14	3.9%	0.099	-98.27
Burroughs/BW	-9.17	2.2%	0.024	-82.52
Glaxo-Wellcome	-8.04	2.4%	0.016	-80.35
Abbott	-5.11	3.1%		-66.42
BMS	-3.81	4.1%		-64.71
Roche	-4.20	3.6%		-62.93
Alcon	-8.71	1.7%	0.037	-60.95
Glaxo	-7.35	1.9%	0.095	-58.79
Eli Lilly	-4.04	3.4%		-56.49
Pharmacia/Upjohn	-3.01	3.4%		-42.08
Sanofi	-7.81	1.2%	0.091	-39.06
Ciba-Geigy	-5.00	1.7%		-35.03
Warner-Lambert	-3.45	2.4%		-34.50
Boehringer	-8.56	1.0%	0.078	-34.26

TABLE 10.3
cont.

Sponsor	Months of Advantage per NME	Portion of Sample Sponsored	Probability for Statistically Significant Firm Effects ($p < 0.10$)	Aggregate Firm Advantage (in months of review time, 1977–2000)
Zeneca	−5.40	1.4%		−32.40
Syntex	−4.27	1.7%		−29.91
Rhone	−5.50	1.2%		−27.52
Sandoz	−3.64	1.7%		−25.45
Organon	−3.18	1.4%		−19.07
Bayer	−1.94	2.2%		−17.43
Johnson & Johnson	−0.47	6.0%		−11.67
Hoechst	0.40	2.4%		4.03
Novartis	1.36	1.0%		5.44
Aventis	4.06	1.2%		20.29
Pfizer	3.01	4.1%		51.19
Wyeth-Ayerst	5.78	2.4%		57.83
Schering-Plough	13.45	1.9%		107.59

simple terms, by multiplying a company's average approval time differential by the number of products it developed during the sample period. This simple calculation probably over-estimates the advantage of the largest firms (such as Merck), but it does not affect the rank-ordering that emerges from the data. These statistics appear to echo the intuition of observers of the global pharmaceutical industry and the FDA in the late twentieth century: Merck stands far and above the other firms in its average speed of NME approval, even when its size, its experience, over-time trends, and the therapeutic target of the drug are taken into account. What is perhaps more surprising is the set of firms that did not perform as well during this period—Pfizer, Wyeth-Ayerst, Hoechst (which includes Hoechst Marion Roussel), and Schering-Plough. The rank-ordering of firms supplies one glimpse into firms' variable reputations during the late twentieth century.[63]

An Analysis of Priority Ratings. Additional insight into firm differences can be gained from examining which drugs get priority ratings. Priority ratings are the highest pre-review scores that the Administration assigns to new drugs at the time of their NDA submission, before the review process begins. In the system developed in the late 1970s and 1980s, the highest rating was "1A" (with alternatives of B and C, which denoted progressively less innovative or critical therapies). The system was later changed to a binary coding, with "1P" representing priority drugs and "1S" representing other, "standard" drugs. While priority ratings officially designate the perceived therapeutic innovation promised in a new molecule, they are also the product of lobbying efforts by sponsors and, more recently, by patient advocacy groups. At their core, priority ratings reflect FDA judgments about product quality or risk, but these judgments, too, are influenced by firm reputations.

Priority ratings are not fully determined by technical considerations, then, but are partially endogenous to the political and organizational factors shaping U.S. pharmaceutical regulation and firm-level development. There is, in addition, a crucial didactic reason for analyzing priority ratings. They are established before NDA review and remained fixed over the entire review. Any factor affecting FDA priority ratings therefore exercises its influence before Administration reviewers commence their official scrutiny of the application. Whatever political, organizational, and scientific mechanisms shape priority ratings are necessarily distinct from those that generate longer or shorter reviews, after the ratings have been set. Table 10.4 reports summary data from analyses of which factors were statistically associated

[63]It is important to underscore that the estimate in the rightmost column of table 10.3 is a linear extrapolation and linearity is used as a demonstrative assumption. Still, the persistence of Merck's advantages, combined with the large number of new molecules that the company sponsored in the late twentieth century, suggests that it enjoyed some appreciable and enduring regulatory advantages. If for instance Merck's aggregated advantage was one-third of the amount estimated in table 10.3, the company would still have benefited from a sum total of five years' marketing lead relative to firms such as Pfizer during this period.

TABLE 10.4
Variables Associated with Probability of Receiving a Priority Rating,
NMEs Submitted 1977–2000

Percentage of NMEs receiving Priority Status in Sample: 29.2%

Variable	Associated Shift for One-Unit Increase Variable	Lower 95% C.I. for Associated Shift	Upper 95% C.I. for Associated Shift	Standard Deviation of Variable	Associated Shift for One SD Increase in Variable
Firm sales (logged, deflated)	-0.3%	-2.7%	2.2%	2.2	-0.6%
Previous firm NME submissions	1.1%	0.2%	1.9%	6.3	6.7%
Number of previously approved NMEs for primary indication	-0.8%	-1.6%	0.0%	10.6	-8.3%
Year of NME submission (trend)	1.3%	0.3%	2.4%	5.1	6.7%

Notes: C.I. = "confidence interval." Shift estimates and associated confidence intervals are retrieved from random-effects logistic regression with priority rating as dependent variable and listed variables as regressors. NMEs in sample = 414; random effects estimated for 144 primary indications. Larger effects observed if random effects are estimated for sponsoring firm.

with which drugs received the highest priority ratings of the various classifications over the past twenty years.

Examination of aggregate patterns suggests that large firms were no more likely to receive priority ratings than smaller firms were, at least in the late twentieth century. Indeed, the estimated association between firm sales and ratings is slightly negative. Whatever advantages large firms may have in FDA regulation, they are not more likely to receive priority ratings for their drugs. Firms with more submissions were, however, more likely to receive priority ratings, which suggests that these ratings have served to reflect the Administration's judgments about likely product quality and safety, uncertainty over which is reduced by solid firm reputations. Consistent with the formal rationale for assigning priority ratings—which are supposed to accrue to those drugs that target "unmet medical need"—later entrants to a disease-specific therapeutic category are less likely to receive priority status, while orphan drugs are more likely to receive it.

Priority ratings offer one other window into the aggregate patterns of regulatory decision making in the late twentieth century. They are a convenient means of parsing the set of drugs developed and approved into two sets: those where the Administration knowingly subjected itself to pressure for their speedy approval by assigning high status to them, and those where the Administration did not subject itself to such pressure. Examining priority drugs, there is no observable relationship between firm size and the speed of approval in the late twentieth century. The statistical advantage of larger firms appears in those drugs that did not receive high priority ratings, where the weight of the FDA's own imprimatur did not weigh upon the decision, and where the force of organizational skill and reputation exercised a much greater effect.[64]

DUAL CREDIBILITY AND PRODUCT DEVELOPMENT

Each new molecule that is launched economically and prescribed therapeutically reflects and masks a long, costly saga of experimentation and claims-making. Commercial sponsors are carriers of reputations, and the relationship between these firms and their regulator is one in which particular intentions are under constant and enduring surveillance. Ultimately, neither FDA officials, nor their most esteemed advisers, nor company functionaries know with perfect confidence how a new drug will fare in widespread clinical use and in a national or global marketplace. The vast system of compulsory experimentation put in place by the Administration's regulations and

[64]The estimated elasticity of the relationship between firm sales and NME approval time helps to illuminate this relationship. For the set of nonpriority drugs approved from 1977 to 2000, the estimated elasticity is -0.69, meaning that a 10 percent increase in firm sales is associated with a 7 percent reduction in approval time ($p < 0.0001$). When priority drugs are examined separately, this elasticity estimate falls to -0.10, and is statistically insignificant ($p = 0.63$).

the Kefauver-Harris Amendments greatly reduces this uncertainty, but can never resolve it. Coursing through the development process and driving much of its ultimate outcomes is the politics of dual credibility: the mutual gaze of firm and regulator. American pharmaceutical regulation relies throughout upon the judgment not simply of the technical features of a new drug application or a marketed therapy, but of the remarks and displayed emotions of the sponsor and its governor. In this relationship, whether brief or enduring, the Administration benefits from a combination of esteem and fear.

American Pharmaceutical Regulation in International Context: Audiences, Comparisons, and Dependencies

GOVERNMENT REGULATION of the development and market entry of therapeutic medicines is a global phenomenon. Many countries—including most member states of the European Union today—possess their own regulatory agencies dedicated to pre-market review and post-market surveillance of medicines. Over the course of the late twentieth century, these agencies spread persistently across continents, economies, and contexts. Many of the world's pharmaceutical regulatory agencies—in Australia, Taiwan, South Korea, Brazil, China, and other countries—have been created or fundamentally transformed since 1989. At present, dozens of nations (comprising at least three-quarters of the world's population) have their own legislation governing ethical drugs; evaluating safety and efficacy during the "pre-market" life of medicines; and governing their sale, advertising, manufacture, and distribution after regulatory approval and marketing. Indeed, the multiplication of national regulation has been so continual and varied that industrial and intergovernmental voices have since the 1970s attempted to achieve "harmonization" of the unwieldy mix.[1]

The international plethora of organizations, rules, and laws dedicated to the governance of pharmaceuticals creates opportunities for meaningful and illuminating comparisons. There is considerable variation across these country-specific settings—in legislation, in powers delegated to state regulators as opposed to professional bodies and industry-based organizations, in administrative structure, in the relative power of domestic drug companies, in the dependence of the state regulator upon national medical and pharmacy professions, in the strength and scattering of organized patient advocates and consumer safety activists. Genuine distinctions among the status and reputations of these national regulatory agencies persist and help to account for the variable authority and power of the agencies themselves.

From the vantage of reputation, however, these various regulatory bodies create and animate a different kind of politics. These regulators and the governments of which they form a part are crucial audiences and referents for each other, and for the Food and Drug Administration. They are audiences because they form a peer group of sorts. National regulators engage in

[1]Until the creation by the "Benelux" countries (Belgium, Netherlands, Luxembourg) of a supranational registration system in 1973, pharmaceutical regulation in the West was almost exclusively a national-level phenomenon. In contemporary China, much decision making for pharmaceutical regulation is carried out at the provincial level; in India, there is considerable state-level variation in the organizational capacity and policy of drug regulation.

the same sort of problem solving and learning activity that the FDA is charged with, and politicians, citizens, firms, and organized publics in these nations are audiences to which these regulators are held at least partially accountable. These agencies are referents because audiences in the United States (Congress, a consumer advocacy group, a pharmaceutical industry trade association) can point to foreign regulators as an example of how the Administration has failed, succeeded, delayed, accelerated, over-regulated, under-regulated, or something else. To the extent that national regulators create audiences for one another, the cozy assumption that these agencies can be compared as if they were "data points" in an experiment must be thrown out. Since the agencies are watching and learning from one another's decisions, and since they adopt and reject one another's standards and precedents, they cannot be considered independent of one another.[2]

The power of the Administration's organizational reputation in the twentieth century has generated other sorts of dependencies as well. While the official boundaries and personnel of a regulatory agency may lie neatly within the confines of a nation, the reputation of that agency does not. Beliefs, information, and symbols flow across national and geographic borders. And no agency has functioned as a more persistent net exporter of ideas, symbols, concepts, forms, standards, and institutions than the FDA. This fluidity of organizational symbols—the Investigational New Drug process (with "Phase 1," "Phase 2," and "Phase 3" trials), the New Drug Application form and procedure, the person of Frances Kelsey, the concepts and elaboration of "Good Manufacturing Practices" and "Good Laboratory Practices," the adverse event report—means that what happens at the FDA affects pharmaceutical regulation, production, and use the world over. While in recent years observers have begun to attribute greater and greater international status to the regulators of the European Union, it is fair to say that the U.S. Food and Drug Administration was in the twentieth century the dominant national regulator in the governance of global pharmaceutical markets.[3]

It would be unfortunate to re-enact a form of "American exceptionalism" by pointing to the uniqueness of the FDA and its organizational reputation. Historians and other students of politics and institutions in the United States have in recent years demonstrated pervasive dependence of

[2] I have attempted to incorporate these considerations of international politics and transnational dependence throughout this book—see chapters 3, 4, 5, 9, and 10 for examples—but some of the patterns deserve explicit and separate treatment as the creatures of reputation-based politics.

[3] Experienced European observers often argue that arrangements in the Netherlands also provided a highly emulated model. Graham Dukes, who served as Medical Director of the Netherlands Commission for the Evaluation of Medicines from 1972 to 1982, remarks that "the Netherlands model, alongside the longer experience with functioning evaluation systems in Scandinavia, provided the essential foundations for what were later to become the provisions on control of medicines applicable to all member states of the European Community, provisions which developed rapidly from 1965 onwards"; *The Law and Ethics of the Pharmaceutical Industry* (Amsterdam: Elsevier, 2006), 107; see also 89, 131, 138.

American developments upon prior and simultaneous changes on other continents and in other nations. In the governance of pharmaceuticals, too, there are meaningful patterns of dependence whereby the Administration's officials have looked to other nations for guidance and precedent, and have borrowed procedures and concepts from foreign regulatory organizations. These patterns must not be forgotten. Yet to characterize the FDA as just another pharmaceutical regulator would be to commit both anachronisms and understatements. Indeed, a truly historical and transnational perspective on global pharmaceutical regulation places greater emphasis upon the Administration, not less. Given the agency's image and its power over the world's most profitable pharmaceutical market, the FDA influences the international politics and political economy of pharmaceuticals more than any other regulatory agency. This influence comes in many forms, from the attention given to its public actions to the silent adoption of its less visible assumptions and ingrained patterns of behavior. The status and cultural power of the Administration testifies not principally to American dominance in global affairs, but rather to an increasingly globalized world of therapeutics and medicine. Within that world, the FDA has become a setter of standards for technological, scientific, economic, and cultural development in medicine. This capacity to define standards and assumptions flows, again, from the Administration's reputation and power.

In the international reach of the FDA's concepts and approaches—even and perhaps especially when these concepts and approaches are resisted or contested—the "third face" of regulatory power emerges again into view. In the global pharmaceutical realm, the third face of regulatory power is the capacity to define legitimate science and the standards of evaluation not merely within professions and industries, but among other governments that define science and standards within the boundaries of their authority. It is the power to establish a certain handful of procedures as the default setting that any nation revising or launching a scheme of pharmaceutical regulation will start with. The core point is that nations copy not only the Administration's drug-specific decisions—whether or not to revise labeling on an approved drug, whether or not to ask for more clinical trials, whether or not to approve or register a new drug for marketing—but also the Administration's procedures, rules, and symbols. Hence, the FDA's conceptual power extends internationally. Such power stems not from global legal authority but rather from political, economic, and scientific leverage exercised through the mechanisms of reputation and legitimacy.[4]

---

[4]In recent decades, an important literature on transnational or "global" history has arisen, and its effect has been to fundamentally transform narratives of nationhood and national institutional development. For some exemplary readings, see Daniel Rodgers, *Atlantic Crossings* (Cambridge, MA: Harvard University Press, 1998); Matthew Connelly, "Seeing Beyond the State: The Population Control Movement and the Problem of Sovereignty," *Past & Present* 193 (Dec. 2006): 197–233; "*AHR* Conversation: On Transnational History," *American Historical Review* 111 (5) (Dec. 2006): 1441–64. For a recent attempt at transnational understandings of twentieth-century pharmaceutical history, see Sophie Chauveau and Viviane Quirke,

The copying of standards and structures does not, of course, necessarily equate to the copying of behavior. Much of the spread of the American model in international pharmaceuticals can be described as a form of isomorphism, namely the aim of foreign governments to look "rational" and legitimate by adopting institutions that do not constrain and shape behavior as fully as they do in the pioneer country. Yet standards and structures are not costless. Even when copied FDA standards are followed imperfectly or meet with partial compliance, they still constrain behavior. The necessity for drug sponsors to complete three sequentially phased trials, or to complete bioavailability studies, or to complete a form (the French Autorisation de Mise sur le Marché (AMM), or the "Schedule Y" of India) that closely resembles the FDA's new drug application form or its investigational new drug application—these necessary and methodical steps of drug development in Europe, Asia, and other settings impose agendas upon drug companies, upon clinical researchers, and upon government officials themselves.[5]

COMPARISONS AND DEPENDENCIES AMONG DEVELOPED NATIONS

In matters of pharmaceuticals, the FDA is most frequently compared with national regulatory authorities in Europe and with agencies in Australia, Canada, Japan, and New Zealand. In the main, these regulators govern pharmaceutical development, production, and marketing in "advanced industrialized" nations: those countries with larger economies, democratic and competitive political systems, and historically enduring republican and democratic institutions.

Any discussion of the relations and comparisons among the FDA and these regulators must first acknowledge a salient fact. In the late twentieth and early twenty-first centuries, the United States was the only nation among those called "advanced and industrialized" in which the government did not provide some form of universal health insurance for its citizens. It is, moreover, the only such nation in which the government does not directly constrain pharmaceutical prices by regulation or bargaining. Put differently, all of the "Western" agencies to which the FDA is compared govern pharmaceutical marketing in countries where drug prices are regulated through nationalized

---

"The American 'Model' and the British and French Pharmaceutical Industries in the Twentieth Century," presented at the Helsinki Congress of the International Economic History Association, August 2006.

[5] The classic account of institutional isomorphism in sociology appears in John W. Meyer and Brian Rowan, "Institutionalized Organizations: Formal Structure as Myth and Ceremony," *American Journal of Sociology* 83 (2): 340–63. See more generally the collection of essays in Walter W. Powell and Paul J. DiMaggio, eds., *The New Institutionalism in Organizational Analysis* (Chicago: University of Chicago Press, 1991), and the notion of "organizational repertoires" in Elisabeth Clemens, *The People's Lobby: Organizational Innovation and the Rise of Interest Group Politics in the United States, 1890–1925* (Chicago: University of Chicago Press, 1997).

or government-provided health insurance. In many of these nations, the government is the principal (sometimes the only) purchaser of the products being regulated. Relatedly, in many of these countries (especially in Europe), there was no genuine system of patent protection for innovations for most of the twentieth century. Many observers have surmised that the dual role of these governments—as buyer and as entry regulator—creates significant constraints for safety and efficacy regulation. Drug regulators in these other countries are said to be more attentive to issues of price, so that even an otherwise "safe and effective" drug will be turned down or later withdrawn when a cheaper alternative is available. Governments are said to make trade-offs on matters of price and affordability, on one dimension, and safety and efficacy on other dimensions.[6]

These readings have plausibility and evidence, but it is possible to over-simplify matters. In most advanced industrialized nations with universal, government-provided health insurance, the regulation of drug safety and efficacy is often undertaken by administrative bodies different from those that constrain prices or establish national formularies. It is not clear that these different administrative bodies coordinate their activities and deci-sions, and it is sometimes clear that they do not at all act in concert. The partial separation of "welfare" state from "regulatory" state in these na-tions implies not that pharmaceutical regulators act with autonomy, but rather that they pay little attention to questions of price and affordability in making their decisions and plans.[7]

---

[6]To make the comparison more precise, there are several forms of government-provided health insurance at the national level in the United States. These include (1) provision of care for military veterans through the Veterans' Administration (VA) health system, (2) provision of health insurance for the poor through Medicaid (whose funding burden is shared by the states), (3) and provision of health insurance for the aged and infirm by Medicare. Since the creation of "Medicare Part D" in 2002, the American government has insured non-hospitalization drug purchases as well as bills for physicians' visits, procedures, and hospitalization. A crucial and controversial plank of Medicare Part D, however, expressly forbids the federal government from bargaining over prices with pharmaceutical companies. Jonathan Oberlander, *The Politi-cal Life of Medicare* (Chicago: University of Chicago Press, 2003). Of course, many U.S. poli-cies affect pharmaceutical prices indirectly; the contrast is most stark when direct price regula-tion is examined.

Even with these caveats, the cross-national difference persists and has been the subject of considerable scholarship in political science, sociology, history, and economics. For an in-depth historical analysis of the United States, see Jacob Hacker, *The Divided Welfare State* (New York: Cambridge University Press, 2002), especially his "Introduction: American Exceptional-ism Revisited." Sven Steinmo, *Taxation and Democracy: Swedish, British and American Ap-proaches to Financing the Modern State* (New Haven: Yale University Press, 1993). For a plausible claim that British regulators balance the needs of the national health system and the regulatory demands of the domestic market, see Stephen Ceccoli, "Divergent Paths to Drug Regulation in the United States and the United Kingdom," *Journal of Policy History* 14 (2) (2002): 140.

[7]In the United Kingdom, the Pharmaceutical Price Regulation Scheme constrains profits from drug sales as a percentage of return on capital, hence the regulation of prices is indirect and harkens to "rate of return" regulation used in the United States and Europe for power and

Local and royal governments in Europe have regulated food and drugs for hundreds of years, and many nations can point to still-functioning drug statutes that date from the early nineteenth century. Norway adopted national pharmaceutical regulation in 1928 and Sweden followed in 1935. Sweden's institutions were of particular interest to FDA officials, as they included explicit recognition of efficacy and the establishment of a royal medical board—the Board of Pharmaceutical Specialties—that advised the crown and established an official pharmacopoeia that limited the set of legally marketed drugs. Following these Nordic countries and the United States, the Fifth Republic government of France adopted in 1945 a law governing the pharmacy profession, establishing pharmacists as experts entitled to assess firms' compliance with safety regulations and to ensure that scientific tests on drugs were completed. The closest thing to an administrative system of drug evaluation came in the institutions established under the Netherlands Medicines Act of 1958. This law established mandatory review of safety and efficacy for new and already-marketed drugs, and positioned a Board of Experts to carry out evaluations in consultation with nongovernment experts and laboratories. Even the progressive Dutch government, however, lacked anything like the FDA's Bureau of Medicine and Bureau of Pharmacology. The Netherlands erected a system of drug evaluation, but it was not an administrative system characterized by embedded organizational capacity.[8]

The other notable regulator of therapeutics in the pre-thalidomide era lay in the French government, which like the FDA relied upon pharmacological expertise and procedures for pre-market examination of drugs. A decade and more before the thalidomide crisis, French officials regarded their laws as more stringent than any existing in Germany (which was the French government's primary reference point and competitor in matters pharmaceutical and chemical). The Stalimon episode—which occurred when a tin compound marketed as an oral medication for furunculosis caused nearly one hundred

---

utility companies. In Canada, price regulation is carried out by the Patented Medicines Prices Review Board, which uses an index of drug prices in other industrialized nations. Wictorowicz, "Emergent Patterns in the Regulation of Pharmaceuticals," 627–8; Ellen Immergut, "Institutions, Veto Points and Policy Results: A Comparative Analysis of Health Care," *Journal of Public Policy* 10 (4) (1990): 391–416.

[8]Some of these features of the Swedish and Dutch systems, and their differences with the American system at mid-century, are examined in chapter 3. For an accessible summary of Swedish institutions as of the late 1970s, see Ake Liljestrand (Department of Drugs, National Board of Health and Welfare), "Requirements in Sweden," in J. Z. Bowers and G. P. Velo, eds., *Drug Assessment Criteria and Methods: Proceedings of the International Symposium on Scientific Criteria and Methods for Drug Assessment held in Rome, Italy, 5–7 July 1979* (Amsterdam: Elsevier/North-Holland Biomedical Press, 1979), 29–38. FDA officials would later note the progressivity of the Swedish efficacy standard; J. Richard Crout, address at FDA 2006 Science Conference, April 18, 2006; Washington, DC. Philip R. Lee and Jessica Herzstein, "International Drug Regulation," *Annual Review of Public Health* 7 (1986): 217–35; Bernard L. Oser, "The Scientists' Forum," *FDCLJ* 13 (1958): 196–7. The Dutch title of the 1958 legislation is *Wet op de Geneesmiddelenvoorzienung*; see Dukes, *Law and Ethics of the Pharmaceutical Industry*, 107–8.

deaths and dozens of significant injuries—induced the French government
to further tighten requirements several years before thalidomide. In the process, French experts examined U.S. models (they were also looking at U.S.
and FDA models from the late 1940s through the 1950s). Yet even the pharmacological progressivity of pre-thalidomide French arrangements paled in
comparison to the procedures and protocols developed at the FDA Pharmacology Bureau and Division of Medicine. Requirements for pre-marketing
safety evaluation in pre-thalidomide France rested almost entirely on animal
tests (as compared to the increasing reliance on clinical tests at the FDA).
French officials in pharmacology and in regulation kept a close eye on American developments, in part seeking information from an understanding that
French testing requirements were years behind the clinical test requirements
of American authorities. The gaze that French officials cast across the Atlantic was significant; in Europe, only the Netherlands had a drug regulatory
scheme as stringent as that of the French.[9]

As of 1961, when reports of thalidomide's connection to birth defects
emerged, European nations (most notably Great Britain) lacked a unified
administrative scheme for regulating the development and marketing of ethical drugs. In West Germany, a 1961 statute revamped the existing Bundesgesundheitsamt (BGA, or Federal Health Office) into a pre-market registration agency. Companies introducing new drugs were required to procure a
manufacturing license from the BGA and to submit summaries of chemical
and pharmacological studies for registration. Among European countries,
the German system was advanced for its time, yet it left considerable authority and social control in the hands of the powerful German medical profession. Physicians' and pharmacists' societies promulgated standards of drug
evaluation, leaving the BGA as a passive recipient of these standards. Registration, moreover, did not translate into regulatory power. The BGA never
possessed a genuine veto over product development or marketing; its powers
over drug companies were limited to bargaining with firms over approved
products with identifiable safety problems. When the thalidomide episode
hit the Western world, Sweden and the Netherlands were the only nations
with a formal efficacy requirement for pre-market registration, although the
United States had essentially adopted such a requirement informally.[10]

---

[9] For a summary of pre-market safety testing in France on the eve of the thalidomide disaster,
see J. Cheymol (Directeur de l'Institut de Pharmacologie, Faculté de Médecine, Paris), *Détermi-
nation de l'Innocuité des Nouvelles Préparations Pharmaceutiques avant leur Mise en Vente—
Exigences et Méthodes*, WHO/EURO-203/9, 14 avril 1961; AWHO. Assay procedures for
animal tests had been elaborated by the *Commission des Essais* for several drug categories, including hypnotics, local anesthetics, anti-coagulants and some antibiotics. Pre-thalidomide
French institutions had been shaped by the Stalinon crisis of the late 1950s; Christian Bonah and
Jean-Paul Gaudilliere, "Faute, accident ou risque iatrogène? La régulation des évènements indé-
sirables du médicament à l'aune des affaires Stalinon et Distilbène," *Revue Francaise des Affaires
Sociales* 3 (4) (2007): 123–51. Dukes, *Law and Ethics of the Pharmaceutical Industry*, 106.

[10] As Arthur Daemmrich concisely describes the limitations of the German law, "the BGA
lacked any mechanism to slow or prevent a medicine from reaching the market. Instead, the

Before the thalidomide episode, then, American drug regulation exhibited bureaucracy, protocol, and veto power; contemporary European drug regulation shared few of these traits. In the United States, often termed the "stateless society" of the West, pharmaceutical regulation was administratively centralized and characterized by much higher organizational capacity than in Europe. This procedural and organizational distinction between American and European institutions would have struck observers of European and American politics as rather odd. While Sweden had an efficacy requirement, no other country exhibited anything like the New Drug Application process that was conceived in the 1950s FDA, and no other nation habitually employed inspectors to examine pharmaceutical research and development, production, sales and marketing with stiff criminal penalties for legal violations. In some cases, such as France and Germany, the power that might have resided in the bureaucratic state was instead exercised by professions and their organized associations, along with industrial groups. In Sweden and Germany, too, there was considerable reliance upon decentralized arrangements whereby regulation of drugs was left to local health boards (Sweden) or state governments (Länder, in Germany).[11]

In global perspective, the thalidomide episode triggered a nation-by-nation examination of institutions for drug development, approval, and surveillance. While the regulatory legacy of the episode is best remembered today in the United States, the thalidomide tragedy also occasioned governments worldwide to scrutinize their procedures and capacities for regulating drugs. What was a global phenomenon of self-examination was not, of course, uniform across nations in its procedures and results. There were incredibly varied responses to the thalidomide affair, and some countries were as likely to reject the American model as to emulate it. Yet nation by nation, introspection was quickly accompanied by extended gazes at the United States and the FDA, for it was widely perceived that American regulators

---

government was placed in a reactive posture whereby officials could only advise companies to voluntarily withdraw drugs that proved dangerous once they were widely available"; *Pharmacopolitics: Drug Regulation in the United States and Germany* (Chapel Hill: University of North Carolina Press, 2004), 38. For a contemporary description of these weaknesses in the years immediately following the 1976 law, see Franz Cross, "Drug Legislation in the Federal Republic of Germany," in Bowers and Velo, *Drug Assessment Criteria and Methods*, 55–6; also Ute Stapel, *Die Arzneimittelgesetze 1961 und 1976* (Stuttgart: Deutcher Apotheker Verlag, 1988).

[11] In an otherwise informative article, Mary Wictorowicz overstates the "fragmented" character of U.S. pharmaceutical regulation; "Emergent Patterns in the Regulation of Pharmaceuticals: Institutions and Interests in the United States, Canada, Britain and France," *Journal of Health Politics, Policy and Law* 28 (4) (Aug. 2003): 640. She and others rightly characterize American pharmaceutical regulation as involving greater administrative discretion than in other nations, but she also characterizes Canadian and European arrangements as entailing more "bargaining" between firms and the government. The difference on this dimension, if one exists, is that in the United States, bargaining between the regulator and the regulated occurs more informally and on a drug-by-drug basis, due to the FDA's strong veto power over market entry; see chapter 6 and Lars Noah, "Administrative Arm Twisting in the Shadow of Congressional Delegations of Authority," *Wisconsin Law Review* 1997 (5): 873–941.

had gotten matters "correct" in the thalidomide affair. Whether or not the Administration was copied, it quickly became the "global standard" to which other nations referred in constructing new models and institutions.

Thalidomide imposed its greatest and most visible human misery upon the citizens of West Germany, and no sooner had the West German Bundesrepublik passed new legislation in 1961 than it was forced to revisit its own institutions. Germany's response to thalidomide moved the nation not toward an American system of administrative discretion and control, but in several directions at once. Professional societies in medicine and pharmacology responded to the episode not defensively, but aggressively by lobbying for greater control over the testing and marketing of drugs. Legislation passed in 1964 imposed two new requirements upon new drugs. First, all new medicines were required to undergo pre-market testing before marketing. The 1964 statute left these evaluations in the hands of licensed industrial sponsors, and standard-setting for these tests was determined entirely by medical and pharmacology societies, not at all by the BGA. Second, the 1964 statute initiated a prescription requirement for all drugs with novel ingredients. This plank of the law reflected the power of the German medical profession, as well as the particular narrative of thalidomide and the conscious design of the 1964 statute to prevent its reoccurrence. Thalidomide had been marketed as Contergan in Germany, and was most commonly purchased by parents as a sedative for their children, as a tranquilizer and sleep aid for adults, and as an anti-nausea drug by pregnant women.[12]

The end result of the 1964 law was a regime of pharmaceutical regulation that was legally more strict than its predecessor, but no stronger administratively. The German legislative response had been to accord greater discretion and trust to the national pharmaceutical industry and the state-legitimated professions. Yet when American correspondents visited the country in 1962, they also perceived a society concerned about centralized control and committed to federalism. The 1964 law left considerable authority in the hands of the Länder governments, keeping the BGA as an information-gathering body without standard-setting or punitive authority. So too, German citizens appeared to balance a distrust of central state authority with a greater willingness to rely upon the incentives of companies. Those interviewed "pointed out that the Government itself could never duplicate the great variety of facilities available to the industry." Combined with a corporatist political structure that enmeshed professions and industry within the state apparatus, West Germany's cultural commitments to federalism and state distrust seemed to preclude the possibility of greater BGA power after thalidomide. The BGA was politically and culturally constrained from ac-

---

[12]Wilhelm Bartmann, *Zwischen Tradition und Fortschrift: aus der Geschichte der Pharmabereiche von Bayer, Hoechst und Schering von 1935–1975* (Stuttgart: Franz Steiner Verlag, 2003), III.2, 222–4. Stapel, *Die Arzneimittelgesetze 1961 und 1976*; cited in Daemmrich, *Pharmacopolitics*. Beate Kirk, *Der Contergan-Fall: eine unvermeidbare Arzneimittelkatastrophe?* (Stuttgart: Deutsche Apotheker Verlag, 1999). Abraham and Lewis, *Regulating Medicines in Europe*, 54 (citing an unpublished paper by Leigh Hancher and co-author).

quiring a reputation for protection, or a capacity for strong authority over the German pharmaceutical market.[13]

In the two English-speaking nations most afflicted by thalidomide—Australia and Great Britain—new institutions assumed the form of advisory bodies. The Australian Drug Evaluation Committee (ADEC) first met in July 1963, with the formal charge of advising the government on issues of drug safety and effectiveness, and occasionally with the intent of evaluating new medicines. Yet the Committee did not evaluate each new drug that came to its attention and did not establish standards of evidence or procedure for the introduction of new medicines. For decades after thalidomide, the principal activities of Australian regulators lay in post-market surveillance.[14]

In 1963, the British government established a Committee on the Safety of Drugs (CSD), a weak and advisory regulatory agency which set standards for the pharmaceutical industry to follow when initiating clinical trials, introducing drugs to market and following drug experience after initial marketing. The CSD's work depended heavily upon its liaison with the Association of British Pharmaceutical Industries (ABPI). The arrangement by which companies submitted new drug applications to the Committee was voluntary. Until 1968, nothing in British law or regulation required the CSD's approval for new drugs to be marketed. In dimensions of organizational capacity and reputation, too, the CSD depended heavily upon British drug companies. Five of the twelve committee members came from the industry, and upon his retirement the Committee's original chairman, Sir Derrick Dunlop, moved to a senior position within the ABPI. When manufacturers submitted new drug protocols to the Committee, the Committee could not draw upon independent physicians or pharmacologists to review them. Instead, the Committee was compelled to trust the data in the submissions that came to them. Early patterns of review suggest that the Committee did just this, refusing to approve 2–6 percent of the applications submitted.[15]

[13]Stapel, *Die Arzneimittelgesetze 1961 und 1976*; cited in Daemmrich, *Pharmacopolitics*. Crosby S. Noyes (foreign correspondent, *Washington Star*), "Thalidomide's Shadow: Germany Shuns Controls," *Washington Star* (evening edition), August 28, 1962, p. 2. "And it is argued that the improvement of testing procedures should be left to the industry which has itself the liveliest and most direct interest in insuring the safety and effectiveness of its profits."

[14]John McEwen, "Australian Drug Evaluation Committee (ADEC) 40th Anniversary," *International Journal of Pharmaceutical Medicine* 18 (4) (2004): 225–6; A. M. Walshe, "The Adverse Drug Reporting Reaction Scheme and the Australian Drug Evaluation Committee," *Medical Journal of Australia* 2 (2) (July 13, 1968): 82–5.

[15]The ABPI and the Proprietary Association of Great Britain promised not to market any drug or launch any clinical trial without the Committee's approval; see the remarks of Dunlop in "Pharmaceuticals," *Times of London*, November 9, 1970, I. These and other characterizations of the British regulatory system rely heavily upon the insightful characterizations of sociologist John Abraham and his collaborators. See Abraham, *Science, Politics and the Pharmaceutical Industry: Controversy and Bias in Drug Regulation* (London: University College Press, 1995); Abraham and Graham Lewis, *Regulating Medicines in Europe: Competition, Expertise and Public Health* (London and New York: Routledge, 2000), especially chap. 3 (51); Abraham, "Scientific Standards and Institutional Interests: Carcinogenic Risk Assessment of Benoxaprofen in the UK and US," *Social Studies of Science* 23 (1993): 420–23.

From audiences in British medicine, the stark differences between British and American organizational capacity were inescapable and significant. When concerns arose in the early 1960s about oral contraceptives and their associated risks of stroke, the Food and Drug Administration entered into extended bargaining with Searle over the contents of a "Dear Doctor" letter. The FDA's postmarket regulation of oral contraceptives was limited, to be sure, but the *British Medical Journal* saw an apparatus in Washington that was entirely lacking in London.

> It is of course impossible to know how much of the contents of the Searle letter is due to its consultations with the FDA. Certainly the fact that it was prepared in association with a Government agency lends it a weight and authority to which it could hardly lay claim otherwise. This is perhaps a welcome reminder that the FDA has a wider function than merely registered drugs—it can also exercise a useful effect on the amount and quality of information which the pharmaceutical houses disseminate to the profession. It can insist, for instance, on the notification of side-effects in promotional and package literature. We have, by contrast, no official provision in this country for insuring that dangers and disadvantages of preparations are so notified—this is left entirely to the judgment of the industry.[16]

The principal post-thalidomide moves toward an American model in European drug regulation came in two steps: one of voice in two global organizations, the other of piecemeal action in a beacon country. In 1965 and again in 1975 and 1978, the European Economic Community issued directives on the regulation of pharmaceuticals. The 1965 instruction called upon all Member States to "approximate" their institutions of drug regulation, and in doing so strongly suggested that an administrative gatekeeping process be established in each country. No "proprietary medicinal product" could be marketed in a member state, the EEC declared, unless it had been authorized by a "competent authority" of that nation. The EEC further gestured to American-style administrative processes when it called for the establishment of formal "application" processes in each country that contained specific "particulars and documents." The Community also requested evaluations that rested upon three sorts of investigations: chemical and biological tests, followed by "pharmacological and toxicological tests," concluding with "clinical trials." No one in 1965 could mistake these recommendations as anything other than a formal gesture to the NDA and IND processes at the Administration.[17]

As a rough comparison, the FDA refused or induced withdrawal of 10–25 percent of NME applications submitted during the 1970s; see chapter 6.

[16] "Today's Drugs: Oral Contraceptives and Thrombophlebitis," *BMJ* (Sept. 15, 1962): 727. *Medical Tribune*, August 20, 1962, p. 23.

[17] "Council Directive 65/65/EEC of 26 January 1965 on the approximation of provisions laid down by Law, Regulation or Administrative Action relating to proprietary medicinal products," *Official Journal of the European Community* 22 (Feb. 9, 1965): 369–73. Peter Beaconsfield, "Drug Safety and the Law: Harmonisation and Its Obstacles in the EEC," *Pharmaceuti-*

As the EEC directives were taking shape, officials of the World Health Organization in Geneva also issued a series of instructions to their member governments and international bureaucrats. The twin governing bodies of the WHO—its World Health Assembly (WHA) and its Executive Board—traded reports, requests, and resolutions, each building toward minimum standards for drug quality control and for safety and efficacy evaluation of drugs. These echoed the American model of drug evaluation in numerous ways, not least by recognizing the primacy of national-level health authorities and drug clearance regimes. The WHO Assembly's efforts to improve adverse reaction reporting among member nations drew explicitly upon FDA models and resources, including a heavy reliance upon the FDA's data processing facilities. After a half-decade of studying the problem of quality control, the Assembly in July 1969 issued recommendations for member adoption of "Good Manufacturing Practices" guidelines. In part because WHO officials favored FDA models of drug registration, manufacturing control, and adverse event surveillance, many of the Organziation's recommendations to member states called for the implicit emulation of American structure and protocol. The WHO Director-General's report of 1970, *Safety and Efficacy of Drugs: Principles for Drug Control*, was particularly noteworthy in this respect. The report called for "regulations to impose requirements on manufacturers or institutions undertaking drug research," including extensive preclinical requirements and "an outline of the proposed procedures in human subjects." These were gestures to regulating preclinical experiment, requiring prospective designs for clinical trials before they began, and regulating therapeutic research generally, and the FDA was by 1970 far ahead of the world's other agencies. So too, the report's insistence that a national regulatory agency have strong pharmacology capacities was also a direct gesture in the direction of the FDA. One year later, the WHO Assembly called for the "stimulation of national regulations for drug control" and the establishment of "national drug regulatory agencies" with required training of staff, again gesturing toward pharmacology and pharmaceutical control.[18]

---

cal Journal, June 1, 1974, 502–4. Though I have not been able to establish the point, it is possible that the 1965 directive was also influenced by the mimicry of American arrangements in Finland, which in its 1964 Drug Law created a "New Drug Application" procedure; Juhana Idanpään-Heikkilä, "Restrictions in Prescribing the New Medicines, Price Evaluation of New Medicines, and Some Other Requirements Applied in Finland," in Bowers and Velo, *Drug Assessment Criteria*, 40.

[18]The WHA's recommendations for minimum requirements for drug evaluation and monitoring came in Assembly resolution WHA15.41 (May 1962), Assembly resolution WHA16.36 and Executive Board resolution EB 33.R21; all in *Handbook of Resolutions and Decisions of the World Health Assembly and the Executive Board*, vol. 1: 1945–1972 (Geneva, WHO: 1973), 138–9. The quality control resolutions appear in WHA17.41, WHA18.36, WHA19.47 and WHA22.50 (July 1969), the last of which elaborated and recommended the "Good Practice" concept; *Handbook*, 133. Report of the WHO Director-General, *Safety and Efficacy of Drugs: Principles for Drug Control* (EB47/9), 27 November 1970, AWHO; recommendations

The second shift toward an American model came when the British Parliament passed the Medicines Act of 1968. The British pharmaceutical industry was the most powerful in Europe at the time, and Britain's initiative for new law marked a symbolic formal response to the EEC directive from three years earlier. The 1968 Act governed drug regulation in the United Kingdom until 1995, when British drug laws were superseded by those of the European Union. The Act created an administrative drug licensing scheme that required drug manufacturers to receive government approval before launching clinical trials and before marketing a new drug. The stop point in British regulation was the government's Licensing Authority, at the time entitled the Medicines Division of the Department of Health. Companies applied to the Licensing Authority for the legal rights to market a medicinal product, and the Authority could grant or deny these applications. No drug could be advertised or marketed without Medicines Division approval of both the medicine and its "data sheet" that embedded information about the drug's indications and adverse events. Hence, the 1968 legislation vaulted the powers of British government over pharmaceutical marketing as well as production and market entry. When the application involved a new active substance (NAS)—when in other words it would have been called a new molecular entity in the United States—it was always referred to the Committee on the Safety of Medicines (CSM), which superseded the CSD. The Committee's advice was not compulsory for the Medicines Division but was almost always followed.[19]

In ways that British politicians and officials would admit, and in many ways that they would not, the Medicines Act and associated institutional changes formed a self-conscious move toward a more administrative, FDA-style system. By September 1971, when the apparatus for carrying out the Medicines Act was in place, the United Kingdom had joined the United States as the only country to require administrative approval for a clinical trial as well as for drug marketing. What was established as an "IND application" in the United States was now, in British regulation, a "clinical trial certificate." From the 1960s through the 1970s, British officials also regularly corresponded and met with FDA leaders; in these exchanges the most frequent topic of discussion was the Administration's standards for

for regulation of research appear on p. 2, and suggestions on "technical structure" appear on p. 5. See also the executive board resolution of the same title, EB47.R29 (25 January 1971); AWHO. The Director-General's report of 1970 followed a run of the WHO *Technical Report Series* that seems to have been occasioned by the global thalidomide crisis; WHO *Technical Report Series* Nos. 287 (1964), 341 (1966), 364 (1967), 403 (1968), and 426 (1969).

[19]Abraham and Lewis, *Regulating Medicines in Europe*, 53–4. Charles Medawar, *Power and Dependence: Social Audit on the Safety of Medicines* (London: Social Audit, 1992), 74–5; Ceccoli, "Divergent Paths," 144–7. P. A. Andrews, G. M. Thompson, and C. Ward, "A Regulatory View of the Medicines Act in the United Kingdom," *Journal of Clinical Pharmacology* 24 (1984): 6–18. E. M. Tansey and L. A Reynolds, "The Committee on the Safety of Drugs," *Wellcome Witnesses to Twentieth-Century Medicine* [serial] (1) (April 1997), 103–35.

clinical experimentation. Moreover, Britain largely copied its nomenclature and regulations of post-marketing surveillance from the American system. The risks of drugs were tabulated as "adverse drug reactions" (the term used in FDA regulations) and as in the United States, such reports were legally mandated from drug producers but only voluntarily collected from physicians. Imitating the FDA's Office of Drug Surveillance, Britain created a drug surveillance office within the Medicines Division.[20]

Despite the formal mimicry of American arrangements, British institutions for new drug licensing operated quite differently in practice and in reputation. The Medicines Division had but a fraction of the Administration's organizational capacity, and it also lacked reputation for independence from the ABPI. Derrick Dunlop would defend the more informal character of his country's regulatory style, pointing to the "vast bureaucratic food and drug administration" in the United States and how American critics saw virtue in British patterns of "self-regulation." Yet Dunlop made these arguments defensively, as the 1968 changes had come in part from dissatisfaction with his Committee's operations after 1964. Minister of Health Richard Crossman and other parliamentarians had been pressing for new legislation, and an influential 1967 report by a committee chaired by Lord Sainsbury had criticized the British system, calling for a "new body" of regulation and declaring that "some limitation on the freedom of marketing of medicines is now essential."[21]

British journalists, too, gestured to the distinctive features of the American system. In a news analysis, *Times* writer Michael Leapman wondered whether Americans in the 1970s—reeling from a General Motors recall of

[20]On exchanges, see "Investigational drug regulation of the [FDA] of the U.S.A. with special reference to points affecting non-American investigators," 24 February 1969; William J. Gyarfas to Medical Research Council, January 8, 1969; FD 7-1748, UKNA. The Medical Research Council also kept copies of the IND circulars published by Kelsey's Investigational New Drug branch; FD 7-1748, UKNA. On a series of semiannual meetings in the 1970s between FDA officials and British and Canadian regulatory leaders, see Richard A. Merrill, "FDA and Mutual Recognition Agreements: Five Models of Harmonization," *FDLJ* 53 (1998): 133.

For early references to "adverse drug reactions" and the establishment of the Office of Drug Surveillance three years earlier in the United States, see *FR* 32 (130) (July 7, 1967): 10008. Organized drug surveillance had started earlier within the Division of Medicine; see chapter 8. Medawar, *Power and Dependence: Social Audit on the safety of Medicines*, 74–5. The 1968 Act also established a Medicines Commission, which advised the Minister of Health on appointments (in particular those to the CSM), and acted as a review body to which pharmaceutical companies could appeal where the Medicines Division had refused or revoked a license; Abraham and Lewis, *Regulating Medicines in Europe*, 54. For provisions for inspection authority that echoed the powers given to the FDA in 1962, see Medicines Act 1968, chap. 111.

[21]Lord Sainsbury (Chairman), *Report of the Committee on Enquiry into the Relationship of the Pharmaceutical Industry with the National Health Service, 1965–7* (London: HMSO, 1967), 92–3, quoted in Medawar, *Power and Dependence*, 75. Dunlop argued that his committee's lack of legal power had not "proved a serious embarrassment"; "Pharmaceuticals," *The Times of London*, November 9, 1970, I. Abraham and Courtney Davis, "Testing Times: The Emergence of the Practolol Disaster and Its Challenge to British Drug Regulation in the Modern Period," *Social History of Medicine* 19 (1) (2006): 131.

6.5 million cars, worried about continued Ralph Nader reports, and increasingly attached to "natural food" movements—were "worrying themselves to death." Among the anxieties that had recently buffeted the nation, wrote Leapman, only the FDA's warning on bathing infants in hexachlorophene solution was warranted. "It is indeed a tribute to the [American] nation's vigilance that generally, as in the case of hexachlorophene, possible dangers are detected before they have apparently done any substantial harm."[22]

In the enactment and slow administration of the Medicines Act, British regulators revealed their consistent deference to and reliance upon the ABPI, in particular the Glaxo and Wellcome companies. The ABPI, characterized as "one of the more vociferous trade organizations in British industry" by *The Times*, reacted caustically to the Sainsbury Committee report and defensively to the 1968 legislation. Wellcome Foundation chairman Sir Michael Perrin, one of the most influential men in British business and philanthropy, warned consistently of American-style "Government interference in what should be the direct accountability between research in an industrial company, the Board of Directors who were responsible for its business, and the ultimate users of its products." This vision of corporate responsibility as a substitute for government regulation surfaced repeatedly in the administrative implementation of the Act. The ABPI held out its Code of Pharmaceutical Marketing Practice as the basis of industry practice and as a model for governance. Underlying the Code, however, was a vision of regulation in which "every company in its simple self-interest would obviously wish to market only products that are both effective and safe." So extensive was this ethic that the Association could openly avow that "it has not been found necessary to apply sanctions to secure compliance" with provisions of the Code. In the early 1970s, under Dunlop's leadership, British regulators then continually approved drugs that were rejected or delayed by the FDA. These included the infamous beta-blockers to which FDA critics in the United States gestured. Ironically, one of these drugs—practolol (Eraldin)—would soon qualify among many observers as the nation's "greatest modern drug disaster."[23]

In the early 1970s, then, the arrangements of British pharmaceutical regulation formally aped some of the most visible features of the FDA, even as they persisted in deference to organized drug manufacturers. This was in

[22]Leapman, "Hazards of Consumer Safety Drive," *Times of London*, December 10, 1971, 9.

[23]Perrin was one of the most influential personalities in the British pharmaceutical industry. "The Wellcome Foundation Limited: Sir Michael Perrin's Statement," *The Times*, February 1, 1968, 26. *The Times* was generally supportive of Wellcome Foundation and ABPI statements about pharmaceutical regulation; see the editorial "Safety of Drugs," *The Times*, September 8, 1967, 11. The ABPI's *Code of Practice for the Pharmaceutical Industry* was first issued in 1958 and was continually revised through the remainder of the century. On the departures of the 1968 statute from the Sainsbury report's recommendations, see Ceccoli, "Divergent Paths," 145. Abraham and Davis ("Testing Times," 140–41) note that the British pharmaceutical industry was greatly valued in the 1970s for its positive contribution to the nation's balance of trade; for a contextualized account of the practolol episode, consult the entire article.

part a reflection of institutional ability; the incapacity of the British government, remarked one former CSM member, meant "decentralization to industry." The most influential critics of these patterns came from Parliament and from the British medical profession. In a 1990 review in the *British Medical Journal,* two noted physicians stated that from 1972 to 1988, the Medicines Act had been significantly "breached over 1200 times." The authors laid the responsibility for this pattern of failure not upon the legislation itself but upon the administrative institutions of British drug regulation. "Health ministers, by not enforcing the regulations concerning promotion, have abrogated their responsibility to the ABPI, but the evidence suggests that the code has failed to deter promotional excesses."[24]

The British reforms of the late 1960s and early 1970s nonetheless impelled domestic institutions toward greater formal similarity with American arrangements and, more slowly and informally, toward greater regulatory stringency and administrative activity. In meaningful respects, movements in Britain were facilitated by numerous and frequent meetings with FDA officials. In England, Germany, France, and the "Benelux" countries (Belgium, Netherlands, Luxembourg), the laments of domestic and pan-European audiences generated demands for more meaningful movement toward the American model through the 1970s and early 1980s. A European Commission directive from 1965 required all member states to establish formal drug approval procedures in national regulatory agencies, and to evaluate old and new medicines in accordance with modern licensing standards by 1990. In the United Kingdom itself, the directive led to a Committee on the Review of Medicines that assessed the safety and efficacy of thousands of drugs that had been grandfathered under the 1968 law. The British Committee was an explicit and openly avowed copy of the FDA's Drug Efficacy Study and its review and removal of pre-1962 drugs. A significant and underappreciated irony of this period is that, even as the drug lag debate raged in the United States, pressuring American officials to consider the virtues of European models of regulation, there was a quiet but substantial move among European governments to emulate the FDA in their regulation of medicines.[25]

[24] A. Herxheimer and J. Collier, "Promotion by the British Pharmaceutical Industry, 1983–8: A Critical Analysis of Sself-Regulation," *BMJ* 300 (Feb. 3, 1990): 307–11; quoted in Medawar, *Power and Dependence,* 77.

[25] Abraham and Lewis, *Regulating Medicines in Europe,* 60. On legitimacy dynamics, consult Meyer and Rowan, "Institutionalized Organizations: Formal Structure as Myth and Ceremony." This isomorphism also held for EU directives on pre-market evaluations of safety and efficacy of medicines, directed at Member States; Abraham and Lewis, *Regulating Medicines in Europe,* 54–5; K. Schmitt-Rau, "The Drug Regulatory System in the FRG," *Journal of Clinical Pharmacology* 28 (1988): 1064–70. In a 1985 report, the National Academy of Sciences noted extensive international adoption of American standards, concepts, and procedures in the preceding decade: "Most industrialized countries have consistent national policies and institutional arrangements for evaluating the safety and efficacy of drugs. These appear to have been strengthened in recent years, influenced to some extent by the United States Food and Drug

As in Great Britain, Sweden moved haltingly and incrementally in the late 1960s and early 1970s toward a more administrative and "rational" system of drug regulation. In 1968, the royal medical board and the national board of social affairs were merged to create the National Board of Health and Welfare. Within this body, a Drug Division was created in 1971, and in 1976, its offices were moved from Stockholm to Uppsala. Hence, it was four decades after Sweden's official efficacy standard that a state organization was wholly conducting both new drug evaluation and pharmacovigilance. In the 1970s, Drug Division authorities began to request individual "case report forms" from manufacturers, routinely examined pharmacokinetic data, and had adopted a "minimum of two controlled trials" standard like that used in the United States. Indeed, by the end of the 1970s, the Drug Division in Sweden was operating in some respects more conservatively than in the United States.[26]

As Sweden and Great Britain forged what officials in both countries called more "rational" and "orderly" systems, the European Economic Community continued to press its member states for more comprehensive regimes of drug regulation. As in 1965, the Second Directive on pharmaceuticals of 1975 was aimed at "approximation" and "harmonization"—the reduction of implicit and explicit trade barriers among European nations. Yet the Second Directive had a decidedly nonliberal feel, and its long-term effect was anything but deregulatory. In article after article, the Directive of 1975 elaborated meticulous provisions for agencies and companies to follow. These provisions varied in their length and in their consequences, with a seemingly negative association between the two. At the most exhaustive and ineffectual, the Directive set out minimum scientific qualifications of license-seeking manufacturers. These education and training requirements were imposed not upon agencies, but upon the industry and upon commercial holders of marketing licenses. Observers saw the requirements as embedding so many

---

Administration's example and assistance to other countries"; *Assessing Medical Technologies* (Washington, DC: National Academies Press, 1985), 229. On British mimicry of American arrangements in general, see Jonathan Liebenau, "The 20th Century British Pharmaceutical Industry," in Liebenau, Gregory J. Higby, and Elaine C. Stroud, eds., *Pill Peddlers: Essays on the History of the Pharmaceutical Industry* (Madison: American Institute of the History of Pharmacy, 1990), 126–8; [quoting Liebenau], Chauveau and Quirke, "The American 'Model' and the British and French Pharmaceutical Industries in the Twentieth Century," 11–12. On the Benelux merger of 1973 and institutions at the time from a European perspective, see the reports of C. J. van Boxtel: "L'Enregistrement des Medicaments au Benelux," paper presented at international meetings of the Syndicat National de 'Industrie Pharmaceutique, Paris, October 14–16, 1974; "Erfahriung mit eines Germainsamen Arzneimittelmarkt in den Beneluxländern," presented to the Hauptversammlung des Bundesverbandes der Pharmazeutischen Industrie, Berlin, June 1970; attachments to van Boxtel to V. Fattorusso, June 27, 1975; P5/288/1, AWHO.

[26]Liljestrand, "Requirements in Sweden," 31–4. The Swedish Medical Products Agency regards the 1971 reforms and 1976 transfer as the full administrative modernization of Swedish regulatory arrangements. Lakesmedelsverket, *Swedish Medical Products Agency—A Center of Regulatory Excellence* (Uppsala: MPA, 2006), 6.

loopholes, however, that neither standardization in firms' scientific capacities nor high-quality license applications was achieved. Other features of the Second Directive—protocols for chemical and pharmacological studies, manufacturing controls and associated tests, patient brochures, and standards for clinical trials and the reporting of data (including individual case histories) that came from them—carried a more robust effect. The Community's adoption of the brochure was a nod to the patient package inserts of the United States; what Cornell pharmacologist Walter Modell mocked as a "stuffer" in 1973 had by 1980 become a near-global practice. And the push for disaggregated test data formed a piecemeal rejection of the "summary data" approach that British regulators then used, and it composed a gesture toward the documentation requirements of the FDA. It would take two decades more—and the International Conference of Harmonization—for European regulators to fully embrace individual case reports as part of the Common Technical Document, but the Community's preference had been clearly stated. By 1983, finally, the Community officially pushed its member agencies to engage in the regulation of bioavailability and bioequivalence, something that the FDA had been doing since 1971 at latest.[27]

In 1976, following the EEC's overtures and several years of studying foreign institutions and the American model in particular, West Germany struck at the established arrangements of its early 1960s legislation and passed new legislation that handed significant new authorities and capacities to the Federal Health Office (Bundesgesundheitsamt; BGA). Spurred by this legislation and increasingly attentive to European and American audiences, German regulators began to visit greater scrutiny upon new drug applications; of 850 applications submitted from January 1978 to June 1980, over 100 were rejected or withdrawn, and most of the others submitted were returned with requests for more data. Like the 1968 Medicines Act, the third Arzneimittelgesetz (Medicines Law) of 1976 formed an additional step toward an American-style system, though with important exceptions. As in the United States, all medicines required German government pre-approval on the basis of safety and efficacy criteria, and applications to the BGA were required to include clinical, pharmacological, and toxicological data. The BGA also created "authorization commissions," similar to advisory committees established in the United States. Unlike the United States, the BGA did not establish standards for drug evaluation. Due in part to national physician lobbying, the critical role of standard-setting remained the province of the

[27]See Articles 21 through 24 of the "Second Council Directive 75/319/EEC of 20 May 1975 on the approximation of provisions laid down by Law, Regulation or Administrative Action relating to proprietary medicinal products," *Official Journal* L 147 (June 9, 1975): 13–22. Further standards were spelled out in Council Directive 75/318/EEC on the same date; *Official Journal* L 147 (June 9, 1975): 1–12. For the 1983 amendments (83/570/EEC), including bioavailability requirements (Article 3), see *Official Journal* L 332 (Nov. 28, 1983): 1–10. Abraham and Lewis, *Regulating Medicines in Europe*, 83–5. On the limits of the moves toward harmonization, see David Vogel, "The Globalization of Pharmaceutical Regulation," *Governance* 11 (1) (January 1988): 3.

Federal Chamber of Physicians (Bundesärztekammer). FDA advisory committees, moreover, would continue to shape policy through their influence on the issuance of rules and guidance documents. Jurisdictions were much narrower in post-1976 Germany, where the authorization commissions decided upon approval only, case by case.[28]

The French government followed in 1978, establishing a new drug review process in the national Ministry of Health and Welfare. The introduction of medicines into the French health system now compelled the granting of an Autorisation de Mise sur le Marché (AMM), which could be granted only after manufacturers had filed a complete application for AMM (Demande d'AMM) with the Ministry. As in Great Britain, the process was superintended by a standing committee—the Commission d'Autorisation de Mise sur le Marché (CAMM). Formally, the Demande d'AMM process in France mimicked the NDA process at the Administration, but as elsewhere in Europe, formal imitation concealed immense procedural reliance upon both industrial sponsors and professions. French standards for toxicity, pharmacodynamics (dose-response over time, often involving blood studies) and pharmacokinetics borrowed heavily from American concepts; following the FDA, French regulations from 1979 required manufacturers to submit individual case reports from clinical trials. Yet the central agent in the French review system was not a state medical officer, but a consultant rapporteur whose full-time employment lay outside the government. The Commission regulated the qualifications and behavior of these experts. And more than in Great Britain, the French ministry in the late twentieth century appears to have relied heavily upon the data summaries of industrial sponsors in their review of the Demandes. In critical respects, then, the Ministry of Health and Welfare had delegated responsibilities for data gathering and evaluation to industrial sponsors and to the professions. As in Germany and Great Britain, but even more so, French arrangements bespoke the understandings of what political scientists have called *corporatism*: the joint governance and self-regulation of industrial sectors through trade associations and professions who helped to populate and shape the state apparatus.[29]

[28]NAS, *Assessing Medical Technologies*, 236. Daemmrich, *Pharmacopolitics*, 40–42. For evidence of German consideration of the FDA model among government officials and in the pharmacology community in the years before the 1976 reforms, see the untitled report of Franz Gross (Pharmacologist, University of Heidelberg), 3 January 1973; Bestand B 189, Akten 11563, BK. The German BGA could bypass recommendations of the approval commissions. I thank Nils Kessel and Christian Bonah for this reference.

[29]Within the Ministry, the Direction de la Pharmacie et du Medicament (DPhM) governed new medicines, and the DPhM's Division de l'Enregistrement du Medicament (DEM) reviewed all Demandes d'AMM. The AMM had existed since 1967, but the 1978 reforms transformed its protocol and its use. Emmanuelle M. Voisin, Francoise Cheix, Marie-Danielle Campion, and Peter Hoyle, "New Drug Registration in France," *FDCLJ* 46 (1991): 707–25. For a wide ranging and casual discussion of the difference of French arrangements with those of the U.S. and other European countries, see Phillippe Urfalino, *Le grand méchant loup pharmaceutique: Angoisse ou vigilance?* (Paris: Les éditions Textuel, 2005), 45–80. For a more particular, historical focus on France, see Sophie Chauveau, *L'Invention Pharmaceutique: La Pharmacie*

The cross-Atlantic differences in national pharmaceutical regulation were stark, and they bespoke what political scientists have called the differing "national styles" of regulation. Simply put, American law and procedure created dual, opposing identities for the "sponsor" and the regulator," whereas a less legalistic, less adversarial understanding prevailed in most of Europe. Yet these international differences were not fixed categories but mobile targets. At the precise historical moment when observers began to draw up lists of cross-national differences, England, West Germany, and France began to drift further toward their perceptions of the FDA model. Corporatist arrangements remained in all three countries, even in nations like Britain less known for corporatism. Yet underlying these patterns was a continual, barely perceptible but significant movement toward American symbols. The slow and partial convergence of European formal arrangements to American institutions was influenced in part by multilateral and bilateral discussions involving the FDA itself, shaped in part by explicit instructions from the European Community and the World Health Organization, and structured as much as anything else by an appreciative understanding of American institutions as more "modern," "rigorous," and "scientific."[30]

. . .

Among notable pharmaceutical regulators outside of Europe and the United States—Australia, Canada, and Japan—there was varied acceptance of the American idiom during the 1970s. Australia continued to rely upon its national drug evaluation committee for assessments, and emphasized post-market surveillance more than pre-market review, joining with the World Health Organization's efforts to create systematic post-marketing drug surveillance regimes. Many of the ADEC's approval decisions were made after watching those of European and American regulators, and Australian licensing agreements for cancer drugs depended upon a set of bilateral relationships with the FDA and the National Cancer Institute in the sharing of clinical trial information and protocols for cancer drug testing and utilization.[31]

Francaise entre l'État et le Société au XXe siècle (Paris: Institut d'edition Sanofi-Synthelabo, 1999), 565–601; Chauveau, "Médicament et Société en France au 20e Siècle," Vingtième Siècle. Revue d'histoire 73 (1) (Janvier-mars 2002): 169–85. An accessible English introduction is Paul Lechat, "Present Requirements for Drug Control in France," in J. Z. Bowers and G. P. Velo, eds., Drug Assessment Criteria, 59–63. Wictorowicz, "Emergent Patterns," 637–8; Hancher, Regulating for Competition. For a classic clarifying essay on corporatism, see Philippe Schmitter, "Still the Century of Corporatism," Review of Politics 36 (1) (1974): 85–131. I thank Christian Bonah and Sophie Chauveau for helpful discussions on this point.

[30]NAS, Assessing Medical Technologies, 235. On the role of the WHO, consult Stuart Nightengale, "Drug Regulation and Policy Formulation," Milbank Memorial Fund Quarterly: Health and Society 59 (3): 412–44.

[31]L. Sanson, "The Australian National Medicinal Drug Policy," Journal of Quality in Clinical Practice 19 (1999): 31–5. Ian W. Boyd, "The Role of the Australian Adverse Drug Reactions Advisory Committee (ADRAC) in Monitoring Drug Safety," Toxicology 181–182 (2002): 99–102. See the interviews of Martin Tattersall (then Chairman, ADEC) and Stan Goulston (Former President, Royal Australasian College of Physicians); "Drug Evaluation in Australia,"

National legislation in Canada governing food and drugs predated that in the United States by over three decades. The food and drug law of 1874 established criminal penalties at common law for public health fraud. In the twentieth century, the Ministry of Health and Welfare began to examine new drug applications in the wake of the thalidomide episode in 1963. The reviews were undertaken by the Drug Directorate of the Ministry's Health Protection Branch (HPB). The procedures and behavior of Canadian regulators—including clinical trial standards, and the adoption of good laboratory practices and good manufacturing practices—were broadly influenced by bilateral arrangements between the United States and Canada, and by tripartite meetings between U.S., Canadian, and British regulators. The Drug Directorate was renamed Therapeutics Product Programme (TPP) in 1997. Later, the HPB was established as Health Canada and the TPP became the Therapeutic Products Directorate. In Canada, as in other countries, the regulation of pharmaceuticals is split among numerous government bodies, leading to a system of institutional fragmentation more commonly observed in the United States. Post-market regulation is undertaken not by the TPP but by the Pharmaceutical Advertising Advisory Board (PAAB), which enforces the nation's Code of Marketing Practice.[32]

Among those nations most often called "industrialized," Japan seemed to present the most enduring contrast to the institutions of the United States in drug regulation. For years, the Ministry of Health and Welfare—whose Bureau of Pharmaceutical Affairs administered the post-war Pharmaceutical Affairs Law of 1948 (re-enacted in 1960)—was considered one of the most stringent regulators of drug safety, perhaps the only agency as stringent as the FDA. Yet until the 1980s, the Ministry was also known for the absence of demanding efficacy regulations and clinical trial standards; a Laetrile-like drug was marketed for decades in Japan with the official licensure of the Ministry. So too, Japan's system of explicit state sponsorship of industry— the organization of pharmaceutical producers (called *Kiko*) was half-public and half-private and was supervised by the Ministry—created a less for-

---

The Health Report with Norman Swan on (Australian) Radio National, December 21, 1998. Senator Grant Tambling, address on the 200th meeting of the Australian Drug Evaluation Committee, December 3, 1998, Sydney University. For the basis of contemporary regulation, see the Therapeutic Goods Act of 1989, particularly Section 23 (applications).

[32]Robert E. Curran, "Regulatory Control in Canada Under the Food and Drugs Act," *FDCLJ* 17 (May 1962): 312–22; Wictorowicz, "Emergent Patterns," 630. On the tripartite meetings, see Merrill, "FDA and Mutual Recognition Agreements," 133; Linda Horton, "Mutual Recognition Agreements and Harmonization," *Seton Hall Law Review* 29 (1999): 692–735. A memorandum of understanding on GLPs was signed between the Health Protection Branch and the FDA in 1979; FDA Compliance Policy Guide 7156a.05, Chapter 56a, October 1, 1980, "MOU with Health Protection Branch Regarding Good Laboratory Practices (FDA 225-79-8400)." An earlier memorandum for joint inspection of manufacturing plants was signed in 1973; FDA Compliance Policy Guide 7156a.01, Chapter 56c, October 1, 1980, "Agreement with Canada Concerning Exchange of Drug Plant Inspection Information (FDA 225-75-2027)."

mally adversarial relationship between national industries and the state, a relationship as corporatist as any in Europe. With the move toward efficacy regulation, Japan eventually (and ironically) became one of the more rigorous state regulators in the industrialized world, adopting requirements for clinical trials demonstrating comparative efficacy trials in the 1990s. Administratively, Japanese health officials have long desired an FDA-like agency, and in recent years created a unified structure for the governance of pharmaceuticals from preclinical trials to post-marketing surveillance.[33]

Further Institutional Mimicry: Nonlegislative Standards and Structures. While national legislatures in Europe pushed systems of pharmaceutical evaluation toward greater formality in the 1970s, administrative structures, procedures, and concepts also flowed across the Atlantic and Pacific. In Britain, Germany, and France, the landmark statutes of 1968 to 1978 were implemented rather slowly, with several years of delay in the establishment of the most basic institutions. In these and other countries, the slowness of administrative change in regulatory structures dashed the hopes of harmonization proponents, who saw regulatory progress as an essential mode of trade liberalization in the pharmaceutical sector.

In the development of standards for drug testing and evaluation, these cross-national flows of concepts and symbols served to generate similarities and further contrasts. In the United Kingdom, the Association of British Pharmaceutical Industries (ABPI) developed standards for clinical testing in the mid-1970s and published these in 1977. Ian Shedden, who was Lilly's Vice President for Clinical Research and Regulatory Affairs, was also from 1973 to 1976 a member of the ABPI's Research and Development Committee, which elaborated the ABPI guidelines on the carcinogenicity testing of new drugs. It was not until the late 1970s that British officials began to adopt American-style monitoring of clinical trials. By the late 1980s and early 1990s, as talk of a pan-European agency for drug regulation became more concrete, many pharmaceutical industry observers believed that Britain offered the most stringent and demanding pharmaceutical regulation in the European Union.[34]

---

[33]C. N. Roberts, "Objectives and Achievements of Pharmaceutical Regulations in Japan," in Stuart R. Walker and John P. Griffin, *International Medicines Regulation: A Look Forward to 1992* (Dordrecht: Kluwer Academic, 1989); Ames Gross, "Regulatory Changes in Japan's Pharmaceutical Industry," *Pacific Bridge Medical—Japan Medical Publications* (Bethesda, MD: Pacific Bridge Medical, November 1998). On the adoption of comparative efficacy trials, see Kouseishou, *A Guideline for the Statistical Analysis of Clinical Trials* (Tokyo: Japanese Ministry of Public Health, 1992) (in Japanese). Chihiro Hirotsu, "Impact of the ICH E9 Guideline Statistical Principles for Clinical Trials on the Conduct of Clinical Trials in Japan," *DIJ* (2003). "FDA-style Agency for Japan," *Nature Biotechnology* 17 (Jan. 1999): 7.

[34]ABPI, *Guidelines for Preclinical and Clinical Testing of New Medicinal Products, Part I— Laboratory Investigations* (London: ABPI, 1977). Cited in John Abraham, "Scientific Standards and Institutional Interests: Carcinogenic Risk Assessment of Benoxaprofen in the UK and US," *Social Studies of Science* 23 (1993): 387–444. NAS, *Assessing Medical Technologies,*

Still, through the 1980s and 1990s, in Great Britain and elsewhere in Europe, there were continued gazes at the Administration. West Germany also adopted good laboratory practices and good manufacturing practices from the American model. In an explicit adoption of American practice, both Germany and Sweden in the 1980s began employing a professional medical statistician in their drug regulatory agencies. This effort lay both decades (and dozens of statisticians) behind that of the FDA. A working party of the Royal Statistical Society would lament in 1991 that whereas the Administration employed over fifty biostatisticians in the regulation of drugs, the British government employed not one. Not only the United Kingdom but also "the European Community at large" regulated new medicines "without appropriate input from experienced statisticians." At the core of these problems was the lack of statistical guidance in prospective trial design.[35]

The movement of the world's drug agencies toward a more "rational," administrative, and comprehensive model of pharmaceutical assessment and regulation meant that the contrasts that had rendered the Administration "exceptional" had, by the 1990s, waned. As early as 1987, Upjohn regulatory affairs director Otto Kreuzer declared that the FDA "can no longer be considered the toughest or most demanding regulatory agency" in global pharmaceutical regulation. Kreuzer might have overstated his case, but into the 1990s this sort of claim would appear with increasing frequency in the pages of medical journals, of trade newsletters, and of business journalism.[36]

EUROPEANIZATION AND HARMONIZATION: THE CEMENT OF MIMICRY

In the past two decades, several vast energies of institutional convergence have shaped the regulatory institutions of Europe, Japan, and the United States, at one level, and the institutions of dozens of nations with smaller pharmaceutical markets, at another. The solidification of the European Union created a legal structure within which authorities could fashion a single continental agency with a centralized drug registration procedure. At the same time, regulatory agencies and representatives of multinational pharmaceutical enterprises were holding symposia where "harmonization" of the world's premarket regulatory processes was openly discussed and planned. In some measure, the initiative for harmonization stemmed from broad recognition of the plausible claim that the variety of uncoordinated national regulatory

---

235. Frances O. Kelsey, "The Bioresearch Monitoring Program," *FDCLJ* 46 (1991): 63; Hancher, *Regulating for Competition*; Wictorowicz, "Emergent Patterns," 636.

[35] Statistics and Statisticians in Drug Regulation in the United Kingdom," *Journal of the Royal Statistical Society, Series A* (Statistics and Society) 151 (3) (1991): 413–19.

[36] Otto A. Kreuzer, "International Drug Registration," *FDCLJ* 43 (1988): 559; Kreuzer's article was originally presented at a Food and Drug Law Institute conference in December 1987.

procedures amounted to a waste of resources, as companies needlessly duplicated dozens of new drug applications and hundreds of clinical tests for each new medicinal product. In other ways, the harmonization initiative was part of a broader and global "neoliberal" paradigm of the streamlining and weakening of regulatory states. In this sense, harmonization was facilitated by the growing agenda power of multinational drug companies and their representation in Western politics and in organizations like PhRMA.[37]

Less visibly but meaningfully, the worldwide reforms of the 1990s cemented the status of the U.S. Food and Drug Administration as a "global standard." Particularly in Europe but also in Japan and several other East Asian nations, weak regulatory states attempted to copy the formal institutions of American regulation, even as they lacked the resources, informal institutions, and organizational image so central to the Administration's power.[38]

The rise of a pan-European structure of drug regulation constituted a slow, painful, and halting process. By the 1980s, the work of the EEC in creating coordinated multistate procedures with mutual recognition of drug approvals and assessment standards was seen by industrial and neoliberal audiences as a failure. The Association of British Pharmaceutical Industry (ABPI) issued a "Blueprint for Europe" in 1988 that surveyed the lessons of the previous decades and outlined the essential components of viable reform. The "Blueprint" embedded and elaborated two core ideas: the notion that a singular procedure should govern registration of medicines throughout Europe, and the proposal that state regulators should be constrained by deadlines, in particular a 210-day clock that limited the time elapsed in review of a license application. These ideas composed the basis for a set of new regulatory institutions whose operation officially began in 1995.[39]

Regulatory arrangements governing new drugs in Europe are now quite

[37]For some accessible and helpful attempts, see Vogel, "The Globalization of Pharmaceutical Regulation"; Abraham and Lewis, *Regulating Medicines in Europe*, especially chapters 4 and 5; Boris Hauray and Philippe Urfalino, "La formation d'une Europe du médicament par transformation conjointe," presented at the 7th Congress of the Association française de science politique (AFSP), Lille, September 18–21, 2002; Urfalino, *Le grand méchant loup pharmaceutique*, 82–113.

[38]I borrow the term global standard from French observers Boris Hauray and Philippe Urfalino. "La FDA, l'Agence américaine leader depuis les années 1960 dans l'évaluation des médicaments constitue la référence mondiale"; "La formation d'une Europe du médicament par transformation conjointe," p. 9, n. 8. See also Urfalino's remarks in *Le grand méchant loup pharmaceutique*, 47–9; and F. Badey, "Les États-Unis et la santé. La FDA, une centenaire sémillante," *Seve: Les Tribunes de la Sante* 19 (2008): 83–9.

[39]The process by which Europe went from the building blocks of the EEC Directives to the EMEA and several procedures of registration is a complicated one. For accessible narratives, see Abraham and Lewis, *Regulating Medicines in Europe*, chap. 4, and Hauray and Urfalino, "La formation d'une Europe de medicament par transformation conjointe." On the shared notion of failure for coordination of national agencies, see Vogel, "Globalization of Pharmaceutical Regulation," 4. "ABPI's 'Blueprint for Europe'," *Scrip* 1330 (29 July 1988): 7–8; referenced in Abraham and Lewis, 87.

complex. One way of simplifying them is to ask which quasi-state organization gets to make the essential decisions on whether to authorize a new drug for marketing. In the "decentralized" procedure of registration, the agent of choice is a national agency as it was before 1995, when there was the expectation (some would say the aspiration) that once one member state had reviewed a drug and cleared it for marketing, the other states would follow this decision. Since 1995, all other member states are required to authorize the drug within ninety days or to formally refuse authorization on the basis of "public health" criteria. Two other critical differences since 1995 are that the various national agencies operate under statutory deadlines of 210 days, and (perhaps more powerfully) that if an aggrieved firm wishes to contest the rejection of its drug it can do so by appeal to the Committee on Proprietary Medicinal Products (CPMP). The Committee is composed of fifteen members (one each from the member states) and its opinions become binding by decision of the European Commission. In this way, the European Union allows the decisions of one member state to supersede the laws and decisions of another on commodities within the common pharmaceutical market.[40]

In the "centralized" procedure, which originated in 1995, a drug sponsor applies to the London-based European Agency for the Evaluation of Medicinal Products (EMEA). This agency is organizationally separate from the national regulators and has many of the official functions that have long been carried out by the FDA. Agency officials examine the application and the statistical analyses making the case for authorization. They may commission new tests, and they may inspect facilities used for production of the new drug in question. They may call upon the member states or other non-public experts as rapporteurs in assisting the evaluation. Quite often (usually on Day 120 of the clock), EMEA officials advance a list of questions to the sponsor, and this juncture often induces the firm to withdraw the application (possibly to be refilled later). Upon the European Agency's evaluation, the application goes to the CPMP, which issues a favorable or unfavorable decision on the application. Additional steps remain in the process, and there are avenues of appeal, but the central choices are rendered by the Agency and its supervising Committee.[41]

At the turn of the century, most observers agreed that despite its progress and growth, the European Agency appeared weak in comparison with its American counterpart. The Administration and Congress had created a "strong pharmaceutical state" in the United States only in part through formal institutions. The FDA's parchment institutions—the NDA process, phased clinical trials, the architecture of bioequivalence and bioavailability,

---

[40]Abraham and Lewis, *Regulating Medicines in Europe*, 88–97, 107–8. Dukes, *Law and Ethics of the Pharmaceutical Industry*, 126; Dukes also discusses incentives for "forum shopping" in the decentralized procedure.

[41]Richard Kingham, Peter Bogaert, and Pamela Eddy, "The New European Medicines Agency," *FDLJ* 49 (1994): 301–21. Abraham and Lewis, *Regulating Medicines in Europe*, 97–107.

the emergence of good laboratory practices, good clinical practices, and good manufacturing practices and associated regulations—were to some degree epiphenomenal reflections of an underlying reality: an organizational capacity and an organizational reputation that generally reinforced one another. In Europe and other Western nations, political leaders in the late twentieth century simply lacked the bona fide ability to stitch together an FDA-like organization with the human talents and the broad esteem and autonomy possessed by the Administration. Instead, Western and European imitators did the next best thing: they emulated structurally what they could not attain behaviorally. As two British observers remarked in 2000, the European Agency was only an attempted emulation, not a successful one.

> Europeanization of medicines regulation is occurring, and at an accelerating pace. Yet a European "superstate" of medicines regulation, akin to the American FDA, remains a "virtual reality" without the resources to develop a substantial independent base of regulatory scientists. While Europeanization of medicines regulation is real and perhaps more rapid than in any other sector, it remains fundamentally dependent on the expertise and resources derived from the national agencies. In these respects the combined regulatory power of the Commission, the EMEA and the CPMP is much less autonomous than that of the FDA, even though the EU *en bloc* now represents the largest market for pharmaceuticals in the world.[42]

To the extent that the European Agency has morphed features of the Administration, moreover, it has copied the FDA of the 1950s, 1960s, 1970s, and 1980s, and less the organization of the past two decades.

The other disconnect between institutional form and policy reality in Europe rests in the growing power of multinational business, particularly drug companies, in world politics. Pharmaceutical firms have always wielded power in its various faces, but in the late twentieth century these firms accumulated vast resources through the immense profits reaped from sales of their products. They also adapted with new organizational models that provided them with enhanced legitimacy and superior capacities for political mobilization. In Europe, drug companies formed a crucial component of valued export sectors in the economies of European nations whose leaders were anxious about their international trade balances. In ways that few nation-states could equal, moreover, multinational companies and their organizations could apply political pressure to numerous political, economic, and professional agents at once.

At this writing, the ideational rivalry of the EMEA and the FDA is an ongoing story. As the European Agency has matured, and as the larger European Union has developed and become more institutionally stable, EMEA officials have become more assertive in challenging decisions and standards of the FDA, and they have become more aggressive in pointing to their procedures as models for other nations to follow. In the aftermath of several

---

[42] Abraham and Lewis, *Regulating Medicines in Europe*, 144.

high-profile safety-based drug withdrawals, moreover, broader professional and political concerns have been raised about the FDA in the 1990s and early twenty-first century. These have led international observers, particularly non-Western nations, to attach greater legitimacy to the decisions and forms of the European Agency.

One enduring political legacy of the EEC, and eventually the EMEA, is that it created an organization large enough to join in multilateral negotiations with FDA officials in planning for global harmonization. The International Conference on Harmonization (ICH) predates the formation of the European Union, and its evolution is well known among participants and observers of the contemporary pharmaceutical world. The ICH emerged from meetings in the early 1990s among regulatory officials from Europe, the United States, and Japan. At the time, these three markets accounted for nine in every ten dollars of drug research and development, and 75 percent of global medicines production. Although participants in the Conference—there have been numerous meetings of "the Conference," and its membership has experienced considerable turnover—were concerned to coordinate enforcement activities, most of its labor has been directed at simplifying and standardizing the drug development and registration process. The Conference aimed to create a Common Technical Document (CTD) which could constitute (or form the basis for) an application to any of the world's regulatory agencies.[43]

In many ways, the evolution and the architecture of the Common Technical Document have reduced the uniqueness of the FDA's New Drug Application form and the regulated experiments that it summarizes. Yet in the standardization of rhetoric and information achieved in its Common Technical Document, the ICH has in fact accelerated and cemented the global reach of the Administration's core conceptual innovations from the twentieth century. The Document summarizes information that is produced according to regulations and precedents that have been shaped by the FDA more so than by any other organization on the planet. The Document organizes data in categories and sequences that meaningfully echo and rely upon the 1956 New Drug Application form and the philosophy that generated it.

WHO AND DRUG REGULATION IN DEVELOPING NATIONS: THE ECHO OF AMERICAN PROTOCOL

Outside of the ICH markets, many countries have begun to erect and modify their national drug registration procedures. Much of this endeavor has been encouraged and helped along by the World Health Organization

[43] Vogel ("The Globalization of Pharmaceutical Regulation," 11–16) offers a concise summary of developments in the ICH to 1998. For a critical examination, see John Abraham and Tim Reed, "Progress, Innovation and Regulatory Science in Drug Development: The Politics of International Standard-Setting," *Social Studies of Science* 32 (3) (June 2002): 337–69. With the vast advance of information technology in the 1990s, ICH efforts refocused upon the electronic Common Technical Document (eCTD).

(WHO) and the FDA itself. As the market for pharmaceutical production and research has exploded in the last three decades, these countries have seized upon the creation of "institutions" to convey the credibility of their manufacturing and research sectors. In several cases from East Asia, national officials have imported procedures and structures wholesale from the Administration. Even as the Chinese government continues to delegate significant authority to its provincial governments in the regulation of drugs, its central state has established a state Food and Drug Administration (sFDA). Since the 1980s, the government has operated a registration procedure that is now entitled the "New Drug Approval" process, and since 1999, the agency has openly adopted "Good Clinical Practice" and "Good Laboratory Practice" standards from the United States. South Korea has established a Korea Food and Drug Administration (KFDA) and has also adopted GLP, GMP, and other American standards. In other cases, particularly those such as Brazil and Singapore where national officials have adopted new institutions in the past few years, non-Western states have looked more to the European Agency as a model.[44]

Perhaps the most important single organization serving to spread FDA standards, concepts, and protocols in the developing world is not the Administration itself, but the Geneva-based WHO. The Organization has concerned itself with issues of global pharmaceuticals since its inception in 1948, and increasingly since the mid-1950s, as "quality control" became a central issue for users of pharmaceuticals in developing countries. Before and after the thalidomide tragedy, the World Health Assembly, the WHO Executive Board, and a series of WHO study groups bandied proposals and declarations back and forth about the creation and encouragement of institutions for quality control and "good practice" in the manufacture, preparation, and storage of ethical drugs in their member nations. As early as 1956, a WHO study group authored the notion that every member state should have a "national control authority" with central laboratory facilities, and the Organization repeated this recommendation in 1961 and 1962. This was more of a departure than it might seem now, because several large member states at the time, not least India and West Germany, had left regulation to provincial or state laboratories (where these existed at all). WHO officials knew that a national drug control authority would have required considerable standardization and administrative capacity that was lacking in most national capitals. So too, the idea that the central agent of quality control regulation should be a government agency was a conscious depar-

[44]Stuart Nightengale, "Drug Regulation and Policy Formulation," *Milbank Memorial Fund Quarterly: Health and Society* 59 (3): 412–44. NAS, *Assessing Medical Technologies*, 237. Rongling Deng and Kenneth I. Kaitin, "The Regulation and Approval of New Drugs in China," *DIJ* 37 (2004): 29–39; Young-Ok Kim, et al., "Safety Evaluation for New Drug Approval in Korea," *DIJ* 35 (1) (January-March 2001): 285–91. Howard Lee, "Good Review Practices: The First Step Forward for the Korea Food and Drug Administration," *DIJ* 39 (2005): 185–92. Gerald B. N. Wong and John C. W. Lin, "Drug Regulation by Singapore's Health Sciences Authority: The Role of the Centre for Drug Evaluation," *DIJ* 37 (2003): 15S–25S.

ture from numerous models in Germany, France, the United Kingdom, and even partially the United States, where nongovernment pharmacopoeia served to generate standards and dissolution or disintegration tests for regulatory use.[45]

WHO officials wanted member states to possess not merely a regulatory laboratory, but an agency with inspection capability and procedures for regulating drug manufacture and pharmacy preparation. In this respect, the FDA's decades-old "good manufacturing practices" regulations provided an appropriate model from which to base recommendations. From 1969 onward, WHO recommendations for improvements in quality control became progressively inseparable from recommendations for "good manufacturing practices." By the late 1970s and 1980s, WHO officials were using good manufacturing practice guidelines to foster changes in European regulatory systems, including Sweden's.[46]

The WHO's movement toward an American model was by no means a linear or foreordained development. For one thing, attention to issues of quality control—post-approval regulation of manufacturing, compounding, and storage—preceded attention to issues of registration by a decade. What FDA officials had conjoined in the 1940s and 1950s (pre-market approval and quality control regulations), WHO officials had implicitly separated. WHO officials did not systematically devote attention to standards for pharmacological and clinical evaluation in pre-market until after the thalidomide crisis. In 1963, the World Health Assembly issued a call for shared information among member states on adverse reactions, drugs rejected during regulatory review, and registration standards. Then in the late 1960s and early 1970s, WHO officials and bodies began offering suggestions about the relation between drug evaluation and "drug registration" systems in member states. For another matter, the WHO's borrowing of American concepts about bioavailability undermined its own quality control standards, as

[45]The WHO Study Group on the Use of Specifications for Pharmaceutical Preparations in December 1956 at WHO headquarters in Geneva; WHO Technical Report Series 138 (1957). The Geneva meeting was followed by a European Technical Meeting on the Quality Control of Pharmaceutical Preparations, Warsaw, 29 May 1961; WHO Technical Report Series 249 (1962). C. A. Morrell, "Organization of a Government Office and Laboratory for the Quality Control of Pharmaceutical Preparations," EURO-203/29, 27 March 1961; AWHO. A. Calo, "Méthodes Officielles par les Laboratoires de l'Etat pour le Contrôle de le Qualité des Préparations Pharmaceutiques," EURO-203/14, 5 mai 1961; AWHO. WHO officials were well aware that their suggestion for national drug control authorities departed from institutions in France, India and other countries; WHO Technical Report Series 138 (1957): 6–8.

[46]WHO Expert Committee on Specifications for Pharmaceutical Preparations, Twenty-Fifth Report, WHO Technical Report Series 567 (1975). On the WHO's continuing push for good manufacturing practices in the 1970s and years following, see Assembly declaration WHA28.65, and Official Records of the World Health Organization, 226 (1975), Annex 12. See also Certification Scheme on the Quality of Pharmaceutical Products Moving in International Commerce, WHO/PHARM/82.6 (Geneva, WHO: 1982). Reference to WHO GMP standards in Article 4 of Memorandum of Agreement between the Swedish National Board of Health and the Food and Drug Administration, October 1972; FDA Compliance Policy Guides, 7156c.01 (signed Charles C. Edwards and Bror Rexed, Director-General NBHW, Sweden).

demonstrations of varying bioavailability showed that previous tests for chemical stability were insufficient to guarantee quality control.[47]

The Organization's regulatory standards were, moreover, influenced by nongovernmental entities, not least the American Pharmaceutical Manufacturers Association (PMA) and the U.S. Pharmacopeia. From the early 1970s through the 1980s, the PMA was an important source of diffusion for good manufacturing practices at the WHO, and often served as a conduit through which FDA concepts and standards flowed. Debates about quality control were then, and are now, often connected to debates about generic medicines and whether they can be trusted as much as their brand-name predecessors. The story of the international diffusion of generic drugs standards and drug manufacture standards merits a separate treatment, but the economic issues at stake cannot be separated from these regulatory standards. Many brand-name manufacturers favored the international adoption of good manufacturing practices, quite possibly for the same reason they favored stricter regulation of generic drugs in the United States: larger, brand-name firms were better able to meet manufacturing regulations, and at lower cost, than smaller companies and generic drug firms. The imposition of good manufacturing practices was also a strategy for raising the fixed and variable costs of rival and generic producers.[48]

More broadly, WHO reports and recommendations—each of them echoed by WHO offices in the country of each member state—began to solidify the status of the FDA as regulatory exemplar. In "Guidelines for the Organization of a National Regulatory Agency" issued in 1971, WHO recommendations—carried to member states by WHO officials—began to extol the virtues of single, centralized government organizations for the registration and post-market control of drugs. These organizations were to possess staff trained in pharmacology, and by the 1980s they were expected to have laboratories grounded in "good laboratory practice" standards that bore the clear imprint of the FDA's 1974 rules. These incantations continued through the succeeding two decades, as WHO officials and reports continued to

[47]WHA, "Évaluation Clinique et Pharmacologique des Préparations Pharmaceutiques: Norms pour les Médicaments," WHA16.38 (23 mai 1963); "Évaluation Clinique et Pharmacologique des Préparations Pharmaceutiques," WHA16.36 (23 mai 1963). A 1975 report discussed a particularly linearized, phased model of drug development as "the assembling of information... a cumulative process"; WHO *Technical Bulletin Report* 1975 (p. 15 and Annex 5). In considering standards for bioavailability tests, WHO officials relied heavily and thoroughly on existing FDA rules, along with standards adopted in the UK, Switzerland, and Canada; WHO, "Dissolution Test for the International Pharmacopoeia," undated (probably 1988), P5-445-4, AWHO.

[48]International Federation of Pharmaceutical Manufacturers' Associations, *Good Manufacturing Practices in the Pharmaceutical Industry*, Proceedings of a Symposium held in Geneva, Switzerland, September 1971 (Geneva, WHO, 1972). WHO, "Guidelines for Dissolution Testing," WHO/PHARM/84.5 (Geneva, WHO, July 1978). WHO, "Good Manufacturing Practices in the Quality Control of Drugs," WHO/PHARM/84.6 (Geneva, WHO, 1983). This WHO report was based on a tape and a slide show sent to WHO officials by the American PMA in 1983.

regard the FDA as a model agency on issues of transparency into the 1990s. The timing of these broadcasts was significant, as the 1970s and 1980s saw numerous institutional revisions of drug laws in developing countries. Many member states had implicitly or explicitly delegated drug registration decisions either to local and regional boards or to pharmacopoeial bodies (as in much of Europe). Because the "recommended drug laws" were the basis of much emulation, the WHO reports served to militate against decentralized models of drug regulation that were based on national pharmacopoeia.[49]

ECHOES OF THE AMERICAN REGULATORY MODEL: GOVERNANCE OF
TRADITIONAL AND ALLOPATHIC MEDICINES IN MODERN INDIA

One country where FDA models have had marked implications for the development of pharmaceutical institutions and practice is modern India. India provides a distinctive window into the international diffusion of FDA standards because of its democratic political system, its massive and exploding population, its rapid economic development in recent decades (particularly in the sector of manufacturing and clinical trials), its decentralized system of pharmaceutical regulation, and its co-existence and mixture of traditional with modern medical and healing practices. Much of traditional Indian medicine corresponds to several dominant healing traditions that are religiously and culturally premised (primarily but not exclusively Ayurvedic, Unani, and Siddha healing traditions). Clinical trial procedures have both shaped and constrained the development of traditional medicines, and the practitioners and makers of traditional medicine have adapted and partially rationalized their products. In crucial ways the presence of FDA standards in India represents a flexible application of external rules to local conditions. The resulting standards were neither entirely American nor entirely Ayurvedic, but represented something of a feasible middle ground.[50]

[49]Resolution of the Executive Board of the WHO (47th Session) "Safety and Efficacy of Drugs: Principles for Drug Control," EB47.R29, 25 January 1971; based on a Report of the WHO Director-General, EB47/9, 27 November 1970, AWHO. "Good Laboratory Practices in Governmental Drug Control Laboratories," WHO/PHARM/84.512/Rev.2 (Geneva, WHO: 1985). WHO Expert Committee on Specifications for Pharmaceutical Preparations, "Structure and Management of a National Drug Control Laboratory; note from the Secretariat," WHO/PHA/EC/81.12, AWHO. For a case where WHO reports singled out the FDA as uniquely laudable on the dimension of transparency, see "ISDB assesses the transparency of drug regulatory agencies," *Essential Drugs Monitor No. 24–1997* (WHO/DAP—WHO/EDM, 1997).

[50]The study of twentieth-century India (economy and polity), of Ayurvedic medicine and pharmaceuticals, and of pharmaceuticals and polypharmaceuticals in modern India all lie far afield from my expertise. They are also the subject of numerous separate treatments. My aim here is to suggest that late twentieth-century developments in Indian pharmaceutical regulation have been shaped by concepts and standards adopted and reappropriated from the FDA. The following section is meant to be merely suggestive and to stimulate imagination and further research. For helpful conversations I am indebted to B. Suresh (President, Pharmacy Council of India and President, Indian Pharmaceutical Association), Patricia Barton, Jean-Paul Gaudiellere,

National pharmaceutical regulation in modern India was shaped by the passage of the Drugs and Cosmetics Act of 1940 in the late years of the independence movement. The Act was followed by the Drugs and Cosmetics Rules of 1945. In crucial ways, these acts represented a conscious (albeit partial) adoption of British and American institutions. In 1941, after the legislation was passed but before its administrative institutions were established, Indian medical professionals supported the creation of a "food and drug administration." The rules of 1945 outlined a more elaborate vision for regulation, and with amendments they have governed pharmaceutical development, production, marketing, and utilization since mid-century. In these rules, the most notable feature of the 1940s Indian system adopted from an American model was a licensing system for imported drugs commenced in April 1947, officially superintended by a Drugs Controller located in Delhi. Still, most quality control and regulation decisions in twentieth-century India were delegated to the state-level drug control authorities. So too, the administrative capacity of the Indian system was highly decentralized. The principal government laboratory of the mid-twentieth century, for instance, was located not in Delhi but in Calcutta. And much of the Indian government's pharmacological expertise was housed in the Haffkine Institute of Mumbai, which carried out a large proportion of the Indian government's drug testing in the middle twentieth century.[51]

A series of institutional reforms in the 1970s created the structural backdrop for modern pharmaceutical market and industry in India. The principal spur came in a 1971 government price control law for drugs that invalidated patent protection in pharmaceuticals, chemicals, and agricultural chemicals. The 1971 patent law led to the realm of "polypharmaceuticals" in India. Indian pharmaceutical companies could now freely make generic versions of popular drugs and sell them to countries whose markets lacked patent protections for "pioneer" producers. As a result, India slowly but surely became a critical source of production for many low-cost generic drugs.

P. Hari, Frank May, Mitchell Weiss and others; as usual, all errors and omissions are entirely my own.

[51] The Indian government in 1930 and 1931 appointed a "Drugs Enquiry Committee" headed by Lieutenant Colonel Sir Ram Nath Chopra. The Chopra committee recommended "a drugs and pharmacy legislation on the lines of those existing in Great Britain and America"; *Indian Medical Gazette* (June 1947), 351; *Gazette of India*, December 22, 1945. One call for a "food and drug administration" in the wake of the 1940 legislation came in "The Future of Medical Organization in India," (editorial), *Indian Medical Gazette* (January 1941): 41. "The Drugs and Cosmetics Rules, 1945," were designed to extend to "the whole of India." (Part I); Notification from the Department of Health, New Delhi, December 21, 1945. On the import license rules, see *Indian Medical Gazette*, (April 1947), 217. The national drug control laboratory in Calcutta was converted from the Biomedical Standards Laboratory in the same city in 1947, and was then headed by B. Mukherji, a member of the American ASPET and the Swiss Biological and Medical Society; *Indian Medical Gazette*, (April 1947), 216. For comparative state and regional statistics on pharmacological testing, see D. W. Soman (Director-General, Haffkine Institute), *Report of the Haffkine Institute for the Year 1955* (Bombay, 1955); in Nehru Memorial Library, Delhi.

Social and government efforts to stimulate the rise of domestic production and industry were expressed in a government commission publication—"The Report of the Committee on Drugs and Pharmaceuticals," or the Hathi Committee Report of 1975. The Hathi committee report called for a number of institutional changes, including registration and quality control measures. Much of the Hathi committee's report came to statutory fruition in the 1978 Drug Control law, which both set up a national registration system and enabled a schedule of price controls set forth in 1979. As of 1978, something of a new drug registration system existed in India, though one that continued the highly decentralized character of pre-1970 arrangements. These reforms modernized India's regulatory infrastructure only to a degree. The basic and enduring issue was one of incredible gulfs of scientific and administrative capacity across states. As an industry survey admitted in 1984, it was "well known that in most states the quality control administration does not exist for all practical purposes." Symbolically, in those few states where administrative and scientific capacity were in evidence (Gujarat and Maharashtra, for instance), the relevant state agencies called themselves "food and drug administrations."[52]

During and since the 1970s, various commentators and observers have lamented the problem of "drug quality" in India. Scholars and government

[52]Ministry of Petroleum and Chemicals, *Report of the Committee on Drugs and Pharmaceuticals* (Delhi, 1975). For portraits of Indian pharmaceutical production and regulation on the eve of the Hathi Committee report, see R. V. Rangarao, *Indian Drug Industry: Its Status and Perspective* (New Delhi: Center for Studies in Science Policy, Jawaharlal Nehru University, 1974); in Nehru Memorial Library (NML), Delhi. A series of policy reports and dissertations from Nehru University scholars and students covered the Indian pharmaceutical industry in the 1970s and 1980s and are available at this library and at the Jawaharlal Nehru University (JNU) library. Many of these have summary statistics on Indian drug regulation at the state level.

European and international health organization portraits of Indian regulation also emphasized the decentralized and federal character of the country's institutions and organizations; L. F. Dodson, "Assignment Report on Drug Laboratory Techniques and Biological Standardization: Proposals for Strengthening Government Controls over Biological and Pharmaceutical Products in India," 15 January 1968; SEA/HIM-24, AWHO. T. Canback, "Assignment Report on Drug Laboratory Techniques and Biological Standardization (WHO Project—India 0222)," 10 November 1970; SEA/Drugs 8, AWHO.

Partially in response to the Hathi Committee report, a National Drug Policy (NDP) was passed in 1978 and was followed by the government's Drug Price Control Order (DPCO). The Government outlined its response to the report in *Government Decisions on the Report of the Hathi Committee*, Centre for Research on Indian Economy (Bombay), 29 March 1978; JNU Library, Delhi. The Government explicitly declined to implement the Hathi committee's report for a National Drug Authority; *Government Decisions*, 19–20. On the weak status of drug control in the states in the 1970s and 1980s, consult P. L. Narayana, *The Indian Pharmaceutical Industry: Problems and Prospects* (Delhi: National Council of Applied Economic Research, 1984), 53–54. "The expert committees that have studied this problem in the past have drawn attention to the absence of Drug Control Administration in many states. Most states do not possess even laboratory equipment or trained staff to exercise the necessary quality checks." For a similar judgment, see the *Report of the Committee on Category II Drugs* (Vijay L. Kelkar, Chairman), New Delhi, August 1987 ("Kelkar Committee Report"); reprinted in D. K. Mittal, *Drugs and Pharmaceutical Industry* (New Delhi: Anmol Publications, 1993), 173.

reports have often documented the issue of drug quality as a regulatory problem, as Indian state control agencies relaxed standards so that small producers could meet the requirements. The upshot of this policy, among other developments, is that a perceived crisis of Indian drug quality has developed, one that was particularly acute in the 1980s. The Government announced a new National Drug Policy (NDP) in 1986 and a new Drugs Price Control Order (DPCO) in 1987. Following these two measures, Indian officials in 1988 established new registration and quality control procedures and strengthened rules governing clinical trials and animal toxicity tests. The 1988 rules officially pegged the stages in the drug development system of India to the three-phase system in use in the United States, and they instituted a requirement that human clinical trials receive written permission for their initiation from the Drugs Controller General of India (DCGI). The 1988 rules also detailed the data requirements for new drug applications and clinical trial applications. As with the IND form used in the United States, Indian clinical trial approval required an advance protocol for all proposed trials, sample case report forms to be used, and the names and qualifications of investigators.[53]

The changes of 1986 to 1988 issued from the multiple directions that Indian politics, industry, and science were taking at the time. Observers detected the scent of liberalization in the rules, which created an opening for foreign companies to conduct clinical trials in India. Yet consumer advocates and left parties exacted concessions from the government in its rulemaking. From 1988 until 2005, clinical trials in India were governed by a restrictive rule that cast its gaze upon the United States and the FDA's three-phase system of clinical experiment. Under the "Schedule Y" regulations handed down by the Drugs Controller General, no clinical trials could be conducted on Indian subjects unless trials of an identical phase had already been completed and regulated in another country (often the United States). Hence, for all drugs discovered outside the nation, a Phase 1 trial with Indian subjects required the existence of an FDA-regulated Phase 2 trial. This "phase lag" requirement was premised upon critics' laments that in a global world of clinical trials, Indian patients would be used as guinea pigs, assuming the risk of

[53]On quality control as a regulatory problem, consult Saradindu Bhaduri, *An Economic Analysis of R&D and Technology Generation in the Indian Pharmaceutical Industry* (Ph.D. diss., Jawaharlal Nehru University, 2001), 88; C. S. Daniel, *Indian Drug and Pharmaceutical Industry: An Analysis of Problems and Policies since Independence* (M. Phil. diss., Jawaharlal Nehru University, 1986); both in JNU Library, Delhi. Daniel found that, in the mid-1980s, Indian state regulatory agencies possessed about one-quarter to one-fifth of the personnel needed for inspections. For related discussions, see Dukes, *Law and Ethics of Pharmaceutical Industry*, 56–7, and 335. From the 1970s to the present, various essays published by Indian medical authorities in the *Indian Journal of Pharmacology* have served as a social barometer for the problem of drug quality; see for instance A. Y. Khan and N.M.K. Ghilzai, "Counterfeit and Substandard Quality of Drugs: The Need for an Effective and Stringent Regulatory Control in India and Other Developing Countries," *Indian Journal of Pharmacology* 39 (4) (Aug. 2007): 206–7.

earlier studies for the development of drugs that would eventually be used by patients in wealthier markets. Indian politicians thus adopted a new drug application and investigational drug procedure in 1988, complete with a phased system of experiment. Yet the adoption was premised upon terms that were locally and politically negotiated, and that were designed to protect the ethical and personal interests of India's citizens.[54]

As concerns the regulation of manufacturing, the fragmentary character of the India system robustly endured reforms in 2004 and 2005 that "harmonized" the country's regulations. For allopathic drugs there would appear to be two production sectors, which in reality overlap greatly. On one hand there is a highly diffuse industry for drug manufacturing; some 20,000 small manufacturing units produce drugs in India, almost all of them at relatively low cost. This has led to growing national and international concerns about the quality and variability of India's drug supply. Recent reports suggest that India produces 35 percent of Asia's substandard and counterfeit drugs, and that one in ten drugs produced in the country is of substandard quality. The decentralized system of quality control regulation furthers this problem. Of India's twenty-eight states, only fifteen have functional drug testing laboratories, and only seven of these are considered adequately staffed and equipped.[55]

On the other hand, some of India's larger generic drugs manufacturing companies—particularly Ranbaxy, Dr. Reddy's, Cipla, Hetero, and others—have become especially adept at navigating the FDA's generic drug approval system. For these companies, the regulatory system is rather robust, in part because the generic drug sector in India accounts for valued exports, wealth, and jobs. In recent years since 2000, Ranbaxy has been the largest single generic sponsor for ANDAs at the Administration, and the company is widely celebrated in international business circles for its speed of ANDA filing and its success with these applications. Yet even Ranbaxy, perhaps the most legitimated name in Indian pharmaceuticals, has been unable to escape the quality control problems that have plagued the lower-tier market. In November 2004, WHO officials withdrew essential medicines approval for

---

[54] "Requirement and Guidelines on Clinical Trials for Import and Manufacture of a New Drug" (Schedule Y), Sections 1.1–1.2, *The 1988 Drugs and Cosmetics Rules*, Ministry of Health and Family Welfare (Department of Health), New Delhi, 21 September 1988. On the political context of India at the time, see Ramachandra Guha, *India After Gandhi: The History of the World's Largest Democracy* (New York: Harper Perennial, 2007), chapters 24 and 25. On the phase lag rule and its relaxation in 2005, see Sonia Shah, *The Body Hunters: Testing New Drugs on the World's Poorest Patients* (New York: New Press, 2006), 117. The phase lag was partially changed in January 2005, when a revised Schedule Y was published that permitted "same phase" trials of drugs in India while similar trials were under way overseas. Still, as of 2007, initial Phase 1 studies were permitted only for drugs developed domestically.

[55] Khan and Ghilzai, "Counterfeit and Substandard Quality of Drugs," 206; citing the Government of India's Mashelkar Committee Report, August 2003. G. Mudur, "India to Introduce Death Penalty for Peddling Fake Drugs," *BMJ* 327 (2003): 414. Another source of policy refraction lies in the placement of pharmacy governance in the Ministry of Science and Technology, while pharmaceuticals are controlled by agencies in the Ministry of Health.

anti-retroviral drugs produced by Ranbaxy, Cipla, and Hetero, and in November 2008, FDA officials barred a series of Ranbaxy imports over quality control issues.[56]

One of the most striking adaptations of the American regulatory model has occurred in India's governance of Ayurvedic medicines. The traditional healing system of Ayurveda includes many practices, but Ayurvedic drug products processed from herbs have been so long legitimated that they possess their own pharmacopoeia and textbooks. In the 1980s, as a result of quality control concerns and communication with WHO officials, the Government of India officially applied good manufacturing practices (GMPs) and phased clinical trials to drugs from the Ayurvedic, Siddha, and Unani traditions. These moves were resisted by traditional Ayurvedic practitioners in India, who feared that their remedies would be disproven in clinical trials or delegitimated by quality control testing. The adoption of GMPs and phased clinical trials represented the transport of a concept and a nomenclature. Molecular treatments developed from Ayurvedic remedies are now expected to pass through the phased clinical trial system much as allopathic medicines do. Yet Ayurveda's encounter with the American regulatory model also represents the selective appropriation of FDA concepts by Indian government officials. If medicines are listed in recognized Ayurvedic literature or in *The Ayurvedic Pharmacopoeia of India*—which has status as a legal document under the 1940 Drugs and Cosmetics Act—then they need not clear pre-clinical (animal) tests before entering into human testing. A crucial hurdle in the toxicology requirements for drug testing—one that was central to the American regulatory system of the 1950s and 1960s—is culturally superseded for Ayurvedic drugs in India. Good manufacturing practices are, moreover, enforced selectively and variably because the policing institutions are state food and drug administrations, which vary widely in their capacities and approaches. Due to pressure from what observers call the "Ayurvedic lobby," each state food and drug administration in India now has an Ayurvedic drugs control officer. Here, too, Indian government's mimicry of FDA standards and procedures remains incomplete and, in telling ways, fragmentary and negotiated. Indian observers report that the competence of these controller officials varies widely, as do applied standards of enforcement.[57]

The past decade has witnessed two geographically disparate but related programs to further modernize traditional medicine, particularly Ayurvedic treatments. The first, the "golden triangle initiative" under way in India, is

---

[56]Bhupesh Bhandari, *The Ranbaxy Story: Rise of an Indian Multinational* (New York: Penguin Global, 2005), 172–3, 216–19.

[57]T. V. Padma, "Outlook India: Ayurveda," *Nature* 436 (July 28, 2005): 486. *The Ayurvedic Pharmacopoeia of India*, Vols. 1–4 (New Delhi: The Controller of Publications, 2004). The government has also established regional drug testing laboratories for Ayurvedic, Siddha, and Unani medicines, under Rules 160 A to J of the Drugs and Cosmetics Rules of 1945. In many respects, the regulation of Ayurvedic drugs is more stringent in Sri Lanka, representing a much smaller market, than in India, a disparity due not least to India's far-flung and little coordinated system of manufacturing regulation.

an attempt to link three streams of society and three administrative agencies. The streams are "Modern Science, Modern Medicine and Traditional Medicine"; the corresponding agencies are the Council for Scientific and Industrial Research (CSIR), the Indian Council for Medical Research (ICMR) and the Department of Ayurveda, Yoga & Naturopathy, Unani, Siddha and Homeopathy (AYUSH). The triangle is an attempt to facilitate the isolation of lead molecules from Ayurvedic remedies (by the CSIR) that can be approved for clinical trials (by the ICMR) and then regulated by the Government (AYUSH). By combining modern molecular synthesis, the globalized regime of clinical trials, and traditional medicine, the golden triangle uses FDA-inspired standards to convert part of Ayurvedic medicine to a molecular model and to gain greater global legitimacy in a rapidly developing alternative medicine market. The second program, in the United States, is an attempt to apply the development standards for traditional molecular treatments to "botanical drugs." In the 1990s, CDER officials at the Administration began working on a guidance document that would elaborate standards for "botanical drugs," essentially the sort of molecules like those isolated by India's golden triangle initiative. CDER officials completed their first draft guidance in 2000 and finalized it in 2004. The botanical drug products guidance represents an attempt to incorporate recognition of the validity of Ayurvedic and other healing traditions within the parameters of the Administration's structures and protocols. Significantly, the products regulated are not considered dietary and herbal supplements, as are some traditional Ayurvedic products, but as "new drugs" of a different order.[58]

CONCLUSION: ORGANIZATIONAL IMAGE, GLOBAL REGULATION, AND IMPLICATIONS FOR COMPARATIVE STUDY

At the core of international comparisons lies the idea that two cases are at least partially independent. One country has decided to do things one way, and another country has chosen or fallen into a different path. If the scholar or observer seeks to understand why the German welfare state is more "generous" than that of the United States, or why the Japanese tax ministry has greater authority over setting policy than does the American Internal Revenue Service (IRS), the standard method is to compare two or more nations on the dimension of interest (welfare state size and generosity), and assess the differences between them in dimensions of political culture, institutions, economic development, the organization of interests, and similar factors otherwise known as "independent" (or causal) variables.[59]

[58]The AYUSH and ICMR agencies lay within the Ministry of Health, whereas the CSIT is located in the Ministry of Science and Technology. FDA/CDER, "Guidance for Industry: Botanical Drug Products," June 2004.

[59]The key concept is that of *conditional* independence. Assuming scholars have properly taken account of ("controlled for") other factors affecting the outcome of interest—condition-

A reputation-based perspective on international regulation points to a fundamental problem with these sorts of comparisons: the independence is violated because nations are forever comparing, contrasting, adopting, and rejecting the models of others. A broad literature in "transnational" history and politics—heavily influential in scholarship in U.S. history at this writing—has shed doubt about these methods of inference, emphasizing the fluidity of ideas, persons, and resources. The lens of organizational image supplements these analyses by pointing to a particular model that has been adopted—the standards, forms, and concepts of the FDA in a particular epoch of time (the 1950s through the 1980s and perhaps beyond)—and by helping to identify legitimacy as one of the central mechanisms at work. It is critical to emphasize that much of the evidence for the FDA's organizational reputation in world politics comes not from imitation but from contrast and outright rejection. The knowledge of one regulator's standards can induce other national officials to resist as well as copy the global standard. Just as important, the presence of a common referent—particularly one that is a living, breathing agency of government and not simply a parchment institution—leads national and regulatory officials to justify their actions by reference to the regulator's behavior. Hence, one avenue for dependence among the national "cases" of regulation comes from explicit copying or rejection of standard models—the architecture of Phase 1, 2, and 3 trials, the reliance upon randomized clinical studies with a placebo control, the administrative processes of investigational new drug registration, and the new drug application.

A second avenue for dependence among nations is in the audiences that lie outside regulatory bodies. In the United States, Congress has consistently observed events and structures in the United Kingdom and has gestured to the FDA to copy or avoid these examples. The editorial page of the *Wall Street Journal* will note the approval of a new cancer therapy in Europe and use this fact to badger the Administration into approving the same drug. Or, similarly, AIDS activists point to approval of medicines overseas as justification for trials here. At the core of the "drug lag" controversy was a comparison between U.S. and European regulators, particularly those in England, France, West Germany, and Switzerland. These comparisons were active, a product in part of explicit, calculated arguments made by American critics and by British and German authorities themselves who decided that, while they needed to emulate the FDA in some respects, the adversarial process set up in the United States should be avoided.

The facility of these comparisons is made possible by the fact that, in large

---

ing on those factors, that is—a causal inference is said to be (more) valid if the causal factor appears in one country independently of its appearance in another. Gary King, Robert Keohane, and Sidney Verba, *Designing Social Inquiry* (Princeton: Princeton University Press, 1994). The easiest way to accomplish this is by randomization. Scholars are also apt to use proposed "natural experiments" in which an historical process with a high degree of randomness influences different countries in different ways.

Table 11.1

Cross-National Dependencies in Global Pharmaceutical Regulation in the Twentieth Century [cells contain year of first adoption by row state of column institution]

	Unified State Regulatory Agency	Pre-market Review	Efficacy Standard	Standardized New Drug Application	Regulated R&D Process (phased studies)	Bioequiv. and Bioavail. Regulation	Good Laboratory Practices	Good Mfg Practices	Guidelines for Clinical Evaluation	Advisory Committee System
Netherlands/ BENELUX	1958	1958	1958	1958	1975	1983				
Norway	1928	1928			1975	1983				
Sweden	1934	1934	1934	1971/1976	1975	1983				
United States	1906/1927	1938	1947–1962 [informal] 1962 [formal]	1947–1956	1962	1970	1974	1956	1971	1963–1965
United Kingdom	1963/1971	1963	1963	1971	1963	1983			1974/1977	1970
France		1945	1978	1967	1995	1983			1978	1978

Table 11.1
cont.

	Unified State Regulatory Agency	Pre-market Review	Efficacy Standard	Standardized New Drug Application	Regulated R&D Process (phased studies)	Bioequiv. and Bioavail. Regulation	Good Laboratory Practices	Good Mfg Practices	Guidelines for Clinical Evaluation	Advisory Committee System
Germany/ W. Germany	1961	1961	1976	1961	1978	1983				1976
Japan	1962	1948		1962				1975	1992	
Canada	1963	1963					1979			
Australia	1963	1963	1963	1989/1990	1989/1990	1990		1991		1968
European Union	1995	1995	1965	1965	1975	1983				
China	1979	1985	1985	1985	1999	1999	1999	1999	1999	none
South Korea	1953						1995		1994	

Note: Shaded cell denotes those institutions adopted first in the United States that were substantially copied by other nations or regions. BENELUX stands for Belgium, Netherlands, and Luxembourg, who unified their pharmaceutical regulations in 1973.

measure, regulators in different countries are reviewing identical molecules (particularly where bioequivalence standards have been satisfied), and in some cases, identical clinical trial data. This permits an immediate comparison of decisions. Every time a drug causes problems in Europe, Japan, or elsewhere, it is easy enough for professionals and journalists to compare its regulation with how the FDA treated it. Just the same, the approval of medicines in Europe or Canada can create reputational pressure for the FDA to accelerate the same medicines to market, and the safety-based withdrawal of a drug in Japan or New Zealand can create similar pressure for tighter post-marketing regulation in the United States.

Such comparisons are popular—they are undertaken daily by social scientists, academic physicians, and by politicians and journalists—but they fail to take account of the fact that the American regulatory model has become a global exemplar. In order to address the basic question of why countries have adopted the model of a central approval agency over the model of health board licensing (as in Sweden), a perspective centered upon organizational image delivers important explanatory power. Organizational reputation helps to account for a crucial puzzle—why it is that for so much of modern policymaking, especially of the welfare and social policy variety, the United States is known for historical decentralization, but in the regulation of food and drugs, the model of centralized governance adopted so broadly has been not a European model, but a particular American model embedded in a single organization. Compelling evidence for the appeal of this model rests in the very popularity of the Administration's title (see table 11.1), which has been adopted by China's State Food and Drug Administration (SFDA), the state food and drug administrations of India (perhaps best exemplified by the Maharashtra State FDA), and the FDAs of Saudi Arabia and South Korea.

CHAPTER TWELVE

Conclusion: A Reputation in Relief

Quem patronum rogaturus, cum vix justus sit securus?

—*Dies Irae*, Requiem Mass

WHETHER OR NOT their members find comfort in the fact, regulatory organizations are carriers of reputations. The organizations and the individuals attached to them are known alternatively for bumbling or for dramatic success, for gentility and laxity or for vigor and fierceness, for risk-aversion and methodical scrutiny or for sleeping at the wheel. Those reputations reflect, encode, and simplify complicated histories. And ultimately, those reputations feed back to shape the organizations they represent. A reputation becomes a tool of regulation, a tool with which federal officials herd citizens, firms, and medical researchers into more appropriate, legal behavior. Reputations become organizational assets, deployed at one time to secure greater legal authority, at another to fend off a budget cut, at another to lobby for policy change. Reputations become targets for those dissatisfied with the agency's decisions, or for inveterate ideological opponents of the agency's existence or authority. Reputations became markers of the authority and power that a federal agency possesses, and that competing entities—a national medical association, an organization of pharmaceutical producers, another governmental body—do not. Reputations create their own realities.

Organizational reputations provide a model for the understanding of regulatory agencies and bureaucracies generally. In looking for a model with which to understand the evolution and behavior of the U.S. Food and Drug Administration in something so vital as its regulation of therapeutic products, it is particularly useful and especially flexible. I hope to have shown that the usual metaphors—benevolent pursuit of public interest, persistent capture by producers, distributive politics—all fail to clarify, illuminate, and even predict the complex realities of American pharmaceutical regulation and, most likely, of the global governance of pharmaceuticals in the twentieth century.

Reputations embed status, symbols, culture, and history. They allow for the partially rational pursuit of ends, all the while recognizing the inherent (sometimes strategic) ambiguity of essential facts, organizational self-presentation, and policies. The politics of reputation entails conscious management of image and the often unconscious shaping of the very assumptions, goals, and information that regulators, companies, doctors, scientists, patients, activists, journalists, and politicians carry with them on a daily basis.

A focus on reputation in politics allows us to rethink the current devotion in the social sciences to notions of "path-dependence" or institutional stability. A wide set of arguments in political science, economics, history, and sociology have attempted to understand why institutions as diverse as constitutions, social welfare states, financial transparency regimes, professional groups, legislative committees, and international organizations prove highly resistant to efforts of reformers to change them. The response from the social sciences has been to point to "feedback" effects of institutions—the way that welfare policies condition citizenship among the very people who vote to sustain those policies, the way that civil service reform paves the way for creation of government workers' unions; the way that constitutions make their own reform highly incremental and hence preserve their stability.[1]

A perspective on organizational and institutional image suggests another mechanism, one that has eluded much of modern social science. At times the crucial stasis in institutions and organizations is generated not by the known (or knowable) cost of changing the rules but by the little-noticed impossibility of changing images, symbols, mind-sets, and assumptions. A form of cognitive reliance upon existing symbols, rituals, and rhetoric attaches to organizational and political reputations, such that it generates a form of history-dependence that is little recognized in our understanding of institutions.

In thinking about the complicated history of American pharmaceutical regulation, a reputation-based standpoint also presents a combination of insights, predictions, and interpretations that are hard to come by using existing theories and conceptual structures. Among the patterns for which a reputation-based perspective offers a unique and credible account are the following.

- Why the United States has the most bureaucratically intensive form of drug regulation among advanced industrialized countries, even as other nations have more administrative governments and larger public sectors.

- Why the creation of new regulatory legislation in 1938 was premised upon a report and proposal from the very agency that would receive authority and discretion in the legislation.

- Why the Administration was able to incorporate efficacy judgments, case report forms, and protocol considerations in new drug review more than a decade before congressional statute permitted it.

- Why the effectiveness, drug testing, and drug control provisions of 1962 were passed but the patent and pricing provisions of the Kefauver proposal were not.

[1]Kathleen Thelen, "Historical Institutionalism in Comparative Politics," *Annual Review of Political Science* (1999) 369–404. Pierson, *Politics in Time: History, Institutions, and Social Analysis* (Princeton: Princeton University Press, 2004). Eric Schickler, *Disjointed Pluralism: Institutional Innovation and the Development of the U.S. Congress* (Princeton: Princeton University Press, 2001). Douglass North, *Institutions, Institutional Change and Economic Performance* (New York: Cambridge University Press, 1990), chap. 10. Peter Hall and Rosemary Taylor, "Political Science and the Three New Institutionalisms," *Political Studies* 44 (1996): 936–57.

- Why many Administration officials approach drug approval as irreversible in decision even as it is reversible at law.
- Why drugs approved in divisions with longer-tenured directors are less likely to receive labeling revisions in subsequent years, even though these drugs do not have a different adverse event profile after approval.
- Why the twentieth-century FDA received nearly unparalleled judicial deference in its regulation of drugs, and why the Department of Justice was less likely to decline case referrals from the FDA than from other agencies.
- Why the Administration's standards in phased experiment, bioavailability, bioequivalence, and surrogate endpoints have diffused throughout the world, reducing the cross-national variation in pharmaceutical regulation.
- Why drugs are approved more quickly when they target diseases that receive greater public attention in national media and congressional hearings, and why these same drugs are more likely to be referred to advisory committees before the final approval decision.[2]

Taken individually, these patterns may admit of idiosyncratic explanation. Taken together, it is difficult to account for them without reference to organizational reputation and the directive, gatekeeping, and conceptual regulatory power that it supports.

It would be hasty and undeserved to claim too much for a reputation-based account of government regulation. It does not offer "covering laws" in the sense of the unified field theories that characterized twentieth-century physics. Indeed, no such theory exists for accurate generalization across the manifold agencies of government, and especially over historical time in regulatory politics. At its core, a unified theory of government agencies has as much wisdom and appeal as a unified theory of creatures that swim; there are simply too many types, too many species out there, and generalization is best attempted within these categories and not across them. What the vantage of reputation offers is not a chance to generate singular laws of all regulation, but an opportunity to approach regulation in its complexity, as a contest played out among diverse audiences. Such an approach permits us to detect politics where we otherwise would miss it, to see forces at work that occupy the attention and anxiety of regulators, that buffet the strategies and miscues of firms, and that attract the conscious and unconscious attention of journalists and politicians, if not scholars.

. . .

[2]Previous chapters provide a treatment of these different patterns, including the United States in comparison with other nations (Introduction, chapters 3 and 11), the 1938 Act (Chapter 2), the incorporation of modern drug regulation before 1962 (chapter 3), the Kefauver bill and 1962 legislation (chapter 4), judicial deference to FDA drug regulation (chapters 5 and 6), patterns of drug review and advisory committee consultation (chapters 6 and 7), patterns of relabeling (chapter 9), and the diffusion of FDA concepts across international boundaries (chapter 11).

Unfortunately, there is growing concern that the FDA may have lost the confidence of the public and Congress—much to our detriment. When Americans are nervous about eating spinach or tomatoes or cantaloupes, that's not good for our health and it is terrible for our farmers. When nearly two-thirds of Americans do not trust the FDA's ability to ensure the safety and effectiveness of pharmaceuticals, the result is Americans may hesitate to take important medications that protect their health. This is unacceptable.

—Former Senator Tom Daschle, January 8, 2009

The regulatory power of the Food and Drug Administration in the modern pharmaceutical world flows from many sources, but from none more than organizational image. The image of the Administration is multidimensional and is suspended among numerous audiences, but its basic features—a demonstrated capacity for citizen protection, a vigilance against threats to drug safety and medicinal effect, an enduring commitment to scientific principles of assessment, unremunerated work of regulation, appropriate flexibility to pivotal constituencies—have forcefully supported the accrual of directive, gatekeeping, and conceptual power to a small organization. The image often overstates the underlying pattern of behavior but, like any reputation, sustains fictions that have powerful influences of their own.

At this writing, the reputation and the power of the Food and Drug Administration in the governance of pharmaceuticals have waned appreciably. They have not disappeared, it is important to recognize, and much of the system whose history I have examined and interpreted here still exists in stable form. Any commodity that can be defined as a "new drug" must still gain the approval of the Administration, and for this reason must demonstrate bioavailability, safety, effectiveness, and other properties in a series of experiments whose parameters are defined by the gatekeeper itself. The sponsors of the drugs and the claims attendant to them are criminally as well as civilly liable to the directives of the Administration. Drug companies, medical researchers, and foreign governments still structure their discussions and their activity upon concepts framed by FDA officials.

Yet the rise of libertarian models and conservative politics in the United States, the accretion of power to the global pharmaceutical industry, and the globalization of economic regulation have all weakened the authority and force of the Administration's capacities and actions. These developments cast light on the late twentieth-century system of American pharmaceutical regulation, and they help to cast that regime into starker historical relief, thereby illuminating its features.

DRUG WITHDRAWALS AND THE GOLD STANDARD: THE RIGHTWARD SHIFT OF THE FDA

The story of pharmaceutical politics (and the FDA's decline) in the past few decades demands a book or two in its own right. For now, the lens of a reputation-based perspective offers a sketch for this narrative. The sketch is one of weakened organizational image, accompanied by waning power in its distinct facets.[3]

The politics of American pharmaceutical regulation has been transformed for many reasons. Not the least of these appears in broader trends in American politics itself. A much more conservative paradigm governed the period from the 1970s to the early twenty-first century, and for regulatory agencies it culminated less in the Reagan administration than in the "Republican revolution" of 1994, when Republicans achieved their first majority in the House of Representatives since the 83rd Congress (1953–54). Combined with a Republican Senate, a centrist Democratic president in Bill Clinton who felt chastised by the 1994 elections, and newly energized anti-regulatory voices coming from within and outside of Washington, House Republicans launched a thorough and visceral attack on the FDA, targeting its pharmaceutical policies in particular. House Speaker Newt Gingrich called the FDA the "number one job-killer" in 1994, and in the ensuing years House and Senate committees held hearings on "FDA reform."[4]

The passage of the Food and Drug Administration Modernization Act (FDAMA) in 1997 reflected many congressional Republicans' wishes, albeit imperfectly. The law changed the FDA's mission statement in pharmaceutical policy—emphasizing "timely," "efficient," and "prompt" review of new drugs—and it re-authorized the prescription drug user fees that had begun five years before (and in so doing, tightened the deadlines governing NDA review). Most symbolically, the bills that preceded the 1997 Act flirted with the evisceration and privatization of FDA gatekeeping power—by authorizing experiments with "third party" review (this made its way into statute for medical device regulation) and by calling for the FDA to decide on a new drug submission within thirty days once the same drug had been approved by selected foreign regulators.[5]

With the election of George W. Bush as the nation's forty-third president, both elective branches of government were generally governed by Republicans from 2001 to 2006. The brand of Republicans governing the nation in

[3]The argument here is related to but distinct from the perceptive essay of James T. O'Reilly, "Losing Deference in the FDA's Second Century: Judicial Review, Politics, and a Diminished Legacy of Expertise," *Cornell Law Review* 93 (2007–2008): 939–1002. O'Reilly's focus is on judicial deference, not reputation per se, and his treatment is less concerned with nonjudicial audiences.

[4]Hilts, *Protecting America's Health*, 296. Hilts offers an apt summary of this period, including documentation of the organized conservative assault on the Administration at the level of think tanks and foundations. Among many of the hearings in question, see *The Need for FDA Reform: Hearing before the Subcommittee on Health and Environment of the Committee on Commerce, House of Representatives*, 104th Congress, Second Session, February 27, 1996 (Washington, DC: GPO, 1997).

[5]The altered mission statement in FDAMA tasked the agency with promoting the public health "by promptly and efficiently reviewing clinical research and taking appropriate action on the marketing of regulated products in a timely manner"; Public Law 105-115, and its preamble. On some of the bills introduced in 1996, see Karen Young Kreeger, "FDA Reform Debate Heating Up As Senate, House Propose Bills," *The Scientist* 10 (10) (May 13, 1996): 1.

the 1990s and early twenty-first century was generally more unified and ideologically driven than in previous decades. Two other audiences for American pharmaceutical regulation—the national pharmaceutical industry and various disease advocates—were also better organized and more politically vocal than before. President Clinton's health-care reform plan, proposed and debated at length in 1993 and 1994, galvanized and unified American and global drug companies against government regulation and helped set in motion a broader conservative trend in domestic politics. The Pharmaceutical Manufacturers Association renamed itself the Pharmaceutical Research and Manufacturers Association in 1994, and patient advocacy groups (an increasing number of them funded partially or wholly by pharmaceutical industry interests) exploded.[6]

The Administration's response to these poverties was one that continued and accentuated its response to the challenges from cancer and AIDS. The model of deregulation that was applied in American pharmaceutical policy was less direct and statutory and more erosive and subterranean. In contrast to other realms of policy—environmental policy, telecommunications, antitrust, labor, and consumer product safety—deregulation in American pharmaceutical policy has taken a different, less visible form. In a way that is telling and perhaps cognizant of the agency's reputation, it has proceeded behind the scenes, under the radar, in moves of administration—Daniel Troy's reversal of agency's position on pre-emption, the issuance of guidelines for medical journal article distribution, the slow but persistent move to greater reliance on user fees—rather than in direct public acts of legislation. Regulation in the libertarian-leaning 1990s and under President George W. Bush largely failed to keep pace with changing technologies and strategies of pharmaceutical marketing.[7]

[6] For particular evidence that the health-care battles of 1993 and 1994 animated conservative and antigovernment opposition from health insurance and pharmaceutical companies, see Theda Skocpol, *Boomerang: Health Care Reform and the Turn Against Government* (New York: Norton, 1997); Anna D. Sinaiko, "A Special Interest in Health: The Pharmaceutical Research and Manufacturers of America's Influence on Health Care Policy in the United States," senior thesis, Princeton University (1998).

In 2004, one study reported "3,100 disease-specific advocacy groups with at least some involvement in political issues." A crucial difference between the patient advocacy groups of the late 1980s and early 1990s came in the reduced reliance of earlier groups upon pharmaceutical industry funding. This question demands further research; Carpenter, "The Political Economy of FDA Drug Approval," *Health Affairs* (Jan./Feb. 2004) 23 (1) (2004): 56–8.

[7] The notion of subterranean politics is one I take from Jacob S. Hacker, "Privatizing Risk without Privatizing the Welfare State: The Hidden Politics of Social Policy Retrenchment in the United States," *American Political Science Review* 98 (May 2004): 243–60. Hacker's model aptly summarizes the intent of many conservatives with regard to pharmaceutical regulation, but it is worth noting that 1990s officials at the FDA also tried to advance several informational initiatives, including the "medication guide" proposals of 1995 and 1998, that were shot down from outside of the agency. The FDA also tried to implement "medication guides," but was thwarted. FDA, "Proposed Rule: Prescription Drug Product Labeling; Medication Guide Requirements," *FR* 60 (164): August 24, 1995; "Final Rule: Prescription Drug Product Labeling; Medication Guide Requirements," *FR* 63 (230): December 1, 1998.

In articulating a new vision, the agency published several transformative guidance documents drafted and issued in the 1990s that elaborated the idea of "risk management." To some extent, these documents reflected new understandings of drug risk that had taken hold in pharmacoepidemiology, but in many other ways they reflected a political vision of drug regulation that counseled the acceptance of more risks in the act of drug approval and increasingly aimed to "manage" these risks once the product was on the market. Similarly, the agency in 1997 floated a new guidance document that heralded significant policy change for direct-to-consumer advertising. No longer would television and other broadcast advertisements for prescription drugs have to include a complete listing of adverse reactions and side effects; the new guidance effectively permits companies to display a drug's brand name in the same advertisement as it touted the drug's benefits. At some level, "direct-to-consumer" advertising had existed for years, but in other ways and more implicitly, the 1997 policy change brought direct-to-consumer advertising to the airwaves and (indirectly) the Internet.[8]

Changes in Drug Review. At the level of everyday regulatory practice, the Administration's behavior began to encode and reflect these political transformations. In many respects, the changes pre-dated the user fee legislation of 1992. When Paul Leber and his colleagues in the Neuropharmacological Drug Products Division reviewed the new drug application for the antidepressant sertraline (Zoloft), they noticed a clear change in the political climate that confronted them.

> It is noteworthy that several [European] national drug regulatory authorities, presumably provided with the same body of information that is contained in the NDA submitted to us, have not been willing to allow Sertraline's marketing in their respective countries [due to] the "lack of robustness" of the clinical evidence supporting its efficacy in the treatment of depression. This turn of events may seem somewhat surprising in view of the fact that the agency [FDA] is traditionally more conservative than its European counterparts. . . . Many of these foreign regulatory initiatives have potential merit, but, given the perceived urgency we express as an institution for expediting the public's access to new, potentially promising drugs, I do not believe we can successfully introduce more demanding requirements domestically, at least until there is a significant "sea change" in our society's collective attitude toward Federal regulation of new drug approvals.[9]

---

[8] *Managing the Risks of Medical Product Use: Creating a Risk Management Framework*, Report to the FDA Commissioner from the Task Force on Risk Management (Rockville, MD: FDA, May 1999). Some of these initiatives were supported by David Kessler and his successor, Jane Henney, and implemented by career official Janet Woodcock, appointed to head CDER in May 1994 and re-appointed to the position in March 2008. On the DTCA policy changes, see Julie Donohue, Marisa Cevasco, and Meredith B. Rosenthal, "A Decade of Direct-to-Consumer Advertising of Prescription Drugs," *NEJM* 357 (7) (2007): 673–81.

[9] Paul Leber, "Recommendation to Approve Zoloft (Sertraline)," FDA memo to Robert Temple (Director, Office of Drug Evaluation), December 24, 1991, 1–2; cited in Abraham and

Leber's memorandum expressly stated regulatory liberality as an organizational commitment, and it reflected an underlying calculus of reputation. The reason that new requirements for drug testing would not fly, in Leber's statement, had less to do with expected political opposition and more to do with the "perceived urgency we express as an institution." Some years later, in an interview, Leber argued that partisan and ideological politics had changed regulatory standards at the FDA. The procedural "liberal" had articulated the standards of a regulatory conservative. "We're acting more as a political body than a scientific one. The standards are dictated by the existing political parties. We're making decisions that we wouldn't have made 20 years ago."[10]

At an aggregate level, the user fee laws shaped drug review with a mechanism that was similar to the "December effect" that had governed NDA approval from the 1970s through the early 1990s. The user fee law created a form of contractual accountability to at least two of the agency's audiences: the Congress and the political wing of the American pharmaceutical industry (PhRMA). The renewal of user fee legislation in 1997, 2002, and 2007 put industry representatives explicitly at the table with top-level FDA officials. In a very real sense, it was this miniature audience to which FDA drug-reviewing divisions would be held answerable. The divisions' spectators appeared not as the "industry" or the "drug companies" writ broadly, but as the political organizations representing American pharmaceuticals writ structurally.[11]

The temporal structure of new drug review shifted to reflect these realities. Whereas drug reviews reflected a temporally smooth but variable process in the years before 1992, the review process after PDUFA was governed by drug review deadlines. Under the various commitments outlined in 1992, 1997, and 2002, the FDA committed to review 90 percent of priority NDAs within six months by 1997, and committed to review 90 percent of standard NDAs within 10 months by 2002. Whereas new drug approvals had been concentrated in the month of December during the era of "drug lag criti-

---

Sheppard, "Complacent and Conflicting Scientific Expertise in British and American Drug Regulation: Clinical Risk Assessment of Triazolam," *Social Studies of Science* 29 (6) (Dec. 1999): 830–31.

[10]Leber quoted in Michael Day, "US Drug Safety Regime "Flawed,"" *New Scientist* (Nov. 9, 1996): 10; cited in Abraham and Sheppard, "Complacent and Conflicting Scientific Expertise," 831.

[11]The industry officials included PhRMA representatives and, later, those from the Biotechnology Industry Organization (BIO). Some statistics on the frequency of meetings between FDA and PhRMA officials over user fee reauthorization in 2007 appear in the testimony of FDA official Theresa Mullin before the House Energy and Commerce Subcommittee on Health, April 17, 2007. For an argument that the debates over re-authorization in 2002 reflected the political influence of drug companies achieved through campaign contributions, see Robert Dreyfuss, "Popping Contributions: The New Battle for the FDA," *The American Prospect*, November 30, 2002. On the most recent round of negotiations before re-authorization, see FDA, "Prescription Drug User Fee Act; Public Meeting," *FR* 72 (9) (January 16, 2007).

cism," the December effect all but disappeared in the user fee era, only to be replaced by a different sort of discontinuity: a piling of approvals in the deadline months (at present, this is the tenth month of review). For standard NMEs, the rate of first-cycle approval in the deadline months after PDUFA was eight to twelve times higher than at other times in the review clock.[12]

As this pattern solidified, two other transformations took place more quietly. First, the "approvable letter" by which the Administration notified a sponsor that a drug had nearly met the conditions for approval—conditioned upon submission of new data, changes in labeling, or some other revision to an NDA—was transformed in its symbolism. What once had been celebrated by companies and investors as heralding the imminent approval of a product became, in the user fee era, a form of bad news. The finality of NDA approval that was expected to arrive with a review deadline would, with an "approvable letter," be postponed. For the Administration's drug reviewing divisions, the approvable letter became a tool for prolonging the evaluation process in light of the burdens imposed by new political and legal expectations. A second transformation was the added burden placed upon noncontractual promises that sponsors of approved NDAs made to continue studying their product in post-marketing trials. These "Phase 4 commitments" were frequently made but infrequently observed, in part because there was no enforceable legal contract binding the companies to complete them, in part because the Administration lacked tools to enforce these commitments.[13]

As the changes in behavior multiplied, agency observers and critics began to question the policies and whether the Administration had become too lenient on the companies and products under its purview. *Los Angeles Times* reporter David Willman penned a series of influential newspaper articles linking the regulatory changes to a slew of new drug safety problems. Willman's series was entitled "How a New Policy Led to Seven Deadly Drugs," and its subtitle pointed to a fundamental change in the Administration's public identity: "Once a wary watchdog, the Food and Drug Administration set out to become a 'partner' of the pharmaceutical industry." For these articles, Willman garnered a Pulitzer Prize in 2001, and in celebrating Willman's reporting, the Pulitzer Committee cast doubt upon the organizational subject of his writing. Willman had won the Pulitzer, the prize committee said, for "his pioneering exposé of seven unsafe prescription drugs that had been approved by the Food and Drug Administration, and an analysis of the policy reforms that had reduced the agency's effectiveness." Along with other investigations, Willman's reporting helped generate momentum for

---

[12]Daniel Carpenter, et al., "Deadline Effects in Regulatory Drug Review: A Methodological and Empirical Analysis," Robert Wood Johnson Foundation Working Paper, October 2009.

[13]On Phase 4 studies and their difficulties as a regulatory tool, see chapter 9. The Administration was given the authority to issue fines to uncompleted Phase 4 studies in the Food and Drug Administration Amendments Act of 2007, which re-authorized the user fee program for another five years.

the market withdrawal of Rezulin in 2001. Along with investigations by Sidney Wolfe's Health Research Group at Public Citizen, moreover, one of Willman's cases (alosetron, marketed by Glaxo Wellcome as Lotronex for irritable bowel syndrome) generated a particularly strident critique of the agency from *Lancet* editor Richard Horton. Horton's essay, entitled "Lotronex and the FDA: A Fatal Erosion of Integrity," was among the first and most notable forays by a medical journal editor into the drug safety debate of the early twenty-first century, and Horton's editorial influentially highlighted the agency's growing image problem. In a line that would become a common refrain in medical journal essays, newspaper op-eds, congressional speeches, and other public expressions of doubt, Horton argued that "The FDA urgently needs to re-establish the public's trust."[14]

VIOXX, THE GOLD STANDARD, AND THE CONTOURS OF A REPUTATION

We depend on the FDA. We depend on it every day. It clearly has to be considered one of the great brands, if you will, in America, in the world. It's the gold standard.

A brand really is nothing more than a promise. It's an expression of trust. And Americans place it, place their trust in the Food and Drug Administration.
—Republican Secretary of Health and Human Services Michael O. Leavitt, 2006

I no longer believe that the FDA and the EPA are the global "gold standard" for public safety, and I have little confidence that public safety is placed above corporate interests.
—*Newsweek* reader Robin McStay of Weaverville, California, in a Letter to the Editor, February 2008[15]

A different aperture into the emerging politics of U.S. pharmaceutical regulation, as well as a view of the expectations that have hovered over the agency for several decades, comes from the more recent policy tragedy of Vioxx. In September 2004, the global pharmaceutical firm Merck abruptly announced the immediate and total market withdrawal of its anti-arthritis drug rofecoxib (Vioxx). Vioxx was the first in a class of new anti-arthritis drugs called COX-2 inhibitors. The official reason for Vioxx's withdrawal was a tripling of the heart attack rate in patients taking Vioxx, compared to other medications and to placebo, in a clinical trial testing the drug's treatment potential for colon polyps.

Quite aside from its profound effect upon the Administration's image and subsequent policy changes, the Vioxx tragedy is filled with irony and some

[14]Willman, "How a New Policy Led to Seven Deadly Drugs," *LAT*, December 20, 2000; Horton, "Lotronex and the FDA: A Fatal Erosion of Integrity," *Lancet* 357 (9268) (May 19, 2001): 1544–5.

[15]Leavitt, "Remarks as Delivered at FDA Centennial," June 30, 2006. Leavitt was the Cabinet appointee of President George W. Bush and had previously served as the Republican governor of Utah. McStay remark in "Letters," *Newsweek*, February 18, 2008, 22.

measure of predictability. Several factors that were evident in the "old regime" of pharmaceutical regulation quite plausibly shaped the agency's decision making in the case of Vioxx and related drugs. The first and most notable is that Merck was perhaps the single most trusted corporate name at the FDA in the late twentieth century. Through the 1970s and 1980s, and culminating in the celebrated and purportedly science-driven tenure of executive Roy Vagelos, Merck had maintained a general and network-specific relationship of trust with the Administration. A highly uncertain environment like that presented by the early review of COX-2 inhibitors meant that the FDA as a learning organization was relying not only upon data specific to the sponsor's application, but upon the general image and information attached to the sponsor itself. This reliance was all the more accentuated by Vioxx's quick clinical development; the rofecoxib molecule Vioxx was patented in 1994 and submitted as a new drug application in the fall of 1998. Even by modern standards, its clinical development and testing were quite rapid.

The second contextual factor concerned the target population for the drug. Osteoarthritis was in the 1990s among the most publicized medical conditions in the United States, and Vioxx was the first investigational new drug in a highly celebrated line of therapies to attack this condition while also presenting a more acceptable gastrointestinal safety profile. The Administration's quick decision on the Vioxx submission, then, was associated with arthritis's political clout and also of its early status in its pharmacological class. A telling (albeit non-experimental) signal comes from comparing asthma and arthritis. In the 1990s, as Vioxx was being developed, arthritis in all of its forms was responsible for a fraction (about one-tenth to one fifth) of asthma's associated hospitalizations and deaths (a burden which falls disproportionately on the young and poor). Yet when social and political factors were observed, arthritis received considerably more media coverage than asthma did in American newspapers of the same time period, and arthritis drugs were approved much more quickly than asthma drugs were (on average) from the 1970s through the 1990s.[16]

The primary point of conflict over Vioxx was not its initial approval, however, but the tortuous process by which its safety risks were debated once it reached the market and was prescribed to millions of patients. Several large-scale studies in 2000 and 2001 showed evidence that rofecoxib was related to heart attacks, leading epidemiologists in the FDA's Office of Drug Safety (particularly David Graham) to recommend a black-box warning for the drug or even the market removal of its highest dosage form. The

---

[16]See data in Carpenter, "The Political Economy of FDA Drug Approval." The saga of Vioxx was part of a larger social story about the management of arthritis. With an aging population in the United states, there was a particular expansion in the use of nonsteroidal anti-inflammatory drugs in the 1980s and 1990s, and these drugs were associated with serious gastrointestinal adverse effects. This fact was well known in the 1980s; Bernard S. Bloom, "Direct Medical Costs of Disease and Gastrointestinal Side Effects during Treatment for Arthritis," *American Journal of Medicine* 84 (2) (Supp. 1) (Feb. 22, 1988): 20–24.

Administration's drug reviewing center (CDER) decided instead to place information from the VIGOR study in the "Warnings" section of the label. The dispute over Vioxx quickly became a debate about the relative value of pharmacology versus epidemiology, and the value of randomized controlled trials versus observational studies in drug regulation. The failures of Graham and his colleagues to gain acceptance of their recommendations in 2001 and 2002 demonstrated the continued centrality of pharmacology (and the methodology of prospectively designed, randomized, controlled trials) at the Administration. And beyond the methodological and professional divide, there was an organizational fissure. Vioxx and other drug safety debates pitted drug reviewing medical officers (such as Temple and Lourdes Villalba) symbolically and structurally against post-marketing surveillance officers (such as Graham and Andrew Mosholder, who pointed to increased suicidality risks among adolescent users of new antidepressant drugs). These fissures were opened to public view when Graham testified before the Senate finance Committee in November 2004, and openly declared that "FDA and its Center for Drug Evaluation and Research are broken" and that "the FDA, as currently configured, is incapable of protecting America against another Vioxx. We are virtually defenseless."[17]

In the months and years that followed the Vioxx withdrawal, something of a public drama unfolded in the United States and around the world. Blame was cast upon numerous institutions, not least Merck itself, which was reported to have set aside $10–$15 billion to cover the expected costs of lawsuits. Yet, as national anxiety seemed to heighten and as recrimination accelerated, another story emerged, one with roots that predated the Vioxx tragedy. Voices from various quarters in American society and politics were echoing a common refrain: the U.S. Food and Drug Administration had lost some of its scientific and consumer protection luster.

The language of this extended lament became starkest in the wake of the unexpected resignation of FDA Commissioner Lester Crawford in September 2005. Hillary Clinton, Senator for New York and a frequent FDA critic, welcomed the news of Lester Crawford's departure by expressing her hopes for superior leadership: "the FDA has a real opportunity to restore its battered reputation and nominate a leader with vision and drive to ensure that

---

[17]In November 2000, a Merck-sponsored clinical trial named VIGOR (Vioxx Gastrointestinal Outcomes Research) found a fivefold increase in heart attack risk with high-dose rofecoxib. Bombardier, et al., "Comparison of Upper Gastrointestinal Toxicity of Rofecoxib and Naproxen in Patients with Rheumatoid Arthritis," *NEJM* 343 (2000):1520–28. This study was later subject to considerable controversy over the alleged suppression of data by the authors; see Gregory D. Curfman, Stephen Morrissey, and Jeffrey M. Drazen, "Expression of Concern," *NEJM* 353 (26) (Dec. 29, 2005): 2813–14. Graham appeared before the Senate Finance Committee at the invitation of Senator Charles Grassley of Iowa and his testimony made headlines and nightly news in a variety of settings; "Testimony of David J. Graham, MD, MPH," before the Senate Finance Committee, November 18, 2004. Revealing memoranda about how Merck Research Laboratories personnel perceived the FDA and its drug safety officers at this time are available in the Drug Industry Digital Archive, UCSF.

the FDA upholds its gold standard of drug regulation." Clinton's Democratic colleagues in the Senate also used the language of a gold standard. Senator Edward Kennedy of Massachusetts, with a long history of consumer protection activism and someone who was fast becoming one of the most consistent advocates for biotechnology firms in Congress, stated that "the FDA gold standard has been tarnished." Senator Patty Murray from Washington concluded that, during Crawford's tenure, "the FDA's reputation as the gold standard in public health has been tarnished."[18]

The idea that the FDA had established a "gold standard" in consumer protection, or in public health, or in scientific evaluation of drugs, was repeatedly voiced in the 1990s and early twenty-first century. The language awkwardly combined at least two metaphors from the vernacular of global political and scientific history: the gold standard as a financial regime in which the supply of money was pegged to the underlying aggregate value of gold reserves, and the gold standard as a definitive test of a scientific hypothesis, particularly as applied to randomized, controlled clinical trials.[19]

The language of consumer protection and of gold standard decision making seemed confined to no quarter of American political economy. In arguing that the Vioxx withdrawal was uncharacteristic of the U.S. system, a spokesman for the pharmaceutical industry's main lobbying group—the Pharmaceutical Research and Manufacturers of America (PhRMA)—stated that the FDA served as the "gold standard" of drug safety regulation. When Republican President George W. Bush launched his "Emergency Plan for AIDS Relief" in 2004, his proposal to have inexpensive fixed-dose combination AIDS drugs distributed in less developed countries relied upon a rapid FDA approval process. Randall Tobias, a former Eli Lilly CEO whom Bush appointed as U.S. Global AIDS Coordinator, talked about the assurance that quick FDA review of these drugs would provide: "With FDA review, we will have a gold-standard assurance that a combination product will be safe and effective." Libertarian critics of the agency also acknowledged the "gold standard" reputation, even as they drew attention to the other side of the coin: the delays for new therapies caused by the gold standard, delays that they considered unacceptable. Two years earlier in 2002, when the Admin-

---

[18]Senator Clinton was the spouse of former President Bill Clinton. Marc Kaufman, "FDA Commissioner Steps Down After Rocky Two-Month Tenure," *WP*, September 24, 2005, A7. Diedtra Henderson, "FDA Chief Quits: Tenure Marked by Turmoil," *BG*, September 24, 2005. For Kennedy's remark, see Patricia Guthrie, "U.S. Senate Passes FDA Revitalization Act," *Canadian Medical Association Journal* 177 (1) (July 3, 2007): 23. Connecticut representative Rosa DeLauro used slightly different language, but no less celebratory of the FDA's past in regulating drugs: "The FDA's regulatory role in protecting public health 'has been bedrock,'" DeLauro said, but "This foundation is jarred." Henderson, "FDA chief answers his critics in House," *BG*, July 27, 2005, D3.

[19]For some discussion of the "gold standard" concepts as applied to Administration's clinical experiment standards, see Jennifer Kulynych, "Will FDA Relinquish the 'Gold Standard' for New Drug Approval? Redefining 'Substantial Evidence' in the FDA Modernization Act of 1997," *FDLJ* 54 (1999): 127–49.

istration approved the abortion pill mifepristone (trade name RU-486), anti-abortion critics lamented that the agency had violated its own "gold standard norms."[20]

Indeed, the equation of the Administration itself (or its procedures or decisions) to a gold standard dates from the 1990s and perhaps earlier. In signing new FDA reform legislation in 1997, President Bill Clinton stated that "The FDA has always set the gold standard for consumer safety." Even inveterate FDA critic Sidney Wolfe, longtime head of Public Citizen's Health Research Group, would use the language, applying it to the FDA of a by-gone era. "At one time, ten years ago, I would have said—and did say—that the FDA was the gold standard, that no country was doing a better job, either in the approval of drugs in the first place, or, secondly, in finding out [about safety problems] as quickly as possible once they came on the market. That's no longer the case."[21]

In the aftermath of the Vioxx withdrawal, related congressional hearings at which FDA scientists revealed unsavory details of the agency's internal politics, and the resignation of Crawford, media outlets, medical journals, and other commentators began to size up the agency. These narratives commonly described a regulatory tragedy, an organization that had fallen from lofty heights. Medical journals began asking "what's wrong with" or "what ails" the agency, while others reported that its credibility had been tarnished. The chief medical officer of the drug company Pfizer openly argued that loss of public trust in the Administration was bad for business: "There has been a loss of confidence in the F.D.A., and we can't afford to have that," said Joseph M. Feczko. "When our medicines come out, we want people to understand they have gone through a rigorous review process." The influential Institute of Medicine released a 2006 report—*The Future of Drug Safety*—which noted "a perception of crisis that has compromised the credibility of the FDA and the pharmaceutical industry."[22]

[20]PhRMA spokesman Jeff Trewhitt statement in Alexandra Marks, "How Drug Approval Woes Crept Up on FDA," *Christian Science Monitor*, November 26, 2004. "Citizen Petition and Request for Administrative Stay of FDA Approval of Mifeprex for Medical Abortion," August 20, 2002. Andy Coghlan, "U.S. Accelerates HIV Drug Approval," *New Scientist*, May 17, 2004; Jim Lobe, "Bush's AIDS Relief Plan Will Delay Drugs, Reward Big Pharma," *Foreign Policy in Focus*, May 26, 2004; Stephen Walker, "S.O.S. to the FDA," *WSJ*, August 23, 2003.

[21]"Remarks by the President at Food and Drug Administration Bill Signing," November 21, 1997; Executive Office of the President. For Wolfe remark, see Public Broadcasting System, "Frontline: Safe and Effective?" broadcast of November 13, 2003. It is possible, though I am unable to document the point precisely, that Wolfe himself authored the "gold standard" metaphor, making its frequent use by conservative politicians and pharmaceutical industry representatives all the more ironic, as well as perhaps politically savvy.

[22]Meredith Wadman, "Troubling Reports Tarnish Credibility of US Drug Agency," *Nature Medicine* 12 (11) (Nov. 2006): 1223. Philip B. Fontanarosa, Drummond Rennie, and Catherine D. De Angelis. "Postmarketing Surveillance—Lack of Vigilance, Lack of Trust," *JAMA* 292(21) (Dec. 1, 2004): 2647–50; R.Horton, "Lotronex and the FDA: A Fatal Erosion of Integrity," *Lancet* (2001) 357: 1544–5. Feczko quoted in Robert Pear and Gardiner Harris, "Passage of Drug Safety Bill Was Common Goal for Two Very Different Senators," *NYT*, May 11, 2007.

All of these debates occurred in a time of intense political polarization in the United States, and they came at the same time that the administration of President George W. Bush remained in office and was observed to appoint a large number of ideologically conservative individuals to office. In ways that reflected the ideological direction the Bush administration was headed, as well as the political and social circles in which conservatives of the time trafficked, Bush appointees to the FDA came from two institutions that had served as homes of criticism and resistance to the Administration in the 1970s: M. D. Anderson Hospital and the American Enterprise Institute in Washington. It was at Anderson where Commissioner Andrew von Eschenbach worked before coming to his post, and it was from the Institute that Bush appointed two of the agency's top policy commissioners of the time— Scott Gottlieb and Randall Lutter. Gottlieb's appointment in 2005 as Deputy Commissioner for Medical and Scientific Affairs brought particular criticism, as the young physician had worked principally as a biotechnology stock analyst before his arrival to the agency. Perhaps the most consequential Bush appointment was general counsel Daniel Troy, who among other things initiated a set of opinions averring that Administration approval decisions often preempted state-level "failure to warn" lawsuits against drug manufacturers. The Bush administration's management of the FDA, particularly its operations in pharmaceutical regulation, led to a noticeable drop in the FDA's public credibility. Perhaps the low point of the Bush administration's governance of the FDA came in Commissioner Lester Crawford's decision in August 2005 to deny over-the-counter (OTC) marketing status to levonorgestrel (marketed by Barr Laboratories under the trade name "Plan B"). Crawford's decision on levonorgestrel—widely known as the "morning-after pill" and opposed by many religious conservatives because they considered it an abortifacient and an incentive for sexual promiscuity—overturned the recommendations of FDA reviewers and of the agency's advisory committee on the subject. The rejection led Susan Wood, then Assistant Commissioner for Women's Health and Director of the Office of Women's Health, to announce her resignation just days later. Wood's resignation received national media attention, and the Crawford decision brought wide censure in the media and from medical journals, less for its outcome than for the fact that Crawford had interfered with science and, perhaps less noticeably but no less significantly, with the autonomy of the FDA's drug-reviewing divisions. Political interference in science in the case of "Plan B" came not only in Crawford's rejection of data, but more symbolically in his having overturned a decision that had been reached through established administrative procedures.[23]

[23]In discussing polarization, I am referring to an elite-level phenomenon among national politicians; see Barbara Sinclair, *Party Wars: Polarization and the Politics of National Policy Making* (Norman: University of Oklahoma Press, 2006); Nolan McCarty, Keith T. Poole, and Howard Rosenthal, *Polarized America: The Dance of Ideology and Unequal Riches* (Cambridge, MA: MIT Press, 2006). The Bush administration's more ideological appointment pattern

Perhaps in response to this criticism, officials in CDER and other FDA offices began to apply more rigorous scrutiny to new drugs. Seven months after Vioxx was pulled from the market, FDA officials asked Pfizer to withdraw one of the other COX-2 inhibitors (valdecoxib, trade name Bextra) from the American health system. Pfizer promptly terminated marketing of Bextra but announced that it "respectfully disagrees" with the Administration's request. Beginning in early 2005, the number of black-box warnings added by CDER to drugs soared. Among 314 new molecular entities submitted to the agency between January 1, 1993 and December 31, 2004, thirty-seven received a new black-box warning by December 2007. But of these thirty-seven new boxed warnings, fully twenty-three (or 62 percent) were added in the three-year period from January 2005 to December 2007, as opposed to the twelve (38 percent) that were added in the twelve-year period from January 1993 to January 2005.[24]

Tellingly, when Merck submitted its NDA for a next-generation COX-2 inhibitor (etoricoxib, trade name Arcoxia), CDER officials rejected the application in April 2007. The rejection was an indication both of Merck's regulatory misfortune and, in the eyes of many observers, of a new reticence about large-market drugs at the FDA. "Some say the FDA action on Arcoxia is the latest demonstration of its renewed attention to drug safety," wrote one journalist. Famed cardiologist Steven Nissen of the Cleveland Clinic, who had urged the FDA to reject the drug, observed of CDER officials that "They're acting more decisively on drug safety issues primarily, I think, because they're feeling the heat from the Congress." FDA leaders, as Nissen interpreted their actions, "want to be able to regain the confidence of the Congress—which they don't have right now." Arcoxia's rejection came in the first months of a Democratically controlled Congress that followed the 2006 midterm elections, and it came as the user fee re-authorization was under active consideration on Capitol Hill, attached to a drug safety reform bill pushed by Senators Edward Kennedy and Michael Enzi.[25]

It is tempting, but too clever by half, to view the Administration's more

---

was undoubtedly strategic, and the coupling of politicization with poorer administrative performance has been described in other agencies as well ; David E. Lewis, *The Politics of Presidential Appointments: Political Control and Bureaucratic Performance* (Princeton: Princeton University Press, 2008). On Gottlieb and Wood, see Alicia Mundy, "Wall Street Biotech Insider Gets No. 2 Job at the FDA," *Seattle Times*, August 24, 2005; Marc Kaufman, "FDA Official Quits Over Delay on Plan B," *WP*, September 1, 2005, A8. A summary review of the drug by two members of the advisory committee that voted for the approval of its OTC status appears in Frank Davidoff and James Trussell, "Plan B and the Politics of Doubt," *JAMA* 296 (14) (October 11, 2006): 1775–8.

[24]The 23 drugs are (alphabetically by trade name): Abilify, Actos, Aptivus, Atripla, Avandia, Baraclude, Bextra, Celebrex, Celexa, Cymbalta, Definity, Elidel, Emtriva, Evista, Geodon, Hepsera, Ketek, Mobic, Optimark, Remeron, Seroquel, Strattera, and Zyprexa. Many of these drugs were "class relabelings" in which an entire category of molecules (such as atypical antipsychotics) were re-labeled based upon data from one or more drugs in the class.

[25]Diedtra Henderson, "FDA Rejects Vioxx-like Painkiller," *BG*, April 28, 2007, B6.

stringent posture in recent years as a straightforward response to the criticism it received in the wake of the Vioxx withdrawal. Vioxx undoubtedly helped to change the audience structure facing the FDA, but the matter is probably more complicated. Besides the fact that such interpretations will need to be guided by historical evidence in the years to come, there is also the very real possibility that Vioxx is not the only (or even primary) reference case for FDA officials. In March 2008, Administration official Richard Pazdur cast doubt on his own division's choice five years earlier to approve the lung cancer drug gefinitib (marketed by AstraZeneca under the trade name Iressa). Despite strong skepticism from the CDER statistical reviewer and from industry watchers, the FDA approved Iressa in May 2003, in part for two reasons. First, the *Wall Street Journal* ran several editorials urging the agency to approve it (the most vocal on September 24, 2002). So strong and visible was this pressure that FDA officials are reported to have complained to AstraZeneca about the editorials, worried of a link between the company and the editorial page. Second and more important, lung cancer patient advocates strongly supported approval, and several representatives of the groups offered robust and emotional testimony for the drug at a critical FDA advisory committee meeting in September 2002. As one journalist wrote following the meeting, "These patients—all of whom took Iressa through a compassionate use program—seemed to be the wild card that really helped AstraZeneca in the end. The company has allowed more than 18,000 patients access to Iressa outside its clinical trials, creating a very vocal and persuasive lobbying voice in the drug's favor."[26]

Iressa had been approved on the basis of a clinical trial showing approximately a 10 percent response rate to the medication (a "response" in the pivotal trial was defined by tumor shrinkage of 50 percent or more). It was, however, the only drug of its type available to advanced stage non-small-cell lung cancer patients, so there was some rationale for approval even in the face of slim evidence. Yet in subsequent and larger clinical trials, researchers failed to find an appreciable survival benefit to Iressa. Whatever the ultimate efficacy of the drug, Pazdur later remarked that he felt burned procedurally by his earlier decision. As a *Wall Street Journal* reporter related his reaction, "Dr. Pazdur says he awoke in the middle of the night, agonizing over what to do." The agency then strongly restricted the use of Iressa in 2005. In internal discussions inside and outside of his division, Pazdur then pointed to Iressa as a clear demonstration of a drug whose approval was based on faulty research design and poor quality data. Pazdur's reaction reflected his concern for the integrity of scientific review, but it was also a decision based upon reputation and precedent. He and other FDA officials were bothered

---

[26] Adam Feuerstein, "AstraZeneca Scores Comeback Victory on Iressa," www.thestreet.com/_yahoo/tech/adamfeuerstein/10044113.html (accessed November 12, 2003). I gathered similar impressions from an interview with Philip Crooker, regulatory affairs director, AstraZeneca, 19 May 2003.

by the fact that a possibly ineffective drug got through the agency's approval process on the basis of patient lobbying and emotive factors.[27]

Along with deregulation, there has been a continuing concern among FDA reviewers and center directors to demonstrate legitimacy among multiple audiences, to avoid being pigeonholed or cast according to type. Pazdur himself has been criticized by name in *Wall Street Journal* editorials, just as he has been praised by other observers of cancer therapeutics. And the necessity of reputation management has been as clearly voiced by Pazdur as by any other FDA official in recent years. In 2002, upon the approval of oxaliplatin (trade name Eloxatin), a new platinum-based chemotherapy treatment, Pazdur noted the symbolic value of his division's decision, as his group had rejected a different drug named Erbitrux earlier in the year. "We want to send a message," Pazdur said, speaking of his staff's long nights and overtime spent in reviewing the drug, whose NDA he regarded as unusually strong. He explicitly regarded his division's quick approval (the agency announced that the seven-week review was the fastest to date for a cancer drug) as a message to other drug developers. "The point that we want to get across was the value in doing randomized trials." More recently, observers have described Pazdur as acutely conscious of the multidimensional criticism to which he is subject, and the cancer chief has admitted that "we need to demonstrate regulatory flexibility."[28]

THE COMPLICATED USES OF A REPUTATION: TOBACCO REGULATION AND STATE TORT PREEMPTION

The imagery of gatekeeping—its representation of the agency's capacity to protect citizens through pre-market review of drugs, and its summary of the Administration's power—still enables and constrains American pharmaceutical regulation. Two disputes over the past decade—one representing an initiative from the left, the other an initiative from the right—have featured gatekeeping imagery as a central trope in policy discussion and legal debate. The first came in Commissioner David Kessler's furtive and initially unsuccessful attempt to regulate tobacco. Kessler pressed the idea more aggressively in 1994 and the years following, after investigative journalists for the American Broadcasting Corporation (ABC) network revealed that cigarette

---

[27] Anna Wilde Mathews, "Powerful Medicine: FDA Cancer Czar Stirs Debate on Agency's Role; Anemia-Drug Tussle Puts Pazdur on Spot; Father's Early Death," *WSJ*, March 10, 2008.

[28] Andrew Pollack, "Colorectal Cancer Drug Wins Quick Approval From F.D.A.," *NYT*, August 13, 2002; "Pazdur's Cancer Rules—The FDA's Oncology Chief Gets His Revenge," *WSJ* (editorial), July 6, 2005. The *Journal's* editorialist mocked the Eloxatin decision that "In other words, the less revolutionary drug (Eloxatin) got approved first because its makers had jumped through the right bureaucratic hoops [randomized clinical trials]." Mathews, "Powerful Medicine: FDA Cancer Czar Stirs Debate on Agency's Role"; whether or not he intended that term, Pazdur's verb "demonstrate" is telling.

manufacturers had been manipulating the level of nicotine, the most addictive ingredient in cigarettes. As former Surgeon General C. Everett Koop noted at the conclusion of the ABC report, the reports called for FDA regulation of cigarettes, for they had established the plausibility of the "cigarette as a delivery device for the use of nicotine which is, under ordinary circumstances, a prescription drug." Kessler used and appropriated these arguments, and he began drawing analogies between the cigarette industry and the world of pharmaceuticals. As in the world of pharmaceuticals, he claimed, tobacco companies were trying to affect bodily function through the manipulation of nicotine. And he noted that "the research undertaken by the cigarette industry is more and more resembling drug development."[29]

In proposing to regulate the cigarette as a drug or medical device—the proposed rule was released in 1995 along with an extensive justification of the agency's jurisdiction—Kessler knew he was appropriating a legal, political, and conceptual architecture established for other purposes. The key aim was not to simply regulate cigarettes more generally, but to bring these commodities under the directive, gatekeeping, and conceptual powers of his organization in the realm of pharmaceuticals. The fight against Kessler's proposal was undertaken quickly and aggressively, and it has been well documented. Kessler's proposed extension was challenged in federal court, and in a significant decision in *FDA v. Brown & Williamson Tobacco Corp*, the U.S. Supreme Court in 2000 decided that the Administration lacked the statutory authority to regulate cigarettes absent an explicit congressional statute granting this authority. In recent years, anti-tobacco and public health advocates have tried a different route, seeking to introduce and pass legislation granting the FDA the power to regulate tobacco as a drug. In an odd twist that reflects the precarious legal and political situation in which tobacco companies find themselves in twenty-first century America, a number of cigarette makers expressed considerable support for the idea. Yet in the summer of 2007, as the bill was debated, the Administration's reputation again became a silent entrant into the controversy. Michael Siegel, a public health professor at Boston University, worried that the FDA's positive public face would place an imprimatur upon the cigarette. "It would still be a deadly product. They are not going to make it a safe product by taking out particular smoke constituents. The problem is the public is going to perceive the product is safe because the FDA has assumed jurisdiction." On the positive side, Matthew Myers, president of the National Center for Tobacco-Free Kids, said that "If the FDA only prevented tobacco companies from manipulating their products to make it easier to start and harder to quit, it will make a major contribution to the public health." What Myers most admired about the bill was the discretion it gave to the bill's career scientists. "This bill wisely doesn't try to predict what a cigarette will look like once

---

[29] Allan M. Brandt, *The Cigarette Century: The Rise, Fall and Deadly Persistence of the Product that Defined America* (New York: Basic Books, 2007), 361, 363.

FDA begins to take action. Instead, it says to the scientists at the FDA, 'You have the power to require changes in tobacco products in whatever ways you believe.'"[30]

In 2009, with the arrival of President Barack Obama and his administration, and with hefty Democratic majorities in the House and Senate, Congress passed the Family Smoking Prevention and Tobacco Control Act (Public Law 111-031). The Act added a new Chapter Nine to the Federal Food, Drug and Cosmetic Act that confirmed the FDA's authority to regulate tobacco and thus bypassed the Supreme Court's decision in the *Williamson* case. The law also created a new Center for Tobacco Products within the FDA. The Act struck into law some reforms long desired by anti-tobacco activists, not least required submission of data and research documents on tobacco products, new labeling on cigarettes and smokeless tobacco products (such as chewing tobacco), and new restrictions on advertising and promotion. Perhaps its most marked addition to current regulation came in Section 910, which authorized the Administration to review all "new tobacco products" (a legal category created in the 2009 Act itself) to assess whether permitting the product to be marketed "would be appropriate for the protection of the public health." In manifold ways, the pre-market review section explicitly copied an architecture for review of new products that had evolved for American pharmaceuticals between 1937 and 1963.[31]

The other, more recent initiative came from conservative and libertarian voices, and it sought to extend the FDA's power over pharmaceuticals on a federalist dimension. In 2001, FDA general counsel Daniel Troy wrote an agency legal opinion that proposed the idea of state tort preemption. Drug companies are commonly sued in state courts for "failure to warn" patients of drug risks; under preemption these suits would be invalid unless the plaintiff could prove that the drug sponsor had withheld or misrepresented safety risks to the Administration. The invalidity of state "failure-to-warn" suits would be premised upon the agency's gatekeeping authority, the idea being that once the Administration has declared a drug safe and effective, this position binds state and local governments, including their judicial

---

[30]The proposed rule would rely not upon the definition of tobacco products as "drugs" but as "restricted devices" under Section 520(e) of the Federal food, Drug and Cosmetic Act; other sections of the Act were also invoked. FDA, "Regulations Restricting the Sale and Distribution of Cigarettes and Smokeless Tobacco Protects to Protect Children and Adolescents," *FR* 60 (155) (Aug.11, 1995): 41314. FDA, *Regulation of Cigarettes and Smokeless Tobacco Under the Federal Food, Drug and Cosmetic Act; Volume One: Proposed Rule, Jurisdictional Analysis & Appendices and Related Notices* (Washington, DC: GPO, August 1996). The Court's decision appears at 529 U.S. 120 (2000), 153 F.3d 155, affirmed. Andrew Bridges (AP), "Bill's backers think FDA could engineer a safer cigarette," *BG*, July 17, 2007, A4. I thank Allan Brandt for several insightful discussions about the politics and ironies of this case.

[31]The quoted language appears at Section 910 (c)(2)(A) of the Act. An accessible legislative history appears in C. Stephen Redhead and Vanessa K. Burrows, "FDA Tobacco Regulation: History of the 1996 Rule and Related Legislative Activity, 1998–2008" (Washington, DC: Congressional Research Service, May 28, 2009).

branches. Troy's policy shift, which was published in an agency rule on la-beling and reflected some writings in the conservative "law and economics" community in the 1980s and 1990s, was followed by subsequent lawsuits and legal defenses that attempted to gain judicial recognition of the concept. As many observers noted, Troy's opinion and the subsequent agency policy were novel, and as recently as the late 1990s FDA officials explicitly rejected the doctrine.[32]

The particulars of preemption have been under debate in the federal courts for several years now, and the third in a trilogy of Supreme Court cases—*Wyeth v. Levine*—was heard in oral argument before the Court in November 2008. From the vantage of reputation and power, what is per-haps most interesting about it is that a conservative and pro-business legal movement was officially drawing upon a federal agency's reputation to ad-vance a legal position. And the decisive act that was claimed to obviate tort suits is the same act that stands at the center of FDA regulatory power and reputation—pre-market approval of new drug applications and the labeling embedded in them.[33]

The Supreme Court's decision in *Wyeth v. Levine*, announced in March 2009, stunned business conservatives and legal observers alike. The court ruled 6 to 3 for the plaintiff Levine and against the drug company, explicitly rejecting the idea that the Administration's enabling act preempted state failure-to-warn litigation. On the whole, the rationale of the Court (as ex-pressed in Justice John Paul Stevens' majority opinion) reflected a judgment about statutory interpretation. The Federal Food, Drug and Cosmetic Act simply did not express, explicitly or implicitly, the idea that state lawsuits would be preempted by the Act. And the Court majority noted that other federal legislation granting pre-market approval power to the agency—the Medical Device Amendments of 1976—had included an explicit preemption provision. The *Wyeth v. Levine* decision was in this respect a complete de-feat for business conservatives and for Daniel Troy, the legal architect of the preemption opinions that led to the case.[34]

In the literal fine print of the decision, however—in footnote 11 of the majority opinion —Justice Stevens shot a hole in the argument that the FDA's labeling could be relied upon to ensure safety. Drawing upon a series of reports issued in the early twenty-first century that cast doubt on the Administration's scientific capacities, the footnote drew attention to "seri-ous scientific deficiencies" at the agency, and a lack of "clear and effective

---

[32]For accessible summaries of the recent controversy, consult Gary Young, "FDA Legal Strategy would Pre-Empt Tort Suits," *National Law Journal* 128 (44) (March 5, 2004): 3; Terry Carter, "The Pre-emption Prescription," *ABA Journal*, November 2008.

[33]Along with several other authors, I filed an amicus curiae brief arguing against the pre-emption doctrine in the summer of 2008.

[34]Indeed, in a decision released just one month before —*Riegel v. Medtronic, Inc.* (No. 06-179)—the Court ruled that the explicit preemption clause in the 1976 Amendments did invali-date a series of state failure-to-warn lawsuits.

process for making decisions about, and providing management oversight of, postmarket safety issues." The argument of Daniel Troy and the organized pharmaceutical industry that the FDA labeling process could reliably warn patients and consumers about drug hazards was explicitly rejected.[35]

In two quite diverse ways, then, the Administration's organizational image and the gatekeeping metaphor has become a tool of policymaking, in one case becoming newest and primary weapon in a decades-long fight against tobacco, in another case entering into the very fabric of American federalism.

. . .

At this writing, as the Wyeth majority's opinion suggests, the Administration's image has been badly withered. Its technical reputation has suffered as top scientists have fled the agency or have complained publicly about being overruled or ignored. Its moral reputation has been damaged, among other things, by the impression that Administration officials have too often favored one set of interests (organized pharmaceutical companies) at the expense of others. Its performative reputation has been sullied by awkward Commissioner resignations, odd appointments, and infighting. Its procedural reputation was trashed in the Plan B affair, when the subdelegation norms that govern most drug approval decisions were ignored and when reviewing divisions were overruled by political appointees. Whether these doubts about the agency are founded in plausible and accurate readings of its behavior is separable and, in some ways, irrelevant. In the politics of reputation, symbolic complexes persist well past the claims and events that gave rise to them. Even the "gold standard" metaphor has come under attack. In February 2008, Commissioner Andrew von Eschenbach would appeal again to the metaphor in an interview with the *Wall Street Journal*.

> This agency is the world's gold standard. And people, you and I, will go home tonight and we will have dinner and we will not have to worry about having that dinner. I will give my grandchildren the medication they need when they are sick, and I have confidence and trust in those medications. But that doesn't mean that I'm not looking at tomorrow and realizing that if we don't make the kind of changes that are necessary today, we're not going to be able to continue to assure that tomorrow.

Yet just the previous week, a *Newsweek* reader named Robin McStay of Weaverville, California would contest the metaphor and profess greater confidence in the regulatory institutions of Europe.

> I no longer believe that the FDA and the EPA are the global "gold standard" for public safety, and I have little confidence that public safety is placed above corporate interests.... For my household, with one toddler and a baby on the way, I buy

[35] Majority opinion, *Wyeth v. Levine* (No. 06-1249), footnote 11 (p. 22 of decision).

TABLE 12.1
"Rating the FDA"

"Based on what you know or have heard, how good a job do you think the FDA (Food and Drug Administration) does on ensuring the safety as well as the efficacy of new prescription drugs?"							
	Positive*	Excellent	Good	Negative**	Fair	Poor	Not Sure
2004 %	56	14	43	37	27	10	7
2006 %	36	7	29	58	35	23	6
2007 %	45	7	37	49	29	20	6
2008 %	35	5	30	58	33	25	7

Base: All Adults
Source: WSJ.com/Harris Interactive survey, April 2008.

products that meet EU standards whenever possible, though I have to shop online, and pay more.

A month later, a *Boston Globe* reader argued that "the FDA is not what it used to be" and, in a rare reference to the symbol of the agency's public triumph, wrote that "What we need now are people like Frances Kelsey." A front-page story in *Reader's Digest*, one of the most commonly read print publications in the United States, especially among elderly audiences, asked "Can We Trust the FDA?"[36]

For more and more American citizens, the answer to that question has become negative. Survey responses are difficult to trace over time, but a series of Harris polls from 2000 to 2006 revealed a stunning drop in respondents' self-reported trust in the agency (see table 12.1). Whereas 61 percent of U.S. respondents expressed confidence in the agency in 2000, by 2006, that figure had fallen to 36 percent. An April 2008 survey produced further disturbing evidence. The perception that the FDA "does a good job ensuring the safety and efficacy of new prescription drugs" was shared by 35 percent of respondents, compared to 45 percent of respondents to the same question in 2007 and 56 percent in 2004. As telling was the fact that the survey respondents considered drug regulation to be the agency's the most important task (61 percent).[37]

[36] "Letters," *Newsweek*, February 18, 2008, 22. Perhaps not coincidentally, Von Eschenbach hailed from M. D. Anderson, a source of older opposition to FDA standards; see chapters 6 and 8. Roslyn Talerman, "FDA Not What It Used to Be," *BG*, March 18, 2008, A18. "Can We Trust the FDA?" *Reader's Digest*, April 2008, cover, 118 (story).

[37] Beckey Bright, "Americans Growing Less Confident in FDA's Job on Safety, Poll Shows," *WSJ* online, May 24, 2006 (accessed May 27, 2006). "Confidence in FDA Hits New Low, According to WSJ.com/Harris Interactive Study," April 23, 2008 (Rochester, NY: Harris interactive, 2008). Other writers, drawing upon figures aggregated across quite different surveys from

. . .

There is a haunting line in the Latin poem *Dies Irae* that bespeaks the fear and deep sense of dependence felt by its speaker. In the funeral (*Requiem*) mass in which this line has been sung for centuries, its words anticipate the wrath that will come on the Day of Judgment. "Quem patronem rogaturus, cum vix justus sit sicurus?" asks the soprano voice. "To what protector shall I appeal, when even the just are hardly safe?"

For much of the twentieth century, various audiences in the world of pharmaceuticals asked such a question. Their purpose was not eschatology but policy. They dreaded not an end time of judgment, but a world in which a society would stand at the mercy of those with the power or the knowledge of healing. The poet's question—to which protector shall I appeal?— was asked not of a god but of national institutions. The audiences included communities of physicians and other healers, nations and world organizations launching new health systems, and millions of women around the globe who were considering a new oral contraceptive. No three audiences asked the question more than the constitutional branches of American government—the U.S. Congress, successive presidents and their administrations, and the federal judiciary and its Supreme Court.

The protector to whom American and global society appeals is one endowed with vast power. That power, as I hope to have rendered clear, vastly outstrips the authority and resources given to the agency. By deference of the courts and the decisions of a national legislature, a diminutive agency has acquired broad authority over some of the most powerful companies on the planet, so much so that fear and vigilance have become regulatory tools for an agency without extensive policing capacity. A single organization has been endowed with the ability to shape, accelerate, and even cut off the pipeline of new products in several different industrial sectors, and with the capacity to mold the scientific methods and research agendas of thousands upon thousands of scientists and physicians throughout the world. The agency's decisions have reverberated across national and professional boundaries, and

---

the 1970s to 2006, have put the decline much larger, from confidence ratings of 80 percent or higher in the 1970s to 36 percent in 2006. Alastair J. J. Wood, "Playing 'Kick the FDA' —Risk-free to Players but Hazardous to Public Health,' *NEJM* 358 (17) (April 24, 2008): 1774–5; *FDA Science and Mission at Risk: Report of the Subcommittee on Science and Technology* (Rockville, MD: Food and Drug Administration, November 2007); Peter Barton Hutt, "The State of Science at the Food and Drug Administration," *Administrative Law Review* 60 (Spring 2008): 431–86. In this article, Hutt joins other critics from a number of perspectives— including regulatory conservatives—who have begun to turn against the user fee system, largely because of its symbolic residue. Arguing that "user fees have completely distorted the current FDA budget," Hutt proposes their elimination and a return to full reliance upon appropriations. Hutt's reasons are telling; they had less to do with what he saw as the actual effects of user fees on the FDA and much more to do with what he saw as the *perceived* effects. "In the long run, however, funding the FDA by a tax on the regulated industry is not an appropriate solution to the agency's needs and should be abandoned. This approach has clearly contributed to the decline in the FDA's public credibility."

its standards and definitions shape not only the development of therapies and protocols in Cambridge, Houston, and La Jolla, but also the governance of traditional healing systems in India and Sri Lanka.

Should a government agency, in a democratic republic—one governed by a constitution and the rule of law—have these powers? A more compelling answer to this question demands a separate, still empirical but more philosophical inquiry. I believe, however, that a pharmaceutical regulator should carry directive, gatekeeping, and conceptual powers, limited of course by constitutional and legal constraints and, perhaps most important, by the politics of organizational reputation itself. In the modern pharmaceutical world, the sponsors and producers of medicines are powerful entities, rendered all the more powerful by political and economic transformations of the past century. The multifaceted regulatory power of the Administration, its gatekeeping authority, and the harsher faces and moments of its image, allow a miniature agency to check and constrain a very large and politically dominant industrial sector.

The Administration's gatekeeping power enacts a system of incentives that induces the production of far more information (and higher quality information) from drug companies and medical researchers than would otherwise have occurred. The FDA's power is essentially the capacity to demand of market aspirants that they test their drug in a setting which they do not entirely control, that they take 100, or 1,000, or 10,000 patients, flip a coin and assign research subjects to their treatment or a control group based on chance alone. The production of such information in large quantities provides a vast public good, one useful at once for those who will utilize the therapy and for those who will not, one beneficial for those who prescribe drugs and those who bear the costs of drug utilization, and a stock of information helpful for those who will develop therapies of the future.

The conceptual face of regulatory power may seem insidious, but it allows for the standardization necessary to scientific progress. Medical research and intellectual advancement depend upon a minimally common vocabulary, a set of terms that can be assumed for the sake of devoting cognition and effort to other questions. By defining the sorts of numbers that are debated in drug approval and utilization, and by laying out standards by which drugs are deemed equivalent to one another or distinct, the Administration renders a whole host of health decisions and economic exchanges much easier and more predictable.

There are risks, to be sure, in trusting this multidimensionality of power to a single organization. Yet the very source of this power—organizational image—has consistently served as a force in constraining the behavior and aspiration of the Administration. Whether in the cautionary voice of academic pharmacologists, in the American public's fear of an unproven sleeping pill, or in the protests of oncologists or AIDS sufferers, the collected voices that constitute the Administration's audiences restrained the agency and affected the thinking and, quite plausibly, the emotions of its officials.

In many ways, this politics of reputation carries its own regrettable moments and inefficiencies. Yet for the Administration, as with many other agencies, the politics of reputation enacts another form of representation and constraint.

For those dedicated to constitutional politics and the best traditions of American government, the duality of reputation and regulatory power is both defensible and promising. Regulatory power in its directive, gatekeeping, and conceptual faces coheres well with the Federalists' vision of "strong" government that was necessary for the protection of liberty in its republican understanding. Alexander Hamilton and other republicans believed in the capacity of government to create and facilitate systems of economic exchange and scientific learning. Critical to these functions was the information that government bodies gathered, commanded, ordered, and provided. At its best, the power of the Food and Drug Administration in the pharmaceutical world reflects the aspirations of the progressive vision of the early twentieth century in which the agency was forged. It reflects not only the advancement of modern science, but the traditions and theories of republican government. For pharmaceuticals as for other realms of activity governed by the state, the central criterion of sound governance is not mass or breadth, but legitimated vigor.

PRIMARY SOURCES
AND ARCHIVAL COLLECTIONS

American Medical Association, Archives and Manuscripts Division, Chicago, Illinois

- Records of the Council on Drugs
- Historical Health Fraud and Alternative Medicine Collection

Bentley Historical Library, University of Michigan, Ann Arbor, Michigan

- Records of the College of Pharmacy
- Records of the Office of the University Vice President
- Records of the Department of Internal Medicine, University of Michigan School of Medicine
- Royal Samuel Copeland Papers

Bundesarchiv Koblenz, Koblenz, Germany

Chesney Medical Archives, Johns Hopkins Medical Institutions, Johns Hopkins University, Baltimore, Maryland

- Eugene Maximilian Karl Geiling Papers

Countway Medical Library, Archives and Special Collections, Harvard Medical School, Boston, Massachusetts

- Maxwell Finland Papers
- Edward H. Kass Papers

FDA Library, U.S. Food and Drug Administration, Rockville, Maryland

- Assorted Files and Reports
- Accession Files

Headquarters of the World Health Organization, Geneva, Switzerland

- WHO Archives
- WHO Library

Historical Collections, Baker Business Library, Harvard Business School, Boston, Massachusetts

- Baker Old Class Serial Collection

Hoskins Special Collections Library, University of Tennessee, Knoxville, Tennessee

- Senator Estes Kefauver Papers
- Senator Estes Kefauver Collection

Jawaharlal Nehru Memorial Library, New Delhi, India

- Documents and Reports of the Government of India

John F. Kennedy Presidential Library, Boston, Massachusetts

- Presidential Papers of John F. Kennedy
- Kennedy Pre-Presidential Papers

• Records of the U.S. Department of Health, Education and Welfare
• Records of the U.S. Bureau of the Budget
• Still Photograph Collections

J. Richard Crout Papers, private collection in possession of J. Richard Crout, Bethesda, Maryland

Julius Hauser Professional Papers, private collection in possession of Hauser family, Baltimore, Maryland

J. Willard Marriott Library, University of Utah, Salt Lake City, Utah

• Louis Goodman Papers

Kalamazoo Public Library, Kalamazoo, Michigan

• Upjohn Company Files

Library of Medicine and Science, Rutgers University, Piscataway, New Jersey

Mandeville Special Collections Library, University of California, San Diego, La Jolla, California

• Charles Edwards Collection
• Robert Hamburger Collection
• Records of the Vice President for Health Sciences, UCSD

Manuscript Division, Library of Congress, Washington, DC

• William A. Blackmun Papers
• Frances Oldham Kelsey Papers
• Thurgood Marshall Papers
• Harvey Washington Wiley Papers

Mayo Foundation Archives, Mayo Clinic, Rochester, Minnesota

• Barker Collection
• Dr. Philip S. Hench Collection
• Dr. John S. Lundy Collection
• Records of the Mayo Clinical Society
• Records of the Committee on Medical Education and Research
• Records of the Committee on the Safety of Therapeutic Agents
• Records of the Mayo Clinic Laboratory Society
• Records of the Mayo Clinic Oncology Committee
• Records of the Mayo Clinic Research Administrative Committee
• Records of the Mayo Clinic Research and Laboratory Committee
• Records of the Mayo Clinic Sciences Committee

Mayo Foundation History of Medicine Library, Mayo Clinic, Rochester, Minnesota

• Mayo Authors Publications Series

M. D. Anderson Cancer Center Research Medical Library, University of Texas M. D. Anderson Cancer Center, Houston, Texas

• Charles LeMaistre Collection

• Kenneth Clark Collection

National Academies Archives, Washington, DC

• Records of the Drug Efficacy Study

National Archives and Records Administration, Washington, DC,
and College Park, Maryland

• Records of the Secretary of Agriculture, RG 16
• Records of the Food and Drug Administration, RG 88
• Records of the Post Office Department, RG 28
• Records of the Committee on Agriculture, Records of the House
  of Representatives, RG 146
• Records of the Committee on Manufactures, Records of the Senate, RG 46
• Records of the National Institutes of Health, RG 433
• Records of the Presidency of Richard M. Nixon, 1969–1974 [NA II]

National Archives of the United Kingdom, Kew, London, England

• Records of the Committee on the Safety of Drugs
• Records of the Committee on Medicines

National Library of Medicine, History of Medicine Division, Archives and Modern
Manuscripts Program, Bethesda, Maryland

• John Adriani Papers
• Harry F. Dowling Papers
• James L. Goddard Papers
• James Harvey Young Papers
• FDA Oral History Series
  –William W. Goodrich Oral History
  –Frances Kelsey Oral History
  –Ralph Weilerstein Oral History
  –J. Richard Crout Oral History

New York Public Library, New York, New York

• Records of the AIDS Coalition to Unleash Power (ACT-UP), New York

Othmer Library in the History of Chemistry, Chemical Heritage Foundation,
Philadelphia, Pennsylvania

• Orlando Aloysius Battista Oral History
• David P. Holveck Oral History
• Miguel Angel Ondetti Oral History

Parke-Davis Regulatory Affairs Office and Company Library, Parke-Davis
Company (later Pfizer Corporation), Ann Arbor, Michigan

• Assorted files from the Regulatory Affairs Office

Public Policy Collection, Seeley G. Mudd Library, Princeton University,
Princeton, New Jersey

• American Civil Liberties Union Archives
• Roger Baldwin Papers

- George S. McGovern Papers
- William Fitts Ryan Papers
- H. Alexander Smith Papers
- Adlai Stevenson Papers

Riggs/Carson Library, Keck Graduate Institute of Applied Life Sciences, Claremont, California

- Assorted Files

Rush Rhees Library, University of Rochester, Rochester, New York

- Louis C. Lasagna Papers

Schlesinger Library, Radcliffe College, Harvard University, Cambridge, Massachusetts

- Barbara Seaman Papers

St. Louis Mercantile Library, University of Missouri–St. Louis

- Mallinckrodt Company Advertising Scrapbooks

University Library, Jawaharlal Nehru University, New Delhi, India

- Theses and Dissertations
- Documents and Reports of the Government of India

University of Chicago, Archives and Special Collections Library, Chicago, Illinois

- Lowell T. Coggeshall Papers
- Morris Fishbein Papers
- President's Papers, 1925–1945
- President's Papers, Appointments

University of Pennsylvania, Archives and Special Collections, Philadelphia, Pennsylvania

- Alfred Newton Richards Papers

University of California, San Francisco Library, Archives and Special Collections, San Francisco, California

- Thomas Nathaniel Burbridge Papers
- California Medical Association Papers
- Records of the California Society for the Promotion of Medical Research
- Henry Colle Papers
- Otto Ernst Guttentag Papers
- Choh Hao Li Papers
- Healing Alternatives Foundation Collection
- Philip R. Lee Papers
- Chauncey Depew Leake Papers
- McNaughton Foundation Publications, Correspondence
- Sidney J. Riegelman Papers
- William J. Rutter Papers
- San Francisco General Hospital, selected records [Ward 84/86]
- Drug Industry Digital Archive [online collection]

Wellcome Library for the History of Medicine, London, England

- Burroughs-Wellcome Papers
- Records of Wellcome Tuckahoe Lab
- Wellcome Foundation Ltd—Internal Business Correspondence
- Wellcome Oral Histories

Wisconsin State Historical Society, Madison, Wisconsin

- Records of the U.S. Pharmacopoeial Convention
- Robert Fischelis Papers
- Gaylord Nelson Papers

INDEX

Note: Page references in italics indicate figures.

Aaron, Harold, 327–28
Abbott Laboratories: compliance with FDA, 7, 7n.7; Desoxyn, 201–2; Endrate, 180; on NDAs, 169; Nembutal, problems with, 147; Operation Expedite, 642; regulatory affairs offices at, 644; reputation of, 202; as research-intensive, 657n.34
Abbott Laboratories v. Gardner, 360n.80
A-B-C system, 491, 504–5
Abel, John Jacob, 133, 134n.19, 214
abortifacients, 129n.13, 739–41
abortion pill, 739–41
ABPI (Association of British Pharmaceutical Industries), 695, 695n.15, 699–701, 700n.23, 707, 709
Abraham, John, 488–89n.32, 695n.15, 700n.23
Abrams, Frank W., 167n.77
Abramson, Ernst, 138
absorption testing, 131
acetanilid, 80, 80n.13
acne. *See* Enovid
acronym-known drugs, 287–88
ACS (American Cancer Society), 307; campaign against unproved cancer remedies, 417; cancer awareness campaigns by, 400; challenges to, 400–401; vs. NCI, 407–8, 410n.24; relations with FDA, 401; research funding efforts of, 400
Activase (TPA). *See* TPA
ACT-UP (AIDS Coalition to Unleash Power), 396; on AZT pricing, 457; Ellen Cooper criticized by, 443; credibility of, 445, 447; on DDI, 447; pressure applied by, 443, 443n; prominence of, 430n.59, 431; relations with FDA, 444, 447–48; vs. TAG, 456
Acyclovir, 672n.55
Adams, John, 558
ADEC (Australian Drug Evaluation Committee), 695, 705
Adkinson, N. Franklin, 382–83
Administration. *See entries beginning with* "FDA"
administration/making of modern drug review (1963–1985), 468–92; emergence of organization, 468, 480–92, 481nn.21–22, 482, 483–86nn.23–29, 488–90nn.31–34, 492nn.36–38; overview of, 468–69. *See also*

patterns of administration/organization/ interpretation of modern drug review
Administrative Procedure Act (1946), 347
adverse-event reporting (AER), 587, 589–94, 591–92nn.9–11, 593–94n.13, 601, 634, 655–56
Adverse Event Reporting Committee, 593
Advisory Committee on Health Policy, 235
Advisory Committee on Infective Drug Products, 436–38, 437n.70
Advisory Committee on Investigational Drugs. *See* Modell Committee
Advisory Committee on Obstetrics and Gynecology, 342–43, 601
AEI Center for Health Policy Research, 377, 377n.109
AER. *See* adverse-event reporting
African Americans, perceived link with venereal disease, 90, 92n.29
agenda formation, study of, 52
Agendas, Alternatives and Public Policies (Kingdon), 230
agenda-setting, 53n.36; and the Federal Food, Drug and Cosmetic Act, 80–83, 83–84nn.18–19, 85 (table); and problem definition, 380n.115
aggregated medical opinion, 330–31
Agriculture Department. *See* USDA
AIDS Coalition to Unleash Power. *See* ACT-UP
AIDS crisis, 383–84, 428–57; activists/groups, 429–31, 430n.59, 441–47, 444n.80 (*see also* ACT-UP; Delaney, Martin; Kramer, Larry; Project Inform); AIDS as a "gay disease," 429–30, 430n.58; AIDS as a retrovirus, 432–33; documentation of, 428–29; early causal theories, 430, 430n.58; FDA response to, 393–94, 428–29, 440–41, 457–58n.100; fear and uncertainty over causes of, 429; HIV virus's role identified, 430–31; Hudson story, 431–32; Kaposi's sarcoma linked to, 429, 447; mechanism/pathology of AIDS, 432–33; media coverage of, 431, 448; multiplicity/ diversity of organizations representing patients, 431; October 11 demonstration against FDA (1988), 443–45, 444n.80; overview of, 394–95; *Pneumocystis carinii*

Intergovernmental Relations Subcommittee
of the Committee on Government Operations. *See* Fountain committee
Internal Revenue Service, 275n.69
International Conference on Harmonization
(ICH), 515, 703, 712, 712n
international context of American regulation, 686–726; Europeanization and harmonization, 515, 686, 703, 707–12,
712n.43; global regulation, 723, 724–25
(table), 726; independent variables in
comparisons, 722–23, 722–23n.59; India,
governance of medicines in, 716–22,
716–20nn.50–55, 721–22nn.57–58; organizational image, 723, 726; overview of,
686–89, 686n; WHO and regulation in
developing nations, 712–16, 714n.45,
715nn.47–48. *See also* developed nations,
comparisons/dependencies among
international drug lag. *See* "nation of first
approval" metric
International Pharmacopeia, 210
International Union of Pure and Applied
Chemistry, 307
Interstate Commerce Commission (ICC), 25
intimidation. *See* deterrence
intrauterine devices (IUDs), 342
Intron A, 440–41n.75
investigation, definition of, 257
investigational drug regulations, 237n.14
Investigational New Drug Branch: authority
of, 290–91; Frances Kelsey as head of, 280,
306, 469–70, 548, 569; medical officers
in, 290, 470, 471–72 (table), 473, 473n.8;
and the Modell Committee, 303–4
IRB. *See under* human subjects protection
IRB: A Review of Human Subjects Research,
567n.36
Iressa (gefinitib), 743
Irons, Wesley, 183
isoprinosine, 515
isoprotenerol, 615n
ISO standards, 35n
Israel, S. Leon, 321
Italy, thalidomide use in, 241n.20
Ivy, Andrew, 148, 411

Jackson, Charles O., 82, 82n.16, 87, 98n.43
Jacob, Stanley, 287–89, 289n.91, 479
Jain, Anruth K., 601n.26
*JAMA (Journal of the American Medical Asso-
ciation)*, 76–77; advertising in, 207n.148;
criticism of, 604; drug advertising in, 207–

8; on elixir sulfanilamide, 89–90, 94; on
Laetrile-related deaths, 422; Van Winkle
report in, 115–16
Japan: drug regulation in, 22–23, 23 (table),
296, 689; state legitimacy in, 53; thalido-
mide use in, 241n.20; vs. United States,
drug regulation in, 705–7
Javits, Jacob, 255, 259, 259n.49, 548
Jennings, John, 537–38, 538n.99
Jin, Kun, 507n.53
John Birch Society, 418, 423, 427
Johns Hopkins University, 94, 172, 332
Johnson, Anita, 489
Johnson, D. W., 600–601
Johnson, United States v., 116, 150
Johnson, Walter, 15n.20
Johnson and Johnson: INDs terminated
for, 289; off-label promotion by, 619;
Ortho-Novum, 535, 538, 616; as
research-intensive, 657n.34
Joint Center for Regulatory Policy, 364–
65n.88
Jolly, Eugene R. ("Dick"), 127 (table)
Jones, Boisfeuillet, 305–6, 318
Joslin Clinic (Boston), 611
*Journal of the American Medical Associa-
tion. See JAMA*
Junod, Suzanne White, 187n.109
Justice Department, 233, 361, 656

Kabi Pharmacia, 658
Kaiser Permanente, 602n.27
Kallet, Arthur, 222–23, 327–28, 331
Kaopectate with Neomycin, 164–65
Kaposi's sarcoma, 429, 447
Katz, Russell, 542
Katzmann, Robert, 444n.81
Kaufman, Herbert, 43n.17
Kazman, Sam, 379
Kefauver, Estes, 132, 146n.40; on adequate
time for drug review, 477–78; on the AMA,
209; on the automatic approval provision,
254; *Crime in America*, 232; on FDA as
protector, 173; hearings on crime/racke-
teering, 231–32; and Frances Kelsey, 213,
245; vs. Kennedy, 236, 254; and Larrick,
254, 259n.49; personality/style of, 236;
political career of, 231–32; reputation of,
188–89; S.3677 introduced by, 234–35n.11;
Subcommittee on Antitrust and Monopoly
chaired by, 231; Subcommittee on Monopoly chaired by, 231, 231n.5; on *Time*'s
cover, 232n.6. *See also* S.1552

Princeton Studies in American Politics
Historical, International, and Comparative Perspectives